SO-BMG-632

Immunity to

Parasitic Animals

Immunity to Parasitic Animals

VOLUME 2

EDITORS

G. J. JACKSON   The Rockefeller University, New York
ROBERT HERMAN   National Institute of Allergy and Infectious
   Diseases, National Institutes of Health, Bethesda
IRA SINGER   The American Medical Association, Chicago

Foreword by William Hay Taliaferro

APPLETON-CENTURY-CROFTS

Educational Division

MEREDITH CORPORATION

New York

To

William Hay Taliaferro

CONTRIBUTORS

WILLIAM BALAMUTH, Ph.D.
Professor, Department of Zoology, University of California, Berkeley, California

E. BENJAMINI, Ph.D.
Assistant Director and Research Scientist, Laboratory of Medical Entomology, Kaiser Foundation Research Institute, San Francisco, California

ASHTON C. CUCKLER, Ph.D.
Executive Director, Quinton Research Laboratories, Merck & Co., Inc., Merck Institute for Therapeutic Research, Rahway, New Jersey

PHILIP A. D'ALESANDRO, Ph.D.
Associate Professor, The Rockefeller University, New York, New York

ROBERT S. DESOWITZ, Ph.D., D.Sc.
Professor of Tropical Medicine, Section of Tropical Medicine and Medical Microbiology, School of Medicine, University of Hawaii, Honolulu, Hawaii

FRANK A. EHRENFORD, Ph.D.
Research Specialist, Agricultural Department, The Dow Chemical Company, Lake Jackson, Texas

BEN F. FEINGOLD, M.D.
Chief, Department of Allergy, Kaiser Foundation Hospital, San Francisco, California

P. C. C. GARNHAM, M.D., D.Sc.
Emeritus Professor of Medical Protozoology, University of London; Senior Research Fellow, Department of Zoology, Imperial College of Science and Technology, Ascot, England

FRANS C. GOBLE, Sc.D.
  Director of Biology, Research and Development Department, Smith, Miller, and Patch, Inc., New Brunswick, New Jersey

B. M. HONIGBERG, Ph.D.
  Professor, Department of Zoology, University of Massachusetts, Amherst, Massachusetts

IRVING G. KAGAN, Ph.D.
  Chief, Parasitology Section, National Communicable Disease Center, Health Services and Mental Health Administration, Public Health Service, U.S. Department of Health, Education, and Welfare, Atlanta, Georgia

ZBIGNIEW KOZAR, Ph.D.
  Professor, Department of Parasitology and Parasitic Diseases, Veterinary Faculty, University School of Agriculture, University of Wroclaw, Wroclaw, Poland

ROBERT M. LEWERT, Sc.D.
  Professor, Department of Microbiology, University of Chicago, Chicago, Illinois

R. BARCLAY McGHEE, Ph.D.
  Alumni Foundation Distinguished Professor, Department of Zoology, University of Georgia, Athens, Georgia

GILBERT F. OTTO, Sc.D.
  Professor, Department of Zoology, University of Maryland, College Park, Maryland

EDWARD G. PLATZER, Ph.D.
  Guest Investigator, The Rockefeller University, New York, New York

MIODRAG RISTIC, D.V.M., Ph.D.
  Professor of Veterinary Pathology and Hygiene and of Veterinary Research, College of Veterinary Medicine, University of Illinois, Urbana-Champaign, Illinois

ROY E. RITTS, JR., M.D.
  Head, Section of Microbiology, Mayo Clinic and Foundation; Professor of Microbiology, Mayo Graduate School of Medicine, University of Minnesota, Rochester, Minnesota

WASIM A. SIDDIQUI, Ph.D.

Associate Professor, Department of Tropical Medicine and Microbiology, School of Medicine, University of Hawaii, Honolulu, Hawaii. Formerly of the Department of Preventive Medicine, Stanford University School of Medicine, Palo Alto, California

PAUL H. SILVERMAN, Ph.D., D.Sc.

Professor, Department of Zoology, University of Illinois, Urbana, Illinois

LESLIE A. STAUBER, Ph.D.

Professor, Department of Zoology and Bureau of Biological Research, Rutgers University, New Brunswick, New Jersey

RALPH E. THORSON, Sc.D.

Professor, Department of Biology, University of Notre Dame, Notre Dame, Indiana

CLARENCE J. WEINMANN, Ph.D.

Associate Professor of Parasitology, Department of Entomology and Parasitology, University of California, Berkeley, California

AVIVAH ZUCKERMAN, Ph.D.

Professor of Parasitology, Unit of Protozoology, Microbiological Institute, Hebrew University–Hadassah Medical School, Jerusalem, Israel

FOREWORD

The fact that the original edition of my book, *The Immunology of Parasitic Infections*, appeared forty years ago indicates the need for a systematic review and appraisal of the progress that has been made in this subject during the intervening years. Notable achievements have clarified some of the relationships between the invertebrates and their parasites. Our present understanding of immune mechanisms in these forms, however, is greatly handicapped by difficulties in obtaining normal hosts and in applying modern immunologic techniques. In any case, the presence of organized lymphoid tissue and of certain forms of immunity in some primitive fish seems to indicate that cellular, as well as dependent humoral, immunologic mechanisms manifested in higher mammals may operate in all other vertebrates and even in invertebrates provided suitable allowance is made for differences in host structure and function. Furthermore, these immunologic mechanisms seem to rest primarily on the activities of available cells and potential reserves of the connective tissue. This nutritive, scavenging, and reparative system, which cares for natural waste products and injury in the body, is certainly *par excellence* the system able to cope with foreign materials that gain entrance into a host. Such a concept stems from the work of Metchnikov on phagocytes and that of Maximow on inflammation. Other potent factors to be considered include physiologic, nutritional, and genetic conditions inherent in the host, the metabolic requirements of the parasite, and environmental patterns.

Later portions of this new edition reveal the ingenious approaches that have uncovered striking host-parasite relationships in the higher vertebrates. Here, specialized immunologic techniques, using rigidly controlled materials, are serving to amplify our knowledge of immune processes at the cellular and molecular levels.

WILLIAM HAY TALIAFERRO

Distinguished Service Professor Emeritus,
Department of Microbiology,
University of Chicago, Chicago, Illinois

Senior Scientist, Argonne National
Laboratory, Argonne, Illinois

CONTENTS

VOLUME 1

Part 1
Immunity in Zooparasitic
Infections

Part 2
Immunity of Plant Hosts

Part 3
Immunity of Invertebrate Hosts

Part 4
Immunity of Cold-Blooded
Vertebrate Hosts

VOLUME 2

Part 5
Immunity in Avian Hosts

Part 6
Immunity in Mammalian Hosts

Part 7
Immunity: Diagnosis and Prophylaxis

EDITORS' INTRODUCTION

The first book on immunity and parasitology was Taliaferro's.* Much more than a survey of what was known, it set an example. The subject was not an organism, neither host nor parasite, but a course of events, the infection. An infection was charted by following the changes (cellular, serologic, inflammatory, etc.) in experienced as well as inexperienced hosts, and changes in the number, stage, and morphology of the parasites. Cause-and-effect relationships were implied by the temporal juxtaposition of the changes. Substantiation of particular interactions (the establishment of high lytic antibody titers and a rapid decrease in the number of parasites, for instance) was then tried by isolating the implicated host factors or parasites to test them in a fresh, living or nonliving, environment. Taliaferro's analytic way of looking at parasitic infections suggested an experimental approach that is still usefully applied.

The second book on our topic, Culbertson's,† surveyed the early findings and reviewed the experimental work done in the decade following Taliaferro's volume. It was still possible at the time for one author to present the subject. The books since then have dealt with only parts of the topic or have been collected from several authors.**

The present collaboration attempts a width of coverage. Critics may consider the inclusion of chapters on higher plant hosts unjustified since the very applicability of the word "immunity" is doubtful outside the animal kingdom, but these and discussions of other far-out topics were requested for two reasons. The question, "What about plants?" is almost always raised in courses and symposia on the phylogeny of immunity. More importantly, the mention of unrelated mechanisms of resistance may remind experimenters that "dominant" forms of immunity may

---

*Taliaferro, W. H. 1929. The Immunology of Parasitic Infections. New York, The Century Co.

†Culbertson, J. T. 1941. Immunity against Animal Parasites. New York, Columbia University Press.

**Shikhobalova, N. P. 1950. Questions of Immunity in Helminthiasis. Moscow, U.S.S.R. Academy of Sciences.

Resistance and immunity in parasitic infections. 1958. Rice Institute Pamphlet 45 (1).

Garnham, P. C. C., E. A. Pierce, and I. Roitt, eds. 1963. Immunity to Protozoa. Oxford, Blackwell Scientific Publications.

Seminar on immunity to parasitic helminths. 1963. Exp. Parasit., 13 (1).

Haley, A. J., E. H. Sadun, and L. A. Jackowski, Jr., eds. 1963. Immunodiagnosis of helminthic infections. Amer. J. Hyg. Monogr. Ser. No. 22.

World Health Organization. 1965. Immunology and parasitic diseases. W.H.O. Techn. Rep. Ser. No. 315.

Pan American Sanitary Bureau of the World Health Organization. 1967. Immunological aspects of parasitic infections. Pan Amer. Health Org. Sci. Publ. No. 150.

Taylor, A. E. R., ed. 1968. Immunity to Parasites. Oxford, Blackwell Scientific Publications.

not be the exclusive ones within a group of organisms. Consequently, even a chapter on bacterial resistance to viral infection might not have been premature.

Before authors could be invited, the editors had to decide not only on boundaries but also arrange the space within, so that in the forum there might be maximal coverage and minimal overlap. Since immunity is the host's, we chose to divide the book by types of hosts and subdivide it by types of parasites. Nevertheless, some overlap is inevitable and not undesirable in a large work that few will read from front to back at one sitting. Each section on a related host grouping begins with a chapter on the mechanisms of immunity in that group without specific references to parasites. Three chapters are outside the general scheme: Sprent's on evolutionary and certain hereditary aspects of host immunity to parasitic animals opens the first, or "plant, invertebrate, and cold-blooded vertebrate" volume; Kagan's on immunologic testing and Silverman's on vaccination conclude the second, the "bird and mammal" volume.

Within his chapter an author was asked to be comprehensive at the level of a reference work, but, hopefully, interesting in order to pique the curiosity of advanced students in biology and medicine and stimulate other immunologists to use parasitic animals where appropriate in teaching and research. Thus, while this book stresses basic biologic matters, clinicians, as well as researchers, may find much of value to them.

It will soon be apparent to the reader that not all authors mean the same by "immunity," "resistance," "susceptibility," "infection," and so forth. Consequently no attempt is made to index these words. Nor has there been an attempt to persuade authors to adhere to or to avoid any one theory of immunity. The reader will again discover different approaches: the "serologic," the "cellular," and the "ecologic" points of view may be stressed or ignored. To have imposed a false consensus on the participants would not have benefited the state of our knowledge.

The editors would like to thank especially Professor William Trager of the Rockefeller University for his encouragement. During much of the planning and preparation of the book, two of the editors, Drs. Herman and Jackson, were supported in part by the U. S. Public Health Service through grants AI-04842, 2K3AI9522, and 2TAI192 from the National Institute of Allergy and Infectious Diseases.

G. J. JACKSON

ROBERT HERMAN

IRA SINGER

5

Immunity in Avian Hosts

General Mechanisms and Principles of Avian Immunity

R. BARCLAY McGHEE
Department of Zoology, University of Georgia, Athens, Georgia

INTRODUCTION

The intricacies of immunologic mechanisms generally increase concomitantly with the evolutionary development from invertebrates to vertebrates. Within the vertebrates, sophistication has increased along with the evolutionary processes leading to mammals. Mammals have been most extensively studied regarding their immunologic capabilities and have been shown to possess highly specialized responses, including antibody formation and homograft immunity. Knowledge of comparative immunology has suffered, but interest in other groups, including birds, has been developing in recent years. Knowledge gained from experiments on vertebrates other than mammals is now adding significantly to the understanding of basic immunologic processes, and it can be expected to make perhaps even greater contributions as the number of species of vertebrates under investigation increases. One of many examples of how studies of other vertebrates have aided in understanding similar processes in mammals is presented by Good and his co-workers (1964, 1965), who have been interested for many years in the biologic role of the mammalian thymus. The function of this organ eluded investigators until Chang et al. (1955) and Glick et al. (1956) demonstrated the close relationship of the avian bursa of Fabricius (cloacal thymus) and immunologic processes in the chicken.

Recent advances in methodology, increasing interest in organ transplantation, and the hope that greater knowledge of immunology might aid in the control of many diseases of man and animals have instigated rapid expansions in immunologic research. This is especially true about those diseases which appear to be developing drug resistance faster than new drugs can be found (e.g., malaria) or those which have thus far not yielded to drug therapy (e.g., Chagas' disease).

In view of the research in malaria, coccidia, and worms in various avian species, a discussion of avian immunology along with limited comparison of immunologic phenomena with other animals, such as the guinea pig, rabbit, or even man, would seem to be in order. The present discussion will be essentially of chicken immunology, since by far the majority of research programs on birds have been carried out with this species. This probably results from the relative ease of raising and handling of the chicken and because of its importance in the poultry industry. This points to the need for investigation of other avian species, especially in view of certain variations in immunologic responses among the avian hosts studied. Because of these variations, it is somewhat difficult to make broad generalizations in certain areas of avian immunology, and it is important to mention that it is desirable to include the species name studied in any discussion (Rose and Orlans, 1962).

No attempt is made here to include all the references on any given topic under discussion. Rather, enough literature hopefully will be cited to verify and clarify the areas of avian immunology discussed.

CELLULAR MECHANISMS

Present knowledge of immune mechanisms and the immune response leave little doubt as to an association between blood and connective tissue and all types of immunologic mechanisms. Because of the major role of lymphoid tissue in immune processes, discussion of avian immunity should include the embryonic and postembryonic development of the tissue. The relationship between age and onset of immunologic responses will be presented later. Because the cells involved in the various types of immune responses are lymphoidal, there can be no development of immunity in the embryonic animal until the lymphoid tissue has appeared and, to a certain extent, matured.

There are excellent recent general discussions of the ontogeny and phylogeny of immunity (Good and Papermaster, 1964); however, our interests here will be restricted to avian species. Consideration will be given to the types of cells involved in the immune processes in infections in aves, as well as some discussion of the reaction of these cells to various stimuli.

Age and appearance of lymphoid tissue

The major lymphoid organs of aves include the thymus and spleen, plus one peculiar to avian species: the bursa of Fabricius to which there appears to be no homologue in other vertebrates. Since Forbes (1877) pointed out that it is lymphoidal in nature, the question as to the function of this organ has occupied the efforts of a vast number of workers. Forbes' suggestion of its lymphoidal nature has been confirmed by Jolly (1915), Boyden (1922), Calhoun (1933), Ackerman (1962), Ackerman and Knouff (1959), and others (*see* Good and Papermaster, 1964). More will be said about the bursa of Fabricius in a subsequent section; it suffices here to mention that the bursa is a blind, plicated, sac-like lympho-epithelial structure which arises as a posterior diverticulum from the cloaca. A number of workers (Glick et al., 1956; Glick, 1958, 1961; Chang, 1957; Chang et al., 1959; Mueller et al., 1960, 1962; and others) have demonstrated the association of bursa with the development of immunologic mechanisms in such birds as the chicken and pheasant.

The mammalian thymus appears to be the first organ of the mammalian embryo to develop appreciable lymphoid tissues (Good and Papermaster, 1964). Mouse thymus, for example, develops lymphoidal cells and becomes a recognizable lymphoid organ between the 12th and 14th days of gestation (Auerbach, 1961), while the rabbit thymus becomes a lymphoid organ between 18 and 20 days of gestation (Good et al., 1965). The lymphoid tissue of the thymus appears to originate early in the epithelial component of the developing gland in response to an initial inductive stimulus by mesenchymal contact (Auerbach, 1961). In the chicken the thymus is a primary lymphoid organ in which lymphocytogenesis begins around the 9th to 12th day of incubation, becoming a lymphoid organ by the 14th day (Papermaster and Good, 1962; and others). Although the thymus becomes lymphoidal in the developing avian embryo before the bursa, the latter also develops lymphoid tissue early in embryonic development. Although the rudiments of the bursa can be recognized as an epithelial diverticulum of the cloaca by the fifth day of incubation (Boyden, 1922), it is the 15th to 16th day before it is recognizable as a lymphoid organ (Schrier and Hamilton, 1952; Ruth, 1961; Papermaster and Good, 1962). At 18 days of egg incubation it has become well organized, and from this time until about the time of hatching, it apparently contains the only lymphoid tissues (Papermaster and Good, 1962; Yamaguchi et al., 1964). The spleen is still primarily involved in granulocytopoiesis. Significant lymphoid follicle development in the spleen and gut tract does not take place until one to two weeks after hatching. However, in some individuals, lymphoid development of chicken spleen and other peripheral lymphoid tissue appears to be well underway at hatching (Cooper et al., 1966a). Solomon (1963) reports the presence of lymphocytes in very low numbers in the spleens of embryonic chickens within as early as 12 days of incubation, and he states that they were fairly numerous by the 15th day. McGhee (1949) noted the appearance of small lymphocytes in the spleens of duck embryos as early as 26 days of incubation. At hatching (28 days), small nests of lymphocytes were visible and increased with the age of the duckling.

Lymphoid tissue in the bursa appears to arise from the epithelial component, although Jolly (1915) believed it to be mesenchymal in origin. Morphologic and histochemical studies of the developing bursa (Ackerman and Knouff, 1959; Ackerman, 1962) provided evidence that the medullary portion of the lymphoid follicles of the bursa arises as an epithelial bud from the surface endodermal epithelium, with some of the epithelial cells transforming directly into lymphocytes. The lymphocytic cells of the cortical portion of the follicle are derived from two sources: mesenchymal cells, and undifferentiated epithelial cells or lymphoblasts.

The thymus of mammals and the thymus and bursa of birds are thus shown to be primary organs in the development of lymphoid tissue. A number of suggestions indicate that cells from these organs are disseminated to other parts of the animal; Ruth (1960) and Auerbach (1961) suggested that the mammalian thymus gives rise to certain lymphoid cells which are transported to the mesenchymal tissues where subsequent development of lymphoidal tissue occurs. Papermaster and Good (1962) suggested that the bursa and thymus may act together as sources of immunologically competent cells which are then transported to the spleen, liver, bone marrow, and other sites where these cells then undergo proliferation. Nossal (1964) noted seeding of thymic cells (mostly small lymphocytes) from the guinea pig thymus into the rest of the lymphoid tissue. Some of these workers stress that cell seeding is not the only role of the thymus.

Although the interval between the time of appearance of lymphoid tissue in the thymus and bursa and the appearance of lymphoid follicular development in other parts of the body varies from species to species, the development of lymphoid tissue in all other organs appears later than that in the thymus and bursa. In the rabbit, for example, the spleen and lymph nodes begin to show follicular lymphoid development just prior to 28 days of gestation (Good et al., 1965). In the mouse, on the other hand, the thymus is the only organ which is lymphoidal at birth.

Phagocytosis and development of phagocytic ability in aves

The prominent role of phagocytic activity as a defense mechanism in the immunity of vertebrates and in the removal of foreign particulate matter has been stressed in many publications, including those of Kent (1961) and Taliaferro (1963).

Most studies concerning phagocytosis have been carried out on mature animals. There is considerable evidence emphasizing the phagocytic importance in both birds and mammals of such organs as the liver and spleen, and to some degree the bone marrow. These organs are especially well-populated with cells capable of phagocytosis.

Relatively little information is available about the development of phagocytic capability or about the major organs or sites involved in either bird or mammalian embryos. Results of a few investigations indicate that ectodermal cells of the early embryonic avian blastoderm possess phagocytic ability (Kujono, 1918; Heine, 1936; Steinmuller, 1937; Dabrowska, 1950, as reviewed by Kent, 1961). This capability apparently disappears at about two to three days of egg incubation. Thereafter, until hatching, only certain migratory cells, white blood cells, and peritoneal epithelium retained phagocytic ability.

Goodpasture and Anderson (1937) reported the phagocytosis of bacteria dropped onto the chorioallantoic membrane of the chick embryo. McGhee (1942) injected three-day-old chick embryos with canary blood infected with malaria parasites or with India ink and recorded active phagocytosis by all cell types and in all tissue except in cells of the notochord and the embryonic blood corpuscles.

The type of material used influences the results, and this may explain the findings of Perez del Castillo (1957) that the onset of phagocytic ability occurs later than that observed by McGhee. Using a carbon suspension, Perez del Castillo (1957) concluded that phagocytosis in the liver does not take place at all before the 12th day of incubation and that it does not become very marked until the 16th day. Kent (1961), using thorotrast, a compound of particulate consistency composed of thorium dioxide and dextrine, made observations similar to those McGhee obtained with malarial parasites and India ink. Although there was little uptake of thorotrast inside the embryo itself until the organs associated with the lymphoid-macrophage system were differentiated, Kent (1961) noted the appearance of thorotrast in the Küpffer cells lining the liver sinusoids of embryos within as early as four days of incubation. On the fifth day, thorotrast accumulation was noted in the spleen, though this organ was taking up less than the liver at the time. Particles were also seen in the yolk sac membranes as soon as the mesodermal portion was formed. The relative importance of the yolk sac wall decreased as the liver and spleen developed, but thorotrast uptake continued until the time of hatching. In addition, by 14 to 19 days of incubation, small amounts of the compound were beginning to appear in the lungs and bone marrow. Kent further states that the activity in older embryos took place mostly in sites similar to those observed in the young chicken; i.e., mainly in the liver, but also in macrophages in the spleen, lungs, and the bone marrow, as well as in the areolar connective tissue of the mesenteries and body wall.

Karthigasu and Jenkin (1963) studied the rate of clearance of *Escherichia coli* and *Salmonella gallinarum* following their intravenous injections into chick embryos. The former was removed at a much faster rate than the latter at all ages studied. The clearance rate of *E. coli* increased with age of the embryos from 10 through 18 days of embryo development, while that of *S. gallinarum* remained relatively constant. Results indicated that the rate of clearance of smooth strains of *E. coli* was limited by the presence or absence of serum opsonins. They observed that during the early stages of incubation the membranes accounted for a high percentage of the material phagocytosed. The importance of these structures as a phagocytic system decreases toward the hatching period, at which time the liver appears to be the most significant organ. This is in agreement with observations by Kent and others (*see* above).

Cell type involved in the immune response

Extensive lymphoid development in the chick apparently occurs within the period from a week prior to and through the week following the time of hatching. At this age the avian host has become capable of various types of immunologic responses to various antigens, including infectious disease organisms. Response of immunologically competent birds to infectious agents such as protozoa has been shown to depend on both cellular and humoral factors (Taliaferro, 1949, 1963; Goble and Singer, 1960). Of course, serum factors are themselves products of cells and all immunologic activity is ultimately dependent on cells of lymphoidal origin.

The cells involved in the immune processes of birds are generally similar to those of other vertebrates. Included in the functions of these cells are the removal or isolation of foreign material, the performing of reparative processes, and the production of antibodies. Involved cells include the fibroblast, endothelium, fixed and free macrophages, polyblasts, and nongranular and granular leukocytes.

The fibroblasts and true endothelium may function in the formation of connective tissue walls around antigenic material or may function in repair. Fibroblasts of birds differ from those of mammals in that those of the former are capable of reversion to blast cells, with their considerable potential, while those of the latter are apparently differentiated.

Macrophages are defined functionally as cells capable of becoming phagocytic with minimal or no morphologic change. They may be fixed, such as reticular cells, littoral cells of the liver, adrenal, and hypophysis, adventitial cells of the perivascular area, histiocytes of skin, intestine, and lung, and the glial macrophages of the brain.

Polyblasts are phagocytic and considered to be transitional between nongranular leukocytes and macrophages. The nongranular leukocytes include monocytes, lymphocytes (small, medium, and large), and plasma cells.

The granular leukocytes of birds are difficult to classify. Among them there is a "typical" heterophil, and also what Hewitt (1940) classed the pseudoeosinophil. In addition, there is an eosinophil and a more or less typical basophil. Heterophils possess phagocytic abilities, while the function of the eosinophil and the basophil are less clearly understood (Taliaferro, 1949).

Investigators have classified cells involved in phagocytic activity in several ways: Metchnikov (1905) included fixed and free macrophages, polyblasts, and some nongranular leukocytes in this "macrophage system." Aschoff's reticuloendothelial system (1924) included the fixed cells of endothelium, fibroblasts, and macrophages, as well as the inflammatory macrophages. He did not, however, include the nongranular leukocytes. Taliaferro and Mulligan (1937), recognizing the important interplay between the mesenchymal reserve and the free lymphoid cells and intermediates of these types, proposed the term "lymphoid-macrophage system." Their unitarian concept of the origin of hematologic cells is, of course, contrary to those who hold a polyphyletic concept of the origin of such cells. The thorough work of Taliaferro and Mulligan (1937) and Bloom and Taliaferro (1938) lends authority to their concept of the lymphoid-macrophage system. The common use of the term "reticuloendothelial system" to include nongranular leukocytes is incorrect, is foreign to Aschoff's original concept, and should be supplanted by the term "lymphoid-macrophage system."

ACQUISITION OF ANTIBODY BY YOUNG AVES

Embryonic and young vertebrates are generally poor synthesizers of antibody (Freund, 1930; Bridges et al., 1959; and others). Several methods have evolved in various species by which the antibodies are passively transferred from the mother (see Good and Papermaster, 1964). In the rabbit and guinea pig, this transfer of antibodies takes place by way of the yolk sac, and in the human being, apparently by way of the placenta (see Halliday, 1955; Brambell et al., 1948, 1949, 1950, and 1958). In rats and mice two mechanisms appear to be involved. Some antibody is passively transferred to the young in utero but the major portion is obtained through the colostrum immediately after birth. In the horse, pig, and cow, antibodies are not apparently present in fetal or newborn animals but passive reception through means of a massive dose from the colostrum takes place soon after birth.

Passive transfer of antibodies from mother to offspring in aves

It has been noted that tetanus antitoxin (Ramon, 1928), diphtheria antitoxin (Jukes et al., 1934), neutralizing antibody to Newcastle disease virus

(Brandley et al., 1946), immunity to duck hepatitis (Hanson and Alberts, 1960), antibodies to protozoa (Barrow and Miller, 1964), antibody to bacteria (Buxton, 1952), and antibodies to purified proteins such as bovine serum albumin (Patterson et al., 1962a) are passed from the mother to the egg in various avian species, including the hen and duck. Antibodies have been shown to be transferred from the egg contents to the developing avian embryos in many cases.

The titers of antibody in the egg, the interval of time between peak serum titers and peak egg titers, and the persistence of the passively transferred antibodies in the young bird developing from these eggs are influenced by the antigen used in the immunization of the hen, as well as by the route of injection. There will also be a certain amount of variation between individual birds in a given experiment. For example, Buxton (1952) noted transference of both agglutinins and other antibody to the offspring via the yolk using hens immunized with killed or living *Salmonella typhi* or *Salmonella pullorum*, as well as birds naturally infected with the latter organism. When killed bacteria were injected into hens intravenously, the serum titers ranged as high as 1: 5,120, whereas levels in the yolk of eggs laid by hens naturally infected with *Salmonella pullorum* had titers about equal to those of the serum. Antibody transference was observed to continue for up to 280 days after initial injection of hens when killed organisms were used, whereas eggs laid up to 474 days later by the naturally infected birds showed antibody. The sera and egg yolk from these hens also had a nonagglutinating antibody which was of about equal titer in the sera and egg yolk from those hens injected via the intravenous route. In those animals which were inoculated subcutaneously or intramuscularly, on the other hand, the yolk demonstrated much lower titers than did the sera of the hens.

Buxton (1952) also reported a rise in antibody titer in the blood of embryos developing from eggs containing passively transferred antibodies. This increase occurred from about the 11th day of egg incubation until the time of hatching, at which time peak titer was reached, sometimes approximating the titer of the yolk. These passively transferred antibodies decreased rapidly during the first three days after hatching and had disappeared almost entirely by the 17th day. Agglutinating antibody was observed to disappear from the sera of the chicks more rapidly than nonagglutinating antibody.

The work of Buxton showed, furthermore, that antibody is absorbed from the yolk through the vitelline and hepatic portal circulation. Little or no antibody was observed to be transferred via the yolk stalk to the intestine of the developing embryo. Antibodies fed by mouth to chicks immediately after hatching did not produce demonstrable circulating titers (Brierley and Hemmings, 1956).

Hosada et al. (1955), in a detailed study of the transfer of antibodies from hen to egg, observed that antibody to red blood cells appeared in the sera of hens in four days, in egg white at seven days, and in yolk at nine days after stimulation with these cells, and reached maximum titers on the seventh day in serum, ninth day in egg white, and eleventh day in the yolk after the start of injection. Agglutinins transmitted from hen to egg were detectable in the sera of two-week-old chicks but not in the sera of three-week-old birds. Patterson et al. (1962a) noted the appearance of antibodies to bovine serum albumin in the yolk of the eggs of immune birds some four days after appearance in the serum. The peak titer in the yolk appeared at five through eight days after the peak titer was observed in the serum of the parent. Using *Salmonella pullorum* or *Brucella abortus*, Brierley and Hemmings (1956) found the titer of egg yolk was directly related to the serum titer of the hen. In the chicken and duck these passively transferred antibodies disappeared after about one month (Patterson et al., 1962a; Brandley et al., 1946). Chickens hatching from eggs laid by hens immune to Newcastle disease virus showed demonstrable amounts of passive immunity for about one month of life (Brandley et al., 1946). The persistence of antibodies for this length of time has been observed to interfere with active immunization efforts to certain agents such as Newcastle disease virus (Brandley et al., 1946; Richey and Schmittle, 1962).

Although Buxton (1952) obtained evidence for his hypothesis that some of the antibody transferred to yolk may have been synthesized by follicular epithelium, Patterson et al. (1962b) observed that in the chicken, gamma-globulin is preferentially transferred by the follicular epithelium of the ovary to the developing ova some four to five days preceding ovulation at the time when the developing ovum is undergoing rapid growth. The concentration of gamma-globulin in the yolk of the egg reaches many times the concentration of the other serum protein components, such as albumin, for example.

Karthigasu et al. (1964), in studying bacterial opsonins, concluded that although both 7S and 19S antibodies are passed from the hen to the yolk and are detectable in the yolk sac contents of the developing embryo, only the 7S type was found in the serum of the developing chick embryo. Shortly after hatching, both types of antibody were found. The hen follicular epithelium seems to pass both types of antibody, but these workers suggested that the selectivity of the yolk sac membrane of the embryo allows only the passage of the smaller globulins.

The transmission of antibodies from mother to offspring appears to have some degree of specificity both for the gamma-globulin fraction of the serum and for gamma-globulins of the animal's own species. In the rabbit (Brambell et al., 1949) the yolk sac wall is selective for rabbit antibody; that of other species is transferred to a lesser extent. Although it has been shown that such foreign proteins as bovine gamma-globulin, rat serum, hemocyanin, and albumin fractions, as well as other materials, are transferred in substantially unmodified form from hen's blood into the egg (Knight and Schectman, 1954), the follicular epithelium of the chicken ovary is also selective in that these substances are passed in relatively small quantities, and, as mentioned previously, chicken gamma-globulin concentration in the yolk of the egg reaches many times the concentration of other chicken serum proteins. In addition, while fowl immunoglobulins to *Salmonella pullorum* or *Brucella abortus* injected experimentally into the yolk sac remnant of the newly hatched chick give rise to circulating titers in the chick blood several days later, the rabbit, cow, and horse immunoglobulins so injected do not do so (Brierley and Hemmings, 1956). Furthermore, immune pigeon serum gives rise to lower concentrations in the hatched chick than does the chicken serum. Thus there is considerable evidence that the yolk sac splanchnopleure has a rather high selectivity in the passage of avian immunoglobulins.

In addition to mechanisms having been evolved to insure passage of antibodies from mother to offspring, an adaptation appears to have been developed on the part of the embryos which assists the young bird in retaining these passively transferred antibodies as long as possible. In the adult hen the halflife of I^{131}-labeled chicken serum albumin (CSA) is 66 hours and that of labeled chicken gamma-globulin (CGG) is 35 hours, while in the newly hatched chick the halflife of labeled CSA is 42 hours and CGG is 72 hours (Patterson et al., 1962b). This species demonstrates, as do most mammals, a gamma-globulin sparing effect during the first days of life.

Thus it is established that in birds, as well as in mammals, mechanisms have evolved to transfer passively immunoglobulins from mother to offspring. Such antibody probably aids in the protection immediately after hatching until the young bird becomes capable of making its own antibodies.

Age and antibody synthesis

Albumin, alpha-, beta-, and gamma-globulins, as well as fibrinogen, appear in various fluids and tissues of certain embryonic animals at a very early age (Brambell et al., 1948). The gamma-globulin fraction has been shown to contain specific immunoglobulins, and although there is some evidence of antibody synthesis in certain embryonic animals (Silverstein, 1964), the majority of immunoglobulins found in the blood of embryonic animals is passively transferred from the parent (Good and Papermaster, 1964). The literature indicates that in general, embryonic, recently hatched, and very young animals are relatively poor synthesizers of antibody (Buxton, 1954). One of the earlier workers in this area (Rywosch, 1907) noted the inability of chicken embryos or newly hatched animals to synthesize antibody when injected with *Escherichia coli*. Grasset (1929) observed no immunity to diphtheria toxoid in developing embryos or in newly hatched chicks. Weinberg and Guelin (1936) observed no antibody synthesis by either chick embryos or recently hatched chicks when injected with *Clostridium sporogenes*. Burnet (1941) obtained negative results using influenza virus injected into 12-day chick embryos (reviewed by Good and Papermaster, 1964), and Beveridge and Burnet (1946) could detect no antibody response to bacteriophage in chick embryos of various ages. Numerous other investigations indicated very little or no antibody response by avian embryos to a variety of antigens.

Solomon and Tucker (1963), using the elimination of red blood cells in an immune manner, a technique they claim to be much more sensitive for antibody detection than usual serologic methods, obtained some evidence that the chick embryo may sometimes (in two out of 16 birds) be capable of a very weak immune response just prior to hatching. Newly hatched chicks were observed to become sensitized to foreign red cells. Wolfe and Dilks (1948), using serum protein antigens, found a significant albeit low antibody production by newly hatched chicks. Antibody-producing ability developed gradually as the chickens aged. Between four and five weeks of age there appeared to be a rather sudden maturation of antibody-producing ability, since the average antibody titers of birds stimulated at five weeks were much greater than those of birds stimulated at four weeks. The increase was attributed in part to the fact that almost all birds responded at five weeks of age, whereas some of the younger birds did not respond with production of detectable antibody. Increase in antibody-producing ability continued in the chicken until at least 20 to 25 weeks of age (Wolfe et al., 1957b). Every animal over 13 weeks of age was observed to respond to injection of bovine serum albumin. These workers also noted a direct correlation between the size of the spleen and antibody-producing ability in young chickens.

Results of similar studies in mammals are comparable to those noted with birds in that antibody production begins at or near birth and increases during early life. Fetal and new-born individuals of many species usually respond very poorly if at all to a variety of immunizing agents (Baumgartner, 1934; Osborn et al., 1952; Smith and Bridges, 1958). The widespread failure to detect antibody production led some to the conclusion that mammals of these ages were incapable of an immune response. Recent research shows, however, that given the proper antigen and proper conditions, some embryonic mammals such as sheep (Silverstein, 1964) and human beings (Uhr et al., 1960; 1962) are capable of producing detectable antibodies. The ability to produce antibodies in mammals appears at the same time plasma cells are first found (Deichmille and Dixon, 1957b; Bridges et al., 1959).

A number of interesting experiments designed to elucidate further the ability and conditions of formation of antibody by isolated mesenchymal cells have taken advantage of the inability of antibody response by the young mammal or bird. Recent experiments have demonstrated the production of antibody by adult chicken spleen cells when put into developing chick embryos. Exposure to antigen before transplantation into the developing chick embryo or young chicks was a prerequisite for such antibody production (Truka, 1957; Sibal and Olson, 1958; Papermaster et al., 1959; Sibal, 1961; Gold and Benedict, 1963). This can be done with a variety of antigens when adult splenic cells are exposed to the antigens either *in vivo* or *in vitro*. The antibody produced in the embryo after transplantation of these cells is principally 19S, thus indicating a primary response (Gold and Benedict, 1963). Rabbit spleen cells treated in a similar manner and transplanted into avian species do not produce antibody (Truka, 1957).

These studies of antibody synthesis in embryonic and early postnatal animals indicate that in both birds and mammals, embryos are, in general, relatively immunologically deficient, and that maturation occurs sometimes near birth or during the first weeks after birth. Some degree of maturation continues in the chicken for the first several months of post-hatching life.

Age and immune tolerance

As pointed out by Silverstein (1964), a general discussion of the ontogeny of the immune response should include information gathered from studies of immunologic tolerance since this phenomenon is so closely related to the response of the developing organism and its maturing cell systems. Results from these investigations support the aforementioned conclusions regarding immunologic maturation.

Excellent reviews on immunologic tolerance and transplantation immunity have appeared relatively recently (Hasek et al., 1961; Smith, 1961), and only a limited discussion of the subject will be presented here. A given amount of antigen injected into an animal may result in either an immune response or unresponsiveness, depending to a great extent on the age of the animal. The time near birth or hatching appears to be the time of a rather abrupt ending of the stage when tolerance can be most easily induced. This adaptive period appears to end slightly before birth in the sheep and rabbit, at one or two days after birth or hatching in the mouse, dog, chicken, and turkey, and may persist for several days after birth or hatching in the rat and duck (Hasek et al., 1961).

The ease of obtaining experimental embryonic animals almost assured the avian embryo a primary spot in immunologic tolerance studies. Burnet et al. (1950) used chick embryos in early attempts at inducing tolerance. Unfortunately, this work was not successful, nor were later attempts by Cohn (1957). Success was subsequently obtained by a number of workers using a variety of antigens. Wolfe et al. (1957a) observed unresponsiveness in chicks injected a few hours after hatching with bovine serum albumin and challenged several weeks later. Stevens and co-workers (1958), using human serum albumin, observed maximum tolerance in embryos injected at 14 days of incubation. Friedman and Gaby (1960), using *Shigella paradysenteriae* soluble antigen, produced maximum tolerance in embryos injected at 14 days before hatching. Hirata and Schechtman (1960) obtained similar results when human gamma-globulin and bovine serum albumin were used as antigens. They observed maximum unresponsiveness in groups injected from 13 to 16 days of incubation through one to three days post-hatching. Thus it appears, based on information obtained from tolerance studies, that the time very near hatching (a few days before through a few days after) is a time of major changes in the immunologic capabilities of chickens. This is during the time when antibody producing ability begins to appear. The typical immune response apparently appears at about two to eight days of age, depending on the antigen and route of injection (Solomon and Tucker, 1963).

BURSECTOMY, THYMECTOMY, AND ANTIBODY PRODUCTION

The thymus of mammals and birds as well as birds' bursa of Fabricius have long attracted the interest of biologists. Although numerous contributions dealing with these organs have appeared in the literature, their biologic role remained an enigma until recently. The similarity of the thymus and bursa has long been noted in referring to the latter as the "cloacal thymus." Recent interest in both developed almost simultaneously, with work on the bursa greatly stimulating and enlightening some of the investigations of the thymus. The elucidation of the biologic role of the thymus is mostly due to the persistent interest of Metcalf (1960), Miller and co-workers (*see* Miller et al., 1965), and Good and associates (*see* Good et al., 1965). The credit for clarification of the biologic role of the bursa of Fabricius belongs to Glick and associates (Glick et al., 1956, 1958). According to Good et al. (1965), investigators had attempted for several years to demonstrate, in experimental animals, an immunologic role of the thymus. Such a role for this organ was suspected by many workers for various reasons, including those arising from clinical observations on patients with diseased thymuses (Good and Papermaster, 1964). However, efforts to demonstrate rigorously an immunologic function were largely unfruitful. In the meantime, Glick and co-workers (1956) discovered that removal of the bursa profoundly lessened antibody response. Following this, it was found that removal of the thymus in mammals at an early age markedly influenced the future immunologic capabilities of the animal. Such mammals as mice, rats, and rabbits thymectomized at an early age generally show markedly impaired immune responses (i.e., production of less humoral antibody, delay of homograft rejection, and impaired development of hypersensitivities) when tested a few weeks later (Miller et al., 1965; Good et al., 1965; Jankovic et al., 1962). Some progress has been made with similar investigations on the avian thymus (Aspinall et al., 1963; Graetzer et al., 1963a; Warner et al., 1962; Archer and Pierce, 1961; Good et al., 1965).

Thus the immunologic role of the mammalian and avian thymuses, as well as of the avian bursa of Fabricius, becomes more apparent. We shall briefly review the more important aspects of this relationship. Excellent discussions of these organs and their role in the immune response can be found in recent articles by Warner and Szenberg (1964) and Good et al. (1964, 1965).

The bursa is a lymphoepithelial organ, peculiar to birds and present in all species thus far studied. It is a pear-shaped structure which arises as a dorsal posterior diverticulum from the cloaca. The parenchyma is composed almost entirely of lymphoid follicles which are closely related to the lining epithelium (Forbes, 1877; Jolly, 1915; Ackerman and Knouff, 1959). Ackerman and Knouff hold that the lymphocytes and lymphoid follicles arise from undifferentiated endodermal epithelial cells.

The development of the bursal primordium begins around the end of the first four to five days of egg incubation (Jolly, 1915), and it evidently becomes a lymphoid organ around the 14th to 15th day of incubation (Ackerman and Knouff, 1959, 1964). In 17-day embryos, the bursa is relatively large and filled with lymphoidal follicles (Meyer et al., 1959). It grows most rapidly in the first two to five weeks after hatching (Glick, 1959, 1960b) and becomes fully developed in the young post-hatched bird around the time of sexual maturity (Davy, 1866; Forbes, 1877; Jolly, 1915; Riddle, 1928). Regression of the organ, in some species beginning as early as 30 to 40 days of age (Glick, 1960b), parallels marked enlargement of the testes and production of considerable quantities of sex hormones (Glick, 1959). In most older animals, the bursa becomes atrophied and eventually involutes completely.

In the chick, it begins its development about the fifth day of incubation (Boyden, 1922; Ackerman and Knouff, 1959) as a proliferation of the endoderm on the caudal border of the cloaca adjoining the anal plate. It continues to grow and enlarge until the chick has reached the age of one to four months (Jolly, 1915). Soon after this time, involution of the organ begins and by the end of the first year it has almost completely disappeared. Thus it is obvious that the period of most rapid growth and development of the bursa coincides with the period when the young bird acquires the ability to develop antibody to many antigens.

The considerable interest in the relationship between the bursa and antibody formation is largely due to the discovery by Glick and his associates (1956) that following surgical removal of the bursa from chicks during the first two weeks of post-hatching life, the adults became deficient producers of antibody to *Salmonella typhimurium*. These observations have since been verified repeatedly and extended. The discovery by Meyer et al. (1959) that 19-nortestosterone would either completely prevent or arrest the development of bursal tissue when given early enough during embryonic development was of considerable interest and simplified the study of this organ. The fact that hormonal bursectomy is much easier and quicker to perform, and probably more thorough than the surgical technique, has greatly facilitated the expanded studies of the role of this organ in the immune response.

The earlier workers observed that birds surgically or chemically bursectomized slightly before, at, or up to 12 to 15 days after hatching usually exhibit the greatest deficiency in antibody production when inoculated at some four to six weeks later with any number of antigens, including red blood cells, bovine serum albumin, and various bacterial antigens. Similar effects were observed in reduction of resistance to various infections. Birds bursectomized at or near hatching showed no measureable antibody to a variety of antigens when challenged four to six weeks later (Glick et al., 1956; Glick, 1958; Chang et al., 1957, 1959; Graetzer et al., 1963b; Mueller et al., 1960; Wolfe et al., 1962). Bursectomy at one week post-hatching markedly decreased antibody formation on challenge, while bursectomy at 2, 3, 4, and 5 weeks of age showed progressively less effect until, finally, removal of the bursa at 10 to 12 weeks of age had little or no effect on the ability of the host's immunologic response. Some later reports state that with techniques apparently more sensitive than those used by the above workers, antibody may still be detected in some chickens bursectomized within 24 hours of hatching (Cooper et al., 1966b; Pierce et al., 1966). The levels are apparently quite low, however. Mueller et al. (1960) made the interesting observation that chicks bursectomized at five weeks of age and inoculated with a single dose of antigen at 22 weeks of age showed little antibody response, but if the inoculation was done at 34 weeks of age, bursectomy had little effect on the ability on the animals to produce antibody. This indicated to them that recovery was taking place, that some other tissue was taking over, or that possibly the bursa was not completely destroyed. Similar evidence of recovery was noted in thymectomized rabbits (Good et al., 1965), in which case the appendix was partially responsible for recovery.

Although there can be no argument that removal of the bursa in the embryonic or newly hatched chick interferes with the ability of the animal to form circulating antibody, ablation of the bursa during this time appears to have little or no effect on the development of the capacity for rejection of skin homotransplants. Aspinall et al. (1963) found that neither steroidal nor surgical removal of the bursa had any effect on homograft rejection. Warner et al. (1962) stated that they found no effect of bursectomy on homograft immunity to solid grafts, and Szenberg and Warner (1964) apparently found the same. However, chickens hatched from eggs previously treated with 19-nortestosterone show a deficient homograft response to massive intraperitoneal injection of adult homologous spleen cells, which is manifested by splenomegaly, histologic changes characteristic of the graft-versus-host reaction, and a runting syndrome (Papermaster et al., 1961, 1962). The role of the bursa in the delayed type of hypersensitivity reaction does not yet appear to be clearly understood. Some workers (Jankovic et al., 1963) report that bursectomy shortly after hatching does not suppress the development of the delayed hypersensitivity reaction, while others (Szenberg and Warner, 1962) report the elimination of the capacity to elicit delayed hypersensitivity reactions to tuberculin in bursectomized birds. The time and method of bursectomy appear to be important and further work in this area would be enlightening.

In addition to the bursa, the thymus plays a role in the development of immunologic processes. Apparently the thymus is the major primary lymphoid organ of mammals. Destruction of the thymus in young mammals results in impairment of antibody production (Archer and Pierce, 1961; Ackerman and Knouff, 1964; Good et al., 1965), prevention of development of capacity for homograft rejection, and in general causes hypoplasia of lymphoid tissue. Thymectomy in birds apparently has little or no effect on such immunologic responses as reaction to vaccination, formation of humoral antibody, degree of immunity, or resistance to disease (Bandheim, 1965). Warner and Szenberg (1962) noted that neonatal thymectomy had no effect on production of antibody in chicks injected with human gamma-globulin or other antigens. Isakovic et al. (1963) obtained inconsistent results in studies of thymectomy effects on antibody production in chickens. They did note, however, that 6 percent of those birds without a thymus failed to respond, whereas 100 percent of the controls responded. Cooper et al. (1965), using thymectomy in combination with irradiation, have recently shown that antibody production in the chicken is "somehow" dependent on the presence of the thymus, at least in some individuals.

In birds the thymus apparently is involved with delayed hypersensitivity and homograft immunity. Warner and Szenberg (1962) reported that some chickens in which the thymic cortex had been destroyed did not normally reject homografts. Aspinall et al. (1963) noted that thymectomy one to three days after hatching delayed homograft rejection in some chickens. Cooper et al. (1965) found that thymectomy had little consistent effect on homograft rejection, but if thymectomy was followed by irradiation, the process was prolonged. Apparently the age of the bird at the time of thymectomy is important here, as it was in bursectomy.

Observations of the bursectomy effects on humoral antibody and of thymectomy effects on homograft immunity and hypersensitivity have prompted some workers to suggest that in mammals the thymus appears to be the primary lymphoid organ functioning in the development of all types of immunologic processes, but in the chicken there may possibly be two or more primary levels of lymphocytopoiesis with each level controlling different types of immune response. The original concept of a dissociation of immunologic processes was suggested by Warner et al. (1962). Cooper et al. (1966a) have presented evidence to support this theory by making use of thymectomy or bursectomy followed by irradiaton. These workers state that the thymus-dependent tissues of the chicken are basic to ontogenesis of cellular immunity, while the bursa-dependent part is basic to antibody formation.

Results with other avian species may differ somewhat from those observed using the chicken. Vojteskova et al. (1963), for example, found no effect of thymectomy or bursectomy on homograft survival in ducks. Additional work in this area with other species of aves might be informative.

There is, as might be expected, considerable evidence linking the bursa with resistance of birds to certain infections. A general consensus exists that birds without a bursa are unhealthy and may die early of disease and other causes. Bursectomy has been shown to render chickens more susceptible to such pathogens as *Leptospira icterohaemorrhagiae* (Kemenes and Pethes, 1963) and *Salmonella typhimurium* (Chang et al., 1959).

Although bursectomy results in lowering of plasma cell numbers (Isakovic and Jankovic, 1964; Cooper et al., 1966a), these cells are still readily detectable (Carey and Warner, 1964). In general, germinal centers appear to be reduced in bursectomized chickens (Warner et al., 1962; Pierce and Long, 1965; Pierce et al., 1966). Bursectomy results in lower serum levels of 7S gamma-globulin (Ortega and Der, 1964; Pierce et al., 1966) as well as of 19S immunoglobulins (Pierce et al., 1966). Although bursectomized chickens produce no detectable or less specific antibody, they still have appreciable levels of gamma-globulin (Carey and Warner, 1964; Pierce et al., 1966). There are fewer small lymphocytes in the peripheral blood of thymectomized chickens (Warner and Szenberg, 1962). These workers also recorded the depletion of small lymphocytes in the spleen and cloaca of such birds. Warner et al. (1962) noted that thymic atrophy resulted in the absence of germinal centers in the spleen, whereas Jankovic and Isakovic (1964) and others noted germinal centers and normal plasma cell levels in thymectomized chickens. There is a marked proliferation of plasma cells in thymectomized chicks seven days after injection of antigen, and although plasma cells are present in bursaless chickens, there is apparently no proliferation upon immunization.

Kerstetter et al. (1962), using bovine serum albumin and a fluorescent dye in the ring-necked pheasant, found antigen in cell clones in the bursa itself and indicated that the bursa is capable of antibody synthesis. Mass cultures of cells derived from the bursa as well as other embryonic tissues of the 16-day chick embryo have been observed to synthesize and release into the nutrient medium a protein which has the characteristics of chicken gamma-M globulin (Marinkovic and Baluda, 1966). Dent and Good (1965) found that neither bursal nor thymic cell suspensions produced specific hemolysins or hemagglutinins to sheep red blood cells.

While the discussion to this point can leave little doubt that the bursa of Fabricius plays a fundamental role in the development of birds' ability to produce antibody, we are still left with the question of the manner in which these observed effects are brought about. Since the immunologic capability of the bursaless bird can be partially restored by surgical transplantation of bursal tissue into such animals (Isakovic et al., 1963), the question arises as to whether a cellular or humoral mechanism or a combination of the two is involved. The work of Glick (1960a) suggested the possibility of a noncellular, perhaps hormone-like, mechanism when he found that saline extracts of bursal tissues increased measurably the antibody titers of bursaless chickens. Further evidence that the bursa elaborates a noncellular agent has recently appeared. Jankovic and Leskowitz (1965) and St. Pierre and Ackerman (1965) have demonstrated the restoration of immunologic reactivity to bursectomized chickens by implanting into them bursal tissue in millipore diffusion chambers which are believed by the authors to be cell-impermeable. Although the impermeability of the chambers to cells appears to be questioned by some, this work, as well as that of Glick, suggests a noncellular material is involved. Similar techniques indicate that the mammalian thymus ensures the development of normal immunologic capacity by means of humoral mechanisms, at least in part (see Miller et al., 1965). Other evidence suggests that the bursa and thymus seed other organs with lymphoid cells (Woods and Linna, 1965).

OTHER FACTORS INFLUENCING ANTIBODY PRODUCTION

In addition to the importance of the thymus and bursa of Fabricius, the previous discussion has emphasized the importance of age and hence the maturation of lymphoid tissue in the immune response of aves. After the animal has become old enough to be competent immunologically, still other factors influence the type and intensity of the immune response. In birds, as well as in mammals, the route of injection, the nature of the antigen used, the quantity of antigen used, and the species of animal under investigation have been observed to play important roles in antibody formation.

Not all species of birds appear to be equally good producers of precipitins. There is also some variation among strains or among individuals of a given species (Mueller, 1960). Chickens have been found to be excellent precipitin producers to animal serum proteins such as bovine serum albumin (Wolfe and Dilks, 1948; Goodman et al., 1951; Makinodan et al., 1952). On a quantitative basis chickens produce as much as 90 mg of antibody nitrogen per ml of antiserum after a single intravenous injection of 10 mg of bovine serum albumin per kg of body weight (Abramoff and Wolfe, 1956), as compared to the rabbit which produces only about 26 mg of antibody nitrogen per ml of antiserum after a single intravenous injection of 7.5 mg per kg body weight of the same antigen (Condie and Good, 1956). In addition, a larger percent of chickens injected with bovine serum albumin responds with good titers than do rabbits. For example, only 80 to 95 percent of normal adult rabbits were found to respond (Dixon and Maurer, 1955), while 100 percent of the chickens over 13 weeks of age were found to respond to the same antigen (Wolfe et al., 1957b). The owl, pheasant, and partridge are classed as "good" precipitin producers by Wolfe and Dilks (1949), but average titers were found to be well below those of chickens comparably treated. Turkeys and ducks under comparable conditions were observed to produce quite low precipitin titers and a number of individuals did not respond at all (Wolfe and Dilks, 1949). No precipitins were detected in the sera of guinea fowls and pigeons in the same experiment. Chickens are also reasonably good producers of agglutinins, of neutralizing antibodies to various viruses, and are fair producers of hemolysins. Ducks have been noted to be especially poor producers of hemolysins or agglutinins to various avian red blood cells (McGhee, 1963, unpublished). Similar species differences have been noted for mammals. For example, rabbits are good precipitin producers, whereas the ground squirrel and fox were much poorer producers under similar conditions (Wolfe and Dilks, 1949).

The quantity of antigen injected may well determine whether the host will respond at all. If a response is produced, such quantities may be a factor in the time of appearance of antibodies in the circulating blood. When smaller quantities of an antigen such as bovine serum albumin are given (e.g., 40 mg per kg body weight), antibody appears earlier and the peak titer is reached earlier than when large quantities (200 mg per kg body weight) are given (Brown and Wolfe, 1954). On the other hand, the ultimate maximum antibody content is greater when larger amounts of antigen are used for stimulation. If the quantity of antigen given becomes too large, however, the bird may not respond at all. Virtually all of the chickens given 40 mg of bovine serum albumin per kg body weight responded with good titers (Wolfe et al., 1957a), but adult chickens given 2.61 mg of the same antigen per kg body weight responded with detectable antibody production in only about one half of the individuals tested. However, the response to a different antigen, namely human gamma-globulin, remained unaffected in these birds (Mueller, 1960). The secondary response may also be dependent on the amount of antigen used for both the primary and secondary injections. Primary injections of approximately 1 mg per kg body weight of bovine serum albumin failed to produce a secondary response upon challenge (Blazhovec, 1963). The optimal quantity of bovine serum albumin for antibody stimulation in chickens for either a single injection (Wolfe and Dilks, 1948) or for both primary and secondary stimulation (Blazhovec, 1963) appears to be around 40 mg per kg body weight. A single injection of this amount is more effective than four injections of 10 mg each.

Other variables involved in the secondary response include the age of the animal at the time of primary stimulation and the interval of time between primary and secondary stimulation. Chickens injected with 40 mg per kg of bovine serum albumin at 20 days of age do not exhibit a secondary response when challenged at 6, 12, and 22 weeks of age. A primary injection at six weeks of age yields an occasional response to reinjection at 12 and 22 weeks. Virtually 100 percent of those birds given primary injections at 12 weeks of age and challenged at 22 weeks of age displayed good secondary responses. Chickens given a primary injection at 14 weeks of age give larger mean titers when reinjected at 50 weeks of age than do those given primary injections at 41 or 47 weeks of age (Blazhovec, 1963). Hence the capacity for anamnestic response in the chicken is apparently developed sometime between the ages of 6 and 12 weeks of age (Wolfe et al., 1960, 1961) and reaches a peak shortly thereafter (Blazhovec, 1963).

In conjunction with the quantity of antigen, the route of injection exerts considerable influence upon antibody response. When a single stimulatory injection of smaller quantities of antigen is given, the response is quicker, and peak titer is reached earlier than when the injection is administered by the intravenous route (Brown and Wolfe, 1954). On the other hand, when large amounts of antigen are used, there are indications of better titers when the subcutaneous route is utilized.

Chickens, as well as rabbits, respond earlier to human gamma-globulin than to bovine serum albumin (Abramoff and Wolfe, 1956). In general, animal proteins appear to produce the best responses. Two plant proteins used were not as antigenic as several of animal origin. However, hemoglobin, thyroglobin, and certain polysaccharides elicit no antibody response in chickens (Schmidt and Wolfe, 1953). Antigenicity also appears to be correlated with an increase in molecular weight (Woods, 1963).

The immunologic response observed in aves is, as in mammals, tempered by previous and present serologic and antigenic experiences. Chickens grown under germ-free conditions are characterized by underdevelopment of the lymphoid-macrophage system, have fewer plasma cells and secondary nodules, and generally have lower gamma-globulin levels in the serum. Such animals, in comparison to normally grown controls, require an additional induction period of one day to produce detectable antibody levels to a given antigen such as bovine serum albumin (Wostman and Olson, 1964). Both groups, however, reach peak antibody titer at about the same time. Decline in the antibody titer of germ-free chickens, however, is slower than that for conventional chickens.

When two antigens such as human gamma-globulin and bovine serum albumin are administered simultaneously, in conventional chickens the peak titer is about one-half that of the normal controls in the chicken. Although hemoglobin itself does not stimulate detectable antibody production in the chicken, when it is given simultaneously with bovine serum albumin, the response to bovine serum albumin is lowered (Abramoff, 1955). Bovine serum albumin is prevented from eliciting a secondary response when simultaneously injected with human gamma-globulin following a previous sensitization with bovine serum albumin. The primary response to human gamma-globulin was also lowered in this instance. One should be aware of the possibility of other antigen contaminants in a given system under investigation along with their possible effects on the primary and secondary responses of the host.

The time of appearance of antibodies may depend on the antigen, the quantity given, and the route of injection, as mentioned above. In response to injection of 40 mg per kg of an antigen such as bovine serum albumin or an active infection with a pathogen such as *Salmonella*, antibody may be detected within one to several days (Buxton and Davies, 1963). The peak titer to a single injection of bovine serum albumin is usually reached at about eight days post-injection (Abramoff and Wolfe, 1956; Abramoff, 1960) and will have returned to minimal levels or sometimes even have disappeared by the 18th day post-injection. Precipitating antibody may be detected in the sera of chickens some 300 to 470 days after the last injection but may at that time be quite low (Gilden and Rosenquist, 1963). These authors obtained evidence for continued antibody synthesis during this period of time, rather than a gradual release of previously synthesized antibody. Hence, they conclude that antigen or parts of antigen must have been stored in relevant cells.

The specificity of both primary and secondary immunologic responses in aves appears to be quite marked. For example, nonspecific responses have not been observed in experiments designed to study this phenomenon using closely related antigens unless the antigens actually had some identical chemical constituents (Abramoff and Wolfe, 1956; Gilden, 1963). These experiments were carried out with a considerable number of birds and a number of different antigens.

The importance of the spleen in acquired immunity and antibody production in mammals (Taliaferro and Taliaferro, 1950) and in resistance to infection in birds (Taliaferro and Mulligan, 1937) has been known for some time. The effect of splenectomy on precipitin production in fowls against the soluble antigen bovine serum albumin was first noted by Wolfe et al. (1950), who reported a significant reduction in antibody nitrogen in splenectomized animals. Splenectomized chickens were less responsive to small injections of antigen than were nonsplenectomized controls. The spleen was observed to increase in size upon injection or antigenic stimulation, and peak titer of antibody in the latter instance can be observed to be reached about two days after peak spleen size (Norton et al., 1950). This increase is actual, since calculations have been done on a dry weight basis by a number of workers. There is an increase of plasmocytes in the spleen which coincides with the rise of antibody in the circulating blood (Makinodan et al., 1954b).

More direct evidence for the role of the spleen in antibody formation in aves was obtained by Mitchison (1957), who succeeded in the transference of antibody-producing ability from immunized chickens to chicks by the transference of splenic tissue, but not by similar transfer of bone marrow. More recently, spleen cells have been observed to produce antibody *in vitro* after *in vivo* stimulation with either primary or secondary injections of antigen (Patterson et al., 1963b; 1964).

IN VITRO REACTIONS INVOLVING AVIAN ANTISERA

Although a number of types of antibodies including agglutinins, lysins, opsonins, precipitins, and neutralizing antibodies are known to be produced by various species of birds, the vast majority of studies have been concerned with the precipitin reaction involving chicken antibody to serum proteins (e.g., bovine serum albumin).

It is generally agreed that an increase in the NaCl concentration in the precipitating system up to the range of salting out of the proteins (14 to 18 percent) results in increases in the precipitate nitrogen for the chicken, as well as the pheasant, owl, and turkey (Goodman et al., 1951, 1952; Makinodan et al., 1960; Clarkson, 1963). The rate of the reaction is also markedly increased. The optimum concentration of NaCl is approximately 8.0 percent instead of the normal physiologic concentration of 0.85 to 0.9 percent (Goodman et al., 1951). Increased concentration of anions, such as iodide and sulfate, up to 0.26 M also produce increases in precipitate (Goodman et al., 1954). Similar observations have been made recently in immunoelectrophoresis studies involving chicken antibody (Weiner and Goldman, 1964; Tempelis and Lofz, 1965). Lines formed in the medium could be washed out by rinsing in 0.85 percent NaCl. Where lines were formed at the lower salt concentration, they were much lighter and more diffuse than at the high concentration.

The increased NaCl concentration effect on the chicken antiserum-bovine serum albumin system appears to be in contrast to observations on the rabbit system. Workers consistently report decreased amounts of precipitate nitrogen formed in systems using increased salt concentrations with rabbit antisera (Aladjem and Lieberman, 1952). This holds true when either the euglobulin or pseudoglobulin fraction is involved in the reaction. Indeed, using the pseudoglobulin fraction in the virtual absence of salt, the precipitation reactions not only persist but yield larger quantities of precipitate nitrogen.

While there is general consensus that increased salt concentration in those serologic reactions involving chicken antisera produces an increase in precipitate nitrogen, there appears as yet to be no agreement as to the explanation of this phenomenon. Early suggestions were that alpha-globulin was coprecipitating with the gamma fraction (Deutsch et al., 1949). However, Goodman and Ramsey (1957) and Banovitz and Wolfe (1959), as well as others, claim that no significant amounts of alpha-globulin are involved. A number of researchers have demonstrated the specificity of the antigen-antibody reactions at the higher salt concentrations. Other explanations include the salting out of certain insoluble complexes (Goodman et al., 1951), and the insistence by some that there is a coprecipitation of normal serum components, including macroglobulin (Makinodan et al., 1960; Williams and Donermeyer, 1962).

Later evidence indicates that there are at least two different antibodies involved (Banovitz et al., 1959; Orlans, et al., 1961; Orlans, 1962; Aitken and Mulligan, 1962; Benedict et al., 1963a-d; Hersh and Benedict, 1966). In this regard, the results obtained by Aitken and Mulligan (1962), for example, tend to confirm those of Orlans et al. (1961). Based on observations of the former investigators of the ratio of antibody-to-antigen nitrogen relative to precipitation at 1, 4, and 8 percent NaCl concentrations, they postulated that: 1. There might be a nonspecific precipitation occurring; 2. There might be a contaminant in their antigen (BSA); or 3. The reaction might be a reflection of the presence of a "heavy" and a "light" antibody. In the last instance they postulated, as did Orlans et al. (1961), that in the higher salt concentration there was more precipitation of the light antibody complexes. In their opinion, the third alternative, i.e., the "light" and "heavy" antibody hypothesis, best explained their results.

Orlans (1962) demonstrated through the use of rabbit antibody to antigen-antibody complexes in precipitating chicken serum that there were indeed two antibodies present in immune chicken serum. In view of the persistence of antibody in the supernatant following precipitation in the higher concentrations of antigen-antibody levels, she concluded that precipitation at the higher salt concentrations was not a salting out of antibody and that the explanation of the phenomenon must be sought in terms of more complex interactions of fowl serum. Hersh and Benedict (1966) believe the answer lies in polymer formation. They found that chicken gamma-G 7S globulin polymerizes to form a molecule with an extrapolated sedimentation coefficient of approximately 14S in a solution of 1.5 M NaCl, whereas rabbit gamma-G antibody has the same sedimentation coefficient in both high and low NaCl concentrations.

These observations of maximum activity of fowl antisera at about 8.0 percent NaCl concentration as opposed to 0.9 percent or lower for the rabbit system have both practical as well as academic implications. It makes it possible to investigate antigens which are insoluble at the optimal salt concentration for activity of mammalian antibody, but which may be soluble at the higher salt concentration required for avian antibody activity. A demonstration of such an application has been performed using the plant protein, edestin, which is a globulin from hemp seed (Munoz and Becker, 1952). This protein is insoluble in 0.15 percent salt solution but is soluble in 10 percent NaCl.

Another interesting phenomenon of certain avian antisera, not characteristic of mammalian antibody, is the rise in titer of the former upon standing (Wolfe, 1942; Cover et al., 1960). This increase can be detected as early as 11 hours after harvesting chicken antisera (Wolfe, 1942; Wolfe and Dilks, 1946), and the majority of sera reach a peak titer five to eight days later, remaining at peak titer for as long as 12 days or more. After the initial increase *in vitro*, there is usually a gradual decline in titer (Gengozian and Wolfe, 1957). In an occasional serum, the maximum titer may be maintained for several months. This *in vitro* rise in titer is quite variable from individual to individual and from species to species. The rate of decrease is dependent, moreover, upon the individual serum. Pheasants and owls show some evidence of *in vitro* rise in titer in their antisera, although it may not be quite so marked as that seen in chicken sera. Partridge, turkey, and duck sera show no change upon standing insofar as titer is concerned (Wolfe and Dilks, 1949).

Antibody produced by the chicken has been shown to be superior to that of the mammal in a number of instances involving certain serologic tests. For example, Furesz and Moreau (1963) found that young roosters were consistently superior to monkeys in their response to a one dose antigenicity test for Salk polio vaccine. Patterson et al. (1963a) found roosters to be superior to guinea pigs as a source of anti-insulin antibody because: 1. The relatively low toxicity of insulin for chickens permits a larger antigenic stimulus; 2. The chicken is a very rapid producer of precipitins; and 3. Larger amounts of antiserum could be obtained from a single bleeding.

ELECTROPHORETIC STUDIES OF AVIAN SERA

Total blood proteins of serum increase with age (Brandt et al., 1951; Schechtman and Hoffman, 1952; Marshall and Deutsch, 1950; Kaminski and

Durieux, 1956; Weller and Schechtman, 1962). There is a constant change not only in the relative proportions but also in appearance and disappearance of certain components in embryonic sera.

Sensitive immunologic techniques have detected very slight alpha- and beta-globulin activity in chick embryos as early as two to three days of incubation (Kaminski and Durieux, 1956; Schechtman and Hoffman, 1952). The fifth day of egg incubation was the earliest age at which any significant amounts of serum components have been clearly resolved using electrophoretic techniques (Weller and Schechtman, 1962). Chick embryo serum collected at five days of incubation can be resolved into fractions termed gamma-E and alpha-2-E ("E" meaning embryonic, since these are clearly resolved only in embryonic sera). At this age there is a slow moving continuum designated "S" and another continuum which moves ahead of the alpha-2-E component and forms a long fingerlike projection. This continuum will eventually become the alpha-1 and albumin fractions. The components are in extremely low concentrations, but they increase each day until by the seventh day, the gamma fraction is replaced by a band which migrates at the same rate as human beta. The S continuum decreases with increasing age. Albumin first appears as a distinct component on the ninth day and has identical mobility with albumin of the adult. Prealbumin appears and then disappears during this time. By day 10, the alpha-2-E fraction makes up 40 percent of the serum protein and is thus the major component. On succeeding days there is considerable change in the relative percentages of the components. The most dramatic changes include a steep decline of alpha-2-E on the 14th to 15th days and the doubling of the albumin at 10 through 14 days. At 15 days a new alpha-1-globulin appears, remains until hatching, and becomes permanent. At about the time of hatching, alpha-2-E is replaced by alpha-2-adult. About the 18th day of incubation, alpha-3 appears and gradually increases until maturity. There is a gradual increase of the gamma-beta complex from 10 days until hatching, a period when passively transferred antibody is being rapidly absorbed from the yolk by the developing embryo.

Thus, while the concentrations and relative percentages may change further with age, the young chick at hatching has the basic components of the adult chicken or mammal. There is an additional substance, designated the delta fraction, that moves behind the gamma fraction (Richards and Orlans, 1965). Laying hens also have an additional component which is not present in non-laying females, males, or immature chicks (Brandt et al., 1951). Trager and McGhee (1950) recorded a rise in the euglobulin fraction of the sera of the laying hens which were at the same time observed to be more resistant to malaria.

The origin of serum proteins in developing embryos is an interesting question on which there appears to be a dearth of information. Sabin (1917) believed serum proteins came from disintegrating blood cells as has been observed in adult mammals (Sabin, 1939; White and Dougherty, 1946). Schechtman and Hoffman (1952) obtained evidence of a relationship between the appearance of alpha- and beta-globulins and the rate of cell destruction in the developing chick embryo, a suggestion which lends some support to Sabin's suggestion.

While some authors (e.g., Moore, 1945) point out that an increase in gamma-globulin levels in the blood does not necessarily mean an increase in specific antibody content, it is generally accepted that in birds, as in mammals, such is the case. An increase in antibody titer is accompanied by increased levels of gamma-globulin in serum. Moreover, birds maintained in germ-free conditions have relatively low gamma-globulin levels until exposed to some immunizing agent (Wostman and Olson, 1964; Thorbecke et al., 1957). Specific adsorption of avian antisera with homologous antigen before electrophoresis considerably reduces the gamma-globulin component (Deutsch et al., 1949; Banovitz and Wolfe, 1959).

In a number of immunized mammals, antibodies with a sedimentation coefficient of 19S are synthesized initially, followed by the synthesis of 7S gamma-globulin antibody (Stelos and Taliaferro, 1959; Bauer and Stavitsky, 1961; Uhr et al., 1962). A similar response is noted in chickens (Benedict et al., 1962; 1963a-d), and turkeys (Dreesman et al., 1963). There is a change in response from predominantly 19S to predominantly 7S antibodies, but a high concentration of the latter may develop slowly and only after prolonged repeated stimulation.

COMPLEMENT

As pointed out by Heidelberger (1951), complement, next to antibody, is one of the most important auxiliary substances concerned with immunity. Although immunologists are apparently not in agreement on a definition of complement, it is known that its functions include promotion of phagocytosis, combination with antigen and antibody, and mediation of dissolution of certain agents. Practically speaking, it serves as a valuable diagnostic test.

Although widely distributed among the vertebrates, guinea pig and human complement have been the systems most extensively investigated. They have been found to be very similar and easily replace each other in serologic reactions (Rice and Crowson, 1950). While it has been known for several decades that many birds possess natural hemolysins for red blood cells of other animals due to an antibody and a heat-labile component, relatively little work appears to have been done on avian complement. Studies include these observations on natural hemolysins plus certain other information, including a few experiments on cross-activation involving whole complement.

McGhee (1952) observed that duck complement contains the four basic components known from mammalian systems. Further, he found that resolution of duck complement into the various components can be accomplished with methods almost identical to those used for mammalian systems, indicating similar chemical and physical characteristics. As in most animals (Rice and Crowson, 1950), the first component of complement was found in the duck in the highest titer, with the second and sometimes the third component being the limiting ones. In general, titers in this animal were lower than those recorded for mammals. As in mammals, titers of avian complement depend on the species involved. Chicken and turkey complements appear to be of relatively low hemolytic titer and are somewhat unstable (Rice and Crowson, 1950), while the complements of ducks (McGhee, 1952) and geese (Zia and Liu, 1950) are higher in titer, but still somewhat lower than that in the mammal.

Fowl complement has many characteristics in common with that of the classical guinea pig system. Fowl complement, like guinea pig complement, is inactivated by heating at 56°C for 30 minutes (McGhee, 1952; Rose and Orlans, 1962), or by treatment with 0.02 M EDTA. It remains unchanged for at least six months at −70°C. Fowl complement is still lytic at 12 to 18 months at −20°C. The lytic activity increases slightly in fowl complement upon thawing after freezing. The deterioration of high concentrations of fowl complement kept at room temperature or at 37°C for short periods is not marked; but in dilute solutions even a short period at 37°C caused considerable reductions in titer. As with guinea pig complement, this deterioration was not so pronounced in the presence of additional protein, e.g., in a weak bovine serum albumin solution.

In spite of all these similar chemical and physical characteristics between avian and mammalian complements, fowl serum will not fix guinea pig complement. The marked anticomplementary effect of fresh fowl serum on guinea pig complement and its reduction by heating to 56°C are well known (Bushnell and Hudson, 1927).

There is excellent evidence from mammalian and avian systems for complement fixation *in vivo*. Complement titers in immunized rabbits are reduced on injection of antigen (Stavitsky et al., 1949). Complement titers may be depressed in human and guinea pig serum sickness and anaphylaxis (Rutstein et al., 1942). McGhee (1952) observed similar reduction in complement in ducks undergoing infections with *Plasmodium lophurae*. There was reduction in total complement as well as in all components on the terminal day of infection, suggesting *in vivo* antigen-antibody reaction and fixation of complement.

Attempts to determine the ontogeny of complement in avian embryos are limited to the work of Sherman (1919), who could detect no complement (C′) in chick embryos until hatching. In a series of unpublished observations, McGhee determined whether pooled plasma from chick embryos from 10 days of incubation until several days after hatching contained any components of complement. He found, as did Sherman (1919), that the full quota of complement is not present until immediately after hatching. Components one and three appeared in minute amounts on days 18, 19, and 20. In one group of embryos, two pools of plasma were harvested: one from chicks of 21 days incubation inside intact shells, and one from chicks which were pipping the shell. Those pipping the shell had the full complementary activity in the plasma, while those that had not begun to peck at the shell did not.

CONCLUSION

Though differing in some respects, immune processes in those birds studied are, in general, comparable to those found in the higher invertebrates. Those differences that do occur emphasize the need for further comparative studies. Vertebrates possess complement, but they differ both qualitatively and quantitatively with respect to this substance. Lymphoid tissue is characteristic in all groups, but in birds, it is found in an additional organ not present in mammals—the bursa of Fabricius. It may well be that the still somewhat unclear function of this peculiar organ is submerged in other tissues in the more highly evolved animals.

A distinct advantage of studying immune processes in aves lies in the fact that embryonic development is extracorporeal and, therefore, subject to greater ease of manipulation and observation than that which occurs in intrauterine sites. Thus, much of our knowledge of immune tolerance and ovarian transfer of antibody has been harvested from research on avian embryos.

Sufficient differences do exist between the immune systems of aves and other vertebrates to justify additional intensive studies of avian immunity, not only for the special interests inherent in the system but also from the standpoint of a better understanding of the phylogeny of immunity.

REFERENCES

Abramoff, P. 1955. Antibody studies in chickens: (a) Effect of simultaneous injection of two antigens and (b) non-specific anamnestic response. Dissertation Abstracts, 15: 2605.
———— 1960. Competition of antigens. I. The effect of a secondary response to a heterologous antigen administered at the same time. J. Immun., 85: 648-655.
———— and H. R. Wolfe, 1956. Precipitin production in chickens. XIII. A quantitative study of the effect of simultaneous injection of two antigens. J. Immun., 77: 94-101.
Ackerman, G. A. 1962. Electron microscopy of the bursa of Fabricius of the embryonic chick with particular reference to the lympho-epithelial nodules. J. Cell. Biol., 13: 127-146.
———— and R. A. Knouff. 1959. Lymphocytopoiesis in the bursa of Fabricius. Amer. J. Anat., 104: 163-205.
———— and R. A. Knouff. 1964. In The Thymus in Immunobiology. Good, R. A. and Gabrielson, A. E., eds. New York, Harper and Row, Publishers, pp. 123-146.
Aitken, I. D., and W. Mulligan. 1962. Quantitative precipitin studies on fowl antisera to bovine serum albumin and to bovine gamma globulin. Immunology, 5: 295-305.
Aladjem, F., and M. Lieberman. 1952. The antigen-antibody reaction. I. The influence of sodium chloride concentration on the quantitive precipitin reaction. J. Immun., 69: 117-130.
Archer, O., and J. C. Pierce. 1961. Role of the thymus in the development of the immune response. Fed. Proc., 20: 26.
Aschoff, L. 1924. Das reticulo-endotheliale System. Ergebn. Inn. Med. Kinderheilk., 26: 1-118.

Aspinall, R. L., R. K. Meyer, M. A. Graetzer, and H. R. Wolfe. 1963. Effect of thymectomy and bursectomy on the survival of skin homografts in chickens. J. Immun., 90:
872-877.

Auerbach, R. 1961. Experimental analysis of the origin of cell types in the development
of the mouse thymus. Develop. Biol., 3: 336-354.

Bandheim, U. 1965. Der Einfluss der Thymektomie beim Hühn auf die antikörperbildung gegen Newcastle Disease and Hühnenpocken Virus. Zbl. Veterinaermed. [B],
12: 143-154.

Banovitz, J. S., and H. R. Wolfe. 1959. Precipitin production in chickens. XIX. The
components of chicken antiserum involved in the precipitin reaction. J. Immun., 82:
489-496.

———— J. Singer, and H. R. Wolfe. 1959. Precipitin production in chickens. XVIII.
Physical chemical studies on complexes of bovine serum albumin and its chicken antibodies. J. Immun., 82: 481-488.

Barrow, J. H., Jr., and A. C. Miller. 1964. Fluorescence of an antibody specific for *Leu-
cocytozoon* in the globulins of (duck) egg white. J. Parasit., 50: 45.

Bauer, D. C., and A. B. Stavitsky. 1961. On the different molecular forms of antibody
synthesized by rabbits during the early response to a single injection of protein and
cellular antigens. Proc. Nat. Acad. Sci. USA, 47: 1667-1680.

Baumgartner, L. 1934. The relationship of age to immunological reactions. Yale J. Biol.
Med., 6: 403-434.

———— 1937. Age and antibody production. III. Quantitative studies on the precipitin
reaction with antisera produced in young and adult rabbits. J. Immun., 33: 477-488.

Benedict, A. A.. and R. J. Brown. 1962. Chromatographic and ultracentrifugal differences between primary and secondary chicken antibodies. Bact. Proc., 62: 86.

———— R. J. Brown, and R. Ayergar. 1962. Physical properties of antibody to bovine
serum albumin as demonstrated by hemagglutinations. J. Exp. Med., 115: 195-208.

———— R. J. Brown, and R. Hersh. 1963a. Inactivation of high and low molecular weight
chicken antibodies by mercaptoethanol. Proc. Soc. Exp. Biol. Med., 113: 136-138.

———— C. Larson, and H. Nik-Kahn. 1963b. Synthesis of chicken antibodies of high
and low molecular weight. Science, 139: 1302-1303.

———— C. Larson, and H. Nik-Kahn. 1963c. Synthesis of high and low molecular weight
chicken antibodies. Fed. Proc., 22: 325.

———— R. T. Hersh, and C. Larson. 1963d. The temporal synthesis of chicken antibodies. The effect of salt on the precipitin reaction. J. Immun., 91: 795-802.

Beveridge, W. I. B., and F. M. Burnet. 1946. The cultivation of viruses and rickettsiae
in the chick embryo. Med. Res. Counc. Spec. Rep. Ser. (London), 256.

Blazhovec, A. A. 1963. Factors affecting the primary and secondary response to BSA in
the chicken. Dissertation Abstracts, 24: 1754.

Bloom, W., and W. H. Taliaferro. 1938. Regeneration of the malarial spleen in the
canary after infarction and after burning. J. Infect. Dis., 63: 54-70.

Boyden, E. A. 1922. The development of the cloaca in birds with special reference to
the origin of the bursa of Fabricius, the formation of a unrodeal sinus, and the regular occurrence of a cloacal fenestra. Amer. J. Anat., 30: 163-201.

Brambell, F. W. R. 1958. The passive immunity of the young mammal. Biol. Rev., 33:
488-531.

———— W. A. Hemmings, and W. T. Rowlands. 1948. The passage of antibodies from
the maternal circulation into the embryo in rabbits. Proc. Roy. Soc. (Biol.), 135:
390-403.

———— W. A. Hemmings, M. Henderson, H. J. Parry, and W. T. Rowlands, 1949. The
route of antibodies passing from the maternal to the fetal circulation in rabbits. Proc.
Roy. Soc. (Biol.), 136: 131-144.

———— W. A. Hemmings, M. Henderson, and W. T. Rowlands, 1950. The selective
admission of antibodies to the foetus by the yolk-sac splanchnopleur in rabbits. Proc.
Roy. Soc. (Biol.), 137: 239-252.

Brandley, C. A., H. E. Mosses, and E. L. Jungherr. 1946. Transmission of antiviral
activity via the egg and the role of congenital passive immunity to Newcastle disease
in chickens. Poult. Sci., 25: 397-398.

Brandt, L. W., R. E. Clegg, and A. C. Andrews. 1951. The effect of age and degree of
maturity on the serum proteins of the chicken. J. Biol. Chem., 191: 105-111.

Bridges, R. A., R. M. Condie, S. J. Zak, and R. A. Good. 1959. The morphologic basis of
antibody formation development during the neonatal period. J. Lab. Clin. Med., 53:
331-351.

Brierley, J., and W. A. Hemmings. 1956. The selective transport of antibodies from the yolk sac to the circulation of the chick. J. Embryol. Exp. Morph., 4:34-41.

Brown, E. S., and H. R. Wolfe. 1954. Factors influencing the antibody production of chickens injected with a soluble antigen. Poult. Sci., 33: 255-261.

Burnet, F. M. 1941. Growth of influenza virus in the allantoic cavity of the chick embryo. Aust. J. Exp. Biol. Med. Sci., 19: 291-295.

———— J. D. Stone, and M. Edney. 1950. The failure of antibody production in chick embryos. Aust. J. Exp. Biol. Med. Sci., 28: 291-297.

Bushnell, L. D., and C. B. Hudson, 1927. Complement fixation and agglutination tests for *Salmonella pullorum* infection. J. Infect. Dis., 41: 388-394.

Buxton, A. 1951. Transfer of bacterial antibodies from the hen to the chick. Nature (London), 168: 657-658.

———— 1952. On the transference of bacterial antibodies from the hen to the chick. J. Gen. Microbiol., 7: 268-286.

———— 1954. Antibody production in avian embryos and young chicks. J. Gen. Microbiol., 10: 398-410.

———— and J. M. Davies. 1963. Studies on immunity and pathogenesis of Salmonellosis. II. Antibody production and accumulation of bacterial polysaccharide in the tissues of chickens infected with *Salmonella gallinarum*. Immunology, 6: 530-538.

Calhoun, M. L. 1933. The microscopic anatomy of the digestive tract of *Gallus domesticus*. Iowa State Coll. J. Sci., 7: 261-282.

Carey, J., and N. L. Warner. 1964. Gamma-globulin synthesis in hormonally bursectomized chickens. Nature (London), 203: 784-785.

Chang, T. S. 1957. The significance of the bursa of Fabricius of chickens in antibody production. Dissertation Abstracts, 17: 2117.

———— B. Glick, and A. R. Winter. 1955. The significance of the bursa of Fabricius of chickens in antibody production. Poult. Sci., 34: 1187.

———— M. S. Rheins, and A. R. Winter. 1957. The significance of the bursa of Fabricius in antibody production in chickens. I. Age in chickens. Poult. Sci., 36: 735-738.

———— M. S. Rheins, and A. R. Winter. 1959. The significance of the bursa of Fabricius of chickens in antibody production. 3. Resistance to *Salmonella typhimurium* infection. Poult. Sci., 38: 174-176.

Clarkson, M. J. 1963. Immunological responses to *Histomonas meleagridis* in the turkey and fowl. Immunology, 6: 156-168.

Cohn, M. 1957. The problem of specific inhibition of antibody synthesis in adult animals by immunization of embryos. Ann. N.Y. Acad. Sci., 64: 859-876.

Condie, R. M., and R. A. Good. 1956. Inhibition of immunological enhancement by endotoxin in refractory rabbits. Immunochemical study. Proc. Soc. Exp. Biol. Med., 91: 414-418.

Cooper, M. D., R. D. A. Peterson, and R. A. Good. 1965. Delineation of the thymic and bursal lymphoid systems in the chicken. Nature (London), 205: 143-146.

———— R. D. A. Peterson, M. A. South, and R. A. Good. 1966a. The functions of the thymic and bursal lymphoid systems in the chicken. Nature (London), 205: 143-146.

———— M. L. Schwartz, and R. A. Good. 1966b. Restoration of gamma globulin production in agammaglobulinemic chickens. Science, 151: 471-473.

Cover, M. S., W. J. Benton, and M. A. Whelan. 1960. The thermostability of chicken serum to be used in the PPLO agglutination test. Ann. N.Y. Acad. Sci., 79: 567-573.

Davy, J. 1866. On the bursa of Fabricii. Proc. Roy. Soc. (Biol.), 15: 94-102.

Deichmille, M. P., and F. J. Dixon. 1957a. The metabolism of serum proteins in neonatal rabbits. J. Gen. Physiol., 43: 1047-1069.

———— and F. J. Dixon. 1957b. Synthesis of serum proteins in the neonatal and developing rabbit. Fed. Proc., 16: 410-411.

Dent, P. B., and R. A. Good. 1965. Absence of antibody production in the bursa of Fabricius. Nature (London), 207: 491-493.

Deutsch, H. F., J. C. Nicol, and M. Cohn. 1949. Biophysical studies of immune chicken serum. J. Immun., 63: 195-210.

Dixon, F. J., and P. H. Maurer. 1955. Immunologic unresponsiveness induced by protein antigens. J. Exp. Med., 101: 245-257.

Dreesman, G., A. A. Benedict, and R. W. Moore. 1963. Physical characteristics of turkey anti-ornithosis direct and indirect complement-fixing antibodies. Fed. Proc., 22: 325.

Forbes, W. A. 1877. On the bursa of Fabricii in birds. Proc. Zool. Soc. (London), pp. 304-318

Freund, J. 1930. Influence of age upon antibody formation. J. Immun., 18: 315-324.

Friedman, H., and W. L. Gaby. 1960. Immunological unresponsiveness in mice following neonatal exposure to *Shigella* antigens. J. Immun., 85: 478-482.

Furesz, J., and P. Moreau. 1963. Use of roosters in the antigentity testing of Salk polio-myelitis vaccine. J. Immun., 90: 193-200.

Gengozian, N., and H. E. Wolfe. 1957. Precipitin production in chickens. XV. The effect of aging of the antisera on precipitate formation. J. Immun., 78: 401-408.

Gilden, R. V. 1963. Antibody responses after successive injections of related antigens. Immunology, 6: 30-36.

———— and G. L. Rosenquist. 1963. Duration of antibody response to soluble antigen: Incorporation of sulphur-35 methionine into normal and antibody globulin. Nature (London), 200: 1116-1117.

Glick, B. 1958. Further evidence for the role of the bursa of Fabricius in antibody production. Poult. Sci., 37: 240-241.

———— 1959. The experimental production of the stress picture with cortisone and the effect of penicillin in young chickens. Ohio. J. Sci., 59: 81-87.

———— 1960a. Extracts from the bursa of Fabricius a lympho-epithelial gland of the chicken—stimulate the production of antibodies in bursectomized chickens. Poult. Sci., 39: 1097-1101.

———— 1960b. Growth of the bursa of Fabricius and its relationship to the adrenal gland in the white Pekin duck, white Leghorn, outbred and inbred New Hampshire. Poult. Sci., 39: 130-144.

———— 1961. Influence of dipping eggs in male hormone solutions on lymphatic tissue and antibody response in chickens. Endocrinology, 69: 984-985.

———— T. S. Chang, and R. G. Jaap. 1956. The bursa of Fabricius in antibody production. Poult. Sci., 35: 224-225.

Goble, F. C., and I. Singer. 1960. The reticuloendothelial system in experimental malaria and trypanosomiasis. Ann. N.Y. Acad. Sci., 88: 149-171.

Gold, E. F., and A. A. Benedict. 1963. Transfer to neonatal chickens of the primary antibody response initiated *in vitro*. Nature (London), 200: 696-697.

Good, R. A., and B. W. Papermaster. 1964. Ontogeny and phylogeny of adaptive immunity. Advances Immun., 4: 1-115.

———— A. P. Dalmasso, C. Martinez, O. K. Archer, J. C. Pierce, and B. W. Papermaster. 1962. The role of the thymus in development of immunologic capacity in rabbits and mice. J. Exp. Med., 116: 773-796.

———— R. D. A. Peterson, C. Martinez, D. E. R. Sutherland, M. J. Kellum, and J. Finstad. 1965. The thymus in immunobiology, with special reference to autoimmune disease. Ann. N.Y. Acad. Sci., 124: 73-94.

Goodman, M., and H. R. Wolfe. 1952. Precipitin production in chickens. VIII. A comparison of the effect of salt concentration on precipitate formation of pheasant, owl, and chicken antisera. J. Immun., 69: 423-434.

———— and D. S. Ramsey. 1957. Specificity of reaction of chicken antiserum in high NaCl concentrations. Fed. Proc., 16: 416.

———— H. R. Wolfe, and S. Norton. 1951. Precipitin production in chickens. VI. The effect of varying concentrations of NaCl on precipitate formation. J. Immun., 66: 225-236.

———— H. R. Wolfe, and R. Goldberg. 1954. Precipitin production in chickens. XII. The effects of variation in ionic species and concentration on precipitate formation. J. Immun., 72: 440-445.

Goodpasture, E. W., and K. Anderson. 1937. Problem of infection as presented by bacterial invasion of the chorio-allantoic membrane of chick embryos. Amer. J. Path., 13: 149-174.

Graetzer, M. A., H. R. Wolfe, R. L. Aspinall, and R. K. Meyer. 1963a. Effect of thymectomy and bursectomy on precipitin and natural hemagglutinin production in the chicken. J. Immun., 90: 873-880.

———— W. P. Cote, and H. R. Wolfe. 1963b. The effect of bursectomy at different ages on precipitin and natural hemagglutinin production in the chicken. J. Immun., 91: 576-581.

Grasset, E. 1929. Recherches sur la sensibilité du tissu embryonnaire aux antigenes. Essais d'immunisation comparée de l'embryon de poule et de la poule adults. C. R. Soc. Biol. (Paris), 101: 1102-1104.

Halliday, R. 1955. The adsorption of antibodies from immune sera by the gut of the young rat. Proc. Roy. Soc. (Biol.), 143: 408-413.

Hanson, L. E., and J. O. Alberts. 1960. Immunological characteristics of duck hepatitis virus. Poult. Sci., 39: 1257-1258.

Hasek, M., A. Lengerova, and T. Hraba. 1961. Transplantation immunity and tolerance. In Advances in Immunology, Vol. 1. New York, Academic Press Inc., pp. 1-66.

Heidelberger, M. 1951. National Academy of Sciences Conference on Complement. Proc. Nat. Acad. Sci. USA, 37: 185-189.

Hersh, R. T., and A. A. Benedict. 1966. Aggregation of chicken gamma-G immunoglobulin in 1.5 M sodium chloride. Biochem. Biophys. Acta, 115: 242-244.

Hewitt, R. 1940. Bird Malaria. American Journal of Hygiene Monograph Series No. 15, Baltmore, The Johns Hopkins' University Press.

Hirata, A. A., and A. M. Schechtman. 1960. Studies on immunologic depression in chickens. J. Immun., 85: 230-239.

Hosoda, T., T. Kaneko, K. Mogi, and T. Abe. 1955. Transfer of antibodies in the hen to her eggs and to the offspring. Bull. Nat. Inst. Agric. Sci. (Japan); Series G, Animal Husbandry, 10: 125-129.

Isakovic, K., and B. D. Jankovic. 1964. Role of the thymus and the bursa of Fabricius in immune reactions in chickens. II. Cellular changes in lymphoid tissues of thymectomized, bursectomized and normal chickens in the course of antibody response. Int. Arch. Allerg., 24: 296.

———— B. D. Jankovic, L. Popeskovic, and D. Milosevic. 1963. Effect of neonatal thymectomy, bursectomy, and thymo-bursectomy on haemagglutinin production in chickens. Nature (London), 200: 273-274.

Jankovic, B. D., and K. Isakovic. 1964. Role of the thymus and bursa of Fabricius in immune reactions in chickens. I. Changes in lymphoid tissues of chickens surgically thymectomized at hatching. Int. Arch. Allerg., 24: 278-295.

———— and Sidney Leskowitz. 1965. Restoration of antibody producing capacity in bursectomized chickens by bursal grafts in millipore chambers. Proc. Soc. Exp. Biol. Med., 118: 1164-1166.

———— B. H. Waksman, and B. G. Arnason. 1962. Role of the thymus in immune reactions in rats. I. The immunologic response to bovine serum albumin (antibody formation, Arthus reactivity, and delayed hypersensitivity) in rats thymectomized or splenectomized at various times after birth. J. Exp. Med., 116: 159-176.

———— M. Isvaneski, D. Milosevic, and L. Popeskovic. 1963. Delayed hypersensitive reactions in bursectomized chickens. Nature (London), 198: 298-299.

Jolly, F. 1915. Recherches sur la bourse de Fabricius et sur les organes lymphoepitheliaux. Arch. Anat. Mic., 16: 363-547.

Jukes, R. H., D. T. Fraser, and M. D. Orr. 1934. The transmission of diphtheria antitoxin from hen to egg. J. Immun., 26: 353-360.

Kaminski, M., and J. Durieux. 1956. A comparative study of constituents of chicken and embryo serum and egg white. Exp. Cell. Res., 10: 590-618.

Karthigasu, K., and C. R. Jenkin. 1963. The functional development of the reticuloendothelial system of the chick embryo. Immunology, 6: 255-263.

———— C. R. Jenkin, and K. J. Turner. 1964. The nature of the opsonins in adult hen serum and developing chick embryos to certain gram-negative bacteria. Aust. J. Exp. Biol. Med. Sci., 42: 499-510.

Kemenes, F., and G. Pethes. 1963. Further evidence for the role of the bursa of Fabricius in antibody production in chickens. Z. Immunitätsforsch., 125: 446-458.

Kent, R. 1961. The development of the phagocytic activity of the reticuloendothelial system in the chick. J. Embryol. Exp. Morph., 9: 128-137.

Kerstetter, T. H., Jr., I. O. Buss, and H. A. Went. 1962. Antibody-producing function of the bursa of Fabricius of the ring-necked pheasant. J. Exp. Zool., 149: 233-237.

Knight, P. F., and A. M. Schechtman. 1954. The passage of heterologous serum protein from the circulation into the ovum of the fowl. J. Exp. Zool., 127: 271-304.

Makinodan, F., H. R. Wolfe, M. Goodman, and R. Ruth. 1952. Precipitin production in chickens. VII. The relation between circulating antibody and anaphylactic shock. J. Immun., 68: 219-226.

———— R. F. Ruth, and H. R. Wolfe. 1954a. Precipitin production in chickens. X. Cellular changes in the spleen during antibody production. J. Immun., 72: 39-44.

———— R. F. Ruth, and H. R. Wolfe, 1954b. Precipitin production in chickens. XI. Site of antibody production. J. Immun., 72: 45-51.

———— N. Gengozian, and R. E. Canning. 1960. Demonstration of a normal serum macroglobulin co-precipitating with bovine serum albumin (BSA—chicken anti-BSA). J. Immun., 85: 435-446.

Marshall, M. E., and H. F. Deutsch. 1950. Some protein changes in fluids of the developing chick embryo. J. Biol. Chem., 185: 155-168.

Marinkovich, V. A., and M. A. Baluda. 1966. In vitro synthesis of M-like globulin by various chick embryonic cells. Immunology, 10: 383-397.

McGhee, R. B. 1942. Reproductive habits of *Plasmodium cathemerium* in embryos and the resistance of embryos to this parasite. M.S. thesis, Athens, Georgia, University of Georgia.

——— 1949. The course of infection of *Plasmodium gallinaceum* in duck embryos. J. Infect. Dis., 84: 98-104.

——— 1952. The effect of a malarial infection on the titer of complement and its components in ducks. J. Immun., 68: 421-427.

——— 1963. Unpublished observation.

Metcalf, D. 1960. The effects of thymectomy on the lymphoid tissues of the mouse. Brit. J. Haemat., 6: 324-333.

Metchinkov, E. 1905. Immunity in Infective Diseases. Cambridge, Cambridge University Press.

Meyer, R. K., M. A. Rao, and R. L. Aspinall. 1959. Inhibition of the development of the bursa of Fabricius in the embryos of the common fowl by 19-nortestosterone. Endocrinology, 64: 890-897.

Miller, J. F. A. P., D. Osoba, and P. Dukor. 1965. A humoral thymus mechanism responsible for immunologic maturation. Ann. N.Y. Acad. Sci., 124: 95-104.

Mitchison, N. A. 1957. Adaptive transfer of antibody production in poultry by spleen tissue. Folia Biol. (Praha), 3: 72-76.

Moore, D. H. 1945. Species differences in serum protein patterns. J. Biol. Chem., 161: 21-32.

Moore, M. A. S., and J. J. T. Owen. 1966. Experimental studies on the development of the bursa of Fabricius. Develop. Biol., 14: 40.

Mueller, A. P. 1960. Experimental studies on the immune response of chickens to soluble antigen. Dissertation Abstracts, 21: 710.

——— H. R. Wolfe, and R. K. Meyer. 1960. Precipitin production in chickens. XXI. Antibody production in bursectomized chickens and in chickens injected with 19-nortestosterone on the fifth day of incubation. J. Immun., 85: 172-179.

——— H. R. Wolfe, R. K. Meyer, and R. L. Aspinall. 1962. Further studies on the role of the bursa of Fabricius in antibody production. J. Immun., 88: 354-360.

Munoz, J., and E. L. Becker. 1952. The use of chicken antiserum in the immunochemical studies of edestin. J. Immun., 68: 405-412.

Norton, S., H. R. Wolfe, and J. F. Crow. 1950. Effect of injections of soluble antigen on the spleen size and antibody production in chickens. Anat. Rec., 107: 133-147.

Nossal, G. J. V. 1964. Studies on the rate of seeding of lymphocytes from the intact guinea pig thymus. Ann. N.Y. Acad. Sci., 120: 171-181.

Orlans, E. 1962. Fowl antibody: II. The composition of specific precipitates formed by antisera to sera albumin, haemoglobin, and myoglobin and some properties of non-precipitating antibody. Immunology, 5: 306-321.

——— M. E. Rose, and J. R. Marrack. 1961. Fowl antibody: I. Some physical and immunological properties. Immunology, 4: 262-277.

Ortega, L. G., and B. K. Der. 1964. Studies of agammaglobulinemia induced by ablation of the bursa of Fabricius. Fed. Proc. 23: 546.

Osborn, J. J., J. Dancis, and J. F. Julia. 1952. Studies of the immunology of the newborn infant. I. Age and antibody production. Pediatrics, 9: 736-744.

Papermaster, B. W., and R. A. Good. 1962. Relative contributions of the thymus and the bursa of Fabricius to the maturation of the lymphoreticular system and immunological potential in the chicken. Nature (London), 196: 838-840

——— S. G. Bradley, D. W. Watson and R. A. Good. 1959. Antibody production in neonatal chickens following injection of adult cells mixed with antigen *in vitro*. Proc. Soc. Exp. Biol. Med., 102: 260-264.

——— D. I. Friedman, and R. A. Good. 1961. Modification of the homograft response in young chicks with 19-nortestosterone. Fed. Proc., 20: 36.

——— D. S. Friedman, and R. A. Good. 1962. Relationship of the bursa of Fabricius to immunological responsiveness and homograft immunity in the chicken. Proc. Soc.

Patterson, R., J. S. Youngner, W. O. Weigle, and F. J. Dixon. 1962a. Antibody production and transfer to egg yolk in chickens. J. Immun., 89: 272-278.

——— J. S. Youngner, W. O. Weigle, and F. J. Dixon. 1962b. The metabolism of serum proteins in the hen and chick, and secretion of serum proteins by the ovary of the hen. J. Gen. Physiol., 45: 501-513.

———— J. A. Calwell, E. Cary, and R. N. Stauffer. 1963a. Avian anti-insulin antibody. Fed. Proc., 22: 672.

———— I. M. Suszko, and J. J. Pruzansky. 1963b. Immunofluorescent studies of the *in vitro* production of antibody by chicken spleen cells. J. Histochem. Cytochem., 12: 18.

———— I. M. Suszko, and J. J. Pruzansky. 1964. *In vitro* production of chicken globulins and precipitating antibody. Immunology, 7: 440-448.

Perez del Castillo, E. E. 1957. In Physiopathology of the Reticuloendothelial System. Oxford, Blackwell Scientific Publications, p. 312.

Pierce, A. E., and P. L. Long. 1965. Studies on acquired immunity to coccidiosis in bursaless and thymectomized fowls. Immunology, 9: 427-439.

———— R. C. Chubb, and P. L. Long. 1966. The significance of the bursa of Fabricius in relation to the synthesis of 7S and 19S immune globulins and specific antibody activity in the fowl. Immunology, 10: 321-337.

Ramon, G. 1928. Sur le passage de la toxine et de l'antitoxine tetanique de la poule à l'oeuf et au poussin. C. R. Soc. Biol. (Paris), 99: 1476-1478.

Rice, C. E., and C. N. Crowson. 1950. The interchangeability of the complement components of different animal species. 2. In the hemolysins of sheep erythrocytes sensitized with rabbit amboceptor. J. Immun., 65: 201-210.

Richards, C. B., and E. Orlans. 1965. Serum delta-globulin in the young fowl (0-29 days old) and in other avian species. Nature (London), 205: 92-93.

Richey, D. J., and S. C. Schmittle. 1962. The effect of congenital passive immunity levels on the response of chicks to Newcastle disease vaccination. J. Immun., 89: 344-347.

Riddle, O. 1928. Growth of the gonads and bursa of Fabricii in doves and pigeons with data for body growth and age at maturity. Amer. J. Physiol., 86: 248-365.

Rose, M. and E. Orlans. 1962. Fowl antibody: III. Its haemolytic activity with complements of various species and some properties of fowl complement. Immunology, 5: 633-641.

Ruth, R. 1960. Ontogeny of blood cells. Fed. Proc., 19: 579-585.

———— 1961. Derivation of antibody-producing cells from ectodermal-endodermal epithelia. Anat. Rec., 139: 270.

———— M. A. Graetzer, W. E. Briles, and H. R. Wolfe. 1964. Depression of the immune response to isoantigens after removal of the bursa of Fabricius. Fed. Proc., 23: 190.

Rutstein, D. D., and W. H. Walder. 1942. Complement activity in pneumonia. J. Clin. Invest., 21: 347-352.

Rywosch, M. 1907. Über Hamolyse and Baktercidie des embryonalen Hühnerblutes. Zbl. Bakt. [Orig.], 44: 468-474.

Sabin, F. 1917. Preliminary note on differentiation of angioblasts and the method by which they produce blood vessels, blood plasma, and red blood cells as seen in the living chick. Anat. Rec., 13: 199-204.

———— 1939. Cellular reactions to a dye-protein with a concept of the mechanism of antibody formation. J. Exp. Med., 70: 67-82.

Schechtman, A. M., and H. Hoffmann. 1952. Serological studies on the origin of globulins in the serum of the chick embryo. J. Exp. Zool., 120: 375-390.

Schmidt, N. H., and H. R. Wolfe. 1953. Precipitin production in chickens. IX. A quantitative study of antibody response to nine different purified substances. J. Immun., 71: 214-219

Schrier, J. E., and H. L. Hamilton. 1952. An experimental study of the origin of the parathyroid and thymus glands in the chick. J. Exp. Zool., 119: 165-187.

Sherman, H. W. 1919. Antibodies in the chick. J. Infect. Dis., 25: 256-258.

Sibal, L. R. 1961. Effect of endotoxin on antibody production by chicken spleen cells transferred to chick chorioallantois. J. Immun., 87: 362-366.

———— and N. H. Olson. 1958. Production of antibodies by adult hen spleen cells transferred to chick embryos. Proc. Soc. Exp. Biol. Med., 97: 575-579.

Silverstein, A. M. 1964. Ontogeny of the immune response. Science, 144: 1423-1428.

Smith, R. T. 1961. Immunological tolerance of nonliving antigens. *In* Advances in Immunology, Vol. 1. Taliaferro, W. H., and Humphrey, J. H., eds. New York, Academic Press, Inc., pp. 67-124.

———— and R. A. Bridges. 1958. Immunological unresponsiveness in rabbits produced by neonatal injection of defined antigens. J. Exp. Med., 108: 227-250.

Solomon, J. B. 1963. Actively acquired transplantation immunity in the chick embryo. Nature (London), 189: 1171-1173.
———— and D. F. Tucker. 1963. Ontogenesis of immunity to erythrocytic antigens in the chick. Immunology, 6: 592-601.
Stavitsky, A. B., R. Stavitsky, and E. E. Ecker. 1949. Loss of hemolytic complement and of granulocytes following reinjection of an antigen into the rabbit. J. Immun., 63: 389-407.
Stelos, P., and W. H. Taliaferro. 1959. Comparative study of rabbit hemolysins to various antigens. II. Hemolysins to the Forssman antigen of guinea pig kidney, human type A red cells, and sheep red cells. J. Infect. Dis., 104: 105-118.
Stevens, K. M., H. C. Pietryk, and G. L. Ciminera. 1958. Acquired immunological tolerance to a protein antigen in chickens. Brit. J. Exp. Path., 39: 1-7.
St. Pierre, R. L., and G. A. Ackerman. 1965. Bursa of Fabricius in chickens: Possible humoral factors. Science, 147: 1307-1308.
Szenberg, A., and N. L. Warner. 1962. Dissociation of immunological responsiveness in fowls with a hormonally arrested development of lymphoid tissues. Nature (London), 194: 146-147.
———— and N. L. Warner. 1964. Immunological reaction of bursaless fowls to homograft antigens. Ann. N.Y. Acad. Sci., 120: 150-161.
Taliaferro, W. H. 1949. The cellular basis of immunity. Ann. Rev. Microbiol., 3: 159-194.
———— 1963. Cellular and humoral factors in immunity to protozoa. In Immunity to Protozoa. Garnham, P. C. C, Pierce, A. E., and Roitt, I., eds. Oxford, Blackwell Scientific Publications, pp. 22-38.
———— and H. W. Mulligan. 1937. The histopathology of malaria with special reference to the function and origin of the macrophages in defence. Indian Med. J. Mem., 29: 1-138.
———— and L. G. Taliaferro. 1950. The dynamics of hemolysin formation in intact and splenectomized rabbits. J. Infect. Dis., 87: 37-62.
Tempelis, C. H., and M. F. Lofz. 1965. An adaptation of the immunoelectrophoretic method for the use of chicken-precipitating antisera. J. Immun., 95: 418-421.
Thorbecke, G. J., H. A. Gordon, B. Wostman, M. Wagner, and J. A. Reyniers. 1957. Lymphoid tissue and serum gamma globulin in young germ-free chickens. J. Infect. Dis., 101: 237-251.
Trager, W., and R. B. McGhee. 1950. Factors in plasma concerned in natural resistance to an avian malaria parasite (Plasmodium lophurae). J. Exp. Med., 91: 365-379.
Truka, Z. 1957. Tvorba protilatek isolovanymi bunkami slezioy slepice po smosemos antigenem in vitro prenosem na kurata. čzesk. Mikrobiol., 2: 344-349.
Uhr, J. W. 1960. Development of delayed-type hypersensitivity in guinea pig embryos. Nature (London), 187: 957-959.
———— J. Dancis, and C. G. Neumann. 1960. Delayed-type hypersensitivity in premature neonatal humans. Nature (London), 187: 1130-1131.
———— J. Dancis, E. C. Franklin, M. S. Finkelstein, and E. W. Lewis. 1962. The antibody response to bacteriophage ΦX-174 in new born premature infants. J. Clin. Invest., 41: 1509-1513.
Vojteskova, M., M. Masnerova, and J. Viklicky. 1963. Homograft response in ducks after thymectomy and/or bursectomy and with or without transplanted homologous thymus and/or bursa of Fabricius. Folia Biol. (Praha), 9: 424-432.
Warner, N. L., and N. A. Szenberg. 1962. Effect of neonatal thymectomy on the immune response in the chicken. Nature (London), 1962: 784-785.
———— and A. Szenberg. 1964. The immunological function of the bursa of Fabricius in the chicken. Ann. Rev. Microbiol., 18: 253-268.
———— A. Szenberg, and F. M. Burnet. 1962. The immunological role of different lymphoid organs in the chicken. I. Dissociation of immunological responsiveness. Aust. J. Exp. Biol. Med. Sci., 40: 373-388.
Weiner, L. M., and M. Goldman. 1964. Salt requirements in agar gel immunoelectrophoresis using chicken antisera. Fed. Proc., 23: 141.
Weinberg, M., and A. Guelin. 1936. Recherches sur l'immunité active de l'embryon. C. R. Soc. Biol. (Paris), 122: 1229-1231.
Weller, E. M., and A. M. Schechtman. 1962. Ontogeny of serum proteins in the chicken. Develop. Biol., 4: 517-531.

White, A., and T. F. Dougherty. 1946. The role of lymphocytes in normal and immune globulin production and the mode of release of globulin from lymphocytes. Ann. N.Y. Acad. Sci., 46: 859-880.

Williams, J. W., and D. D. Donermeyer. 1962. The interaction of bovine serum albumin and its chicken antibodies. J. Biol. Chem., 237: 2123-2130.

Wolfe, R. 1942. Precipitin production in chickens. I. Interfacial titers as affected by quantity of antigen injected and aging of antisera. J. Immun., 44: 135-145.

———— and E. Dilks. 1946. Precipitin production in chicken. II. Studies on the *in vitro* rise in interfacial titers and the formation of precipitins. J. Immun., 52: 331-341.

———— and E. Dilks. 1948. Precipitin production in chickens. III. The variation in the antibody response as correlated with the age of the animal. J. Immun., 58: 245-250.

———— and E. Dilks. 1949. Precipitin production in chickens. IV. A comparison of the antibody response of eight avian species. J. Immun., 61: 251-257.

———— S. Norton, E. Springer, M. Goldman, and C. A. Herrick. 1950. Precipitin production in chickens. V. The effect of splenectomy on antibody formation. J. Immun., 64: 179-184.

Wolfe, H. R., C. Tempelis, A. Mueller, and S. Reibel. 1957. Precipitin production in chickens. XVIII. The effect of massive injections of bovine serum albumin at hatching on subsequent antibody production. J. Immun., 79: 147-153.

———— A. P. Mueller, J. Ness, and C. Tempelis, 1957b. Precipitin production in chickens. XVI. The relationship of age to antibody production. J. Immun., 79: 142-146.

———— A. Amin, A. P. Mueller, and F. R. Aronson. 1960. The secondary response of chickens given a primary inoculation of bovine serum albumin at different ages. Int. Arch. Allerg., 17: 106-115.

———— A. Amin, A. P. Mueller, and F. R. Aronson. 1961. The secondary response of chickens given a primary inoculation of bovine serum albumin at different ages. Arch. Inst. Hessarek, 13: 49-59.

———— M. A. Carroll and W. P. Cote. 1962. The effect of bursectomy of the chicken on the formation of precipitins and haemagglutinins. Fed. Proc., 21: 22.

Woods, R. 1963. Factors affecting the immune response of chickens. Dissertation Abstracts, 24: 1768-1769.

———— and J. Linna. 1965. The transport of cells from the bursa of Fabricius to the spleen and the thymus. Acta. Path. Microbiol. Scand., 64: 470.

Wostmann, B. S. and G. B. Olson. 1964. Precipitating antibody production in germ-free chickens. J. Immun., 92: 41-48.

Yamaguchi, Y., Y. Suzuki, K. Takahashi, S. Azitsu, and K. Sumita. 1964. The role of thymus and bursa of Fabricius in the development of lymphoid tissue and immunologic capacity. Jap. J. Bact., 19: 447-457.

Zia, S. H., and Feng-Ling Liu. 1950. Study of the serum complement activity of common domestic fowls. Peking Natural History Bulletin, 18: 189-194.

Avian Malaria

R. BARCLAY McGHEE

Department of Zoology, University of Georgia, Athens, Georgia

INTRODUCTION

In order to appreciate fully the phenomenon of immunity of aves to malaria, one must be aware of the biology of the species of the genus *Plasmodium* not only in the various families of birds but also in the mammalia, the reptilia and, if present, amphibia. In all the various hosts, the general principles of development, transmission, and physiology, in so far as they have been determined, are similar. Indeed, one may classify exoerythrocytic schizogony regardless of the host into two types: the *P. elongatum* type in which the nonerythrocytic stages are in the hematologic cells, and the *P. gallinaceum* type in which the exoerythrocytic stages are found in various cells of the body other than blood cells, i.e., in the endothelial cells, macrophages, and the parenchymal cells of the liver (Thompson and Huff, 1944). There are, of course, some differences in the development of the pre-erythrocytic stages of the human, simian, and rodent malarias in the liver cells compared to the development of similar stages in the macrophages and, later, in the endothelium of avian species.

Individuals working in the field of immunology may choose to work with a species of avian malaria, *Plasmodium berghei* of the rodent, *P. cynomolgi* of the monkey, or even the various plasmodia of man. Any general discussion of immunity of birds to malaria must, therefore, include reference to some of the work carried out with other hosts that bears some promise of having application to avian malarias and their hosts.

Distribution of plasmodia in various classes of animals

Amphibia. Except for an unconfirmed report by Fantham, Porter, and Richardson (1942) of two species of plasmodia, one in the bullfrog *Rana catesbeiana*, and one in the toad *Bufo americana*, no species of *Plasmodium* has been observed in amphibians. The author has examined hundreds of blood films of both the above genera of amphibia without finding malaria organisms. A relative of plasmodia, *Babesiosoma stableri*, has been described in *Rana pipiens* and has been transferred to Fowler's toad, *Bufo fowleri* (Schmittner and McGhee, 1961). The finding that this species of intraerythrocytic protozoan is transmissible to toads provides a host-parasite complex admirably suited for intensive study of the mechanism of immunity in a poikilothermic animal.

Reptilia. According to Garnham (1966), there are 24 species of reptilian malarias in lizards and one species in a snake. The bulk of data concerning the development of these malarias was reported by Thompson and Huff (1944). Despite the work of these and other investigators (for example, Ball and Pringle, 1965) the invertebrate vectors of these species of plasmodia are still unknown. Jordon (1964), however, observed oocysts in a few mosquitoes which fed on infected lizards.

Avian malaria. Although many species have been described as occurring in birds, there are only 25 species that are generally accepted (Garnham, 1966). As will be pointed out later, morphology, which is the major criterion for identification of a given species, changes markedly when the parasite exists in a different host species. Indeed, the criterion of infectivity for a formerly common laboratory host, the canary, is erroneous at times. For instance, *P. lophurae* is differentiated, in part, from *P. circumflexum* (Hewitt, 1940) by its inability to infect canaries readily. Both the author (unpublished, 1952) and Jordon (1957) found that canaries are easily infected by both organisms, which are morphologically markedly alike.

The malarial species which have been commonly used in the study of avian immunity are: *Plasmodium gallinaceum* (Brumpt, 1935), a parasite of the jungle fowl which is transmissible to domesticated chickens; *Plasmodium lophurae* (Coggeshall, 1938), isolated from a fire-backed pheasant (*Lophurae igniti igniti*) and transmissible to a variety of animals (McGhee, 1957;

Jordon, 1957); *Plasmodium cathemerium* (Hartman, 1927), isolated from a variety of passerine birds and used mostly in the canary and duckling; *Plasmodium relictum* (Grassi and Feletti, 1891), also found in many passerine birds and infective for the canary, duckling, and pigeon; *P. circumflexum* (Kikuth, 1931), a parasite of passerines infective for canaries and chicks (McGhee, 1957); and *P. fallax* (Schwetz, 1930), a parasite of an African guinea fowl infective for chicks and turkeys.

Rodent malaria. The discovery of *Plasmodium berghei* by Vincke and Lips (1948) and the ability of this parasite to infect a variety of rodent hosts has provided a valuable tool for research in the biology of the malarias. The elucidation of the mosquito and the pre-erythrocytic cycles was carried out by Yoeli (1965) through an adroit combination of field and laboratory efforts. Other species infecting rodents are *P. vinckei* (Rodhain, 1952) and *P. chabaudi* (Landau, 1965). The possibility exists, however, that the latter species may be merely *P. vinckei* which has been changed due to an intercurrent eperythrozoon infection (Ott and Stauber, 1967).

Primate malaria. The accidental infection of human laboratory workers by a strain of the monkey malaria, *P. cynomolgi*, has stimulated investigations on the role of simian malaria as a possible agent of human infections (Eyles, 1963). Several new species of monkey malaria have been described, and the total number of species now exceeds ten (Garnham, 1966).

Human malaria. The four species of human malaria (*P. vivax*, *P. malariae*, *P. falciparum*, *P. ovale*) are well known and need no extended description.

Comparative view of the various plasmodia

Insofar as we now know, plasmodia are alike in that: 1. They undergo development in two hosts, a vertebrate and a mosquito; 2. They do not, as was one time presumed, enter the erythrocyte directly following their injection via the mosquito salivary juice, but rather enter into an exoerythrocytic cycle which occurs in cells other than the red blood cell; and 3. They spend some stage of their life cycle in the erythrocyte of the circulating blood stream. In this cell they undergo schizogony and initiate the sexual cycle. Inasmuch as the general cycles are similar, it follows that there is the possibility that the immune mechanisms are likewise similar. It is for this reason that malaria of lower animals has stimulated many investigators to study these "lower forms" of malaria, primarily as a means of applying their findings to the problems of human malaria. Others study avian malaria and its immunology because the intricate obligatory relationship between the host and parasite is intriguing, and the results are sometimes personally rewarding though quite often frustrating.

As pointed out, the life cycle of malaria is not one which can be studied in one host or even in one environment. Immunity in a broader sense is indicative of the protection of populations as well as individuals, populations of invertebrates as well as vertebrates. Any approach to immunity should, therefore, consider not only the intrinisic aspects of immunity (the classical "natural" and "acquired" immunity), but should also consider the extrinsic factors which might protect, expose, or modify the incidence of the parasite population in a given vertebrate or invertebrate population.

We shall, therefore, first consider factors influencing extrinsic immunity and later, the various aspects of intrinsic immunity.

EXTRINSIC IMMUNITY: GENERAL CONCEPTS OF THE ECOLOGY OF DISEASE

Despite the utilization of ecologic methods for the prevention and spread of disease, epidemiologists have been slow to incorporate principles of ecology in any consideration of the general disease processes. Nor have the ecologists made any attempts, beyond discussing the various interrelationships of animals, to systemize or categorize disease into the general ecologic concept. In this system, the malaria parasite would be a parasite in one host and, in another, a commensal. The parasitologist is well aware that he is dealing with populations of animals, that the density of these populations, especially regarding parasites, plays a most important role in disease production, and that mortality rates are important in either the two hosts or in the parasite itself.

One of the attempts to fit disease organisms into the general ecologic picture is that of Pavlovsky's "doctrine of nidality," a concept which holds that the disease itself occupies a habitat (Dogiel, 1964). As expanded in a later work of Pavlovsky (1966), the concept of natural nidality as related to transmissible disease is characterized by the presence of a host, a vector, and a disease-producing organism in a cyclical sequential transmission, and that such a circulation takes place under optimal environmental conditions. In other words, the natural nidus of a disease is related to a specific geographic landscape; for example, marshy conditions which might well be the habitat of malaria-bearing mosquitoes, susceptible avian hosts, and necessarily, the plasmodium. The recognition of the particular landscape involved in the successful cycling of a given disease enables one to predict the possibility of occurrence of a disease situation; the basis of the so-called landscape epidemiology. This concept is rather easily visualized in the case of a single host disease or parasite but becomes more complicated when two or even three hosts are involved. Audy (1958) emphasizes the adaptation of parasites to two or more species which form adjacent links in a food chain. Such a chain could be visualized as linking the mosquito to the vertebrate in a more or less obligatory manner inasmuch as the mosquito must have blood to produce its offspring most successfully.

Thus malaria might be considered as having a habitat—this habitat includes the dual existence of the causative agent in the mosquito and the vertebrate host. In order to understand this habitat and to gain some insight into the phenomenon of extrinsic immunity, one must survey the habitats, niches, populations, and the various limitations of environment on not only the parasite, but also the bird and the adult and larval stages of mosquitoes. General considerations of the parasite in its respective hosts will be reserved for the discussion of intrinsic immunity, but the general features of ecology of the two hosts will be considered at this point.

The habitats of the avian vertebrate host are as varied as could be imagined, ranging from the open sea to the American desert, and include hosts living an almost continuous existence on or under ground, as well as those having an almost nonterrestrial existence as seen in the chimney swift, *Chaetura pelagica*. Birds may be completely gregarious and live in the same site, or they may be individualistic and stoutly defend their territory from any intrusion from the same species of bird. They may even, as in the case of the red-winged blackbird (*Agelaius phoeniceus*), segregate in flocks of the same sex at certain times of the year. Their range may be extremely wide as in the case of the red-tailed hawk (*Buteo jamaicensis*), or it may be restricted to a quarter-mile of stream bank as in the case of the Louisiana water thrush (*Seiurus motacilla*). This range and habitat, of course, would affect the chances of the bird becoming infected with the parasite of avian malaria; one would not expect to find the same incidence in the road-runner (*Geococcyx californianus*) of the American desert as in the red-winged blackbird, a semigregarious dweller of the marsh. If any general statement were to be made, it would be to the effect that the infection of the vertebrate has to be related to an overlapping of its habitat with that of the invertebrate host, the mosquito. This implies at least a relationship to an aquatic environment.

In addition to overlapping habitats, the population level of the vertebrate must be of a density such that the chances of transmission of the parasite are high. The sudden drop of natality, a rise in mortality, or dispersal from a given habitat could singly or collectively seriously endanger the survival of the parasite. Thus we see an anomalous condition of high mortality providing some degree of extrinsic immunity to a host population.

The same concept applies to the mosquito host. First, the species which is capable of transmitting the parasite must be present in the community in which the suitable vertebrate host has a habitat. Secondly, the conditions for the developing larvae must be suitable. In order for proper growth and transformation to occur, the temperature of the pond or marsh water should be within certain limits, as must be the pH, the salinity, and the available planktonic foodstuffs. If these conditions are met and if other factors such as predators and parasites are overcome, the population density of larval, and subsequently, pupal and adult mosquitoes, will assuredly be high.

The adult mosquito, fortunately for the malaria parasite, has a different niche than do the larvae. The larvae feed as carnivores on plankton, the adult females feed, in part, on the blood of vertebrates. The habitats of the mosquito and vertebrate hosts overlap at this point. The overlap may be temporary, for example, the overlapping of the habitats of the human being and of the tsetse fly at the water holes of Nigeria during the dry season (Godwin, 1965), or it may be a permanent overlapping as in the case of a nonmigrating water bird and the mosquito.

The variety of habitats, of species, and of parasites makes difficult any comprehensive discussion of ecology and its relation to malaria. Moreover, with few exceptions, no intensive research has been done on the subject relative to the epidemiology of avian malaria.

One such effort is the excellent work of Herman (1938) dealing with the infection of the red-winged blackbird by the avian malaria parasite, *Plasmodium circumflexum*. Works by other authors may be classed as ecologic studies, but the one cited is in the author's opinion most inclusive and most informative. Herman chose a bird host, the red-winged blackbird (*Agelaius phoeniceus*), which has a rather well-defined habitat, and a malaria parasite (*Plasmodium circumflexum*) which appears to be very narrowly host-specific with regard to its mosquito vectors, *Culiseta* (=*Theobaldia*) *melanura* and *C. annulata*.

The vertebrate host ranges from Canada to Florida on the eastern reaches of the Appalachian Mountains. It is a migratory bird in the more northern states, but overwinters in flocks from Georgia southward. In the northern areas the bird is considered one of the harbingers of spring since its voice is one of the first to be heard in March. They usually nest in marshy regions and seem to have a preference for fixing their nests near the water in cattail plants. Despite their preference for marshes as a site for nesting, they are usually upland birds and reside in such areas in non-nesting seasons (Allen, 1914). Nesting season reaches its height in June and the young leave the nest about 10 to 12 days after birth. They nest in a semigregarious situation, and in the area studied by Herman (1938), fifteen nests were discovered on a pond 1,500 feet long and 100 feet wide.

The mosquito vector is *Culiseta* (=*Theobaldia*) *melanura*, a species which belongs to a rather small genus but which has a world-wide distribution. *Culiseta melanura* is found in the eastern and central United States and Canada, and as far south as the Gulf of Mexico. Larvae occur mostly in small permanent ponds, particularly those in marshy areas. The species apparently overwinters in the larval form in the northern parts of the United States. Other mosquitoes which occurred in the area (*Aedes sollicitans, A. canadensis, A. canator, A. vexans, Culex pipiens, C. apicalis*) were not suitable hosts for the development of *P. circumflexum*.

Rather than relying on the usual method of parasite survey, i.e., that of examining thin blood films, Herman utilized the susceptible canary into which blood from captured birds was inoculated. In this way, he detected a 60 percent incidence of infected birds. Forty percent of the adults and twenty percent of the juveniles were harboring *P. circumflexum*. A surprising finding was that no fledglings prior to leaving the nest were found to be infected. Some of these birds were later recaptured after departing the nest and the group was found to be thirty percent infected. These birds became infected after leaving the nest, and it follows that young blackbirds are insusceptible, at least at a very early age. This resistance or extrinsic immunity is in all probability a function of the ecology of the bird at that time. Herman suggests that perhaps the infection is acquired during migration. Even more importantly, he found that *Culiseta melanura* was not breeding in the particular pond under study and that the nearest population center of this mosquito was five miles away. This factor, plus the fact that the young blackbirds had a decided tendency to wander from the nesting area, would lead one to suppose that the infection was contracted from infected mosquitoes in other habitats during the fledgling period of wandering.

Herman also found that although adult birds were infected with *P. cathemerium*, no young birds were so infected. In this instance the problem becomes more puzzling; the vector of this malaria, *Culex pipiens*, was quite numerous in the same pond frequented by the birds. He interpreted this to be a factor of population density of *P. cathemerium* in the blackbird. The parasites were difficult to find in peripheral blood films; infections in mature birds were characterized by few parasites. It may be that there were insufficient populations of this parasite at this time of year or in this location to produce infections in the young.

While certain data, such as the density of mosquitoes and their seasonal peaks, are lacking in this interesting study, one can nevertheless draw certain conclusions regarding the extrinsic immunity of these birds to malaria. The pond under study served as a habitat for the developing red-wing blackbirds and, in this particular area, the population of these birds had a high density. As shown by blood inoculation, the populations of *P. circumflexum* in the birds were likewise high. A susceptible mosquito population in this area was, however, nonexistent. Herman did not investigate the cause of this lack of vectors, though it would have been interesting to have done so. Obviously the pond was not a satisfactory habitat for the insect, and a check of the environmental aspects of the pond would have done much toward explaining the lack of infection of fledglings. The fledglings by virtue of the extreme restriction of their habitat, i.e., to the nest, were not exposed to infection. As they left the nest and wandered, their habitat was extended to the point where it overlapped that of the infected mosquito and they then became ecologically susceptible.

The problem of extrinsic immunity may be approached through the doctrine of nidality in considering the habitat of the disease, but one must at the same time have knowledge of the habitats of the parasite, the invertebrate host, and the vertebrate host. The various habitats must overlap in order for the disease or the parasite to continue to exist. In addition the population levels within each habitat are important, for if the population levels of any or all of the various components of the system (bird, mosquito, or parasite) fall, the hosts become extrinsically immune.

Too little work has been done on this problem of extrinsic immunity, or perhaps better termed "biocenotic immunity" (Dogiel, 1964), to draw any firm conclusions. It is a subject, however, that has many fascinating aspects and one that should be more actively pursued.

INTRINSIC IMMUNITY

Intrinsic immunity, in contrast to extrinsic immunity, deals with a given host and its parasite (or parasites), exclusive of ecologic factors. Regarding malaria, studies concern plasmodia and their invertebrate or vertebrate hosts. The investigations of vertebrate hosts usually focus on either the exoerythrocytic or erythrocytic stages. Because of the relative recency of the elucidation of the pre-erythrocytic cycle of malaria, the bulk of studies have inclined toward the erythrocytic stages. Moreover, little is known about the development of acquired immunity to the parasites in their exoerythrocytic cycle. Although occurring prior to erythrocytic schizogony, immune processes, both innate and acquired, occur concomitantly. It is easier, however, to consider first immunity to exoerythrocytic development and then to follow this by a discussion of innate and acquired immunity to erythrocytic stages of development.

The exoerythrocytic stages

Innate immunity.   In a series of experiments, Huff (1954) examined the development of seven species of malarias in nine species of birds in relation to the distribution of exoerythrocytic stages. Infections were induced by the injection either of blood or of sporozoite stages of the avian malaria studied. In earlier studies (Huff and Coulston, 1944), it had been found that mature exoerythrocytic stages were not demonstrable prior to 36 hours in the various organs of birds injected with the sporozoites of *P. gallinaceum*. The parasites in this infection occurred in the spleen; other organs and the blood were infected after 48 hours. Huff (1954) confirmed his earlier observations and expanded the findings. Exoerythrocytic stages were not widespread until approximately 10 days after injection of erythrocytic stages. The same sequence of events occurred when turkeys served as the experimental host. In ducklings, exoerythrocytic stages were observed in only two of ten animals injected with sporozoites. This is in contrast to the infections in duck embryos in which heavy infections of all organs examined were observed following the intravenous injection of sporozoites (McGhee, 1949). Exoerythrocytic stages were well distributed in chick embryos. No parasites were observed in partridges, and only two of 17 pheasants were observed to have exoerythrocytic stages following sporozoite injections (Huff, 1954).

Plasmodium fallax infections in turkeys were similar to those produced by *P. gallinaceum* in chicks, except there was no predilection of exoerythrocytic stages for splenic tissue. Sporozoites were infective for some chicks, but no erythrocytic stages resulted, whereas in blood-induced infections, a majority of the erythrocytes was infected. Only two of 17 birds receiving sporozoites were found to have exoerythrocytic stages in the organs. Two of 24 animals injected with blood stages were found to harbor exoerythrocytic stages. No parasites occurred in the red blood cells. The degree of blood infection following sporozoite injection varied from none in partridges to heavy in guinea fowls (the presumed natural host of *P. fallax*). Surprisingly, no exoerythrocytic stages were found in guinea fowls injected with sporozoites. None was found in pheasants despite other experiments which demonstrated the development of cryptozoites in injected pheasants. Ducklings, pigeons, and canaries were only slightly susceptible to infection with sporozoites.

Sporozoites of *P. lophurae* (Huff et al., 1947) were infective for chicks, ducklings, turkey poults, canaries, and guinea keets. Blood-induced infections with this parasite resulted in the finding of exoerythrocytic stages in turkeys but not in chicks (*see also* Manresa, 1953).

Only one canary of six injected with sporozoites and only one of 14 injected with the erythrocytic stages of *Plasmodium relictum* were found to harbor exoerythrocytic stages (Huff, 1957). Although parasitemias were produced in canaries by injection of blood containing *P. cathemerium* and *P. circumflexum*, few exoerythrocytic stages were found in those injected with *P. cathemerium* and none was found in those injected with *P. circumflexum*.

The results indicated that possibly the change of host cell preference of the sporozoite from macrophage to endothelium to erythrocyte was the result of: (1) depletion of some nutritive materials necessary for the parasite survival or (2) immunity on the part of the host cell, or both. Attempts to alter this natural sequence by either successive infections of two different hosts, by passive immunization, or by active immunization failed to alter the sequence of development, indicating that acquired immunity *per se* seemed to have little effect (Huff, 1959).

The reason for the predilection of parasites for various cells during various stages of development is not clear, but it is probable, as postulated by Huff (1959), that the parasite introduced by the mosquito into a susceptible host is involved in its own evolutionary development. Attempts to interfere with or to change such an evolutionary pattern would be difficult to achieve. It was noted (Huff, 1959) that in turkeys injected with cultured exoerythrocytic stages of *P. fallax*, the pattern of development was essentially that of sporozoites in the same host. With the exception of *P. elongatum*, the development of the sporozoite to erythrocytic stages is similar—so similar in fact that one could probably not differentiate the various exoerythrocytic stages on morphologic grounds. Exoerythrocytic forms begin their development in cells of the lymphoid-macrophage system, progress from there to endothelium, and eventually, to the circulating erythrocytes. In *P. elongatum* on the other hand, infection occurs in all the stages of erythropoiesis and in lymphocytes.

One possible explanation of the host cell preference is that of acquired or natural immunity. Some cells, at one time amenable to infection, become refractory, and the site of infection changes. Another possible explanation may be found in the condition obtaining in chick and duck embryos infected with the exoerythrocytic stages of *P. gallinaceum*. Infections produced from the grafts of tissues containing exoerythrocytic stages (Zuckerman, 1946) or produced by intravenous injection of sporozoites (McGhee, 1949) were similar in that the *P. elongatum* type as well as the *P. gallinaceum* type of infection resulted. Both investigators reported the infection of all the cells of the erythrocytic series.

In the embryo, in contrast to the hatched chick, the spleen is one of the major sites of erythropoiesis. As pointed out by Huff (1954), the spleen is the organ first infected. In the embryo, therefore, initial exoerythrocytic development takes place at one of the major sites of blood cell formation. Infection at any stage would conceivably flush the cell and its parasites into the circulating blood stream. This condition occurs in the infected chick and duck embryo. In the hatched chick, however, this route of infection is largely closed. The bone marrow is, at best, lightly infected and then not until the parasites appear in the blood stream (Porter, 1942; Coulston et al., 1945).

In the embryo and in the hatched bird, *P. elongatum* develops in the bone marrow and would be in a position to infect all the blood cells and their precursors. The production of exoerythrocytic stages from blood stages may well be related to acquired immunity, as suggested by Huff (1959). The limits of cell penetration by erythrocytic merozoites are unknown. It includes, of course, penetration of endothelium unless this cell is, contrary to present beliefs, phagocytic. The removal of merozoites either through humoral or cellular antibody or both, as well as the removal of sensitized infected and perhaps uninfected erythrocytes, make this habitat untenable for the erythrocytic stages. Meanwhile, endothelial tissues may be infected, but they would be returning most new merozoites to the circulating blood stream. Upon the onset of acquired immunity, those parasites in the endothelium and their progeny, now in adjacent endothelium, would again be at least partially sheltered from antibody in the plasma. The speculation noted above presupposed the invasion of a cell ontogenetically rather far removed from the erythrocytes.

Innate immunity has a more direct effect upon the development of sporozoites. Beckman (1945) clearly demonstrated that sporozoites may develop for a period in a foreign host but are later destroyed. Raffaelle (1955) found that the sporozoites of *P. gallinaceum* will survive for over 100 minutes in rat skin. The same investigator reported the infection of *Aedes aegypti* with *Plasmodium berghei*, and the infection of chicks by this normally mammalian parasite following the bite of these mosquitoes. Raffaelle postulated that there is a change of such a magnitude as a result of the parasite's sojourn in the culicine mosquito that the potentiality to infect an avian host, rather than the usual mammalian host, becomes an actuality. In view of the difficulty encountered in producing infections in *Anopheles* mosquitoes with this parasite, and in view of the fact that the parasite rather reluctantly invades the erythrocytes of duck embryos and not those of chicks, it is to be hoped that this experiment will be repeated. If repetition of the experiment is accomplished, the significance of this finding is considerable, indicating that an invertebrate host's supporting the existence of a malaria parasite may determine its ability to overcome the natural defenses of the vertebrate host.

Further indications of immunity to sporozoite infections were provided by the studies by Haas et al. (1949), who protected chicks from infection by the injection of blood extracts. The factor responsible for this protection was in the protein fraction of the blood. Inasmuch as the degree of resistance was measured by the infection of the erythrocytes, it is difficult to determine whether this phenomenon reflects natural or acquired resistance to infections. Antimalarial activity of erythrocyte extracts had been reported previously by Jacobs (1948), and Haas et al. (1949) suggested that the two factors may be similar.

Only one attempt to discover the effect of sex on the development of malaria induced by sporozoite injection has been carried out (Bennison and Coatney, 1948). Female chicks were found to be more susceptible than the males, but the administration of sex hormones did not ameliorate the infections.

Acquired immunity. The relationship of acquired immunity to exoerythrocytic parasites has proved difficult to demonstrate. Chickens hyperimmunized to erythrocytic forms of *P. gallinaceum* permitted the development of apparently normal cryptozoites as if no immunity were present (Huff and Coulston, 1946). The same results were observed with the sporozoites of *P. relictum* in hyperimmunized pigeons (Huff and Coulston, 1946). The cryptozoites of malaria once in the cytoplasm of the host cell seemed to be protected from natural and perhaps the acquired immune processes of the host. Later in the infection, however, degenerate exoerythrocytic stages were observed, and Huff (1959) believed that these forms were a result of antibody action. Prior to this stage, it appears that acquired immunity plays no role, or only a very small one, in the development of the pre-erythrocytic stage of malaria.

The erythrocytic cycle

Although the exoerythrocytic and erythrocytic stages of malaria are being dealt with separately, it is merely for the sake of convenience; both innate and acquired immune reactions may be common to both. In both, there are the same dynamic conditions relative to the host-parasite relationship. In both cycles, the degree of immunity, either innate or acquired, is only relative and may never be expected to be complete for any two animals. The immune reaction may be affected by the presence or absence of some or all necessary foodstuffs, by the existence of natural parasiticidal antibodies, or, eventually, by specific acquired antibodies. If innate immunity is effective, acquired antibody reactions may be either slight or nonexistent. Although there appear to be remarkable overall similarities as to immunity to the various species of malaria, what is true for the host-parasite reactions for one host may not be so for another. Thus, results should not be extrapolated to include several species of malaria when dealing with such a complex subject. Modifying Garnham's statement slightly, one may truly say the malaria parasites provide most interesting variations on the theme of immunity (Garnham, 1963).

Innate immunity. The study of innate immunity, although considered difficult to approach, has yielded some rather precise information in relatively recent years. Allison (1963) has shown that one type of resistance to human malaria brought about by the altered hemoglobin of sickle cell anemia is specifically due to an inherited recessive gene. Other findings, while not so precise, have shed considerable light on the phenomenon.

One of the oldest but still applicable concepts of immunity is that of atrepsis, which simply indicates a lack of some basic material necessary for the survival of the parasite in an inhospitable environment (Erlich, 1908). It has been long recognized that glucose is indispensible for the growth and multiplication of the malaria parasite (Bass and Johns, 1912). Hegner and MacDougall (1926) and MacDougall (1927) noted that in birds in which the blood sugar levels had been elevated by intravenous injection of glucose, the parasitemias were much greater. Bass and Johns (1913) noted more severe malarial infections in diabetic humans. Although no study has been done of diabetes in the bird and the severity of malaria, Tolbert and McGhee (1960) made rats diabetic by the administration of alloxan and found that although the blood sugar levels were extremely high, the malaria infection was severely curtailed. Rigdon and Marvin (1953) showed that the injection of insulin into infected birds produced no effect on the parasitemia. It should be noted, however, that injection of insulin or the production of a diabetic condition produces profound changes in the metabolic activity of the host. Diabetic conditions, for example, depress the levels of coenzyme A. The loss of this essential food material (Trager, 1952) could in itself account for the decreased levels of parasitemia.

Somewhat in line with the above work was the subjugation of infected birds to low oxygen tensions (Gajewski and Tatum, 1944) with a resultant relapse in infected birds. Both these birds and those treated with epinephrine were thought to be adversely affected regarding phagocytosis as a result of hyperglycemia. A deficiency of biotin (Trager, 1943a) results in greater levels of parasitemia in animals infected with *P. lophurae*. Vitamin A deficiency seems to have no effect on the levels of infection in ducklings parasitized with *P. lophurae* (Rigdon, 1947).

One of the observations relative to acquired immunity to avian malaria was the decrease in mean numbers of merozoites subsequent to the crisis in canaries infected with *P. cathemerium* (Boyd, 1939). The same sort of reduction may be produced in birds made deficient in pantothenic acid, which may be corrected by the issuance of an adequate diet during the infectious periods (Huff et al., 1959). The dependence of *P. lophurae* in culture on pantothenate (Trager, 1943b) and the aviral properties of an analog of this substance (Marshall, 1946) both point to the exciting possibilities concerning natural immunity and malaria therapy inherent in this too little studied area of malariology.

Riboflavin deficiency appears to be necessary for the survival of some species of malarial parasites. Riboflavin deficiency in chicks made them more susceptible to infection, and more deaths occurred in deficient animals. In monkeys, ascorbic acid deficiency modified and extended the course of infection of *P. knowlesi*. Deficiency of folic acid or protein (Seeler et al., 1944) also decreased the resistance of chickens to infection by *P. lophurae*. Trager (1947) showed a lipoprotein inhibited growth of *P. lophurae* in culture and in the intact animal.

The phenomenon of age resistance is well known in avian malaria, and infections in younger animals are usually more severe than in older ones (Coggeshall, 1938; Terzian, 1941; Hewitt, 1942). This aspect of immunity has been investigated in avian embryos beginning with the work of Wolfson (1940). McGhee (1949, 1957) has shown that many parasites will readily develop in both chicken and duck embryos. In fact, no parasite of those tried, including *P. berghei* from rodents, failed to develop when injected into duck embryos. *Plasmodium gallinaceum* produced heavy infections in duck embryos, but hatched ducklings were normally immune to infection.

In carrying the study of the relation of age and resistance further, Trager (1948) showed that adult egg-laying ducks were quite resistant to malaria produced by *P. lophurae*. Trager and McGhee (1950) injected plasma from ovulating ducks into normally highly susceptible ducklings and observed a heightened resistance. In a few cases the plasma of drakes with hypertrophied testes also produced resistance. A euglobulin fraction was isolated from the blood of the egg-laying ducks, and injection of this material into susceptible ducklings conferred some resistance to malaria infections. A specific delimitation of age factors and that of hormonal factors in the above work is difficult. It appeared that follicle stimulating hormone (FSH) and luteinizing hormone (LH) were active in the donor ducks, and it may well be that the resistance was due to primary or secondary effects of these hormones.

Studies concerning the natural resistance of hosts to infection have concentrated on the role of the serum and phagocytic cells, and the host cell has been to a great extent neglected. The idea of host cell resistance is not new, however, and may be ascribed to Erlich (1908), who assumed that immunity to certain diseases might be due to a deficiency in nutritional materials. The problems in studying the specific role of the erythrocyte in resistance are quite apparent. They include the difficulties of securing a medium in which erythrocytes of various animal species might coexist and, once such a medium has been found, separating the two coexisting cells. These difficulties are illustrated in the work of Huff and Coulston (1946), who, although securing patent parasitemias of *Plasmodium gallinaceum* in ducks after transfusions of chicken erythrocytes, were unable to state which species' cells were infected with any degree of certainty. By utilizing the malarious chicken embryo blood stream as a medium and mammalian erythrocytes as the test cells, these difficulties have been overcome to a certain extent, although the results generate doubts as to the efficacy of this immature host's defense mechanisms (McGhee, 1949).

Chick embryos were inoculated with the parasite *P. lophurae* on the 10th day of incubation. On the second or third day after inoculation, 0.2 ml of washed erythrocytes from various species of animals were injected into another vein. Four hours later, blood films were stained and examined for the presence of parasites in the introduced erythrocytes.

Positive infections were observed in the red cells of the mouse, rabbit, and pig (Fig. 1). These susceptible erythrocytes are similar with respect to sodium: potassium ratios and in concentrations of organic acid-soluble phosphorus (OAP). The erythrocytes which are nearest in chemical composition to those of the susceptible animals are those of the guinea pig and rat (McGhee, 1950). Rappaport and Guest (1941) demonstrated a higher concentration of organic acid phosphate in weanling rats than in adults, and it was found that OAP concentrations in newly-born rat and guinea pig erythrocytes were well within the range of the amounts found in cells susceptible to infection by *P. lophurae*. Upon injection of erythrocytes from these two animals into infected embryos, it was found that those of the baby rat were indeed susceptible, but that the erythrocytes of the baby (and fetal) guinea pig, fetal human, and baby sheep were not (McGhee, 1953c). Thus, although the hypothesis relating OAP to susceptibility was not entirely applicable, the age of the rat was reflected in the susceptibility of its erythrocytes.

In order to ascertain the age at which the erythrocytes of rats acquired complete resistance to infection by the parasite *P. lophurae*, washed red blood cells of rats of various ages were introduced into the circulating blood stream of infected chick embryos. The rate of penetration of cells from a 13-day-old rat was 1.4 percent, compared to 3.0 percent in a less than one-day-old rat erythrocyte. By the time the rat reached 30 days of age, the merozoite penetration rate was reduced to 0.1 percent, and by 40 days only two of the injected red blood cells were observed to contain parasites, a penetration rate of 0.01 percent.

For comparison, washed erythrocytes from less than 1-day-old mice, 2-day-old mice, and adult mice were similarly injected into embryos infected with *P. lophurae*. Inasmuch as cells from all ages of mice were susceptible (as indicated by infection of the intact animals), the differences were not so marked as that observed in rats. The rate of penetration of baby mouse erythrocytes was 0.18 percent; that of the cells of the 21-day-old mice was 0.43 percent, and that of adult mice was 0.35 percent.

Thus the erythrocytes from four species of birds, from two species of rodents, one artiodactyla and one lagomorph—animals widely divergent in their taxonomic status but somewhat similar in chemical makeup of their erythrocytes—were found to be susceptible to infection by an avian malaria

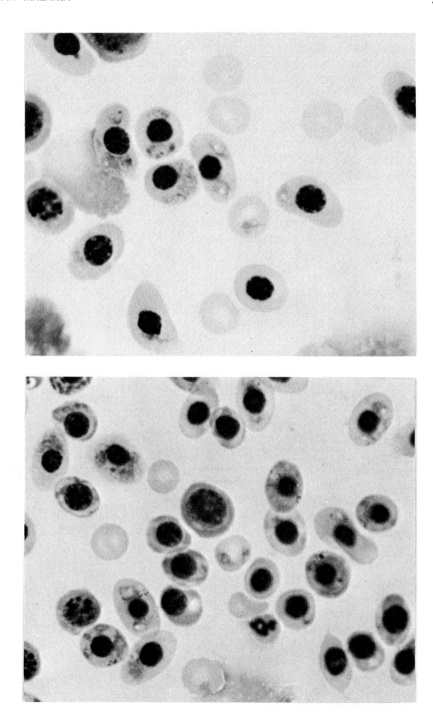

FIG. 1.   Infection of erythrocytes of the mouse in the circulating blood stream of chick embryos infected with *Plasmodium lophurae*. × 1,600.

parasite (Fig. 2). The erythrocytes of two of these animals, the rat and the mouse, were more susceptible when taken from young animals. It remained, therefore, to discover, if possible, the mechanisms of susceptibility. To do this, it became necessary to use a cell which was more susceptible than those of the mouse and less toxic than those of the pig, rabbit, or baby rat. The duck cell met these requirements well and could be easily distinguished from the chick erythrocyte by the shape of its nucleus. They were nontoxic and remained in the embryo circulation for periods of up to 30 hours without too much evidence of degeneration.

Examination of washed adult duck erythrocytes in infected chick embryos revealed a rather unexpected aspect of cell susceptibility (McGhee, 1953a). Hitherto, all cells tested had, at best, been only lightly infected, but now as many as 15 percent of the duck erythrocytes were infected after only four hours. At the end of a 4-hour period, there was no material change in the rel-

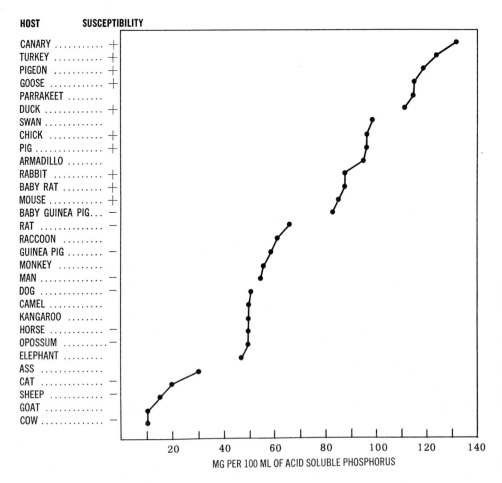

FIG. 2. The relation of acid-soluble phosphorus concentration of the erythrocyte to susceptibility to infection by the avian malaria parasite, *Plasmodium lophurae.*

ative numbers of parasites in chick embryo cells, whereas the percentage of parasitized duck cells steadily increased. Subsequent experiments served to emphasize the extreme susceptibility of duck erythrocytes. At the end of the 24-hour period, the relative numbers of parasites in duck erythrocytes either approached or actually exceeded those in chick cells. If a calculation of the deposition of available merozoites was made, it would appear that nearly all merozoites either entered duck cells or, presumably, died during the 4-hour period. In a series of studies made on infected chicken embryos not receiving duck cells, it could be demonstrated that in low-grade infections the number of surviving merozoites was approximately 28 percent. Later during infections, the percentage of surviving merozoites decreased until the time that the infection averaged 45 parasites per 100 erythrocytes, when the survival rate of merozoites over a 4-hour period was zero. When, however, duck cells were introduced, the survival values of merozoites remained at a constant level, regardless of the chick cell infection. Moreover, in low-grade infections, instead of the usual percentage of infective units penetrating chick erythrocytes, the invasion rate was nearly zero. These data suggest that the duck erythrocytes were so constituted that in some way the merozoites managed to infect them differentially in preference to the chick cells.

The ability of a parasite usually found in a nucleated avian erythrocyte to penetrate, grow, and reproduce in an anucleated mammalian cell indicates that the presence of a host cell nucleus is not necessary for the life of this parasite.

The similarities existing in infected cells in relation to their chemical makeup (except that of the guinea pig) indicate a certain predilection of the parasite toward these similar cells.

The decrease of susceptibility of rat erythrocytes coincident with aging of the animal suggests that perhaps hemoglobin might also enter into the picture of susceptibility, inasmuch as about the same time sequence is followed in the replacement of fetal by adult hemoglobin.

The preferential invasion of duck erythrocytes is particularly pertinent to an examination of mechanisms of susceptibility. If we visualize the situation that occurs when we introduce duck cells, we find the following picture: Following its release from the mother segmenter, the merozoite floats around in the blood stream, hitting approximately four chicken cells to every one duck cell, yet when it contacts this latter cell penetration ensues. There must be, therefore, some peculiarity of the surface of the duck erythrocyte that makes it much more acceptable to penetration (or attachment) by the merozoite.

In the belief that the entry and growth of a parasite or parasites in the erythrocytes might alter the susceptibility of the cell, parasitized duck erythrocytes were washed and injected into infected chicken embryos (McGhee, 1953). The results indicated that when infections (in the duck erythrocytes) were of low magnitude, the amount of invasion of these cells was virtually unaltered, but when the parasitemia in the introduced duck cells was in the vicinity of 84 parasites per 100 erythrocytes, no further penetration ensued. At this time the merozoite death rate approached that of uninjected, but similarly infected, chicken embryos. A differential count relative to numbers of parasites per erythrocyte in the introduced duck cells indicated that as the level of infection increased, the number of multiply infected erythrocytes likewise increased. Thus, when the infection rate was 2 to 13 parasites per 100 erythrocytes, there were no quadrupally or triply infected cells and only approximately 4 percent doubly infected erythrocytes. When, however, the infection was 170 parasites per 100 erythrocytes a few (2 percent) of the cells contained four parasites, 12 percent were triply infected, and 50 percent were doubly infected.

Four hours after the introduction of these variously infected duck erythrocytes, blood films were made and the cells again counted relative to the numbers of parasites per erythrocyte. In no instance was there a relative increase in the numbers of the introduced cells with four or five parasites, although in the lower grade infections there was some increase in those cells having two parasites. It would appear, therefore, that when the duck erythrocyte contained two or more parasites, it became altered in such a way that subsequent invasion by merozoites was rendered more difficult. That additional invasion was possible, is, of course, indicated by the presence of some cells with four parasites.

Two experiments were done with a view toward altering the surface of the erythrocyte (McGhee, 1953b). The first of these consisted in treating uninfected duck erythrocytes with steapsin, a process which removes one of the hydrocarbon chains from the surface of the cell. Erythrocytes so treated were no less susceptible than untreated cells from the same source. Secondly, duck red blood cells were treated with rabbit anti-duck-erythrocyte serum. The amount of antibody used was necessarily less than one unit, since greater amounts produced excessive intravascular agglutination in the embryos and resulted in the death of the host animal. In those embryos receiving duck cells that were exposed to less than one unit of antibody, there was a drastic reduction of the introduced cell after 4 hours. The amount of invasion of the remaining cells, however, was reduced to approximately one-tenth of that normally found.

Three experiments aimed at changing the hemoglobin of the cell were performed. One batch of uninfected duck erythrocytes was subjected to carbon monoxide for 15 minutes in order to produce carbon monoxyhemoglobin. These erythrocytes, following their injection into infected embryos, were invaded by merozoites and the parasites developed in them just as well as in untreated embryos.

Duck erythrocytes were lysed with distilled water and the ghosts injected into embryos. After four hours it was impossible to find any duck cells. When duck cells were only partially lysed, however, sufficient erythrocytes could be found even at 24 hours to gain some idea of the amount of invasion. Penetration took place but was drastically reduced over that in unlysed duck cells.

Finally, duck erythrocytes were treated *in vitro* with phenylhydrazine. When they were treated with 5 mg of the chemical and then washed and injected into embryos, there was no reduction in the amount of parasite invasion. When 10 mg of phenylhydrazine was used to one ml of washed erythrocytes, there was a sharp reduction in invasion. Duck cells treated with 20 mg of phenylhydrazine per ml of washed cells did not differ materially from those treated with 10 mg. However, when the dosage was increased to 40 mg, no invasion of treated cells resulted.

On the surface, it appears as if the destruction of hemoglobin removes the factors of susceptibility, but it might be well to examine these results more closely. In the smaller dosage, only about 20 to 30 percent of the hemoglobin is altered and the vital functions of the erythrocytes are apparently unchanged. No information is available concerning the effect of greater concentrations upon cell materials other than hemoglobin, but since phenylhydrazine is a general cytoplasmic toxin, probably substances other than hemoglobin are destroyed. One cannot be sure, therefore, that the destruction of hemoglobin is the factor solely responsible for the replacement of susceptibility with resistance.

Attempts were made to determine whether the susceptibility of erythrocytes of several species to *P. lophurae* represented a general phenomenon or if it represented a special case peculiar to *P. lophurae* (McGhee, 1957). A series of experiments were carried out involving the susceptibility of four species of birds and three species of mammals to invasion by four species of avian malarias: *P. lophurae*, *P. cathemerium*, *P. gallinaceum*, and *P. circumflexum*. All bird cells were susceptible to all species of avian malaria, but not to the same degree. In addition to the ability to infect bird erythrocytes, *P. lophurae* also invaded erythrocytes of the rabbit, mouse, and baby rat. *Plasmodium circumflexum* was quite similar to *P. lophurae* in its penetration of bird erythrocytes, but in the case of mammalian cells, it was only able to infect those cells of the baby rat. Infection of avian cells was, in general, less by *P. cathemerium*. In so far as mammals were concerned, only the erythrocytes of adult rats were subject to infection by this parasite, and then only in one instance when the number of segmenting parasites was extremely high.

Of the four species of malaria, *P. gallinaceum* was most restricted in its invasiveness. If the invasion of erythrocytes by malaria parasites is the result of forceful entry, one would expect the apparent difference between cell susceptibility to *P. gallinaceum* and *P. cathemerium*. One would assume that from the results obtained, the cell surface of chicken erythrocytes is weakest, whereas those of the pigeon, duck, and canary are stronger in their resistance to *P. gallinaceum*. *Plasmodium cathemerium* is, however, practically unable to invade chicken cells, but it invades those of the duck, pigeon, and canary quite well.

In summary:
1. The taxonomic status of an animal has no bearing on the susceptibility or resistance of its erythrocytes to infection. Generally speaking, however, there are distinct similarities in cytochemistry of the susceptible cells.
2. When duck erythrocytes were the experimental cells, there was preferential invasion over that of the host chicken cells.

3. Infection of erythrocytes somehow alters the cell to the point that susceptibility decreases.

4. Cells of a single species of animal are not susceptible to the same degree of invasion by various parasites.

5. Drastic alteration of the cell by various means alters susceptibility.

All these findings indicate that invasion of the erythrocyte is accomplished by some chemical pathway. It is the author's belief that this invasion is accomplished by an enzyme of the parasite, and that this enzyme, in addition to facilitating penetration, produces other effects on the host cell and thereby on the host animal.

Host Specificity. The strictness or looseness of host specificity may be understood only as related to a given group of hosts. *Plasmodium relictum* and *P. cathemerium* are found in a wide variety of wild birds, but successful infections of mammals have not been forthcoming (Beckman, 1945). A more rigid host specificity has been noted for *P. vaughani* and *P. polare* (Manwell, 1938). *Plasmodium circumflexum* occurs in a wide variety of birds, is infective for canaries (Jordon, 1957), and is capable of infecting the erythrocytes of the same host species as does *P. lophurae*. *Plasmodium lophurae* has the widest host distribution of any avian malaria parasite studied, although the conditions of susceptibility have been demonstrated experimentally only. Jordon (1957) reported successful experimental infections of pheasants, coots, domestic pigeons, and canaries.

In view of the invasion and development of *P. lophurae* in various mammalian cells, McGhee (1951) attempted to infect the intact animal. Since it seemed that erythrocytes of infant mice were more susceptible to infection and since younger animals would possibly contain less natural antibody in their blood stream, this age of mouse was used in the preliminary experiments. When embryo blood containing vast quantities of parasites was injected intravenously into new-born mice, varying degrees of infection of the recipient mouse erythrocytes were observed within 24 hours. No infections were observed subsequent to eight days after injection.

Using a system of alternating the passages of parasites between the rather resistant mouse and the nonresistant chick embryos, it was possible to select parasites that were able to survive for longer and longer periods in the mouse. It was possible after the fourth adaptive infection to discard the embryo passage and rely entirely on mouse-to-mouse passage. Transfers were made thereafter every tenth day and resulted in low grade infections through the tenth direct passage. At this time the parasitemia rose markedly and reached peaks as high as 2,200 parasites per 10,000 mouse erythrocytes.

In adult mice infections of a transient nature were observed only after massive doses of parasites were introduced intravenously and intraperitoneally.

To determine whether *P. lophurae* had adapted itself to the erythrocytes, the serum, or both, two sets of embryos, one infected with the regular stock passage and the other with parasites derived from the tenth mouse passage, were treated with 0.2 ml of washed mouse erythrocytes. Infections in the two groups were comparable at the time of injection. There was no significant difference in the number of mouse cells infected. The rate of increase of the parasites was not as great in the infections derived from the mouse-adapted parasites, although the mean merozoite count for each group was the same. In considering the morphology of *P. lophurae* in the mouse, it was necessary to study the parasites from the initial and final passages, and, in addition, those parasites from the earlier and later stages of the infection in the established strain. During the adaptive passages, either in the embryo-mouse alternation or in mouse passage alone, there was a decided tendency on the part of the parasites to assume more and more the characteristics of *P. lophurae* in the bird. The early trophozoites were similar in all infections, and the characteristic ring forms generally associated with mammalian malaria were absent. Banding was common in initial infections, while in later passages the parasites tended to be more compact although banding was occasionally observed (Fig. 3).

Following adaptation of the parasite to baby mice, infections were maintained in this host for a period of three years (McGhee, 1956). From the third through the seventh month there was a rapid increase in the monthly average numbers of parasites. From the seventh through the fourteenth month until the termination of the infection the average level of parasitemia fluctuated roughly between 2,500 and 3,000 parasites per 10,000 erythrocytes.

A further check on the adaptation of this parasite was made comparing infections in individual mice after the parasite's existence for one and three years in mice. The course of infection was more severe in later than in earlier infections. Principal differences lay in the height of parasitemia, the rate of rise, and the duration of parasitemia. In three-year infections, the rise in parasite numbers was more regular and reached an average peak of 1,600 parasites per 10,000 erythrocytes. After three years it was possible to find parasites in the blood stream of 22-day-old mice, whereas the greatest duration of parasitemia in one-year infections was 14 days.

The success in infecting mice encouraged attempts to see if similar infections might be produced in rats (McGhee, 1953c). Baby rats were given large doses of infected embryo blood. The erythrocytes in the intact animal were quite susceptible as indicated by a greater severity of infection in the baby rat than in the baby mouse. Certain infections reached peaks of 1,280 parasites per 10,000 erythrocytes as compared with 280 parasites per 10,000 erythrocytes in the mouse. Peaks were attained on the third or fourth day and were followed by a sharp decline in the number of parasites. In general, the morphology of *P. lophurae* in rat erythrocytes was similar to the same parasite in the mouse.

The discovery of *Plasmodium berghei*, a malaria parasite of rodents, provided the opportunity of investigating its capabilities of producing infections in foreign hosts (McGhee, 1954). First, chick embryos were injected intravenously with large doses of mouse blood containing the parasites of *P. berghei*. No infection ensued. However, when duck and goose embryos were injected, it was possible to find avian erythrocytes infected.

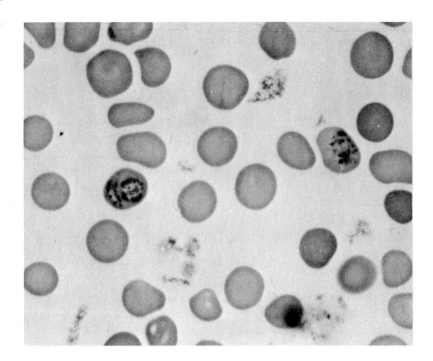

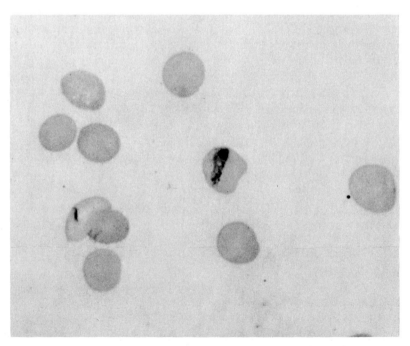

FIG. 3. Infection of the intact mouse with the avian malaria parasite, *Plasmodium lophurae*. Band forms are represented in doubly and singly infected erythrocytes. × 1,600.

There were two distinctly different morphologic types of young parasites, depending on whether invasion was accomplished in erythroblasts or orthochromic erythrocytes. In the latter, cell development was abnormal, but in the young erythrocytes it proceeded normally until segmentation. Attempts to establish the infection in embryos through a second passage were unsuccessful.

These experiments show rather dramatically the remarkable ability of certain malarias to infect a number of hosts other than those with which they are generally associated. I have no doubt that other examples might be found and that, if properly handled, human malaria might be infective for some avian embryos or immature mammals (*see* Weinman, 1966).

Acquired immunity. In a given host infected with a given parasite, modifications of a general scheme of development of acquired immunity might take place, but these variations are usually a question of degree and are related to the virulence of the infecting organism. The problems of both innate and acquired immunity have been the object of intensive research efforts by Taliaferro and his associates, and any discussion of these topics would be futile without drawing heavily on their works. Spatial limitations do not allow a full exposition of these carefully performed and penetrating works, so the reader is urged to consult the original papers.

The appearance of erythrocytic stages of malaria, whether from sporozoite or blood injection, is soon followed by changes in the lymphoid-macrophage system. If erythrocytic stages of the parasite are injected into the skin of previously uninfected birds, they are confronted first with a migration of lymphocytes and heterophils into the area, followed by the appearance of macrophages and active phagocytosis of the infected and non-infected red blood cells. In canaries, at least, inoculation of hyperimmune birds showed little effect on the speed or activity of the defense cells. In animals in which a greater amount of antigen is produced (as in *P. knowlesi* in monkeys), the degree of inflammation increased concomitantly with hyperimmunity (Taliaferro and Bloom, 1945).

Examination of other organs associated with the lymphoid-macrophage systems pointed out the major role of the spleen in defense reactions (Taliaferro and Taliaferro, 1955; Taliaferro, 1956). Early in the course of the infection, there is an increase of phagocytosis in this organ, chiefly as a result of engulfment of parasites by the already present macrophages of the Schweigger-Seidel sheaths. Later phagocytosis occurs predominantly in the red pulp. As will be discussed later, phagocytosis is concerned not only with the disposition of parasites and parasitized cells, but also with lymphocytes and non-infected erythrocytes.

Constant call on the supply of macrophages and the elimination of the lymphocytes by their transformation to macrophages and by the lymphocytocidal activities of the parasites result in a depletion of the mesenchymal reserves and a marked decrease in the lymphatic nodules of the infected bird (Taliaferro, 1963). Lymphoid depletion is followed in turn by hyperplasia and an eventual return to a condition approaching normalcy. Phagocytosis progresses and there is a later development of erythropoiesis. There is an infiltration of the red pulp of the spleen by large lymphocytes which are apparently the hemocytoblasts responsible for the production of erythrocytes, granulocytes, and plasma cells. These plasma cells, thought by many to be the source of antibody, begin to appear contemporaneously with acquired immunity. In animals immunized or hyperimmunized to infection, there is generally no need of the intense activity described for the spleen. There is, as a result of the parasiticidal activity of antibody, no depletion of the mesenchymal reserves and consequently no period of hyperactivity as indicated by the hyperplasia in previously uninfected animals.

In the liver, phagocytosis is principally by the Küpffer cells. Although there is phagocytosis in the bone marrow, it is not as extensive or intensive as it is in the liver and spleen. Macrophages in the bone marrow contain relatively fewer inclusions than the large cells of the spleen. The hemocytoblasts seem to be at least one source of macrophages, since cells practically indistinguishable from them may be observed engulfing parasitized erythrocytes. This latter phenomenon has also been observed by the author (unpublished, 1967). Reactions in the other tissues are minimal.

The importance of the mesenchymal reserve has been emphasized by Taliaferro (1963), Singer (1954), and numerous other authors (*see* the review by Goble and Singer, 1960). Although there seems to be some question as to the effectiveness of the methods used, depletion of mesenchymal reserves by blockage by various substances (Krichewski and Meersohn, 1932; Gingrich, 1932, 1934; Trager, 1941; McGhee, 1959) seems to be indicated provided sufficient material is injected to saturate the system effectively. Radiation has been observed to produce opposite effects by different investigators (Rigdon and Rudisell, 1949; Thompson et al., 1948). Taliaferro and Taliaferro (1948) indicate little effect on innate immunity in chickens treated with nitrogen mustard, an effective lymphocyte-killing substance.

Gajewski and Tatum (1944) and Hughes and Tatum (1955) found that hypoxic conditions associated with those at 19,000 to 20,000 feet of altitude resulted in lowered resistance and consequent relapses with avian malaria. At conditions equivalent to little more than one-half of this altitude, however, hypoxia produced a stimulating effect on the lymphoid-macrophage system (Geigy and Freyvogel, 1953; Herbig-Sandreuter, 1953).

Despite the diversity of findings relative to the depression or stimulation of the lymphoid-macrophage system, this system is of utmost importance in controlling malaria infections both from the standpoint of cellular defense and the synthesis of antibody.

The demonstration of humoral antibodies has proved a more difficult task due probably to the fact that such antibodies in birds infected with malaria are not very effective and in all probability are present in relatively small amounts. It should be kept in mind that the fulminating infections produced in the laboratory are almost never encountered in nature. Herman (1942) reported the finding of one heavily infected canary, and McGhee (unpublished, 1945) found a moribund barn owl (*Tyto alba*) in the New Hebrides Islands with an infection in over 90 percent of its red blood cells. It is probable, therefore, that in nature innate immunity is primarily operative and that acquired immunity is not important to the extent that it is in laboratory infections.

It is generally believed that serologic reactions are manifestations of the presence of antibodies specific for the antigens used. If so, agglutinins both innate (Trager et al., 1950) and acquired (Stauber et al., 1951) to *P. lophurae* are present in ducklings. Opsonins have been demonstrated by Zuckerman (1945) and protective antibodies have been demonstrated. Eaton (1939) demonstrated complement fixation to a soluble antigen extracted from blood infected with *P. knowlesi*, and Davis (1948) found a similar reaction to antigen from duck blood infected with *P. lophurae*.

Although not in the purview of this subject, McGregor and Gilles (1960) have shown that the antibody fraction lies in the 7S fraction of gamma-cans, and that the serum of such individuals may be used for partially immunizing normally susceptible individuals. Cohen and McGregor (1963) have shown that the antibody fraction lies in the 7S fraction of gamma-globulin. Their work establishes the reality of humoral immunity in malaria. No comparable work has been done using birds, but as Taliaferro has noted, immunity depends to a large extent on the quantity and quality of antigen present.

In ducks undergoing severe infections with *P. lophurae*, intravascular hemolysis is noted prior to and during the crisis. Hemolysis and a precipitous drop in parasite numbers suggest an intense antigen-antibody reaction. Immune hemolysis is accompanied by a fixing of complement. Ducks undergoing severe cases of malaria were tested regarding the proportions of complement and its four components (McGhee, 1952). In ducks undergoing infections there was a reduction in the total complement levels. The presence of an *in vivo* hemolysis was always coincident with a decrease in complement and affected all components on the terminal day of infection. In subterminal hemolysis, C'1 and C'3 were little affected in most instances, while C'2 and C'4 were sharply reduced. The drop in complement, the hemolytic reaction, and the destruction of parasites all suggest the intense antigen-antibody combination of acquired immunity.

While always difficult and often impossible to demonstrate, it is generally agreed that humoral antibodies exist in avian malaria infections. Early attempts to find circulating antibodies were unsuccessful, and a belief arose that none was present (Moldovan, 1912; Sergent and Catanei, 1937). Coggeshall and Kumm (1937), however, were successful in passively immunizing monkeys to infections of *P. knowlesi*. This work was followed by Manwell and Goldstein producing passive immunization in canaries to *P. circumflexum* (1938). In a summary of such work up to 1942, Hewitt (1942) stated that humoral antibodies probably exist in avian malaria infections. Taliaferro and Taliaferro (1945) showed a cross-immunity existing between birds infected with *P. gallinaceum* and *P. lophurae*.

Zuckerman (1945) was able to show by the use of tissue culture techniques, the presence of an opsonin directed against infected and noninfected chicken erythrocytes. Trager et al. (1950) demonstrated a specific heat-stable agglutinin to the freed erythrocytic stages of *P. lophurae* in the plasma of affected ducklings. Labeled fluorescent antibodies have also been used to detect antibodies (Ingram et al., 1961), and the Coombs' test was used by Zuckerman (1960a) in her investigations of autoimmune phenomena in rats infected with *P. berghei*.

The possible occurrence of autoantibody reactions in malaria infections presupposes the existence of humoral antibodies and will be discussed under the various aspects of immunopathy.

The difficulty in obtaining immunity passively and the apparent necessity of having parasites present in the individual to produce immunity has been regarded as a special kind of immunity of premunition (Sergent, 1963). The belief in this type of immunity has somewhat discouraged attempts to produce a suitable vaccine against malaria. The work of McGregor and Gilles (1960), however, suggests that a sterile immunity may exist in humans. Corradetti (1963) has shown that in a special strain of albino rat, sterile immunity to reinfection with *P. berghei* obtains. As of now, sterile immunity has not been clearly demonstrated in avian malaria. It may well be that the level of effective antigen may play an important role in the sterile immunity observed in rats to *P. berghei* and in monkeys to *P. cynomolgi* (Garnham, 1963).

Identification of the antigens of malaria has been made difficult by the presence of host material. Sherman (1964) recognized this complication and dealt with it, in large measure, through the use of immunoelectrophoresis. He first obtained two major components of hemazoin and a soluble protein. Using Ouchterlony and immunoelectrophoretic methods, he obtained four to six precipitating antigens of *P. lophurae*. Spira and Zuckerman (1964) used gel diffusion and demonstrated 12 to 16 bands for *P. gallinaceum*.

McGhee (unpublished, 1965) noted that following the injection of filtered malarious plasma and, after a suitable period of time, a subsequent injection of malarious blood, the mortality rate in recipient ducks was 50 percent rather than the usual 100 percent.

Immunopathology.   Most investigators feel that products of the parasite and of the affected cell induce allergenic reactions. Brown (1913) was of the opinion that a pigment liberated at time of merozoite release was hemolytic. Abrami and Senevet (1919) regarded paroxysms as indications of anaphylactic shock due to the liberation of a sensitizing agent. In human, rodent, or avian malaria there is a loss of erythrocytes to such an extent that one must agree that uninfected as well as infected cells are removed from the circulation. Terzian (1941) speculated on the mechanism of erythrocyte removal, as did Coffin (1941). Coffin, although suspecting the presence of autoantibodies, could not overlook the possibility of an isoantibody being responsible for anemia. Zuckerman (1960a) studied infections of *Plasmodium berghei* and concluded that the excessive removal of uninfected erythrocytes was a result of autoantibody reaction. To demonstrate the presence of this substance, she used a modification of Coombs' test only to find later that the same positive test could be obtained in animals rendered anemic by bleeding or by treatment with phenylhydrazine hydrochloride (Zuckerman and Spira, 1961). At about the same time and unaware of Zuckerman's latest research, the author discovered that if ducklings were given subcutaneous injections of a *P. lophurae* modified by continued passage in duck embryos, a severe anemia developed despite an extremely low parasitemia.

Concomitantly with the anemia there was a reduction, sometimes to the point of extinction, of polychromatophil erythroblasts both in the circulating blood and in the bone marrow. Subsequent investigations (McGhee, 1964) indicated that the same blood dyscrasia could be induced in ducklings injected intravenously with duckling-adapted *P. lophurae* and controlled with quinine. If, however, ducklings were infected with *P. relictum* (a parasite contrasting with *P. lophurae* in its preference for young erythrocytes), there was a stimulation of the bone marrow and a rise in the percentages of circulating polychromatophil erythroblasts. Having demonstrated a lack of concentration of parasites and the absence of an accompanying viral infection, the author concluded, as did Zuckerman, that as far as the *P. lophurae* infections were concerned, the phenomenon was an autoimmune state.

As well as dyscrasia of the peripheral blood, there were marked changes in the bone marrows of such infected birds. Over a period of ten days and correlated with the levels of parasitemia, there were several decided changes in the percentages of the various cell types. The percentage of heterophil granulocytes increased, but they were eventually reduced to extremely low numbers. The relative numbers of hemocytoblasts were unchanged, but there was a steady increase in the numbers of basophil erythroblasts. As seen in the peripheral circulation, there was a marked reduction of polychromatophil erythroblasts until in some ducklings, there was none visible in bone marrow preparations. Mature erythrocytes were not drastically reduced in number until the later stages of the infection, but at approximately ten days the number dropped markedly. The greatest change was in the number of macrophages. They increased from less than one per 100 cells to as high as 16 percent of the total cell population by the eighth day.

Active phagocytosis of all cell types, excepting the hemocytoblasts, was evident. By counting the percentage of various classes of cells within the macrophages and by comparing these with the differential count of the bone marrow, it was possible to determine selectivity in cases in which it existed relative to the type of cell engulfed.

Phagocytosis from days seven through ten was selective for heterophil granulocytes. At no time was there a selective phagocytosis for basophil erythroblasts, although many were detectable within the macrophage cytoplasm. The percentage of these cells in macrophages increased as the differential count in the bone marrow increased. A strong selectivity for mature erythrocytes was evident. Every count revealed a higher percentage in macrophages than in the bone marrow.

At no time was there any preferential engulfment of infected erythrocytes. A comparison of the number of parasitized erythrocytes within and without the macrophages was always fairly constant. Throughout this study, however, certain macrophages were noted that were filled with hemazoin alone. As is well known, malaria pigment resists digestion and its appearance in these macrophages may have represented an accumulative process. Very few of the macrophages contained more than four or five inclusions. Generally, these phagocytes were rather small and perhaps would fall into the polyblast category rather than that of a full-fledged macrophage. No intensive examinations of spleens were carried out; perhaps there the phagocytosis was selective for infected erythrocytes.

When chicks were infected with *Plasmodium lophurae* and the infection controlled with quinine hydrochloride, somewhat similar findings resulted (Sloan and McGhee, 1965). Anemias disproportionate to infections were apparent. There was, however, no real reduction in the percentage of polychromatophil erythroblasts in the circulating blood or in the bone marrow. Instead, there was an increased proportion of this type of cell, and examination of the bone marrow further revealed that phagocytosis was rather specifically directed toward the mature erythrocytes. Again, however, there was no selection for infected over noninfected erythrocytes. A somewhat similar observation with regard to the changes in cell types in the peripheral circulation of chicks was made by Zuckerman (1960b).

Anemia in malarious ducklings is far in excess of that which would be expected from the rupture of erythrocytes by the emerging parasites. One obvious reason for loss of many of the infected and noninfected erythrocytes is their engulfment by macrophages. This nonselective phagocytosis is not a new observation; it was recorded by Taliaferro and Cannon (1936) in monkey malaria, by Cox et al. (1966) for *Plasmodium berghei* in rats, and by Schroeder et al. (1965) for *Babesia rodhaini* in rats.

Active phagocytosis implies a presence of active macrophages. As stated above, the percentages of macrophages increase markedly in the bone marrow. If these cells arise from existing bone marrow cells, i.e., hemocytoblasts, this represents a depletion in cells, of which some would have been destined to become erythrocytes. Adherence to the monophyletic school of cell derivation would give rise to the assumption that macrophages would be produced from hemocytoblasts. Yet throughout, the numbers of cells of this type remained more or less constant. Increased cytokinesis as evidenced by mitotic figures was evident for the basophil erythroblasts, and it is possible that macrophages may in some instances be derived from these cells. The virtual disappearance of the polychromatophil erythroblast can be explained in part by selective phagocytosis. In addition, however, the diversion of earlier stem cells to macrophages may result in a block of erythropoiesis and affect further the production of polychromatophil erythroblasts and mature erythrocytes.

If the effects of parasiticidal antibody, erythropoiesis stasis, cell destruction by parasite emergence, and widespread engulfment of both infected and noninfected cells of the erythrocytic series are combined, then the phenomenon of anemia out of proportion to that expected by cell rupture may be explained.

It is difficult to explain the difference in the selectivity for phagocytosis of erythrocytes in the chicken as opposed to that in the duck. The above account does not elucidate the mechanism inherent in phagocytosis of uninfected erythrocytes. It could fit into any of the hypothetical models proposed to explain autoantibody reactions (Zuckerman, 1964). In addition to (1) the sharing of common antigens, (2) the coating of target cells with parasite antigen, and (3) the sensitization of target cells with antibody, it may also be postulated that (4) the phagocytosis of blood cells might be due to a nonspecific reaction. Such phagocytosis made possible by proliferation of macrophages by the original antigenic stimulus might continue even when the quantity of antigen is greatly reduced or lost.

Concerning (2) and (3) above, the possibility is always present that a virus may be accompanying the parasite and becomes fixed to the erythrocyte, which later might be subjected to an antibody reaction. Such a possibility exists in one series of *P. lophurae* infections and will be discussed in a subsequent section.

One of the hypotheses advanced for the autoantibody-like reaction in malaria bears on the presence of parasite antigens fixed on noninfected erythrocytes. Soluble antigens which increase in proportion to infection have been found in the serum of white Pekin ducklings infected with *P. lophurae* (Davis, 1948) and in malarious monkeys (Eaton, 1939). Corwin and McGhee (1966) subjected ducklings to a regimen of filtered malarious plasma and observed marked anemia and polychromatophil erythroblast reduction in the peripheral circulation. Injection of uninfected ducklings with whole uninfected blood, with immune plasma, or with saline solution produced no marked changes in the blood picture. Thus, it was possible to induce anemia and blood dyscrasia in the absence of the malaria parasite.

One of the objections to classifying the malaria syndrome as involving autoimmunity has been the inability of investigators to detect hemolysin or other antibody material in the blood by serologic means. The use of Coombs' test and the detection of erythrocyte-bound globulin in rats infected with *P. berghei* seemed to be a most promising lead until Zuckerman and Spira (1961) also found a similar reaction in rats made anemic either by bleeding or by administraton of phenylhydrazine. Cox et al. (1966) also demonstrated a hemagglutination and observed erythrophagocytosis associated with *Plasmodium berghei* infections in rats. However they also found hemagglutinin titers, albeit lower than in infected rats, in uninfected animals. Uninfected erythrocytes were primarily phagocytosed. Kreier et al. (1966) demonstrated an agglutinin for trypsinized autologous and homologous erythrocytes of rats undergoing *Plasmodium berghei* infections. The agglutinin was eluted from the erythrocyte and was identified as a globulin. These latter investigators did not, however, introduce anemic control animals; the findings are subject to the same restrictions as in the earlier works of Zuckerman and Cox et al. They suggested that these agglutinins are induced as a result of some parasite substance modifying the uninfected erythrocytes. Recently Kreier (personal communication, 1967) reported he and his colleagues have been able to detect globulin bound to erythrocytes of chickens infected with *Plasmodium gallinaceum*. In these studies, they were still able to demonstrate bound globulin after adsorption of the serum with reticulocytes. Publication and confirmation of these data will contribute measurably to our knowledge of the immune process in malaria.

The demonstration of antibody on uninfected erythrocytes in malarious birds raises the question of what model (*see* Zuckerman, 1964) best explains the reaction. Although it is quite possible that there may be a sharing of antigens between the parasite and the host cell, it would seem that most workers lean toward the view that there is some alteration of the host cell by the parasite antigen or by other products of the infectious agent. Kreier (1967) postulates the presence of proteolytic or parasite exoenzymes as the factors responsible for the erythrocyte change.

The above suggestion that an enzyme of the parasite is responsible for the induction of antigenicity in host erythrocytes suggests a plausible solution for the removal of uninfected cells and bears on an earlier hypothesis of the author (McGhee, 1952) that penetration of the erythrocyte by the merozoite is accomplished by physiochemical means. Sherman (1966) and Trager (1956) suggested the possibility of an enzyme of penetration.

Our thinking in the past has been clouded by Schaudinn's observation (1899) of the physical entry of the erythrocyte by force. From that time until now, no similar observation of cell entry has been observed. At one time Trager and McGhee (unpublished) examined microcultures of *Plasmodium lophurae* and were able to see the actual progress of segmentation of this avian malaria parasite. If one looked at mature parasites with several nuclei but no cytoplasmic cleavage, the following events took place: There was suddenly a convulsive rounding up of the host cell. During this short stage the parasite, because of the concentration of host cytoplasm, became invisible. The reaction was so violent and so sudden that quite often a bit of cytoplasm was left behind in the process and trailed as a tail. Shortly thereafter, the process reversed and the host erythrocyte resumed its usual shape. During this obscure phase, cytokinesis had taken place and one could now see the individual merozoites dancing in the cytoplasm. Again the host cell rounded up, but now did not return to its former shape. Rather, the merozoites exploded from the cell along with hemoglobin. In one instance (Trager, 1956), a merozoite entered an adjacent erythrocyte with extreme rapidity. This same type of entry has been seen by Dr. A. B. Weathersby (personal communication, 1966) who observed the entry of exoerythrocytic merozoites into erythrocytes in brain capillaries.

Our previous thinking had been to the effect that the liberation of the merozoites from the host cell has been accomplished by crowding of the host erythrocyte until it burst. Even cytochemists believe this; for example, Ponder (1948) said, "In these cases the destruction of the cells is almost certainly mechanical." The findings reported above do not necessarily disprove this, but if one examines the literature, certain interesting facts present themselves. The segmenting parasites of *Plasmodium gallinaceum* and *P. circumflexum* are large and exceed the size of the gametocytes. The segmenters of *Plasmodium nucelophilum*, *P. rouxi*, *P. elongatum*, and *P. vaughani*, on the other hand, are smaller than the gametocytes of the same species. Yet the gametocytes in the peripheral circulation do not destroy the erythrocyte whereas the small segmenting parasites do. The hypothesis of strict mechanical destruction is, therefore, invalid. It is much more logical to assume that the egress of the merozoites is accomplished by some elaboration on the part of the parasites, i.e., a substance that weakens the erythrocyte ultrastructure.

Schaudinn's observations in 1899 suggest the merozoite enters the erythrocyte by force. Those of Trager, Weathersby, and McGhee suggest an entry by means of an enzyme. The observations presented as to the comparative susceptibility of various erythrocytes to various species of parasites show that there is no "stronger" or "weaker" parasite or erythrocyte and indicate a selectivity of penetration (McGhee, 1957). This selectivity is even more pronounced when the parasite preferentially invades duck over chick erythrocytes.

We may, therefore, conclude that while there is some reason to accept the concept of mechanical exit and entry of erythrocytes by the parasite, the more logical concept would be that this is accomplished by means of an enzyme of release and penetration. Conceivably these may be the same substance. The red blood cell itself is constructed as follows: On the outside of the membrane and comprising a depth of 20 Å is the antisphering substance, a protein, crystalbumin. Directly under this are lipids and cross-sections of proteins. The entire membrane comprises approximately 130 Å. The proteins have been isolated from human erythrocytes and have been given the name elanin and stromatin. Elanin is thought by Calvin et al. (1946) to be the site of the Rh factor. The fatty components consist of cephalin, cholesterol, and lecithin. The parasite, therefore, must contain a substance that will act with one or more components to gain entry into the hemoglobin-rich interior of the erythrocyte. The presence of these organic materials may be further demonstrated by the fact that proteolytic enzymes lyse erythrocytes, whereas lipases alter the permeability of the membrane. If the liberation of merozoites is accomplished through the auspices of an enzyme, it stands to reason that some of this substance would be poured into the blood stream. In the event that it had fixed onto a cell surface later in contact with a merozoite, entry would be effected. In addition, however, other cells, not penetrated by the merozoite, would likewise be exposed to this enzyme. All this suggests the presence of an enzyme present in the blood stream of malarious birds; an enzyme which becomes fixed to erythrocytes. Such erythrocytes could conceivably become antigenic and be subject to antibody action and subsequent phagocytosis.

Under these circumstances the levels of antigen (i.e., enzyme) would profoundly modify the course of infection. If the parasitemia remains low, the quantity of enzyme per erythrocyte would of necessity be low, cell removal would be rather slow, and the production of anemia a matter of days. Such a condition is seen in ducklings undergoing controlled infections of *P. lophurae* (McGhee, 1964). On the other hand, if the numbers of parasites increase to large proportions, the liberation-penetration enzyme levels likewise would increase and fix to susceptible areas of uninfected and infected erythrocytes. The antigen-antibody reaction and the binding of complement under these circumstances are more severe and a conspicuous crisis is engendered. The end result of the latter case is either the death or the rapid recovery of the afflicted animal.

One should bear in mind that despite the apparently insidious nature of the autoimmune-like process, it does serve to dispose of the parasite eventually. The above reasoning could explain the work of Rigdon and Varnadoe (1945), repeated by Becker et al. (1949), which indicated that as long as ducks were transfused with red blood cells, there was no crisis, only continued parasitemia. Such transfusions would dilute the enzyme and prevent the wholesale destruction of cells by antibody and complement.

At the present time, therefore, we feel that there is an enzyme liberated by the segmenting parasite, an enzyme that fixes at random on all the cell types of the circulating blood stream. The fixation of this enzyme, in all probability onto a protein of the ultrastructure of the erythrocyte, performs as a hapten and stimulates the production of antibodies and the formation of macrophages. The continued fixing of antigen and continued removal of erythrocytes so exposed produces an anemia which is only relieved with the elimination of the majority of the parasites.

Work is now in progress to confirm or deny this hypothesis. If it proves to be true, the implications of these findings could be significant in a better understanding of the pathology of malaria infections.

Interactions between malaria and other parasites. As a general practice, the investigator conducting research on avian malaria is concerned more with attempting to insure a single infective agent rather than studying the relationships of combinations of parasites. Huff (1963) experimentally infected a canary with both *Plasmodium cathemerium* and *P. relictum.* Wolfson (1945) studied ducklings infected with *P. cathemerium* and *P. lophurae* and came to the conclusion that the parasites developed independently of each other; the effects on the host were not magnified or diminished by the dual infections. The author was able to infect ducklings with both *P. lophurae* and *P. relictum* (McGhee, 1964). The latter parasite (as is true of *P. cathemerium*) preferentially invades young red blood cells while *P. lophurae* attacks, as a rule, the mature erythrocyte. The combined infections acted more as if the infecting agent were *P. lophurae* alone in that there was no flooding of the peripheral blood stream with immature red blood cells. Taliaferro and Taliaferro (1945) infected chickens hyperimmunized with either *P. lophurae* or *P. gallinaceum* with the alternate parasite and were able to show some cross-reactions between the two parasites.

Rats with latent infections of *Hemobartonella muris* when injected with

P. berghei responded by displaying both parasites in the blood stream (Hsu and Geiman, 1952). Such rats had a longer incubation period for *P. berghei* than was noted in *Hemobartonella*-infected rats and eventually developed a higher peak of parasitemia. *Eperythrozoon coccoides* and *P. berghei* infections in white mice result in an antagonistic relationship (Peters, 1965).

A much more insidious relationship may exist between malaria and viruses, especially if the virus is cryptic or dependent on the parasite for survival. Fowl pox in canaries infected with *P. cathemerium* seriously affected the parasite even to the point of apparently being responsible for the loss of gametocytes in the particular laboratory strain. Ornithosis virus plus *P. lophurae* in the duckling causes a heightened susceptibility of the affected ducklings, but if the virus has run its course before the introduction of parasites, the disease is not so severe (Jacobs, 1957). Pigeons infected with *P. relictum* do not attain the titers of encephalitis virus obtained in unaffected birds (Barnett, 1956). In ducklings, splenic necrosis due to virus infection interferes with the development of *P. lophurae* (Trager, 1959). Treatment of chicks infected with Rous chicken sarcoma either by infection with *P. lophurae* or by injection of malarious plasma resulted in some interference in the development of the tumor (Trager and McGhee, 1953). Somewhat similar findings were reported by Nadel et al. (1954) in leukemic mice infected with *P. berghei.*

Concomitant infection of chicks with *Eimeria acervulina* and *E. mitis* decreased the immunity of chicks to infection with *P. juxtanucleare* (Al-Dabagh, 1961).

Any serious deviation of the malaria parasite from its usual type of infection should be carefully scrutinized for the presence of an accompanying virus. The profound anemia in ducklings with a low level of parasitemia induced by subcutaneous injection of duck embryo-adapted *P. lophurae* was one such example (McGhee, 1960). Despite various tests, no virus could be demonstrated. Later, Corwin and McGhee (1966) found that malarious plasma filtered through a Seitz filter with a pore size of 0.1 μ produced a blood and bone marrow dyscrasia (McGhee, 1967) similar to that seen in malarious birds. Again the presence of a virus was suspected, and now it appears that there is a filterable agent present in the malarious plasma used (McGhee and Loftis, 1968); an agent which is responsible, at least in part, for some of the symptoms seen in ducklings infected with this particular strain of *P. lophurae.* Continuous transfer of the agent has been achieved and moderate to severe anemias have resulted. In ducklings so treated and later challenged with malaria, the infection runs as severe a course, but there is a compensatory hyperplasia of polychromatophil erythroblasts not seen in unimmunized ducklings. Approximately 50 percent of the ducklings survive as compared to practically 100 percent mortality in nonimmunized ducklings.

Thus, the injection of ducklings with the filterable agent and subsequent immunization to its effects bring about the survival of many ducklings. An immunity to malaria is simulated, while in reality it merely relieves the host animal of an additional deleterious factor interfering with its survival. This simulation of immune and autoimmune effects may be more common than is realized and should be considered in all work with autoimmune processes and specific parasitic protista.

REFERENCES

Abrami, P. and G. Senevet. 1919. Pathogenie de l'acces palustre. La crise hemoclassique initiale. Bull. Soc. Med. Hop. Paris, 43: 530-537.

Al-Dabagh, M. A. 1961. Synergism between coccidia parasites (*Eimeria mitis* and *E. acervulina*) and malarial parasites (*Plasmodium gallinaceum* and *P. justanucleare*) in the chick. Parasitology, 51: 257-265.

Allen, A. A. 1914. The red-winged blackbird; A study in the ecology of a cat-tail marsh. Abst. Proc. Linn. Soc. N. Y., 24-25: 43-128.

Allison, A. C. 1963. An inherited factor in blood conferring resistance to protozoa. *In* Immunity to Protozoa. Garnham, P. C. C., Pierce, A. E., and Roitt, I., eds. Oxford, Blackwell Scientific Publications.

Audy, R. R. 1958. The localization of disease with special reference to the zoonoses. Trans. Roy. Soc. Trop. Med. Hyg., 52: 308-334.

Ball, G. C., and G. Pringle. 1965. *Plasmodium fischeri* n. sp. from *Chamaeleo fischeri*. J. Protozool., 12: 479-482.

Barnett, H. 1956. Experimental studies of concurrent infection of canaries and of the mosquito *Culex tarsalis* with *Plasmodium relictum* and western equine encephalitis virus. Amer. Soc. Trop. Med. Hyg., 5: 99-109.

Bass, C. C., and F. M. Johns. 1912. The cultivation of malarial plasmodia (*Plasmodium vivax* and *Plasmodium falciparum*) *in vitro*. J. Exp. Med., 16: 567-579.

———— 1913. Cultivation of malaria plasmodia, *Plasmodium falciparum*, in the blood of a diabetic without the addition of dextrose. Amer. J. Trop. Dis., 1: 240-249.

Becker, E. R., A. A. Marousek, and C. E. Brodine. 1949. Observations on *Plasmodium lophurae* infections in Pekin ducks transfused with duck and chick erythrocytes. National Malaria Society, 8: 290-297.

Beckman, H. 1945. Infectivity of sporozoites of *Plasmodium cathemerium* $^3H_2$ exposed *in vitro* to hen and canary bloods. Proc. Soc. Exp. Biol. Med., 67: 172-176.

Bennison, B. E., and G. R. Coatney. 1948. The sex of the host as a factor in *Plasmodium gallinaceum* infections. Science, 107: 147-148.

Boyd, G. H. 1939. A study of the rate of reproduction in the avian malaria parasite, *Plasmodium cathemerium*. Amer. J. Hyg., 29: 119-129.

Brown, W. H. 1913. Malaria pigment (hematin) as an active factor in the production of the blood picture of malaria. J. Exp. Med., 13: 290-298.

Brumpt, E. D. 1935. *Plasmodium gallinaceum* n. sp. de la poule domestique. C. R. Acad. Sci., (Paris) 200: 783-785.

Calvin, M., R. S. Evans, V. Behrendt, and C. Calvin. 1946. Rh Antigen and Hapten. Nature of antigen and its isolation from erythrocyte stroma. Proc. Soc. Exp. Biol. Med., 61: 416-419.

Coffin, G. S. 1941. Active immunization of birds against malaria. J. Infect. Dis., 89: 1-7.

Coggeshall, L. T., 1938. *Plasmodium lophurae* a new species of malaria pathogenic for domestic fowl. Amer. J. Hyg., 27: 615-618.

———— and H. W. Kumm. 1937. Demonstration of passive immunity in experimental monkey malaria. J. Exp. Med., 66: 177-184.

Cohen, S., and D. A. McGregor. 1963. Gamma globulin and acquired immunity to malaria. *In* Immunity to Protozoa. Garnham, P. C. C., Pierce, A. E., and Roitt, I., eds. Oxford, Blackwell Scientific Publications, pp. 123-159.

Corradetti, A. 1963. Acquired sterile immunity in experimental protozoal infections. *In* Immunity to Protozoa. Garnham, P. C. C., Pierce, A. E., and Roitt, I., eds. Oxford, Blackwell Scientific Publications, pp. 69-77.

Corwin, R. N., and R. B. McGhee. 1966. Anemia in ducklings treated with malarious plasma. Exp. Parasit., 18: 281-289.

Coulston, F., W. Cantrell, and C. G. Huff. 1945. The distribution and localization of sporozoites and pre-erythrocytic stages in infections with *Plasmodium gallinaceum*. J. Infect. Dis., 76: 226-238.

Cox, H. W., W. F. Schroeder, and M. Ristic. 1966. Hemagglutination and erythro-phagocytosis associated with the anemia of *Plasmodium berghei* infections in rats. J. Protozool., 14: 327-333.

Davis, B. D. 1948. Complement fixation with soluble antigens of *Plasmodium knowlesi* and *Plasmodium lophurae*. J. Immun., 58: 269-281.

Dogiel, V. A. 1964. General Parasitology. London, Oliver and Boyd.

Eaton, M. D. 1939. The soluble malarial antigen in the serum of monkeys infected with *Plasmodium knowlesi*. J. Exp. Med., 69: 517-532.

Erlich, P. 1908. The Harden Lectures, 1907. London.

Eyles, D. E. 1963. The species of simian malaria: Taxonomy, morphology, life cycle, and geographical distribution of the monkey species. J. Parasit., 49: 866-887.

Fantham, H. B., A. Porter, and L. R. Richardson. 1942. Some haematozoa observed in vertebrates in eastern Canada. Parasitology, 34: 199-226.

Gajewski, J. E. and A. L. Tatum. 1944. A study of mechanisms of relapse in avian malaria. J. Infect. Dis., 74: 85-92.

Garnham, P. C. C. 1963. An introduction to protozoal immunity. In Immunity to Proto-zoa. Garnham, P. C. C., Pierce, A. E., and Roitt, I., eds. Oxford, Blackwell Scientific Publications, pp. 3-21.

———— 1966. Malaria Parasites and Other Haemosporidia. Oxford, Blackwell Scientific Publications, pp. 742-743.

Geigy, R. and T. Freyvogel. 1953. On the influence of high altitudes on the course of infection of chicken malaria (*P. gallinaceum*). Acta Tropica, 11: 167-171.

Gingrich, W. 1932. Immunity to superinfection and cross immunity in malaria infections in birds. J. Prevent. Med., 6: 197-246.

———— 1934. The effect of an increased burden of phagocytosis upon natural and acquired immunity to bird malaria. J. Parasit. 20: 332-333.

Goble, F., and I. Singer. 1960. The reticuloendothelial system in experimental malaria and trypanosomiasis. Ann. N.Y. Acad. Sci., 88: 149-171.

Godwin, D. G. 1965. Personal communication.

Grassi, B. and R. Feletti. 1891. Malaria-Parasiten in den Vögelin. Zbl. Bakt., 9: 402-409, 429-433, 461-467.

Haas, V. H., A. Wilcox, and N. Coleman. 1949. Modification of *Plasmodium gallinaceum* infections by certain tissue extracts. J. Nat. Malar. Soc., 8: 85-99.

Hartman, E. 1927. Three new species of bird malaria, *Plasmodium praecox*, *P. catheme-rium* and *P. inconstans*. n. sp. Arch. Protistenk., 60:1-7.

Hegner, R., and M. MacDougall. 1926. Modifying the course of infections with bird malaria by changing the sugar content of blood. Amer. J. Hyg., 6: 602-609.

Herbig-Sandreuter, A. 1953. Untersuchungen über den Einfluss der Hohenklimas auf Hühnenmalaria (*Plasmodium gallinaceum*, Brumpt). Acta Tropica, 10: 1-27.

Herman, C. W. 1938. Epidemiology of malaria in Eastern Redwings (*Agelaius phoeni-ceus*). Amer. J. Hyg., 28: 232-243.

———— 1942. A fatal case of spontaneous malaria in a canary. J. Amer. Vet. Med. Ass., 101: 789.

Hewitt, R. 1940. Bird Malaria. Baltimore, The Johns Hopkins Press.

———— 1942. Studies on the host-parasite relationships of untreated infections with *Plasmodium lophurae* in ducks. Amer. J. Hyg., 36:6-42.

Hsu, D. Y. M., and Q. M. Geiman. 1952. Synergistic effect of *Haemobartonella muris* on *Plasmodium berghei* in white rats. Amer. J. Trop. Med. Hyg., 1: 747-760.

Huff, C. G. 1954. Changes in host-cell preferences in malarial parasites and their relation to splenic reticular cells. J. Infect. Dis., 94: 173-177.

———— 1957. Organ and tissue distribution of the exoerythrocytic stages of avian malaria parasites. Exp. Parasit., 6: 143-162.

———— 1959. Further studies on host cell preferences by exoerythrocytic stages of avian malaria. Exp. Parasit., 8: 163-170.

———— 1963. Experimental research on avian malaria. In Advances in Parasitology, Vol. 1. Dawes, B., ed. New York, Academic Press, Inc., pp. 1-65.

———— and F. Coulston. 1944. The development of *Plasmodium gallinaceum* from sporo-zoite to erythrocytic trophozoite. J. Infect. Dis., 77: 224-248.

———— and F. Coulston. 1946. The relation of natural and acquired immunity of various avian hosts to the cryptozoites and metacryptozoites of *Plasmodium gallinaceum* and *Plasmodium relictum*. J. Infect. Dis., 78: 99-117.

———— F. Coulston, R. L. Laird, and R. C. Porter. 1947. Pre-erythrocytic development of *Plasmodium lophurae* in various hosts. J. Infect. Dis., 81: 7-13.

———— D. F. Marchbank, and T. Shiroishi, 1959. Susceptibility and resistance of avian and mosquito hosts to strains of *Plasmodium relictum* isolated from pigeons. J. Protozool., 6: 46-51.

Hughs, F. W., and A. L. Tatum. 1955. The effects of hypoxia on infections with *Plasmodium cathemerium*. J. Infect. Dis., 77: 158-176.

Ingram, R. L., L. B. Otken, and J. R. Jumper. 1961. Staining of malaria parasites by the fluorescent antibody technic. Proc. Soc. Exp. Biol. Med., 106: 52-54.

Jacobs, H. R. 1948. Increased resistance of ducklings to *Plasmodium lophurae* following injections of clotted blood. Quart. Bull. Northwestern Univ. Med. School, 22: 253.

———— 1957. Effect of ornithosis on experimental fowl malaria. Proc. Soc. Exp. Biol. Med., 95: 372-373.

Jordon, H. B. 1957. Host resistance and regulation of the development of *Plasmodium lophurae* in pheasants, coots and domestic pigeons. J. Parasit., 43: 395-408.

———— 1964. Lizard malaria in Georgia. J. Protozool., 11: 562-566.

Kikuth, W. 1931. Über verschiedene Stämme von Vogelmalaria. Zbl. Bakt., 122: 213-214.

Krichewski, I. L., and J. S. Meerson. 1932. Über die Bedeutung des retikuloendothelialen Apparates bei Infektionkrankheiten, Die Rolle des Retikuloendothelial systems bei Vogelmalaria. Z. Ges. Immunitätsforsch. Exp. Ther., 76: 499-506.

Kreier, J. 1967. Personal communication.

———— O. Shapiro, D. Dillay, I. P. Szilvassy, and M. Ristic. 1966. Autoimmune reactions in rats with *Plasmodium berghei* infection. Exp. Parasit., 19: 155-162.

Landau, I. 1965. Description de *Plasmodium chabaudi* n. sp. parasite de rongeurs africains. C. R. Acad. Sci. [D] (Paris), 260: 3758-3761.

MacDougall, M. 1927. The effect of changes in the sugar content of the blood on bird malaria. Amer. J. Hyg., 7: 625-647.

Manresa, M. 1953. The occurrence of phanerozoites of *Plasmodium lophurae* in inoculated turkeys. J. Parasit., 39: 452-455.

Manwell, R. 1938. The identification of the avian malarias. Amer. J. Trop. Med., 18: 565-575.

———— and F. Goldstein. 1938. Life history and immunity studies of the avian malaria parasite, *Plasmodium circumflexum*. Proc. Soc. Exp. Biol. Med., 39: 426-428.

Marshall, E. K. 1946. Chemotherapy of malaria 1941-1945. Fed. Proc., 5: 298-304.

McGregor, I. A., and H. M. Gilles. 1960. Studies on the significance of high serum gamma globulin concentration in Gambian Africans. Gamma globulin concentrations of Gambian children in the fourth, fifth and sixth year of life. Ann. Trop. Med. Parasit., 54: 275-282.

McGhee, R. B. 1949. Pre-erythrocytic development of *Plasmodium gallinaceum* in duck embryos. J. Infect. Dis., 84: 105-110.

———— 1950. The ability of the avian malaria parasite, *Plasmodium lophurae*, to infect erythrocytes of distantly related species of animals. Amer. J. Hyg., 52: 42-47.

———— 1951. The adaptation of the avian malaria parasite, *Plasmodium lophurae*, to a continuous existence in infant mice. J. Infect. Dis., 88:86-97.

———— 1952. The effect of a malaria infection on the titer of complement and its components in ducks. J. Immun., 68: 421-428.

———— 1953a. The infection by *Plasmodium lophurae* of duck erythrocytes in the chicken embryo. J. Exp. Med., 97: 773-782.

———— 1953b. Factors affecting the susceptibility of erythrocytes to an intracellular parasite. Ann. N. Y. Acad. Sci., 56: 1070-1073.

———— 1953c. The influence of age of the animal upon the susceptibility of mammalian erythrocytes to infection of the avian malaria parasite, *Plasmodium lophurae*. J. Infect. Dis., 93: 4-9.

———— 1954. The infection of duck and goose erythrocytes by the mammalian malaria parasite, *Plasmodium berghei*. J. Protozool., 1: 145-148.

———— 1956. A study of changes occuring in *Plasmodium lophurae* after three years of continuous existence in mice. J. Protozool., 3: 122-126.

———— 1957. Comparative susceptibility of various erythrocytes to four species of avian plasmodia. J. Infect. Dis., 100: 92-96.

———— 1959. Modification of the course of infection of *Plasmodium lophurae* by the injection of components of the erythrocyte. J. Parasit., 45 (Suppl.): 48.

———— 1960. An autoimmune reaction produced in ducklings in response to injections of duck embryo blood infected with *Plasmodium lophurae*. J. Infect. Dis., 107: 410-418.

———— 1964. Autoimmunity in malaria. Amer. Jour. Trop. Med. Hyg., 13: 219-224.

———— 1967. Erythrophagocytosis in ducklings injected with malarious plasma. *In* Progress in Protozoology. International Congress Series No. 91. Amsterdam, Excerpta Medica Foundation, p. 71.

———— and W. E. Loftis. 1968. A filterable, proliferating factor simulating autoimmunity in malarious and nonmalarious ducklings. Exp. Parasit., 22: 299-308.

Moldovan, I. 1912. Über die Immunitätsverhältnisse der Vogelmalaria. Zbl. Bakt., 61: Infect. Dis., 79: 272-277.

Moldovan, I. 1912. Über die Immunitätsverhältnisse der Vogelmalaria. Zbl. Bakt., 61: 105-111.

Nadel, E. M., J. Greenberg, and G. R. Coatney. 1954. The effect of malaria (*Plasmodium berghei*) on leukemia L$_{1210}$ in mice. J. Infect. Dis., 95: 109-113.

Ott, K. J., and L. A. Stauber. 1967. *Eperythrozoon coccoides*: Influence on course of infection of *Plasmodium chabaudi* in mouse. Science, 155 (3769): 1546.

Pavlovsky, E. N. 1966. Natural Nidality of Transmissable Diseases. Urbana, University of Illinois Press.

Peters, W. 1965. Competitive relationship between *Eperythrozoon coccoides* and *Plasmodium berghei* in the mouse. Exp. Parasit., 16: 158-166.

Ponder, E. 1948. Hemolysis and Related Phenomena. New York, Grune and Stratton.

Porter, R. J. 1942. The tissue distribution of exoerythrocytic schizonts in spororoite induced infections with *Plasmodium cathemerium*. J. Infect. Dis., 71: 1-17.

Raffaele, G. 1955. Alcune osservazione sulla vitalita degli sporozoiti. Riv. Malar., 34: 215-226.

Rappaport, S., and I. Guest. 1941. Distribution of acid-soluble phosphorus in the blood cells of various vertebrates. J. Biol. Chem., 138: 269-282.

Rigdon, R. H. 1947. Effect of vitamin A deficiency in *Plasmodium lophurae* in ducks. J. Infect. Dis., 79: 272-277.

———— and N. H. Marvin. 1953. The effect of insulin on *Plasmodium lophurae* infections in ducks. Amer. J. Hyg., 45: 185-190.

———— and H. Rudisell. 1945. Effect of radiation on malaria. An experimental study in the chick and duck. Proc. Soc. Exp. Biol. Med., 59: 167-170.

———— and N. B. Varnadoe. 1945. Transfusions of red cells in malaria. An experimental study in ducks. Amer. J. Trop. Med., 25: 409-415.

Rodhain, S. 1952. *Plasmodium vinckei* n. sp. Un deuxième *Plasmodium* parasite, de rongeurs sauvages au Katanga. Ann. Soc. Belg. Med. Trop., 32: 275-278.

Schaudinn, F. 1899. Über den Generationswechsel der Coccidien und neuere Malariaforschung. Sitzangsber. Ges. Naturf. Freunde., 7: 159.

Schmittner, S. M., and R. B. McGhee. 1961. The intraerythrocytic development of *Babesiosoma stableri* n. sp. in *Rana pipiens pipiens*. J. Protozool., 8: 381-386.

Schroeder, W. F., H. W. Cox, and M. Ristic. 1966. Anaemia, parasitemia, erythrophagocytosis, and haemagglutinins in *Babesia rodhaini* infection. Ann. Trop. Med. Parasit., 60: 31-38.

Schwetz, J. 1930. Sur un plasmodium avaire à formes de division allongées *Plasmodium fallax*, n. sp. Arch. Inst. Pasteur d'Algerie, 8: 289-296.

Seeler, A. O., W. H. Ott, and M. E. Gundel. 1944. Effect of biotin deficiency on the course of *Plasmodium lophurae* infection in chicks. Proc. Soc. Exp. Bio. Med., 55: 107-109.

Sergent, E. 1963. Latent infection and premunition. Some definitions of microbiology and immunology. *In* Immunity to Protozoa. Garnham, P. C. C., Pierce, A. E., and Roitt, I., eds. Oxford, Blackwell Scientific Publications, pp. 39-47.

———— and A. Catanei. 1937. Le serum d'oiseau paludien (à *Plasmodium relictum*) n'est ni infectant ni prémunissant. Arch. Inst. Pasteur d'Algerie, 15: 18-19.

Sherman, I. 1964. Antigens of *Plasmodium lophurae*. J. Protozool., 11: 409-417.

———— 1966. In vitro studies of factors affecting penetration of duck erythrocytes by avian malaria (*Plasmodium lophurae*). J. Parasit., 52: 17-22.

Singer, I. 1954. The cellular reactions to infections with *Plasmodium berghei* in the white mouse. J. Infect. Dis., 94: 241-261.

Sloan, B. H., and R. B. McGhee. 1965. Autoimmunity in chickens infected with *Plasmodium lophurae*. J. Parasit. 50 (Suppl.): 36.

Spira, D., and A. Zuckerman. 1964. Recent advances in the antigenic analysis of plasmodia. Milit. Med., 131: 1117-1123.

Stauber, L. A., H. Walker, and A. P. Richardson. 1951. The *in vitro* agglutination of erythrocyte-free avian plasmodia. J. Infect. Dis., 89: 31-34.

Taliaferro, W. H. 1956. Functions of the spleen in immunity. J. Trop. Med. Hyg., 5: 391-410.

——— 1963. Cellular and humoral factors in immunity to protozoa. *In* Immunity to Protozoa. Garnham, P. C. C., Pierce, A. E., and Roitt, I., eds. Oxford, Blackwell Scientific Publications, pp. 22-38.

——— and P. R. Cannon. 1936. The cellular reaction during primary infections and super-infections of *Plasmodium brasilianum* in Panamanian monkeys. J. Infect. Dis., 59: 72-125.

——— and W. Bloom. 1945. Inflammatory reactions in the skin of normal and immune canaries after the local injection of malarial blood. J. Infect. Dis., 77: 109-138.

——— and L. G. Taliaferro. 1948. Reduction in immunity in chicken malarias following *naceum* and *Plasmodium lophurae*. J. Infect. Dis., 77: 224-248.

——— and L. G. Taliaferro. 1945. Immunological relationships of *Plasmodium galli-* treatment with nitrogen mustard. J. Infect. Dis., 82: 5-30.

——— and L. G. Taliaferro. 1955. Reactions of the connective tissue in chickens to *Plasmodium gallinaceum* and *Plasmodium lophurae*. I. Histopathology during initial infections and superinfections. J. Infect. Dis., 97: 99-146.

Terzian, L. 1941. Studies on *Plasmodium lophurae*. A malarial parasite in fowls. I. Biological characteristics. II. Pathology and effects of experimental conditions. Amer. J. Hyg., 33: 1-22.

Thompson, P. E., and C. G. Huff. 1944. A saurian malaria parasite, *Plasmodium mexicanum*, with both elongatum and gallinaceum types. J. Infect. Dis., 74: 48-67.

——— D. A. McGinty, D. L. Bush, and M. L. Wilson. 1948. Radioiron in ducks and canaries and its effect on their initial malaria infection. J. Infect. Dis., 83: 23-32.

Tolbert, M. G., and R. B. McGhee. 1960. The effect of alloxan diabetes on *Plasmodium berghei* infections in albino rats. J. Parasit., 46: 552-558.

Trager, W. 1941. The effect of intraperitoneal injections of carbon ink in the course of *Plasmodium lophurae* infection in chickens. Amer. J. Hyg., 34: 141: 149.

——— 1943a. The influence of biotin upon susceptibility to malaria. J. Exp. Med., 77: 557-582.

——— 1943b. Further studies on the survival and development *in vitro* of a malarial parasite. J. Exp. Med., 77: 411-420.

——— 1947. The relation to the course of avian malaria of biotin and a fat-soluble material having the biological activities of biotin. J. Exp. Med., 85: 663-683.

——— 1948. The resistance of egg-laying ducks to infection by the malaria parasite, *Plasmodium lophurae*. J. Parasit., 28: 457-465.

——— 1950. Studies on the extracellular cultivation of an intracellular parasite (avian malaria). I. Development of the organisms in erythrocyte extracts, and the favoring effect of adenosinetriphosphate. J. Exp. Med., 92: 349-353.

——— 1952. Studies on the extracellular cultivation of an intracellular parasite (avian malaria). II. The effects of malate and of coenzyme A concentrates. J. Exp. Med., 96: 439-450.

——— 1956. The intracellular position of malaria parasites. Trans. Roy. Soc. Trop. Med. Hyg., 50: 419-420.

——— 1959. A new virus of ducks interfering with development of malaria parasite, *Plasmodium lophurae*. Proc. Soc. Exp. Biol. Med., 101: 578-582.

——— and R. B. McGhee. 1950. Factors in plasma concerned in natural resistance to an avian malaria parasite (*Plasmodium lophurae*). J. Exp. Med., 91: 365-379.

——— and R. B. McGhee. 1953. Inhibition of chicken tumor I by plasma from chickens infected with an avian malaria parasite. Proc. Soc. Exp. Biol. Med., 83: 349-352.

——— L. A. Stauber, and S. Ben-Harel. 1950. Innate and acquired agglutinins in ducks to the malaria parasite, *Plasmodium lophurae*. Proc. Soc. Exp. Biol. Med., 75: 766-771.

Vincke, I. H., and M. Lips. 1948. Un nouveau plasmodium d'un rongeur sauvage du Congo, *Plasmodium berghei* n. sp. Ann. Soc. Belg. Med. Trop., 28: 97-102.

Weathersby, A. B. 1966. Personal communication.

Weinman, D., D. C. Cavanaugh, and R. S. Desowitz. 1966. *Plasmodium falciparum* in *Mus musculus*. Trans. Roy. Soc. Trop. Med. Hyg., 60: 562.

Wolfson, F. 1940. Successful cultivation of avian plasmodia in duck embryos. Amer. J. Hyg., 32: 60-61.

——— 1945. An experimental study of mixed infections with *Plasmodium cathemerium* and *Plasmodium lophurae* in ducks. Amer. J. Hyg., 41: 123-135.

Yoeli, M. 1965. Studies on *Plasmodium berghei* in nature and under experimental conditions. Trans. Roy. Soc. Trop. Med. Hyg., 59: 255-276.

Zuckerman, A. 1945. *In vitro* opsonic tests with *Plasmodium gallinaceum* and *P. lophurae*. J. Infect. Dis., 77: 28-59.

———— 1946. Infections with *Plasmodium gallinaceum* in chick embryos induced by exoerythrocytic and blood stages. J. Infect. Dis., 79: 1-11.

———— 1960a. Auto-antibody in rats infected with *Plasmodium berghei*. Nature (London), 185: 189-190.

———— 1960b. Blood loss and replacement in plasmodial infections. IV. *Plasmodium gallinaceum* and *Plasmodium lophurae* in untreated and pre-bled mature chickens and in untreated chicks. J. Infect. Dis., 107: 133-148.

———— 1964. Autoimmunization and other types of indirect damage to host cells as factors in certain protozoan diseases. Exp. Parasit., 15: 138-183.

———— and D. Spira. 1961. Blood loss and replacement in plasmodial infections. V. Positive antiglobulin tests in rat anemias due to the rodent malarias *Plasmodium berghei* and *Plasmodium vinckei*, to cardiac bleedings, and to treatment with phenylhydrazine hydrochloride. J. Infect. Dis., 108: 339-348.

Coccidiosis and Histomoniasis in Avian Hosts

ASHTON C. CUCKLER

Merck Institute for Therapeutic Research, Rahway, New Jersey

INTRODUCTION

Coccidiosis and histomoniasis are important diseases of poultry, and if they are not controlled by chemotherapeutic or immunologic means, great economic losses may occur. In addition to the practical importance of these diseases, the development of immunity to coccidiosis has theoretical interest as a model for the study and demonstration of immune mechanisms involving protozoan parasites. Much of the early work on coccidiosis immunity was confused because the many species of coccidia in chickens and turkeys were not then recognized. However, a solid basis for further studies was provided by the classical studies of Smith (1910), who apparently was the first to recognize a host-reaction to intestinal coccidia, and of Johnson (1927), who recognized that resistance to coccidiosis in older birds was due to previous infection. Then too, Tyzzer (1929) realized for the first time that there were several species of coccidia in chickens and that the resistance developed after infection was rigidly species-specific. Although only a single species of protozoan has been recognized as causing histomoniasis until recently, the demonstration of immunity development following recovery from this parasitic infection has been difficult to obtain. Classical investigations of this disease have been carried out by Smith (1895) and by Tyzzer (1919), who recognized the parasite as a protozoan and described it and the pathology it causes in turkeys and other gallinaceous birds.

The purpose of this report is to review the literature since the publication of the classical studies cited above and to summarize information on the host-parasite relationships and on the development of immunity following infection with these parasites.

HOST-PARASITE RELATIONSHIPS IN COCCIDIOSIS

Description of life cycle

The typical life cycle of a coccidium of the genus *Eimeria* involves sexual and asexual reproduction in the host and the subsequent development of the oocyst outside the host. The details of the life cycle of *Eimeria tenella* (Railliet and Lucet, 1891) Fantham, 1909, which causes cecal coccidiosis in chickens, were first described in the classic paper by Tyzzer (1929). When freshly passed in the feces of the infected chicken, the oocysts of *Eimeria* contain a single cell (the sporont) and are not infective for another host. Outside of the body the oocysts undergo a "ripening" or sporulation process (sporogony). This requires suitable conditions of temperature, moisture, and oxygen, and the sporont, which is diploid, undergoes reduction division by formation of a polar body. The sporont, which now contains two chromosomes (Walton, 1959), divides into four sporoblasts, each of which develops into a sporocyst. When sporulation is completed, each sporocyst contains two sporozoites for a total of eight in each oocyst. Sporulation is completed in one to two days and the oocyst becomes infective for another individual of the host species.

When the sporulated oocysts are swallowed by a susceptible chicken, the oocysts pass through the crop and into the gizzard. Here the oocyst wall breaks open releasing the sporocysts, which then pass on to the small intestine where the sporozoites are activated and emerge from the sporocyst. Pancreatic juice causes the excystation of *E. tenella*, and Ikeda (1955) reported that trypsin was the responsible enzyme. This has been confirmed by Farr and Doran (1962), who used trypsin and bile salts for releasing sporozoites from mechanically liberated sporocysts.

The sporozoites, which are motile, pass through the striated border and epithelial cells of the host cecum and, according to Patillo (1959), move along the basement membrane to the lamina propria. Macrophages then engulf the sporozoites and carry them to the glands of Lieberkühn. Here sporozoites leave the macrophages and enter the glandular epithelium, where they develop below the host cell nucleus. After the penetration of a suitable epithelial cell, the parasite grows and becomes a trophozoite. The nucleus of the trophozoite divides by asexual multiple fission (schizogony), and each first generation schizont, according to Tyzzer (1929), forms about 900 first generation merozoites, each 2 to 4 μ long. In two to three days, these break out of the epithelial cell and each merozoite enters a new host cell.

The parasite grows, rounds up, and becomes the second generation schizont, which by simultaneous segmentation of the nucleus produces some 200 or 300 second generation merozoites, each about 16 μ long when they break out of the infected cell. A small number of these second generation merozoites enter new cells and develop into small third generation schizonts, which produce only a few (4 to 30) moderate-sized (7 μ long) third generation merozoites. The majority of the second generation merozoites enter new host cells and initiate the sexual phase (gametogony) of the life cycle. Some become microgametocytes which produce large numbers of microgametes; others become macrogametocytes. The microgametocytes break out and fertilize the numerous macrogametes formed from each of the macrogametocytes. The fertilized macrogamete (zygote) forms a double-layered wall and is transformed into an oocyst. The oocysts break out of the cecal wall, and the first ones pass out in the feces in six to seven days. The passage of oocysts continues for several days, and in the absence of reinfection, the host spontaneously becomes free of parasites, since the asexual cycle does not continue indefinitely, as occurs with *Plasmodia* infections.

Potential oocyst production of different species

The potential oocyst production of various species of coccidia is of importance since it influences the development of immunity in a flock, as well as the epidemiology of the disease and the possible economic losses. As might be expected, the reproductive potential of coccidia varies greatly from species to species. This is due primarily to the number of generations of schizonts formed and also to the number of merozoites produced in each generation. Other factors which influence the production of oocysts are the number of oocysts inoculated, the size of the host, the number of susceptible cells available, the effectiveness of the host's defense mechanisms, the localization and penetration of the parasites in the epithelium, the virulence and pathogenicity of the various stages of the life cycle, and the consequent hemorrhaging and sloughing of intestinal tissues. All of these factors are of importance and influence the reproductive capacity of the various species of coccidia in poultry.

In general, the greatest yields of oocysts are obtained with smaller rather than heavier inoculations of oocysts. Studies by Brackett and Bliznick (1952) showed that a bird infected with *E. acervulina* Tyzzer, 1929 produced about 40 times more oocysts than did a bird of similar age infected with *E. necatrix* Johnson, 1930. A chicken infected with *E. tenella* produced some 60 million oocysts, about one-seventh the number produced by *E. acervulina*. *E. brunetti* Levine, 1942 and *E. maxima* Tyzzer, 1929 are less prolific producers of oocysts when heavy inoculations are given. However, under ideal conditions in which light inoculations are given, the maximum number of oocysts produced per oocyst inoculated is highest with *E. brunetti* and *E. tenella*, and lowest with *E. maxima*. Brackett and Bliznick (1950, 1952) showed that with graded infections of coccidia in two- to three-week-old chickens, there was a linear relationship between the number of oocysts produced and the number inoculated into the chickens. The smallest inoculations provided the highest yield of oocysts for each oocyst inoculated, demonstrating a "crowding effect." Comparable results were reported by Rose and Long (1962). After inoculations of 500 oocysts each of *E. tenella*, *E. maxima*, and *E. necatrix*, the "reproductive index" (number of oocysts produced per oocyst fed) was 64,000, 30,000, and 12,000, respectively. Although a single oocyst of *E. tenella* is theoretically capable of producing about 2.5 million second generation merozoites, each of which can develop into a macrogametocyte or microgametocyte, it is obvious that the actual number produced is considerably below the theoretical yield.

Development of protective immunity

Numerous investigators have reported that chickens which had recovered from coccidiosis were resistant to reinfection. Beach and Corl (1925) were apparently the first to show that chickens which survived an acute infection with a large dose of sporulated oocysts were resistant to subsequent infection with "similar" coccidia. Johnson (1927) demonstrated that a high degree of resistance to infection with cecal coccidia was produced in chickens within 15 days after previous inoculation and that the resistance lasted for at least six and one-half months. He also stated that "no reciprocal relationship between small intestine and cecal infection was indicated." This observation was further elaborated by Johnson (1928), who stated that "one species does not produce immunity to another, insofar as the cecal and the two relatively harmless small intestine coccidia are concerned." Tyzzer (1929) showed that acquired resistance in chickens was highly selective and specific for the species of coccidia against which the birds were immunized and that the degree of resistance varied with the size of infective dose of oocysts.

Tyzzer et al. (1932) found that repeated doses of small numbers of *E. necatrix* oocysts protected birds against doses of oocysts which were invariably fatal for control chickens. They also demonstrated there was no cross-immunity between *E. tenella* and *E. necatrix*. The specificity of immunity development was used by Levine (1938, 1942) to isolate, differentiate, and establish two previously unrecognized coccidial species, *E. hagani* Levine, 1938 and *E. brunetti* Levine, 1942, in the chicken. More recently, Edgar and Seibold (1964) have also used this method to recognize *E. mivati* Edgar and Seibold, 1964, the ninth species of *Eimeria* described from chickens. Similarly, Moore and Brown (1951, 1952) and Moore et al. (1954) were able to isolate and identify three species of coccidia (*E. adenoeides*, Moore and Brown, 1951; *E. innocua*, Moore and Brown, 1952; and *E. subrotunda*, Moore et al., 1954), which had not been previously recognized in the turkey.

Since numerous reports had shown that poultry may acquire protective resistance to coccidiosis by oral inoculation of known numbers of sporulated oocysts, the possibility of using this method for controlling coccidiosis mortality was examined by several investigators. Jankiewicz and Scofield (1934) found that chickens became highly resistant or "totally immune" to further infection with *E. tenella* following three doses of oocysts at intervals of five days. Dickinson (1941) stated that the protection produced from inoculations with approximately 5,000 sporulated *E. acervulina* oocysts daily for 10 days was "as solid as the protection from daily dosages many times that amount." Farr (1943) reported that a high degree of resistance to cecal coccidiosis was developed in chickens given 1,000 *E. tenella* oocysts daily for 15 consecutive days. A similar degree of protection was provided by giving the same total number of oocysts in doses of 1,000, 5,000, and 9,000 at intervals of five days. Birds which were resistant to reinfection with *E. tenella* maintained their resistance for at least six months. A single "heavy" inoculation did not protect birds against reinfection with this species of coccidia. Studies by Horton-Smith (1949) indicated, however, that the development of immunity was a more prolonged process after the administration of small numbers of oocysts than after the administration of a single large dose of oocysts.

Because of the difficulties in repeatedly handling and dosing chickens with many small batches of oocysts, a number of investigators used various means to attenuate the virulence of the sporulated oocysts before using them in single or multiple large batches for immunizing chickens. Jankiewicz and Scofield (1934) heated sporulated oocysts for 15 minutes at 48° C and concluded that chicks given three doses of such oocysts at five-day intervals were highly immune when challenged one month later. The similar administration of oocysts heated prior to sporulation provided only partial protection from coccidiosis when the birds were challenged. Albanese and Smetana (1937) reported that x-irradiation attenuated the virulence of oocysts, and Waxler (1941) found that chickens infected with x-ray attenuated oocysts resisted a subsequent heavy re-exposure to infection by normal oocysts, as well as the birds' surviving the severe infection produced by untreated oocysts. Hein (1963) reported that the administration of two doses of x-irradiated oocysts (*E. tenella*) in the drinking water (at 0 and 13 days of age) produced a high degree of immunity in young chicks against reinfection when challenged with a large dose of normal oocysts. The immunized birds showed no evidence of clinical disease after vaccination or reinfection.

Several investigators explored ways to develop practical methods for immunizing chickens to coccidiosis under field conditions. Goldsby and Eveleth (1950) exposed chicks to an immunizing dose of cecal oocysts and controlled the multiplication of the coccidia by means of chemicals in the feed. They found that sulfaquinoxaline was the most effective agent for this purpose. Dickinson et al. (1951) also administered sulfaquinoxaline in the feed to chickens 48 hours after they were exposed to subclinical inoculation with five of the most common species of coccidia (*E. tenella, E. necatrix, E. acervulina, E. praecox,* and *E. maxima*). The medication was given continuously for 14 days, followed by nonmedicated feed. When the birds were challenged at 57 days of age, it was evident that substantial immunity had developed in the flock. Studies initiated by Edgar et al. (1951) and continued by Edgar et al. (1953-1954) provided a "practical" planned method for immunizing chickens against cecal coccidia and several species of intestinal coccidia. This coccidial "vaccine" was a mixture of sporulated oocysts of 3, 5, or 7 species of coccidia. Its use is recommended when the chickens are three to five days old, and they are given the oocysts in their feed or water. The birds are then fed a prophylactic level of one of the coccidiostats in their feed.

Edgar (1958) summarized data from experiments involving several thousand chickens reared on litter which, at three days of age, were exposed to three to five species of coccidia in the feed or water. The birds were fed low levels of one of several coccidiostatic drugs continuously in the feed. They developed sufficient immunity to withstand severe challenge by four to eight weeks of age. Stuart et al. (1963) found in laboratory trials that depending upon the coccidiostat used, the "vaccine" permitted immunity development with certain species but not with others. Bickford (1961) provided an appraisal of the field use of coccidiosis vaccination for flock-replacement chickens grown for egg production. He found that coccidiosis outbreaks occurred in the vaccinated flocks, but the incidence of these decreased with the use of seven species of coccidia in the "vaccine." Although the presently available product has limitations in that outbreaks of coccidiosis occur in 7 to 23 percent of the vaccinated flocks, Bickford concluded that "vaccination is an effective method of preventing coccidiosis in replacements."

Dickinson et al. (1959) and Bankowski et al. (1959) reported that satisfactory immunization was achieved by feeding mixtures of coccidia (*E. tenella, E. necatrix, E. acervulina, E. maxima,* and *E. praecox*) to 5- to 10-day-old birds, and 36 hours later feeding 0.05 percent sulfaquinoxaline for six days, followed by regular ration. Extensive use of this method indicated there was excellent control of coccidiosis and a substantial degree of immunity developed to all species of coccidia.

Carefully controlled field experiments by Reid (1960) indicated that some coccidiostats delayed the development of flock immunity because the coccidiostat may interrupt the life cycle of the parasite and reduce the population of oocysts in the litter. In Reid's studies, the use of a "vaccine" permitted rapid and solid immunity development when the birds were four weeks of age.

Studies by Long (1967) showed that marked resistance to reinfection with *E. mivati* developed after a single infection, but the resistance was not complete until after the third infection.

Numerous investigators (Tyzzer, 1929; Moore, 1954; Clarkson, 1958, 1959a, 1959b; and Clarkson and Gentles, 1958) have reported that repeated infections with turkey coccidia will produce immunity to reinfection with the immunizing species. However, as with other coccidia, the immunity is species-specific and there is no evidence of cross-immunity developing. Coccidiosis is primarily a disease in young turkeys (two to three weeks of age) and a marked age resistance has been noted particularly for the highly pathogenic species, *E. adenoeides* and *E. meleagrimitis* Tyzzer, 1929.

IMMUNITY TO COCCIDIOSIS

Coccidia, unlike many other protozoa, can not multiply indefinitely in a susceptible host, and therefore, coccidiosis is primarily a self-limiting disease in young animals. Although it was often recognized that older animals were less susceptible to infection than the young, this was generally attributed to their age rather than to immunity. Beach and Corl (1925) and Johnson (1927), on the basis of observations on natural outbreaks of the disease, believed that chickens which had recovered from coccidiosis were resistant to reinfection. Because of the difficulties in keeping chickens free from coccidial infections, it was not until Tyzzer (1929) established pure infections by several species of coccidia that the acquired resistance to coccidia was demonstrated to be rigidly species-specific with regard to the parasite. Tyzzer also concluded, and Horton-Smith (1949) confirmed, that the degree of immunity to the different species varied with the magnitude of the number of oocysts used and the severity of the infection. Furthermore, those species which penetrate deeply into the intestinal mucosa provided greater immunity than those parasites which developed in the superficial intestinal epithelium. Horton-Smith (1947) showed that chickens reared in isolation for six months were fully susceptible to acute infection with *Eimeria tenella*, which is characteristically associated with coccidiosis in young chicks.

Since Taliaferro's classic *The Immunology of Parasitic Infections* in 1929 and Culbertson's *Immunity Against Animal Parasites* in 1941, there have been many important developments in parasite immunology. Several excellent reviews on coccidiosis have appeared recently. Davies et al. (1963) provided an up-to-date textbook, *Coccidiosis*. Horton-Smith and Long (1963) reviewed coccidiosis in chickens and turkeys with special emphasis on the development of immunity. Levine (1961 and 1963) and Horton-Smith et al. (1963b) provided comprehensive reviews on the development of immunity to coccidia in domestic animals.

Nature of innate resistance

Herrick (1934) concluded that heredity is a factor in resistance to coccidiosis. He reported that chicks from resistant parents were about 100 percent more resistant to *E. tenella* than chicks from unselected parents. Schildt and McGibbon (1953) found that in seven inbred strains of White Leghorn chicks, only 9 percent of the least resistant chicks lived, while 62 percent of the most resistant strain survived after infection with 100,000 *E. tenella* oocysts. Moultrie et al. (1953-1954) selected coccidiosis-resistant and coccidiosis-susceptible strains and found that after selection for eight generations, 85 percent of the resistant chicks survived a standardized dose of *E. tenella* oocysts, whereas only 28 percent survived in the susceptible strain. Champion (1954) and Rosenberg et al. (1954) reported that selective breeding was effective in establishing lines of chickens which were either resistant or susceptible to coccidiosis. Both investigations suggested that the characteristics for resistance or susceptibility were controlled by multiple genetic factors which presumably act in an additive manner. They also concluded that sex-linkage, cytoplasmic inheritance, or passive transfer through the egg did not have a significant role in the relative resistance or susceptibility to *E. tenella* infection.

Moore and Brown (1951) and Clarkson (1958) found that turkeys acquire an age-resistance to *E. adenoeides* which is not associated with previous infection with the parasite. Clarkson and Gentles (1958) reported that natural outbreaks of coccidiosis occurred primarily in young (1.5- to 5.5-week-old) turkeys. These reports are in agreement with observations from turkey growers, who find that coccidiosis is generally a problem only in the young flock. Studies by Warren et al. (1963) showed that in addition to infections with *E. meleagrimitis* being less pathogenic for older than younger birds, the "reproductive index" (numbers of oocysts passed per oocyst administered) decreased with the age of the turkey.

Specificity of immunity

Nine species of coccidia are now known to develop in chickens and each of these species produces a selective and specific immunity in the host. Tyzzer (1929) observed that when chickens were fed a mixture of coccidia species and had been immunized to only one species, the birds were resistant only to that species. Thus, the immunity was selective and specific. For example, birds which recovered from severe infections of *E. tenella* were challenged with a mixture containing oocysts of *E. tenella*, *E. acervulina*, and *E.*

maxima. There was no evidence of infection with *E. tenella*, but extensive infections developed with the other species.

Cross-immunity tests have been used to differentiate coccidian species in the same host. Levine (1938) isolated *E. hagani* from a mixture of oocysts containing *E. maxima* and other species. He demonstrated by cross-immunity tests in birds immunized with *E. acervulina, E. maxima, E. mitis* Tyzzer, 1929, and *E. praecox* Johnson, 1930 that *E. hagani* was different from other species of coccidia which complete their development in the small intestine of the chicken. Levine (1942) conducted similar cross-immunity studies to confirm that *E. brunetti* was antigenically different from *E. hagani, E. maxima, E. mitis*, and *E. praecox*. Edgar and Seibold (1964) also used cross-immunity tests along with morphologic and biologic criteria for the identification of *E. mivati*.

Moore and Brown (1951) showed that antigenic specificity was useful for distinguishing among the cecal coccidia in turkeys. *E. adenoeides*, a very pathogenic parasite, and *E. meleagridis*, which is relatively nonpathogenic, were conclusively differentiated by appropriate cross-immunity tests. Clarkson (1960) also used cross-immunity tests to show that the strains of *E. adenoeides* and *E. meleagridis*, which he isolated in Great Britain, were indeed two distinct species, although their oocysts were indistinguishable.

Duration of acquired immunity

Many studies have demonstrated the development of acquired immunity to coccidiosis, but there have been very few carefully controlled studies to determine the duration of immunity in the absence of reinfection. Studies designed to assess the duration of immunity have been complicated by the problems associated with keeping birds free from reinfection by the parasites being investigated.

Tyzzer et al. (1932) found that birds thoroughly immune to *E. necatrix* were resistant to reinfection 14 days after disappearance of oocysts from the initial exposure. Farr (1943) reported that chickens, which were maintained under conditions to preclude extraneous infection, were highly resistant when challenged six months after initial exposure to infection with *E. tenella*. After a single immunizing dose of 60,000 *E. tenella* oocysts, Horton-Smith et al. (1961) found that birds were highly immune when challenged two or three weeks after exposure. The resistance was detectably diminished when the chickens were challenged four to six weeks after initial infection. When chickens were given three graded weekly doses of *E. tenella* oocysts, they were completely resistant to reinfection for at least three months (Horton-Smith et al., 1963b). Long (1962) showed that chickens infected with 5,000 *E. maxima* oocysts were highly resistant to reinfection three weeks later. However, no immunity was detected when these chickens were again exposed 10 weeks after the initial challenge. When these birds were again challenged 26 weeks after the third infection, they were highly susceptible to infection.

It is apparent that *E. maxima* stimulates a high degree of resistance to reinfection, but the immunity has a short duration.

In cross-immunity studies with coccidia from turkeys, Clarkson (1959a, 1959b) found that turkeys given 16 successive daily doses of *E. meleagridis* oocysts were completely refractory to challenge infection 26 days after initial exposure. Some of these turkeys were inoculated with *E. adenoeides* oocysts and found highly susceptible, indicating there was no cross-resistance between these species of coccidia. Augustin and Ridges (1963) found that turkeys were highly immune to challenge with *E. meleagrimitis* after inoculation of 4,000 oocysts daily for eight days. Moore (1954) indicated that although "solid" immunity had been produced with all species of turkey coccidia, the maximum duration of immunity was not known for any species.

Phase of the life cycle involved in immune response

When highly effective coccidiostatic drugs became available, it was readily recognized that the inhibition of the development of the coccidial infection might also lead to a decrease or suppression of immunity development to subsequent reinfection. Information obtained from the chemotherapy of coccidiosis has indicated that the schizogonous cycle is more important than the gametogonous phase in producing resistance to reinfection with coccidia. Studies by Horton-Smith and Taylor (1945) and Horton-Smith and Boyland (1946) showed that the principal effect of sulfamerazine was on the second generation schizont of *E. tenella*, which begins developing about 72 hours after initial infection. Kendall and McCullough (1952) confirmed that the different developmental stages of *E. tenella* varied in susceptibility to sulfonamide therapy and that the drug was "coccidiostatic" for all stages prior to the second generation schizonts and "coccidiocidal" for the latter. Similar conclusions were reached by Farr and Wehr (1945) and Wehr and Farr (1947) in their studies on sulfamethazine, by Cuckler and Ott (1947) on sulfaquinoxaline, and by Bankowski (1950) in studies on sulfaguanidine. Cuckler and Malanga (1956) showed that nicarbazin suppressed the development of the second generation schizonts and their merozoites. The presence of retarded schizonts resulted in a marked inflammatory reaction in the tissues. This was interpreted as having a stimulatory effect on immunity development and accounted for the relatively high degree of resistance to reinfection with coccidia observed in chickens fed nicarbazin. These observations were confirmed by Ball (1959). Joyner (1959) found a similar retardation of the second generation schizonts of *E. tenella* in chickens fed a high concentration of chlorotetracycline. Horton-Smith and Long (1959) found that glycarbylamide exerted some effect on the stages in the first schizogony but that the second schizont was more susceptible to the action of the drug.

To demonstrate further that the early parasitic stages up to and including the second generation schizonts were primarily responsible for the development of resistance, Horton-Smith et al. (1963a) rectally inoculated coccidiosis-susceptible chicks with large numbers (20 to 90 million) of second generation merozoites. This inoculum produced an infection primarily of the gametogony stages, with high oocyst production. The birds were reinfected three to four times with merozoites until few, if any, further oocysts were produced. Fourteen days after the last merozoite inoculation, the birds were challenged orally with *E. tenella* oocysts, resulting in severe disease, and the surviving birds produced many oocysts. These studies, and a similar experiment with *E. necatrix*, clearly showed that schizogony was more important than gametogony in producing resistance to reinfection with coccidia. These observations also demonstrated the importance of adjusting the anticoccidial drug dosage and period of administration so that schizogony could develop if active resistance to coccidiosis is desired in the chicken flock.

Pierce et al. (1962) were unable to find intracellular stages and few oocysts of *E. tenella* in chickens challenged after repeated exposures to this parasite. In a more extensive experiment, these investigators (Horton-Smith et al., 1963a) found that first generation schizogony had been suppressed in the highly immune birds, although sporozoites were observed in the epithelial cells of the ceca up to 72 hours after challenge. This suggested that the sporozoites were not immobilized by an immune reaction in the cecal lumen or at the surface of the cecal mucosa. Furthermore, sporozoites recovered from the cecal lumen of immune birds produced normal infections when injected into susceptible chickens. When second generation merozoites were inoculated directly or intrarectally into the ceca of immunized chickens, the parasites invaded the mucosa but failed to develop and were not found 30 hours after injection. This was additional evidence that the immune mechanism was not affecting the parasites in the lumen, but it was only effective after the sporozoites or merozoites invaded the cecal tissue and began further development. Studies by Leathem and Burns (1967) confirmed that sporozoites invaded the cecal mucosa of chickens when challenged 14 to 21 days after the last immunizing dose of *E. tenella* oocysts. However, they found that all stages of the life cycle were suppressed and their development retarded in the immune birds. They also demonstrated that the parasites removed from immune or nonimmune birds at 12 and 24 hours and from nonimmune birds at 48 hours after infection produced severe infections when transferred to susceptible birds. However, sporozoites transferred from immune birds 48 hours after inoculation failed to initiate infections in susceptible birds.

Transfer of immunity

Many attempts have been made to transfer immunity to coccidiosis from resistant to susceptible hosts. Tyzzer (1929) was not able to immunize chickens to coccidiosis by injecting them subcutaneously or intraperitoneally with blood or serum from birds that had recovered from severe cecal coccidiosis. He also was unable to protect birds from infection by feeding them blood from immune chickens or by intrarectally inoculating them with immune serum.

The use of *E. tenella* and the paired ceca permitted Burns and Challey

(1959) and Horton-Smith et al. (1961) to determine whether the immunity developed from coccidial infection in one cecum might be accompanied by development of immunity in the other noninfected cecum. Burns and Challey isolated and fistulated one cecum from the intestinal tract in each chicken. In a test group, sporozoites were introduced through the fistula into the cecal pouch and two weeks later the birds in the test and control groups were given sporulated oocysts orally. The effects of the challenge infection in the two groups of birds were compared. The results suggested that resistance to *E. tenella* was not limited to the cecum at the site of the initial infection. The studies by Horton-Smith and his associates were done somewhat differently. One of the paired ceca was ligated and severed from the intestine. The chickens were later given a heavy oral infection of oocysts. The ligated ceca did not develop infections. After intervals of 7, 14, or 21 days, groups of chickens previously infected in this way were challenged with sporozoites injected into the ceca. It was found that resistance to infection had developed in the previously uninfected and ligated ceca. The results suggested that the immunity acquired by the ligated ceca may have been due to humoral antibodies, to the circulation of lymphoid cells, or to a combination of both factors and was not due to local factors alone.

The studies described above led Long and Rose (1962) to investigate whether the factors responsible for the transfer of resistance from the infected cecum to the previously isolated uninfected cecum might also be transferred from immune hens to chicks via the yolk. Antibodies to several viral and bacterial diseases are reportedly transferred from hen to chicks by this means. A carefully planned and executed experiment was conducted by Long and Rose. They concluded that chicks from hens highly immune to *E. tenella* infection were as susceptible as the chicks from the nonimmune control hens. The chicks hatched from eggs produced by the two groups of hens were inoculated with 100,000 *E. tenella* oocysts at 4, 7, or 14 days of age. Although the total number of chicks challenged in the two groups was dissimilar, the percent mortality from coccidiosis was very similar. The comparison of oocyst production in the progeny from the immune and susceptible hens also showed there was little or no difference between the susceptibility of the two groups of chicks to cecal coccidiosis.

Pierce et al. (1963) made extensive attempts to immunize chickens passively to cecal coccidiosis by injection of serum proteins from highly immune birds. Whole serum or γ-globulin from birds immune to coccidiosis failed to confer passive immunity when injected by intravenous or intraperitoneal routes at varying times relative to challenge infection. The birds were given only small numbers of oocysts orally or merozoites intrarectally to avoid infections which might overwhelm the passively transferred immune serum. However, there was no evidence that the birds had acquired resistance to infection.

Similar studies were reported by Augustin and Ridges (1963) with *E. meleagrimitis.* Serum from "solidly immune" turkeys was injected intraperitoneally into poults before and/or after challenge with relatively small numbers of oocysts. On the basis of oocyst production in the immunized poults as compared with the control poults, this passive immunization had no effect on the development of the infection.

In attempts to produce active immunization without infection, Horton-Smith et al. (1963b) and Rose (1963) injected chicks intramuscularly or subcutaneously with antigenic material prepared from *E. tenella* schizonts or oocysts. By the Ouchterlony agar-gel diffusion test, it was shown that precipitins were formed in the sera of the chicks after injection with the ground-up parasites. These precipitating antibodies were identical with those developing in chickens after infection with *E. tenella*. Although the chicks injected with antigens appeared to have antibodies similar to those in chicks immune to reinfection, these antibodies did not provide protection against oral infection with *E. tenella* oocysts. The infections produced in the "immunized" chicks were very similar to those in control chickens which had not previously been infected.

In further attempts to immunize chicks actively with nonliving parasite material, Long and Rose (1965) parenterally injected chickens with schizont antigen and later challenged the birds for immunity by intravenous inoculations of sporozoites. These studies showed that birds injected with schizont antigen as well as those given *E. tenella* oocysts orally, were protected from a challenge infection with sporozoites given intravenously. Furthermore, chickens injected intravenously or intraperitoneally with serum globulin from chickens immune to reinfection with *E. tenella* were shown to have good protection from parenteral infection with sporozoites. The protection provided by immunoglobulin was greatest when this serum fraction was given shortly before challenge with sporozoites. Serum globulin from normal birds provided no protection to intravenous challenge with sporozoites. The demonstrations of protection with the "dead" antigen and of the transfer of immunoglobulin were both considered to be the result of direct contact between the parasites (the intravenously injected sporozoites) and the antibodies in the serum.

Detection of antibodies

Although many attempts have been made to detect circulating antibodies in the sera from chickens recovered from coccidial infection and resistant to challenge exposure, until recently few reports were available of successful results. McDermott and Stauber (1954) and Stauber (1963) demonstrated agglutinating antibodies in sera of chickens recovered from infection with *E. tenella*. By trypsin digestion and differential centrifugation, suspensions of second generation merozoites were prepared from the infected cecal mucosa. These suspensions were used as antigens to produce antisera in chickens and to detect agglutinins in the sera of immune chickens. Antibodies were found which persisted for at least 30 days and the maximum titers were 1 to 320 between the 10th and 15th days after infection.

Itagaki and Tsubokura (1954) reported that the merozoites of *E. tenella* contained hemolytic antigens, which were thermostable but destroyed by formalin. These same investigators (1955) reported that antisera from rabbits agglutinated merozoites of *E. tenella*. This antibody was destroyed by heating the serum to 75°C.

Moore (1959) attempted to use the complement-fixation test to detect antibodies in the sera of chickens following an acute infection of *E. tenella*. The antigens were extracts prepared from infected cecal tissue and oocysts which were concentrated by ethanol precipitation. A progressive increase in antibody response was detected by this technique in birds infected with *E. tenella*.

The possible importance of humoral antibody in resistance to cecal coccidiosis was further emphasized by the studies of Burns and Challey (1959) and Horton-Smith et al. (1961). These investigators demonstrated that resistance acquired by one cecum after primary infection with *E. tenella* could be transferred to the other noninfected cecum which was ligated or surgically isolated from the intestine. The previously noninfected ligated cecum was found resistant to challenge infection with sporozoites. These observations suggested that the acquired immunity in the ligated ceca was transferred through the circulation of humoral antibodies or by lymphoid cells or both.

Studies by Pierce et al. (1962) demonstrated precipitating antibodies in the sera of chickens completely immune to a challenge infection with 100,000 *E. tenella* oocysts. These antibodies were detected by using the gel diffusion technique of Ouchterlony with antigens prepared from the second generation schizonts or from disrupted oocysts. The sera from normal noninfected birds did not show precipitins with these antigens.

Studies by Horton-Smith et al. (1963b) on the lytic effects of sera from chickens immune to *E. tenella* were confirmed and extended by Long et al. (1963) and Rose (1963). Sporozoites and merozoites underwent lysis after incubation for one hour at 37°C when placed in normal sera from birds highly immune to reinfection with *E. tenella*. Inactivated serum did not cause lysis of these developmental forms; the addition of fresh normal chicken serum to the heated immune serum restored the lytic activity of the latter. Although the infectivity of sporocysts was not affected by incubation in immune or normal sera, the sporozoites and merozoites which were not lysed in heated immune sera had a low rate of infectivity when inoculated into susceptible birds. The infectivity of merozoites was not affected when placed in fresh normal serum; sporozoites remained motile and normal in appearance but their infectivity was reduced. Precipitating antibodies were also noted in some of the immune sera which produced lysis of sporozoites and merozoites.

Burns and Challey (1965) confirmed the presence of lysins for second generation merozoites in the sera from chickens immune to *E. tenella*. They found that lysins appeared in the sera of birds by the seventh day after a heavy infection, and on the eighth to tenth days following a light inoculation of oocysts. The lytic activity persisted in the sera for at least three months following infection. Although lysins appeared in the sera of surgically cecectomized or bursectomized birds, the intensity of the response was less than in normal birds. When chickens were infected by intracecal inoculations, the first generation merozoites appeared to be a greater stimulus for production of lysins than the second generation merozoites. The lytic property of the immune sera was associated with the proteins; fractionation of these indicated the activity was in the γ-globulin components. The sera from normal birds lysed sporozoites, but this effect was enhanced in the case of sera from immune birds.

Herlich (1965) found that sera from chicks highly immune to *E. tenella* would immobilize sporozoites and merozoites after one to two hours of incubation. Sporozoites of *E. acervulina* were similarly immobilized by the homologous hyperimmune serum. The *E. tenella* hyperimmune serum had no immobilizing effect on the sporozoites of *E. acervulina* and vice versa, indicating that the *in vitro* serum inactivation of the sporozoites and merozoites correlates with the specificity of the immune response in the chicken. In addition to the loss in motility, the inactivated sporozoites and merozoites either were not infective or showed a great reduction in infectivity when inoculated intrarectally into susceptible chickens. However, the incubation of sporulated oocysts of *E. acervulina* and *E. tenella* in homologous or heterologous hyperimmune serum had no effect on their oral infectivity. Although Herlich observed agglutination of the second generation merozoites, there was no evidence of lysis of sporozoites or merozoites in the immune or hyperimmune sera. Since tissue extracts from the cecal mucosa of chicks hyperimmune to *E. tenella*, as well as from the upper small intestine of birds hyperimmune to *E. acervulina*, failed to immobilize the sporozoites and/or merozoites, it was suggested that these antibodies are not localized in the cecal or intestinal epithelium.

In further studies on the immunity and cross-immunity developed by chickens infected with *E. tenella*, *E. acervulina*, *E. maxima*, and *E. necatrix*, Rose and Long (1962) carried out very extensive experiments to evaluate the protective resistance obtained with graded infections and to relate this to the development of serum precipitins. These studies further confirmed that the initial infection provided substantial protection from reinfection with each of the immunizing species. Although the birds had marked immunity when challenged with the immunizing species, they were fully susceptible to cross-infection with other species when exposed 15 to 16 weeks following initial infection.

Precipitating antibodies were demonstrated in the sera of birds infected with each of the species of coccidia. The precipitins appeared most promptly with *E. maxima* but were delayed and were of lower intensity after *E. necatrix* infection. Detectable precipitins persisted for at least 50 to 60 days in the birds given *E. tenella*, *E. necatrix*, and *E. acervulina*, and persisted even longer for those given *E. maxima*. A secondary rise in precipitins occurred only in the birds challenged with *E. acervulina* and *E. tenella*. In general, sera obtained after cross-infection only showed precipitins with the cross-infecting antigens and not with the antigens from the species used for immunizing. However, in the case of *E. tenella* and *E. necatrix*, there was evidence of common antigens since chickens immunized with *E. tenella* and then infected with *E. necatrix* (or vice versa) produced precipitins that reacted with antigens from both species.

Augustin and Ridges (1963) conducted extensive studies to assess the role of serum factors in the protective immunity developed by turkeys following repeated exposures to *E. meleagrimitis* Tyzzer, 1929. Although this parasite is highly infective and lethal for young turkeys, protective immunity develops after repeated sublethal infections. In *in vitro* tests, these investigators found that serum (devoid of complement) from immune poults formed "tails" of precipitates on the merozoites. The precipitated material appeared to be extruded from a pore at the pointed end of the merozoite, which became immobilized and was eventually destroyed. Although some lysis occurred when merozoites were placed in unheated normal or immune serum, the normal heated serum did not cause formation of precipitates or immobilize and destroy the merozoites. When merozoites were mixed with normal or immune serum and injected directly into the intestines of turkeys, the results indicated immune serum had detrimental effects on the subsequent development of the parasites, as measured by oocyst production.

In further attempts to determine how immune mechanisms affected the development of the parasites, histologic studies showed that oocysts excysted normally when inoculated into immune poults, and the sporozoites entered the epithelial cells. However, in comparison with the previously uninfected turkeys, relatively few first stage schizonts were found, and these appeared retarded in development in the immune turkeys. In gel-diffusion and electrophoretic studies with sera from solidly immune turkeys, precipitating antibodies specific for infected intestinal tissues were demonstrated. The amount of precipitation appeared to be related to the severity of the infection rather than to the stage of parasitic development in the tissue. Since preparations of oocyst homogenates did not form precipitates with immune sera, it was postulated that the antigens were metabolic products from the developing parasites. It was further suggested that if the metabolic product of the sporozoites is a proteolytic enzyme which facilitates entry of the parasites into the cells, specific antibodies against this enzyme would interfere with the tissue invasion and interrupt the development of the parasite. In addition to antibodies specific for the parasites, the sera of immune turkeys contained precipitating antibodies which reacted with extracts of host tissues, particularly infected tissues. This suggested to Augustin and Ridges the possibility that autoimmune antibodies were formed "due to the release of tissue antigen(s) by the proteolytic enzymes from the parasites."

Cellular factors in immunity

In comparative studies on coccidiosis in chickens, Tyzzer et al. (1932) reported that lymphoid and nongranular wandering cells were very numerous in the intestinal mucosa of chickens repeatedly reinfected with *E. necatrix* oocysts. In histologic studies of the ceca of birds given several graded doses of *E. tenella* oocysts, Pierce et al. (1962) found no intracellular stages of the coccidia and few first generation schizonts. After challenge, the submucosa of the immune birds showed many pyroninophilic (plasma) cells, some heterophil leukocytes in the crypts, and numerous globular leukocytes in the deep glands. Horton-Smith et al. (1963a) and Horton-Smith (1963) found a progressive increase in the total number of white cells (lymphocytes and heterophil leukocytes) in birds immunized with *E. tenella*. White cells from peripheral blood of immune and nonimmune chickens were injected intravenously into two lots of susceptible birds which were then injected intrarectally with second generation merozoites of *E. tenella*. The production of oocysts following challenge was similar in the two groups of birds, indicating the blood cells from the immune chickens had no suppressive effect on the development of parasites.

Long and Pierce (1963) and Pierce and Long (1965) provided evidence supporting a cellular basis for the protective immunity in cecal coccidiosis. These investigators conducted elaborate studies to assess the role of the bursa of Fabricius and the thymus on antibody production and the development of protective immunity to *E. tenella* infection. They found that chickens which had been bursectomized by testosterone treatment during embryonic development failed to develop antibodies, and they had low or undetectable serum immunoglobulin after repeated infection with *E. tenella* oocysts. Although these chickens had very few pyroninophilic cells in their ceca and had small spleens and thymus glands, they developed protective immunity and resisted challenge infection with *E. tenella* oocysts. Lytic antibodies developed in partially thymectomized birds, and the numbers of pyroninophilic cells in the ceca of chickens given three immunizing doses of oocysts were not significantly different from the pseudothymectomized control chickens. The oocyst counts after the immunizing infections suggested that the thymectomized birds were more susceptible than the pseudo-operated chickens. However, both groups appeared fully resistant to challenge infections. Pierce and Long concluded that these studies confirmed their earlier results, indicating humoral antibodies had little, if any, significant role in the development of protective immunity to reinfection with *E. tenella*.

HOST-PARASITE RELATIONSHIPS IN HISTOMONIASIS

Histomonas meleagridis (Smith, 1895) Tyzzer, 1920 is the cause of histomoniasis or infectious enterohepatitis in poultry. This parasite is widespread in chickens but usually does not produce apparent disease in this host. It is an important cause of disease in turkeys which become infected from the reservoir of infection in chickens, and in wild gallinaceous birds such as wild turkeys, pheasants, ruffed grouse, and quail. Cushman (1893) described the appearance and symptoms of turkeys with what was undoubtedly enterohepatitis, or "blackhead," but he did not characterize the disease. Theobald Smith (1895) recognized that the cause of this serious disease was a protozoan and named the organism *Amoeba meleagridis*. For many years this organism was confused with other parasites in the turkey, until Tyzzer (1920a, b) redescribed it as a pleomorphic protozoan with both amoeboid and flagellate characteristics, its appearance being dependent upon its location and the stage of the infection. Recently, Lund (1963) described a nonpathogenic organism, *Histomonas wenrichi*, which parasitizes chickens, turkeys, and pheasants but does not invade the tissues of the cecum or liver. Studies by Franker and Doll (1964) and Bradley and Reid (1966) showed that in addition to *Histomonas*, a suitable species of bacteria had to be present to produce typical infectious enterohepatitis. Reid (1967) recently reviewed the etiology and transmission of this disease in poultry.

Life cycle and epidemiology

H. meleagridis is an extracellular parasite which reproduces by binary fission. Although Tyzzer and Collier (1925) reported this parasite was transmissible by oral ingestion of the trophozoites from infected tissues, Lund (1956) found that large numbers of organisms were required to infect turkeys. Horton-Smith and Long (1956a) reported that histomonad suspensions from infected chickens failed to infect chickens orally on full feed. However, starved chickens were more susceptible, and when chickens were deprived of food and fed an alkaline suspension before oral inoculation with histomonads in tissue suspensions, most of the birds developed cecal lesions and some had typical liver lesions. Successful infection appeared dependent upon the pH of the contents of the gizzard and upper intestine. Tyzzer (1934a) found that infections were produced consistently by cloacal injection of homogenates of the livers from turkeys with histomoniasis. Tyzzer and Fabyan (1920) reported the experimental production of enterohepatitis by subcutaneous inoculation of liver homogenates from acutely infected cases in turkeys of various ages. The organisms were carried from the site of inoculation, and they developed lesions principally in the lung, liver, and kidney.

Studies by McGuire and Morehouse (1958) demonstrated that fatal cases of enterohepatitis could be produced by drawing blood from veins draining the infected ceca of donor birds and inoculating it into the wing veins of susceptible turkeys. Typical blackhead lesions developed in the liver, and lesions containing histomonads were also found in the lungs, kidneys, spleen, and certain other organs. The ceca did not develop lesions. Although histomonads were not found in the fresh or stained samples of blood used for inoculation, these parasites were demonstrated in histologic sections of the liver and other tissues showing lesions. These observations showed that *H. meleagridis* might develop in almost any tissue to which it has access.

Graybill and Smith (1920) and Smith and Graybill (1920) showed that embryonated eggs of the common poultry cecal worm, *Heterakis gallinarum*, transmitted histomonads to turkeys and chickens. The transmission of *H. meleagridis* by this parasitic metazoan has been confirmed by many investigators (McKay and Morehouse, 1947; Swales, 1948; Lund and Burtner, 1957). Farr (1961) showed that *H. gallinarum* eggs in fecal samples remained viable on outdoor plots for 230 weeks and were infective when fed to turkeys. Histomonads survived in these heterakid eggs for 151 weeks. Although *H. meleagridis* has never been observed in the egg, Tyzzer (1934a) reported finding this parasite in the gut wall of half-grown heterakid larvae. Swales (1948) was not able to identify the parasite in newly hatched larvae, but Kendall (1959) observed organisms resembling *H. meleagridis* in the cells lining the gut of a *Heterakis* larva. Studies by Gibbs (1962) demonstrated *Histomonas* in sections of male and female worms as well as the uterine eggs.

In studies with a nonpathogenic strain of *Histomonas*, Lund and Burtner (1957) reported that approximately 0.5 percent of the embryonated eggs of the cecal worm, *Heterakis gallinarum*, contained histomonads and would produce an infection of this parasite in susceptible birds. Furthermore, they found that less than half of the heterakids produced eggs containing *Histomonas* and these worms each averaged only two infected eggs.

Studies have shown that certain free-living invertebrates may also transmit histomonads or heterakids, and therefore blackhead, to susceptible turkeys and chickens. House flies and earthworms from poultry yards (Devolt and Davis, 1936; Madsden, 1962; Lund et al., 1966) were natural carriers of heterakids. House flies, flesh flies, grasshoppers, and sow bugs were mechanical transmitters of heterakids and enterohepatitis to turkeys (Frank, 1953; Spindler, 1967).

IMMUNITY TO HISTOMONIASIS

Tyzzer (1934b) reported that strains of histomonads varied considerably in their virulence for chickens and turkeys. Tyzzer (1932) also found that strains which were maintained in culture for two years were not pathogenic for chickens but they stimulated immunity to more virulent cultures. In later summarizing studies, Tyzzer (1936) reported that various culture strains of *H. meleagridis* were not uniform in regard to the rate of decrease in pathogenicity after many generations in cultures. Some strains attenuated by long cultivation retained their immunizing properties, but these were found later to provide only partial protection against challenge with the fully pathogenic strains.

Although Desowitz (1951) found that chickens three weeks of age were more susceptible than five-week-old chickens to histomoniasis, Kendall (1957) concluded turkeys of various ages were equally susceptible to oral exposure to *H. gallinarum* eggs. All turkeys were essentially uniformly susceptible and developed histomoniasis with high mortality. Turkeys which were challenged for immunity after recovery from infection were found to harbor histomonads in the ceca, but they did not develop symptoms or lesions of histomoniasis upon reinfection.

Brackett and Bliznick (1949) found some evidence of resistance to reinfection after drug therapy. Swales (1950) also suggested that immunity developed when treatment was given to turkeys for not more than 3 or 4 days so that the cecal disease was not completely suppressed. However, Sautter et al. (1950) and Devolt et al. (1954) found no evidence of immunity after the use of suppressive drugs. Indeed, Joyner and Kendall (1955) and Horton-Smith and Long (1956b) reported that relapses or reinfections frequently occurred after withdrawal of preventive treatment. Joyner (1963) presented data which were considered to confirm Swales' hypothesis. If enterohepatitis was allowed to develop for 8 to 10 days before treatment was initiated, the surviving birds showed marked immunity when challenged intrarectally with homogenates of infected tissues containing histomonads. Although he had little indication of the nature of the immunity, Joyner considered that his data demonstrated resistance to the acquisition of a new infection and not to development or relapse of one present in tissues. More recently, Joyner (1966) reported that chickens which had recovered from an initial infection of *Histomonas* are better hosts for *H. gallinarum* than chickens fully susceptible to histomonal infection. Immune chickens supported more and larger immature worms than were found in control chickens. The data also suggested that immunity to the nematode may be produced since *Histomonas* infections induced by *Heterakis* are not as effective as pure *Histomonas* in facilitating and improving the acceptance of the *Heterakis* infection.

In studies on immunity to histomoniasis, Clarkson (1963a) produced experimental infections of *H. meleagridis* by intrarectal inoculation of homogenates of infected tissues. When treatment was delayed for at least 8 days, resistance to reinfection developed and turkeys were protected against further infections. Spontaneous recovery occurred in chickens with healing and disappearance of cecal and early liver lesions. Clarkson attempted to transfer immunity from resistant to susceptible chickens or turkeys by repeated intraperitoneal injections of serum from immune birds. When the chickens and turkeys were challenged by intrarectal inoculations of tissue homogenates from infected birds, all chickens developed typical cecal lesions and all turkeys died with typical histomoniasis. These studies on passive immunity indicated that the protective factor was not primarily in the serum.

Using antigens prepared from infected ceca and livers, Clarkson (1963a) demonstrated (by the agar-gel double diffusion technique) precipitating antibodies in the blood of both chickens and turkeys 10 to 12 days after infection. Although precipitins appeared in the blood, Clarkson considered that the immune barrier might be localized and confined to the epithelium of the ceca since antigens derived from *H. meleagridis* were first detected in the cecal contents of turkeys four days after infection. Furthermore, since birds require about seven days to produce serum precipitins (Rosenquist and Wolfe, 1962), the appearance of precipitating antibodies would not be expected in the serum until the 10th to 12th day after infection. It is not conclusive whether the protective immunity was produced by a factor in the serum, by leukocytes, by a local immunity in the cecal tissues, or by a combination of these factors.

Lund (1959) reported discovery of a strain of *Histomonas* which did not produce blackhead in chickens or turkeys. This nonpathogenic strain was used in attempting to immunize turkeys against enterohepatitis produced with pathogenic strains. Several thousand histomonads from cultures were inoculated intrarectally into young poults on two or three consecutive days. When the poults were challenged three to six weeks later by intrarectal inoculation of pathogenic organisms, there was some protection. However, there was little, if any, protection against a challenge of pathogenic histomonads provided by feeding embryonated *Heterakis* eggs. It was suggested that immunization produced an immune barrier at the surface of the cecal mucosa. This was penetrated by heterakid larvae before releasing their histomonads, thus allowing development of blackhead.

Further studies on immunity development were reported by Lund et al. (1966) using an *in vitro* attenuated strain of *H. meleagridis*. After almost six years of *in vitro* cultivation and some 700 serial passages, this strain was nonpathogenic, but it still stimulated immunity. However, with continued *in vitro* cultivation, this was lost so that by the 835th passage the organisms did not induce detectable immunity in chickens. The data suggested these *in vitro* attenuated histomonads provided slight protection against virulent histomonad infections produced with *Heterakis* eggs. Lund et al. (1967) continued the cultivation of *H. meleagridis* through 1,000 passages and found that the organisms had lost much of their ability either to infect or to immunize turkeys and chickens.

CONCLUSION

Although avian coccidiosis is of great economic importance and it has long been known that protective immunity or resistance to reinfection with *Eimeria* species can be acquired, it is only recently that an understanding has begun to emerge regarding the defense mechanisms involved. In addition to the innate resistance associated with genetic factors in the host, it is now evident that turkeys, but not chickens, develop an age resistance to infection with coccidia. The immunity acquired by coccidial infection in the host is highly selective and specific, and the intensity of immunity varies with the species of parasite and severity of infection. In the absence of reinfection, the duration of immunity also varies, but it is clear that protection lasts only for a limited period. The schizogonous cycles, and particularly the second generation schizonts, are primarily responsible for producing resistance to reinfection with coccidia. Generally, it has not been possible to demonstrate the passive transfer of immunity from resistant to susceptible birds. Recent data have shown that resistance could be transferred from an intact infected cecum to the cecum surgically isolated from the intestinal tract but with normal blood supply. This suggested that the immunity was possibly due to circulation of humoral antibodies, lymphoid cells, or both. Specific antibodies have been demonstrated frequently in the sera of birds resistant to coccidiosis, but generally the concentration of these circulating antibodies was not increased after resistant chickens were exposed to reinfection. Similar antibodies have been elicited by injecting susceptible birds with antigenic material from second generation schizonts, but these birds showed no protection when challenged orally with oocysts. However, birds were actively immunized with second generation schizont antigens and were protected from infection when challenged by intravenous injection of sporozoites. Similarly, if challenge infections are given intravenously, it has been possible to protect birds by transfer of serum globulin from resistant to susceptible birds. Although bursectomized chickens did not develop detectable antibodies after repeated infection with *E. tenella* oocysts, these birds developed protective immunity and resisted challenge infection. Thymectomized birds developed lytic antibodies and also were successfully immunized to repeated oral doses of oocysts and resisted challenge infection. These apparently conflicting observations indicate that a combination of humoral and cellular factors are most likely involved in coccidial immunity.

Histomoniasis is a particularly important disease in turkeys, which are uniformly susceptible at all ages. Young chickens are more susceptible than older ones, but all ages are relatively insusceptible to this disease. Birds which recover from infection are generally resistant to reinfection, but resistance cannot be transferred to susceptible birds by injections of sera from immune birds. Although precipitating antibodies have been demonstrated in sera from immune turkeys, it is not evident whether the protective immunity is due to antibodies in the serum, local immunity in the cecal tissues by leukocytes, or a combination of these factors.

REFERENCES

Albanese, A. A., and H. Smetana. 1937. Studies on the effect of x-rays on the pathogenicity of *Eimeria tenella*. Amer. J. Hyg., 26: 27-39.

Augustin, R., and A. P. Ridges. 1963. Immunity mechanisms in *Eimeria meleagrimitis*. *In* Immunity to Protozoa. Garnham, P. C. C., Pierce, A. E., and Roitt, I. eds. Oxford, Blackwell Scientific Publications, pp. 296-335.

Ball, S. J. 1959. Chemotherapy of caecal coccidiosis in chickens: The activity of nicarbazin. Vet. Rec., 71: 86-91.

Bankowski, R. A. 1950. Effect of sulfaguanidine upon the developmental stages of *Eimeria tenella*. Amer. J. Vet. Res., 11: 130-136.

———— D. E. Stover, and S. L. Jamison. 1959. Coccidiosis immunization at a poultry testing project. Proceedings of the 63rd Annual Meeting of the U. S. Livestock Sanitary Association, 11. 226-230.

Beach, J. R., and J. C. Corl. 1925. Studies in the control of avian coccidiosis. Poult. Sci., 4: 83-93.

Bickford, R. L. 1961. Appraisal of coccidiosis vaccination for replacements. Tenth Annual Poultry Health Conference, University of New Hampshire, pp. 35-40.

Brackett, S., and A. Bliznick. 1949. The development of resistance to and the effect of some new chemotherapeutic agents on enterohepatitis induced by oral administration of cecal worm ova to chicken and turkeys. J. Parasit., 35: 16-17.

———— and A. Bliznick. 1950. The occurrence and economic importance of coccidiosis in chickens. Animal Feed Department, Lederle Laboratories Division, American Cyanamid Co., p. 78.

———— and A. Bliznick. 1952. The reproductive potential of five species of coccidia of the chicken as demonstrated by oocyst production. J. Parasit., 38: 133-138.

Bradley, R. E. and W. M. Reid. 1966. Histomonas meleagridis and several bacteria as agents of infectious enterohepatitis in gnotobiotic turkeys. Exp. Parasit., 19: 91-101.

Burns, W. C., and J. R. Challey. 1959. Resistance of birds to challenge with Eimeria tenella. Exp. Parasit., 8: 515-526.

———— and J. R. Challey. 1965. Serum lysins in chickens infected with Eimeria tenella. J. Parasit., 51: 660-668.

Champion, L. R. 1954. The inheritance of resistance to cecal coccidiosis in the domestic fowl. Poult. Sci., 33: 670-681.

Clarkson, M. J. 1958. Life history and pathogenicity of Eimeria adenoeides Moore and Brown, 1951, in the turkey poult. Parasitology, 48: 70-88.

———— 1959a. The life history and pathogenicity of Eimeria meleagrimitis Tyzzer, 1929, in the turkey poult. Parasitology, 49: 70-82.

———— 1959b. The life history and pathogenicity of Eimeria meleagridis Tyzzer, 1927, in the turkey poult. Parasitology, 49: 519-528.

———— 1960. The coccidia of the turkey. Ann. Trop. Med. Parasit., 54: 253-257.

———— 1963a. Immunological responses to Histomonas meleagridis in the turkey and laying fowl. Immunology, 6: 156-168.

———— 1963b. Immunity to histomoniasis (blackhead). Poult. Rev., 3: 43-46.

———— and M. A. Gentles. 1958. Coccidiosis in turkeys. Vet. Rec., 70: 211-214.

Cuckler, A. C., and W. H. Ott. 1947. The effect of sulfaquinoxaline on the developmental stages of Eimeria tenella. J. Parasit., 33 (Suppl.): 10-11.

———— and C. M. Malanga. 1956. The effect of nicarbazin on the development of immunity to avian coccidia. J. Parasit., 42: 593-607.

Culbertson, J. T. 1941. Immunity against Animal Parasites. New York, Columbia University Press, p. 274.

Cushman, S. 1893. The production of turkeys. Rhode Island Agricultural Experimental Station Bulletin, 25: 89-123.

Davies, S. F. M., L. P. Joyner, and S. B. Kendall. 1963. Coccidiosis. Edinburgh and London, Oliver and Boyd.

Desowitz, R. S. 1951. Age as a factor influencing fatal infections of histomoniasis in chickens. J. Comp. Path., 61: 231-236.

Devolt, H. M., and C. R. Davis. 1936. Blackhead (infectious enterohepatitis) in turkeys, with notes on other intestinal protozoa. Maryland Agricultural Experimental Station Bulletin, 392: 493-567.

———— F. G. Tromba, and A. P. Holst. 1954. An investigation to determine whether immunity to infectious enterohepatitis (blackhead) of turkeys develops during Enheptin treatment. Poult. Sci., 33: 1256-1261.

Dickinson, E. M. 1941. The effects of variable dosages of sporulated Eimeria acervulina oocysts on chickens. Poultry Sci., 20: 413-424.

———— W. E. Babcock, and J. W. Osebold. 1951. Coccidial immunity studies in chickens. Poultry Sci., 30: 76-80.

———— W. E. Babcock, and J. G. Kilian. 1959. A program of immunization against avian coccidia. Proceedings of the 63rd Annual Meeting of the U. S. Livestock Sanitary Association, pp. 223-225.

Edgar, S. A. 1958. Control of coccidiosis in chickens and turkeys by immunization. Proceedings of the Association of Southern Agricultural Workers, Little Rock, Arkansas, pp. 203-204.

———— D. F. King, and L. W. Johnson. 1951. Control of avian coccidiosis through breeding or immunization. Poult. Sci., 30: 911.

———— D. F. King, and C. Flanagan. 1953-54. Breeding and immunizing chickens for resistance to coccidiosis. 2. Immunizing phase. 64th and 65th Annual Reports, Agricultural Experimental Station, Alabama Polytechnic Institute, p. 45.

———— and C. T. Seibold. 1964. A new coccidium of chickens, *Eimeria mivati* sp. n. (Protozoa: Eimeriidae) with details of its life history. J. Parasit., 50: 193-204.

Farr, M. M. 1943. Resistance of chickens to cecal coccidiosis. Poult. Sci., 22: 277-286.

———— 1961. Further observations on survival of the protozoan parasite, *Histomonas meleagridis*, and eggs of poultry nematodes in feces of infected birds. Cornell Vet., 51; 3-13.

———— and E. E. Wehr. 1945. Sulfamerazine therapy in experimental cecal coccidiosis of chickens. J. Parasit., 31: 353-358.

———— and D. J. Doran. 1962. Comparative excystation of four species of poultry coccidia. J. Protozool., 9: 403-407.

Frank, J. F. 1953. A note on the experimental transmission of enterohepatitis of turkeys by arthropods. Canad. J. Comp. Med., 17: 230-231.

Franker, C. K., and J. P. Doll. 1964. Experimental histomoniasis in gnotobiotic turkeys. II. Effects of some cecal bacteria on pathogenesis. J. Parasit., 50: 636-640.

Gibbs, B. J. 1962. The occurrence of the protozoan parasite *Histomonas meleagridis* in adults and eggs of the cecal worm. *Heterakis gallinae.* J. Protozool. 9: 288-293.

Goldsby, A. I., and D. F. Eveleth. 1950. Immunizing baby chicks against cecal coccidiosis. Agricultural Experimental Station, North Dakota Agricultural College, Bulletin 361.

Graybill, H. W., and T. Smith. 1920. Production of fatal blackhead in turkeys by feeding embryonated eggs of *Heterakis papillosa.* J. Exp. Med., 31: 647-655.

Hein, H. 1963. Vaccination against infection with *Eimeria tenella* in broiler chickens. 17th World Veterinary Congress, Hanover, 1443-1452.

Herlich, H. 1965. Effect of chicken antiserum and tissue extracts on the oocysts, sporozoites and merozoites of *Eimeria tenella* and *E. acervulina.* J. Parasit., 51: 847-851.

Herrick, C. A. 1934. The development of resistance to the protozoan parasite, *Eimeria tenella*, by the chicken. J. Parasit., 20: 329-330.

Horton-Smith, C. 1947. Coccidiosis—some factors influencing its epidemiology. Vet. Rec., 59: 645-656.

———— 1949. Some factors influencing the origin and course of epidemics of coccidiosis in poultry. Ann. N. Y. Acad. Sci., 52: 449-457.

———— 1963. Immunity to avian coccidiosis. Brit. Vet. J., 119: 99-109.

———— and E. Boyland. 1946. Sulphonamides in the treatment of caecal coccidiosis of chickens. Brit. J. Pharmacol., 1: 139-152.

———— J. Beattie, and P. L. Long. 1961. Resistance to *Eimeria tenella* and its transference from one cecum to the other in individual fowls. Immunology, 4: 111-121.

———— and P. L. Long. 1956a. Studies in Histomoniasis I. The infection of chickens (*Gallus gallus*) with histomonad suspensions. Parasitology, 46: 79-90.

———— and P. L. Long. 1956b. Further observations on the chemotherapy of histomoniasis (blackhead) in turkeys. J. Comp. Path. Ther., 66: 378-388.

———— and P. L. Long. 1959. The anticoccidial activity of glycarbylamide. Brit. Vet. J., 115: 55-62.

———— and P. L. Long. 1963. Coccidia and coccidiosis in the domestic fowl and turkey. *In* Advances in Parasitology, Vol. 1. Dawes, B., ed. New York, Academic Press, Inc., pp. 68-107.

———— P. L. Long, and A. E. Pierce. 1963a. Behavior of invasive stages of *Eimeria tenella* in the immune fowl (*Gallus domesticus*). Exp. Parasit., 13: 66-74.

———— P. L. Long, A. E. Pierce, and M. E. Rose. 1963b. Immunity to coccidia in domestic animals. *In* Immunity to Protozoa. Garnham, P. C. C., Pierce, A. E., and Roitt, I. eds. Oxford, Blackwell Scientific Publications, pp. 273-295.

———— and E. L. Taylor. 1945. Sulfamezathine in the drinking-water as a treatment for cecal coccidiosis in chickens. Vet. Rec., 57: 35-36.

Ikeda, M. 1955. Factors necessary for *E. tenella* infection of the chicken. II. Influence of the pancreatic juice on infection. Jap. J. Vet. Sci., 17: 225-230.

Itagaki, K., and M. Tsubokura. 1954. Studies on coccidiosis in fowls. III. On the hemolysis by merozoites. Jap. J. Vet. Sci., 16: 159-165.

———— and M. Tsubokura. 1955. Studies on coccidiosis in fowls. IV. On the agglutination of merozoites. Jap. J. Vet. Sci., 17: 139-143.

Jankiewicz, H. A., and R. H. Scofield. 1934. The administration of heated occysts of *Eimeria tenella* as a means of establishing resistance and immunity to cecal coccidiosis. J. Amer. Vet. Med. Ass., 37: 507-526.

Johnson, W. T. 1927. Immunity or resistance of the chicken to coccidial infection. Oregon Agricultural Experimental Station Bulletin No. 230, 1-31.

———— 1928. Coccidiosis of the chicken. Oregon Agricultural Experimental Station Bulletin No. 238, 5-16.

Joyner, L. P. 1959. The effects of chlorotetracycline on the development of *Eimeria tenella*. Vet. Rec., 71: 43-46.

———— 1963. Immunity to histomoniasis in turkeys following treatment with Dimetridazole. J. Comp. Path., 73: 201-207.

———— 1966. Infections with *Heterakis gallinarum* in chickens following recovery from histomoniasis. Parasitology, 56: 171-177.

———— and S. B. Kendall. 1955. The use of 2-amino-5-nitrothiazole in the control of histomoniasis. Vet. Rec., 67: 180-183.

Kendall, S. B. 1957. Some factors influencing resistance to histomoniasis in turkeys. Brit. Vet. J., 133: 435-439.

———— 1959. The occurrence of *Histomonas meleagridis* in *Heterakis gallinae*. Parasitology, 49: 169-172.

———— and F. S. McCullough. 1952. Relationships between sulphamezathine therapy and acquisition of immunity to *Eimeria tenella*. J. Comp. Path., 62: 116.

Leathem, W. D., and W. C. Burns. 1967. Effects of the immune chicken on the endogenous stages of *Eimeria tenella*. J. Parasit., 53: 180-185.

Levine, N. D. 1961. Protozoan Parasites of Domestic Animals and of Man. Minneapolis, Burgess Publishing Co., pp. 74-81 and 202-230.

———— 1963. Coccidiosis. Ann. Rev. Microbiol., 17: 179-198.

Levine, P. P. 1938. *Eimeria hagani* n. sp. (Protozoa: Eimeriidae) a new coccidium of the chicken. Cornell Vet., 28: 263-266.

———— 1942. A new coccidium pathogenic for chickens, *Eimeria brunetti* n. sp. (Protozoa: Eimeriidae). Cornell Vet., 32: 430-439.

Long, P. L. 1962. Observations on the duration of the acquired immunity of chickens to *Eimeria maxima* Tyzzer, 1929. Parasitology, 52: 89-93.

———— 1967. Studies on *Eimeria mivati* in chickens and a comparison with *Eimeria acervulina*. J. Comp. Path., 77: 315-325.

———— and A. E. Pierce. 1963. Role of cellular factors in the mediation of immunity to avian coccidiosis (*Eimeria tenella*). Nature (London), 200: 426-427.

———— and M. E. Rose. 1962. Attempted transfer of resistance to *Eimeria tenella* infections from domestic hens to their progeny. Exp. Parasit., 12: 75-81.

———— and M. E. Rose. 1965. Active and passive immunization of chickens against intravenously induced infections of *Eimeria tenella*. Exp. Parasit., 16: 1-7.

———— M. E. Rose and A. E. Pierce. 1963. Effects of fowl sera on some stages in the life cycle of *Eimeria tenella*. Exp. Parasit., 14: 210-217.

Lund, E. E. 1956. On transmission of *Histomonas* in turkeys. Poult. Sci., 35: 900-904.

———— 1959. Immunizing action of a nonpathogenic strain of *Histomonas* against blackhead in turkeys. J. Protozool., 6: 182-185.

———— 1963. *Histomonas wenrichi* n. sp. (Mastigophora: Mastig amoebidae), a nonpathogenic parasite of gallinaceous birds. J. Protozool., 10: 401-404.

———— P. C. Augustine, and D. J. Ellis. 1966. Immunizing action of *in vitro*-attenuated *Histomonas meleagridis* in chickens and turkeys. Exp. Parasit., 35: 403-407.

———— and R. H. Burtner. 1957. Infectivity of *Heterakis gallinae* eggs with *Histomonas meleagridis*. Exp. Parasit., 6: 189-193.

———— E. E. Wehr, and D. J. Ellis. 1966. Earthworm transmission of *Heterakis* and *Histomonas* to turkeys and chickens. J. Parasit., 52: 899-902.

———— P. C. Augustine and A. M. Chute. 1967. *Histomonas meleagridis* after one thousand *in vitro* passages. J. Protozool., 14: 349-351.

Madsen, H. 1962. On the interaction between *Heterakis gallinarum, Ascaridia galli,* "blackhead" and the chicken. J. Helminth., 36: 107-142.

McDermott, J. J., and L. A. Stauber. 1954. Preparation and agglutination of merozoite suspensions of the chicken coccidium *Eimeria tenella*. J. Parasit., 40 (Suppl.): 23-24.

McGuire, W. C., and W. F. Morehouse. 1958. Blood-induced blackhead. J. Parasit., 44: 292-295.

McKay, F., and N. F. Morehouse. 1947. Studies on experimental blackhead infection in turkeys. J. Parasit., 33 (Suppl.): 11-12.

Moore, E. N. 1954. Species of coccidia affecting turkeys. Proceedings of the 91st Annual Meeting of the American Veterinary Medical Association, pp. 300-304.

—— and J. A. Brown. 1951. A new coccidium pathogenic for turkeys, *Eimeria adenoeides* n. sp. (Protozoa: Eimeriidae). Cornell Vet., 41: 125-136.

—— and J. A. Brown. 1952. A new coccidium of turkeys, *Eimeria innocua* n. sp. (Protozoa: Eimeriidae). Cornell Vet., 42: 395-402.

—— J. A. Brown, and R. D. Carter. 1954. A new coccidium of turkeys, *Eimeria subrotunda* n. sp. (Protozoa: Eimeriidae). Poult. Sci., 33: 925-929.

Moore, T. D. 1959. Antibody response of chickens to an acute infection of *Eimeria tenella*. Dissertation Abstracts, 20: 1536.

Moultrie, F., S. A. Edgar, and D. F. King. 1953-1954. Breeding and immunizing chickens for resistance to coccidiosis. 1. Breeding chickens for resistance to coccidiosis. 64th and 65th Annual Reports Agricultural Experimental Station, Alabama Polytechnic Institute, pp. 44-45.

Patillo, W. H. 1959. The invasion of the cecal mucosa of the chicken by sporozoites of *Eimeria tenella*. J. Parasit., 45: 253-257.

Pierce, A. E., and P. L. Long. 1965. Studies on acquired immunity to coccidiosis in bursaless and thymectomized fowls. Immunology, 9: 427-439.

—— P. L. Long and C. Horton-Smith. 1962. Immunity to *Eimeria tenella* in young fowls (*Gallus domesticus*). Immunology, 5: 129-152.

—— P. L. Long, and C. Horton-Smith. 1963. Attempts to induce a passive immunity to *Eimeria tenella* in young fowls (*Gallus domesticus*). Immunology, 6: 37-47.

Reid, W. M. 1960. The relationship between coccidiostats and poultry flock immunity in coccidiosis control programs. Poult. Sci., 39: 1431-1437.

—— 1967. Etiology and dissemination of the blackhead disease syndrome in turkeys and chickens. Exp. Parasit., 21: 249-275.

Rose, M. E. 1963. Some aspects of immunity to *Eimeria* infections. Ann. N. Y. Acad. Sci., 113: 383-399.

—— and P. L. Long. 1962. Immunity to four species of *Eimeria* in fowls. Immunology, 5: 79-92.

Rosenberg, M. M., J. E. Alicata, and A. L. Palafox. 1954. Further evidence of hereditary resistance and susceptibility to cecal coccidiosis in chickens. Poult. Sci., 33: 972-980.

Rosenquist, G. L., and H. R. Wolfe. 1962. Effect of splenectomy at different ages on precipitin production in chickens. Immunology, 5: 211-221.

Sautter, J. H., B. S. Pomeroy, and M. H. Roepke. 1950. Histomoniasis (enterohepatitis) in turkeys. II. Chemotherapy of experimental histomoniasis. Amer. J. Vet. Res., 11: 120-129.

Schildt, C. S., and W. H. McGibbon. 1953. Coccidiosis resistance varies within breeds. What's new in farm science. University of Wisconsin Bulletin, No. 500, p. 27.

Smith, T. 1895. An infectious disease among turkeys caused by protozoa (infectious enterohepatitis). U. S. Department of Agriculture, Bureau of Animal Industry Bulletin No. 8, pp. 7-38.

—— 1910. A protective reaction of the host in intestinal coccidiosis of the rabbit. J. Med. Res., 23: 407.

—— and H. W. Graybill. 1920. Blackhead in chickens and its experimental production by feeding embryonated eggs of *Heterakis papillosa*. J. Exp. Med., 32: 143-152.

Spindler, L. A. 1967. Experimental transmission of *Histomonas meleagridis* and *Heterakis gallinarum* by the sow-bug, *Porcellio scaber*, and its implications for further research. Proc. Helminth Soc. (Washington), 34: 26-29.

Stauber, L. A. 1963. Some aspects of immunity to intracellular protozoan parasites. J. Parasit., 49: 3-11.

Stuart, E. E., H. W. Bruins, and R. D. Keenum. 1963. The immunogenicity of a commercial coccidiosis vaccine in conjunction with Trithiadol and zoalene. Avian Dis., 7: 12-18.

Swales, W. E. 1948. Enterohepatitis (Blackhead) in turkeys. II. Observations on transmission by the cecal worm (*Heterakis gallinae*). Canad. J. Comp. Med. Vet. Sci., 12: 97-100.

—— 1950. The use and limitations of drugs in poultry practice. Canad. J. Comp. Med., 14: 355.

Taliaferro, W. H. 1929. The Immunology of Parasitic Infections. New York, The Century Co.

Tyzzer, E. E. 1919. Developmental phases of the protozoan of "blackhead" in turkeys. J. Med. Res., 40: 1-30.

———— 1920a. The flagellate character and reclassification of the parasite producing "blackhead" in turkeys. *Histomonas* (n.g.) *meleagridis* (Smith). J. Parasit., 6: 124-131.

———— 1920b. Observations on the transmission of "blackhead" in turkeys—the common fowl as a source of infection. J. Med. Res., 41: 219-237.

———— 1929. Coccidiosis in gallinaceous birds. Amer. J. Hyg., 10: 269-383.

———— 1932. Problems and observations concerning transmission of blackhead infection in turkeys. Proc. Amer. Phil. Soc., 71: 407-410.

———— 1934a. Studies on histomoniasis or "blackhead" infection in the chicken and the turkey. Proc. Amer. Acad. Arts Sci., 69: 187-264.

———— 1934b. Loss of virulence in the protozoan of "blackhead," a fatal disease of turkeys, and the immunizing properties of attenuated strains. Science, 78: 522-523.

———— 1936. A study of immunity produced by infection with attenuated culture-strains of *Histomonas meleagridis*. J. Comp. Path. Ther., 49: 285-303.

———— and J. Collier. 1925. Induced and natural transmission of blackhead in the absence of *Heterakis*. J. Infect. Dis., 37: 265-276.

———— and M. Fabyan. 1920. Further studies on "blackhead" in turkeys with special reference to transmission by inoculation. J. Infect. Dis., 27: 207-239.

———— H. Theiler, and E. E. Jones. 1932. Coccidiosis in gallinaceous birds. II. A comparative study of species of *Eimeria* of the chicken. Amer. J. Hyg., 15: 319-393.

Walton, A. C. 1959. Some parasites and their chromosomes. J. Parasit., 45: 1:20.

Warren, E. W., S. J. Ball, and J. R. Fagg. 1963. Age resistance by turkeys to *Eimeria meleagrimitis* Tyzzer, 1929. Nature (London), 200: 238-240.

Waxler, S. H. 1941. Immunization against cecal coccidiosis in chickens by the use of x-ray attenuated oocysts. J. Amer. Vet. Med. Ass., 99: 481-485.

Wehr, E. E., and M. M. Farr. 1947. Effect of sulfamethazine on the coccidian parasite, *Eimeria tenella*, of chickens. Proc. Helminth Soc. (Washington), 14: 1-20.

Avian Immunity to Metazoan Parasites

FRANK A. EHRENFORD
The Dow Chemical Company, Lake Jackson, Texas

INTRODUCTION

Since poultry are a major protein food source in economically advanced
countries, and since they promise to become a principal source for much of

the world, increased interest and research in poultry diseases are very appropriate because along with the basic husbandry problems of breeding, feeding, and housing, there are the losses caused by infectious diseases. As well as the infectious diseases caused by viruses, bacteria, fungi, and protozoa, there are those caused by the metazoa or helminths. Despite much knowledge and know-how about controlling the helminth diseases of poultry, these internal parasites continue to take their toll of biologic taxes, which are only another form of fiscal taxes. Should any animal husbandman tolerate a 10, 15, 20, or even occasionally, a 90 percent reduction in yield?

New or better methods of disease control are needed—some of these may be provided by immunology. Scattered, specific investigations have been made in the area of poultry helminth diseases, but most of these studies have amounted to little more than probes. Studies with continuity and depth are needed. If an early overall summary by Culbertson (1941) is compared to what is available nearly three decades later, surprisingly little research work has accumulated on domestic birds with regard to immunity. Perhaps this situation is due to poultry science being one of the newer research areas, especially from the standpoint of immunology. The apparent research lag may not be too serious a problem, because advances in the knowledge of immunologic phenomena and techniques derived from mammalian investigations should provide guidelines which may immediately be applied to poultry research. The goal of detecting, isolating, and purifying specific protection-inducing antigens, as compared to those which are diagnostic, seems much closer now than five years ago, but this illusion should not detract from the thrill of the chase. There are a multitude of technical problems to solve, and while many exciting clues have been found, the pursuit for knowledge in helminth immunologic research will probably not advance uniformly or rapidly.

In economically underdeveloped countries, little progress has been made toward developing the poultry industry as a principal source of food. Much can be learned from practices in the United States and Israel, both of which have highly developed poultry industries. In fact, Israel presents a remarkable example of starting from nothing and developing a highly functional poultry industry in 20 years, and, in the face of a tremendous population growth, achieving international first place in per capita supply and the export of poultry products, besides providing assistance to several dozen countries in techniques, training, and materials (Proceedings Poultry Congress, 1968). Each region or country will need to develop its own approaches to poultry raising because of economic, ecologic, parasitic, and poultry differences.

Although immunity to helminths infecting poultry is the main subject of concern here, it is worthwhile to consider briefly other aspects of disease control pertaining to aviculture, since by doing so a better perspective will be gained. The broad picture of disease control is essential in reaching an intelligent assay of the areas which merit attention.

Historical and economic factors

During the last 15 years, poultry production in the United States has changed from small individual flocks numbering in the hundreds to large cooperative operations consisting of as many as tens of thousands of birds. This has resulted in increases from millions to something like two billion birds annually. This increase occurred during the period of a human generation. Similar increases might occur elsewhere.

Because of a gradual increase in efficiency based on better economic analyses and practices, it has been duly recognized that beef and pork are expensive to produce, about 10 to 15 times as much as poultry, which is a relatively inexpensive source of protein. Cockrill (1964) considers poultry the most adaptable of domestic food animals to climate and regional conditions. He indicates an important point—that disease is the limiting factor in poultry production. Poultry consumption will surely increase in various parts of the world, and it is in those areas where the results of much research on poultry disease problems will be most needed for production of an efficient and dependable protein food source.

Although food production is the primary need, it should also be carefully noted that related disease problems, particularly parasitic ones, cannot be overlooked for long. They must be sought for, recognized, and dealt with early. Parasite problems tend to be hidden and hence often overlooked. When they are not completely hidden, they appear to be minor factors in comparison with other infectious diseases. On the other hand, parasite problems may not show up until husbandry practices bring them on. The most obvious problem of this sort is the one created by the crowding of animals brought about by the intensified use of land, a point emphasized by Card (1961). Constant close proximity of hosts tips the biologic balance in favor of the parasites, as well as of infectious disease of any kind. Also, other factors such as genetic selection for meat and egg production probably tend to encourage the perpetuation of birds which are susceptible to various infectious diseases, including helminths.

Some idea of the relative importance of helminth parasites is indicated in a ranking of diseases based on Poultry Conference Reports in the United States from 1960 to 1965; those due to helminths were fairly low, ranging from a high of 13 percent to a low of less than 1.0 percent. *Ascaridia* infections are the most common at 5.5 percent (range 2 to 13), *Capillaria* at 1.0 percent (range 0 to 4.2), tapeworms at 1.0 percent (range 0 to 2.3), and *Heterakis* at 0.8 percent (range 0 to 1.3). Despite the fact that the figures appear so small, buildups with epidemic characteristics occur, which are serious. Consequently, there is a steady drain on meat and egg production.

Agriculture Handbook No. 291 (1965), based on experience in the United States, presents a comprehensive viewpoint of the husbandry losses in poultry due to parasites (protozoan and metazoan). The helminths cause about

22 percent of these losses. In comparison with coccidiosis alone, which is considered a major disease, helminths cause a 36 percent loss. These are impressive figures, especially since poultry practices are relatively advanced where they occur.

On the other hand, the toll of helminth parasites outside the United States is formidable. Correa (1963), in Guatemala, indicates a 150,000 dollar loss on 700,000 birds (about 21 percent) of which a large part was due to helminths. Polakova (1965), in Czechoslovakia, finds that *Ascaridia* alone caused a loss of 96,200 kg in a million hens during one year (about 8 percent). These examples clearly show that helminths still play an important part in poultry husbandry in most areas of the world, both in highly developed economies as well as those less developed. Other aspects of the morbidity and mortality problems are discussed by Card (1961), Biester and Schwarte (1965), and Soulsby (1965).

Metazoa of importance

Depending upon the species of host fowl, there will be different kinds of worms involved in producing morbidity and mortality. In addition, the helminths of importance will vary according to the region or country in which the husbandry exists. In other words, the kind of bird and the regional ecosystems will determine the major parasites.

Knowledge of the culprit parasites will, of course, come from surveys based on necropsies. Fecal examinations would contribute useful but less accurate data, since immature forms may be present, and consequently no eggs or larvae would be available for diagnostic purposes. In addition, slaughterhouse records would add usable information. Trained people are mandatory for these important, specific diagnoses, since the information derived provides the basis for assessing the extent of problems and eventually the plans for instituting specific control measures. When control methods are in force, surveillance must be maintained in order to support the desired standards.

There is no comprehensive worldwide compilation of economically important internal parasites available. Publications on regional parasite incidence are limited and discontinuous, but compilations of limited value may be made for gaining some perspective on the relative size and extent of the parasitic problems. Introductory backgrounds regarding specific helminth parasites and their pathology are provided by Gardiner (1956) and Wehr and Farr (1956) for the continental United States, by Ershov (1956) for the U.S.S.R., by Alicata (1964) for Hawaii, by Segal et al. (1968) for the Vietnam-Thailand-Laos-Cambodia area, by Soulsby (1968) for Africa and in general, and by Soulsby (1965) and Biester and Schwarte (1965) on a worldwide basis.

An abbreviated classification of some of the important helminths will be

considered in the interests of establishing the scope of the subject. Taxonomically, the Metazoa are divided into the phylum Nemathelminthes, which includes the class Nematoda (roundworms) and the class Acanthocephala (thorny-headed worms), and the phylum Platyhelminthes, which includes the class Cestoda (tapeworms) and the class Trematoda (flukes). A majority of the disease problems stemming from helminths are caused by nematodes. Considering chickens alone, probably eight genera (including *Ascaridia* and *Heterakis*) cause most of the troubles. Among the cestodes six genera are of importance; among the trematodes six genera produce significant degrees of debility.

A further complicating feature of helminth disease is the concomitant morbidity produced by mixed infections consisting of three or four species. When domestic fowl are considered in the broad sense (chickens, turkeys, ducks, geese, and guinea hens) the list of culprit parasites increases markedly and includes the thorny-headed worms. The total species in a problem area may easily increase to one dozen.

Ecologic factors

The influence of the environment will vary according to geographic location and climate; besides, the soil, water sources, and local fauna may be reservoirs of helminth parasites to which the particular poultry involved may be susceptible. The type of husbandry system employed will more or less modify the influence of the birds' environmental factors.

In the life cycle of the parasite, the two environments it must contend with under natural conditions are the environments external and internal to the host. A third, artificial environment for the parasite is the laboratory *in vitro* environment, which appears to be equally or more hazardous than natural surroundings.

Studies concerned with factors external to the host, such as moisture films, particle size, and relationships in the soil, have been discussed and summarized by Lee (1965). An interesting and refreshing approach to ecologic concepts in nematology is given by Wallace (1962). The plant and animal parasitic nematodes, although living in entirely different environments, may prove to have surprisingly close affinities which could lead to novel approaches in animal nematode immunology. Seemingly remote information can become very useful when applied to real problems in the cultivation of similar organism stages, e.g., in the culture of larvae. Carrying the thought further, larvae, adults, and eggs or metabolic products of the plant nematodes might be used for antigenic materials against the poultry parasitic forms. Demski (1966) initiated a probe along these lines, using *Rhabditis* to sensitize against *Dictyocaulus* with positive results.

Read (1950) has reported on internal host factors of the digestive tract which is external to the host in the anatomic and embryologic senses.

Secondly, internal host factors from the parenteral viewpoint, in which the host and the parasite interact more intimately, are discussed by Stauber (1960).

Methods of control

In the attempts to control infectious disease problems, it soon becomes apparent that all direct and indirect preventive methods need to be used to some degree. No single method gives complete control. The larger or more important the problem, the more supporting control methods are used. Besides a protective vaccine, and in support of it, the following types of control must be considered:

Chemical (Direct)
1. Chemotherapy against parasite stages in the host. When used in conjunction with a vaccine, it may enhance its function.
2. Chemicals applied to the environment outside the host to control nonparasitic stages of the life cycle.

Physical (Direct and Indirect)
1. Barriers such as wire floors and fences.
2. X-ray attenuation of organism stages, particularly the infective stage.
3. Litter removal, an important factor in maintaining infection rate, according to Reid et al. (1964), when it is not done properly.

Biologic (Direct and Indirect)
1. Alternate hosts such as ducks and geese to absorb some of the helminths which would otherwise go to the principal host. Alternate hosts are more effective if the parasites do not injure or kill them.
2. Vector control: earthworms, insects, or other carriers such as wild birds.
3. (a) Alteration of the parasite by passage through other hosts, or by modified culture techniques to provide antigenic material.
   (b) The use of intact parasitic organisms or fractions thereof for antigens.
4. Raising resistant birds through genetic manipulations.

Political (Direct and Indirect)
1. Regulations preventing the importation of infected birds into a country.
2. Regulations on transportation of infected birds from area to area within a country.

The life cycles of helminths are of great importance in reaching an understanding of the problems of control, since certain points in the cycles are susceptible to control measures and since stages of the parasite outside the host should be considered as a source of substances for inducing immunity. More-

over, stages in the life cycle may introduce other parasites, e.g., *Heterakis* sometimes carries *Histomonas*. It is of interest to note that while the eggs of *Heterakis* were considered important as carriers of *Histomonas*, it has recently been shown (Lund et al., 1966), that earthworms are probably the principal vehicle. Another view, that of Spindler (1967), indicates that sow bugs may be significant vectors. Probably both earthworms and sow bugs are vectors under field conditions. It would be advantageous to determine the main vector since the methods of control would be different; the resulting savings in control cost could be substantial.

In conducting surveys of any size, the quality of laboratory work is of great importance, since it is of critical consequence to obtain accurate diagnoses and identification of both known and new species. One cannot place too much emphasis on this matter. One aspect of the problem is covered on the identification of parasite species by Reid (1959) who points out the need for trained people; another, from the broader aspects of economics, by Sadler (1961); and still another, from the general viewpoint of the necessity of teamwork, by Nestler (1962).

IMMUNOLOGY

Contributions to the literature on immunology have increased substantially since 1964, including basic studies concerned with the nature of the immune response and the tissues involved. Graetzer et al. (1963) reported on the various lymphoid organs, particularly the bursa of Fabricius, and how they are involved in immunity. Claflin et al. (1966) showed a relationship between the thymus and bursa in antibody response. Dreesman et al. (1965) showed that antibody species may be related to the nature of the immunizing antigen, as shown by serum globulins. Glick and Whatley (1967) showed that the bursa produces an immunoglobulin serum fraction, IgM. Marinkovich and Baluda (1966) reported *in vitro* production of 19S IgM-like globulin in tissue cell cultures. Delhanty and Solomon (1966) reported that four different types of serum antibodies are produced by the responses of young and adult chickens: two IgM's, possibly one IgA, and one IgG.

Recently, many new aspects of genetics, serology, immunochemistry, and related fields have been covered. Excellent discussions and summaries approaching immunology from different viewpoints and also considering the various problems involved in mammalian immune phenomena are available in Soulsby (1957, 1961), Smyth (1962), Soulsby (1962a, b), and Tromba (1962), as well as elsewhere. Gordon (1957) provides a comprehensive coverage of the expected developments in sheep husbandry—many of the same principles are directly applicable to poultry husbandry. More specialized discussions on possible mechanisms of immunity depending on the types of helminths are given in regard to nematodes in sheep (Soulsby, 1966), on schistosomiasis (Kagan, 1966), and on cestodes (Weinman, 1966). Perusal of these discussions will provide much material which may suggest applications to the immunology of poultry helminths.

Nutritional factors

Present day practices in poultry husbandry do not appear to consider rations except insofar as they are related to meat and egg production. We know that a well-nourished healthy animal is more tolerant of disease. Is it true, then, that in the dominating press for economic advantage, all other factors are to be considered minimal or even inessential? Can the chicken outrun the parasites, as it were, and get to the market before their effects are felt? The answer to the latter is negative, and it is amply supported by data presented in the Agriculture Handbook No. 291 (1965).

The effect of nutrition upon immunity may be profound. At least that is what mammalian studies on the host-parasite relationship have demonstrated with proteins and carbohydrates. Earlier, no effect of diet with respect to resistance of chickens to *Heterakis* was found by Clapham (1934). However, increased dietary protein appears to have an appreciable effect on increased resistance to *Ascaridia*, as shown earlier by Ackert and Beach (1933). Also, pteroylglutamic acid with a liver extract had a suppressive effect on the development of *Ascaridia*, according to Sadun et al. (1950), whereas glycine and leucine were found to have no value in increasing resistance to *Ascaridia* (Reidel, 1954, 1955). Diets low in phosphorus and calcium reduced the growth and number of *Ascaridia* in chickens, as shown by Gaafar and Ackert (1953).

According to Reidel and Ackert (1951) the type and source of proteins have a significant effect on the resistance of ascarid-infected chickens. The effect of vitamins has been studied: Vasilev (1961) found that vitamin B_{12} enhanced resistance to *Ascaridia*, and Krone (1963) found an increased resistance to *Heterakis* with vitamin A. Leutskaya (1964) confirmed earlier work showing that vitamin A increased antibody response to *Ascaridia*, but this could also have been due to age differences in the hosts. Additional in-depth studies along this line would yield new useful information, as well as explaining some apparently contradictory reports. With our limited knowledge of the effects of nutrition on resistance to helminthoses, it is a peculiar omission to find rations currently based only on growth requirements of the host and its egg production to the exclusion of other considerations. It would be ironical to find ultimately that the worms have been supported in nutritional luxury.

Biochemical factors

Investigations have followed several lines of endeavor in the last five years. Studies on resistance to helminths have assumed that a lack of metabolic elements (consisting of nutritional elements in the physiologic milieu required by the parasite) due to developmental or physiologic immaturity of the host might be unfavorable to the worms. Rogers (1962) presents a provocative summary of some of the particular biochemical factors and requirements of helminths in their associations with the host.

Genetic defects in the susceptible host animal and alterations in metabolism have also been considered. Genetic manipulation to increase resistance to parasites could provide a durable long-lasting protection. However, it is well to remember that the worms also have adaptive faculties, and a partially worm resistant breed today could, in time, become relatively susceptible through parasite adaptation. Ample evidence is provided from the area of chemotherapy to show that insects, protozoa, and helminths can adapt to and survive various lethal chemical treatments.

The identification of antigens has centered around proteins and protein complexes with lipids and carbohydrates, as well as polypeptides. The specific determination of the proteins involved becomes the intriguing task of the biochemist, the molecular biologist, and the immunochemist. A multiple, many faceted approach is provided by Cheng (1963). In addition, a good discussion and summary of techniques is given by Sober et al. (1965).

Another useful discussion of the quantitative problems in methodology concerned with determining the degree of protective and nonprotective antigens with related antibody is given by Singer (1965). The problems of determining the specific chemical identity of both antigen and antibody are major goals. However, it appears that antigenicity, in part, is related to certain types of proteins with certain substituent groups, so that when these chemical structures are present antigenicity results (Sela, 1966). The use of polystyrene to make protein conjugates is another chemical modification which is of interest (Steele, 1965). With this sort of evidence available, it seems practical to consider making weak antigens strong and, perhaps, making good antigens more potent with various immunogenic chemical substituents, possibly by procedural modifications similar to those reported by Adler (1967). Another approach toward increasing the potency of protective antigens has been achieved by means of adjuvants. Here again, is a neglected area. There has been no extensive effort to find new or improved adjuvants, nor for enhancing weak protective antigens.

Natural versus acquired immunity

Good and Papermaster (1964) found that the antibody-producing capability of chicks up to four weeks of age was very low, but between four to five weeks, a sudden development occurred. They considered that immunologic maturity in the chicken was reached at about five weeks and that this event was correlated with spleen size. Maturation of immunologic capability continues throughout life and is derived from thymus-lymphoid tissue and the bursa.

408   IMMUNITY IN AVIAN HOSTS

So-called age resistance is a form of natural resistance and is specifically related to factors such as tissue resistance, an increase in a cellular component, or to a more mature immunogenic capacity of the host. Clapham (1934) was unable to demonstrate age resistance with *Heterakis* in chickens, but subsequently Daugalieva (1966) showed that it occurs. The difference in results probably is due to a more comprehensive experimental time interval in the latter study. In turkeys, an age resistance was shown with a tapeworm, *Raillietina* (Kireev, 1965). Ackert et al. (1935b) and Darski (1962) found that lightweight breeds suffered more debility from *Ascaridia* than heavier breeds, and that cocks had a greater incidence and intensity of infection than hens. He also found that an increase in the age of the birds was related to a decrease in intensity and incidence of infection. The inverse relationship between breed weight and morbidity found by Darski was apparently confirmed by Jaffe (1966), who observed a greater antibody response in birds with larger bursas. (Jaffe's data assume a direct relationship of body weight and bursal size.)

The environment in which birds are kept has an important bearing (independently of host resistance) on the worm parasite population, which will become established without adequate control measures. In regard to numbers as well as variety of worms, farm flocks have the most, floor layers have less, and cage layers have the least. This kind of parasitic helminth array was observed for *Heterakis* (Dixon and Hansen, 1965).

Another approach toward developing acquired immunity is that of using another organism to instill immunity against a more pathogenic one. Phrased another way, are there any host-protective interactions between different genera or species of parasitic organisms? One such interaction was studied among three species which commonly appear in chickens: *Heterakis*, *Ascaridia*, and *Histomonas*. Based on the varying sizes of adult *Heterakis*, there was evidence of resistance (Madsen, 1962a). In another instance, histomoniasis was followed by heterakiasis; the prior protozoan infection decreased resistance to *Heterakis* (Joyner, 1966). This finding is not surprising since the debilitating effects of histomoniasis very probably reduced protective response to the helminth infection. Although Clapham (1934) in using *Heterakis* was unable to show appreciable protection against reinfection, Shikhobalova (1956a) demonstrated protection against reinfection with *Syngamus*. The important features involved in these two examples are (1) *Heterakis* may be a weak stimulator of resistance because of its location, or because it is better adapted to the host, and (2) *Syngamus* appears to be a more potent antigen producer than *Heterakis* even though both worms engage in minimal tissue penetration. Cross-protection was demonstrated between *Syngamus skrjabinomorpha* and *S. trachea* (Shikhobalova, 1956b). From the suggestive evidence at hand, it seems logical to expect that there would be some combination of worm species which would induce strong protection.

Another aspect of increasing resistance was reported by Benoit et al. (1957) in which DNA extracted from the testicular tissue of donor ducks was used to bring about a hormone-mediated somatic transformation in recipient ducks. While this procedure would hardly fit true mutation, it does have suggestive merit. An interferon or related system is suggested by the study. In fact, Brown and Nakano (1967) have provided the next step by showing that polyadenylic and polycytidylic acids enhance antibody formation when given in close conjunction with an antigen.

Acquired resistance using normal or natural worms has been demonstrated by Lund (1958, 1967) with *Heterakis*. Malviya and Deo (1966), using *Ascaridia*, were able to show complete resistance to challenge. The mechanism of "self-cure" has been observed in chickens (Graham et al. 1932, Lund, 1958, and Bhattacharjee, 1960).

Another way of reaching the acquired resistant state is by x-ray attenuation of the infective stage of the subject worm. Varga (1964a,b) used *Ascaridia* but did not obtain a high degree of protection; with *Syngamus* a substantial degree of protection was achieved (Varga, 1964c, 1965, 1966; Zeigler, 1966). Although x-ray attenuation is quite a remarkable concept, it has marked disadvantages if used in mass production: the system necessary for the supply of infective larvae to be attenuated poses a problem in production, and the viability of the attenuated living material is of short duration, thus requiring a constant fresh supply.

Other means of attenuation, such as chemical or thermal, need investigation. Another way to modify the immune response was used by Kendall (1965): in this instance, resistance was reduced by diethylcarbamazine to a non-avian worm, *Dictyocaulus*. Failure to enhance resistance might have been due to wrong timing in administration, inappropriate drug dose level, or even using a chemical substance inimical to the immune response.

The manners in which investigations are carried out are multiple. Some are naturalistic in design, others are quite artificial, even bizarre. Madsen (1962b) showed this has considerable influence on experimental outcomes, e.g., with natural hosts and infective dosage as compared to artificial hosts and infective dosage, a low infective dose may be ineffective, whereas a very high dose may mask any response. Frequently, animals are infected with unnaturally high numbers of organisms, the results of which could easily mask any significant responses. Infective doses should be somewhere in the neighborhood of those found in natural populations.

Genetic factors

The influence of genetics on the physical, physiologic, immunologic makeup is generally accepted. Earlier studies used this approach with respect to developing chickens resistant to nematodes, but it has not been followed extensively. An early attempt was made by Ackert and Wilmoth (1934) in introducing cockerels highly susceptible to ascarids to a resistant flock, which resulted in a definite depression of resistance in the following generation. Shikhobalova (1956a) found that cockerels were more resistant to *Syngamus* than pullets.

Berghen (1966) found serum protein changes in *Capillaria* infections indicating that pigeons were susceptible though chickens were resistant. This change consisted of an increase in globulins, which indicated antibody formation, while albumins remained at normal levels. Ackert and Eisenbrandt (1935) found turkeys more resistant to *Ascaridia* than chickens. However, based on worm populations, the number of *Ascaridia* was two and one-half times greater in turkeys than in chickens, according to Dixon and Hansen (1965). These conflicting results may not be in strong disagreement if experimental conditions were equated. No differences were found in resistance to *Ascaridia* between imported standard breeds of chickens and native Egyptian strains (Reid, 1955).

It is apparent that age resistance depends on cellular and humoral factors, since the physiology of young birds (chicks) differs from that of older birds (layers and breeders). Besides the age difference, it would appear that the habits of the younger birds as compared to the older ones would have considerable effect on exposure to the parasites, e.g., the relatively sedentary layers are essentially isolated from internal parasite contact, whereas the breeders might not be. Consequently, any resistance classified as "age resistance" needs to be qualified by more specific designation or explanation of behavioral and environmental circumstances.

It was also shown by Stone and Irwin (1963), that artificial selection relative to blood groups in poultry flocks favors the heterozygote, the result of which may turn out to have some important bearing on antibody formation.

Methodology for determining inherited differences in birds has provided a useful basis for selecting resistant strains. A technique of determining genetic differences in birds using rabbits immunized to chicken blood plasma has been suggested by Berry and Dolyak (1961). Another approach, which appears to be an accurate and simple procedure, is that of inoculating white cells from the blood or spleen of adult chickens on to the chorioallantoic membrane of 9- to 11-day-old chicks (Sharon, 1965). The resulting pathology was indicative of genetic differences: the stronger the reaction, the greater the differences. This technique could be used in conjunction with metazoan tolerance studies to develop resistant breeds.

Raising helminth-resistant birds would be an efficient way to avoid the effects of worms. Resistant breeds would reduce or negate the necessity for control measures involving chemical and physical resources, as well as the need for vaccines. How well meat production and egg laying features can be reconciled with worm resistance should be an intriguing study.

The negative effects of breeding poultry for market production have yet to be delineated. A clue to the insidious manner in which antagonistic factors may be operating relative to parasite acquisition or resistance is provided by Kamrin (1967). Inbreeding is given as an example of how birds may develop an immune tolerant state (ITS) which is defined as suppression of the immunologic system so that it will not readily reject foreign tissues or cells. In the ITS there is a marked change in behavior expressed in increased physical activity in two ways: following a stimulus object consistently, and an escape activity in response to situations. In practical terms, inbreeding may result in birds highly susceptible to worm infections, as well as poor weight gainers, because of their behavioral responses to environmental stimuli.

A classical example of a practical application of genetic resistance is provided by Brahma cattle, which were selected for their greater tick resistance and hot weather tolerance in comparison to Hereford and Angus. A similar selection for parasite resistance could be made in poultry breeds in which suggestive evidence indicates appreciable breed differences. When a substantial degree of resistance occurs along with other desirable features, some method of enhancing the natural resistance might be sought, thereby utilizing a natural advantage.

Passive immunity

Passive immunity generally is not regarded with much favor since it has been found in mammals that the protection given by this method is usually not of long duration. There is also the possibility of sensitivity developing if multiple injections are used. However, in view of the husbandry practices that provide birds for the market at ages which are in the range of passive protection (60 to 90 days), it seems that a method using passive immunity may well have application to helminth problems for their first several months. Vatne (1963) showed that sera from birds experimentally infected with *Heterakis* and *Ascaridia* provided significant protection in recipients challenged with infective eggs of *Heterakis*. Evidence of protection was based on larva length and numbers surviving. Using *Escherichia coli*, Malkinson (1965) demonstrated a transfer of passive immunity from hens to chicks. A study, which appears to be contradictory, showed that passive immunization of chickens with *Ascaridia* brought about an increase in the number of worms in the immunized birds (Egerton and Hansen, 1955). Apparently the level of antigen was just enough to somehow stimulate overcompensation by the worms; the study, however, has not been reproduced.

Antibody transmission through the egg would provide a basic mechanism for the practical application of passive immunity. Orlans (1967) has provided interesting evidence, using red blood cells, that a passive immunity may be transferred from egg yolk to chick. If this technique can be applied to specific worm parasites, an important goal would be achieved. Extending this idea further, it may be possible to inoculate the egg with protective antibodies to enhance passive immunity in either degree or duration. The most critical period of chick susceptibility is from the time of hatch to about 90 days age. If the egg could be inoculated with an appropriate specific antibody known to protect for about 90 days, the objective would be won. Other approaches might employ an adjuvant to enhance egg antibody potency or a formulation to prolong existing egg antibody life after hatching.

Another phenomenon to be investigated is "crop feeding" such as found in pigeon squabs. Although this particular mechanism of possible passive antibody transmission would be more limited in terms of practical application than the egg method, it might reveal an oral transmission of antibody.

Specific versus general immunity

All the examples of resistance and immunity which have been mentioned in the present discussion are quite specific and apparently do not extend beyond the generic level. This specificity extends into mammalian immunology where it is wide-spread. Does this substantial weight of evidence deny the possibility of developing a vaccine against two or three species? Very possibly yes, but it is also worth trying to find evidence to the contrary. This probably will be done by not following in the footsteps of classical immunology. Various degrees of innovation are necessary.

The use of a less pathogenic parasitic nematode to produce immunity against a more pathogenic one is a possibility. Protection derived from this method may stem from common antigens, which would be sufficiently group-specific at the generic level. Or it might be that metabolic products of the vaccinating nematode are toxic to the challenge organism. If the idea of broad protection is carried further, unrelated species from a different environment entirely (e.g., plant nematodes) might be used to produce antigens for stimulating protection against animal nematode species, as was suggested by Wallace (1962). Such an approach has been tried by Demski (1966), using free-living *Rhabditis* as a vaccine and challenging with the lungworm, *Dictyocaulus*, thereby attempting to utilize a mechanism of presensitization. This method produced some positive results which were encouraging.

The use of a less harmful parasitic nematode to protect against a more pathogenic one is an interesting concept. Protection achieved by this type of preparation possibly stems from a common antigen which might be group-specific at the generic level. Another aspect is that of interference of one species by another, such as *Trichuris muris* and *Aspicularis tetraptera* in the mouse (Keeling, 1961). This interspecific antagonism seemed to be due to metabolic products which were produced by the interfering parasite, and not immunity of the host. But perhaps these metabolic products could be used as antigens to produce immunity against the target species.

Humoral versus cellular factors

Resistance of older birds to *Ascaridia* is attributed by Ackert et al. (1939) to the presence of thermostable growth-inhibiting substances in the mucoscretion of goblet cells of the intestinal tract. The maximum resistance to *Ascaridia* in older birds is reached in about 93 days, according to Ackert et al. (1935a). Clapham (1939) found older chicks more resistant to *Syngamus* than younger birds. Also, Shikhobalova (1956b) demonstrated an antibody response in chicks vaccinated with *Syngamus*. In this case, the resistance is probably not due to goblet cells but some other factors since *Syngamus* locates in the esophagus. Egerton and Hansen (1955) found evidence of a humoral factor based on the weight gains of birds immunized with both normal and protective sera, which increased tolerance to the toxic metabolic products of *Ascaridia*.

Jaffe (1966) found two populations of immunologically competent cells: one derived from the thymus and responsible for cell-mediated reactions; the second, from the bursa and responsible for the population of immunologically compotent cells. The possibility of a third antibody was mentioned. The interrelationships are not clear, but a working hypothesis based on the functions of the thymus has been stated by Persich (1966).

Another concept has been proposed by Todd and Hansen (1951) by which a differentiation is made between immunity to infection and immunity to disease. Egerton and Hansen (1955) gave evidence supporting their proposal to include a concept of the "tolerant" state. Here is an example of the important but little understood relationship existing between the host and the parasite. Though it is known that there are products formed by the host, products formed by the parasite, and products formed as a result of interaction between the two (the last products possibly containing the antigens which are responsible for stimulating protective antibodies), identification of the mechanisms involved and the active materials will tax ingenuity.

Avian and mammalian immunity compared

Most research in immunology has been done with mammals. Sufficient methodology now exists to permit research with birds and reptiles in order to compare immunologic phenomena and determine which features are common or unique. More knowledge of basic immunologic phenomena would have considerable value in extending our concepts of the mechanisms involved.

Initial studies have established some very interesting facts. Peyer's patches in the intestines of mammals appear to be the equivalent of the bursa in chickens (Cooper et al., 1966). The lymph nodules in chicken spleen are equivalent to mammalian lymph nodes and the spleen, and evidence also indicates that the bursa of chickens produces a humoral agent which acts to confer immune reactivity, at least in part (St. Pierre and Ackerman, 1966). Jaffe (1966) also indicated that the bursa, as well as the thymus, produces immunologically competent cells. From these few studies, it is suggested that there may be a closer similarity than previously thought between the avian system of immunity and the reticuloendothelial system of mammals.

Persich (1966), in a concise and informative summary on mechanisms of immunity, gives a chronology of the salient features of various theories of immunity. Especially noteworthy is an explanation of the role of the thymus in poultry immunity, indicating that it serves as an important transitory precursor to initiating the establishment of the immunity system of the adolescent and adult chicken. In other words, the thymus acts to trigger the immunologic competence of the chick, a process which appears to take several weeks after hatching. If this is true, it suggests that there may be no passive transfer of maternal immunogens through the egg. However, the story is just beginning to unfold and doubtless there will be phenomena found which we are not aware of presently.

In vitro culture of helminths

Since a parasitic worm is difficult to study when it is inside the host, it is convenient to study the organism outside the host where it can be seen. However, it is well to remember that in removing the organism from its normal habitat, an artificial situation is created in which the complex natural host-parasite relationship is broken. Perhaps what we seek in the way of protective antigens is produced, at least in part, during the intimate union of host and parasite.

However, *in vitro* studies can give some useful information, as shown by the elegant and fascinating work of Roche and Layrisse (1966) on the method of feeding of the canine hookworm, *Ancylostoma caninum*. Nutritional requirements of the parasites may be discovered by such studies, from which some indirect clues may be provided regarding metabolic pathways that would be subject to immunochemical attack.

Culturing techniques will provide the following immunologic tools:
1. Metabolic products or excretions as immunogens.
2. The production of adult and larva helminth material for vaccine application.
3. The determination of physiologic patterns and systems, e.g., the metabolic pathways.
4. Means for attenuating parasites by physical or chemical methods for the possible production of a vaccine.

Thorson (1963) has suggested a method by which vaccines may be made: (1) Find and characterize the active enzyme or protein mosaic, (2) Produce the mosaic in practical quantity, (3) Determine the biochemical structure, (4) Synthesize the protective antigen-antibody mosaic. As he points out, all steps are feasible, but the end product, the vaccine, will take some time to realize. *In vitro* culture could be useful here. Tromba (1962) suggested that study of the functions of cells and tissues of helminths *in vitro* will provide leads toward protective antigens which might be distinct and different from those used for diagnostic purposes.

Extensive background is provided on physiology and biochemistry of parasitic helminths by Rogers (1962), Cheng (1963), and von Brand (1966). Here the helminths infecting chickens have been studied along with those infecting mammalian hosts, though only briefly. The interesting aspects of artificial culture, however, strongly suggest attaining some success in finding a vaccine. In general, secretions or other metabolic substances have amply demonstrated an ability to induce strong protection, whereas living and dead worms and fractions from nonintact worms demonstrate weaker or no detectable protection-inducing capacity (Weinstein, 1960). Additional discussions of excretory products by other parasites are given by Stauber (1960). The collection of parasite metabolites would be possible if there were appropriate culture or maintenance techniques for helminths. If excretory products are of prime importance as immunogens, it seems self-evident that *in vitro* culture should be vigorously supported by more extensive investigations. Taylor and Baker (1968) have summarized the methodology in this area and have provided a basis for expansion and innovation.

New host-parasite systems

A new approach or a further deployment of ideas is needed in the area of poultry research. Mammals are widely used for several pilot model host systems in research. Poultry-parasite systems are infrequently considered and thus infrequently used. A notable exception is the use of avian malaria, in which results of experimental antimalarial chemotherapy in avian hosts were extrapolated to human uses. Insufficient attention has been directed toward the reverse, i.e., applying knowledge of mammalian phenomena to avian uses. While details may differ, we need to know whether or not there are basic phenomena common to both.

The prophylactic approach should receive serious consideration—finding means for protecting the host against entry of the parasite or stopping development in the early larval stages before extensive tissue contact occurs are important. The goal is to block adult maturation with the ensuing major disease process, and at the same time preventing the passage of the parasite to other hosts. Smyth (1969) presents a fascinating discursive summary on certain host-parasite phenomena. He also shows that other organisms, which include single-celled animals, can provide much useful basic information when studied at the cellular and subcellular levels. The resulting information can be applied to multicellular parasites.

CONCLUSION

It is to be hoped that this presentation will stimulate interest and generate more activity in an area presently begging for attention. It was not intended to be fully discursive—there is much less knowledge about immunology in the avian area than in the mammalian. Rather than attempt an inflated treatment of poultry immunology based on mammalian analogies, this brief treatment indicates essentially the current status of the field. At the present time the science of immunology as applied to poultry is in its developing period; most pertinent data are less than ten years old.

It should be apparent that a tremendous amount of work needs to be done on the immunology of poultry to helminths, both protective and diagnostic, for practical and theoretical reasons. There is abundant room for workers in several scientific disciplines. They need to assist each other and to team up to help in building a background of information characterizing metazoan immunologic phenomena at the subcellular level, at the cellular level, at the organism level, and at the population level of both bird host and parasite.

Avian metazoan immunology is a tempting frontier of research. It is one of the least exploited areas of contemporary scientific investigations. New techniques, new concepts, and opportunities for original research both basic and applied—these attractive features in relation to an increasingly important worldwide food source should give ample summons to those seeking a scientific area in which to test their intellectual and technical mettle.

At the present state of knowledge, immune phenomena seem to be based on specific factors, based on the particular host and the particular parasite. Frequently, the host is in different states of maturation. Frequently, the studies are made in the laboratory in nondefinitive hosts. Small wonder then, that much of the data from apparently related studies are not decisive. From this background, a clear research target emerges, namely, the task of studying in depth the several sorts of worms and their effects on the various kinds of birds. Once patterns are discovered, the approaches to creating resistant birds would become more apparent.

Basic patterns of similar physiology will no doubt emerge from what are classified as different parasites. Basic metabolic pathways will be elucidated, similarities and differences will appear, and these will provide bases for enhancing or providing absolute immunity. The goal of fully effective poultry vaccines will require cooperation and data from the area of mammalian immunology as well.

REFERENCES

Ackert, J. E., and T. D. Beach. 1933. Resistance of chickens to the nematode, *Ascaridia lineata,* affected by dietary supplements. Trans. Amer. Micr. Soc., 52: 51-58.
———— and J. H. Wilmoth. 1934. Resistant and susceptible strains of white Minorca chickens to the nematode, *Ascaridia lineata* (Schneider). J. Parasit., 20: 323-324.
———— and L. L. Eisenbrandt. 1935. Comparative resistance of bronze turkeys and white leghorn chickens to the intestinal nematode, *Ascaridia lineata* (Schneider). J. Parasit., 21: 200-204.
———— D. A. Porter, and T. D. Beach. 1935a. Age resistance of chickens to the nematode, *Ascaridia lineata* (Schneider). J. Parasit., 21: 205-213.
———— L. L. Eisenbrandt, J. H. Wilmoth, B. Glading, and I. Pratt. 1935b. Comparative resistance of five breeds of chickens to the nematode, *Ascaridia lineata* (Schneider). J. Agric. Res., 50: 607-624.
———— S. A. Edgar, and L. P. Frick. 1939. Goblet cells and age resistance of animals to parasitism. Trans. Amer. Micro. Soc., 58: 81-89.
Adler, H. E. 1967. The antiglobulin procedure for the detection of antibodies of avian origin. Avian Dis., 11: 69-78.
Agriculture Handbook No. 291. 1965. Internal parasites of livestock and poultry. Washington, D. C., U. S. Government Printing Office.

Alicata, J. E. 1964. Parasitic infections of man and animals in Hawaii. Honolulu, Hawaii University, Tech. Bull. No. 61.

Benoit, J., P. Leroy, C. Vendrely, and R. Vendrely. 1957. Des mutations somatiques dirigées sont-elles possibles chez les oiseaux. C. R. Acad. Sci [D] (Paris), 244: 2320 and 245: 448.

Berghen, P. 1966. Serum protein changes in *Capillaria obsignata* infections. Exp. Parasit., 19: 34-41.

Berry, J. E., and F. Dolyak. 1961. Immunogenetic relationships between breeds of chickens. Poult. Sci., 40: 1363-1364.

Bhattacharjee, M. L. 1960. Beitrag zur Biologie and Epidemiologie von *Trichostrongylus tenuis* des Geflügels. Dissertation, Giessen. (*In* Helminth. Abstr., 1965. 34: 229.)

Biester, H. E., and L. H. Schwarte. 1965. Diseases of Poultry. Ames, The Iowa State University Press, 5th ed.

Brown, W., and M. Nakano. 1967. Antibody formation: stimulation by polyadenylic and polycytidylic acids. Science, 157: 819-821.

Card, L. E. 1961. Poultry Production. Philadelphia, Lea and Febiger, 9th ed.

Cheng, T. C., ed. 1963. Some biochemical and immunological aspects of host-parasite relationships. N. Y. Acad. Sci., 113: 1-510.

Claflin, A. J., O. Smithies and R. K. Meyer. 1966. Antibody responses in bursa-deficient chickens. J. Immun., 97: 693-699.

Clapham, P. A. 1934. Some observations on the response of chickens to infestation with *Heterakis gallinae*. J. Helminth., 12: 71-78.

———— 1939. On the larval migration of *Syngamus trachea* and its causal relationship to pneumonia in young birds. J. Helminth., 17: 159-162.

Cockrill, W. R. 1964. International trends in veterinary medicine. *In* Advances in Veterinary Science, Vol. 9. Brandly, C. A., and Jungherr, E. L., eds. New York, Academic Press, Inc., pp. 252 and 325.

Cooper, M. D., D. Y. Percy, M. F. McKneally, A. E. Gabrielsen, D. E. R. Sutherland, and R. A. Good. 1966. A mammalian equivalent of the avian bursa of Fabricius. Lancet, 1: 1388-1391.

Correa, W. M. 1963. Avian diseases in Guatemala. Poult. Sci., 42: 559-561.

Culbertson, J. T. 1941. Immunity against Animal Parasites. New York. Columbia University Press.

Darski, J. 1962. Some factors influencing the infectiveness and fertility of *Ascaridia galli* in chickens. Acta. Parasit. Polonica, 10: 411-418. (*In* Helminth. Abstr., 1964. 33: 7.)

Daugalieva, E. K. 1966. Age immunity against *Heterakis* in chickens. Vestn. Sel. Khoz. Nauki, Alma-Ata, 12: 62-65. (*In* Helminth. Abstr., 1967. 36: 411.)

Delhanty, J. J., and J. B. Solomon. 1966. The nature of antibodies to goat erythrocytes in the developing chicken. Immunology, 11: 103-113.

Demski, G. 1966. Increasing the resistance to parasitic infections. I. Sensitization with *Rhabditis axei* (Cobbold, 1884) against infections with bovine lungworm *Dictyocaulus viviparus* (Bloch, 1782). Arch. Exp. Vet. Med., 20: 599-607. (*In* Helminth. Abstr., 1967. 36: 430.)

Dixon, C. F., and M. F. Hansen. 1965. Helminths of poultry in Kansas. Poult. Sci., 44: 1307-1315.

Dreesman, G., C. Larson, R. N. Pinkard, R. M. Groyon, and A. A. Benedict. 1965. Antibody activity in different chicken globulins. Proc. Soc. Exp. Biol. Med., 118: 292-296.

Egerton, J. R., and M. F. Hansen. 1955. Immunity and tolerance of chickens to the roundworm, *Ascaridia galli* (Schrank). Exp. Parasit. 4: 335-350.

Ershov, V. S., ed. 1956. Parasitology and parasitic diseases of livestock. Moscow, State Publishing House for Agricultural Literature.

Gaafar, S. M., and J. E. Ackert. 1953. Studies on mineral deficient diets as factors in resistance of fowls to parasitism. Exp. Parasit., 2: 185-208.

Gardiner, J. L. 1956. Tapeworms of chickens and turkeys; roundworms. *In* Yearbook of Agriculture, Animal Diseases. Washington, D. C., U. S. Government Printing Office, pp. 484-490.

Glick, B., and S. Whatley. 1967. The presence of immunoglobulin in the bursa Fabricius. Poult. Sci., 46: 1587-1588.

Good, R. A., and B. W. Papermaster. 1964. Ontogeny and phylogeny of adaptive immunity. *In* Advances in Immunology, Vol. 4. Taliaferro, W. H., and Humphrey, J. H., eds. New York, Academic Press, Inc., pp. 1-115.

Gordon, H. M. 1957. Helminthic diseases. *In* Advances in Veterinary Science, Vol. 3. Brandly, C. A., and Jungherr, E. L., eds. New York, Academic Press, Inc., pp. 288-351.

Graetzer, M. A., W. P. Cote, and H. R. Wolfe. 1963. The effect of bursectomy at different ages on precipitin and natural haemagglutinin production in the chicken. J. Immun., 91: 576-581.

Graham, G. L., J. E. Ackert, and R. W. Jones. 1932. Studies on an acquired resistance of chickens to the nematode *Ascaridia lineata* (Schneider). Amer. J. Hyg., 15: 726-740.

Jaffe, W. P. 1966. Avian immunobiology. Poult. Sci., 45: 109-118.

Joyner, L. P. 1966. Infection with *Heterakis gallinarum* in chickens following recovery from histomoniases. Parasitology, 56: 171-177.

Kagan, I. G. 1966. Mechanisms of immunity in trematode infections. *In* Biology of Parasites; Emphasis on Veterinary Parasites. Soulsby, E. J. L., ed. New York, Academic Press, Inc., pp. 277-299.

Kamrin, B. B. 1967. The effect of the immune tolerant state on early behaviour of domestic fowl. Anim. Behav., 15: 217-222.

Keeling, J. E. D. 1961. Experimental trichuriasis. I. Antagonism between *Trichuris muris* and *Aspicularis tetraptera* in the albino mouse. J. Parasit., 47: 641-646.

Kendall, S. B. 1965. The effect of large doses of diethylcarbamazine on the development of resistance to reinfection with *Dictyocaulus viviparus*. J. Comp. Path., 75: 443-448.

Kireev, N. A. 1965. Age susceptibility of turkeys to *Raillietina* infection. Veterinariya, 42: 60-62. (*In* Helminth. Abstr., 1967. 36: 57.)

Krone, G. 1963. Untersuchungen über den Einfluss unterscheidlicher Vitamin-A-Dosen im Kükenalleinfutter auf die *Heterakis gallinae* infektion. Dissertation, Berlin. (*In* Helminth. Abstr., 1966. 35: 101.)

Lee, D. L. 1965. The Physiology of the Nematodes. San Francisco, W. N. Freeman and Co.

Leutskaya, Z. K. 1964. Content of different forms of vitamin A in the liver and liver mitochondria after immobilization with antigen of *Ascaridia galli* of chickens deprived of Vitamin A. Dokl. Akad. Nauk SSSR, 159: 464-465. (*In* Helminth. Abstr., 1965. 34: 107.)

Lund, E. E. 1958. Studies on "self cure" and acquired resistance to *Heterakis* infections in chickens and turkeys. J. Parasit., 44: 27.

——— 1967. Acquired resistance to experimental *Heterakis* infections in chickens and turkeys: Effect on the transmission of *Histomonas meleagridis*. J. Helminth., 41: 55-62.

——— E. E. Wehr, and D. J. Ellis. 1966. Earthworm transmission of *Heterakis* and *Histomonas* to turkeys and chickens. J. Parasit., 52: 889-902.

Madsen, H. 1962a. On the interaction between *Heterakis gallinarum, Ascaridia galli,* "blackhead" and the chicken. J. Helminth., 36: 107-142.

——— 1962b. The so-called tissue phase in nematodes. J. Helminth., 36: 143-148.

Malkinson, M. 1965. The transmission of passive immunity to *Escherichia coli* from mother to young in the domestic fowl (*Gallus domesticus*). Immunology, 9: 311-317.

Malviya, H. C., and P. G. Deo. 1966. Effect of heavy primary infection on the subsequent light infection of *Ascaridia galli* (Schrank, 1788) Freeborn, 1923, in chickens. Indian Vet. J., 43: 689-691.

Marinkovich, V. A., and M. A. Baluda. 1966. *In vitro* synthesis of gamma-M-like globulin by various chick embryonic cells. Immunology, 10: 383-397.

Nestler, R. B. 1962. Disciplinary interrelationships: Are they being given proper consideration? Poult. Sci., 41: 745-750.

Orlans, E. 1967. Fowl antibody: a comparison of natural, primary and secondary antibodies to erythrocytes in hen sera: their transmission to yolk and chick. Immunology, 12: 27-37.

Persich, A. R. 1966. The mechanism of immunity in the light of current research. Amer. J. Med. Techn., 32: 77-84.

Polakova, M. 1965. Zamovenost drobeze askaridiozon a vliv invaze *A. galli* na vaher slepic. Vet. Med. (Praha), 38: 615-624. (*In* Helminth. Abstr., 1966. 35: 9.)

Proceedings Poultry Congress. 1968. Proceedings of the Third European Poultry Conference. Jerusalem, Israel. (Publication planned, 1970.)

Read, C. P., Jr. 1950. The vertebrate small intestine as an environment for parasitic helminths. Rice Institute Pamphlet No. 37, pp. 1-94.

Reid, W. M. 1955. Comparative resistance of imported standard breeds and native Egyptian strains of poultry to *Ascaridia galli*. Poult. Sci., 34: 30-35.

———— 1959. Egg characteristics as aids in species identification and control of chicken tapeworms. Avian Dis., 3: 188-197.

———— R. L. Kemp, and A. K. Prestwood. 1964. Infections with the tapeworm, *Raillietina cesticillus*, in Georgia poultry flocks. Avian Dis., 8: 347-358.

Reidel, B. B. 1954. The relationship of glycine to the resistance of chickens to the roundworm, *Ascaridia galli*. Poult. Sci., 33: 742-746.

———— and J. E. Ackert. 1951. Quantity and source of proteins as factors in the resistance of chickens to ascarids. Poult. Sci., 30: 497-502.

Roche, M., and M. Layrisse. 1966. The nature and cause of "hookworm anemia." Amer. J. Trop. Med. Hyg., 15 (Part 2): 1032-1102.

Rogers, W. P. 1962. The Nature of Parasitism: The Relationship of Some Metazoan Parasites to Their Hosts. New York, Academic Press, Inc.

Sadler, W. W. 1961. Adequacy of criteria used to evaluate the results of poultry disease research. Avian Dis., 5: 348-350.

Sadun, E. H., C. K. Keith, M. J. Pankey, and J. R. Totter. 1950. The influence of dietary pteroylglutamic acid and A.P.A. liver extract on survival and growth of the nematode, *Ascaridia galli*, in chickens fed purified and natural diets. Amer. J. Hyg., 51: 274-291.

Segal, D. B., J. M. Humphrey, S. J. Edwards, and M. D. Kirby. 1968. Parasites of man and domestic animals in Vietnam, Thailand, Laos, and Cambodia. Exp. Parasit., 23: 287-293.

Sela, M. 1966. Immunological studies with synthetic polypeptides. *In* Advances in Immunology, Vol. 6. Taliaferro, W. H., and Humphrey, J. H., eds. New York, Academic Press, Inc., pp. 29-129.

Sharon, R. 1965. Immunologic reaction as a means for determining purity of chicken strains. Poult. Sci., 44: 1612-1614.

Shikhobalova, N. P. 1956a. Immunity in chicks, acquired as a result of infection with *Syngamus*. Trud. Gel'mint. Lab., 8: 259-266. (*In* Helminth. Abstr., 1956. 25: 334.)

———— 1956b. Demonstration of precipitates in the blood of chicks infected with *Syngamus skrjabinomorpha*. Trud. Gel'mint. Lab., 8: 259-266. (*In* Helminth. Abstr., 1956. 25: 334.)

Singer, S. J. 1965. Structure and function of antigen and antibody proteins. *In* The Proteins: Composition, Structure and Function. Neurath, H., ed. New York, Academic Press, Inc., pp. 270-347.

Smyth, J. D. 1962. Introduction to Animal Parasitology. Springfield, Ill., Charles C Thomas, 1st ed.

———— 1969. Parasites as models. Parasitology, 59: 73-91.

Sober, H. A., R. W. Hartley, Jr., W. R. Carroll, and E. A. Petersen. 1965. Fractionation of proteins. *In* The Proteins: Composition, Structure and Function. Neurath, H., ed. New York, Academic Press, Inc., pp. 7-10 and 65-74.

Soulsby, E. J. L. 1957. Some immunological phenomena in parasitic infections. Vet. Rec., 69: 1129-1136.

———— 1961. Symposium on recent advances in the treatment and control of internal parasites. Immune mechanisms in helminth infections. Vet. Rec., 73: 1053-1058, 1069-1074.

———— 1962a. Immunity to helminths and its effect on helminth infection. *In* Animal Health and Production. Grunsell, C. S., and Wright, A. I., eds. Washington, D. C., Butterworth Co.

———— 1962b. Antigen-antibody reaction in helminth infections. *In* Advances in Immunology, Vol. 2. Taliaferro, W. H., and Humphrey, J. H., eds. New York, Academic Press, Inc., pp. 265-308.

———— 1965. Textbook of Veterinary Clinical Parasitology. Vol. 1, Helminths. Philadelphia, F. A. Davis.

———— 1966. The mechanisms of immunity in gastrointestinal nematodes. *In* Biology of Parasites; Emphasis on Veterinary Parasites. Soulsby, E. J. L., ed. New York, Academic Press, Inc., pp. 255-276.

———— 1968. Helminths, arthropods and protozoa of domestic animals. Monnig's Veterinary Helminthology and Entomology. Baltimore, The Williams and Wilkins Co., 6th ed.

Spindler, L. A. 1967. Experimental transmission of *Histomonas meleagridis* and *Heterakis gallinarum* by the sowbug. *Porcellio scaber*, and its implications for further research. Proc. Helminth. Soc. (Washington), 34: 26-29.

Stauber, L., ed. 1960. Host Influence on Parasite Physiology. New Brunswick, N.J., Rutgers University Press.
Steele, A. S. V. 1965. The immunising effects of polystyrene-protein conjugates. J. Path. Bact., 89: 691-701.
St. Pierre, R. L., and G. A. Ackerman. 1966. Influence of bursa implantation upon lymphocytic nodules and plasma cells in spleens of bursectomized chickens. Proc. Soc. Exp. Biol. Med., 122: 1280-1284.
Stone, W. H., and M. R. Irwin. 1963. Blood groups in animals other than man. In Advances in Immunology, Vol. 3. Dixon, F. J. Jr., and Humphrey, J. H., eds. New York, Academic Press, Inc., pp. 344-345.
Taylor, A. E. R., and J. R. Baker, 1968. The Cultivation of Parasites In Vitro. Oxford, Blackwell Scientific Publications.
Thorson, R. E. 1963. Seminar on immunity to parasitic helminths. II. Physiology of immunity to helminth infections. Exp. Parasit., 13: 3-12.
Todd, A. C., and M. F. Hansen. 1951. The economic import of host-resistance to helminth infection. Amer. J. Vet. Res., 12: 58-64.
Tromba, F. G. 1962. Immunology of nematode diseases. J. Parasit., 48: 839-845.
Varga, I. 1964a. Immunization experiments with irradiated larvae. I. Studies on the effect of X-rays on eggs and larvae of Ascaridia galli. Acta Vet. Hung., 14: 95-103. (In Helminth. Abstr., 1966. 35: 57.)
——— 1964b. Immunization experiments with irradiated larvae. II. The resistance-inducing effect of treatment with irradiated larvae of Ascaridia galli in chickens. Acta Vet. Hung., 14: 399-410. (In Helminth. Abstr., 1966. 35: 57.)
——— 1964c. Immunization experiments with irradiated larvae. III. The effect of X-rays upon eggs and larvae of Syngamus trachea. Acta Vet. Hung., 14: 411-418. (In Helminth. Abstr., 1966. 35: 57.)
——— 1965. Immunizálási Kiserlétek besugárzott Syngamus trachea-lárvákkal csirkékben. Magy. Allatorv. Lap., 20: 205-210. (In Helminth. Abstr., 1966. 35: 57.)
——— 1966. Naposcsibék immunizálása besugárzott Syngamus trachea-lárvákkal. Magy. Allatorv. Lap., 21: 197-200. (In Helminth. Abstr., 1966. 35: 394.)
Vasilev, I. 1961. (Effect of vitamin B_{12} and some antibiotics on the resistance of chickens to Ascaridia galli.) Izv. Tsent. Khelmint. Lab. (Sofia), 6: 33-42. (In Helminth. Abstr., 1968. 37: 294.)
Vatne, R. D. 1963. Aspects of the biology of Heterakis gallinarum (Nematoda) in chickens and their host-parasite relations. Dissertation Abstracts, 24: 1767-1768. (In Helminth. Abstr., 1964. 33: 164.)
von Brand, T. 1966. Biochemistry of Parasites. New York, Academic Press, Inc.
Wallace, H. R. 1962. The future of nematode ecology. J. Parasit., 48: 846-849.
Wehr, E. E., and M. M. Farr. 1956. Parasites affecting the ducks and geese. In Yearbook of Agriculture, Animal Diseases. Washington, D. C., U. S. Government Printing Office, pp. 500-502.
Weinman, C. J. 1966. Immunity mechanisms in cestode infections. In Biology of Parasites; Emphasis on Veterinary Parasites. Soulsby, E. J. L., ed. New York, Academic Press, Inc., pp. 302-320.
Weinstein, P. 1960. Excretory mechanisms and excretory products of nematodes: An appraisal. In Host Influence on Parasite Physiology. Stauber, L., ed. New Brunswick, N. J., Rutgers University Press, pp. 65-92.
Ziegler, K. 1966. Vakcinace kuřat proti syngamóze. Vet. Med. (Praha), 39: 569-578. (In Helminth. Abstr., 1968. 37: 296.)

6

Immunity in Mammalian Hosts

General Mechanisms and Principles
of Mammalian Immunity

ROY E. RITTS, JR.

Section of Microbiology, Mayo Clinic, Rochester, Minnesota

INTRODUCTION

The purpose of this chapter is to review briefly the new information in immunology that would be relevant to current studies in parasitology. There has been no attempt to present an exhaustive review of each possible topic, and several important areas such as immunologic tolerance and transplantation immunology have not been discussed except inasmuch as they bear on the selected topics. However, the bibliography has been chosen to be widely representative of newer data and, in addition to specific references, contains citations of excellent review articles or published symposia.

The complex subject of mammalian immune response to parasitic animals adds a frustrating and, seemingly, an almost perversely obfuscating dimension to immunology. Immunity to parasites violates no general principle of immunology, but it introduces new difficulties resulting from host-parasite interactions.

There are a number of complicating factors in immunity to parasitic animals that arise from the nature of the parasites themselves. Primarily, parasites constitute exceedingly complex antigenic mosaics. Cellular and multicellular constituents, excretions and secretions, body coverings and various other specific anatomic parts are capable of contributing antigenic stimuli to the host. Further, the variety of morphologic forms within the life cycle of the parasites, the varying methods and sites of invasion, and variation in host organ or tissue localization of the different forms add complicating factors to the problem. Thus, the host response must be examined not only with respect to individual antigenic stimuli, but also with respect to the overall expression of immunity to the particular form of the specific infecting parasite. There may be a humoral antibody response which is capable of "neutralization" of the organism in tissues, or which may even prevent the establishment of infection in general. Other antibody responses may result in sensitizing phenomena. A cellular delayed-type hypersensitivity response may occur as the primary reaction to parasitic antigens, or it may occur along with the early humoral response. Immunologic reactivity is the result of the combination of responses engendered by the various antigenic stimuli presented to the host at any time.

Such immunologic responses do not necessarily confer immunity. In fact, many of the antibodies seen in parasitic infections do not appear to contribute in any way to immunity, though some are responsible for allergic inflammatory responses which are capable of exacerbating the infection. Similarly, the delayed-type cellular response, either as an isolated event or in combination with a humoral response, may be the primary pathogenic mechanism of some infections.

ANTIBODY-ELICITING IMMUNOGENS

Antigens can be generally characterized by their common biochemical and physical properties. This type of characterization provides an operational definition of more practical and theoretical value than the mere statement that they are materials capable of inducing and reacting with antibody or immunologically competent cells.

It is generally understood that antigens possess chemical groupings which are different from all other substances normally coming into contact with the host's immunologically competent cells. It is true in theory that antigens are foreign to the host, but many "self" or autoantigens such as thyroglobulin can hardly be termed "foreign." However, it is clear that under normal circumstances these "self" substances are, in a sense, foreign to the host's immune mechanisms, since they are normally anatomically sequestered from the immunologically competent cells. Another parameter of foreignness is the configuration of the immunogen. Even very slight alterations in the steric arrangement of side-chains in a molecule can account for differences in antigenicity. The classic demonstrations by Landsteiner (1962) have indicated that even levo- and dextrorotatory isomers of a hapten, as well as the transfer of nitro groups from a *meta* to a *para* position on a benzene ring, can be distinguished by the immunologic mechanism.

Although it is well-known that very small molecular weight chemicals (haptens) may be immunogenic when conjugated *in vivo* or *in vitro* with protein carriers or other materials, there is a general molecular size limitation associated with immunogenicity. For proteins and carbohydrates, the immunogenicity is roughly proportional to the molecular weight. The lower limit for immunogenicity is in the order of molecular weight 3,800 (e.g., pancreatic glucagon) for proteins, but it is many hundred-fold higher for carbohydrates. Dextran (molecular weight approximately 100,000) is only weakly antigenic even under extraordinary experimental conditions, but its polymers (molecular weights of 500,000 to 600,000), although essentially chemically similar to dextran, are much more potent immunogens.

In addition to foreignness and relatively large size, it is thought that to be immunologic a substance must be soluble or digestible *in vivo*. Biologically inert materials such as cellulose apparently are unable to induce an immune reaction.

The route by which a putative immunogen is introduced into the host may be the determining factor in the kind of response thus engendered. For example, 2,4,6-trinitrochlorobenzene (picryl chloride) gives rise to a potent delayed-type hypersensitivity when given in minute amounts intracutaneously or when painted upon the skin with oil or acetone as the vehicle. Prior feeding of this hapten before attempted sensitization confers a durable tolerance (i.e., specific immunologic unresponsiveness). Also, when this hapten is appropriately conjugated to bovine serum albumin or chicken red-cell stromata *in vitro* (as opposed to the *in vivo* conjugation via disulfide linkages, as occurs in the skin) and given intravenously or subcutaneously, antipicryl antibodies are produced (Chase et al., 1963).

Because of the variety of antigenic stimuli presented to the host by parasitic animals, it is worth noting that multiple simultaneous administration of apparently unrelated immunogens may result in diminished antibody production. When they are given at the same time, ferritin and hemocyanin reduce the antibody response to bovine γ-globulin, and the γ-globulin similarly reduces the antiferritin antibody level. Conversely, it is well-known that "triple vaccine," consisting of tetanus toxoid, diphtheria toxoid, and heat-killed *Bordetella pertussis*, induces greater antibody production than do single doses of each immunogen. In this situation, *B. pertussis* is very likely acting as a potent adjuvant for the mixture, as well as an efficient immunogen. In any experimental study of immunity to parasitic animals, it is crucial that identifiable immunogens are used insofar as possible and that their effects are fully determined by altering the route of administration.

ANTIBODIES

Although a detailed discussion of the formation and structure of antibody is beyond the scope of this introduction, it seems pertinent to note that there appear to be relatively few attempts reported in recent literature to characterize the immunoglobulin responses seen in parasitic infections.

It is thought that when an immunogen is introduced into an organism, the critical factor is its eventual primary contact with macrophages. Intravenous administration of soluble antigens is followed by typical patterns of equilibration, metabolic decay, and "immune elimination," depending upon the state of immunity in the host (Talmage et al., 1951). Whether the antigenic stimuli in acquired infections behave similarly is doubtful, since except in overwhelming infections, most antigenic substances will be slowly elaborated in the tissue. The local inflammatory reaction with its attendant cellular response thus appears to be the first contact of the immunogen with the immune mechanism.

The role of macrophages is thought to involve considerably more functions than that of being only a vehicle for the antigen. A variety of experimental approaches and observations indicate that the antigen requires "activation" before being presented to the lymphocytic-plasma cell antibody-producing mechanism. Some antigens are thought to be nonimmunogenic when presented directly to lymphocytes, but the precise mechanism by which macrophages confer the immunogenic properties upon the antigenic materials is conjectural. Most conjecture involves the possibility of the antigen being associated in some way with macrophage RNA. Whether this effect is due to merely an adjuvant-like quality of RNA, a chemical change in the antigen, or a modification of the information contained in the RNA is not understood (Adler et al., 1966; Mannick and Egdahl, 1964; Gallily and Feldman, 1967; Fishman and Adler, 1967). It is possible that failure of macrophage-antigen interaction may be the basis of immunologic tolerance. That is, the direct presentation of an antigen to the plasma cell precursors without the intervention of the contribution from macrophages causes the immunologic mechanism to regard the antigen as "self" material.

The next step in antibody formation is thought to be the stimulation by "activated" antigen of small lymphocytes, causing them to differentiate into large, rapidly dividing "immunoblasts." The latter are reported to undergo asymmetrical division, forming the antibody-producing plasma cell and a large lymphocyte which eventually becomes the small lymphocyte with "memory storage." These "memory" cells are thought to persist for ten or more years in humans. There is evidence that antibodies are principally formed on the endoplasmic reticulum in plasma cells, but a small proportion seem to be formed in lymphocytes as well (dePetris et al., 1963; Harris et al., 1966; see also Harris, 1966, for a review). One of these lymphocytes, probably the smaller one, participates in the genesis of delayed-type hypersensitivity. However, the results of using selected dosages of drugs such as 2-mercaptoethanol and 5-mercaptopurine in tolerance experiments suggest that a cellular dissociation of early antibody-mediated sensitivity and the delayed cellular reactivity takes place (Schwartz, 1965). This dissociation may, however, be merely a dose or sensitivity response to the various cellular types in the stages of their differentiation.

Whether or not one cell can produce more than one type of antibody is not known, although there are claims and denials that it can. However, there appear to be no contrasting studies performed under the same conditions with identical immunogens. It is clear that most antibody-producing cells can synthesize both light and heavy chains and thus could produce a complete immunoglobulin. It is of some interest that 2 percent of cells apparently possess the ability to synthesize both κ and λ light chains and about 1 percent contain the heavy chain of both γG and γA-immunoglobulins, although there is some suspicion about the latter finding (Williamson and Askonas, 1967; see also Porter, 1966, for a review).

The elucidation of antibody structure has been one of the most active areas of recent investigations. Reduction of disulfide linkages has shown γG-globulin to be made up of two heavy (molecular weight approximately 50,000) and two light (molecular weight approximately 25,000) chains, with the former units retaining most of the immunologic specificity (Fleischman et al., 1963). Enzymatic cleavage of bivalent γG-globulin has yielded two fragments, each retaining specificity for the immunogen. These are called Fab (antigen-binding fragments). A third fragment serves as the core piece to which Fab are attached and is immunologically inert. This piece can be crystallized and therefore is termed Fc (Porter, 1959). End-group analysis has convincingly shown that the aminoacid sequence, especially in the Fab region, establishes the conformation of the active site, and it is thus responsible for the immunospecificity of the molecule (Cold Spring Harbor Symp. Quant. Biol., 1967).

BIOLOGIC CONSEQUENCES OF IMMUNE REACTIONS

While there are two main categories of immunologic responses, i.e., antibody-mediated early hypersensitivity and immunocompetent cellular-mediated, delayed-type response, there is a spectrum of possible biologic responses ranging from protective effects to tissue injury, and occasionally no overt reaction occurs at all. The latter responses depend on the type, amount, and localization of the immunogen and on which immunologic response is evoked.

Early-type (or immediate-type) sensitivities

These were so named because the reactions provoked in a sensitized host by a specific antigen were noted to give gross response in minutes or hours, whereas the cellular-mediated or delayed-type hypersensitivities required a day or frequently two days to manifest a maximum response. These temporal terms are rather firmly fixed in the lexicon of immunology and are reasonably accurate biologic descriptions. Nonetheless, because of some clear overlaps and exceptions, the operational designations of "antibody-mediated" or "cellular-mediated" will be employed. Table 1 illustrates the major differences between these two inflammatory reactions.

Table 1

Comparison between Antibody-mediated and Cellular-mediated
Immunologic Responses

Properties of the Responses	Antibody-mediated Response	Cellular-mediated Response
Basic mechanism	Reaction mediated by immunoglobulin participation either in complex, by direct action, or by initiating release of pharmacologically active substances.[a]	Reaction mediated by very few specifically sensitized or competent lymphocytes which in the presence of Ag, are chemotoxic for other round cells.[b]
Passive transfer	By serum; γG-globulin (anaphylaxis) and γE-globulin (reagin) are active. Also by antibody-producing cells.	By leukocytes, or in man, by "transfer-factor" from leukocytes. Not by serum.[c]
Appearance of reaction in sensitive host	Wheal and erythema Anaphylaxis (generally in minutes) Arthus reaction (in hours to 1 day) Serum sickness (in days to 1 week)	Generally within 24-72 hours, although with some materials, even weeks or months are needed.
Character of the reaction	Depends on type. Local reactions are marked by initial erythema and edema, often with central ischemia and flare (atopy) or eventual necrosis (Arthus). Vascular cuffing, polymorphoneutrophils, and thrombi are usual.	Local reaction is characteristically indurated by dense accumulation of round cells, often perivascularly.
In vitro correlates or animal demonstrations	Specific antibody measurement Schultz-Dale reaction[e] Passive cutaneous anaphylaxis[g] Prausnitz-Küstner reaction[i]	Lymphocyte transformation[d] Macrophage inhibition[f] Cytotoxicity of antigen for explanted cells[h]

[a] Cochrane and Ward (1966): Austen and Humphrey (1963); Dixon et al. (1958).
[b] Leskowitz (1967); Ward et al. (1969).
[c] Chase (1945); Bloom and Chase (1967); Lawrence et al. (1963).
[d] Oppenheim (1968); Mellman and Rawnsley (1966).
[e] Kabat et al. (1963); Noah (1964).
[f] George and Vaughan (1962); David et al. (1964); Bloom and Bennett (1966).
[g] Ovary (1964).
[h] Lubaroff and Ritts (1964).
[i] Sherman (1965).

Antibody-mediated reactivities are further classified on the basis of the specific antibodies and mechanisms involved. There are four such gross mechanisms: inactivation, cytotoxicity, pharmacologic activation, and the formation of immune complexes.

Immune inactivation. This category is based on the fairly recent observation that antibodies may inactivate biologically active proteins such as enzymes and hormones (Cinader and Lepow, 1966). Despite the laboratory observation that the antigenic determinants are frequently remote from the active enzyme-receptor site of such molecules, thus permitting biologic activity even after antibody combination, there are several instances in man where antihormone antibodies create a deficiency state. Presumably, in these cases the sites are close enough that steric masking of the active site is caused by antibody attachment to the molecule. This mechanism has been observed in "insulin resistance" (Pope, 1966) and in pernicious anemia, in which there appear to be antibodies directed against gastric mucosa, parietal cells, and intrinsic factor (Irvine, 1966) and against nearly all of the blood-clotting factors (Margolius et al., 1961).

Cytotoxic reactions. The precise mechanism involved in this immune response is not clear. There appear to be several ways in which cell lysis or cell inactivation may occur. An antibody directed against a specific cell or portion thereof is capable of direct inactivation. However, it is thought that in most circumstances, the antibody-antigen complex activates complement, which acts as the primary mediator of cytotoxicity (Nelson, 1965; Muller-Eberhard, 1968; Waksman, 1958; Cochrane and Ward, 1966). Indeed, a recent observation suggests that complement, even in the absence of continued immunologic stimulation (i.e., antibody), is capable of maintaining or inducing an immunologic inflammatory reaction (Johnston et al., 1969).

Many manifestations of the cytotoxic immune response are noted in man. Often these are of an autoimmune nature. They may be exogenously induced by drugs complexing to tissues, as in sedormid purpura (Ackroyd, 1952), or by prior infection, which is frequently of viral etiology (Baldini, 1966). An endogenous source of the immunogen is well-recognized in hemolytic anemias and erythroblastosis fetalis. In the latter case, Rh immunization can be prevented by passive transfer of Rh^+ cells and anti-Rh serum in Rh^- male volunteers. Passive transfer of anti-Rh γG-globulin to Rh^- mothers after parturition of Rh^+ babies prevents the immunization and the later possibility of incompatibility (Freda et al., 1967).

Pharmacologically mediated hypersensitivities. These are displayed by the allergic or "atopic" and the anaphylactic reactions (*see* Spector and Willoughby, 1968). In the immunologic manifestations of these hypersensitivities, the "allergen" or immunogen reacts with antibody which probably passively coats reactive cells, with the consequent release of a number of active materials from the cells. These very active pharmacologic substances include histamine, serotonin, bradykinin, slow-reacting substances (SRS-A), heparin, and acetylcholine. The cells which are thought to be primarily involved are the tissue mast cells and the circulating platelets and basophils.

Anaphylaxis, or the systemic shock syndrome, is normally a man-made condition. Anaphylaxis is sometimes observed in nature, particularly in those individuals who are very sensitive to the venoms of insects, but the mechanism of anaphylaxis requires a fairly large and rapid systemic dissemination of the immunogen in the sensitive host. Cutaneous anaphylaxis is frequently observed and is pharmacologically similar to the systemic reaction. The clinical manifestations of anaphylaxis depend upon the host species, each having a different array of "shock organs" or "target tissues" (Austen and Humphrey, 1963). In general, the pharmacologically active mediators cause acute vasoconstriction followed by vasodilation and increased vascular permeability, collapse and smooth muscle contraction. There also may be increased secretory activity of mucosal tissues in the gut and nasopharynx. The predominance of the response with respect to a given organ system may vary with each species. For example, man exhibits profound pulmonary and circulatory effects (James and Austen, 1964).

Cutaneous anaphylaxis produces the typical histamine "triple response" with redness, wheal (often with pseudopodia), and a spreading flare, which rarely last more than 2 to 3 hours. The response reaches its maximum intensity within a few minutes (rarely more than 30 minutes). These skin reactions are generally boggy at the periphery, and histologically, they reveal few or no cellular infiltrates. Extensive edema, more recently thought to be localized within epithelial cell vacuoles rather than interstitially, may only be an initial event.

The atopies or allergies are, in a general sense, mechanistically similar to anaphylaxis. Operationally, the natural "dose," the route of administration of the allergen, and the apparently hereditary familial susceptibility differentiate it from systemic anaphylaxis, and immunologically, the antibody involved is quite different. The antibody involved in allergies, termed reagin, is γE-globulin (Ishizaka et al., 1966). It is nonprecipitable, heat-labile, and skin-sensitizing, and it does not fix complement (Sherman, 1965; Osler et al., 1968). This γE-immunoglobulin is thought to fix to the surface of cells in minute amounts. The cells are triggered to release pharmacologically active substances when the allergen complexes to the antibody. An intermediate activation of an enzyme has been postulated to occur after the allergen-reagin interaction, but clear demonstration of such a mechanism is not available.

Immune complexes (Arthus reactivities).   A major biologic consequence of antigen-antibody interaction is the immune inflammatory reaction produced by this toxic complex. Soluble circulating antigen-antibody complexes eventually form microprecipitates which are found in and adjacent to the walls of blood vessels. The complexes fix and activate complement, which causes a consequent polymorphonuclear cell response. The cells release cathepsin and permeability factors which affect basement membranes in the kidney and venules and in the arteriole elastic layers (Cochrane, 1967). In generalized form, the observed syndrome resulting from disseminated complexes is serum sickness (Dixon et al., 1958).

The Arthus reaction requires 6 hours to develop to maximum intensity and generally fades in 24 hours. In severe reactions, central necrosis occurs. Serum sickness may occur and persist for many days or weeks, and it may conceivably occur with the first dose of a foreign protein if the halflife of the protein is appreciably longer than the induction time for its antibody. In this circumstance, there is still antigen present in the host when antibody has formed. This would require an extremely potent immunogen and responsive host, for it is estimated that about 1,000 times more antibody is required to elicit a toxic-complex reaction than to elicit anaphylaxis.

The Arthus reaction is marked by edema, cellular proliferation, and, frequently, extravasation of red blood cells. It is distinguishable from delayed-type reactivities by its bogginess, rapid development, and occasional hemorrhagic quality. The central necrosis, when it occurs, may mimic that seen in the severe Cochard delayed-response, but in the latter, dense cellular induration is nearly always present. Histologically, the edema and cellular proliferation are obvious, and the numerous red cells, platelet thrombi and fibrinoid disorganization, and necrosis of the vasculature are prominent features.

Delayed-type hypersensitivity

The sequence of events leading to the manifestations of delayed-type hypersensitivity are essentially similar to those in the case of early-type hypersensitivity. The induction period of 7 to 10 days after initial antigenic exposure, the anamnestic response, and the eliciting of the response are operationally consonant with the gross events seen in early-type reactivities. Indeed, both types of biologic reactivities may result from one immunogen, and the resultant skin reaction may manifest a combination of each.

However, the mediator of delayed reactivity is the lymphocyte. The specificity of the reaction is just as precise as that of early-type reactions in spite of the absence of an antibody mechanism. Passive transfer of lymphocytes from a sensitized host to a normergic recipient will confer delayed-type reactivity (Chase, 1945; Bloom and Chase, 1967). It should be emphasized that in transfer studies, antibody synthesis is similarly transferred if it is operative in the donor animal at the time of the cell transfer. Thus, if both early and delayed reactivities to a common antigen are observed in the donor, they will be simultaneously transferred. The transfer of serum in this instance will passively confer only early-type hypersensitivity to the recipient. An additional complication of passive transfer experiments is that circulating antigen from the donor animal may be transferred and cause direct, active immunization of the recipient. This possibility is always present and is especially germane to experiments which employ infection, particularly with parasites, as the immunogenic stimulus.

Species differences. Curiously, man differs from other animals in his greater ability to respond in a delayed fashion, even though this mechanism is thought to represent a primitive host defense mechanism and is seen in lower forms of animals in the absence of antibody synthesis. Man appears capable of responding in a delayed fashion to quantitatively less inciting antigen than, for example, the guinea pig. The guinea pig in turn is much more reactive than many other rodents, such as the mouse (in which cellular hypersensitivity is induced with difficulty) or the Syrian hamster (in which several examples of delayed reactivities cannot be induced at all).

This species difference between man and other animals is especially notable in cellular transfer studies. In man, lysates of peripheral leukocytes are capable of transferring delayed-type hypersensitivity. A material derived from these cells has been called transfer factor and has a molecular weight of less than 10,000. It is a dialyzable material, and it is not affected by DNase, RNase, or trypsin (Lawrence et al., 1963). It may be eluted from lymphocytes by exposing them to the specific antigen, yet the presence of the antigen does not inhibit the cells' capacity to transfer hypersensitivity (Bloom and Chase, 1967). However, in other animals there has been no convincing or controlled study in which anything other than whole, viable leukocytes could transfer this reaction. Indeed, pretreatment of animal donor leukocytes with mitomycin C or D, which blocks RNA- or DNA-dependent RNA synthesis, prevents the transfer of delayed-type hypersensitivity. Studies of this kind have been confined to hypersensitivity reactions to bacterial antigens or various benzene-containing chemical haptens. It would be interesting to test parasitic antigens under similar circumstances, although there is no *a priori* reason to assume the results would be any different.

In vitro correlates. Aside from the practical difficulties in conducting some studies in man, a primary obstacle to our understanding of this important immunologic reaction has been the lack of suitable or reproducible *in vitro* correlates of delayed-type hypersensitivity. Recently, new techniques have been introduced which promise to be important tools for furthering our understanding of this phenomenon, even though each has some defects.

Lymphocyte transformation is the *in vitro* expression of the lymphocyte to undergo blast formation in the presence of an antigen to which its donor responds in a delayed fashion. Lymphocytes which are transformed by plant mitogens nonspecifically or by antigens or other cells in mixed lymphocyte cultures undergo rapid synthesis of protein, RNA, and DNA. Thus, the standard assay of transformation is based on the cellular uptake and incorporation of H^3-thymidine under appropriately controlled conditions. Morphologically, there is enlargement of the nucleus and cytoplasm accompanied by pyroninophilia, the appearance of hydrolase-rich granules and polyribosomes, and sometimes mitosis (Claman and Brunstetter, 1969).

There are a number of nonspecific substances (e.g., phytohemagglutinin, concanavalin A, endotoxin) which are capable of inducing lymphocytes to undergo blast transformation (Mellman and Rawnsley, 1966; Oppenheim, 1968). These are useful agents in this *in vitro* test because they can offer some measure of the host's capacity to respond with delayed-type hypersensitivity as a general biologic phenomenon. Absence of transformation in response to nonspecific stimuli has become a routine indicator of the absence of delayed hypersensitivity response in immune deficiency diseases of man (Cooperband et al., 1968).

In practice there is little or no cross-reactivity observed when cells are transformed by specific antigen. A host with skin-test sensitivity to histoplasmin but not tuberculin will yield cells that are transformable by the former antigen but not the latter. Occasionally, a blast transformation will occur in the absence of a positive skin test when routine amounts of the antigen are used. In some cases, much larger skin-test doses reveal the presence of reactivity, but because toxic dose levels are approached and because often no skin reactivity is seen at all, there is some controversy about the sensitivity of this procedure. Some workers feel that blast transformation is so sensitive that it is detectable much earlier than skin-test reactivity.

A second *in vitro* correlate of delayed-type hypersensitivity is the macrophage migration inhibition test (George and Vaughan, 1962). Lymphocytes from delayed-hypersensitivity-reactive donors elaborate a migratory inhibitory factor (MIF) in the presence of the specific antigen. MIF is active without the presence of antigen. It is not a complete immunoglobulin, but it has a molecular weight of 60,000 to 75,000 (David et al., 1964). When injected into skin, it produces a histologic reaction similar to a typical delayed-type hypersensitivity response (Bloom and Bennett, 1966).

Skin tests. Both the prototypical tuberculin reactivity and the skin-contact hypersensitivity or allergy are delayed-type hypersensitivities and are demonstrable by blast transformation or inhibition of macrophage migration. The reactions of the sensitive host are delayed 24 to 72 hours after injection, and the hallmark of the skin reaction is induration resulting from dense accumulation of white blood cells. In skin-contact tests, spongiosis, vesiculation, and often necrosis are observed in the epidermis, and the histocyte and small round cell infiltrates predominate in the dermis, especially around small veins. Polymorphonuclear leukocytes are sparse and generally do not appear prominent unless necrosis is observed (Waksman, 1960).

Granulomatous hypersensitivity reactions. Granulomatous hypersensitivities have been recently introduced as a distinct category of immune inflammatory response (Epstein, 1968). Typical epithelioid and giant cells characterize this reaction, as do the months or years it apparently takes to become manifest. Such reactions are prototypical of certain infections and allergies, notably tuberculosis, the tuberculoid form of leprosy, beryllium hypersensitivity, several diseases of uncertain etiology (such as Boeck's sarcoidosis, Crohn's disease, and Wegner's granulomatosis), and perhaps a group of interstitial pneumonitides caused by inhalation of organic particles (such as farmer's lung, bagassosis, and pigeon-breeder's disease). It is convenient to separate these responses, at least on a basis of temporal and histologic criteria, but they appear to be extremely delayed or modified delayed hypersensitive reactions much in the way that serum sickness, though often more delayed in time, is similar to the Arthus reaction in concept.

MECHANISMS OF IMMUNITY

Immunity is classically and routinely discussed in terms of native or innate nonspecific immunity as opposed to acquired specific immunity. This custom will not be followed here because of the author's conviction that "innate immunity" in reality consists of the inflammatory response and phagocytosis found in all mammals, plus those single, or occasionally several, factors that have to do with susceptibility or resistance of a certain species of animals to a particular organism. Usually these factors are specific tissue enzymes of the particular host which appear to preclude generalized infection or the establishment of a single infection in a given tissue. Frequently, experimental nutritional deficiencies are shown to exert an influence on susceptibility. Other cases of native immunity said to be related to a "natural" antibody have usually revealed that the "normal" and specific immunoglobulin was acquired as a result of an unexplained infection or was a cross-reacting antibody. These susceptibility and/or resistance factors will not be considered in further detail. However, one should bear in mind that experimental studies in immunology always need to be controlled with respect to the various possible "innate" factors.

Coombs and Smith (1968) have lucidly outlined four essential modes by which immunity can be effected. *Mode A* involves the reaction of serum antibody with or without cofactors such as complement. In this mechanism, the immunoglobulin may neutralize a toxin (e.g., antitoxin), coat an organism and thus inhibit its growth, or block attachment of an organism to cells (e.g., inhibition of virus hemadsorption). The immunoglobulin may activate complement which may create a local membrane reactivity, or the antibody may combine with its antigen (if soluble) to induce an Arthus inflammatory response. Taliaferro and Sarles (1939) suggested that antibodies to the excretory and other soluble antigens of migrating larval helminths may neutralize or block the enzymes of their secretions so as to inhibit larval development. Trypanosomes are also lysed by antibody and complement (Lourie and O'Connor, 1937).

Mode B involves the elaboration of a specific serum immunoglobulin, cofactors, and nonsensitized (or "nonallergized") cells. Phagocytosis is the prototypical response of this mode, although phagocytosis, as a general rudimentary mechanism, may not necessarily require specific antibody or the activation of complement. However, with the elaboration of complement, a chemotoxic gradient is established, and specific antibody enhances this powerful immune defense reaction. Nonetheless, it has been observed that even in the presence of antibody- or opsonin-enhanced phagocytosis, some organisms, notably streptococci (Wilson et al., 1957), tubercle bacilli (Suter, 1952), and leishmania (*see* Stauber's chapter, pp. 752-753) are not killed and may even multiply. Further, if microorganisms are able to resist enzymatic destruction while in the cellular milieu, they are protected from the effects of antibody and again may even multiply. Under such circumstances, microorganisms may even be widely disseminated in the host by leukocytes.

Mode C involves the passive sensitization of macrophages ("passively allergized cells") by cytophilic antibody (Boyden and Sorkin, 1960; Nelson and Boyden, 1967; Rowley et al., 1964). Such sensitized cells are thought to be active on serous surfaces where opsonins are absent. Coombs (1968) speculates that disengagement of helminths from the gut may be caused by reaginic sensitization of mast cells followed by subsequent degranulation and the release of mediators. This would increase vascular permeability and thus facilitate localization of antibody and other factors at the site of attachment. It is of interest that immunoglobulin concentration in the gut appears to be quite high, and it may even be the primary mechanism in the self-cure reaction (Soulsby and Stewart, 1960). Immune serum exerts a variable but slight adverse *in vitro* effect on adult parasites. However, such *in vitro* studies with purified γA-immunoglobulin, which is known to be secreted in the gut, apparently have not been performed to date.

Mode D involves the actively sensitized cells. As was discussed previously, there is abundant evidence that antigens are capable of transforming uncommitted lymphocytes into immunologically competent cells which mediate delayed-hypersensitivity responses. There is some speculation that these small transformed cells may on occasion assume macrophagic properties, but there is rather clear evidence that they are able to inhibit macrophage migration at least in tissue culture (Bloom and Bennett, 1966; David et al., 1964). How this latter mechanism operates *in vivo* is uncertain. Mackaness (1967) contended that these "immune macrophages" are essentially identical to those immunocompetent cells participating in delayed-type hypersensitivity. This reasoning is consistent with the observations of Nelson and Boyden (1963, 1967), who demonstrated that this form of specific cellular immunity associated with "cytophilic antibody" (Boyden and Sorkin, 1960) is operative only in animals demonstrating delayed-type hypersensitivity. However, it is clear that "cellular immunity" wanes when antigen disappears, but the specific delayed-type response persists for many years. Further, the induction of delayed-type hypersensitivity to any specific antigen appears to confer upon the host's macrophages a heightened, nonspecific ability for phagocytosis of many (heterologously antigenic) microorganisms. Thus, there seem to be conflicts in identifying the "cellular immunity" of Mode D with delayed-type hypersensitivity.

CONCLUSION

Nearly every facet of current immunologic advances is relevant to parasitic infections. An apparent γE-reagin has been demonstrated in helminth infestation (Ogilvie, 1964, 1967). Passive cellular transfers have conferred immunity to *Trichostrongylus colubriformis* in guinea pigs (Dineen and Wayland, 1966). Nonetheless, the structural and chemical complexity of parasite immunogens, the anatomic sequestration of some stages of their life cycle, and the practical difficulty of *in vitro* maintenance of parasitic animals make the attainment of effective immunization against these organisms a monumental feat. It is clear that great progress has been made, as has been reported by the World Health Organization Expert Committee on immunology and parasitic diseases (1965), but that in terms of the desired end, today's accomplishments are only a beginning.

REFERENCES

Ackroyd, J. F. 1952. Sedormid purpura. *In* Progress in Allergy, Vol. 3. Kallós, P., ed. Basel, S. Karger, p. 531.

Adler, F. L., M. Fishman, and S. Dray. 1966. Antibody formation initiated *in vitro*. III. Antibody formation and allotypic specificity directed by ribonucleic acid from peritoneal exudate cells. J. Immun., 97:554-558.

Austen, K. F., and J. H. Humphrey. 1963. *In vitro* studies of the mechanism of anaphylaxis. *In* Advances in Immunology, Vol. 3. Dixon, F. J., and Humphrey, J. H., eds. New York, Academic Press, Inc., pp. 3-96.

Baldini, M. 1966. Idiopathic thrombocytopenic purpura. New Eng. J. Med., 274: 1245.

Bloom, B. R., and B. P. Bennett. 1966. Mechanism of a reaction *in vitro* associated with delayed-type hypersensitivity. Science, 153:80-82.

——— and M. W. Chase. 1967. Transfer of delayed-type hypersensitivity. A critical review and experimental study in guinea pig. *In* Progress in Allergy, Vol. 10. Kallós, P., and Waksman, B. H., eds. Basel, S. Karger, p. 151.

Boyden, S. V., and E. Sorkin. 1960. The absorption of antigens by spleen cells previously treated with antiserum *in vitro*. Immunology, 3:272.

Chase, M. W. 1945. Cellular transfer of cutaneous hypersensitivity to tuberculin. Proc. Soc. Exp. Biol. Med., 59:134-135.

——— J. R. Battisto, and R. E. Ritts, Jr. 1963. The acquisition of immunological tolerance. *In* Conceptual Advances in Immunology and Oncology. New York, Harper and Row, Hoeber Medical Division, p. 399.

Cinader, B., and I. H. Lepow. 1966. Neutralization of biologically active molecules. *In* Antibodies to Biologically Active Molecules. Cinader, B., ed. Oxford and New York, Pergamon Press.

Claman, H. N., and F. H. Brunstetter. 1969. Human thymus cell cultures with phytohemagglutinin and antilymphocyte serum. *In* Proceedings of the Third Annual Leucocyte Culture Conference. Rieke, W. O., ed. New York, Appleton-Century-Crofts, pp. 199-212.

Cochrane, C. G. 1967. Mediators of the Arthus and related reactions. *In* Progress in Allergy, Vol. 11. Kallós, P., and Waksman, B. H., eds. Basel, S. Karger, p. 1.

——— and P. A. Ward. 1966. The role of complement in lesions induced by immunologic reactions. *In* Immunology, Vol. 4. Grabar, P., and Miesher, P., eds. Basel, Benno Schwabe, p. 443.

Cold Spring Harbor Symposia on Quantitative Biology. 1967. Structure of antibodies. Cold Spring Harbor Symp. Quant. Biol., 32:9-132.

Coombs, R. R. A. 1968. Immunity. *In* Immunity to Parasites. Sixth Symposium of the British Society for Parasitology. Taylor, A. E. R., ed. Oxford, Blackwell Scientific Publications, p. 3.

——— and H. Smith. 1968. The allergic reactions and immunity. *In* Clinical Aspects of Immunology, 2nd Ed. Gell, P. G. H., and Coombs, R. R. A., eds. Oxford, Blackwell Scientific Publications, p. 423.

Cooperband, S. R., F. S. Rosen, and S. Kibrick. 1968. Studies on the *in vitro* behavior of agammaglobulinemic lymphocytes. J. Clin. Invest., 47:836-847.

David, J. R., S. Al-Askari, H. S. Lawrence, and L. Thomas. 1964. Delayed hypersensitivity *in vitro*. I. The specificity of inhibition of cell migration by antigens. J. Immun., 93:264-273.

DePetris, S., G. Karlsbad, and B. Pernis. 1963. Localization of antibodies in plasma cells by electron microscopy. J. Exp. Med., 117:849-862.

Dineen, J. K., and B. M. Wagland. 1966. The cellular transfer of immunity to *Trichostrongylus colubriformis* in an isogenic strain of guinea pig. Immunology, 11:47-57.

Dixon, F. J., J. J. Vasquez, and W. O. Weigl. 1958. Pathogenesis of serum sickness. Arch. Path. (Chicago), 65:18.

Epstein, W. L. 1967. Granulomatous hypersensitivity. In Progress in Allergy, Vol. 11. Kallós, P., and Waksman, B. H., eds. Basel, S. Karger, p. 86.

Fishman, M., and F. L. Adler. 1967. The role of macrophage RNA in the immune response. Cold Spring Harbor Symp. Quant. Biol., 32:343.

Fleischman, J., R. R. Porter, and E. M. Press. 1963. The arrangement of the peptide chains in γ-globulin. Biochemistry, 88:220.

Freda, V. J., J. G. Gorman, and W. Pollack. 1967. Suppression of the primary Rh immune response with passive Rh IgG immunoglobulin. New Eng. J. Med., 277:1022.

Gallily, R. and M. Feldman. 1967. The role of the macrophage in the induction of antibody in x-irradiated animals. Immunology, 12:197-206.

George, M., and J. H. Vaughan. 1962. In vitro cell migration as a model for delayed hypersensitivity. Proc. Soc. Exp. Bio. Med., 111:514-521.

Harris, T. N. 1966. Symposium: Recent advances on the biology and function of the lymphocyte. Introductory remarks. Fed. Proc., 25:1711-1741.

———— K. Jummeler, and S. Harris. 1966. Electron microscopic observations on antibody-producing lymph node cells. J. Exp. Med., 123:161-172.

Irvine, W. J. 1965. Immunologic aspects of pernicious anemia. New Eng. J. Med., 273:432.

Ishizaka, K., T. Ishizaka, and M. M. Hornbrook. 1966. Physicochemical properties of human reaginic antibody. IV. Presence of a unique immunoglobulin as a carrier of reaginic activity. J. Immun., 97:75-85.

James, L. P., and K. F. Austen. 1964. Fatal systemic anaphylaxis in man. New Eng. J. Med., 270:597.

Johnston, R. B., Jr., M. R. Klemperer, C. A. Alper, and F. S. Rosen. 1969. The enhancement of bacterial phagocytosis by serum: The role of complement components and two cofactors. J. Exp. Med., 129:1275.

Kabat, E. A., P. Liacopoulos, M. Liacopoulos-Briot, B. N. Halpern, and E. H. Relyveld. 1963. Studies on the sensitizing properties of human antisera and purified antibodies. J. Immun., 90:810.

Landsteiner, K. 1962. The Specificity of Serological Reactions. New York, Dover Publications, Inc., pp. 168, 172, 174, 186, 192, 262-265.

Lawrence, H. S., S. Al-Askari, J. David, E. C. Franklin, and B. Zweiman. 1963. Transfer of immunological information in humans with dialysates of leucocyte extracts. Trans. Ass. Amer. Physicians, 76:84-91.

Leskowitz, S. 1967. Mechanism of delayed reactions. Science, 155:350.

Lourie, E. M., and R. S. O'Connor. 1937. Trypanolysis in vitro by mouse immune serum. Ann. Trop. Med. Parasit., 30:365.

Lubaroff, D. M., and R. E. Ritts, Jr. 1964. In vitro cytotoxicity in delayed-type hypersensitivity and immunological tolerance. Proc. Soc. Exp. Biol. Med., 116:823-827.

Mackaness, G. B. 1967. The relationship of delayed-type hypersensitivity to acquired cellular resistance. Brit. Med. Bull., 23:52.

Mannick, J. A., and R. H. Egdahl. 1964. Transfer of heightened immunity to skin homografts by lymphoid RNA. J. Clin. Invest., 43:2166-2177.

Margolius, A., Jr., D. P. Jackson, and O. D. Ratnoff. 1961. Circulating anticoagulants. Medicine, 40:145-202.

Mellman, W. J., and H. M. Rawnsley. 1966. Blastogenesis in peripheral blood lymphocytes in response to phytohemagglutinin and antigens. Fed. Proc., 25:1720-1722.

Muller-Eberhard, H. J. 1968. Chemistry and reaction mechanisms of complement. In Advances in Immunology, Vol. 8. Dixon, F. J., and Kunkle, H. G., eds. New York, Academic Press, Inc., pp. 2-80.

Nelson, D. S., and S. V. Boyden. 1963. The loss of macrophages from peritoneal exudates following injection of antigens into guinea pigs with delayed-type hypersensitivity. Immunology, 6:264.

———— and S. V. Boyden. 1967. Macrophage cytophilic antibodies and delayed hypersensitivity. Brit. Med. Bull., 23:15.

Nelson, R. A., Jr. 1965. The role of complement in immune phenomena. In The Inflammatory Process. Zweifach, B. W., Grant, L., and McCluskey, R. T., eds. New York, Academic Press, Inc., pp. 819-872.

Noah, J. W. 1964. Anaphylactic histamine release and the Schultz-Dale reaction. In Immunological Methods. Ackroyd, J. F., ed. Oxford, Blackwell Scientific Publications, pp. 285-309.

Ogilvie, B. M. 1964. Reagin-like antibodies in animals immune to helminth parasites. Nature (London), 204:91.

———— 1967. Reagin-like antibodies in rats infected with the nematode parasite *Nippostronglyus brasiliensis.* Immunology, 12:113-131.

Oppenheim, J. J. 1968. Relationship of *in vitro* lymphocyte transformation to delayed hypersensitivity in guinea pigs and man. Fed. Proc., 27:21-28.

Osler, A. G., L. M. Lichtenstein, and D. A. Levy. 1968. *In vitro* studies of human reaginic allergy. *In* Advances in Immunology, Vol. 8. Dixon, F. J., and Kunkle, H. G., eds. New York, Academic Press, Inc., pp. 183-231.

Ovary, Z. 1964. Passive cutaneous anaphylaxis. *In* Immunological Methods. Ackroyd, J. F., ed. Oxford, Blackwell Scientific Publications, pp. 259-283.

Pope, C. C. 1966. The immunology of insulin. *In* Advances in Immunology, Vol. 5. Dixon, F. J., and Humphrey, J. H., eds. New York, Academic Press, Inc., p. 209.

Porter, R. R. 1959. The hydrolysis of rabbit γ-globulin and antibodies with crystalline papain. Biochem. J., 73:119.

———— 1966. A discussion of the chemistry and biology of immunoglobulins. Proc. Roy. Soc. [Biol.], 166:114-243.

Rowley, D., K. J. Turner, and C. R. Jenkins. 1964. The basis for immunity to mouse typhoid. 3. Cell-bound antibody. Austr. J. Exp. Biol. Med. Sci., 42:237.

Schwartz, R. S. 1965. Immunosuppressive Drugs. *In* Progress in Allergy, Vol. 9. Kallós, P., and Waksman, B. H., eds. Basel, S. Karger, p. 246.

Sherman, W. B. 1965. The atopic diseases. *In* Immunological Diseases. Samter, M., ed. Boston, Little, Brown and Co., pp. 503-505.

Soulsby, E. J. L., and D. F. Stewart. 1960. Serological studies of the self-cure reaction in sheep infected with *Haemonchus contortus.* Austr. J. Agric. Res., 2:595.

Spector, W. G., and D. D. Willoughby. 1968 The Pharmacology of Inflammation. New York, Grune and Stratton, Inc., pp. 1-23.

Suter, E. 1952. The multiplication of tubercle bacilli within phagocytes cultivated *in vitro* and effect of streptomycin and isonicotinic acid hydrazide. Amer. Rev. Tuberculosis, 65:775-776.

Taliaferro, W. H., and M. P. Sarles. 1939. The cellular reactions in the skin, lungs and intestine of normal and immune rats after infection with *Nippostrongylus muris.* J. Infect. Dis., 64:157-192.

Talmage, D. W., F. J. Dixon, S. C. Bukantz, and G. J. Dammin. 1951. Antigen elimination from blood as early manifestation of immune response. J. Immun., 67:243-255

Waksman, B. H. 1958. Cell lysis and related phenomena in hypersensitivity reactions including immunohematologic diseases. *In* Progress in Allergy, Vol. 5. Kallós, P., ed. Basel, S. Karger, p. 349.

———— 1960. A comparative histopathological study of delayed hypersensitive reactions. *In* Cellular Aspects of Immunity. Ciba Symposium. Boston, Little, Brown, and Co., p. 280.

Ward, P. A., H. B. Remold, and J. R. David. 1969. Leukostatic factor produced by sensitized lymphocytes. Science, 163:1079.

Williamson, A. R., and B. A. Askonas. 1967. Biosynthesis of immunoglobulins; the separate classes of polyribosomes synthesizing heavy and light chains. J. Molec. Biol., 23:201.

Wilson, A. T., G. G. Wiley, and P. Bruno. 1957. Fate of non-virulent Group A streptococci phagocytized by human and mouse neutrophiles. J. Exp. Med., 106:777.

World Health Organization Expert Committee Report. 1965. Immunology and Parasitic Diseases. W.H.O. Tech. Rep. Ser. No. 315, pp. 1-64.

Amoebas and Other Intestinal Protozoa

WILLIAM BALAMUTH
Department of Zoology, University of California, Berkeley, California

WASIM A. SIDDIQUI
Department of Preventive Medicine, Stanford University School of Medicine,
Palo Alto, California

INTRODUCTION

All major groups of Protozoa have colonized the alimentary canal of higher vertebrates, but considerable selectivity is evident with respect to the specific regions inhabited and the extent of the host-parasite interaction. In the mammalian intestinal tract, the lumen is most frequently involved and the large intestine is affected more than the small intestine. The flagellate *Giardia* stands out as essentially the sole inhabitant of the small intestine, occurring either free in the lumen or clamped onto the mucosal surface, and occasionally evoking mild diarrhea and interference with fat absorption. Other flagellates (e.g., *Trichomonas—see* next chapter) are lumen-dwellers of the large intestine and are accompanied by a variety of ciliates and amoebas.

Tissue invasion is relatively rare among intestinal protozoa and signifies truly pathogenic capacities. Intestinal Sporozoa (i.e., Coccidia—*see* chapters by Cuckler and by Kozar) grow exclusively in the mucosa and deeper tissues, often producing serious disease. The few species which have been reported in humans are not important pathogens, and in fact may not actually be typical human parasites. The most outstanding instances of tissue invasion by intestinal protozoa are contributed by the amoeba, *Entamoeba histolytica*, and the ciliate, *Balantidium coli*, both of which occur in the large intestine. *B. coli* is normally commensal in swine. It occasionally reaches humans and other primates where it may cause extensive ulceration and undermine the mucosa in a way similar to the action of *E. histolytica*. However, its low frequency as a pathogen lessens its interest for us and relatively few immunologic studies have been conducted. On the other hand, *E. histolytica* has been the object of intensive, and often controversial, investigation. This species will be the primary subject of the present discussion. As a widespread protozoan whose natural host is apparently the human and whose presence is associated with typical intestinal disease and frequent spread to other sites, *E. histolytica* provides a valuable model for a detailed study of an intestinal protozoan.

INTESTINAL AMOEBAS

Our knowledge of parasitic amoebas has greatly increased during the past two decades, both in regard to their basic biology and to the details of host-parasite interaction. Amoebas have captured footholds in the alimentary canal of practically all major groups of invertebrate and vertebrate animals, being encountered most frequently in arthropods and vertebrates. In contrast to the great taxonomic diversity of free-living forms, relatively few genera have become adapted to a parasitic existence—mainly some hartmannellid forms (e.g., *Hartmannella* spp.) and members of the artificial assemblage grouped with the family Endamoebidae (e.g., *Entamoeba* spp.). Species of the genus *Entamoeba* occur commonly in tetrapod vertebrates; they are distinguished primarily on the basis of nuclear morphology, locomotor pattern, and contents of their cysts. Host specificity is apparently well-defined, at least at the level of host class, but it is remarkable that the "*histolytica*" characteristics (trophozoite nucleus possessing a delicate, central nucleolus; relatively rapid, slug-like motility; and quadrinucleate cysts with elongated, bacilliform chromatoid bars) are also the very features which occur most frequently in the *Entamoeba* spp. of various vertebrates; examples are *E. ranarum* of frogs, *E. invadens* and *E. terrapinae* of reptiles, and *E. histolytica* of primates. Selection apparently has had a role in preserving these key indices of a successful, adaptable genome. Several other genera (*Endolimax, Iodamoeba, Dientamoeba*) and other species of *Entamoeba* are also found in mammals, but their commensal nature (with the possible exception of *D. fragilis*) eliminates them from further consideration here (*see* Kudo, 1966, for details of morphology and host distribution).

The *"Entamoeba histolytica* complex" and human amoebiasis

E. histolytica is a cosmopolitan parasite encountered in all regions of the world, although epidemiologic factors result in a higher incidence in underdeveloped tropical areas. Some investigators have questioned whether this amoeba is actually pathogenic, since most infected individuals appear to be asymptomatic carriers. Another possibility is that so-called *E. histolytica* may actually comprise a group of similarly appearing amoebas, only one of which is capable of inducing disease. Considerable progress has been made recently in providing answers to these questions, largely as a result of improved techniques of *in vitro* experimentation.

Several genetically distinct variants of *E. histolytica* are now known. One morphologic variant has been known for a half century, namely, the so-called small race *E. histolytica*; this type cohabits the colon lumen with the more typical large races, while having a genetically determined smaller size of both trophozoite and cyst stages. Cyst sizes have been shown to be less subject than trophozoites to nutritional influences, and most workers agree that a diameter less than 10 μ separates living cysts of the small race from wild-type *E. histolytica* (*see* Neal, 1966, for a review). The small race has also been shown to be antigenically distinct (Goldman et al., 1960), and of significance for our present discussion is the preponderant evidence that the small race is essentially nonpathogenic in humans and in experimentally infected hosts (Hoare, 1961). This combination of features supports the conclusion of numerous, but not all, investigators that the small race qualifies as a distinct species, bearing the name *E. hartmanni*. The present authors accept this conclusion as both desirable and valid.

Special attention has been paid within the past decade to two ecologic variants of the *E. histolytica* pattern that are morphologically indistinguishable from *E. histolytica*—a type widespread in polluted fresh water named *E. moshkovskii*, and an occasional isolate from humans which is adapted to grow well over the temperature range of 20° to 37°C (e.g., Laredo and Huff strains). These variants, while derived from diverse sources, share both this eurythermal property and a lack of pathogenicity for mammalian hosts, and recent biochemical studies disclose special enzymic similarities of their glucokinases (Reeves et al., 1967). Support is growing for the view that these eurythermal isolates may constitute a distinctive "physiologic species" that presumably mutated from wild-type *E. histolytica*.

In summary, the best available evidence indicates that *E. histolytica* (*sensu stricto*) is the causal agent of a typical form of colitis. Experimental tests have satisfied the essential demands of Koch's postulates (Thimann, 1963), in that these amoebas have been isolated from lesions in the human, cultivated *in vitro*, and subsequently have induced disease of varying severity following introduction into a wide variety of mammalian hosts (e.g., monkeys, dogs, cats, rabbits, and rodents). However, one cannot deny the existence of considerable variability in strain virulence; indeed, virulence can be experimentally increased by serial animal passage (Thompson et al., 1954; Neal and Vincent, 1956), and becomes lessened following prolonged cultivation (Thompson et al., 1954; Vincent and Neal, 1960).

Biology of *Entamoeba histolytica*

Much remains to be learned about *E. histolytica*, but it is gratifying that considerable progress has been made during the past decade, and prospects are even better for the years immediately ahead. The life cycle is completely known, axenic cultivation has finally been achieved, and the nature of the host-parasite interaction and antigenic composition of the amoeba are being actively studied.

Life Cycle. Like other amoebas, *Entamoeba* has a simple life cycle devoid of any sexual phenomena. Two stages alternate—the trophozoite (feeding stage) grows at the expense of the host and multiplies by binary fission, and the cyst (dormant stage) represents the means of transmission via oral contamination. The essential features of the life cycle are well-known, especially through the pioneering *in vitro* and *in vivo* studies of Dobell (1928, 1931). Excystation takes place in the lower small intestine or colon, liberating a quadrinucleate amoeba that undergoes repeated division until eight small trophozoites are formed. In the case of typical avirulent strains, the amoebas adopt a commensal existence in the lumen of the large intestine, feeding on bacteria and edible detritus. No evidence of action against host tissue is demonstrable in these cases and no host reactions are evinced. In the case of invasive strains, however, the trophozoites move to the mucosal surface and initiate lytic and ingestive activities. Restriction to the mucosal surface may elicit no sign of disease because of the marked regenerative capacity of intestinal epithelia. On the other hand, penetration of the epithelium is usually followed by spread through subepithelial tissue and extension beyond the muscularis mucosae into the submucosa. Characteristic abscesses and ulceration result from these activities, and extensive involvement of the intestinal wall ensues. These activities provide the basis for the variable degrees of amoebic colitis and, in extreme cases, frank dysentery.

From submucosal sites amoebas may gain access to the hepatic portal circulation and lymphatics and be transported to the liver, lung, brain, and other metastatic foci. The liver is the parenteral organ most frequently involved. In these sites, colonization often occurs unaccompanied by bacterial contamination. Details of the pathology involved have been described in adequate detail (Anderson et al., 1953); it may be noted here that host cellular reactions are minimal and involve no typical leukocytic infiltration or fibrous encapsulation of abscessed areas. In contrast to the more fulminating nature of typical shigellosis, amoebiasis presents the hallmark of a slowly developing chronic disease. The broad range of host-parasite interaction—

extending from a commensal existence in the intestinal lumen to a deep-seated parenteral involvment of diverse organs—might be expected to evoke a corresponding range in intensity of immune reactions, and this aspect will be discussed below.

Cysts are not formed in host tissues. Under still undefined conditions in the intestinal lumen, trophozoites remaining there periodically round up and eliminate food particles, becoming precysts. A developmental process ensues, involving segregation of considerable glycogen, condensation of ribonucleoprotein to form the typical bacilliform chromatoid bars, and secretion of a thin cyst wall. Repeated nuclear division yields a mature quadrinucleate cyst, and this stage is eliminated with feces and is ready to reinfect a suitable host.

Nutrition.   Knowledge of a parasite's nutritional demands has both basic and practical importance. Recognition of specific nutritional requirements identifies the role of the host in meeting the parasite's needs, and in turn points the way toward effective blocking of essential metabolic pathways. Nutritional studies require an *in vitro* approach, proceeding from successful isolation outside the host through the level of axenic cultivation (pure cultures) and ultimately to the development of a chemically defined, minimal culture medium. *E. histolytica* was first cultivated more than 40 years ago, but only in the past decade have pure cultures been achieved, and a defined medium has not yet been developed. An extensive literature has accumulated, the highlights of which are available in reviews by Balamuth and Thompson (1955) and Neal (1967). The present discussion will be limited to a few summary findings deemed relevant to the nature of the basic host-parasite interaction.

The evidence indicates that *E. histolytica* is an obligate anaerobe like most inhabitants of the large intestine. A wide variety of media prepared from natural materials has been used successfully for cultivation with microbial associates. In these media the amoebas thrive on diverse bacteria (or hemoflagellates) and readily ingest particulate carbohydrate and protein substances. They behave similarly in the intestinal lumen, where they also accept host cells (e.g., erythrocytes and sloughed epithelium) when available. The failure of several early attempts at axenic cultivation caused speculation that *Entamoeba* lacked certain essential enzymes which were supplied by the associates. However, Stoll (1957) and Diamond (1961) independently achieved axenic cultivation of *Entamoeba*, the latter author succeeding with *E. histolytica* for the first time and subsequently simplifying his formulation (Diamond and Bartgis, 1965). Undefined components in Diamond's medium include peptone, liver extract, and serum. The development of a chemically defined medium must await future studies (Jackson and Stoll, 1964; Balamuth and Kawakami, 1963).

Reports of specific nutritional requirements based upon use of bacterized cultures are obviously subject to some question. Still, convincing evidence has been published to support the claims of requirements for exogenous carbohydrate and sterol in the diet of *E. histolytica*. The former has been tacitly recognized from earliest days by the inclusion in bacterized cultures of particulate rice starch or other carbohydrate; Balamuth and Howard (1946) showed that addition of purified starch to depleted, waning cultures caused a dramatic increase in amoeba growth even though the bacterial population continued to decline. Diamond (1961) found that carbohydrate was an essential component of his axenic media, and several workers (e.g., Bragg and Reeves, 1962b) have shown that *E. histolytica* carries out anaerobic glycolysis. Sterols or other lipids must frequently be supplied in the diets of many protistan parasites, and *E. histolytica* is no exception. A recent impressive demonstration (Latour et al., 1965) involved the use of a basal, lipid-deficient medium. Tests showed that among numerous compounds only cholesterol and β-sitosterol could satisfy the requirement for added lipid.

Physiologic activities related to pathogenesis.   As noted above, *E. histolytica* plays the highly contrasting roles of a lumen-dwelling commensal and a tissue-penetrating pathogen capable of evoking serious disease. Several studies to account for this pathogenesis have focused on the amoeba's enzymatic capacities. Enzymes identified in *E. histolytica* include the series involved in anaerobic glycolysis (e.g., Bragg and Reeves, 1962b), amylase, acid phosphatase, and hyaluronidase. The last is of special interest in view of its role in spread through tissues, but unfortunately it could not be demonstrated in all pathogenic strains (Jarumilinta and Maegraith, 1960), and thus it cannot be regarded as an essential factor in invasiveness.

Tissue-dwelling trophozoites usually lie in a zone of liquefaction (hence the species name *histolytica*), suggesting extensive proteolytic action. Maegraith and collaborators (*see* Maegraith, 1963) followed hydrolysis by intact amoebas and homogenates of various protein substrates *in vitro*, and reported the presence of gelatinase, pepsin, and trypsin, but not chymotrypsin. They also showed that epithelial suspensions from human and guinea pig colon were readily digested by amoebas. Both pathogenic and nonpathogenic strains of *E. histolytica* shared these capacities, whereas those free-living amoebas tested neither contained trypsin nor lysed epithelial cells *in vitro*. Neal (1960) provided a more detailed account of techniques in his study of enzymic proteolysis. He could not correlate relatively high proteolytic activity with greater invasiveness *in vivo*, although declining proteolytic activity generally served as an index of declining pathogenicity. Neal discovered that mammalian sera contained a strong inhibitor of casein and gelatin hydrolysis. These interesting findings indicate that proteolytic activity, though essential, is not sufficient by itself to account for pathogenicity. The *in vivo* picture is probably highly complex, with multiple enzymatic activities of the parasite interacting with local and general host defense mechanisms and the current physiologic status of the host.

Physiologic status of the host

Of concern here are those properties of the host, apart from the specific immune reactions to be discussed later, that influence the biologic activities of *E. histolytica*. Two general features merit some attention because of the light they cast on the sensitive host-parasite interaction—these are the nutritional state of the host as reflected by the composition of the diet and the ecologic setting of the large intestine, especially as this is influenced by the resident bacterial flora.

Influence of diet. Controlled experiments on human populations are not feasible, but a few relevant observations have been made. South Africa is of interest in this connection, owing to a relatively high incidence of fulminating amoebiasis distributed unequally among the white, the Indian, and the African (Bantu) populations in the Durban area. Elsdon-Dew's extensive work (1958) has included epidemiologic studies. The Bantu population is most seriously affected, but only after becoming urbanized and industrialized. Sanitation clearly plays a role, but Elsdon-Dew's studies point to an abrupt change in diet as a primary factor: i.e., the replacement of the usual maize, milk, and some meat under natural conditions by a high carbohydrate diet ("bun and lemonade diet") in the cities. A low incidence of amoebiasis in factory workers fed by their employers was ascribed to substantial protein in the diet.

Laboratory experiments on animal hosts have provided more convincing evidence under controlled conditions. Thompson (1958) summarized experiments on 400 dogs conducted over a period of 10 years. Extending earlier work by the Faust school (e.g., Faust, 1932), he found that canned salmon allowed uniformly severe infections to be maintained, but the inclusion of cod liver oil and yeast compensated for vitamin deficiencies and greatly lessened mortality. Villarejos (1962) showed the striking inadequacy of canned salmon alone. Uninfected dogs maintained on this diet developed varying degrees of colitis suggesting a chronic nonspecific inflammation of the intestinal mucosa; in contrast, uninfected dogs fed on horse meat did not show these symptoms. Dietary modifications have also been shown to heighten susceptibility of rabbits and guinea pigs to amoebic infection. In his work with guinea pigs, Lynch (1957) showed that a synthetic diet was necessary to produce a severe fulminating disease. Significantly, he reported that this diet caused marked atrophy of the cecal mucosa, and he postulated that this structural change in the host aided invasion by the amoeba.

Dietary cholesterol has been reported independently by Indian (Das and Singh, 1965) and Mexican (Biagi et al., 1962) workers to influence the pathogenicity of *E. histolytica*. In Biagi's study with guinea pigs, elevated intestinal cholesterol and hypercholesterolemia caused distinct enhancement of lesions in the cecum and liver. The Indian investigators obtained similar results for colitis in rats and guinea pigs, and they also reported that the virulence of cultivated strains of *E. histolytica* varied directly with the presence of added cholesterol in the medium. This last finding requires confirmation with critical control of the total cholesterol content in the culture medium, since the egg-serum medium which was used obviously contains adequate cholesterol alone to satisfy any nutritional requirement of the parasite. Nevertheless, the dietary studies on host and parasite agree remarkably well in that the amoeba shows a clear requirement for carbohydrate and cholesterol, among many other substances, and alterations of these components in the host diet modify the physiologic activity (pathogenicity) of the parasite.

Experiments with germ-free hosts.   In ecologic terms, the host offers a wide array of habitats for intruding parasites. Each parasitic infection may be regarded as an ecosystem comprised of both the parasite and the host organ being occupied. This concept has been brilliantly developed for the mammalian digestive tract by Dubos and coworkers (1964, 1965) in their studies on the bacterial flora of germ-free mice and rats. The advent of germ-free hosts now allows controlled experimentation on parasitism in the alimentary canal; for the first time it has become possible to define the biologic agents in organs under study. Dubos' work on bacterial recolonization of the gut of germ-free mice has shown that certain bacteria settle differentially in various regions, in agreement with their distribution in conventional ("contaminated") hosts. The most abundant types prove to be fastidious anaerobes usually overlooked in bacteriologic studies. Dubos has introduced the term "autochthonous flora" to designate those bacteria which become symbiotic with their hosts in the course of evolution. The bacteroides group is the predominant inhabitant of the cecum; this is of special interest in view of the extensive use of *Bacteroides* sp. as a favorable nonbacterial associate of *E. histolytica* (Bragg and Reeves, 1962a).

It has been long recognized that germ-free hosts would be especially valuable in clarifying the factors involved in amoebic colitis. Over the past 15 years, Phillips and his associates have demonstrated unmistakably the relative roles of *E. histolytica* and the enteric flora in producing amoebic enteritis in the germ-free guinea pig. The amoebic inocula in their series of experiments were drawn from monoxenic cultures of the amoeba (NIH strain 200) growing with *Trypanosoma cruzi*; the latter did not survive in the intestinal tract. Three groups of guinea pigs were employed—germ-free, monocontaminated (containing a single bacterial species), and conventional animals. Challenge occurred via intracecal inoculation. The initial report (Phillips et al., 1955) showed that the amoebas could not establish an infection in germ-free hosts; indeed, their maximum survival in the intestine was five days. At the other extreme, 90 percent of conventional hosts developed acute ulcerative amoebiasis, whereas monocontaminated hosts containing *Escherichia coli* or *Aerobacter aerogenes* reacted similarly to conventional hosts.

Subsequent experiments have provided additional data. When greater care was taken in processing amoebic inocula, thereby reducing exposure to oxygen, active lesions were produced in germ-free hosts, although amoebas did not colonize the intestinal lumen (Phillips, 1964). The lesions developed at the site of puncture through the cecal wall, suggesting that traumatization of host tissues was a necessary precondition in these hosts. No fatalities resulted from these infections, even though lesions were even more readily produced when inocula were derived from existing lesions in germ-free animals. In a recent study, Phillips and Gorstein (1966) followed amoebic infections in guinea pigs monocontaminated with each of seven unrelated species of bacteria. Amoebic lesions developed with all bacteria tested, but the severity of disease varied greatly according to the associate. Surprisingly, the presence of *Bacillus subtilis* resulted in the highest percentage of fatalities (7 of 11 hosts), with lesser values for *Clostridium perfringens* (6 out of 12), *Staphylococcus aureus* (8 out of 23), and other species tested. No fatalities occurred with the strain of *E. coli* used in these experiments. The inflammatory responses varied widely from an acute reaction with *B. subtilis* and *S. aureus* to the condition in germ-free hosts of virtually no cellular response or at most a mild inflammatory response.

The experiments just described, and others in the series, support the view that bacteria participate in the etiology of amoebic enteritis. The probable mechanism whereby they accomplish this—and not all bacteria participate to the same degree—is to supply a suitable physical and chemical environment in the intestinal lumen for the establishment of a population of amoebas until penetration of the intestinal wall occurs. In the tissues, the typical invasive activity of the amoebas is often complicated by varying degrees of superimposed bacterial inflammation. The best available evidence leads to the conclusion that the physiologic condition of the host is crucial in determining whether *E. histolytica*—and, surely, many other intestinal parasites—can produce a lasting infection. The site in the host (the large intestine in this case) constitutes a dynamic environment which is subject to constant morphologic and physiologic changes and which supports a microbial flora composed of both normal species and numerous "stray" members that may alter conditions. Genetically diverse strains of amoebas sporadically gain access to this habitat. The interaction which follows is resolved depending upon the state of virulence of the challenging strain of *E. histolytica* and the relative susceptibility of the host. This leads us to consider the immune reactions of the host.

Immune reactions of the host

The presence of immunity in amoebic infections may be demonstrated in the vertebrate host by direct or indirect methods. The direct method involves challenging the host with the parasite *in vivo* and observing the response. Another direct effect of immunity can also be detected by administering immune serum to an animal at the same time that the parasite is introduced. The extent of knowledge about immunity operating in amoebiasis as studied by the direct method is discussed in the following section. Indirect evidence of immunity is provided by serologic reactions, and the voluminous data available on amoebiasis are reviewed in some detail in the section on antigen-antibody reactions.

Natural and acquired immunity. The best available evidence indicates that mammalian amoebiasis is an anthroponosis; namely, under natural conditions it is restricted essentially to humans (Hoare, 1962), even though the same amoeba also occurs in monkeys where it runs a symptomless course

(Dobell, 1931). This fact is of considerable importance to the epidemiologist as well as to the immunologist. However, at present there are no immunologic studies to elucidate the basis of natural immunity in insusceptible mammals. The existence of innate immunity in individual humans is questionable. Rogers (1923) reported spontaneous recovery from amoebic liver abscess in a number of patients. He reported further that recovery occurred spontaneously in 54 percent of cases of pleuropulmonary amoebiasis. Thus, the human body may have some mechanism of resistance against invading amoebas, but its nature is unknown. In reference to the subject of natural immunity in amoebiasis, it may be of interest to mention the work of Maegraith and Harinasuta (1958) on the experimental production of amoebic lesions in the livers of hamsters and guinea pigs. They found that amoebas survived and grew readily in the hamster liver whether injected directly into the liver or following secondary migration from existing intestinal lesions. In the guinea pig neither direct inoculation into the liver nor acute gut involvement led to establishment of amoebas in the liver. Special "preparation" of the host by the production of chronic intestinal lesions was needed before an abscess could be produced even by intraportal inoculation of the parasite. In view of these results, Maegraith (1963) raised the following questions: "Wherein lies the difference between the two animals? Why does the potentially pathogenic parasite so easily accept the conditions offered by the liver cells of the hamster but reject those offered by the guinea pig?" The study of these problems should throw some light on the capacities for interaction of the parasite and the host tissues, and consequently on the nature of so-called natural immunity.

Some degree of natural immunity occurs against the human intestinal protozoa which are normally commensals in the large intestine. The tissues of the human host are apparently completely immune to direct invasion by *Entamoeba coli, Endolimax, Dientamoeba, Trichomonas* and other intestinal flagellates. The immunity is almost complete in the case of *Iodamoeba bütschlii*, though one case has been reported in which it may have broken down when the host was in a profound state of emaciation as a result of malnutrition and malaria (Derrick, 1948). However, given the opportunity, even *E. coli* can attack the tissues of the host—Teodorovich (1963) inoculated sterile cultures of this organism intramurally into the intestine of guinea pigs and produced amoebic lesions, while with a similar technique he produced fulminating infections with nonpathogenic strains of *E. histolytica*.

Nothing is known about acquired immunity to amoebiasis in man (Shaffer et al., 1965). There is no evidence for the development of any resistance to reinfection, so individuals must always be considered susceptible, regardless of a previous history of recovery. The story of acquired resistance against amoebiasis in dogs is very different from that in man. Spontaneous recovery of dogs from experimental amoebiasis was reported by Faust as early as 1932. The occurrence of spontaneous recovery after a long-established infection is a phenomenon which suggests the development of immunity. Swartzwelder and Avant (1952) made an extensive study to assess the degree of resistance to reinfection with *E. histolytica* following elimination of previous infection in dogs. Amoebic infection was established in 39 dogs. The initial induced infection was 85 percent. Despite repeated attempts to reestablish infections in animals whose initial infection had been terminated, only 17 percent could be reinfected. The resistance to infection was active against both homologous and heterologous strains of *E. histolytica.* The tested duration of immunity to reinfection ranged from two and one-half months to nine and one-half months. A small series of animals which received preinoculation blood transfusions from dogs that had become refractory to reinfection with *E. histolytica*, showed a lower infection rate than animals not transfused. Definite conclusions cannot be drawn from this study regarding the possibility of passive transfer of immunity to amoebiasis in dogs by means of blood transfusion. Only ten animals were used for this specific experiment, and the results were not as sharply defined as in the study on actively acquired resistance to reinfection.

In summary, there is no convincing evidence of acquired immunity in human amoebiasis, but it is also clear that no critical studies have been undertaken as yet. In the following section we shall consider the various classes of antibodies induced by *E. histolytica*, and then return to the question of whether certain antigen-antibody reactions in amoebiasis may play a protective role.

Antigen-antibody reactions.   Various immunologic methods have been used for studying the immunology of *E. histolytica*, for example, complement fixation, immobilization, precipitin, fluorescent antibody (FA), hemagglutination (HA), and skin tests. These techniques have been employed (1) to determine their potential value as diagnostic methods, (2) for epidemiologic surveys, and (3) to study the similarities and/or differences between strains and species of *Entamoeba*. These results will be discussed in detail in the following sections, which are divided according to the serologic techniques employed.

Complement-Fixation Test.   The first attempts to devise a complement-fixation test for the diagnosis of intestinal amoebiasis were those of Izar (1914), von Hage (1920), and Scalas (1921). However, it was not until Craig (1927) began a systematic study of the problem that this serologic test was shown to have possibilities as a diagnostic technique. One of the chief difficulties encountered in developing and standardizing this test has been the preparation of a suitable antigen. Even when prepared by the same methods, antigens from different strains of amoebas may vary in sensitivity and specificity. In addition to differences in antigens, numerous procedures have been developed for carrying out the complement-fixation technique. This has led to wide variation in the reported value of the test. Thus, Craig (1933), using the human hemolytic system, reported that the complement-fixation test was 90 percent accurate in intestinal amoebiasis, whereas Paulson and Andrews (1938), using the sheep hemolytic system, believed that its diagnostic accuracy was not over 47 percent.

Incidental to the use of the complement-fixation test for intestinal amoebiasis, results suggested that it was of diagnostic value for patients with accompanying amoebic hepatitis or abscess. Terry and Bozicevich (1948) reported complement-fixation studies on the sera of 15 patients with amoebic hepatitis. Twelve cases showed a positive complement-fixation test on the initial test and all other tests prior to therapy. Hussey and Brown (1950) tested the sera from 124 individuals with *E. histolytica* in their stools and with varying degrees of clinical intestinal amoebiasis. Only three of these sera gave positive reactions. Whereas the complement-fixation test failed to demonstrate the presence of intestinal amoebiasis in most cases, it resulted in a positive reaction in the majority of hepatic amoebiasis patients. Bozicevich (1950) disputed the conclusions of Hussey and Brown as to the negative value of the complement-fixation test for the diagnosis of intestinal amoebiasis. He had conducted 13,000 complement-fixation tests since 1942 and found that in most cases the complement-fixation tests were in agreement with the findings of *E. histolytica* in stools. Bozicevich (1950) also suggested that more dependable tests could probably be carried out with polyvalent antigens than with those derived from a single strain of *E. histolytica*. McDearman and Dunham (1952), using the same commercial form of antigen as Bozicevich (1950), obtained positive reactions in only 15 percent of intestinal amoebiasis in contrast to 85 percent of cases of extraintestinal amoebiasis. Dolkart et al. (1951) concluded from a study of 499 cases that there was no correlation between the occurrence of a positive complement-fixation test and the presence of *E. histolytica* in fecal examination. Elsdon-Dew and Maddison (1952) found only a 63 percent positive correlation with confirmed intestinal amoebiasis, whereas 28 out of 29 cases of liver abscess gave a definite positive reaction.

Immobilization Test.   When amoebas are incubated in the presence of specific antiserum, they are affected to various degrees and in various ways according to the type of observation carried out. This type of reaction, which is commonly exhibited by amoebas, was first described by Cole and Kent (1953) for *E. histolytica*. When placed in homologous antiserum, motile trophozoites soon ceased to form pseudopodia and rounded up. Maximal immobilization was obtained in 20 to 30 minutes, after which the amoebas regained their activity.

The immobilization reaction has been studied by several workers as a method of serologic diagnosis of amoebiasis in man. Cole and Kent (1953) showed that only 38 percent of sera from patients with amoebiasis caused immobilization of the trophozoites. Valentino (1956) confirmed the previous observation of Cole and Kent (1953) and further observed that the immobilizing activity was frequent and strong in sera from patients with intestinal amoebiasis, whereas it was absent, or present to a very low degree, in normal human sera. The immobilization test showed a higher sensitivity than the complement-fixation test. Accordingly, Valentino (1956) called for further investigations on this test in order to ascertain its value in the practical diagnostic field. Biagi and Buentello (1961) also showed that sera from patients with amoebiasis possessed the immobilizing factors. Biagi et al., (1963) studied the value of the immobilization test for the diagnosis of amoebiasis, bearing in mind the possible transfer of the factor(s) responsible for this reaction from mother to child through the placental barrier. For this purpose, tests were carried out with sera obtained from the blood of 150 pregnant women and from the umbilical cord of their offspring during parturition. The sera of those infants in whose mothers the immobilization test was negative were likewise negative, whereas in 86 percent of the infants from mothers with a positive reaction, the test was positive. These experiments provided evidence that the immobilization factor(s) can pass through the placental barrier. However, caution should be exercised in the interpretation of a positive reaction in a newborn baby. Thus, if it is negative in the mother and positive in the infant, it can be assumed that the latter was infected with *E. histolytica*.

Previous investigations had considered that surface antigens were involved in the immobilization reaction, and Biagi et al. (1966) provided data to strengthen this hypothesis. Using the fluorescent-antibody technique, they observed that as immobilization occurred, the fluorescence was localized principally on the surface of the organism. After 45 minutes, it was regularly distributed in the ectoplasm and endoplasm. At 75 minutes all the fluorescent material was present in a large vacuole in the endoplasm, but at 101 minutes it was barely perceptible and at this time resumption of trophozoite motility was observed. Loss of fluorescence was not seen in trophozoites that were not reactivated.

Rabbit antiserum to *E. histolytica* also markedly inhibited the ability of the amoebas to ingest red blood cells *in vitro*, apparently because of the immobilizing effect of the antiserum (Shaffer and Ansfield, 1956).

Zaman (1960) carried out an extensive comparative serologic study with several species of *Entamoeba*, namely, *E. histolytica, E. coli, E. ranarum, E. invadens*, and *E. moshkovskii*, using the immobilization method. He prepared antisera to these species in rabbits and observed the degree of immobilization of the homologous and heterologous species. *E. coli* was found to be unsuitable for comparative immobilization studies due to its normal restricted locomotor activity. However, this species did cross-react with *E. histolytica* in that *E. histolytica* amoebas were partly immobilized by anti-*E. coli* serum. If the results with *E. coli* were omitted, Zaman's results showed that the four remaining species could be divided into two groups. The first group consisted of *E. histolytica* and *E. invadens*, and the second group of *E. moshkovskii* and *E. ranarum*. There was no cross-reaction between these two groups, though cross-reactions did occur within each group. Zaman also studied a series of strains of *E. histolytica* which differed in their virulent or avirulent properties. Immobilization tests showed that virulent strains formed a group distinct from the avirulent strains. However, unlike the results obtained with different species, there was a degree of cross-reaction between the virulent and avirulent strains. These results may be correlated with invasiveness rather than with innate specific differences (Neal, 1966). The relationship between *E. histolytica* and *E. gingivalis*, using the immobilization test, was studied by Sato and Kaneko (1957), who observed a complete absence of cross-reaction between these two species.

The relationship of the three species of *Entamoeba* to the hartmannellid amoebas was described by Adam (1964). Using the immobilization test, she found the two groups were quite distinct and without any degree of cross-reaction. Antisera to *E. histolytica, E. invadens,* and *E. moshkovskii* were prepared and showed no immobilizing effect on four strains of *Hartmannella castellanii.* Similarly, antisera to four strains of *H. castellanii* did not immobilize *E. invadens.*

Precipitin Test.   A precipitate is often formed when a soluble antigen and its antiserum are mixed. If a gel is the supporting medium and the reactants diffuse toward each other through the gel, the precipitate will be formed as one or more bands or lines, and this technique is known as gel diffusion. This technique was first developed by Ouchterlony in 1949, and since then it has been extensively used by microbiologists and immunologists for the qualitative analysis of immunologic systems, especially when comparative studies of antigen and antibody are desired.

Precipitin tests have also been used in the study of amoebiasis for three main purposes: (1) to serve as the diagnostic test for amoebiasis using human sera; (2) to compare the serologic relationship of various pathogenic and nonpathogenic strains of *Entamoeba* and related genera as well as strains of *E. histolytica,* using both human antisera and antisera prepared in experimental animals; and (3) to elucidate the antigenic structure of *E. histolytica* using human, rabbit, or guinea pig antisera. The reports concerning the antigenic structure of *E. histolytica* will be discussed below in the section on the nature of antigens (*see* pp. 461-462).

Precipitins attributed to infections with *E. histolytica* were reported as early as 1924 by Wagener in sera of cats with experimental amoebic dysentery. In 1957, Moan described a simple and rapid precipitin test for significant clinical infection in man with *E. histolytica.* A specific precipitate, observed through a microscope, was the basis of a positive test. However, this test was frequently negative in acute amoebic dysentery and in the asymptomatic carrier state.

More recently the utilization of agar gel as a medium for such reactions has been accompanied by increased interest in the study of precipitins. Nakamura and Baker (1957) studied antibodies related to *E. histolytica* in sera from human patients and from immunized rabbits. Agar-gel plates were employed by those authors, and as many as three antigen-antibody bands were attributed to *E. histolytica.* Maddison and Elsdon-Dew (1961), in certain cases of amoebiasis in man, noted the presence of additional nonspecific antibodies by means of a macrodiffusion procedure using agar gel. This nonspecific fraction was shown to be due to accompanying *Clostridium perfringens (welchii)* antigen. This nonspecific antibody was revealed in 100 percent of amoebic liver abscess cases, 69 percent of cases of amoebic dysentery, and 60 percent of nonamoebic dysentery cases. Nakamura (1961) reported that better results with human sera were obtained when antigen was prepared from newly isolated strains of *E. histolytica.*

An improvement in the application of gel diffusion to analysis of antigen-antibody precipitates was reported by Wadsworth (1957), who used a miniaturized technique known as microdiffusion. It was described as more economical of time and material, as well as possessing greater sensitivity. Atchley et al. (1963), using this microdiffusion technique, tested samples of human sera collected from 16 cases of amoebiasis occurring in African males. Eleven were confirmed cases of acute amoebic dysentery, four of amoebic liver abscess, and one was a cyst-passer with a peptic ulcer but without symptoms of amoebiasis. Additional sera to serve as controls were acquired from 12 individuals in whom no infection of *E. histolytica* was noted. No precipitate bands were observed in microslides with control sera from 12 individuals, but in contrast, 2 to 10 precipitate bands were noted with the sera from all 16 infected persons, including the apparently asymptomatic cyst-passer.

Maddison (1965) reported the results of the precipitin test on a larger series of cases drawn from Durban, Union of South Africa. The cases consisted of (1) 85 African patients with confirmed amoebic liver abscess, (2) 164 African patients with confirmed amoebic dysentery, (3) 57 patients, Africans and Indians, with diseases other than invasive amoebiasis but in whose stools cysts of *E. histolytica* were found, (4) 11 African and Indian patients with bacillary dysentery, (5) 135 African and 107 Indian patients in whom full clinical examination failed to show any symptoms attributable to *E. histolytica*, (6) sera from 24 cases of ulcerative colitis, and (7) control sera collected from 100 white, 109 Indians, and 106 African blood donors. Double-diffusion agar gel and immunoelectrophoretic techniques (Williams and Grabar, 1955) were employed by Maddison. Antibodies apparently directed against specific amoebic components were detected in a high proportion of patients with invasive amoebiasis (97 percent in amoebic liver abscess and 89 percent in amoebic dysentery), a smaller proportion of cyst-passers (37 percent), and a much lower proportion (6 to 27 percent) of random subjects without symptoms attributable to *E. histolytica*. The high incidence of "anti-*C. welchii*" precipitin in patients with diseases other than amoebiasis showed that although this precipitin was demonstrable in 98 percent of patients with amoebic liver abscess, it was not directly related to tissue invasion by *E. histolytica* (Maddison, 1965). While the nonspecific "*C. welchii*" reaction frequently disappeared rapidly under therapy, the apparently specific antiamoebic precipitins persisted in patients following discharge. The presence of antibodies in cyst-passers without clinical symptoms attributable to *E. histolytica* is suggestive of past tissue invasion by the amoeba, or of present subclinical invasion. Similarly, the demonstration of antibodies in the random patients without invasive amoebiasis and in blood donors (control sera) may either be the result of such tissue invasion by *E. histolytica*, or of the presence of nonspecific components in the antigen. Demonstration of antibodies in sera eight months after cure of active amoebiasis indicated that the former may explain their presence in some patients without symptoms of amoebiasis. The detection of antiamoebic precipitins in 14 percent of hospitalized Africans without clinical amoebiasis indicates the danger of the use of positive findings as a diagnostic aid, since these may only reflect past invasive infection. However, negative results in the gel-diffusion test have proved to be of considerable clinical importance in excluding suspected tissue invasion by *E. histolytica* (Maddison, 1965). Similarly, Powell et al. (1965) used the agar-gel diffusion test to diagnose amoebic liver abscess, finding a positive precipitin reaction in 96 percent of proved amoebic liver abscess cases and in 90 percent of clinically diagnosed cases. Also using the agar-gel diffusion technique, Aurenheimer et al. (1966) studied sera from 93 institutionalized persons with demonstrable infection of *E. histolytica*. They found results similar to those previously obtained by Maddison (1965). In only 50 percent of the asymptomatic cases did they find a precipitin reaction; they explained the absence of antibody in the remaining 50 percent of the cases by suggesting that invasion might not have occurred.

Besides the diagnostic value of the precipitin test, this test has also been used by various workers to study serologic relationships among various species of *Entamoeba*, as well as among strains of *E. histolytica*. Sen et al. (1961) prepared anti-*E. histolytica* serum in rabbits and found no reaction with *E. moshkovskii* antigen or antigens from the free-living amoebas, *Naegleria gruberi* and *Schizopyrenus russelli*. Talis et al. (1963) found no common antigens between *E. histolytica* and *E. invadens*. Siddiqui and Balamuth (1965) made an extensive comparative study and found that there was no cross-reaction when heterologous antigens were tested against anti-*E. histolytica* and anti-*E. invadens* sera. The antigens were prepared from *E. histolytica*, *E. invadens*, *E. moshkovskii*, *Hartmannella rhysodes*, and *Mayorella palestinensis*. It is interesting to note that the Laredo strain of *E. histolytica*, a special low-temperature variant, gave some cross-reaction against anti-*E. histolytica* (DKB strain) serum. Goldman and Siddiqui (1965) prepared antisera against the two substrains of *E. histolytica* strain 200 growing with *Trypanosoma cruzi*. The substrains were stable size variants derived from the parent stock by microisolation. No antigenic differences could be demonstrated between the substrains by gel-diffusion and immunoelectrophoretic techniques. Krupp (1966) made an extensive comparative study of 10 strains of *E. histolytica* and one strain of *E. invadens*, employing agar-gel diffusion and immunoelectrophoretic techniques. She found that pathogenic strains (NRS, 200, DKB, BH, and F22) showed no antigenic similarities with nonpathogenic strains (JH, K9, Js, Huff, and Laredo) or with *E. invadens*. The latter showed some immunologic relationship with the Huff strain of *E. histolytica*, and interestingly enough both of these strains grow at room temperature. She also found that there was some degree of difference in the immunoelectrophoretic patterns of the various strains of *E. histolytica* tested. Very recently, Talis (1967) reported a preliminary study on the serologic relationship of *E. histolytica*, *E. invadens*, and *Dientamoeba fragilis*. The anti-*E. invadens* sera reacted with the homologous antigen and with the two strains of *E. histolytica*, but did not react with *D. fragilis*. The anti-*E. histolytica* serum reacted neither with *E. invadens* nor with *D. fragilis* antigens. This is the only reported case of sharing of antigens by *E. invadens* and *E. histolytica* using gel-diffusion techniques; detailed evidence was not submitted.

Fluorescent-Antibody Test.   The fluorescent-antibody (FA) technique provides a means of staining a fixed antigen preparation with a "fluorescent-tagged" antibody. Though the FA technique has been used widely by bacteriologists and virologists, its application to protozoa was initiated by Goldman.

Since 1953, Goldman has been conducting pioneer studies with this technique on various species of *Entamoeba*. Over a period of several years Goldman has attempted to devise a fluorescent-antibody test for human amoebiasis that would allow any strain capable of being cultivated to be used as antigen. Although it was evident very early that antibody-containing sera in amoebiasis cases could be demonstrated by FA technique (Goldman, 1954), practical testing procedures were handicapped by various technical difficulties. The variable staining of individual amoebas on the same smears and the nonspecific green fluorescence which always occurred made the method extremely subjective with regard to reading and interpretation, especially when titers were marginal. Goldman (1966) described a standardized procedure based on the "indirect" FA technique that was designed to overcome these difficulties. Major technical improvements making this possible were the formalin–NH₄OH–Tween 80 fixation method of Maestrone (1963) and the use of Evans Blue as a counterstain (Nichols and McComb, 1962). Using the K9 strain of *E. histolytica* as antigen, Goldman (1966) reported 73.1 percent positive reaction for 52 cases of confirmed intestinal amoebiasis and 91.3 percent for 23 cases of confirmed or unconfirmed extraintestinal amoebiasis. However, 5 out of 16 individuals without amoebic infection were also found to be positive, even at the low titer of the sera. Goldman (1966) further showed that the antigen from the Huff strain of *E. histolytica*, a low-temperature variant like the Laredo strain, showed far fewer positive reactions with antisera from cases of human amoebiasis than did the antigen prepared from a virulent strain like K9.

Jeanes (1964) obtained brilliant fluorescence of amoebas which were exposed to antisera from 3 patients with confirmed hepatic amoebiasis, and very weak fluorescent staining with control sera (6 healthy subjects, 8 patients with nonamoebic liver disorders, and 21 patients with other non-amoebic conditions).

Talis (1966) tested 71 human sera with the indirect FA technique for the presence of antibody to *E. histolytica*. Of the 71 sera, 26 were from cases of amoebiasis (including amoebic liver abscess), 18 from clinically negative cases, 15 from cases with a positive clinical history but negative stools, and 12 from a heterogeneous group with nonamoebic infection. The majority of positive cases reacted at an immunofluorescent titer of 1:80. Nine of the 18 sera from cases diagnosed clinically as free from amoebiasis also gave positive results. Talis suggested that this result might be due to past contact with the amoebas, since no positive results were obtained with sera from sources definitely established as free from amoebiasis.

Goldman (1966) considered the FA technique to be a potentially useful tool in diagnostic epidemiologic studies. In such studies, however, caution must be exercised in interpreting diagnostic titers, and more data are certainly called for to explain the anomalous results found thus far with this technique.

Like other immunologic techniques, the FA test has also been used to study the serologic relationship of various species of *Entamoeba* and strains of *E. histolytica*. The relationship between *E. coli* and *E. histolytica* was first studied by Goldman (1953, 1954). Antisera to both species were prepared, and although some cross-reaction was observed, the heterologous fluorescence was removed by absorption with the appropriate species of amoeba. The use of these antisera with the FA test enabled Goldman (1954) to identify successfully unknown amoebas as either *E. histolytica* or *E. coli*. Amoebas of *Dientamoeba fragilis* and *Endolimax nana* showed virtually negligible fluorescence, while *E. invadens* reacted less than either *E. histolytica* or *E. coli*, but more than *Dientamoeba fragilis* or *Endolimax nana*. *E. moshkovskii* was not significantly stained with an anti-*E. histolytica* serum (Goldman et al., 1960; Goldman and Gleason, 1962). *E. hartmanni* did not significantly fluoresce with anti-*E. histolytica* serum, and conversely anti-*E. hartmanni* serum did not significantly stain *E. histolytica*.

However, the Huff strain of *E. histolytica* showed an intermediate reaction between *E. histolytica* (virulent strain) and *E. hartmanni*. This difference was correlated to the lack of virulence of the Huff strain. This hypothesis was supported by the observation that *E. histolytica* which was taken directly from a cecal ulcer of an experimentally infected guinea pig fluoresced more brightly than amoebas after cultivation *in vitro* for five days or more. The reactions of the Laredo strain have also been studied by the FA technique (Goldman et al., 1962). The fluorescent staining of this strain of *E. histolytica*, which grows at 25° and 37°, was compared with a normal strain of *E. histolytica* growing at 37° and *E. moshkovskii* also growing at 25° and 37°. Five anti-*E. histolytica* sera were used. It was found that the Laredo amoebas grown at 37° fluoresced as brightly as the normal strain of *E. histolytica*, but *E. moshkovskii*, also grown at 37°, stained to a lesser degree. When grown at 25°, the Laredo strain reacted less than *E. histolytica* grown at 37°, and was similar to *E. moshkovskii* grown at 25°. From these data it seems that the Laredo strain resembles *E. histolytica* more closely than *E. moshkovskii*, but it is not completely typical of *E. histolytica*. From these results it was also concluded that the Huff strain of *E. histolytica* resembled the Laredo strain grown at 25°, and resembled *E. moshkovskii* more than typical *E. histolytica*. This is an interesting conclusion, since it was subsequently shown that the Huff strain could also grow at room temperature (Richards et al., 1965). Thus the Laredo strain differs from the K9 strain of *E. histolytica* in two respects—by its low virulence and its ability to grow at room temperature. Siddiqui and Balamuth (1965), using the FA technique, found that there is some degree of serologic relationship in descending order between the IP stain of *E. invadens*, the Laredo strain of *E. histolytica*, the DSR strain of *E. moshkovskii*, and the DKB strain of *E. histolytica* when they were tested against antiserum to an axenic strain

(IP) of *E. invadens.* These results confirmed the observations made earlier by Goldman (1960) and Goldman et al. (1962).

Siddiqui and Balamuth (1965) further found that there was no cross-reaction between free-living amoebas (*Hartmannella rhysodes* and *Mayorella palestinensis*) and three species of *Entamoeba* (*E. histolytica, E. invadens,* and *E. moshkovskii*).

Hemagglutination Test.   The hemagglutination test, though widely used by microbiologists and immunologists, was not employed for the diagnosis of amoebiasis until 1961, when Kessel and collaborators reported the identification of an antibody reacting with amoeba antigen. Preliminary studies by this group (Kessel et al., 1961; Lewis and Kessel, 1961) indicated that the indirect hemagglutination test detected antibodies to *E. histolytica* for long periods of time, even after apparent cure. In one patient with an amoeboma, the HA (hemagglutination) titer dropped only by one half during a four-year follow-up. Variation in reactivity was ascribed to: (1) characteristics of the antigen, (2) duration and frequency of exposure, and (3) efficiency of the host in antibody production. In 1965, Kessel et al. performed indirect HA tests on sera from 455 patients with amoebiasis who harbored *E. histolytica* and from 101 negative cases used as controls. In general, they observed a close positive correlation between the HA test and proved amoebiasis. The HA test was positive in 100 percent of active liver abscess cases, 98 percent of dysentery cases, 66 percent of asymptomatic carriers, and 3 percent of controls. These authors further reported that the indirect HA test remained positive for many years following the initial infection, although the titer of reactivity gradually dropped. Maddison et al. (1965) made an indirect HA test on sera from 410 human cases and compared the results obtained previously by gel-diffusion tests. Both techniques detected antibodies in a high proportion of patients with invasive amoebiasis. There was agreement in 64 of 65 patients with amoebic liver abscess, in 61 of 66 patients with amoebic dysentery, in 16 of 24 asymptomatic cyst-passers, and in 240 of 275 patients with other diseases. Though the specificity of the two tests was similar, there was disagreement in 35 of 275 examinations. To investigate these differences, absorption of sera with sensitized cells was carried out until the HA test became negative. This absorption failed to remove all precipitins and confirmed the impression that different antibodies are involved in the two tests.

Talis (1966) examined 71 human sera by the indirect HA test and compared it with the FA test. The majority of positive cases reacted to both tests, but the titers obtained by the indirect HA method were much higher (1:3,200) than those obtained by the FA test (1:80), indicating that the HA test is more sensitive than the FA test. Milgram et al. (1966) conducted an extensive study on 994 sera using the indirect HA test. Their study indicated a high specificity of the indirect HA test for the sera from patients with extraintestinal amoebiasis and emphasized its value in differentiating amoebic and pyogenic abscesses of the liver. Their results for intestinal amoebiasis were also encouraging. The test was specific but did not detect all cases of intestinal amoebiasis. These authors could not confirm the high positive (66 percent) prevalence of antibodies in carriers obtained by Kessel et al. (1965). The difference between these studies might be due to the different methods of standardization of the test, as well as the place of origin of asymptomatic carriers. In the studies of Milgram et al. (1966) the largest number of carriers were Americans, whereas those of Kessel et al. (1965) were from endemic areas where individuals may have had a previous clinical exposure to amoebiasis.

Healy (1967) provided evidence for the persistence of positive titers for as long as a year or more in follow-up cases of amoebiasis. He measured indirect HA titers on follow-up sera from five patients, three with intestinal amoebiasis and two with amoebic liver abscesses. All five patients were clinically cured and no evidence of reinfection was shown. Initially high titers of 1:1,024 to 1:4,096 were present, but within a period of six months indirect HA titers dropped to a low positive level of 1:128 to 1:256, and these low positive titers were found to persist for a year or more.

Halpern et al. (1967) ran parallel studies with human sera obtained from an endemic amoebiasis area of Durban, Union of South Africa, using HA and agar-gel tests, while the type and source of antigen remained constant (K9 strain of *E. histolytica*). Of these patients, 44, 31, and 34 were checked by HA, agar-gel tests, and microscopic examinations, respectively. Of those examined by HA tests, 86 percent were positive, by agar-gel tests 95 percent were positive, and by microscopic examinations 91 percent were positive. Based on these results, the authors concluded that the serologic identification of *E. histolytica* is practical in a working situation, and that with a proper antigen, valid results seem obtainable by a variety of accepted serologic procedures, such as indirect HA or agar-gel tests.

Skin Test. Tissue response to invasive infection by *E. histolytica* in man is characterized by its noninflammatory nature. Neither the histologic changes nor the clinical findings are indicative of the state of classical hypersensitivity in man. This is probably one of the reasons why investigations by means of skin tests have been infrequent in amoebiasis. Scalas (1923) and Leal (1953), however, reported correlation between infection with *E. histolytica* and demonstrable hypersensitivity in human patients. Heathman (1932) and Menendez (1932) showed a delayed type of hypersensitivity to *E. histolytica* in immunized experimental animals. Heathman (1932) was able to transfer passively the skin-sensitizing antibodies in sera from immunized animals.

Maddison et al. (1968a) made an extensive study employing skin tests in patients with active invasive infections of *E. histolytica* and a comparable asymptomatic group, both of which were drawn from a community in which amoebiasis is highly endemic (Durban, Union of South Africa). An extract of *E. histolytica* (strain DKB) grown in monoxenic culture was used as antigen. A control antigen was prepared from cultures of PPLO grown in the same type of medium as the amoebas. For comparative purpose, parallel tests were run, using HA, agar-gel, and FA techniques. Of the patients with invasive amoebiasis, 81 percent showed positive skin tests, 100 percent were positive in the agar-gel and HA tests, and 90 percent in the FA test. In the asymptomatic group, only 14 percent were positive in skin tests, while 20.5 percent were positive with agar-gel, 32 percent with HA, and 9 percent with FA tests. Based on the results obtained by skin tests, these authors concluded that hypersensitivity was involved in amoebiasis, and that in the active invasive stage it was usually of the immediate type. In no instance of delayed hypersensitivity in the amoebiasis patients had symptoms been present for less than one and one-half months. In the entire group, the duration of symptoms ranged from one week to seven months. Immediate-type skin reactions were demonstrable as early as one week after the appearance of reported symptoms. Though it is evident from the results that the skin test is less sensitive than other serologic tests, its applicability in epidemiologic studies warrants serious consideration.

In this review of the literature on antigen-antibody reactions, critical evaluation has been complicated by the failure of different investigators to use standardized preparations of antigens. Instead, antigens have been drawn from diverse strains of *E. histolytica* grown with miscellaneous bacteria, and different methods have been used to extract antigens. Comparisons between different laboratories and correlations between different serologic tests are rendered correspondingly difficult. However, a few conclusions can be drawn from the preceding discussion of antigen-antibody reactions in amoebiasis:

1. In amoebiasis, humoral antibodies can be detected by most of the standard serologic methods, but the indirect HA test ranks as the most sensitive;

2. For epidemiologic surveys, the precipitin and indirect HA techniques have been widely used and have given satisfactory results;

3. Due to the occurrence of many subclinical cases in which no antibody production can be demonstrated, there is no existing serologic test which can substitute for stool examinations to detect the presence of all amoebic infections;

4. The negative results with the indirect HA and precipitin tests have proved to be of considerable clinical importance in excluding suspected tissue invasion by *E. histolytica*.

As has been pointed out earlier (*see* page 449), there is no evidence for the development of any resistance to reinfection. Therefore, all individuals must be considered susceptible to infection, regardless of their previous history. This suggests, in turn, that antibody response in amoebiasis does not play a protective role, but instead has its principal value in serodiagnosis. This brings us to a consideration of our current knowledge of the biochemical nature of the antibodies involved in amoebiasis.

Nature of antibody.   The liberation of varied antigens from *E. histolytica* induces a complex antibody response. Undoubtedly, amoebic antigens can induce antibodies that will fix complement, agglutinate cells, precipitate proteins, and so forth, depending upon the conditions presented. Many of these *in vitro* reactions may be manifestations of the same antibody under different conditions. On the other hand, one antigen may induce more than one antibody. It is easy to see, therefore, why the antibody response to parasites in general and to parasitic amoebas in particular is complex and still poorly understood.

Smithers (1967) observed that in various parasitic diseases elevated immunoglobulin levels are common. This is also true for amoebiasis. Anderson et al. (1958) reported an increase of α-2-globulins and γ-globulins in a Bantu population with acute intestinal amoebiasis.

Remington (1967), in a review article on characterization of antibodies to parasites, observed: "In marked contrast to the voluminous literature on the immunochemical and physiochemical characterization of antibodies formed in response to infection with a variety of bacteria, viruses and to numerous pure antigens, relatively little is known about the characterization of antibodies formed in response to infection with protozoa and helminths." This statement is readily applicable to the state of knowledge of antibodies in amoebiasis. Though various serologic tests are available for the diagnosis of amoebiasis, we lack knowledge of the nature of the antibodies that participate in these reactions.

Very recently through the work of Maddison, Kagan, and Norman (1968), the first step has been taken to characterize the nature of antibodies formed in response to *E. histolytica* infections in man. Immunoglobulins (IgG, IgA, and IgM) were separated from the sera of two patients (*Patient P:* unproved amoebic liver abscess, passing cysts of *E. histolytica*, blood drawn 2 months after commencement of therapy; *Patient B:* proved acute amoebic dysentery, blood drawn 15 days after initiation of therapy). The techniques used were column chromatography (Sephadex G-200 and DEAE-cellulose) and sucrose-density ultracentrifugation. Anti-whole human serum and anti-human G were prepared in rabbits. Specific anti-IgG, -IgA, and -IgM were obtained commercially. The relative purity of fractions was assayed by gel-diffusion and immunoelectrophoretic techniques against immunoglobulin antisera. Whole serum and fractions of globulins were analyzed by three serodiagnostic methods, i.e., gel-diffusion, hemagglutination, and fluorescent antibody.

A total of four and eight lines of precipitates were formed when whole sera from patients P and B were tested, respectively, with amoeba antigen in gel-diffusion plates. The sera also gave positive results with HA (titers of 1:512 and 1:130,000 in sera from patients P and B, respectively) and FA tests. When immunoglobulin fractions (IgG, IgA, and IgM) of the sera were tested against the amoeba antigen, only IgG fractions of the sera gave the same type of serologic reactions as were obtained by the whole sera. These reactivities were removed by absorption of the whole sera with anti-IgG serum, confirming the above result.

The significance of the work reported above is that it unequivocally demonstrated that only the IgG fraction of the whole globulin was reactive in gel-diffusion, hemagglutination, and FA tests. Since the sera from patients P and B were drawn one month and 15 days, respectively, after the initiation of treatment, this could be a reflection of the type of antibody being produced in relation to the duration of infection. Investigations of sera from patients presenting short clinical histories of amoebiasis and follow-ups on these patients would reveal whether other fractions of immunoglobulin, e.g., IgA and IgM, are produced in the early stages of tissue invasion by *E. histolytica*.

Nature of antigen. The characterization of amoeba antigens by gel-diffusion methods has demonstrated their complexity and has provided a useful assay for their purification. Many workers (Sen et al., 1961; Siddiqui, 1961; Maddison and Elsdon-Dew, 1961; Atchley et al., 1963; Talis et al., 1963; and Goldman and Siddiqui, 1965) have reported from 1 to 10 precipitation bands in the *E. histolytica* antigen-antibody system using Ouchterlony's gel-diffusion method. Krupp (1966) recently evaluated 11 amoebic antigens by immunoelectrophoretic analysis. The number of lines observed in an agar-gel precipitin test represents the minimum numbers of antigenic components that are at equivalence.

The gel-diffusion method has provided an analytical method for immunologists analogous to chromatography for the chemists. It is generally appreciated that finding lines is not an end in itself, but one key step in unravelling the problem leading toward isolation of the antigens responsible for eliciting the antibody response. A set of precipitin lines generally reflects the structure of a number of constituent proteins which are the direct products of the genome of a species. For fractionation and purification of antigens from the complex starting materials, new methods of ever-increasing discrimination are becoming available. Ion-exchange substituted-celluloses, electrophoretic techniques, and density gradient centrifugation have been especially useful. Using these techniques, Lewis and Kessel (1967) have begun a pioneering study on fractionating the amoeba antigens. To separate the components and purify the individual antigens, extracts of the DKB strain of *E. histolytica* were fractionated by gel-filtration on a 2.5 by 45 cm column of Sephadex G-200. Five peaks of protein were obtained, with mobilities approximating those of dextrans, and having molecular weights of 180,000 (peak 1); 80,000 (peak 2); 25,000 (peak 3); 10,000 (peak 4); and 1,000 (peak 5), respectively. In addition to protein, the first two peaks also contained small amounts of carbohydrate, but more than 90 percent of the total carbohydrate accompanied peak number 5. Capability to sensitize tanned red blood cells was found to be primarily in peak 1, in small amounts in peak 2, and absent from peaks 3, 4, and 5. Complement-fixing activity was found in peaks 1, 2, 3, and to a lesser extent in peak 4. Peak 5 was first thought to have no antigenic activity, but further investigations showed small amounts of complement-fixing activity. The data suggest that antigens with the highest molecular weight also sensitized tanned red cells most readily, and that antigens in peaks 3 and 4 were capable of fixing complement strongly but did not contribute to reactivity in the hemagglutination test. A detailed treatment enlarging upon this preliminary report will be a welcome contribution to the research literature.

It may be of interest to mention here briefly a report of Swart and Warren (1962), who compared the antigenicity of physiologically derived substances (PD) *in vitro* of *E. histolytica* with that of its somatic antigens. Included in this report were the methods of separating somatic antigens from PD antigens and the detection of antibodies elicited in rabbits inoculated with either somatic or PD antigens by employing precipitin or immobilizing techniques. The data obtained in this report suggested that *E. histolytica* under *in vitro* conditions does not secrete or excrete any antigenic material into the surrounding medium.

There is now an increasing awareness of the necessity for purifying antigens for study and for providing adequate evidence of physical, chemical, and immunologic homogeneity. Many bacterial antigens are well advanced into the stage of study and identification of epitopes (specific antigenic determinant site, group, or area). As starting material for isolation, bacteria have the advantage of being readily processed in large quantities in a pure state. In the case of characterization of *E. histolytica* antigens, the use of impure products in the past has resulted in many dubious or uninterpretable results. It is known that *E. histolytica* can be cultured axenically (Diamond, 1961). Recently Reeves and Ward (1965) have published a procedure for large-scale cultivation of *E. histolytica*, although bacterial protein contaminates their preparations. A beginning has already been made in the fractionation of amoeba antigens (Lewis and Kessel, 1967), as well as of immunoglobulins produced against *E. histolytica* (Maddison et al., 1968b). The concentrated and coordinated efforts of parasitologists and immunologists are required to unravel the biochemical complexity of amoeba antigens with the goals of identifying the functional antigens(s), their specific sites (epitopes), and finally an understanding of the biosynthetic pathways of epitopes.

INTESTINAL CILIATES

Ciliates are the most complex and animal-like of all protozoa, exhibiting well-coordinated locomotion, definite mouthparts, and the habit of feeding on particulate matter. Numerous parasitic representatives live attached to the external surfaces or enclosed cavities of aquatic invertebrate and vertebrate hosts. In terrestrial vertebrates, ciliates are restricted to the intestinal canal, where they have adapted successfully to anaerobic conditions and to utilization of the host's food supply. The most outstanding example of such adaptation is that of the rumen ciliates, which inhabit the specialized stomach pouch of cattle and break down plant food for the benefit of their hosts. A similar situation is encountered in the cecum and colon of different herbivorous mammals.

Immunologic studies on balantidiasis

Balantidium coli is the only ciliate that occurs in humans. The best evidence suggests that *B. coli* is a natural parasite of swine, inhabiting the large intestine as a harmless commensal. Hoare (1962) reports that over 90 percent of domestic pigs are infected in some countries, and he emphasizes that human balantidiasis should be regarded as an anthropozoonosis. When it becomes established in the human large intestine, it usually invades the intestinal wall, producing severe ulceration with symptoms of diarrhea or dysentery. Monkeys may also harbor *B. coli*, and these hosts usually develop a disease picture like that in humans.

Very little is known about the immunology of human balantidiasis. Krascheninnikow and Jeska (1961), employing the gel-diffusion test, studied the serologic relationship among three species of *Balantidium*, namely, *B. coli*, *B. caviae*, and *B. wenrichi*. These three species, morphologically distinct, were also found to be immunologically distinguishable from each other. *B. coli* and *B. caviae*, though distinct, were found to have four or more antigens and were serologically more closely related to each other than to *B. wenrichi*.

Zaman (1964), using the immobilization test, compared the pig and the human strains of *B. coli*. The results showed that there was no cross-reaction when the human strain was tested against the pig strain antiserum, and vice versa. However, the significance of the clearcut difference between the pig and human strain is not yet clear, as the pig is regarded as the main reservoir for human infections. Zaman (1965), using the pig strain of *B. coli* as an antigen and antiserum produced against it in rabbits, found positive reactions with the FA technique. In contrast to this study, Dzbenski (1966) failed to detect antibodies in sera of naturally infected pigs by the FA test. In the later study, the number of samples was not large enough and, further, the ceca of these pigs when examined at necropsy showed no lesions. On the basis of the last observation, the author concluded that the ciliates live in the intestine as commensals which would be most unlikely to provoke a host antibody response.

REFERENCES

Adam, K. M. G. 1964. A comparative study of hartmannellid amoebae. J. Protozool., 11: 423-430.
Anderson, H. H., W. L. Bostick, and H. G. Johnstone. 1953. Amebiasis—Pathology, Diagnosis and Chemotherapy. Springfield, Ill., Charles C Thomas.
———— A. J. Wilmot, L. Freedman, and J. V. D. Anderson. 1958. Acute African amoebiasis clinical-laboratory studies and response to MA-307. Amer. J. Trop. Med. Hyg., 7: 201-204.
Atchley, F. O., A. H. Aurenheimer, and M. A. Wasley, 1963. Precipitate patterns in agar-gel with sera from human amebiasis and *E. histolytica* antigen. J. Parasit., 49: 313-315.
Aurenheimer, A. H., F. O. Atchley, and M. A. Wasley. 1966. Further studies of amoebiasis by gel-diffusion. J. Parasit., 52: 950-953.

Balamuth, W., and B. Howard. 1946. Biological studies on *Endamoeba histolytica*. I. The growth cycle of populations in a mixed bacterial flora. Amer. J. Trop. Med., 26: 771-782.

——— and P. Thompson. 1955. Comparative studies on amebae and amebicides. *In* Biochemistry and Physiology of Protozoa. Hunter, S. and Lwoff, A., eds. New York, Academic Press, Vol. 2, pp. 227-345.

——— and T. Kawakami. 1963. Nutritional requirements of *Entamoeba invadens*. J. Parasit., 49 (5, sect. 2, abstract): 61.

Biagi-F., F., and L. Buentello. 1961. Immobilization reaction for the diagnosis of amoebiasis. Exp. Parasit., 11: 188-190.

——— E. Robledo, H. Servín, and A. Martuscelli. 1962. The effect of cholesterol on the pathogenicity of *Entamoeba histolytica*. Amer. J. Trop. Med. Hyg., 11: 333-340.

——— I. Gueyara, and L. Rodriguez. 1963. Transmission transplacentaria del factor immovilizante de *Entamoeba histolytica*. Rev. Facult. Med. Mexico, 5: 487-488.

——— B. H. Fernando, and P. S. Ortega. 1966. Remobilization of *Entamoeba histolytica* after exposure to immobilizing antibodies. Exp. Parasit., 18:87-91.

Bozicevich, J. E. 1950. Discussion on amoebiasis panel. Amer. J. Trop. Med., 30: 154-157.

Bragg, P. D., and R. E. Reeves. 1962a. Studies on the carbohydrate metabolism of a gram-negative anaerobe (*Bacteroides symbiosus*) used in the culture of *Entamoeba histolytica*. J. Bact., 83: 76-84.

——— and R. E. Reeves. 1962b. Pathways of glucose dissimilation in the Laredo strain of *Entamoeba histolytica*. Exp. Parasit., 12: 393-400.

Cole, B., and J. Kent. 1953. Immobilization of *Endamoeba histolytica in vitro* by antiserum produced in the rabbit. Proc. Soc. Exp. Biol. Med., 83: 811-814.

Craig, C. F. 1927. Observations upon the hemolytic, cytolytic and complement binding properties of extracts of *Endamoeba histolytica*. Amer. J. Trop. Med., 7: 225-240.

——— 1933. Further observations upon the complement fixation test in the diagnosis of amoebiasis. J. Lab. Clin. Med., 18: 873-881.

Das, S. R., and B. N. Singh. 1965. Virulence of strains of *Entamoeba histolytica* to rats and guinea-pigs, and effect of cholesterol on virulence. Indian J. Exp. Biol., 3: 106-109.

Derrick, E. H. 1948. A fatal case of generalized amoebiasis due to a protozoan closely resembling, if not identical with *Iodamoeba bütschlii*. Trans. Roy. Soc. Trop. Med. Hyg., 42: 191-198.

Diamond, L. S. 1961. Axenic cultivation of *Entamoeba histolytica*. Science, 134: 336-337.

——— and I. L. Bartgis, 1965. Axenic cultivation of *Entamoeba histolytica* in a clear liquid medium. *In* Progress in Protozoology, International Congress Series No. 91. Amsterdam, Excerpta Medica Foundation, p. 102.

Dobell, C. 1928. Researches on the intestinal protozoa of monkeys and man. I. General introduction. II. Description of the whole life-history of *Entamoeba histolytica* in cultures. Parasitology, 20: 327-412.

——— 1931. Researches on the intestinal protozoa of monkeys and man. IV. An experimental study of the *histolytica*-like species of *Entamoeba* living naturally in macaques. Parasitology, 23: 1-72.

Dolkart, R. E., B. Halpern, and J. Cullen. 1951. The diagnosis of amoebiasis, the role of the complement-fixation test and the incidence of the disease in the Chicago area. J. Lab. Clin. Med., 38: 804.

Dubos, R., and R. W. Schaedler. 1964. The digestive tract as an ecosystem. Amer. J. Med. Sci., 248: 267-271.

——— R. W. Schaedler, R. Costello, and P. Hoet. 1965. Indigenous, normal, and autochthonous flora of the gastrointestinal tract. J. Exp. Med., 122: 67-76.

Dzbenski, T. H. 1966. Immuno-fluorescent studies on *Balantidium coli*. Trans. Roy. Soc. Trop. Med. Hyg., 60: 387-389.

Elsdon-Dew, R. 1958. Factors influencing the pathogenicity of *Entamoeba histolytica*. *In* Proceedings of the World Congress on Gastroenterology. Washington, D. C., The Williams & Wilkins Co., pp. 770-773.

——— and S. E. Maddison. 1952. Amoebic complement-fixation reaction. J. Trop. Med. Hyg., 55: 208-211.

Faust, E. C. 1932. Susceptibility, resistance and spontaneous recovery in dogs experimentally infected with *Endamoeba histolytica*. Proc. Soc. Exp. Biol. Med., 29: 659-661.

Goldman, M. 1953. Cytochemical differentiation of *E. histolytica* and *E. coli* by means of fluorescent antibody. Amer. J. Hyg., 58: 319-328.

———— 1954. Use of fluorescein-tagged antibody to identify cultures of *Endamoeba histolytica* and *E. coli*. Amer. J. Hyg., 59: 318-325.

———— 1966. Evaluation of a fluorescent antibody test for amebiasis using two widely different strains as antigens. Amer. J. Trop. Med. Hyg., 15: 694-700.

———— and N. N. Gleason. 1962. Antigenic analysis of *Entamoeba histolytica* by means of fluorescent-antibody. IV. Relationship of two strains of *E. histolytica* and one of *E. hartmanni* demonstrated by cross-absorption techniques. J. Parasit., 48: 778-783.

———— and W. A. Siddiqui. 1965. Comparison of two substrains of *Entamoeba histolytica* by gel-diffusion and immuno-electrophoresis. Exp. Parasit., 17: 326-331.

———— R. K. Carver, and N. N. Gleason. 1960. Antigenic analysis of *Entamoeba histolytica* by means of fluorescent antibody. II. *E. histolytica* and *E. hartmanni*. Exp. Parasit., 10: 366-388.

———— N. N. Gleason, and R. K. Carver. 1962. Antigenic analysis of *E. histolytica* by means of fluorescent antibody. III. Reactions of the Laredo strain with five anti-*histolytica* sera. Amer. J. Trop. Med. Hyg., 11: 341-346.

Halpern, B., J. J. Young, J. Dolkart, P. D. Armour III, and R. E. Dolkart. 1967. The serologic response to patients with amoebiasis compared by gel-diffusion, hemagglutination and phagocytosis techniques with a common *Entamoeba histolytica* antigen preparation. J. Lab. Clin. Med., 69: 467-471.

Healy, G. R. 1968. Use of and limitations to the indirect hemagglutination test in the diagnosis of intestinal amebiasis. Health Lab. Sci., 5: 174-179.

Heathman, L. 1932. Studies of the antigenic properties of some free-living and pathogenic amoebas. Amer. J. Hyg., 16: 97-123.

Hoare, C. A. 1961. Considérations sur l'étiologie de l'amibiase d'après le rapport hôte-parasite. Bull. Soc. Path. Exot., 54: 429-441.

———— 1962. Reservoir hosts and natural foci of human protozoal infections. Acta Trop., 19: 281-317.

Hussey, K. L., and H. W. Brown. 1950. The complement fixation test for hepatic amebiasis. Amer. J. Trop. Med., 30: 147-154.

Izar, G. 1914. Über das Vorkommen specifischer Antikörper in Serum von Amöbenruhrkranken (*Entamoeba tetragena*). Arch. Schiffs- und Tropenhyg., 18: 36-39.

Jackson, G. J., and N. R. Stoll. 1964. Axenic culture studies of *Entamoeba* species. Amer. J. Trop. Med. Hyg., 13: 520-524.

Jarumilinta, R., and B. G. Maegraith. 1960. Hyaluronidase activity in stock cultures of *Entamoeba histolytica*. Ann. Trop. Med. Parasit., 54: 118-128.

Jeanes, A. J. 1964. Immunofluorescent diagnosis of amoebiasis. Brit. Med. J., 2: 1531.

Kessel, J. F., W. P. Lewis, S. Ma, and H. Kim. 1961. Preliminary report on a hemagglutination test for amoebiasis. Proc. Soc. Exp. Biol. Med., 106: 409.

———— W. P. Lewis, C. M. Pasquel, and J. A. Turner. 1965. Indirect hemagglutination and complement fixation tests in amoebiasis. Amer. J. Trop. Med. Hyg., 14: 540-550.

Krascheninnikow, S., and E. L. Jeska. 1961. Agar diffusion studies on the species specificity of *Balantidium coli, B. caviae* and *B. wenrichi*. Immunology, 4: 282-288.

Krupp, I. W. 1966. Immunoelectrophoretic analysis of several strains of *Entamoeba histolytica*. Amer. J. Trop. Med. Hyg., 15: 849-854.

Kudo, R. R. 1966. Protozoology. Springfield, Ill., Charles C Thomas, 5th ed.

Latour, N. G., R. E. Reeves, and M. A. Guidry. 1965. Steroid requirement of *Entamoeba histolytica*. Exp. Parasit., 16: 18-22.

Leal, R. A. 1953. Intradermo-reacao na amebiase (Thesis abstract). Trop. Dis. Bull., 5: 923.

Lewis, W. P., and J. F. Kessel. 1961. Hemagglutination in the diagnosis of toxoplasmosis and amoebiasis. Arch. Ophthal., 66: 471-476.

———— and J. F. Kessel. 1967. Fractionation of *Entamoeba histolytica* antigens by the gel filtration method. Proc. Amer. Soc. Parasit., p. 23 (abstract).

Lynch, J. E. 1957. Histological observations on the influence of a special diet used in experimental amebiasis in guinea pigs. Amer. J. Trop. Med. Hyg., 6: 813-819.

Maddison, S. E. 1965. Characterization of *Entamoeba histolytica*. Antigen-antibody reaction by gel-diffusion. Exp. Parasit., 18: 224-235.

———— and R. Elsdon-Dew. 1961. Non-specific antibodies in amoebiasis. Exp. Parasit., 11: 90-92.

———— S. J. Powell, and R. Elsdon-Dew. 1965. Comparison of hemagglutinins and precipitins in amebiasis. Amer. J. Trop. Med. Hyg., 14: 551-553.

———— I. G. Kagan, and R. Elsdon-Dew. 1968a. Comparison of intradermal and serologic tests for the diagnosis of amebiasis. Amer. J. Trop. Med. Hyg., 17:540-547.

———— I. G. Kagan, and L. Norman. 1968b. Reactivity of human immunoglobulins. J. Immun., 100: 217-226.

Maegraith, B. G. 1963. Pathogenesis and pathogenic mechanisms in protozoal diseases with special reference to amebiasis and malaria. *In* Immunity to Protozoa. Garnham, P. C. C., Pierce, A. E., and Roitt, I., eds. Oxford, Blackwell Scientific Publications, pp. 48-65.

———— and C. Harinasuta. 1958. Experimental hepatic amebiasis. Proc. Sixth Int. Congr. Trop. Med. Malar., 3: 444-458.

Maestrone, G. 1963. Demonstration of leptospiral and viral antigens in formalin-fixed tissues. Nature (London), 197: 409-410.

McDearmen, S. C., and W. B. Dunham. 1952. Complement fixation tests as an aid in the differential diagnosis of extra-intestinal amebiasis. Amer. J. Trop. Med. Hyg., 1: 182-188.

Menendez, P. E. 1932. Serological relationships of *Entamoeba histolytica*. Amer. J. Hyg., 15: 785-808.

Milgram, E. A., G. R. Healy, and I. G. Kagan. 1966. Studies on the use of the indirect hemagglutination test in the diagnosis of amebiasis. Gastroenterology, 50: 645-649.

Moan, J. C. 1957. The serological diagnosis of amoebiasis by means of the precipitin test. Amer. J. Trop. Med. Hyg., 6: 499-513.

Nakamura, M. 1961. A serological study of amebiasis using the agar-gel technique. J. Protozool., 8 (Suppl.): 18-19.

———— and E. E. Baker. 1957. Agar diffusion precipitin technique for the detection of antibodies against *Endamoeba histolytica*. Bact. Proc., p. 95.

Neal, R. A. 1960. Enzymic proteolysis of *Entamoeba histolytica*; biochemical characteristics and relationship with invasiveness. Parasitology, 50: 531-550.

———— 1966. Experimental studies on *Entamoeba* with reference to speciation. *In* Advances in Parasitology, Vol. 4. Dawes, B., ed. New York, Academic Press, Inc., pp. 1-51.

———— 1967. The *in vitro* cultivation of *Entamoeba*. *In* Problems of *In Vitro* Culture (Fifth Symposium of the British Society of Parasitology). Taylor, A. E. R., ed. Oxford, Blackwell Scientific Publications, pp. 9-26.

———— and P. Vincent. 1956. Strain variation in *Entamoeba histolytica*. II. The effect of serial liver passage on the virulence. Parasitology, 46: 173-182.

Nichols, R. L., and D. E. McComb. 1962. Immunofluorescent studies with trachoma and related antigens. J. Immun., 89: 545-554.

Ouchterlony, O. 1949. Antigen-antibody reactions in gels. Acta Path. Microbiol. Scand., 26: 507-515.

Paulson, J., and J. Andrews. 1938. Complement fixation test in amebiasis. A comparative evaluation in clinical practice. Arch. Intern. Med., 61: 562-578.

Phillips, B. P. 1964. Studies on the ameba-bacteria relationship in amebiasis. III. Induced amebic lesions in the germfree guinea pig. Amer. J. Trop. Med. Hyg., 13: 391-395.

———— and F. Gorstein. 1966. Effects of different species of bacteria on the pathology of enteric amebiasis in monocontaminated guinea pigs. Amer. J. Trop. Med. Hyg., 16: 863-868.

———— P. A. Wolfe, C. W. Rees, H. A. Gordon, W. H. Wright, and J. A. Reynolds. 1955. Studies on the ameba-bacteria relationship in amebiasis. Comparative results of the intracecal inoculation of germfree, monocontaminated, and conventional guinea pigs with *Entamoeba histolytica*. Amer. J. Trop. Med. Hyg., 4: 675-692.

Powell, S. J., S. E. Maddison, A. J. Wilmot, and R. Elsdon-Dew. 1965. Amoebic gel-diffusion precipitin test. Clinical evaluation in amoebic liver abscess. Lancet, 2: 602-603.

Reeves, R. E., and A. B. Ward. 1965. Large lot cultivation of *Entamoeba histolytica*. J. Parasit., 51: 321-324.

—— F. Montalvo, and A. Sillero. 1967. Glucokinase from *Entamoeba histolytica* and related organisms. Biochemistry, 6: 1752-1760.

Remington, J. S. 1967. Characterization of antibodies to parasites. *In* Immunologic Aspects of Parasitic Infections. Washington, D. C., Pan American Health Organization Sci. Publ. No. 150., pp. 50-57.

Richards, C. S., M. Goldman, and L. T. Cannon. 1965. Cultivation at 25°C and behavior in hypotonic media of strains of *Entamoeba histolytica*. J. Parasit., 51 (Suppl.): 45.

Rogers, L. 1923. Lettsomian lectures: On amoebic liver abscess; its pathology, prevention and cure. Trans. Med. Soc. London, 45: 130-193.

Sato, R., and M. Kaneko. 1957. A cross immunity test between *E. histolytica* and *E. gingivalis*. Kiseichugaku Zasshi (Jap. J. Parasit.), 6: 5-7.

Scalas, L. 1921. Contributo allo studio della deviazione del complemento nella dissenteria amebica. Riforma Med., 37: 103-104.

—— 1923. L'intradermoreazione nella dysenteria amebica. Riforma Med., 39: 967-969.

Sen, A., S. Mukerjee, and J. C. Ray. 1961. Observations on the antigenic make-up of amebae. Ann. Biochem. Exp. Med., 21: 323-326.

Shaffer, J. G., and J. Ansfield. 1956. The effect of rabbit antisera on the ability of *Entamoeba histolytica* to phagocytose red blood cells. Amer. J. Trop. Med. Hyg., 5: 53-61.

—— W. H. Shlaes, R. A. Radke, and W. L. Palmer. 1965. Amoebiasis: A Biomedical Problem. Springfield, Ill., Charles C Thomas.

Siddiqui, W. A. 1961. Demonstration of antigen-antibody reaction with a monobacterial culture of *E. histolytica*. J. Parasit., 47: 371-372.

—— and W. Balamuth. 1965. Serological comparison of selected parasitic and free-living amoebae *in vitro*, using diffusion-precipitation and fluorescent-antibody technique. J. Protozool., 13: 175-182.

Smithers, S. R. 1967. The induction and nature of antibody response to parasites. *In* Immunologic Aspects of Parasitic Infections. Washington, D. C., Pan American Health Organization Sci. Publ. No. 150, pp. 43-49.

Stoll, N. R. 1957. Axenic serial culture in cell-free medium of *Entamoeba invadens*, a pathogenic amoeba of snakes. Science, 126: 1236.

Swart, D. L., and L. G. Warren. 1962. The origin of antigenic substances in *E. histolytica* Schaudinn, 1903, and serologic manifestation of their antibody inducing properties. J. Parasit., 48: 124-130.

Swartzwelder, J. C., and W. H. Avant. 1952. Immunity to amoebic infections in dogs. Amer. J. Trop. Med. Hyg., 1: 567-575.

Talis B., 1966. Detection of antibodies against *Entamoeba histolytica* in human sera. J. Protozool., 13 (Suppl.): 34.

—— 1967. Antigenic relationships among strains of *Entamoeba histolytica*, *Dientamoeba fragilis* and *Entamoeba invadens*. J. Protozool., 14 (Suppl.): 44.

—— M. Lahav, and S. Ben-Efraim. 1963. Immunological study on some strains of *Entamoeba histolytica*. Bull. Res. Council of Israel, 10 E: 130-136.

Teodorovich, S. D. 1963. Usefulness of single lesion infection in experimental amoebiasis. *In* Progress in Protozoology. Ludvik, J., Lom, J., and Vávra, J., eds. New York, Academic Press, Inc., pp. 592-594.

Terry, L. L., and J. E. Bozicevich. 1948. The importance of the complement fixation test in amebic hepatitis and liver abscess. Southern Med. J., 41: 691-702.

Thimann, K. V. 1963. The Life of Bacteria. New York, The Macmillan Co., 2nd Ed., p. 23.

Thompson, P. E. 1958. Experimental intestinal amebiasis. Proc. Sixth Int. Congr. Trop. Med. Malar., 3: 435-443.

—— D. McCarthy, and J. W. Reinertson. 1954. Observations on the virulence of *Endamoeba histolytica* during prolonged subcultivation. Amer. J. Hyg., 59: 249-261.

Valentino, L. 1956. La renzoine di immobilizzazione nell amebiasi. Rivista dell'Istituto Sieroterapico Italicano (Napoli), 31: 310-317.

Villarejos, V. M. 1962. Role of salmon diet and of rectal intubation in experimental amebic colitis in the dog. Amer. J. Trop. Med. Hyg., 11: 440-447.

Vincent, R., and R. A. Neal. 1960. Duration of invasiveness of *Entamoeba histolytica* maintained *in vitro*. Parasitology, 50: 449-452.

Von Hage. 1920. Über die Diagnose der Amöbenenteritis. Deutsch. Med. Wschr., 46: 682-684.

Wadworth, C. 1957. A slide technique for the analysis of immune precipitates in gel. Int. Arch. Allerg., 10: 355-360.

Wagener, E. H. 1924. A precipitin test in experimental amebic dysentery in cats. Univ. Calif. Publ. Zool., 26: 15-20.

Williams, C. A., and B. Grabar. 1955. Immunoelectrophoretic studies on serum proteins. J. Immun., 74: 158-168.

Zaman, V. 1960. Studies with the immobilization reaction in the genus *Entamoeba*. Ann. Trop. Med. Parasit., 54: 381-391.

———— 1964. Studies on the immobilization reaction in the genus *Balantidium*. Trans. Roy. Soc. Trop. Med. Hyg., 58: 255-259.

———— 1965. The application of fluorescent antibody test to *Balantidium coli*. Trans. Roy. Soc. Trop. Med. Hyg., 59: 80-82.

Trichomonads

B. M. HONIGBERG

Department of Zoology, University of Massachusetts, Amherst, Massachusetts

INTRODUCTION

The members of the zooflagellate order Trichomonadida Kirby (*see* **Honigberg, 1963**), are distributed widely among invertebrate and vertebrate hosts.

Most of these parasites inhabit the hind gut of invertebrates and the large intestine (in many instances also the cecum) of vertebrates. With the exception of the mutualistic species associated with the lower termites (Kirby, 1937, 1941; Hungate, 1955), all the trichomonads found in the lower digestive tract of invertebrate and vertebrate hosts appear to be commensal. Although a few of these forms, for example *Pentatrichomonas hominis*, have been considered by some parasitologists, and especially by medical men, to cause intestinal disturbances (*see* Honigberg, 1963, for references), there is no convincing evidence of etiologic involvement of any of these species in pathologic processes.

Among trichomonads, a few species have invaded sites other than the lower digestive tract, and it is among these that we find frankly pathogenic strains. Such strains exist in *Trichomonas vaginalis*, the urogenital flagellate of man (Honigberg et al., 1966); *Trichomonas gallinae*, a parasite of the upper digestive tract and some other organs of various birds, but most commonly of pigeons (Stabler, 1954); and *Tritrichomonas foetus*, the urogenital trichomonad of cattle (Morgan, 1946; Levine, 1961).

In view of the public health aspects of urogenital trichomoniasis in women and men and because of the veterinary importance of bovine urogenital trichomoniasis, it is not at all surprising that most information on the nutrition and physiology (Shorb, 1964), as well as on immunology and serology of trichomonads, is based upon studies of *T. vaginalis* and *T. foetus*. Some immunologic data are available also on *T. gallinae*, *P. hominis*, and *T. tenax* (a commensal inhabiting the oral cavity of man), presumably because the first is of some importance to poultry breeders and bird lovers and the other two are found in man. In addition, with the exception of *T. tenax*, all the above-mentioned species can be maintained with relative ease in axenic cultures, an important factor in experimental studies of their immunologic characteristics.

Numerous species of trichomonads, many of which can be cultured under axenic conditions, occur in amphibians and reptiles, and there is a certain amount of information available on their nutrition and physiology (Shorb, 1964). However, as far as can be ascertained, data on immunology of these organisms are limited to two reports dealing with *Monocercomonas colubrorum* (Robertson, 1941) and *Tritrichomonas augusta* (Samuels and Chun-Hoon, 1964), respectively.

It has been emphasized by many authors (Trussell, 1947; Frost, 1962; Robertson, 1963) that infections with trichomonads are limited to particular sites in the hosts and that even the most pathogenic strains found in some species do not invade the blood stream; those which may enter blood circulation are said to be promptly lysed by the natural antibodies (Hoffmann, 1966a). These contentions are more applicable to *T. vaginalis* and to *T. foetus* than to *T. gallinae*.

Although various pathogenic strains of *T. gallinae* exhibit predilection for specific sites (Stabler, 1954) in addition to the invariably affected upper digestive tract, it is difficult in many instances to speak of strictly localized infections. In pigeons infected with the highly virulent Jones' Barn strain (Stabler, 1948a, 1951), one can observe on autopsy a wide distribution of the flagellates and of the characteristic caseous lesions in the mouth, oropharynx, and esophagus, as well as the liver, a site always invaded by this strain (Perez-Mesa et al., 1961). While trichomonads have not been found in the blood of living birds, the possibility must be entertained that the Jones' Barn and other pathogenic strains of *T. gallinae* may reach the parenteral sites via the circulatory system.

It has been said also that all trichomonads, including the pathogenic strains, are exclusively extracellular parasites (Hogue, 1938, 1943; Robertson, 1963; *see* Honigberg et al., 1964, 1966, for references). The ability of a relatively virulent strain of *T. vaginalis* to invade the essentially nonphagocytic epithelial cells and fibroblasts in chick liver cell cultures has been demonstrated by Farris (1965). Also, Frost et al. (1961) have shown that on occasions *T. vaginalis* can be found within the cytoplasm of epithelial cells in biopsies taken from the urogenital tract of female patients. There can be no doubt that the Jones' Barn strain of *T. gallinae* invades epithelial cells and fibroblasts in chick liver cell cultures and that it multiplies actively in the phagocytic macrophages in such cultures (Honigberg et al., 1964). Flagellates are lodged also in the hepatic cells of pigeons infected with this strain (Frost et al., 1961). The recent findings of Kulda and Honigberg (1969) indicate that some strains of *T. foetus* actually are able to invade tissue culture cells. In view of the foregoing information, it cannot be assumed that in infections with trichomonads the immune response of the host always is evoked by strictly localized or strictly extracellular parasites.

According to many workers (for example, Lanceley, 1958; Hoffmann, 1966a), the difficulties encountered in immunologic studies of trichomonads are traceable to the fact that these organisms, like all other protozoa, are poor antigens.* Further, many results are vitiated by the presence of presumably natural antibodies in normal sera of various animals. As discussed in different sections of this chapter, such antibodies, mentioned by numerous authors, have been investigated in some detail with regard to *T. foetus* (Kerr and Robertson, 1941, 1954; Robertson, 1941; Morgan, 1944; Pierce, 1955); *T. vaginalis* (Teras, 1961b; Reisenhofer, 1963); and *T. augusta* (Samuels and Chun-Hoon, 1964). Despite all these difficulties, in reviewing the literature one finds that the majority of investigators who employed standard immunologic methods were able to demonstrate antigenic differences not only among various trichomonad species, but also among strains of each species. Agglutination has been employed most often; however, as will become evident from the following account, nearly all known immunologic techniques have been used by different workers.

Trussell (1946) was among the first to indicate that higher titers in var-

* This statement must be viewed with caution since it is evident from various recent reports (*see* Garnham et al., 1963, and elsewhere in this volume) that: 1. Improvements in culture methods of parasitic protozoa have provided adequate quantities of antigens for immunization. 2. Refinements in immunologic techniques have rendered the results with parasitic protozoa comparable to those achievable with bacteria.

ious immunologic tests can be achieved through the use of living trichomonads in immunizing experimental animals. This view has been accepted rather widely among the workers in the field (for example, Lanceley, 1958; Kott and Adler, 1961; Samuels and Chun-Hoon, 1964; Teras, 1961c, 1962a). However, as indicated in a number of reports (Robertson, 1941; Kerr and Robertson, 1943, 1954; Hoffmann and Gorczyński, 1964; Goldman and Honigberg, 1968; Honigberg and Goldman, 1968), specific reactions can be obtained also by employing various kinds of preparations of killed flagellates as antigens. Adjuvants have not been used frequently in experimental immunization of rabbits with trichomonads, although some investigators found their effects advantageous in obtaining specific serologic responses (Samuels and Chun-Hoon, 1964; Goldman and Honigberg, 1968; Honigberg and Goldman, 1968).

The exact methods employed and, probably to a significant degree, the lack of awareness of the existence of many antigenic types within single species might have accounted for the failure of some investigators (Trussell et al., 1942; Schoenherr, 1956) and the only limited success of others to employ serologic techniques in immunologic studies and diagnoses of trichomonads.

Monocercomonas colubrorum (Hammerschmidt)

Monocercomonas colubrorum is a primitive intestinal trichomonad (Honigberg, 1963), widely distributed among lizards and snakes. The available evidence suggests that this flagellate is a harmless commensal. The organism can be isolated and maintained with ease in agnotobiotic cultures and with somewhat greater difficulty in axenic cultures.

All the information on the antigenic attributes of *M. colubrorum* is based on the findings of Robertson (1941), who used one strain of the protozoon. According to this investigator, the strain was maintained in cultures which showed "some slight degree of contamination" with bacteria, but "the contaminants were not present in quantities that in any way disturbed the results."

Normal active rabbit sera had a strong lytic effect upon the flagellates, but agglutination was relatively slight under such conditions. On the other hand, agglutination titers of up to 1:40 were noted in normal rabbit sera inactivated by heating for 30 minutes at 56°C, indicating the presence of natural agglutinating antibodies to *M. colubrorum*. Similar results were reported with other trichomonad species and will be discussed later in connection with *T. vaginalis* (*see* pp. 483–484).

Rabbits were immunized by intravenous inoculations of living flagellates as well as of antigen killed by heat, by treatment with 70 percent alcohol, or by exposure to 5 percent HCl. Living monocercomonads and inactivated anti-*Monocercomonas* rabbit sera were used in immobilization and agglutination tests. In addition, *T. gallinae*, *T. foetus*, and *Herpetomonas* sp. (a trypanosomatid flagellate) were employed with homologous and heterologous rabbit antisera in some experiments.

By means of agglutination, *M. colubrorum* could be differentiated immunologically from *T. gallinae*, *T. foetus*, and *Herpetomonas* sp. Judging from the titers obtained in cross-agglutination experiments (cross-absorption was not employed), the trichomonad from reptiles shared more common antigens with *T. foetus* than either with *T. gallinae* or with *Herpetomonas*. The apparently closer relationship between *M. colubrorum* and *T. foetus* than between the monocercomonad and *T. gallinae* is difficult to explain on the basis of the probable evolutionary kinships among the three genera (Honigberg, 1963). The unexpected results may, as pointed out by Robertson (1941), reflect the fact that "cross-agglutination tests using two sera and two suspensions [of flagellates] are fraught with difficulties owing to the varying sensitiveness of the suspensions." Perhaps they also indicate the unsuitability of the techniques employed by her (*see also* Samuels and Chun-Hoon, 1964) for demonstrating phylogenetic relationships among trichomonad genera and species.

With homologous antisera prepared against living antigens, *M. colubrorum* was immobilized at dilutions up to 1:40. Further, the motility of the flagellates was impaired somewhat even at a 1:160 dilution of antiserum obtained by inoculations of rabbits with an alcohol-killed antigen (the échelon clumping was observed at this dilution). Agglutination titers of 1:5,120 to 1:6,144 were recorded for the monocercomonad in sera prepared by immunizing rabbits with living flagellates, as well as with organisms treated with alcohol or acid or heated for one hour at 100°C. However, the agglutinating activity of sera from animals inoculated with flagellates heated for two hours at 100°C was greatly diminished; the extra hour of heating resulted in a drop in the titer from 1:6,144 to 1:192.

Although monoceromonads killed in various ways were antigenically quite active, larger amounts of dead than of living antigen were employed for the production of antisera characterized by high antibody levels. This requirement has been noted by various authors in regard to other trichomonads. Still, the observations reported by Robertson (1941) suggested that the specific antigen of *M. colubrorum* was thermostable, and similar conclusions were reached on the basis of much more extensive studies involving other trichomonads, especially *T. foetus*.

Trichomonas vaginalis Donné

Among trichomonads, *Trichomonas vaginalis*, a common parasite of the urogenital tract of man, has attracted a great deal of attention. Actually, with the exception of the trypanosomatids and malarial plasmodia, only a very few parasitic protozoa have been the subject of as much morphologic, physiologic, and immunologic research as the species in question. A rather complete account of various aspects of *T. vaginalis* and of human urogenital trichomoniasis up to 1947 was given by Trussell (1947). The more recent developments were summarized by Honigberg (1963), Shorb (1964), and

Honigberg et al. (1966), and much additional information may be found in publications resulting from the several symposia (Reims, France, 1957; Montreal, Canada, 1960; Olsztyn-Kortowo, Poland, 1962; Lublin, Poland, 1964; Białystok, Poland, 1966), devoted primarily or exclusively to various biologic, pathologic, clinical, epidemiologic, and diagnostic studies of *T. vaginalis* and of urogenital trichomoniasis. All the available evidence indicates that in the preponderant majority of cases, *T. vaginalis* is transmitted by sexual intercourse.

Trussell (1947) emphasized the potential and actual pathogenicity of *T. vaginalis* and, more recently, additional convincing evidence for inherent pathogenicity of some of its strains was adduced by numerous biologists, pathologists, and clinicians (Teras, 1954, 1964; Holtroff, 1957; Amino, 1958; Vershinskii, 1958; Frost et al., 1961; Honigberg, 1961; Reardon et al., 1961; Bauer, 1962; Frost and Honigberg, 1962; Laan, 1965; Honigberg et al., 1966; *see* these reports and the aforementioned symposia for additional references).

As far as is known, natural infections with *T. vaginalis* are restricted to humans, among whom both sexes are susceptible. Experimental asymptomatic infections of the genital passages have been established successfully in female monkeys (Trussell and McNutt, 1941; Johnson et al., 1950). The genital tract of spayed or even normal female rats was found to be susceptible to lasting infections with *T. vaginalis* if the animals were pretreated with estradiol benzoate so as to induce permanent heat (Cavier and Mossion, 1956; *see* Combescot et al., 1958, for a résumé of work on this subject). Trichomoniasis accompanied by vaginal secretions and pathologic changes of the vaginal epithelium resulting from intravaginal inoculations of guinea pigs with *T. vaginalis* was reported by Soszka et al. (1962). Of all experimental animals, mice have been employed most frequently for assaying pathogenicity levels among various strains of the parasite (Teras, 1954, 1964; Honigberg, 1961; Reardon et al., 1961; Laan, 1965; Honigberg et al., 1966; *see* these papers for additional references). Although the sites of infection in mice, inoculated either subcutaneously (Honigberg, 1961; Frost and Honigberg, 1962) or intraperitoneally (Teras, 1954, 1964; Reardon et al., 1961; Laan, 1965), are not the normal ones, they provide a suitable environment for the development of lesions, the extent and severity of which accurately reflect the inherent pathogenicity levels of the parasites for the natural hosts (Teras, 1954, 1964; Vershinskii, 1958; Honigberg, 1961; Honigberg et al., 1966). Of special importance to the present discussion is the fact that the intraperitoneal mouse assay has been employed often in immunologic studies of *T. vaginalis* (Arai, 1959; Teras, 1964; Laan, 1965; Nigesen, 1966).

The first immunologic observations on *T. vaginalis* were reported by Riedmüller (1932) who demonstrated weak complement-fixation reactions in sera from guinea pigs inoculated repeatedly via the intraperitoneal route with vaginal material containing the parasites. Soon thereafter, Tokura (1935), using formalinized antigen derived from agnotobiotic cultures for injections of rabbits, was able to show agglutination of living trichomonads exposed to immune sera. His cross-agglutination experiments also pointed to significant immunologic differences between *T. vaginalis* and *P. hominis*. Further, Tokura's (1935) data could be interpreted as suggesting that he observed the lytic effect of active or reactivated immune rabbit sera and of fresh normal carp and eel sera against *T. vaginalis*; thus, without realizing it, he may have been among the first to record the presence of natural antibodies to trichomonads.

The early investigators were handicapped by numerous difficulties in interpreting results based upon the employment of antigens derived from agnotobiotic cultures. Thus, further advances in immunologic studies of *T. vaginalis*, as well as of other trichomonad species, had to await the development of media capable of supporting the growth of these parasites in the absence of bacteria; CPLM (cysteine-peptone-liver-maltose) of Johnson and Trussell (1943) being among the earliest. Axenic cultivation was facilitated also by the discovery of antibiotics, whose usefulness in clearing trichomonad cultures of bacteria soon brought them into universal usage (Adler and Pulvertaft, 1944; Johnson et al., 1945; Quisno and Foter, 1946). Another obstacle in the progress of immunologic studies was the activity of the natural antibodies, a problem discussed in the introduction and in other sections of this chapter. Although, as correctly pointed out by Hoffmann (1966a), media not supplemented with normal animal sera would be preferable for antigenic analysis and serodiagnostic methods, the presence of such sera does not appear to interfere with carefully controlled immunologic tests involving *T. vaginalis* and trichomonads in general.

Trussell (1946) was among the first to compare the effectiveness of living and killed *T. vaginalis* in stimulating production of agglutinating antibodies in rabbits. He also investigated the differences between the titers produced in these animals by intravenous and subcutaneous inoculations. Agglutination titers of 1:640 to 1:5,120 were obtained with the aid of living antigen administered intravenously, while similar injections of killed flagellates resulted in titers ranging between 1:320 and 1:640. Subcutaneous inoculations appeared still less effective. Similar conclusions were reached by Teras (1961c, 1962a), who obtained positive agglutination reactions at 1:5,120 to 1:6,400 dilutions in the majority of sera from rabbits injected intravenously with living flagellates (in one serum the agglutination titer was 1:10,240). When killed flagellates were used, in sera from two rabbits the agglutination titers were said to range from 1:2,560 to 1:5,120 and in one this titer was only 1:640. Although the author (Teras, 1961c) stated that "the highest agglutinin titer (up to 1:10,240) was in the rabbits vaccinated intravenously with living cultures, whereas the agglutinogenic effect of the killed cultures was much smaller (titer up to 1:5,120)," his actual results do not reflect very significant differences in the effects of living and dead antigens. Indeed, the importance of differences represented by a single twofold dilution is questionable. Maximum agglutination titers of only 1:800 were recorded in sera of rabbits inoculated either subcutaneously or intramuscularly with killed flagellates. According to Teras (1961c, 1962a), twice as much antigen was required for the production of agglutinating antibodies to *T. vaginalis* in rabbits inoculated via the subcutaneous or intramuscular route than in animals which received intravenous injections. Irrespective of whether living or killed trichomonads were employed in immunizing the rabbits and regardless of the route of injections, there was a significant drop in the titers by 35 days after the completion of the immunization treatments. Among the more recent investigators many (Lanceley, 1958; Kott and Adler, 1961; Teras, 1963a; Jaakmees, 1965; Laan, 1965; Nigesen, 1966), but by no means all (Hoffmann and Gorczyński, 1964), used living trichomonads and intravenous inoculations for immunization of rabbits with *T. vaginalis*. Recent studies on *T. gallinae* (Honigberg et al., 1969) confirmed the findings of earlier investigators concerning the superiority of this method for the production in rabbits of agglutinating antibodies to trichomonads. They indicated, however, that subcutaneous inoculations of trichomonad homogenates mixed with complete Freund's adjuvant constitute the best way to prepare antisera for use in gel diffusion. As demonstrated by Honigberg and Goldman (1968), such antisera are also very satisfactory for the direct fluorescent-antibody method. These results suggest that subcutaneous administration of mixtures of trichomonad homogenates and Freund's adjuvant might be found equally suitable in the production of rabbit antisera for gel diffusion and fluorescent-antibody experiments involving *T. vaginalis*.

Antigenic identity

The presence of common and unique antigens in *T. vaginalis* and *T. foetus* were demonstrated by cross-agglutination experiments including cross-absorption tests (MacDonald and Tatum, 1948; Schoenherr, 1956; Stępkowski, 1957; Baba, 1957); by hemagglutination* (McEntegart, 1956); by complement fixation (Schoenherr, 1956; Stępkowski, 1957); by precipitin reaction (Schoenherr, 1956), including the gel-diffusion technique (Stępkowski, 1957); and by estimating the phagocytic index in immune blood (Stępkowski, 1961b). The antigenic differences between the bovine and human urogenital parasites were brought out also by the fluorescent-antibody method (direct staining) (McEntegart et al., 1958). According to Baba (1958), 78 percent of mice injected intraperitoneally with heat-killed *T. vaginalis* were protected against an intramuscular challenge with this species, while only 53 and 57 percent of the immunized animals were able to resist similar challenges with *T. foetus* and *T. gallinae*, respectively. Baba (1957) was also able to show antigenic differences between the urogenital trichomonad of man and *T. gallinae* by means of agglutination.

Although MacDonald and Tatum (1948), on the basis of agglutination experiments with nonabsorbed and absorbed rabbit sera, came to the conclusion that *T. vaginalis* and *P. hominis* were antigenically identical, more recent evidence points to the presence of both unique and common antigens

---

* Here and elsewhere in this chapter the term "hemagglutination" refers to passive hemagglutination.

in these species. Thus, Schoenherr (1956), with the aid of agglutination involving reciprocal absorption and of precipitation methods, was able to demonstrate clearcut antigenic differences between the urogenital and the intestinal trichomonads of man. Of interest is the fact that this investigator was the only one to employ fragmented trichomonad antigens in all his agglutination experiments (Zelltrümmeragglutination). Kott and Adler (1961), using nonabsorbed and absorbed antisera in cross-agglutination tests, also demonstrated the presence of common as well as unique antigenic systems in *T. vaginalis*, *T. tenax*, and *P. hominis*. The cross-agglutination and gel diffusion experiments of Oleinik (1964) indicated clear differences between the antigenic constitution of *T. vaginalis*, on the one hand, and those of *P. hominis* and *T. tenax* on the other. They suggested, however, that the two latter species belonged in one serologic type. The rather low titers of the homologous antisera developed against the intestinal (17 strains) and oral (22 strains) trichomonads, which were grown in agnotobiotic cultures, may be considered the possible source of the difficulties encountered by Oleinik (1964) in differentiating the two species by immunologic means. Finally, the agglutination experiments of Samuels and Chun-Hoon (1964) (*see* p. 537) indicated the presence of antigenic differences among *T. vaginalis*, *T. foetus*, *Tetratrichomonas gallinarum* (from the large intestine and cecum of poultry), and *Tritrichomonas augusta* (from the large intestine of amphibians).

It became apparent during the immunologic studies of *T. vaginalis* that there existed antigenic differences among the strains of this parasite (Schoenherr, 1956; Magara, 1957; Amino, 1958; Lanceley, 1958; Teras, 1959, 1963a, 1965, 1966; Kott and Adler, 1961; Nigesen, 1963; Teras and Tompel, 1963; Hoffmann and Gorczyński, 1964; Laan, 1966; Teras et al., 1966a). According to Schoenherr (1956), while some serologic differences among the strains employed by him could be demonstrated by precipitation, the best results were obtained by agglutination. An analysis of the results of his agglutination tests with the fragmented antigens suggests the presence of between three and five antigenic types depending upon the interpretation of the end-point ($\pm$) reactions. At least two such types were demonstrated by Magara (1957) among seven strains with the aid of agglutination, precipitation, and complement-fixation methods. Amino (1958) was unable to show by agglutination technique immunologically distinct types among various strains of *T. vaginalis*, all of which were considered as pathogenic on the basis of the intraperitoneal mouse assay. On the other hand, complement-fixation tests, with titers ranging from 1:400 to 1:3,200, revealed the presence of immunologic strain specificity. The experiments of Lanceley (1958), in which the microagglutination method was employed in a rather superficial investigation of serologic properties of 20 strains and in a more thorough study of four strains, indicated the presence of at least three discrete antigenic types of *T. vaginalis*. One of the four strains possessed three antigenic systems and the remaining three, two systems each. However, among the latter, two seemed to be equipped with the same agglutinogenic system, and one with a different agglutinogenic system. Although the author indicated the presence of three serologic types, the possible existence of four could not be excluded on the basis of the available data, and such a conclusion was reached in reference to Lanceley's results by Hoffmann (1966a). Lanceley (1958) conceded that his report was based on experiments involving a small number of strains and did not include adequate data on the activity of the cross-absorbed sera.

Kott and Adler (1961) reported the existence of eight serologic types among the 19 strains of *T. vaginalis* they examined by means of agglutination and cross-absorption. Their results based on hemagglutination with trichomonad polysaccharides obtained by Fuller's (1938) method and with cell-free extracts of trichomonad homogenates were less clearcut. Four antigenic types, TLR, TN, TRT, and TR, with common and unique antigens, were found among several hundred strains of the urogenital trichomonad of man by the active group of Estonian investigators working under the direction of Professor J. Teras (Teras, 1963a, 1964, 1965, 1966; Teras and Tompel, 1963; Laan 1966; Teras et al., 1966a,b). Cross-agglutination techniques, using both nonabsorbed and cross-absorbed immune sera, as well as a complement-fixation method, were employed in numerous experiments. As far as can be ascertained, among the reports dealing with antigenic types of *T. vaginalis*, those of the Estonian workers were based on the largest number of isolates. The apparently high sensitivity of the agglutination method employed by them in differentiating the types can be seen from the results summarized in Table 1.

The four antigenic types reported by Teras and his collaborators seem to be distributed very widely. For example, the VP type from Czechoslovakia was the same as TLR from Estonia, and LZ from Hungary was identical with TR from Estonia. There can be no doubt, however, that, as pointed out by Nigesen (1963) and Teras et al. (1966a), additional types will be found on further studies. Actually the results of Kott and Adler (1961) and Hoffmann and Gorczyński (1964), to be discussed next, suggest the occurrence of several antigenic types of *T. vaginalis* within quite limited geographic areas.

Table 1

Agglutination of Antigenic Types TLR and TN of *T. vaginalis* with Nonabsorbed and Cross-absorbed Anti-TLR and Anti-TN Rabbit Sera*

Antiserum	Absorbed with Antigen	Titer with Antigen	
		TLR	TN
TLR	None	1:6400	1:320
	TN	1:960	0
TN	None	1:800	1:6400
	TLR	0	1:1600

*Adapted from Teras, J. 1966. Wiad. Parazyt., 12:359.

Hoffmann and Gorczyński (1964) were able to differentiate at least three definite antigenic types among 23 strains of *T. vaginalis*. Their well-planned and carefully executed experiments involved microagglutination and hemagglutination methods, as well as the quantitative Kolmér modification of the complement-fixation test. The results of all three methods showed a high degree of correlation. Inasmuch as the experiments employed all three techniques simultaneously and because of the clear presentation of the data, the results reported by Hoffmann and Gorczyński (1964) will be presented in more detail.

Having established the agglutination (1:20), hemagglutination (1:5), and complement-fixation (1:5) titers of normal rabbit sera, Hoffmann and Gorczyński (1964) set up a series of experiments to observe cross-reactions among four antigens and four antisera prepared against each of the antigens by intravenous inoculations of lyophilized flagellates. The results of these tests are shown in Table 2.

Evidently, among the four strains there were two distinct antigenic types: TA represented one, and the remaining three (1410, 386, and 516) another type (Table 2). The differences among the latter strains were relatively minor, indicating their close kinships. The results obtained with nonabsorbed sera were confirmed fully through the employment of cross-absorbed sera.

Subsequently 23 strains of *T. vaginalis*, isolated from as many persons inhabiting one district of Poland, were cross-reacted with the four above-mentioned rabbit antisera. The results indicated that 13 of the strains were antigenically similar to 1410, 386, or 516; five resembled TA; and the remaining five differed significantly from all the previously recognized antigenic types. It seems probable that additional types could be recognized among the 23 strains through the employment of more sensitive techniques, such as the quantitative fluorescent-antibody method (Honigberg and Goldman, 1968).

Aside from demonstrating the existence of several antigenic types among a population inhabiting a limited geographic area, Hoffmann and Gorczyński (1964) indicated the nearly equal sensitivity of the three serologic methods, i.e., agglutination, hemagglutination, and complement fixation, in the antigenic analysis of *T. vaginalis*. On the other hand, although Teras et al. (1966a) maintained that the differences in intensity of complement-fixation reactions depended upon differences in the serotypes of this parasite, on a significant number of occasions strains (64 out of 99) belonging to all four of the antigenic types recognized by them gave clearly positive reactions with both homologous and heterologous antisera. The results obtained by these workers with agglutination appeared to be more type-specific, only 26 out of 99 strains reacting with the heterologous antisera. The apparent differences between the results reported by Hoffmann and Gorczyński (1964) on the one hand, and by Teras et al. (1966a) on the other, might have depended, at least in part, on the fact that the former employed in all instances antisera

Table 2

Cross-reactions among Four Strains of *T. vaginalis* Obtained by Three
Serologic Methods*

Strains	Antisera											
	Microagglutination				Hemagglutination				Complement Fixation			
	1410	TA	386	516	1410	TA	386	516	1410	TA	386	516
1410	++++	+/-	++	+	++++	+	++	++	++++	+/-	++	+
TA	+/-	++++	+/-	+/-	+/-	++++	+/-	+/-	+/-	+++	+/-	+/-
386	++	++	++++	++	++	++++	++++	+++	++	++	++++	++
516	++	++	++	++++	++	+	+++	++++	++	+	++	++++

++++ = titer for the homologous strain.

+++ = titer 2 times lower than for the homologous strain.

++ = titer 4 times lower than for the homologous strain.

+ = titer 8 times lower than for the homologous strain.

+/- = titer 16 times lower than for the homologous strain.

*After Hoffmann, B., and M. Gorczyński. 1964. Wiad. Parazyt., 10:133.

developed experimentally in rabbits, whereas the latter used sera of patients from whom the 99 strains were originally isolated, these strains having been assigned previously to the four antigenic types by reacting them with experimentally developed rabbit antisera.

According to Kott and Adler (1961), 68 serial passages (over four months) on media containing homologous antisera failed to affect the antigenic identity of two strains of *T. vaginalis*, as determined by agglutination tests. On the other hand, the tests indicated changes in antigenic composition of two other strains as a result of accidental bacterial contamination of cultures. As far as can be deduced from the data published by the authors, prior to the contamination the two strains belonged in distinct serotypes. After the cultures were cleared of bacteria, the strains could be differentiated from their parent populations, but not from each other, by means of cross-agglutination with nonabsorbed and cross-absorbed sera. A population of trichomonads reisolated from the patient who harbored one of the original strains was found to belong to the same antigenic type as the strain obtained in the original isolation and maintained *in vitro* prior to the time of the bacterial contamination. The authors suggested three possibilities to explain the curious antigenic changes: 1. The strains were changed in the same direction as the result of the bacterial contamination; 2. Each of the two cultures contained two antigenic types rather than a single type, one of which disappeared during the period of contamination; 3. A mutant appeared during contamination and replaced the parent strains. The available information precludes any conclusions as to which of the foregoing hypotheses, if any, could explain the antigenic changes. Inasmuch as the identity of the contaminating bacteria was not ascertained, we do not know if the same or different sets of factors were introduced into the cultures. Further, in the absence of results of direct reciprocal absorption involving the two strains, even the second possibility cannot be eliminated. Since antibiotics, undoubtedly used in clearing up the contaminated cultures, are known to affect physiologic attributes of trichomonads grown *in vitro* (Stabler et al., 1964; Honigberg, unpublished data), the possibility of their influence upon the antigenic composition of the strains of Kott and Adler (1961) cannot be dismissed. In general, these and all other immunologic data based on experiments that apparently did not involve clones are difficult to interpret. Only further investigations with clonal cultures of trichomonads could shed some light on the unusual antigenic changes reported by Kott and Adler (1961).

Using agglutination, Kott and Adler (1961) found no changes in the antigenic types of all the noncontaminated strains of *T. vaginalis* during a two and one-half year period of cultivation. Similar apparent immutability of the serotypes of this species upon prolonged maintenance in culture was reported by Teras and Tompel (1963), Laan (1965), and Teras (1965, 1966). The difficulties with accepting such statements in the light of the recent results with *T. gallinae* (Goldman and Honigberg, 1968; Honigberg and Goldman, 1968) will be discussed in the section dealing with the antigenic identity of this species (*see* pp. 511–513).

Antigenic structure

In their experiments with various strains of *T. vaginalis*, Kott and Adler (1961) employed, in addition to agglutination of living flagellates, a hemagglutination test in which polysaccharide fractions of the parasites isolated according to the method of Fuller (1938) served as antigens. As in the direct agglutination tests, hemagglutination experiments involving polysaccharide antigens showed a significant amount of cross-reactivity among some of the antigenic types; however, in hemagglutination discrete types could not be identified by cross-absorption. On the other hand, polysaccharide fractions of three of the strains examined by Kott and Adler (1961), which, on the basis of agglutination, before and after cross-absorption were found to contain both common and unique antigens, showed no cross-hemagglutination. The above results seem to indicate that: 1. Strains of *T. vaginalis* contain immunologically active polysaccharides; 2. In some instances, the polysaccharides represent common antigens in strains which can be assigned to distinct antigenic types on the basis of their agglutination reactions with cross-absorbed sera; 3. In some strains the polysaccharides constitute the unique parts of the antigenic systems.

Another hemagglutination method used by Kott and Adler (1961) involved sensitization of tannin-treated sheep erythrocytes with cell-free extracts of various strains of the urogenital and intestinal trichomonads of man. Antigenic Type II of *Pentatrichomonas hominis* showed no common agglutinogens or polysaccharides (as demonstrated by hemagglutination) with Type I of this species or with strains belonging to all the antigenic types of *T. vaginalis*. Nevertheless, hemagglutination involving cell-free trichomonad extracts revealed the presence of an antigenic system common to both serotypes of *P. hominis* and to all the strains of the urogenital parasite. The authors concluded that this common antigen was not an agglutinogen or a polysaccharide. Unquestionably, better purified antigens and rigorously controlled quantitative immunologic methods will have to be employed for verification of heterogeneity of the antigenic system of *T. vaginalis* implied by the foregoing results.

The more recent preliminary studies of Gorczyński and Jóźwik (1966) confirmed immunogenicity of the polysaccharide fractions of *T. vaginalis* and provided some insight into their chemical composition. Fractions obtained by the sulfuric acid hydrolysis of cold phenol-extracted glycoproteins from five strains of the urogenital trichomonad were employed as antigens in hemagglutination tests. Immune sera developed in rabbits against three other strains of this parasite gave, for the most part, significantly different hemagglutination titers with the five polysaccharide fractions, indicating the presence of various proportions of common and unique antigens among the test strains. The polysaccharide fractions, which represented 70 to 80 percent of the phenol-extracted glycoproteins, were analyzed by paper chromatography for monosaccharides and amino sugars. All five fractions contained glucose and galactose; three also contained mannose or fructose (these two carbohydrates could not be separated chromatographically by the method employed), ribose, and probably deoxyribose; one had all the hexoses but lacked the pentoses; and one lacked mannose or fructose, but had both pentoses. No fucose or amino sugars were found. However, as pointed out by the authors, these sugars might have been missed in the rather small samples used in their relatively insensitive method. It is unfortunate that Gorczyński and Jóźwik (1966) did not employ hemagglutination experiments with the antisera developed against the test strains and that they failed to obtain data on the activity of cross-absorbed sera. There can be no doubt, however, that a combination of immunologic and chemical analyses of trichomonad antigens constitutes a fruitful area for future studies.

Natural antibodies

There are numerous reports which either mention briefly or deal at considerable length with agglutinating and lytic activities of a variety of normal sera against *T. vaginalis*. Tatsuki (1957), using human serum, considered titers up to and including 1:30 as nonspecific in both agglutination and lysis. Observations of Lanceley (1958) led him to ascribe agglutination of several strains of the parasite by homologous and heterologous rabbit antisera to induced antibodies only at titers exceeding 1:40, while Hoffmann and Gorczyński (1964) accepted as specific all microagglutination reactions with immune sera diluted over 1:20.

Using sera derived from forty 15- to 17-year-old, *Trichomonas*-free, sexually inactive boys, Teras (1961b) demonstrated that in most instances the agglutination titers were between 1:40 and 1:80. He concluded that all titers up to 1:80 are nonspecific in the serodiagnosis of *T. vaginalis*. In other reports (Teras, 1959; Teras et al., 1966a; Nigesen et al., 1964; Nigesen, 1966), the Estonian workers were inclined to accept as specific only agglutination reactions with human sera diluted over 1:160. Other investigators (McEntegart, 1952; Kott and Adler, 1961) also considered the presence of antibodies for *T. vaginalis* in normal sera in evaluating the serologic results with this parasite, and Weld and Kean (1958) attempted to explain the ability of such sera to lyse the trichomonads in terms of the CO_2 content of the sera rather than on an immunologic basis.

Reisenhofer's rather extensive study (1963) of the lytic and agglutinating activities of normal human (both male and female), bovine, sheep, horse, swine, and dog sera brought out many interesting differences among them with regard to one strain of *T. vaginalis*. Fresh human sera had strong lytic properties resulting in severe damage to living flagellates at dilutions which ranged from undiluted or 1:2 (99 to 100 percent of organisms) to 1:32 (43 to 44 percent of organisms). Dilutions higher than 1:64 were no longer effective against the parasites. The sex and age of the donors had no effect on the lytic activity, and no differences were observed in this regard between sera from persons who harbored the flagellate and from trichomonad-free individuals. Bovine serum was more active than the human, causing lysis of 100 percent of organisms even at 1:8 dilutions, and a similar high activity was observed with sheep, horse, and dog sera. On the other hand, swine serum was less potent. Heating at 56°C for 30 minutes reduced the lytic activity of all sera, and extension of the inactivation period to 24 hours resulted in a further decrease. In neither instance, however, did heating eliminate completely the ability of the sera to lyse the flagellates. A significant reduction in the lytic effect on the parasites was observed in sera kept for 10 days at 4°C; after 90 days, they were still less potent. Reisenhofer (1963) noted no significant agglutination of *T. vaginalis* in active fresh normal human sera, although some limited clumping did take place at 1:8 and 1:16 dilutions. On the other hand, with bovine sera the strongest agglutination occurred in the undiluted state or at 1:2 dilution, and the reaction was clearly positive even at dilutions reaching 1:64. Activity of all the remaining sera tested fell between those of bovine and human sera, with the highest percentage of agglutination observed at 1:32 dilutions. In the light of these results one wonders if the swine and sheep sera actually were not more active than the bovine, and if the reduced agglutination with the higher concentrations of the former sera did not reflect partial inhibition of the reaction by excess antibody. A rather wide zone of inhibition was demonstrated by Samuels and Chun-Hoon (1964) in experiments involving concentrated normal calf γ-globulin against *T. augusta*; these workers also found sheep serum to be very active against the trichomonad from amphibians. Reisenhofer (1963) found a higher agglutinating capacity for *T. vaginalis* in inactivated than in active human sera; on the other hand, inactivation of bovine sera reduced this capacity. After 90 days (but not after one month) of storage at 4°C, there was a significant rise in the agglutinating potency of active human sera; this rise was less with similarly stored bovine sera. Not all the foregoing results lend themselves to a rational interpretation and the author (Reisenhofer, 1963) makes no attempt at an explanation of these results in immunologic terms. It is clear, however, from her report that two distinct anti-*T. vaginalis* activities, lytic and agglutinating, are exhibited by various animal sera and that the former seems to be dependent upon the presence of the complement. It is also likely that the apparent increase of agglutinating activity of the heat-inactivated human sera could be explained by the early complete lysis of some organisms in the unheated sera. A similar situation was noted by Samuels and Chun-Hoon (1964) in their comparison of the lytic and agglutinating effects of various animal sera on *T. augusta*, and by Robertson (1941) with regard to *M. colubrorum*, *T. gallinae*, and *T. foetus*.

Although Samuels and Chun-Hoon (1964) were concerned mainly with *T. augusta* (*see* pp. 537–540), some of the information contained in their report is pertinent to *T. vaginalis*. According to these investigators, one of the strains of the latter species was agglutinated by normal calf serum in dilutions ranging from 1:8 (78 percent) to 1:512 (19 percent). Inasmuch as the agglutinating activity of this serum for *T. vaginalis* was not reduced significantly by absorption with *T. augusta* and because all its activity was eliminated by absorption with the homologous antigen, the reaction appeared to be species-specific. Of interest to the present discussion are the findings of Samuels and Chun-Hoon (1964) that (as reported by Reisenhofer [1963] on the basis of a less extensive study) sera derived from various animals exhibit differences in their lytic and agglutinating capacities, and that the levels of the two activities need not be equal in the same type of serum.

The available evidence suggests that agglutination and lysis of trichomonads by normal sera is based on antibody activity. The problem of whether one or more natural antibodies are involved in the reactions, if solvable at all, would have to be approached with the aid of purified antigens and strictly quantitative immunologic techniques (for discussion, *see* Samuels and Chun-Hoon, 1964).

Induced antibodies and host resistance

According to Coutts and Silva-Inzunza (1957), individuals in human populations differ in their ability to develop resistance to *T. vaginalis*, with the asymptomatic carriers capable of acquiring relatively high levels of immunity. Although these workers, on the basis of their own investigations and on that of others, entertained the possibility of temporary presence of trichomonads in the host's blood stream, they maintained that, as with *T. foetus* (*see* pp. 533–536), an important role in resistance to *T. vaginalis* is played by local immune mechanisms. Such mechanisms, stimulated by repeated exposure of the urogenital tract epithelium lining to the parasites —for example, in the case of sexual partners of persons infected with *T. vaginalis*—were said to operate at the primary site of infection (*see also* Teras, 1964). Rom and Thiery (1957), aware of the differences in the course of bovine and human urogenital trichomoniasis, especially with regard to the rare occurrence of spontaneous cure in the latter, doubted the existence of local antibodies to the human urogenital parasite. However, in the light of the success achieved by agglutination methods in demonstrating the local antibodies in vaginal secretions of cows infected with *T. foetus*, they employed a similar technique with such secretions of women harboring *T. vaginalis*. Although the results were uniformly negative, they cannot be considered conclusive in view of the very small number of sampled patients (three). Further investigations along similar lines are needed for elucidating the problem of local immunity in *T. vaginalis* infections.

Two lines of study have been followed in regard to immunity to *T. vaginalis*. Some investigators employed living (Kelly and Schnitzer, 1952; Schnitzer and Kelly, 1953; Kelly et al., 1954) or killed (Nakabayashi, 1952; Baba, 1958) parasites in developing active immunity in mice; others concentrated on examining the protective effect in mice of sera obtained from patients infected with *T. vaginalis* and from those who underwent successful treatment for urogenital trichomoniasis (Teras, 1961a, 1963b; Nigesen, 1964, 1966).

According to Kelly and Schnitzer (1952), intramuscular injections of living organisms of an axenic strain of *T. vaginalis* into one hind leg of mice, which resulted in the formation of abscesses at the primary inoculation sites, protected 80 to 100 percent of these animals from developing similar abscesses in the other hind leg upon challenge with living parasites of the same strain. The level of resistance increased during the first week following immunization and remained constant for nine additional weeks. Examinations of the sites of the challenge inoculations revealed living flagellates at four hours postinfection but not thereafter up to 10 days, and during that period there were no indications of pathologic changes leading to the formation of lesions (Schnitzer and Kelly, 1953). Fifteen weeks after immunization there was a slight drop in the level of protection, as evidenced by a small increase in the number of animals which developed typical abscesses upon challenge. No subsequent experiments were carried out to ascertain further changes in resistance. Despite the facts that only a few, if any, living trichomonads could be detected by microscopic examination or by cultivation in the primary lesions after 10 weeks, and that even fewer abscesses were found to contain viable parasites after 15 weeks following the immunizing treatments, the mice remained protected against subsequent infections. Evidently the protective antibodies, whose formation was stimulated by the living antigen, remained active in the host organism for some time after the death of the trichomonads. In addition to the foregoing results, Kelly and Schnitzer (1952) reported that only living flagellates, especially in numbers of 1.25×10^5 or larger, were capable of inducing immunity in mice; formalin-killed parasites proved ineffective in this regard. Further, there appeared to be a significant amount of cross-immunity between *T. vaginalis* and *T. gallinae*, for mice inoculated with the former species remained quite resistant to a challenge with the latter. Finally, of considerable interest was the finding that two weeks after immunization the agglutination titers obtained with sera of the protected mice did not exceed 1:8 to 1:16. It would therefore appear (*see also* other results discussed in this section) that a correlation is lacking between agglutinating and protective antibody levels. The immune response to challenge infections was not affected by splenectomy or by a spleen blockage using Thorotrast (Kelly and Schnitzer, 1952). On the basis of all the available results, the authors concluded that they were dealing basically with an immunity to superinfection which lasted somewhat longer than the trichomonads employed in the primary injections.

In a subsequent series of experiments, Kelly et al. (1954) demonstrated that intramuscular injections of *T. vaginalis* protected 94 to 100 percent of mice against an intraperitoneal challenge, but that immunity against subcutaneous infections was much less. Mice immunized by intraperitoneal inoculations with trichomonads were well protected against subsequent intramuscular infections, but only 30 to 40 percent of animals thus treated appeared to be resistant to subcutaneous challenges. Finally subcutaneous inoculations of parasites failed to confer any immunity to subsequent infections via subcutaneous or intraperitoneal routes; however, they afforded good protection against intramuscular challenge for six weeks, but not for nine weeks, following immunization. The primary subcutaneous lesions were rupturing during the first two weeks, and by six weeks they were mostly healed. It appeared therefore that immunity outlasted the persistence of these abscesses by four but not by seven weeks.

Whereas the above workers found inoculations of killed *T. vaginalis* to confer little if any immunity upon mice, Nakabayashi (1952) reported that formalin-killed urogenital trichomonads protected these animals fairly well against subsequent intraperitoneal inoculations of living parasites. Similar results were published by Baba (1958) who employed heat-killed *T. vaginalis*, *T. gallinae*, and *T. foetus* for immunization of mice. Intraperitoneal injections of large numbers of killed trichomonads in three ascending dosages at four-day intervals (the total dosage was about three times larger than that employed by Kelly et al. [1954] via the same route) protected the experimental animals against intramuscular challenges with living organisms in numbers similar to those used by Kelly et al. (1954). Seventy-six percent of mice immunized with *T. vaginalis* were protected against the homologous parasites, 57 percent against *T. gallinae*, and 53 percent against *T. foetus*. When *T. gallinae* was employed for immunization, 81 percent of mice failed to develop infection upon challenge with the avian trichomonads, while only 50 and 60 percent were protected against inoculations with *T. vaginalis* and *T. foetus*, respectively. In animals injected with *T. foetus*, 80 percent resisted a challenge with the bovine parasite, 61 percent were protected against *T. vaginalis*, and 58 percent against *T. gallinae*. The author (Baba, 1958) concluded that heat-killed antigens had a protective effect against both homologous and heterologous trichomonad species, the most effective immunity being against the former. It seems apparent that a certain, often significant, degree of protection may be conferred upon experimental hosts by high, immunizing inocula of killed antigen. The reports of Kelly and Schnitzer (1952) and Baba (1958) also indicate that the immune reactions are not strictly species-specific; there appears to be a greater or lesser amount of cross-immunity among the several trichomonad species, which evidently contain a number of common antigens. The fact that protection is afforded by antigen introduced at one site against a challenge at another site (Kelly and Schnitzer, 1952; Schnitzer and Kelly, 1953; Kelly et al., 1954; Baba, 1958) may be interpreted as evidence for the presence of circulating protective antibodies, at least in infections of experimental hosts with *T. vaginalis*. On the other hand, we may be dealing here with cellular, rather than with humoral, immune phenomena. Although the true nature of the factors involved in protection of the experimental animals against reinfection with the parasites can be demonstrated only by further investigations, the passive immunity afforded mice by injections of immune sera speaks for the presence of circulating humoral protective antibodies to *T. vaginalis*.

All of the present information on the protective effects in mice of immune rabbit and human sera against experimental infections with *T. vaginalis* comes from the reports of Estonian investigators working under the direction of Professor J. Teras (Teras, 1961a, 1963b; Nigesen, 1964, 1966). Teras (1963b) inoculated mice intraperitoneally with rabbit sera immune to two antigenic types of *T. vaginalis*, TLR and TN (*see* p. 478); the control group received injections of normal rabbit sera. One-half hour after immunization, the animals were challenged, again intraperitoneally, with axenic cultures of strains TLR, TN, and VP; of these, VP belonged in the antigenic type TLR. Necropsy performed on the experimental and control mice 10 days after the challenge inoculations revealed significantly less extensive pathologic changes in the peritoneal cavities of animals pretreated with the immune sera rather than with the normal sera. Whereas through the use of numerical estimates of the abnormal changes (Teras, 1963b) statistically significant differences were found between the control and experimental mice, there seemed to exist no such differences among the groups challenged with trichomonad strains homologous or heterologous to the antisera employed in the immunizing inoculations. Thus, the protective antibodies presumably contained in the immune rabbit sera were not specific as to the antigenic types of *T. vaginalis*. Further, there appeared to be no correlation between the effectiveness of the antisera in protecting mice against infection with the parasites and the agglutination titers of such sera with the homologous and heterologous antigens.

The studies of the protective effects in mice of human sera from persons infected with *T. vaginalis*, started by Teras (1961a), were continued by Nigesen (1964, 1966). While it is not clear whether Nigesen's two reports deal with the same set of experiments, there are sufficient similarities between the earlier (short) and the later (extensive) account to treat them as a unit. It is most unfortunate, indeed, that in this, as in some of their other numerous reports, the Estonian authors failed to mention their previous publications which contain nearly identical information. Nigesen (1966) tested a total of 195 human sera for their protective effects against intraperitoneal infections of mice with axenically cultivated *T. vaginalis*. Among the sera, 73 came from women and 38 from men infected with the parasite. Sixty-seven sera were obtained from parasite-free individuals who had not been exposed to the trichomonads by sexual intercourse with infected mates, while sexual partners of patients affected by trichomoniasis constituted the source of the remaining 12 sera. The control mice were inoculated with physiologic saline solution in place of the sera. Thirty minutes after intraperitoneal injection of the various sera or saline, the mice were given appropriate dosages of trichomonads belonging to antigenic types TLR, TN, TRT, and TR (Nigesen, 1964, 1966). The experimental animals were kept under observation for 10 days. Some of them died during that period and were necropsied on the day of their death. All those which did not succumb during the 10 days were killed and examined for intraperitoneal pathologic changes. The extent of such changes was graded by the method devised by Teras and his collaborators (Nigesen, 1966). Nigesen's 1964 and 1966 reports are in agreement upon the following facts: 1. Sera from the noninfected persons with no history of exposure to the parasite in the sexual partners afforded no protection against intraperitoneal infections of mice with *T. vaginalis*; 2. Sera from infected persons protected the experimental animals against many abnormal changes caused by this parasite, as indicated by a statistical analysis of the numerical indices reflecting the extent and severity of such changes; 3. Sera from the sexual partners of individuals harboring the urogenital trichomonads exerted protective effects in mice similar to those observed with sera of infected persons; 4. There was no clear correlation between the levels of protection afforded by the sera and any of the following parameters: agglutination or complement-fixation titers (Teras, 1961a), clinical manifestations accompanying the infection, and the age and sex of the serum donors.

In addition to numerous close similarities, there are also some differences among the conclusions reached by Nigesen in his two reports. Nigesen (1964) evidently found through the use of all four antigenic types that the protective effects of the sera obtained from patients harboring *T. vaginalis* depended to a large measure upon the antigenic type of the flagellates employed in challenging the experimental animals, for each serum was capable of protecting the mice against at least one of the types. He therefore concluded: "It is apparent from the above [results] that the protective effect of a serum is type-specific." In his subsequent report, Nigesen (1966) stated that as shown by a statistical analysis of the pathogenicity indices, the various sera from patients infected with *T. vaginalis* could be divided into two groups based upon the degree of protection which they afforded mice against the injurious effects of the trichomonads. About 81.5 percent of the sera from women and men had a strong protective effect, and only about 18.5 percent had a weaker one. Although similar differences in the protective potency of the immune sera were noted previously by Teras (1961a), they were not statistically significant, probably, as suggested by Nigesen (1966), because of the relatively small number (nineteen) of samples examined by the former worker. Apparently the above differences were not dependent upon the antigenic type of the trichomonad strains employed in the challenge inoculations. Actually, Nigesen (1966) failed to discuss the reasons for the existence of the two groups of sera, and, as far as the general correlation between the protective activity of the immune sera and the antigenic type of the organisms employed in infections of mice was concerned, he merely referred to the conclusions of Teras (1963b), who denied the existence of any such correlation.

According to Nigesen (1964, 1966), the protective effects of sera from patients infected with *T. vaginalis* became progressively weaker after disappearance of the parasites from the urogenital tract following a course of treatment. These effects became diminished substantially within three months, and in not a single case could they be demonstrated after six months. Apparently, as in other trichomonad infections, the protective antibodies to *T. vaginalis* disappear with relative rapidity in the absence of the antigen.

The acquisition of passive immunity against *T. vaginalis* by mice inoculated with sera from hosts infected with this parasite suggests that circulating protective antibodies may play an important role in human urogenital trichomoniasis.

A section dealing with protective antibodies against *T. vaginalis* would not be complete without a brief mention of the rather astonishing report by Aburel et al. (1963), which as far as can be ascertained describes the only attempts at utilization of active and passive immunity in the treatment of human urogenital trichomoniasis. These workers reported a high degree of success in treatment of 100 women by inoculating their vaginal mucosas with increasing dosages of heat-killed trichomonads obtained from an axenic culture. Although all the patients proved refractory to chemotherapeutic treatments, following vaccination 40 percent lost the infection completely, and alleviation of virtually all the symptoms associated with urogenital trichomoniasis was observed in an additional 49 percent of women. In addition to vaccination, Aburel et al. (1963) injected hyperimmune anti-*T. vaginalis* serum into several areas of the cervix uteri and vagina of three patients who proved refractory to all previous treatments, including vaccination. While all the women apparently showed great improvement and one of them lost the infection altogether, the authors admitted that results based on so few cases could not be considered conclusive.

The available information suggests that circulating protective antibodies may play an important role in human urogenital trichomoniasis. However, it is equally evident from the published reports that the levels of such antibodies in natural and experimental hosts are independent of the agglutination and complement-fixation titers and that the protective activity may be unrelated to the antigenic type of the flagellates used in challenge infections. It appears therefore that future research should be centered on elucidating the nature of these antibodies.

Serodiagnosis

One of the important lines of investigation involving the immunologic characteristics of *T. vaginalis* is represented by the search for serologic methods which can be utilized in routine diagnosis and epidemiologic studies of trichomoniasis. The recent results of this search clearly reflect the presence of a systemic immune response in human infection with the urogenital flagellate, and, as indicated in the preceding section, the infection appears to be accompanied by a generalized systemic resistance. The problem of locally protective or agglutinating antibodies, touched upon by Coutts and Silva-Inzunza (1957) and Teras (1964) among others, has not been investigated to any significant degree. As pointed out elsewhere in this section, the negative results obtained by Rom and Thiery (1957) in their limited attempts at demonstrating the presence of mucoagglutinins in the vaginal secretions of women infected with *T. vaginalis* cannot be considered conclusive. Thus, although local antibodies have been demonstrated in bovine urogenital trichomoniasis and their presence is being utilized with some success in its diagnosis, there is as yet no satisfactory evidence for the existence of such antibodies in infections with *T. vaginalis*. As emphasized by Hoffmann (1966a): "This is unfortunate, because it might be possible in this way to elucidate the cause of the relatively frequent cases of asymptomatic trichomoniasis in men as well as in women."

The method whereby *T. vaginalis* causes systemic response is by no means clear. Wagner and Hees (1937) reported isolating in culture the urogenital trichomonad from the blood of persons infected with this parasite; however, their results have not been confirmed to date. Coutts and Silva-Inzunza (1957) entertained the possibility of periodic invasion of the blood stream by *T. vaginalis*. Hoffmann (1966a) also expressed the view that the urogenital trichomonads enter the circulatory system, and, even when lysed by the natural antibodies present in normal blood, they retain their antigenic characteristics causing the production of specific antibodies. The recent findings of intracellular trichomonads in patients (Frost et al., 1961) and cell cultures (Farris, 1965; Sharma and Honigberg, 1966, 1967) provide further evidence for the occasional intimate association between the urogenital parasites and the host organism which could lead to the formation of specific immune antibodies.

The methods employed in serodiagnosis of *T. vaginalis* will be discussed in the following sequence: complement-fixation, agglutination (including microagglutination), hemagglutination, and fluorescent-antibody techniques.

Complement fixation. As far as can be ascertained, Wendlberger (1936), using alcohol-extracted *T. vaginalis* antigen derived from agnotobiotic cultures, was the first to obtain positive complement-fixation reactions in 22 out of 48 women. All the donors of the positive sera were found to harbor the urogenital trichomonad, and in all of them infection was accompanied by abnormal vaginal discharges, with or without other clinical manifestations. Among the women whose sera failed to inhibit hemolysis, 10 harbored *T. vaginalis*, but only two of these had any abnormal discharges. The author pointed out that since the latter two patients suffered from active gonorrhea, the discharges might have not been caused by the presence of trichomonads. The remaining 16 women, negative on serologic examination, were found not to harbor the urogenital flagellate. On the basis of his findings, Wendlberger (1936) concluded that the immune response was specific for symptomatic cases in which there was a total systemic reaction. He also hypothesized that asymptomatic infections failed to evoke a systemic immune response. Trussell et al. (1942), using suspensions of bacteria-free *T. vaginalis* in saline as antigen, obtained a positive complement-fixation reaction by Kolmér's method with sera from 47.3 percent of 110 women who harbored the trichomonads. Only 16.5 percent of 290 parasite-free patients were found positive by serologic tests. However, whereas among the infected patients who gave a positive complement-fixation reaction many showed some symptoms traceable to trichomoniasis, there was also a significant number of such individuals who were asymptomatic. These latter findings, more in line with those usually observed in bacterial and zooparasitic infections, appeared to contradict the results reported by Wendlberger (1936). Although Trussell et al. (1942) believed that the complement-fixation reaction was specific, they felt that it was unsuitable for diagnostic purposes. Even less satisfactory results in terms of efficiency of the complement-fixation method in human urogenital trichomoniasis were obtained by Stępkowski and Bartoszewski (1959), who, with the aid of formalinized antigen, were able to diagnose as positive only 30 percent of sera from patients found to harbor *T. vaginalis* on microscopic examination.

According to Korte (1957), who subjected sera from 256 women to the complement-fixation test, high titers were found typically in patients with trichomoniasis that was accompanied by severe inflammation. On the other hand, he noted that sera from women with symptoms and pathologic manifestations characteristic of "persistent, chronic, or recurrent" infections had low complement-fixation titers. Korte, who apparently collaborated with Piekarski, claimed that the cases with high titers were readily amenable to treatment whereas those with low titers were refractory. In view of such a correlation, he considered serodiagnosis an important tool in prognosis.

Teras (1962b) was among the first workers to suggest the importance of the antigenic type of trichomonads in the complement-fixation test. Among sera of 114 persons found to harbor *T. vaginalis* on direct examination and by culture methods, 86 percent gave a positive reaction. Serologic investigation of the remaining 16 sera indicated that additional positive results could be achieved through the use of different strains as antigens. The author regarded the complement-fixation reaction as specific in human urogenital trichomoniasis; he thought, however, that further investigations aimed at standardization were essential before the method could have a practical application in diagnosis.

Results which in some respects agree and in others are at variance with those reported by previous investigators can be found in the report by Hoffmann et al. (1963), who conducted an extensive study of the complement-fixation method as applied to human urogenital trichomoniasis. These workers employed the quantitative Kolmér's method with an antigen which consisted of a mixture of 20 strains of *T. vaginalis*, 10 of which were isolated from women and 10 from men. Both phenol-treated suspensions of flagellates and homogenates prepared by freeze-thawing served as antigen. No statistically significant differences were observed between the results obtained with the two types of antigen. The specificity of the complement-fixation reaction was tested first on sera from rabbits immunized with the mixture of trichomonad strains. Titers of 160 Kolmér units were obtained with the immune sera, while the reaction was consistently negative with normal rabbit sera and with sera from experimental animals infected with the etiologic agents of human leptospirosis or syphilis.

Among 715 persons, 275 (about 38 percent) were found to harbor *T. vaginalis*. Of these, a total of 157 (about 57 percent) also gave a positive reaction on serologic examination. Two (40 percent) of five girls less than 15 years old and 93 (about 81 percent) out of 115 mature women had positive sera, with the average titer of 10 and 30.5 Kolmér units, respectively. No boys below the age of 15 were found infected with the urogenital trichomonad, and none gave a positive complement-fixation reaction. On the other hand, positive results were obtained with sera of 62 (40 percent) out of 155 mature men who harbored the parasites, the average titer in this group being 9.6 Kolmér units. Among the 440 people who showed no infection with *T. vaginalis* on direct examination and by the culture method, only 36 (8.1 percent) gave a positive complement-fixation reaction. Among those, 9 percent were young girls, 10 percent were mature women, 3.3 percent were young boys, and 9.4 percent were mature men, with the mean titer for each group being 2.0, 9.6, 2.0, and 9.2 Kolmér units, respectively. In the entire infected group, the mean titer equalled 23.2 Kolmér units, and in the entire parasite-free group, 7.2 Kolmér units. Clinical and epidemiologic study of the *Trichomonas*-free persons whose sera gave a positive reaction revealed that among the females, there were 7 percent of girls whose mothers were infected with the parasite and about 4 percent of mature women who were treated for trichomoniasis within the preceding few years; among the men, the 6 percent without symptoms and 10 percent suffering from chronic urethritis (i.e., the entire 16 percent) were found to have had sexual relations with women affected by urogenital trichomoniasis. Further, the authors thought it likely that some of the serologically positive but apparently parasite-free persons might have actually harbored *T. vaginalis*, for some of the 715 individuals were diagnosed as free of trichomonads on the basis of a single examination, which, as pointed out by numerous investigators, does not constitute sufficient means for revealing a certain proportion of infections. It would therefore appear that a positive serologic test in supposedly noninfected persons must not be considered necessarily as nonspecific. Also, the great differences between the infected and noninfected groups in the percentage of cases found positive on serologic examination and in the average titers are evidence for the specificity of the complement-fixation reaction in urogenital trichomoniasis. It is further evident from the results that a positive reaction is observed more often and has a higher average titer in women than in men infected with *T. vaginalis*.

Table 3 summarizes many of the quantitative data presented by Hoffmann et al. (1963), and it also shows the relationship between the efficiency of the complement-fixation method and the clinical form of human urogenital trichomoniasis. It is evident that the complement-fixation reaction is positive most often in persons suffering from chronic trichomoniasis and least often in those showing symptoms associated with the acute form of infection. The same relationship obtains with individuals in whom the presence of *T. vaginalis* cannot be demonstrated by direct examination.

In the light of their results, Hoffmann et al. (1963) concluded that despite the difficulties encountered in serologic studies of the urogenital trichomonad of man, the various immunologic methods, including complement fixation, deserve further attention because they hold promise for the clinician and the epidemiologist.

The most recent studies of the complement-fixation reaction in human

Table 3

Complement-Fixation Reactions in Persons Infected with *T. vaginalis* and in
Parasite-free Individuals*

	T. vaginalis present								*T. vaginalis* absent							
	Women			Men					Women			Men			
	No.	Positive Reaction		No.	Positive Reaction		No.	Positive Reaction		No.	Positive Reaction	
Symptoms		No.	%		No.	%		No.	%		No.	%
None	46	30	65.2	78	24	30.5	154	10	6.5	208	9	4.3
Acute	13	7	53.8	21	6	28.5	3	0	0.0	26	0	0.0
Chronic	61	58	95.0	56	32	57.0	23	7	30.4	26	10	38.4

* After Hoffmann, B., W. Kazanowska, W. Kliczewski, and J. Krach. 1963. Med. Dośw. Mikrobiol., 15:95-96.

trichomoniasis are described in several reports by the previously mentioned Estonian group of investigators (Jaakmees, 1964b,c, 1965; Jaakmees et al., 1964, 1966; Teras et al., 1964, 1966a). Many of the articles and abstracts give very similar information, and all the data, including the methods, are brought together in Jaakmees's (1965) dissertation, whose contents are summarized below. English-speaking readers will find many of the pertinent facts in the papers by Jaakmees et al. (1966) and Teras et al. (1966a).

In 100 patients (55 women and 45 men) infected with *T. vaginalis*, the Estonian workers (Jaakmees, 1965; Teras et al., 1966a) found by agglutination 43 strains belonging to antigenic type TR, 29 to TRT, 14 to TN, and 13 to TLR. One of the strains reacted with rabbit antisera prepared against all four antigenic types. The dependence of the complement-fixation reaction involving phenol-treated cell-free extracts of the parasites and human sera upon the antigenic type of the infecting strain of *T. vaginalis* was investigated in an experiment summarized in Table 4.

As is evident from Table 4, the complement-fixation reactions in infections with *T. vaginalis* show a certain degree of type specificity; thus,

Table 4

Dependence of the Complement-Fixation Reaction on the Antigenic Type of
T. vaginalis Employed in Tests*

Sera from Persons Infected with Type	No. of Sera	Positive Reactions (+ + + + or + + +) with Antigens					
		TR	TRT	TN	TLR	Homologous	All
TR	43	43	32	33	33	43	24
TRT	29	24	29	23	24	29	20
TN	14	12	12	13	13	13	11
TLR	13	9	12	11	13	13	9
Totals	99	88	85	80	83	98	64

*After Jaakmees, H. 1965. Diss., Cand. Med. Sci., Acad. Sci., Estonian SSR, Inst. Exp. Clin. Med., p. 21.

some positive serologic reactions would be missed if only one antigenic type of the trichomonad were employed in the experiments. However, despite the apparent dependence of the reaction upon the antigenic type, the results do not permit the assignment of the flagellates found in a patient to a given serotype on the basis of the complement-fixing activity of his serum, for equally high titers often are obtained with one serum against both homologous and heterologous types (Jaakmees, 1965; Teras et al., 1966a).

On the basis of the above results, Jaakmees (1965), using all four antigenic types with each serum, investigated the complement-fixing capacities of sera from 382 persons (229 women and 153 men). It was established by direct microscopic examination and with the aid of culture methods that 171 women and 83 men harbored the urogenital trichomonad. Five women and 40 men, found to be parasite-free on several microscopic examinations, had sexual relations with partners infected with *T. vaginalis*. Finally, 83 parasite-free persons (53 women and 30 men) who had no history of sexual contacts with infected individuals constituted the control group.

The control group sera were found uniformly negative for the complement-fixing antibodies in tests using trichomonad extracts as antigen. On the other hand, sera from 170 out of 171 women and of 82 out of 83 men harboring *T. vaginalis* were clearly positive. The single woman with serum capable of only partial inhibition of hemolysis was found to have acquired the infection two weeks prior to the serologic examination.

Table 5 summarizes the results obtained with the sera of infected patients by means of the complement-fixation reaction and shows the effects which the antigenic type of the parasite as well as the clinical form of trichomoniasis may have upon these results.

Table 5

Dependence of the Complement-Fixation Reaction on the Antigenic Type of *T. vaginalis* Employed in the Serodiagnostic Tests and its Relation to the Clinical Manifestations of Trichomoniasis*

Sex	Clinical Manifestations	No. of Sera	Positive Reactions (++++ or +++) with Antigens			
			TN	TLR	TRT	TR
Female	Acute	44	37	37	40	36
	Subacute	46	41	41	44	41
	Chronic	70	61	51	55	57
	None†	11	10	11	11	9
Totals		171	149	140	150	143
Male	Acute and Subacute	12	10	9	9	11
	Chronic	39	32	27	27	30
	None†	32	27	24	27	27
Totals		83	69	60	63	68

* After Jaakmees, H. 1965. Diss., Cand. Med. Sci., Estonian SSR, Inst. Exp. Clin. Med., p. 13 and p. 15.
† "Latent" trichomoniasis.

It is evident from Table 5 that the success of serodiagnosis depends to a significant degree upon the antigenic type of *T. vaginalis* employed in the complement-fixation reaction. If type TN alone were used, about 13 percent of cases would have been missed among the infected women. With TLR, TRT, or TR alone, about 18, 12, and 16 percent, respectively, could not be diagnosed. Among men harboring the urogenital trichomonad, the employment of antigenic types TN, TLR, TRT, or TR alone would give false negative reactions in about 17, 28, 24, and 18 percent of cases, respectively. On the other hand, all the data suggest a lack of correlation between the results obtained by the complement-fixation reaction and the clinical form of trichomoniasis. As pointed out by Trussell et al. (1942), such a lack of correlation would be more in line with the situation obtaining in other parasitic and bacterial infections than the results reported by Wendlberger (1936). However, in view of the findings of Hoffmann et al. (1963), further investigations are needed before a valid conclusion may be reached in regard to the relationship between the clinical manifestations associated with infections by *T. vaginalis* and the results obtained with the aid of the complement-fixation method.

Clearly positive (++++ or +++) complement-fixation reactions were obtained with sera of 28 out of 40 apparently parasite-free men who had sexual partners suffering from trichomoniasis. Weaker reactions (++) were recorded with sera of nine men, while only three sera gave indefinite (±) results. According to Jaakmees (1965), the foregoing findings may depend upon the presence of cryptic infections in the male patients in whom, as suggested by most experts, the urogenital flagellates often are very difficult to find on direct examination or even by culture methods. As a possible alternative explanation of the results, Jaakmees postulated that the antibodies could have remained from previous infections. Such antibodies, present in the host, would account for the positive serologic reactions and also might prevent the parasites from taking hold in the urogenital system despite frequent exposures. Perhaps the very frequency of exposure of the host system to the flagellates is instrumental in the maintenance of the high antibody levels (*see also* Coutts and Silva-Inzunza, 1957; Teras, 1964).

To ascertain the fate of the complement-fixing antibodies in patients who underwent specific treatment, Jaakmees (1965) (*see* also Teras et al., 1964) studied the serologic picture in 24 women and 17 men treated with metronidazole (Flagyl). It has been found that in all cases *T. vaginalis* disappeared from the urogenital tract not later than by the fourth day of treatment. The elimination of the parasite was always followed by a rapid regression of all the clinical manifestations of trichomoniasis. Sera of the treated patients were examined for the presence of the complement-fixing antibodies monthly during the first half, and every three months during the second half of the year following the metronidazole treatment. A continuous reduction in the antibody levels, as evidenced by the decrease in the number of clearly positive reactions, was observed in the sera of patients of both sexes. In the preponderant majority of cases, the specific antibodies disappeared from the blood within a year following the cure; only in eight women could a weak reaction be noted after 12 months. The results indicated that, in general, the drop in the antibody level was faster in men than in women.

The studies on the rate of disappearance of the induced antibodies from sera of patients treated with metronidazole emphasized the fact that, in the absence of the parasites, the immune response of the host was limited to a relatively short period following the infection. On the other hand, they aided in explaining the positive reactions obtained with sera of some of the parasite-free individuals. In addition, according to Jaakmees (1965) and Jaakmees et al. (1966), the investigations threw some light upon the question of dependence of the complement-fixation reaction on the antigenic type of *T. vaginalis* employed in the test. The antibodies were said to disappear at a faster rate in those cases in which their demonstration was dependent on the use of the homologous antigenic type. Further, in some instances, during the period following treatment the obtaining of clearly positive reactions originally independent of the identity of the antigen employed, came to be so dependent. The foregoing results suggested to the authors that the lower the level of the specific antibodies the greater the dependence of the clearly positive complement-fixation reactions on the antigenic type.

On the basis of all the results, the Estonian workers concluded that the complement-fixation reaction constitutes a useful tool in diagnostic and epidemiologic studies of human urogenital trichomonasis, provided that a number of antigenic types of *T. vaginalis* prevalent in a given locality are employed simultaneously as antigens.

Agglutination. Among the early attempts at utilization of the agglutination method for diagnosing human urogenital trichomoniasis, those of Trussell (1946) gave almost completely negative results. Although the author observed titers ranging from 1:640 to 1:5,120 with immune rabbit sera, he recorded only negligible and probably nonspecific titers, mostly 1:10 and 1:20, with a very small percentage (9 percent) of sera from 182 pregnant (90) and syphilitic (92) women, groups typically characterized by a high incidence of infection with *T. vaginalis*.

According to Tatsuki (1957), sera from 84.5 percent of 32 female patients harboring the urogenital trichomonad gave a positive agglutination reaction, with titers ranging from 1:16 to 1:512 and averaging 1:124. Positive agglutination reactions were obtained also with 52 percent of sera from 17 parasite-free women; however, in this group the titers were much lower, with a range from 1:8 to 1:64 and an average of 1:30. Since among 19 boys, only two (10.5 percent) were found to be slightly positive by means of agglutination, Tatsuki (1957) came to consider the results obtained with the parasite-free women as specific and reflecting in some instances the presence of infections that might have been overlooked on direct examination, and in others a history of past infections. According to Tatsuki, all titers exceeding 1:4 were to be considered as specific. Inasmuch as most of the recent investigators have been inclined to reject as nonspecific all the low titers, even up to 1:160 (*see* above), Tatsuki's data are difficult to evaluate; many of his allegedly positive reactions were undoubtedly dependent upon the activity of the natural antibodies. Similar difficulties are encountered regarding the results reported by Arai (1959). Although this latter investigator recorded agglutination titers reaching 1:10,240 with anti-*T. vaginalis* rabbit sera and between 1:10,240 to 1:20,480 with immune mouse sera, the titers observed by him with sera of 92.5 percent of 27 persons infected by the urogenital trichomonad ranged from 1:6 to 1:32. In unsuccessfully treated cases the agglutinating capacity of the sera was retained, but successful medication was followed by a gradual drop of this capacity. Perhaps at least part of the serodiagnostic findings reported by Tatsuki (1957) and Arai (1959) ought to be accepted as valid despite the low agglutination titers, which may merely reflect the relative insensitivity of the methods employed.

Considerably less satisfactory results were reported by Stępkowski and Bartoszewski (1959), who, using formalinized antigen, obtained positive agglutination reaction with sera of only 60 percent of persons found to harbor *T. vaginalis* on direct examination. The authors, while convinced of the specificity of the reaction, considered it to be of only limited practical use in the diagnosis of human urogenital trichomoniasis.

As in several other instances, a considerable amount of work on the application of agglutination to serodiagnosis of urogenital trichomoniasis has been published recently by the Estonian group (Nigesen, 1963, 1966; Nigesen et al., 1964; Jaakmees, 1965; Jaakmees et al., 1964; Teras et al., 1966a,b). The most extensive study was reported by Nigesen (1966) in his doctoral dissertation, but important parts of the investigations are to be found also in the articles by Teras et al. (1966a,b), which are written in English. The following account summarizes the doctoral dissertation of Nigesen (1966), with some additional information taken from Jaakmees (1965) and Teras et al. (1966a,b).

In all experiments the Estonian workers employed axenically grown, living trichomonads washed with and resuspended in physiologic saline. To establish the level of dependence of agglutination upon the antigenic type of *T. vaginalis* used in the reaction, the types of strains from 99 patients were ascertained by reacting them with sera from rabbits immunized by the four basic antigenic types, TR, TRT, TN, and TLR. Forty-three strains were found to belong to type TR, 29 to TRT, 14 to TN, and 13 to TLR (Jaakmees, 1965; Teras et al., 1966a). Of interest from the epidemiologic viewpoint were the observations that 32 of 34 (Teras et al., 1966a) or all of 69 (Nigesen, 1966) married couples found to harbor *T. vaginalis* were infected with strains belonging in the same antigenic type. Whenever a discrepancy was observed it could be traced to extramarital contacts. Having ascertained the antigenic identities of the strains infecting the 99 patients, the authors employed trichomonads belonging to the four types TR, TRT, TN, and TLR, in agglutination tests with the sera from the same persons. The results of the tests are summarized in Table 6.

Table 6 shows that in 97 out of 99 sera from infected individuals the agglutination titers with the homologous antigens were at least 1:320, i.e.,

Table 6

Dependence of the Agglutination Reaction on the Antigenic Type of
T. vaginalis Employed in Tests with Sera from Infected Persons*

Sera from Persons Infected with Type	No. of Sera	Agglutination titer 1:320 or over with Antigens					
		TR	TRT	TN	TR	Homologous	All
TR	43	43	30	27	24	43	15
TRT	29	15	28	19	11	28	6
TN	14	7	8	13	4	13	2
TLR	13	7	8	9	13	13	3
Totals	99	72	74	68	52	97	26

* After Jaakmees, H. 1965. Diss., Cand. Med. Sci., Acad. Sci., Estonian SSR, Inst. Exp. Clin. Med., p. 22.

twice the maximum titer noted in normal human sera, and positive reactions at this serum dilution are considered clearly specific (Nigesen, 1966; Teras et al., 1966a). Significantly fewer clearly positive reactions were obtained with the heterologous antigenic types. Consequently it is apparent that fewer positive cases would have been found by serodiagnosis if only one antigenic type were used in the agglutination test. Whereas the Estonian workers emphasized the need for the employment of several antigenic types in serodiagnosis, they pointed out that the agglutination method was not useful for the identification of the type of the flagellate strain infecting the donor of a given serum, for in many instances the agglutination titer might be equally high in a homologous and a heterologous system.

The major study reported by Nigesen (1966) involved altogether 583 persons. One group included 256 women and 130 men known to harbor *T. vaginalis*; the second consisted of 45 persons who, although negative for trichomonads, were sexual partners of infected individuals; the third, a control group, was represented by 152 individuals found to be free of the parasites on repeated examinations. In all experiments each serum was tested with all four antigenic types of the flagellates. No agglutination reactions with titers exceeding 1:160 were observed with the sera of the control group, and in none of such sera was there any correlation between the antigenic type employed and the titer. Evidently, then, the natural agglutinins present in the normal sera are not type-specific, the results reported by the Estonian workers being in this regard at variance with the findings of Samuels and Chun-Hoon (1964) (*see* pp. 538–539).

Table 7 summarizes the results obtained with the sera from patients infected with *T. vaginalis*.

It is evident from Table 7 that over 94 percent of sera from both men and women infected with *T. vaginalis* gave clearly positive agglutination reactions, whose titers, always exceeding 1:320, proved their specificity. There appears, however, to be little, if any, correlation between the agglutination titers of the sera and the clinical manifestations observed in the donors of these sera (Nigesen, 1966; Teras et al., 1966b). Two possible explanations

Table 7

Agglutination Reaction with Sera from Patients Showing Different Clinical Manifestations of Urogenital Trichomoniasis*

Clinical Manifestations	Women			Men		
		Titer			Titer	
	No.	over 1:320	1:200 to 1:240	No.	over 1:320	1:200 to 1:240
Acute or Subacute	127	122	5	20	20	0
Chronic	115	113	2	70	65	5
None†	14	14	0	40	31	9
Totals	256	249	7	130	116	14

* After Nigesen, U. 1966. Diss., Cand. Med. Sci., Acad. Sci., Estonian SSR, Inst. Exp. Clin. Med., p. 12 and p. 16.
† "Latent" trichomoniasis.

were suggested by Nigesen (1966) for the lower titers noted in agglutination reactions involving sera from seven female and 14 male patients (Table 7). They might have reflected the immunologic differences between the infecting parasites and those employed as antigens in the agglutination tests, or else they represented a relatively recent acquisition of the parasites which had not stimulated as yet a sufficiently large production of agglutinins.

As indicated above, Nigesen (1966) and Teras et al. (1966b) demonstrated the dependence of the agglutination reaction upon the serotype of *T. vaginalis* employed as antigen in the reaction. This dependence was emphasized further by Nigesen (1966), who, utilizing 386 sera from patients infected with the urogenital trichomonad, showed that if just the antigenic type TLR were used in the agglutination test, 35 percent of sera from women and 55 percent of sera from men would have been diagnosed as doubtful or frankly negative. These values would have been 26 and 48 percent with TN alone, 26 and 42 percent with TRT, and 35 and 41 percent with TR. According to the above results the agglutination reaction appears to exhibit a greater dependence upon the immunologic type of the antigen with the sera from men than in those from women.

A study of sera from the 45 parasite-free individuals whose sexual partners suffered from urogenital trichomoniasis revealed the presence of specific agglutinins, with titers at least twice as high as those expected in normal sera. Like the results with the sera of women and men harboring *T. vaginalis*, those obtained with sera of the parasite-free sexual partners of infected individuals depended to a significant degree upon the antigenic type of the trichomonads employed in the agglutination reaction (Nigesen, 1966). If TLR type alone were used, 19 persons would have been diagnosed as negative; if TN only, 13 sera would have given very weak or no agglutination reactions; with TRT or TR, eight and 14 cases, respectively, would have been missed. Inasmuch as in many seropositive partners of patients suffering from urogenital trichomoniasis, the presence of the flagellates could not be demonstrated on numerous microscopic examinations and by repeated attempts at cultivation, Nigesen (1966) suspected that such individuals harbored cryptic infections with *T. vaginalis*, the parasite being lodged in the higher segments of the urogenital tract. The finding of *T. vaginalis* in such sites is reputedly difficult even by the culture methods. Nigesen's (1966) hypothesis differs from the ones expressed by a number of other investigators (Coutts and Silva-Inzunza, 1957; Teras, 1959, 1964; Jaakmees, 1965) in regard to the seropositive but apparently parasite-free individuals.

As an important part of his study of the agglutination reaction in *T. vaginalis* infections, Nigesen (1966) examined changes in the specific antibody level in sera of 24 women and 17 men who underwent treatment with metronidazole. The sera were examined for the presence and level of specific agglutinating antibodies before and for a year and a half after the course of treatment. It was ascertained by a series of microscopic examinations and by repeated attempts at cultivation that in all cases the trichomonads disappeared not later than on the fourth day of the metronidazole regimen. The loss of the flagellates was followed by a rapid alleviation of the clinical symptoms associated with trichomoniasis. There was also a progressive drop in the agglutination titer during the first two months following treatment, but even after six months the reaction was clearly positive in about 50 percent of women and indefinite in the rest. In most female patients the agglutination titer dropped to normal within nine to 12 months, and in all within 16 months following administration of metronidazole. A similar situation existed with the male patients, except that in many cases the titer reached normal levels within six months. The rate of drop of the titers did not seem to show any correlation with the clinical form of trichomoniasis nor with the original pretreatment antibody levels.

In the light of their results, the Estonian workers came to consider the agglutination reaction as a very important tool in diagnosis and epidemiologic studies of urogenital trichomoniasis of man as well as in investigations of efficacy of treatment in infections with *T. vaginalis*.

Hemagglutination. Having ascertained the usefulness of hemagglutination in a system involving polysaccharide extracts of *T. vaginalis* prepared by Fuller's (1938) method and anti-trichomonad rabbit sera, and having established the optimum conditions for the reaction in this experimental system, McEntegart (1952) investigated the efficacy of hemagglutination technique in serodiagnosis of human urogenital trichomoniasis. Sera from 50 "normal" men and 50 "normal" women,* from 50 women infected with the parasites, with or without clinical manifestations, and from 13 normal children were employed in the experiments. All the 163 sera were absorbed with sheep erythrocytes prior to testing to eliminate the possibility of nonspecific hemagglutination. The results of the experiments are summarized in Table 8.

McEntegart hypothesized that some of the positive hemagglutination

---

*Evidently none of the "normal" donors showed any clinical manifestations of trichomoniasis, but they appear not to have been examined for the presence of *T. vaginalis* in their urogenital passages.

Table 8
Results of Hemagglutination Tests with *T. vaginalis**

	Serum from:			
	"Normal" Men	"Normal" Women	Normal Children	Parasitized Women
Total Number	50	50	13	50
Positive at Dilutions:				
1:5†	6	3	4	2
1:10†	10	5	3	5
1:20	3	3	0	15
1:40	0	0	0	12
1:80	0	0	0	10
1:160	0	0	0	2
1:250	0	0	0	3
Positive:				
Number‡	19(3)	11(3)	7(0)	49(42)
Percent‡	38(6)	22(6)	54(0)	98(84)
Negative:				
Number‡	31(47)	39(47)	6(13)	1(8)
Percent‡	62(94)	78(94)	46(100)	2(16)

* After McEntegart, M. G. 1952. J. Clin. Path., 5:279.
† Probably nonspecific reactions.
‡ Numbers and percentages in parentheses adjusted by considering positive reactions at 1:5 and 1:10 dilutions as nonspecific.

reactions observed with low dilutions of sera from supposedly *T. vaginalis*-free donors might have depended upon cross-reactions with the other two trichomonads, *T. tenax* and *P. hominis*, parasitic in man. Although some evidence suggests the existence of common antigens even in phylogentically rather distant species, the instances in which positive immunologic reactions are explained on the basis of the presence of heterologous trichomonad antigens in the hosts cannot be accepted in the absence of actual demonstration of such antigens in the host organism; in not a single instance could the needed evidence be adduced (*see* p. 539 and discussion in Samuels and Chun-Hoon, 1964). Inasmuch as some positive reactions were observed by McEntegart (1952) with sera of children at 1:5 and 1:10 dilutions, he was inclined to consider such reactions as nonspecific (*viz.*, numbers in parentheses in Table 8). However, he felt that because his normal control group was not examined for the presence of the urogenital trichomonad, some of the control sera found positive at the lowest titers could have reflected actual infections. This latter assumption seemed to have been supported by the fact that the 6 percent of positive sera obtained after subtraction of the reactions at the lowest dilutions of serum from the total number of positive results appeared much lower than the over 20 percent of asymptomatic trichomoniasis cases estimated by various surveys to exist among normal populations. In general, the experiments reported by McEntegart (1952) involved relatively small samples and his controls were rather inadequate (*viz.*, the normal group), to warrant a valid interpretation. Still, one is inclined to agree with that author that "possibly improvements in the antigen employed . . . would lead to an increase in the titer obtained with positive sera and . . . make the distinction between true and false positives easier." Undoubtedly the improvement of the antigen would have to include also the employment of several antigenic types.

Hemagglutination tests performed by Lanceley and McEntegart (1953) with sera of five male human volunteers experimentally infected with bacteria-free cultures of *T. vaginalis* gave uniformly negative results. Microscopic examinations failed to reveal the presence of the trichomonads in two cases. In the third case the infection was rather fleeting (three weeks), and in the remaining two, the parasites persisted from 50 to 100 days following inoculation. Mild urethritis was observed in all cases. In the light of the subsequent findings of Hoffmann (1966b), one must view with caution the conclusion reached by Lanceley and McEntergart (1953) that the negative results obtained by them might have been expected, because in bulls infected with *T. foetus*, serologic response is elicited only in unusually severe infections. Even assuming that all the relatively old information pertaining to immunology of the bovine urogenital trichomonad is correct, it seems abundantly clear that the serologic response is in many respects different in *T. foetus* and *T. vaginalis* infections.

The most recent attempts at utilization of the hemagglutination method in serodiagnosis of *T. vaginalis* infections were reported by Hoffmann (1966b). Like the British investigators (McEntegart, 1952; Lanceley and McEntegart, 1953), he employed the polysaccharide fraction of the trichomonad antigen prepared according to the method of Fuller (1938). In each experiment, the appropriate fractions of five freshly isolated strains of *T. vaginalis* belonging to as many different antigenic types were used for sensitization of the sheep red cells. Sera from 380 persons infected with the urogenital flagellate, as well as from 1,242 random individuals, were examined. Hemagglutination at serum dilution of 1:10 was considered as weak positive, and reactions at a titer of 1:20 or higher as positive. Table 9 summarizes the results obtained with the group harboring *T. vaginalis*.

The results (Table 9) indicate a high degree of sensitivity of the hemagglutination reaction among women, for clearly positive results (mean titer 1:46.4) were obtained by this method with sera from over 90 percent of female patients who harbored the urogenital parasite. On the other hand, sera from only 54.6 percent of infected men gave clearly positive reactions, and even among those the mean titer was only 1:28.8. The highest percent of positive results was observed in patients with chronic infection, 98.9 percent in women and 79.7 percent in men, while the hemagglutination test appeared least effective with sera of individuals showing symptoms associated with acute trichomoniasis. Only 50 percent of women and 29.2 percent of men belonging in the latter group could be diagnosed as positive. Inasmuch as persons suffering from acute trichomoniasis would be the most likely to seek medical advice, the lack of sensitivity of the hemagglutination method relative to this group does not seem to constitute a significant drawback.

Table 9
Hemagglutination with Sera from Persons Infected by *T. vaginalis**

| Sex | Clinical Manifestations | No. | Serologic Reactions | | | | mean titer |
| | | | weak positive | | positive | | |
			No.	%	No.	%	
Female	Acute	16	6	37.5	8	50.0	1:17.7
	Chronic	93	1	1.1	92	98.9	1:68.7
	None	77	8	10.4	68	88.3	1:25.4
Totals		186	15	8.1	168	90.3	1:46.4
Male	Acute	24	12	50.0	7	29.2	1:10.0
	Chronic	74	10	13.5	59	79.7	1:48.3
	None	96	46	47.8	40	41.8	1:18.3
Totals		194	68	35.0	103	54.6	1:28.8

* After Hoffman, B. 1966. Wiad. Parazyt., 12:394.

The results obtained with the random group of persons are summarized in Table 10.

There was a certain number of weak positive or even of clearly positive hemagglutination reactions among the sera from the group of random individuals (Table 10). However, irrespective of sex, the percent of positive results in the latter group—38.4 and 20.2 percent for women and men, respectively—was significantly lower than that found among individuals infected with *T. vaginalis*—90.3 percent in women and 54.6 percent in men (Table 9). Inasmuch as sera from a relatively high proportion of women and men over 15 years of age gave positive hemagglutination reactions, Hoffmann (1966b) assumed that some or all of these persons were infected with the urogenital trichomonad, or at least had a history of previous trichomoniasis. To test this hypothesis, the author examined urogenital secretions of 126 women and 94 men in the random group. Thirty-eight women and 11 men were found to harbor *T. vaginalis*. Sera from all the infected individuals gave clearly positive hemagglutination reactions, with titers of 1:20 or higher;

Table 10
Hemagglutination with Sera from a Random Group of Persons*

| Sex | Age | No. | Serologic Reactions | | | | mean titer |
| | | | weak positive | | positive | | |
			No.	%	No.	%	
Female	Under 15 yrs.	83	30	36.1	6	7.3	1:4.4
	Over 15 yrs.	540	204	37.8	233	43.2	1:15.6
Totals		623	234	37.6	239	38.4	1:14.0
Male	Under 15 yrs.	96	43	44.8	0	0.0	1:3.3
	Over 15 yrs.	523	216	41.3	125	23.9	1:9.6
Totals		619	259	41.8	125	20.2	1:8.6

* After Hoffmann, B. 1966. Wiad. Parazyt., 12:395.

however, the parasite-free persons were found to be uniformly negative on serologic examination.

On the basis of his findings, Hoffmann (1966b) concluded that the hemagglutination reaction with the trichomonad antigen, which combines relative simplicity with rather high levels of sensitivity and specificity, holds great promise as a useful tool in serodiagnosis and epidemiologic investigations. When compared with the results of the complement-fixation test obtained by Hoffmann et al. (1963), those reported by him on the basis of hemagglutination appear somewhat superior in terms of a positive correlation between the serologic findings and the ones obtained by direct microscopic examination and the culture methods.

Fluorescent antibody. According to the recent report of Kramář and Kučera (1966), the indirect fluorescent-antibody technique is applicable to diagnosis of trichomonad infections. The authors employed formalinized *T. vaginalis* antigen derived from axenic cultures. Hyperimmune rabbit serum against human γ-globulin conjugated with fluorescein isothiocyanate served as the staining reagent. Sera from five infants under one year of age were used as controls, while the experimental sera came from 17 women and two men known to harbor the urogenital trichomonad and from two women and two men found to be free of the parasites on direct examination. Specific fluorescence of trichomonads was observed with sera from all infected patients; however, none of the sera from uninfected persons and from the infants imparted such fluorescence to the antigen.

If the fluorescent-antibody method were further standardized and tested on a large number of samples, it is entirely likely that it could provide the simplest and most effective tool for diagnostic purposes and epidemiologic surveys of human urogenital trichomoniasis. Certainly this method has proved most useful in studies of amoebiasis (Goldman and Gleason, 1962; Goldman, 1966; Goldman and Cannon, 1967), malaria (Tobie and Coatney, 1961; Kuvin et al., 1962), and toxoplasmosis (Fletcher, 1965; Walton et al., 1966). When one adds to the high sensitivity of the fluorescent-antibody technique for protozoa the simplicity of methodology and relative rapidity of the indirect fluorescent-antibody test, the advantages inherent in its utilization become apparent.

Skin test. Among the early attempts at utilization of the allergic skin reaction for diagnosis of *T. vaginalis* infections, inconclusive results were reported by Wendlberger (1936), who employed alcohol-extracted antigen, and Trussell (1947), who used whole trichomonads for intradermal inoculations. Nearly all persons tested showed an immediate, usually rapidly disappearing, erythrematous reaction which was regarded as nonspecific. Lanceley (1958) also was unable to distinguish between skin reactions obtained by intradermal injections of *T. vaginalis* or of the sterile medium into rabbits that were immunized with this parasite. On the other hand, Adler and Sadowsky (1947) obtained, with the aid of phenol-extracted antigen, a clearly positive skin reaction in 35 (about 81 percent) of 43 patients shown to harbor the urogenital trichomonads by direct microscopic examination. A reaction considered positive was 1 to 2 cm in diameter and appeared within 48 hours after the intradermal inoculation of the antigen. Six (about 14 percent) of the patients infected with the parasite gave indefinite reactions, and the results of the skin test in the remaining two (about 5 percent) were negative.

The few patients who, although shown to harbor the trichomonads, gave indefinite or frankly negative allergic skin reactions might have acquired the infection relatively recently. Such an explanation is supported by the findings discussed earlier in this section in connection with the efficacy of serodiagnostic methods, and also in the views expressed by Adler and Sadowsky (1947), according to whom positive skin reactions were found in those cases of T. vaginalis trichomoniasis in which antigen was absorbed from the site of infection in "amounts sufficient to produce specific sensitization." Further, of some significance in this regard may be the observations of these workers that, although there was no correlation between the reaction intensity and clinical manifestations, the most intense allergic responses were associated with refractory infections.

Among 59 persons whom Adler and Sadowsky (1947) by a single microscopic examination found not to harbor T. vaginalis, 45 (about 76 percent) were also diagnosed as negative by means of the skin test. Seven (about 12 percent) of the other individuals gave an indefinite allergic reaction, and the reaction was clearly positive in the remaining seven. One of the persons belonging in the last group was found to harbor the trichomonads on a second direct examination; another was diagnosed again as negative for the parasites; and no additional microscopic examinations could be made in the remaining five, presumably T. vaginalis-free individuals. It is evident from the above data that a positive correlation between the results of direct examination and of the skin test existed in nearly 80 percent of uninfected persons. Although on a second microscopic examination the authors found the parasites in only one of the cases with a positive skin reaction, there is a distinct possibility that parasite infections might have been revealed in more members of this group by additional examinations and through the use of culture methods.

Inasmuch as a higher percentage of T. vaginalis infection was found by direct examination than by the skin test and since only one additional case was revealed with the aid of the latter method, Adler and Sadowsky (1947) felt that the test could not be recommended for routine diagnostic purposes.

More recently Aburel et al. (1963), using heat-killed T. vaginalis, examined 263 women by direct microscopic method and by the skin test. Of the patients found to harbor the parasites on direct examination, 82 percent gave a positive skin reaction (1 cm in diameter, as read after 24 hours). Three possible alternatives were proposed by the authors in explanation of the lack of an allergic response in the remaining 18 percent of infected individuals: 1. The infecting parasites might have belonged to a different antigenic type than the ones employed in the test (see also Jaakmees, 1965; Jaakmees and Teras, 1966); 2. The infections could have been of relatively recent origin (*see also* Adler and Sadowsky, 1947); 3. The lack of an allergic response possibly depended upon anergy of some patients. Twenty-five percent of women in whom no trichomonads were observed on direct examination (in some instances also by the culture method) gave a positive skin reaction. The authors were inclined to believe that this lack of correlation depended to a degree on the inadequacy of direct examination; also, some of the patients might have had a history of previous trichomonad infections. On the basis of their results, Aburel et al. (1963) concluded that the "intradermal test may . . . considerably reduce the number of direct examinations and cultures required for diagnosis of urogenital trichomoniasis."

Using an extract obtained by suspending dried powdered trichomonads in physiologic saline, Sinelnikova (1961) observed a positive skin reaction (1 to 3 cm in diameter after 24 hours) in 61 percent of women known to harbor *T. vaginalis*. Even less satisfactory results, 41 percent of positive reactions, were recorded in the same group of women with the aid of antigen obtained by hot acid hydrolysis of the parasites. On the other hand, clearly positive skin tests were noted by Sinelnikova (1961) in 77 percent of infected patients when she employed the "corpuscular" antigen, prepared according to the method of Anina-Radchenko (1959), for the intradermal inoculations. This latter worker, using heat-killed organisms suspended in physiologic saline, noted a positive skin reaction in "the majority" of women and men known to be infected with *T. vaginalis*. *Trichomonas*-free persons were found negative by skin tests when injected with all three aforementioned antigen preparations (Anina-Radchenko, 1959; Sinelnikova, 1961).

An extensive study of the skin test as applied to infections with *T. vaginalis* was reported by the Estonian group of workers (Jaakmees, 1964a, 1965; Jaakmees and Teras, 1966). In the course of the investigation, the authors tested 324 persons of both sexes for an allergic skin reaction by intradermal inoculations of an "aqueous lysate" (a phenol-treated extract of flagellates lysed by the addition of distilled water [Jaakmees, 1965]) of four strains of the urogenital trichomonad which belonged to the antigenic types TN, TLR, TRT, and TR. Among the group subjected to the tests, 209 persons were found to harbor *T. vaginalis*, while the presence of the flagellates could not be demonstrated in the remaining 115 individuals on repeated microscopic examinations or by cultivation of the secretions from their urogenital passages. In *Trichomonas*-free persons who were not exposed to the parasites by cohabitation with infected partners, the skin test gave uniformly negative results, but some of the individuals (three out of 40 men and one out of five women) who were thus exposed gave a positive reaction. The authors felt that some of the positive reactions obtained in the parasite-free patients by previous investigators (Adler and Sadowsky, 1947; Theokharov, 1959) could be explained by the above findings. A number of the patients infected with the urogenital trichomonad gave positive skin reactions; however, the percentage of positive results was quite low. According to Jaakmees (1965) and Jaakmees and Teras (1966), the highest numbers of positive skin reactions (erythrematous area from 5 to over 10 mm) were observed among patients suffering from acute or subacute trichomoniasis. Still, even among those individuals, only 21 (28 percent) of 75 women and three (37.5 percent) of eight men could be diagnosed as clearly positive. The results were considerably less satisfactory in patients with chronic or latent trichomoniasis; for example, among 51 women in this group only six (11.8 percent) gave a clearly positive skin reaction.

Although in the light of the foregoing data, the skin test employing the "aqueous lysate" of trichomonads proved generally unsatisfactory for diagnostic purposes, the Estonian workers' experiments provided certain information pertaining to the allergic reaction. They demonstrated for the first time that the reaction appeared to depend upon the antigenic type of *T. vaginalis* employed for the intradermal inoculations. Thus, for example, among the 21 women suffering from acute or subacute urogenital trichomoniasis, positive skin reaction was obtained in all cases with the type TRT, but such reaction was observed in only 10 cases with TLR, and only in 11 with TN and TR. If only one antigenic type were employed in the tests, the number of positive readings might have been significantly lower (Aburel et al., 1963). No correlation could be established between the presence and/or intensity of the intradermal allergic reactions in patients who harbored *T. vaginalis* and the agglutination titers or complement-fixing potency of the sera from these persons. In fact, completely negative results with the skin test were observed in individuals whose sera showed high levels of agglutinating and complement-fixing antibodies. It appears therefore that in urogenital trichomoniasis, "specific allergy does not depend upon [the presence] of complement-fixing antibodies and agglutinins in the sera" (Jaakmees and Teras, 1966).

Having established the inadequacy of the "aqueous lysate" of trichomonads for the skin test, Jaakmees (1965) and Jaakmees and Teras (1966) investigated the suitability for this purpose of a "corpuscular" antigen. This antigen consisted of a cell-free homogenate of the trichomonads suspended in 0.85 percent saline with 0.5 percent phenol. Among 40 parasite-free persons (20 women and 20 men), not one gave a positive skin reaction. On the other hand, all 21 women infected with *T. vaginalis* were found positive by means of the skin test. Regardless of the clinical manifestations associated with trichomoniasis, all patients gave positive skin reactions with at least one antigenic type of *T. vaginalis*. There was no correlation between the agglutination titers and/or complement-fixing potency of the sera from the patients infected with the urogenital trichomonads and the intensity of the allergic reaction observed in such patients.

Although Jaakmees (1965) and Jaakmees and Teras (1966) appeared to have demonstrated the efficacy of the skin test involving the use of "corpuscular antigens" in diagnosis of *T. vaginalis* infections, they were of the opinion that further standardization of the method would be needed before it could be employed satisfactorily in routine diagnosis. It is to be noted that Jaakmees (1965) accepted as clearly positive those reactions which resulted in smaller erythrematous areas (5 to 10 mm) than those considered positive by many workers (*see* above).

It seems clear from the available data that the presence of the urogenital trichomonad in man stimulates the production of specific, perhaps even type-specific, reagins. However, the results obtained by most workers suggest that in the present state of its development, the skin test does not appear to provide any significant advantages over direct examination in routine diagnosis. Perhaps further improvements will render the test effective in demonstrating cryptic infections and in tracing infected sexual partners of parasite-free individuals; it may then prove very useful in epidemiologic investigations.

Conclusions. It is apparent that despite early failures which are still widely quoted in the pertinent literature, recent investigations have placed serodiagnosis of human urogenital trichomoniasis on a much firmer basis. One of the most important advances was the employment of several antigenic types of *T. vaginalis* in the various reactions. Hoffmann (1966b) showed that hemagglutination constituted the most successful immunologic test for urogenital trichomoniasis. This method was employed previously in serodiagnosis of *T. vaginalis* by the British workers (McEntegart, 1952; Lanceley and McEntegart, 1953) with far less success, and Kott and Adler (1961) found hemagglutination less suitable than direct agglutination in their immunologic studies of the trichomonad species of man. According to Hoffmann et al. (1963) and Hoffmann (1966b), a certain degree of correlation existed between the clinical form of *T. vaginalis* trichomoniasis and the efficacy of the complement-fixation test, as well as hemagglutination reactions. On the other hand, no such correlation was found in regard to either the agglutination or complement-fixation methods by the Estonian investigators (Jaakmees, 1965; Jaakmees et al., 1966; Nigesen, 1966; Teras et al., 1966a,b). According to these workers, both of the latter techniques could be employed with complete confidence in serodiagnosis and epidemiologic studies of urogenital trichomoniasis. Only future research may throw some light upon the differences in results reported by the recent investigators and help us in deciding which, if any, of the aforementioned serologic methods can be applied with confidence in such studies. As pointed out before, the fluorescent-antibody technique (Kramář and Kučera, 1966), when properly standardized, also may provide a most useful tool for these investigations. At the present time the skin test does not appear to be very useful.

In many instances, a direct microscopic examination not only may suffice for diagnostic purposes in *T. vaginalis* infections, but may actually constitute the method of choice. On the other hand, well-standardized, highly dependable immunologic methods, often useful for serodiagnostic purposes, could prove of greatest importance in epidemiologic studies and also in following the response of the host system to treatment for trichomoniasis.

The far-reaching implications of infection with *T. vaginalis*, the discussion of which is beyond the scope of this chapter, have been recognized by French, German, Polish, and Russian clinicians and parasitologists (*see* Honigberg et al., 1966, for references), but, for reasons not entirely clear to this writer, these implications have managed to escape the attention of many

American workers. In the light of these implications, immunologic and serologic studies of urogenital trichomoniasis of man seem of great importance. There can be no question that the Estonian and Polish investigators have contributed much to this field. It is unfortunate indeed that the journals in which their reports are published are not readily available to most English-reading scientists.

Trichomonas gallinae (Rivolta)

Natural infections with *Trichomonas gallinae* are restricted to birds. The domestic pigeon, *Columba livia*, is the primary host of this trichomonad, and many other columbiform species are found to harbor it (Stabler, 1954). Numerous pathogenic strains of *T. gallinae* have been reported from the columbids, but outbreaks of canker, the disease caused by this parasite, appear not to be restricted to these hosts. There are reports of infections, accompanied by the typical symptoms, from galliform birds, especially turkeys (Volkmar, 1930; Gierke, 1933; Hawn, 1937; Hinshaw, 1937; Bushnell and Twiehaus, 1940a,b). Chickens also may be infected by this flagellate (Levine and Brandly, 1940), and, according to various investigators (*see* Stabler, 1954), Java sparrows, peregrine falcons, and sea gulls were found to serve as its natural hosts. Many kinds of nestling passerine birds are susceptible to infection with *T. gallinae* and show symptoms characteristic of trichomoniasis when exposed experimentally to virulent strains.

It seems that even among the columbids, in which *T. gallinae* is very common, many strains of the parasite are purely commensal, never causing any symptoms or abnormal changes. On the other hand, some of the strains show different levels of pathogenicity for naturally and experimentally infected avian hosts (Stabler, 1948a, 1951); also the strains found in the galliform birds differ in their pathogenicity (Levine and Brandly, 1939; Levine et al., 1941). According to more recent reports, the differences in pathogenicity levels inherent in the strains of *T. gallinae* maintained in axenic cultures can be demonstrated by means of the subcutaneous "mouse assay" (Honigberg, 1961; Frost and Honigberg, 1962) and in cell cultures (Honigberg et al., 1964; Abraham and Honigberg, 1965).

Antigenic identity

It has been established primarily with the aid of agglutination reactions that *T. gallinae* differs antigenically from *T. foetus* (Morisita, 1939; Robertson, 1941; Schoenherr, 1956; Baba, 1957), *T. vaginalis* (Baba, 1957), *P. hominis* (Schoenherr, 1956), and *Monocercomonas colubrorum*, (Robertson, 1941). Baba (1958) demonstrated significant differences in the proportion of mice protected by intraperitoneal inoculations with killed *T. gallinae, T. vaginalis,* and *T. foetus* against intramuscular infections by homologous and heterologous trichomonad species. When animals immunized with *T. gallinae* were challenged with the homologous and the two heterologous species, the rates of infection were 19 percent, 44 percent, and 40 percent, respectively. Undoubtedly further investigations will reveal antigenic differences between the avian parasites and all other members of the order Trichomonadida.

In experiments involving agglutination, in which fragmented trichomonads served as antigens, Schoenherr (1956) was able to demonstrate certain differences among three strains of *T. gallinae*. Agglutinating antibodies to one of the strains were present in one of the anti-*T. vaginalis* sera. Apparently this particular strain of the urogenital parasite of man possessed common antigens with at least one of the strains of the avian trichomonad. In view of the close phylogenetic relationship between *T. gallinae* and *T. vaginalis* (Honigberg, 1963), it seems likely that a more sensitive method might have revealed such antigens among all the lines of the two species.

More information concerning the antigenic differences among strains of *T. gallinae* was presented recently by Honigberg and Goldman (1968), and Goldman and Honigberg (1968). Three lines of the Jones' Barn strain (Stabler, 1948a, 1951) were used in the experiments. The first involved trichomonads derived from an axenic culture which was kept frozen in liquid nitrogen since its isolation from an experimentally infected pigeon. When used in the immunologic experiments, over a year after its isolation, these parasites killed nonimmune pigeon squabs within eight to nine days. The second line came from the same isolate as the preceding one, but was carried in culture by serial transfers at 37°C for one year. In the process of cultivation, the trichomonads became attenuated. At the time at which they were employed for immunization of rabbits, the parasites caused no symptoms or pathologic changes in nonimmune pigeons and their virulence could not be restored by bird-to-bird transfers (*see* Stabler et al., 1964). From many viewpoints, this line could be considered as a separate strain or substrain. The third line, derived from an earlier isolate of the Jones' Barn strain from a pigeon squab, was attenuated by *in vitro* cultivation for about three years.

Immune sera were obtained from rabbits, each pair inoculated with one sterile cell-free homogenate of each of the three lines. In each case the homogenates were mixed (1:1) with complete Freund's adjuvant. It was shown by means of quantitative fluorescent-antibody methods (Goldman, 1967; Goldman and Cannon, 1967; Honigberg and Goldman, 1968) that all the lines shared a number of antigenic components; that each possessed, in addition, unique antigens; and that the two attenuated substrains contained more antigenic systems than the parent strain. The results obtained with the same three lines by means of the Ouchterlony gel-diffusion technique (Goldman and Honigberg, 1968) confirmed many of those shown before through the employment of the fluorescent-antibody methods. Experiments performed with the aid of the former technique brought out clearly the common antigenic makeup of the three lines of *T. gallinae*. They indicated also that the fully virulent parent strain contained only a weak antigenic system represented by one group of the precipitin lines, which, by contrast, was quite strong, in the secondarily avirulent substrains. The failure of the gel-diffusion technique to reveal any systems unique to each of the three tricho-monad lines could be attributed to the subtlety of the unique antigens and to the relative insensitivity of the Ouchterlony method. The fact that the parental strain was found to possess only a small quantity of certain antigens which apparently increased in concentration concomitant with loss of virulence suggested the possibility that these particular antigens could represent a virulence inhibiting system which constituted part of the normal composition of trichomonad parasites and that its concentration might be inversely proportional to the virulence levels exhibited by various strains (Goldman and Honigberg, 1968). However, an alternate explanation seems possible: the parasites may acquire additional antigens simply as a result of prolonged *in vitro* cultivation, entirely unrelated to retention or loss of virulence. It should be added that experiments with freshly isolated avirulent strains of *T. gallinae* and with substrains of such strains maintained on nonliving media for different periods of time are being conducted at present in the hope of clarifying the problems of the possible relationships between pathogenicity and the antigenic constitution of trichomonads.

The results obtained in the above-mentioned studies on *T. gallinae* are at variance with those reported in regard to strains of *T. vaginalis* by the Estonian workers (Teras and Tompel, 1963; Laan, 1965; Teras, 1965, 1966) on the basis of agglutination tests. According to these investigators, no changes in antigenic types could be found in several strains of the urogenital tricho-monad of man after prolonged periods of axenic cultivation, although the maintenance *in vitro* caused a significant decrease in pathogenicity for mice in those strains that were found to be highly pathogenic soon after their isolation from the patients.

The apparent conflict between the results published on *T. gallinae* (Honig-berg and Goldman, 1968; Goldman and Honigberg, 1968) and on *T. vaginalis* (Teras and Tompel, 1963; Laan, 1965; Teras, 1965, 1966) can be explained in several ways. Aside from the various factors inherent in the different species studied and different immunologic techniques employed, the Estonian investigators did not maintain separate lines of the originally pathogenic strains under conditions, such as very low temperatures, which would preserve their original pathogenicity levels and antigenic composition. Thus they were unable to compare, especially by using absorption, the original isolates with the substrains attenuated by means of prolonged cultivation. If the strains of *T. vaginalis* behaved like those of *T. gallinae* and developed new antigens as well as increased the level of some of the existing antigens during the period of pathogenicity attenuation without losing any of the original antigenic systems, absorption with the attenuated organisms alone would not reveal any differences among the anti-*T. vaginalis* sera. Further, in comparing the results obtained with agglutination and fluorescent-antibody methods, it ought to be kept in mind that agglutination titers based on two-fold dilutions would be incapable of distinguishing less than two-fold differences in reactivity among antisera and that most reactions involving fluorescein-conjugated homologous and heterologous anti-*T. gallinae* sera showed less than two-fold differences. Similar arguments can be adduced against the apparent immutability of the antigenic characteristics of *T. vaginalis* and *P. hominis* (Kott and Adler, 1961) and of *T. foetus* (Robertson, 1941, Kerr and Robertson, 1945; Robertson, 1960) maintained *in vitro* for prolonged time periods.

Natural and induced antibodies

According to Robertson (1941), *T. gallinae* was extremely sensitive to the lytic activity of normal rabbit and guinea pig sera with intact complement. Sera from rabbits (Robertson, 1941) and guinea pigs (Baba, 1957) immunized with living avian parasites via the intravenous and intraperitoneal routes, respectively, showed strong agglutination (Robertson, 1941; Baba, 1957) and immobilization (Baba, 1957) reactions with the homologous living antigen. Specificity of the reactions was demonstrated by cross-agglutination tests which involved living *T. vaginalis* (Baba, 1957), *T. foetus* (Robertson, 1941; Baba, 1957), and *M. colubrorum* (Robertson, 1941).

Protective immune mechanisms

Strong protection against the effects of even the most virulent strains of *T. gallinae* is afforded to birds by previous infections with moderately pathogenic or mild strains of this species (Stabler, 1948b, 1951, 1954). Virulent and mild strains may coexist without any loss of the original pathogenicity by the former. When such mixed infections are transferred to nonimmune pigeons, these hosts succumb promptly. Also, the inherent pathogenicity level of a given strain for nonimmune birds is not affected by prolonged residence in an immune pigeon which may have survived a sublethal attack (Stabler, 1953). Natural loss of infection is said to be followed by a gradual loss of protection against the injurious effects of virulent strains (Stabler, 1954). At no time does there appear to be among the natural hosts any lasting resistance to reinfection.

Until very recently, the nature of immunity against *T. gallinae*, like that against other trichomonad species discussed in this chapter, was obscure. The unpublished results of Stepkowski and Honigberg (1969), however, may provide a plausible explanation for the observations summarized in the preceding paragraph of this section. These investigators used the following five strains or substrains of the avian parasite in gel-diffusion experiments: the fully virulent Jones' Barn (JB) strain; a substrain (JBC) of the latter strain attenuated by 12 months of cultivation in a nonliving medium; a freshly isolated, nonpathogenic SG strain; a substrain (SGC) of SG obtained by 11.5 months of cultivation in a nonliving medium; and an originally nonpathogenic AG strain which had been maintained *in vitro* for about 11 years.

Three major groups of precipitin lines were observed in reactions of all five antigens with the five immune sera which were produced by subcutaneous inoculations of these antigens into rabbits according to the method described by Honigberg and Goldman (1968). Except for AG, which differed from all the others in the composition of all three groups of lines, the remaining strains and substrains seemed quite similar regarding two of the groups. On the other hand, significant differences were observed among the five strains and substrains in the composition of the third major group of precipitin lines, designated as the B lines. Cross-reactions involving all the antigens and antisera revealed that the B group included five distinct subgroups of antigens, which were designated as B_1 to B_5.

Analysis of the results indicated that: 1. The virulent JB strain has, in addition to the complete B_1 antigen complex, traces of some antigens belonging to the B_2 subgroup. Further, some of the components of the B_3 and B_4 complexes appear to be represented by incomplete, hapten-like, antigens. 2. The attenuated JBC substrain has complete B_1 and B_2 antigen complexes; in addition, it seems to contain some incomplete antigens of the B_4 subgroup. 3. Both the SG strain and the SGC substrain, which have some of the B_1 subgroup antigens, are characterized by the possession of the complete B_3 antigen complex. The SGC trichomonads seem to be richer in the B_3 subgroup antigens, but this difference is quantitative rather than qualitative. 4. The AG strain contains complete B_4 and B_5 antigen complexes.

The results of Stępkowski and Honigberg (1969) suggest that the virulent strain of *T. gallinae* has a more limited capacity than the avirulent ones to stimulate the production of antibodies to the B group antigens in the host organism, and that the virulent parasites contain incomplete antigens capable of combining with antibodies produced by the host system against many nonpathogenic strains of the same species. The data also indicate that irrespective of whether a strain is originally nonpathogenic or whether its virulence is lost as a consequence of prolonged cultivation, it has a larger number of complete antigens belonging to the B group.

It has been known for some time (*see* Honigberg, 1961, for references) that mice can be infected with *T. gallinae* via subcutaneous, intraperitoneal, and intramuscular routes. The subcutaneous mouse assay (Honigberg, 1961) reflects faithfully the pathogenicity levels of different strains for their natural hosts. Using subcutaneous inoculations of axenic cultures of the Jones' Barn strain of *T. gallinae*, Warren et al. (1961) studied the protective effects of intraperitoneally injected cell-free, lyophilized, and presumably protein-free supernate of maintenance medium (Simplified Trypticase without serum [Kupferberg et al., 1948]) in which the trichomonads were incubated for four hours at 37°C. The results indicated that this supernate, referred to as "physiologically derived antigen," that contained the substances secreted and excreted by the parasites, was effective in stimulating immune response in the mice; the typical subcutaneous abscesses developed in significantly fewer animals pretreated with the supernate than in the control group.

Warren et al. (1961) concluded that by injection of the supernate, circulating antigens were introduced into the host. These antigens stimulated the production of antibodies which protected the mice against challenge by the living flagellates.

Similar protection was apparently afforded mice treated with triturated bodies of the trichomonads (Warren et al., 1961), and agglutinating antibodies, perhaps similar to those stimulated by the "physiologically derived antigen," were actually demonstrated in sera of animals which received subcutaneous injections of living parasites (Warren and Chandler, 1958). Honigberg (unpublished data) observed that subcutaneous inoculations of either a mild or a virulent strain in one flank failed to protect mice against a subsequent subcutaneous challenge with the latter in the opposite flank. Instead of being absent or smaller, the lesions resulting from the challenge injections were larger, indicating perhaps sensitization. On the other hand, intraperitoneal inoculations of living trichomonads appeared to protect the mice against subsequent introduction of the pathogenic flagellates under the skin of these animals. These data seem to cast some doubt on the assumption that the antibodies found by Warren and Chandler (1958) were the same as those postulated by Warren et al. (1961) on the basis of the results they obtained with the "physiologically derived antigen."

Baba (1958) found a high degree of protection against intramuscular challenges with living homologous antigen in mice immunized by intraperitoneal injections of heat-killed *T. gallinae*. Only 19 percent of the animals developed typical abscesses as a result of the challenge. Significantly less protection was observed in such mice against heterologous antigens, i.e., *T. vaginalis* and *T. foetus*.

Pentatrichomonas hominis (Davaine) and
Trichomonas tenax (O. F. Müller)

Neither *Pentatrichomonas hominis* nor *Trichomonas tenax*, which inhabit the large intestine and the oral cavity of man, respectively, have been proved to contain pathogenic strains (*see* Honigberg, 1963, for references). Only very limited information is available on the immunology of these two species.

The earliest report (Tokura, 1935) on the antigenic attributes of *P. hominis* and *T. tenax* was based on experiments involving flagellates grown in agnotobiotic cultures. The aggulutination titers in sera from rabbits injected intravenously with formalin-killed flagellates were very low (1:6). Apparently with undiluted sera and at very low dilutions (1:2), "group reactions" were noted among *P. hominis*, *T. tenax*, and *T. vaginalis*. These were said to be stronger between the oral trichomonad and the remaining two species than between the intestinal and the urogenital flagellates. In view of his results, Tokura (1935) considered *T. tenax* to occupy an intermediate antigenic position between the other two trichomonads of man. The very low agglutination titers reported by this worker, which do not exceed the titers associated with the natural antibodies to the trichomonad parasites, preclude a meaningful evaluation of his results.

As mentioned above, based on microagglutination tests involving sera from rabbits injected intravenously with formalin-killed flagellates and using living and formalinized organisms as antigens, MacDonald and Tatum (1948) concluded that *P. hominis* and *T. vaginalis* were antigenically identical. This conclusion was borne out apparently also by cross-absorption experiments. On the other hand, Kott and Adler (1961) using agglutination and two hemagglutination methods found that although one of the antigenic types (Type I) of the intestinal trichomonad, which included three strains, shared common antigens with some strains of *T. vaginalis*, it could be differentiated from them by cross-absorption. As evidenced by cross-hemagglutination tests, among the common antigens were the polysaccharides obtained with the aid of Fuller's (1938) formamide extraction method. The second antigenic type (Type II) of *P. hominis*, which included two strains, shared no agglutinogens or immunologically active polysaccharides with Type I of this species or with *T. vaginalis*. However, cross-reactions between Type II on the one hand and Type I of *P. hominis* (as well as strains of the urogenital parasite) on the other were noted in hemagglutination experiments involving erythrocytes sensitized with cell-free extracts of the trichomonads after previous treatment with tannic acid. These results suggested to Kott and Adler (1961) that the antigens revealed by the latter method were neither agglutinogenic nor polysaccharide in character.

Kott and Adler (1961) employed agnotobiotic cultures of three strains of *T. tenax* in agglutination experiments. Before being used in a reaction, the antisera, developed in rabbits by intravenous injections of living flagellates, were absorbed with the bacteria accompanying the protozoa in cultures. Agglutination titers up to 1:2,000 were observed in homologous systems. Cross-agglutination experiments suggested that two of the strains of the oral trichomonad were more closely related to each other than either was to the third strain. Apparently none of the strains shared antigens with *P. hominis* and *T. vaginalis*. Oleinik (1964) obtained somewhat different results with regard to the intestinal, urogenital, and oral trichomonads of man in experiments involving agglutination and gel diffusion. *T. vaginalis* could be differentiated from the other two species, which, however, appeared to be antigenically identical. It was pointed out elsewhere in this chapter that the difficulties with Oleinik's experiments might have depended upon the fact that of the three species, only *T. vaginalis* was maintained under axenic conditions.

It would seem on the basis of the available information (MacDonald and Tatum, 1948; Kott and Adler, 1961) that, as evidenced by cross-agglutination reactions, some strains of *P. hominis* are more closely related to *T. vaginalis* than this latter species is to *T. tenax*. Further, Oleinik's (1964) results appear to point to a close kinship between the intestinal and oral trichomonad, and to suggest the existence of significant antigenic differences between these species and *T. vaginalis*. Such conclusions are not readily reconciled with the information based upon other than immunologic lines of evidence (Honigberg, 1963). Unquestionably, definite information on the antigenic attributes and kinships of *P. hominis* and *T. tenax* must await more extensive studies. Such studies should be facilitated by the development in recent years (Diamond, 1961, 1962; Diamond and Bartgis, 1965) of a medium capable of supporting growth of the oral trichomonad in the absence of bacteria.

Tritrichomonas foetus (Riedmüller)

Much knowledge has been accumulated throughout the years on various aspects of biology, pathogenicity, and immunology of *Tritrichomonas foetus* which inhabits the urogenital tract of cattle, and is considered one of the important protozoan pathogens found in these hosts. Morgan's (1946) monograph summarizes much of the information on *T. foetus* available prior to its publication, and many articles dealing with this parasite may be found in the Reims Symposium (1957) (*see also* Hammond et al., 1956). More recently, Robertson (1963) contributed a short review dealing with the immunologic aspects of *T. foetus* and bovine urogenital trichomoniasis. The interested reader will find much information in all the above publications, which include also a large number of important references regarding this parasite.

The causal relationship between *T. foetus* and urogenital trichomoniasis in cattle was recognized at the end of the last century (Künstler, 1888; Mazzanti, 1900), and the etiologic involvement of this protozoon in abortion in cattle was understood clearly by the 1930's and 1940's (Morgan, 1946).

T. foetus is transmitted from bulls to cows during coitus, and thus the urogenital trichomoniasis may be considered as an almost exclusively venereal infection. In the bull, the parasites are lodged typically in the prepucial cavity (Hammond and Bartlett, 1943), although, on rarer occasions, they also have been found in the urethra and even in the deeper parts of the urogenital tract (Morgan, 1946). Once a bull has been infected, it usually retains the parasite for life. The acute stage of infection, involving inflammation and swelling of the prepuce and accompanied by mucopurulent discharge, usually subsides within two weeks after the exposure of the bull to the parasites. From then on, the infected animal is typically asymptomatic; however, on occasions orchiditis may develop in chronic cases. The severity of the disease varies in the cow. At one end of the spectrum, very mild symptoms prevail; at the other, profound pathologic changes are associated with severe symptoms. Vaginitis, although frequent, is not considered diagnostic. Infections may be restricted to the vagina, but more often the parasites migrate upwards through the cervix into the uterus. The presence of *T. foetus* in the uterus may cause endometritis with resulting temporary or permanent sterility. If conception does occur in the infected cow, the trichomonads can cause a typically early abortion. In other cases, the fetus may die quite early in pregnancy without being expelled from the uterus; pyometra usually develops in such cases, with retention of the corpus luteum and of the cervical plug.

The existence of strains with different inherent pathogenicity levels cannot be doubted. Some indications of such differences are apparent from the early observations of natural and experimental infections in normal hosts (Morgan, 1946). According to the subcutaneous, intramuscular, and intraperitoneal mouse assays reported by Schnitzer et al. (1950), in which one strain of each species, *T. vaginalis*, *T. gallinae*, and *T. foetus*, was employed, the urogenital trichomonad of cattle appeared to be the most pathogenic. Various other accounts dealing with inoculations of *T. foetus* into different experimental animals (*see* Morgan, 1946; and Honigberg, 1961, for references) also tend to point out the relatively high inherent pathogenicity of many strains of this parasite. More recent studies of relative pathogenicity for mice of several axenically cultivated strains indicated low virulence levels of three old stock cultures (Jeffries and Harris, 1967) and of two strains maintained *in vitro* for one and five years, respectively (Purchase and Clark, 1967). It has been emphasized by some workers that prolonged *in vitro* cultivation results in attenuation of pathogenic strains of *T. gallinae* (Stabler et al., 1964) and *T. foetus* (Morgan, 1946) as evidenced by their effects on natural hosts. Similar observations were recorded in mice infected subcutaneously with strains of *T. vaginalis* and *T. gallinae* (Honigberg, 1961), and *in vitro* attenuation might have been the reason for the small lesions reported by Jeffries and Harris (1967) and Purchase and Clark (1967) from these experimental hosts injected with *T. foetus*. The most recent results (Kulda and Honigberg, unpublished) based upon the subcutaneous mouse assay (Honigberg, 1961) of many strains of the bovine trichomonad leave no doubt as to the presence of significant differences in pathogenicity among these strains.

The astonishing claim of transformation of *T. vaginalis* into *T. foetus* following a passage of the former species through mice (Inoki, 1957) unquestionably belongs in the same category with the allegation of Fischer (1938) that bovine urogenital trichomoniasis spreads from women into cattle. Needless to say, in the light of all the available information (*see* Morgan, 1946; and Honigberg, 1963, for references), neither of these statements deserves serious consideration. On the other hand, we must consider seriously the reports claiming that *T. foetus* and *Tritrichomonas suis* belong in the same species. Admittedly there is a great deal of morphologic (Buttrey, 1956; Hibler et al., 1960) and physiologic (Doran, 1957, 1959; Stępkowski, 1966) similarity between these trichomonads from cattle and from swine. Kust (1936a) believed he had found a flagellate similar to *T. foetus* in the urogenital tract and aborted fetuses of pigs. Short-lived experimental infections with *T. suis* could be produced in cows (*see* Levine, 1961, for references), and similar, rather transient infections resulted from introduction of these parasites into the urogenital system of sows (Hammond and Leidl, 1957).

As far as immunologic comparisons of *T. foetus* and *T. suis* are concerned, Sanborn (1955) was able to differentiate between the two species by means of agglutination, while according to Kerr (1958), the mucus agglutination test (*see* pp. 534–535) gave positive results in heifers infected with the parasites from pigs and with the Belfast strain, but not with the Manley strain, of *T. foetus*. Using agglutination and precipitation (including Ouchterlony gel diffusion) methods, Robertson (1960) found that two strains of *T. suis* as well as the Belfast and Manley strains of *T. foetus* shared a number of antigens; the trichomonads from pigs appeared to be more closely related to the Belfast than to the Manley strain of the bovine parasite (*see also* Kerr, 1958). On the basis of her results, Robertson (1960) concluded that *T. foetus* and *T. suis* belonged in a single species. Stępkowski (1961a, 1966) arrived at a similar conclusion with the aid of agglutination, precipitation, and complement-fixation methods, as well as by estimates of the phagocytic activity of leukocytes in immune rabbit blood (*see* p. 520). Only further research may prove unequivocally whether the porcine and the bovine trichomonads represent one species. It appears preferable, at least at present, to retain separate trivial names for the two parasites in question. Whatever the actual identity of the flagellate from pigs, it seems best to exclude it from the following discussion, which thus will be restricted to *T. foetus* from bovine hosts.

The presence of trichomonads, presumed to be *T. foetus*, in the blood stream of cattle has been reported on several occasions (Kust, 1936a,b; Wagner and Hees, 1937; Salzer, 1938), but many more investigators (*see* Morgan, 1946) were unable to find these flagellates in the circulatory system of naturally and experimentally infected bovine hosts. According to Riedmüller (1928) and Witte (1933a,b), living *T. foetus* was present in the pericardial fluid and heart blood of guinea pigs injected intraperitoneally with this parasite. The trichomonad was recovered also from the heart and various organs of aborted fetuses, which usually were examined some time after death (*see* Morgan, 1946, for references). In the latter instances, the possibility of a post-mortem invasion of the blood stream cannot be excluded.

It is apparent from the foregoing discussion that there is hitherto no conclusive proof of the occurrence of *T. foetus* in the blood stream of the natural hosts. However, some considerations presented in this connection in the previous sections of this chapter may also apply to bovine trichomoniasis. Phagocytosis of *T. foetus* by leukocytes has been reported by Wenrich and Emmerson (1933), as well as by Hammond and Bartlett (1945). The former authors suggested that the phagocytic activity represented a defense mechanism of the host, and, according to the latter investigators, reduction in the number of the parasites at various periods during infection depended upon this activity. Ingestion of the flagellates by macrophages is also very common in chick liver cell cultures infected with *T. foetus* (Kulda and Honigberg, 1969). On occasions the trichomonads have also been found in the nonphagocytic epithelial cells in such cultures. The role of phagocytosis in immunity against the bovine urogenital trichomonad has not been investigated to any significant degree; however, Stępkowski (1961a,b) was able to differentiate between *T. foetus* and *T. vaginalis* by comparing phagocytic activity of leukocytes from rabbits immunized with homologous and heterologous antigens. The comparison involved estimates based upon tests which employed antigen-coated collodion particles (Cavelti, 1947), and followed the method recommended by Huddleson et al. (1933). The significant enhancement of phagocytic activity of leukocytes from rabbits immunized with an antigen homologous to that used for coating the collodion particles suggested to Stępkowski (1961b) the formation of specific opsonins in trichomonad infections.

According to Robertson (1963), urogenital "trichomoniasis in cattle is an example of local protozoan infection," but there can be no doubt that the parasites do come into very close contact with the host tissues and that, as she herself pointed out, there is much evidence (*see* pp. 526–532) of "circulating humoral antibody arising from uterine antigen reaching systemic circulation." Thus, even if the infection is considered as purely local, it seems capable of evoking a total systemic response. Only future investigations may ascertain whether, as suggested by Robertson (1963), these circulating antibodies actually play no part in the course of bovine trichomoniasis because they never come in contact with the parasites which are confined to the uterus and vagina.

Antigenic identity

T. foetus and *T. vaginalis* have been shown to contain unique as well as common antigens by means of agglutination, hemagglutination, precipitation (including gel diffusion), complement fixation, fluorescent-antibody method, and phagocytic index in immune blood (*see* p. 476 for references). Further, primarily with the aid of agglutination, the urogenital trichomonad of cattle has been differentiated from *M. colubrorum, T. gallinae, P. hominis, T. gallinarum,* and *T. augusta* (*see* pp. 473, 476, 477, 510, 516, 537, 538 for references).

Robertson's (1941) cross-agglutination experiments suggested a very close antigenic relationship, "amounting almost to identity," between the Glaser and Belfast strains of *T. foetus.* Subsequently, Kerr and Robertson (1945) and Robertson (1960) were able to differentiate clearly between Belfast and Manley strains of this trichomonad by agglutination, skin tests, and precipitation methods, and similar results were obtained by McEntegart (1956) with the aid of hemagglutination. Especially useful for differentiation between the two antigenic types, Manley and Belfast, was the gel-diffusion technique employing the polysaccharide-aminoacid complexes obtained by Feinberg and Morgan's (1953) diethylene glycol extraction method (Robertson, 1960). The complexes obtained in this manner appeared specific for the strains from which they were isolated since their precipitin lines were not shared on the diffusion plates, while the lines associated with substances other than the complexes were shared by both antigenic types. For example, only the "nonpolysaccharide" lines, proved subsequently to involve a protein fraction, resulted from a reaction between anti-Belfast serum and the complete Manley strain antigen. On the other hand, only lines of identity were precipitated in a reaction involving the diethylene glycol fraction extracted from Belfast strain and anti-Belfast serum.

Pierce (1949a) using the agglutination method, found that 17 strains of the bovine urogenital trichomonad isolated in England and Scotland were antigenically very similar either to Manley or to Belfast strain, which thus did not seem to represent antigenic extremes between which all the other strains would fall. The existence of many clearly different antigenic types of *T. foetus* was reported by Florent (1957) on the basis of immunologic studies that included agglutination methods and skin tests. Inasmuch as heifers immunized with a strain of one antigenic type developed resistance to infections with homologous and heterologous strains alike, the author believed that the antigenic differences did not play an important role in the acquisition of immunity and in the epidemiology of the urogenital trichomonad of cattle.

In his immunologic study of *T. foetus*, Stępkowski (1966) employed antitrichomonad sera from rabbits injected intravenously with homogenates of the parasites obtained by freeze-thawing. Agglutination, hemagglutination, complement-fixation, and precipitation methods were used in the antigenic analysis of 10 strains of the parasite. Most information on the antigenic structure of this flagellate was obtained by means of the Ouchterlony gel-diffusion technique. The antigen fraction which uniformly formed a precipitin line with the antiserum was found to be thermolabile, suggesting that it may be a protein compound. In addition, the investigations demonstrated the presence of a thermostable antigen which probably consisted of two fractions. One of the fractions, which, on the basis of its behavior on acid hydrolysis appeared to be firmly bound to a proteinaceous moiety, was common to all strains studied. The second thermostable fraction was highly specific, being restricted usually to a single strain. It appears that the latter antigen may well correspond to the strain-specific "polysaccharide" fraction of *T. foetus* reported by Robertson (1960). Stępkowski's (1966) results suggest also that more than two clearly differentiable antigenic types can be found among strains of *T. foetus*. The strains isolated in Poland, while antigenically distinct from both Manley and Belfast, appear to be closely related to the latter antigenic type.

In the light of the information reported on *T. vaginalis*, one cannot but wonder if more extensive employment of a variety of antigenic types of *T. foetus* in the different methods would not render more meaningful the results obtained in immunologic studies. Perhaps the relatively low efficiency of the serodiagnostic tests (Levine, 1961) could also be increased. Indeed, according to Endress (1939), the strength of the agglutination reaction was dependent upon the strain of the trichomonad employed in the test, and the need for using both the Belfast and Manley strains in herd examinations was emphasized by Pierce (1949a).

Judging from the reports of the English investigators (Robertson, 1941,

1960; Kerr and Robertson, 1945), the two best known antigenic types of *T. foetus*, Belfast and Manley, are not subject to immunologic changes during prolonged *in vitro* cultivation. The difficulty with accepting statements pertaining to the apparent immutability of the antigenic composition of trichomonads grown on nonliving media has been discussed in a previous section of this chapter in the light of the recent results obtained with *T. gallinae* (Goldman and Honigberg, 1968; Honigberg and Goldman, 1968).

Antigenic structure

Various fractions of *T. foetus*, including the polysaccharide fractions extracted by Fuller's (1938) formamide method, gave either very weak or no positive precipitation reactions even with the highest concentrations of immune bovine and rabbit sera (Svec, 1944; MacDonald and Tatum, 1948; Morgan, 1948). Completely negative results with such fractions were recorded also in the skin tests (Svec, 1944; Morgan, 1948).

The findings of Feinberg and Morgan (1953) suggested that immunologic reactivity of the trichloroacetic acid precipitate extracted with acetone and ether ("Tricin") (Kerr, 1944) and of the ethylene glycol (Kerr et al., 1949, 1951) extract of *T. foetus* used in skin tests (*see* pp. 531–532) might have depended upon the presence of some nucleoprotein substances in the preparations. According to preliminary studies (Feinberg and Morgan, 1953), these substances possessed "*T. foetus* specificity."

A serologically active substance was extracted from *T. foetus* by diethylene glycol and analyzed chemically (Feinberg and Morgan, 1953). This substance, which failed to engender the formation of specific agglutinating and precipitating antibodies when injected intradermally and/or intravenously into rabbits, gave specific precipitation reaction with immune rabbit sera (at dilutions up to 1:64,000). The reaction was strain-specific, i.e., the active substance derived from the Manley strain reacted with rabbit anti-Manley serum diluted 1:64,000; with anti-Belfast rabbit sera the titer never exceeded 1:1,000 and was usually less than 1:200. Further, the diethylene glycol-extracted fraction evoked immediate skin reactions in cattle infected with the homologous but not with the heterologous strain. This fraction gave also a positive skin test in rabbits immunized with *T. foetus*, but in such a system the reaction was of the delayed type, appearing 24 hours after inoculation.

It is evident from the foregoing discussion (*see also* Robertson, 1960) that the serologically active substance isolated by Feinberg and Morgan (1953) probably does not represent the complete antigen as it exists in the living or freeze-dried *T. foetus* and might be identified provisionally as a hapten. Still, it is possible that the trichomonad substance, like the human blood group substances, while it has no antigenicity in rabbits, may be strongly antigenic in man and in other animal species (Feinberg and Morgan, 1953).

The investigations of Feinberg and Morgan (1953) gave significant insight into the chemical nature of the diethylene glycol-extracted, specific, serologically active substance. Results obtained by electrophoresis and ultracentrifugation suggested that it consisted of a single electrophoretic component and exhibited a high degree of particle-size homogeneity. The substance, readily soluble in water, contained no proteins when examined by biuret and ninhydrin tests. A strong reaction for carbohydrates was obtained by Molisch test, but reduction of Fehling's solution was not observed until after acid hydrolysis. On chemical analysis, a typical sample of the substance was found to contain 3.2 percent of nitrogen and 1.8 percent of phosphorus. None of the phosphorus was in the free organic form, but 90 percent was liberated in this form after hydrolysis with 2N HCl at 100°C for 72 hours. Maximum liberation of reducing sugars, about 46 percent (expressed as glucose), and of hexosamine, about 9 percent (expressed as glucosamine), was observed after eight to 16 hours of hydrolysis with 0.5N HCl at 100°C. Of the carbohydrates, the most abundant was 6-deoxyhexose (expressed as L-fucose), which accounted for 30 percent of a typical sample of the specific substance. Products of complete hydrolysis of the substance were determined by several chromatographic methods. Fucose and rhamnose were found to compose the 6-deoxyhexose fraction; in addition the carbohydrate moiety contained galactose and xylose. Doubtful spots indicating the possible presence of glucose also were noted, but because of considerable amounts of glycogen-like storage products in trichomonads, it would be "unwise to accept glucose as a component of the specific substance without additional evidence." Glucosamine represented the only amino sugar. There were also in the diethylene glycol-extracted fraction the following aminoacids: lysine, arginine, aspartic acid, glutamic acid, glycine, serine, alanine, threonine, valine, and leucine (isoleucine). The low content of glucosamine (9 percent) in the fraction suggested that most of the nitrogen arose from the aminoacids.

All serologic activity of the substance isolated by Feinberg and Morgan (1953) could be eliminated by subjecting it to the action of a purified enzyme preparation from *Clostridium welchii*, known to destroy the immunologic properties of A, B, and H human blood group mucoids. The latter substances also resemble the serologically active *T. foetus* fraction in their qualitative aminoacid composition.

The foregoing observations suggest that the immunologically active substance extracted from *T. foetus* "consists of a complex carbohydrate to which are firmly bound amino-acids, most probably in the form of a complex amino-acid-containing residue" (Feinberg and Morgan, 1953).

Of some interest to the present discussion are the findings of Robertson (1960) pertaining to the precipitation reaction involving anti-*T. foetus* (Belfast strain) rabbit serum and the enzyme preparations acting on human blood groups B and H isolated by zone electrophoresis by Watkins (1959). The B-hydrolyzing enzyme gave an extremely feeble line characteristic of the polysaccharide-amino complex (Feinberg and Morgan, 1953) and none characteristic of the protein fraction of the trichomonad antigen. On the other hand, as evidenced by the position of the precipitin lines on the gel-diffusion plates, the H-hydrolyzing enzyme reacted with the polysaccharide-aminoacid complex as well as with the protein fraction of the antigen. On the basis of these results and in view of the fact that both enzymes were equally active in regard to the appropriate substrates, Robertson (1960) concluded "that the lines in the diffusion plates produced by the enzyme preparations were not due to the enzymes themselves, but to other antigens separating in the same electrophoretic zone."

Natural antibodies

The occurrence of natural agglutinating antibodies to *T. foetus* in normal sera from a great variety of vertebrates has been reported by numerous investigators (Witte, 1934; Nelson, 1938; Endress, 1939; Morisita, 1939; Zeetti, 1940; Kerr and Robertson, 1941, 1946a, 1954; Robertson, 1941; Schneider, 1941; Byrne, 1942; Morgan, 1944; Pierce, 1949a, 1955). The highest titers (up to 1:1,024) were recorded with horse sera (Schneider, 1941; Morgan, 1944) and the lowest with those of carp, leopard frog, and horned lizard (Morgan, 1944). Chicken sera also were poor in natural agglutininins (Endress, 1939; Schneider, 1941), with titers not exceeding 1:8 (Morgan 1944). Although the figures given by different workers for the actual titers observed with normal rabbit sera varied from 1:4 (Morgan, 1944) to 1:25 (Endress, 1939), they were always lower than those characteristic of normal bovine sera (Endress, 1939; Robertson, 1941; Morgan, 1944). As far as bovine sera are concerned, Endress (1939) stated that one, which appeared to be endowed with the lowest agglutinating capacity among those studied, was active up to 1:25 dilution and that with most normal sera positive agglutination reactions could be observed at much higher dilutions (1:100 to 1:200). According to Morgan (1944), *T. foetus* was agglutinated by normal bovine sera diluted up to 1:128, and Kerr and Robertson (1954) as well as Pierce (1955) reported the agglutinin titers of such sera to be quite constant, ranging from 1:48 to 1:96.

Newborn calves have been shown to possess no natural antibodies to *T. foetus*. However, they have been said to acquire such antibodies within the first 24 hours of life from the maternal colostrum (Kerr and Robertson, 1954; Pierce, 1955). With the aid of fractionation and electrophoresis of the proteins in the colostrum, Pierce (1955) demonstrated that a low-mobility lactoglobulin, comprising 70 to 75 percent of the total whey protein, contained the antibodies. According to that worker, the concentration of the lactoglobulin in the colostrum might be responsible for the significant decline of γ-globulin in sera from cattle approaching calving. The titer of the passive natural agglutinating antibodies rose rapidly in calf sera during the first six days of their life, but thereafter it fell logarithmically within 15 to 55 days (Kerr and Robertson, 1954; Pierce, 1955). The passively acquired antibodies were replaced between the 30th and 60th day after birth by autogenous natural antibodies which reached their maximum levels by about 63 to 113 days.

Pierce (1955) reported that in animals sucking normal colostrum, there was often a period of time intervening between elimination of the passive and appearance of the autogenous antibodies, during which *T. foetus* was not agglutinated by the sera. The natural antibodies could be differentiated from their induced counterparts by the fact that the former agglutinated Belfast and Manley antigenic types to the same titers, while the latter showed specificity for either of these types (Pierce, 1955). However, the natural agglutinins were also found to exhibit a certain amount of type-specificity (Kerr and Robertson, 1954; Pierce, 1955). Either of the two antigenic types absorbed all the homologous antibodies from normal sera but left a reduced amount of the heterologous antibodies. Further, no natural antibodies to *T. foetus* could be absorbed by heterologous species such as *T. vaginalis*. The above observations regarding specificity of the natural antibodies to trichomonads are more in line with those of Samuels and Chun-Hoon (1964) than with the ones of Nigesen (1966). Inoculation of *T. foetus* antigen had no effect upon the disappearance of the titer of the passively acquired natural agglutinins or upon the development of the autogenous antibodies (Kerr and Robertson, 1954). Also, unlike the induced antibodies, the natural ones were incapable of sensitizing the skin of cattle (Kerr and Robertson, 1946a, 1954; Pierce, 1955). The formation of autogenous antibodies was unaffected by inoculation of very young calves (three weeks old or less) with *T. foetus* antigen (Pierce, 1955), although such animals showed immune paralysis in regard to induced agglutinins (Kerr and Robertson, 1954).

According to Pierce (1955), the activity of natural antibodies to *T. foetus* was not affected by absorption with charcoal, kaolin, and cellulose, nor was it diminished by heating at 65°C for 10 minutes. In these characteristics the anti-*T. foetus* agglutinins resembled more the specific natural antibacterial antibodies than the true nonspecific agglutinins against bacteria (Gibson, 1930). On the basis of their physicochemical properties, i.e., precipitation by Na_2SO_4, nondialyzability, thermolability, and susceptibility to trypsin digestion, the natural anti-*T. foetus* antibodies were indentifiable as proteins (Pierce, 1955). Fractionation and electrophoretic studies of bovine sera and colostra by Pierce (1955) indicated that in the former all the antibodies, natural as well as induced, were associated with the γ-globulin complex, and in the latter with the lactoglobulins. This author's findings suggested also that the natural and induced antibodies could be precipitated differentially with Na_2SO_4. As evidenced by testing the globulins with the two antigenic types, Manley and Belfast, of *T. foetus*, the former antibodies were precipitated with 17.5 or 18.5 percent concentrations of Na_2SO_4 while the latter with 12.5 percent concentration of this compound. The antibody levels in sera of cattle could be correlated to a degree with those of the γ-globulin complexes, but the results indicated also that even if young calves produced the three main components of these complexes, they might not have necessarily developed the natural antibodies. According to Pierce (1955), this phenomenon "emphasizes the specificity of the reaction and that the organisms are not agglutinated by a nonspecific serum effect."

Endress (1939) reported lysis of *T. foetus* in normal rabbit and bovine

sera at dilutions exceeding those necessary for a clearly positive agglutination reaction, and it is not quite clear why Morgan (1946) felt that Endress
"confused the immobilization reaction with lysis." Robertson (1941) noted
lysis of the urogenital trichomonad by normal unheated rabbit sera at dilutions reaching 1:24, and some lytic effects were observed by her in sera
diluted to 1:48 and even to 1:96. Agglutination reactions were relatively
weak in such sera (see p. 485 for a plausible explanation). Lytic activity was
reported also in unheated normal guinea pig sera diluted from 1:6 to 1:48,
and a certain amount of such activity occurred at even higher dilutions
(Robertson, 1941). According to Morgan (1946), normal sera from 26 species
of animals, including cattle and horses, lysed *T. foetus*. Different titers were
recorded with the various sera, and in all instances the activity was abolished
by destroying the complement.

Although Pierce (1955) stated that the natural antibody acted as a lysin
in the presence of complement, the question of whether one or two natural
antibodies are involved in the agglutination and lysis of trichomonads has
not yet been resolved (see p. 538 of this chapter and Samuels and Chun-
Hoon, 1964). Although Kerr and Robertson (1954) admitted that means
were lacking for obtaining a rigorous proof of the endogenous origin of
the natural antibody, they adduced some facts in support of such a contention. For example, these workers pointed out that inoculation of *T. foetus*
antigen into calves had no effect upon the disappearance of the titer of the
passive natural antibody derived from the colostrum or upon the development of the autogenous antibody in the sera of such animals. Further, the
remarkable constancy of the fully developed titer in all cattle was evidence
against an explanation involving infection of animals by *T. foetus* or by
organisms which share common antigens with the urogenital trichomonad.
Pierce (1955) favored the hypothesis that the natural antibodies might
represent unmodified γ-globulin molecules having "an accidental genetic configuration complementary to *T. foetus*." This and other hypotheses pertaining to the possible origins and identity of the natural antibodies to trichomonads were considered at some length by Samuels and Chun-Hoon (1964) in
their paper on *T. augusta*, and a discussion of the entire problem is presented
in the section of this chapter dealing with the latter species.

Induced antibodies

Infection with *T. foetus* has been found to stimulate the formation of circulating humoral antibodies as well as of local antibodies, the latter being associated with the vaginal and uterine lining of the cow.

Humoral antibodies. The presence of circulating humoral antibodies to
T. foetus in naturally and experimentally infected cattle and in experimentally infected laboratory animals, including rabbits, guinea pigs, and dogs, has
been demonstrated by complement fixation (Riedmüller, 1932; Witte, 1934;

Endress, 1939; Zeetti, 1940; Schoenherr, 1956; Stępkowski, 1957, 1966), precipitation (Nelson, 1938; Zeetti, 1940; Svec, 1944; Schoenherr, 1956; Stępkowski, 1957, 1966; Robertson, 1960), agglutination (Witte, 1934; Nelson, 1938; Byrne and Nelson, 1939; Endress, 1939; Morisita, 1939; Zeetti, 1940; Kerr and Robertson, 1941, 1943, 1954; Robertson, 1941, 1960; Schneider, 1941; Byrne, 1942; MacDonald and Tatum, 1948; Pierce, 1949a; Feinberg, 1952; Sanborn, 1955; Schoenherr, 1956; Stępkowski, 1957, 1966), immobilization (Kerr and Robertson, 1941; Robertson, 1941; Morgan, 1943; Molinaro et al., 1965), hemagglutination (McEntegart, 1956; Osaki and Oka, 1962; Stępkowski, 1966), and the phagocytic index of leukocytes in immune rabbit blood (Stępkowski, 1961a,b).

In natural infections with *T. foetus*, typically rather low titers of the humoral antibodies have been reported by various investigators (Riedmüller, 1932; Witte, 1934; Endress, 1939; Kerr and Robertson, 1941, 1954; Pierce, 1949a), and it is apparent that tests involving all types of immunologic reactions tend to be positive primarily with sera of animals suffering from severe trichomoniasis, especially in cases associated with abortion, and to a lesser extent with pyometra (Endress, 1939; Kerr and Robertson, 1941; Pierce, 1949a). The formation of circulating humoral antibodies can be also stimulated experimentally by inoculating cattle and laboratory animals with living antigen (Riedmüller, 1932; Witte, 1934; Nelson, 1938; Endress, 1939; Zeetti, 1940; Kerr and Robertson, 1941, 1943; Robertson, 1941, 1960; Schneider, 1941; Svec, 1944; Morgan, 1948; Pierce, 1949a, 1955; Sanborn, 1955; McEntegart, 1956; Schoenherr, 1956) or with various preparations of killed trichomonads (Nelson, 1938; Morisita, 1939; Schneider, 1941; Svec, 1944; MacDonald and Tatum, 1948; Kerr and Robertson, 1954; Stępkowski, 1966). There appears to be no systematic study so far comparing the levels of antibody titers induced by living and killed *T. foetus* antigens. According to Robertson (1941, 1960), living trichomonads were antigenically superior to dried organisms in stimulating the production of agglutinating antibodies, and similar conclusions were reached by Morgan (1943) in experiments involving the immobilization reaction. Still, judging from the results obtained by various investigators, including Kerr and Robertson (1943, 1954), adequate immunologic response can be induced in cattle and laboratory animals by various preparations of killed parasites. In general, the titers observed in sera from experimentally immunized animals were higher than those reported from naturally infected hosts. Agglutination titers as high as 1:10,240 have been reported from experiments involving immune rabbit sera and trichomonads belonging to strains homologous to those employed in immunization (Morisita, 1939; Robertson, 1941). Although the highest titers observed with sera from experimentally infected cattle never exceeded 1:3,000 (Pierce, 1955), they were higher than those recorded from naturally infected cattle (Kerr and Robertson, 1941). As mentioned above, just like the natural antibodies, the induced agglutinins were localized in the γ-globulin complex of the bovine sera and in the lactoglobulins of the colostra (Pierce, 1955).

Irrespective of the form of *T. foetus* antigen employed in immunization of cattle and laboratory animals, various routes have been used for its introduction into the hosts; in all instances specific antibodies appeared in the sera of the immunized animals. These included intraperitoneal (Riedmüller, 1932; Witte, 1934; Zeetti, 1940; Morgan, 1948), intramuscular (Kerr and Robertson, 1941, 1946b, 1954; Svec, 1944; Morgan, 1948), and intravenous (Nelson, 1938; Byrne and Nelson, 1939; Endress, 1939; Morisita, 1939; Kerr and Robertson, 1941; Robertson, 1941, 1960; Schneider, 1941; Byrne, 1942; Svec, 1944; MacDonald and Tatum, 1948; Morgan, 1948; Sanborn, 1955; McEntegart, 1956; Schoenherr, 1956) inoculations. Living and dead antigens were also introduced into the vagina (Byrne and Nelson, 1939; Endress, 1939; Zeetti, 1940; Byrne, 1942; Kerr and Robertson, 1943) and into the uterus (Kerr and Robertson, 1943; Morgan, 1948) of cattle and laboratory animals. Subcutaneous inoculations also were employed (Zeetti, 1940; Florent, 1948). Higher agglutination titers were obtained with sera from rabbits injected intravenously than from those in which *T. foetus* was introduced into the vagina (Byrne and Nelson, 1939; Byrne, 1942; Morgan, 1948). Active infections established in the vaginae of heifers were not accompanied by the production of agglutinating antibodies (Endress, 1939; Kerr and Robertson, 1943), and no positive complement-fixation reactions were obtained with sera from cattle in which *T. foetus* was restricted to the vagina (Riedmüller, 1932). Rather satisfactory results with regard to agglutination were achieved by instilling sterile saline extracts of the urogenital trichomonad into the uterus of cows (Kerr and Robertson, 1943). In the latter experiments, induced agglutinating antibodies were present in sera of six out of eight cows within six to seven days following the introduction of the antigen. Kerr and Robertson (1943) concluded that vaginal infection failed to induce production of humoral antibodies on the basis of the above and other experiments which involved the introduction of living flagellates into the vaginae of heifers after mating (all serologic tests were negative), establishment of living trichomonads in the uteri of pregnant cows (some animals showed elevated agglutination titers), and exposure of cows to a heavily infected bull (positive agglutination reactions were observed in some animals). On the other hand, they believed that the antigen was absorbed from the uterus into the blood circulation and stimulated the production of such antibodies. The foregoing results might explain the finding of elevated antibody titers primarily in cattle suffering from severe trichomoniasis with histories of abortion or pyometra.

As indicated above, positive complement-fixation, precipitation, and agglutination reactions were observed in natural and experimental hosts immunized with living flagellates or with various preparations of killed trichomonads. However, far less success has been achieved through the employment of these reactions in field tests aimed at diagnosis of natural infections with *T. foetus.*

Complement fixation was observed by Riedmüller (1932) with sera from aborting cows, but the results were poorer with sera from animals suffering from trichomonad pyometra (one out of nine cows gave a positive reaction). The titer returned to normal much more slowly (in four to 12 weeks) in animals with histories of abortion than in those with pyometra (in less than three weeks). Witte (1934) reported positive complement-fixation reactions from sera of eight out of ten aborting cows and from six out of nine animals with pyometra; in all cases the titer returned to normal after three and one half to five months. According to Endress (1939), in cattle infected by a bull under controlled conditions the complement-fixation test was more dependable than direct microscopic examination in demonstrating trichomoniasis. In the field test performed by this author, 25 percent of sera from animals from herds known to harbor *T. foetus* gave a positive complement-fixation reaction, while very much lower percentages of positive results were obtained by these means in trichomonad-free cattle. On the other hand, Kerr and Robertson (1941) considered complement fixation inferior to agglutination in herd tests for *T. foetus*.

As far as can be ascertained, precipitation reactions have not been employed for diagnosis of natural infection with the bovine urogenital trichomonad. When used with sera from experimentally immunized cattle, various preparations and extracts of killed parasites gave mostly (Svec, 1944) or completely (Morgan, 1948) negative results.

Although Witte (1934) felt that the relatively high natural agglutinating antibody titer of bovine sera rendered the agglutination test useless for diagnostic purposes, Kerr and Robertson (1941) on the basis of a survey involving a total of 165 cattle, found this test to be of some value. Among 45 animals with completely normal histories none had an elevated titer. Of 25 animals with histories of sterility or abortion all gave clearly positive reactions. The remaining 95 cattle either had suspicious histories or came from a herd with some history of infertility or abortion; forty members of this group had agglutination titers somewhat higher than normal. Thirteen (52 percent) of the frankly positive cases were associated with abortion. The serologic reaction was positive in many cases in which no trichomonads could be demonstrated by direct examination. While the authors emphasized the existence of positive correlation between serologic results and clinically severe cases of bovine urogenital trichomoniasis, they recognized the fact that negative tests did not necessarily reflect the absence of infection with *T. foetus*. At the time of their report, Kerr and Robertson (1941) considered the agglutination reaction to provide a satisfactory herd test to be employed in conjunction with direct examination. The results obtained by Pierce (1949a) through application of the agglutination reaction in field tests were less satisfactory: at best, only 13 percent of cattle from a herd known to be infected with *T. foetus* (an outbreak caused by the Belfast strain) gave clearly positive reactions on serologic examination.

It seems evident from the foregoing account that none of the tests involving complement fixation, precipitation, and agglutination has proved very dependable in serodiagnosis of natural infections with *T. foetus*. Perhaps improvements in the presently employed techniques along lines similar to those found to be successful with *T. vaginalis* could render such tests more useful with regard to the bovine trichomonad. However, it is not surprising that at present serodiagnostic methods have been replaced by other tests (*see* pp. 534–535).

From the theoretical viewpoint, the agglutination experiments reported by Kerr and Robertson (1954) with sera of experimentally immunized cattle are of interest. It was established by these workers that the titers of antibodies to *T. foetus*, passively acquired by calves through feeding on antibody-containing colostra, exhibited a great variability, with an approximate half-life of 14 to 57 days (usually 14 to 20 days). Intramuscular injections of *T. foetus* antigen into animals five months of age or older resulted in the appearance of induced antibodies in the circulation within six to seven days. This period was the same as the one recorded in cattle in which the parasites were instilled in the uterus (Kerr and Robertson, 1943). Finally, the immune paralysis, a phenomenon well known to bacteriologists, was observed in calves inoculated via the intramuscular route during the first three weeks of life (Kerr and Robertson, 1954). The latter finding, among many others, appears to emphasize the basic similarity of the immune host responses to protozoan and bacterial infections.

In addition to complement-fixation, precipitation, and agglutination reactions observed with sera of animals infected with *T. foetus*, several workers (Kerr and Robertson, 1941; Robertson, 1941; Morgan, 1943; Molinaro et al., 1965), reported effects which such sera, when employed at low dilution, had on the motility of the flagellates. The immobilization phenomenon was noted first by Robertson (1941) in anti-*T. foetus* rabbit sera at dilution not exceeding 1:24. Motility of the flagellates was affected by serum dilutions associated with the preagglutination and "flat échelon leaf-like clumping." Subsequently Kerr and Robertson (1941) observed immobilization of the parasites by some sera from cattle with histories of abortion and sterility traceable to urogenital trichomoniasis. All the sera capable of inhibiting motility of the flagellates also gave clearly positive agglutination reactions at higher dilutions. According to Morgan (1943), only some strains of *T. foetus* were suitable for demonstrating the immobilization reaction. Actually, this worker found most strains too sensitive for this purpose. as evidenced by the loss of motility even in saline solution. Kerr and Robertson (1941) also remarked that if "échelon is found in the normal control it signifies that the suspension is so sensitive as to be unsuitable for use, or it indicates that the normal serum has not been treated adequately so as to remove all traces of complement." The experiments reported by Morgan (1943), which involved sera from heifers immunized with living or formalin-killed antigen, showed a great deal of individual variation even with a single strain of the urogenital trichomonad. On the average, the immobilizing antibodies appeared within 17 days after the first injection, achieved the maximum titer in 55 days, and lasted for 177 days. In field tests, Morgan (1943) failed to observe the immobilization reaction with sera from 400 cows and 52 bulls free of *T. foetus*. Ten cows found to harbor the parasites also had negative sera. Only two of

12 animals with a history of trichomonad-induced abortions and two of 29 cows suffering from trichomonad pyometra appeared to contain the immobilizing antibodies, and even in the positive sera, motility of the parasites was affected only at 1:1 dilutions. Judging from the relatively high titer (up to 1:128) reported by Morgan (1943) from heifers inoculated with living parasites and from his discussion in which he employed the term "agglutinins" for the immobilizing antibodies, it seems possible that this author failed to distinguish clearly between the agglutinating and immobilizing antibodies. Actually, Pierce (1949a) quoted Morgan as using the agglutination reaction. The foregoing considerations notwithstanding, it appears nearly certain that Morgan observed immobilization, at least at lower dilutions of the immune sera.

There can be no doubt that like all the other serologic tests involving reactions which are dependent upon the humoral anti-*T. foetus* antibodies, the immobilization test also has little practical value in diagnosis. Although the existence of antibodies capable of affecting motility of the urogenital flagellates of cattle as entities quite distinct from the agglutinating antibodies appears to have been well established for over a quarter of a century, the nature of these antibodies and of the reaction in which they participate were not studied until very recently by immunochemical methods (Molinaro et al., 1965).

Molinaro et al. (1965) demonstrated immobilization of *T. foetus* by native 7S globulins from immune rabbit sera, as well as by bivalent 5S fragments resulting from pepsin digestion. On the other hand, univalent fragments obtained by papain or pepsin treatment of the immunoglobulins failed to affect motility of the flagellates. It was found also that immobilization of the trichomonads by 5S pepsin fragments could be reversed by the addition to the suspension of reducing agents (such as cysteine), which are known to cleave the bivalent 5S fragment into two univalent 3.5S moieties. Thus, bivalency of the antibody appears necessary for immobilizing activity. Further, inasmuch as the loss of motility by the trichomonads took place in the absence of complement, Molinaro et al. (1965) concluded that the antibody action was mechanical.

The fact that the end points of agglutination and immobilization occur at entirely different protein concentrations (0.12 to 0.25 versus 4.0 immunologic equivalents [moles per immunologic valence] per tube) suggests the possibility that the motility-inhibiting antibody differs from the agglutinating antibody (Molinaro et al., 1965). In addition, immobilization of *T. foetus* has been found to be independent of its agglutination (Kerr and Robertson, 1941; Robertson, 1941; Molinaro et al., 1965); the flagellates are immobilized but not agglutinated in antibody excess. The immunochemical results help to explain to a large measure the occurrence of immobilization at low dilutions of sera, the great variability of individual responses among naturally infected cattle, and the relatively higher titers observed in experimentally immunized natural and laboratory hosts.

Although Morgan (1948), using a variety of fractions of *T. foetus*, obtained uniformly negative results with the intradermal test, there is over-whelming evidence that the induced humoral antibodies sensitize the skin. An immediate allergic skin reaction, which reaches its peak in 30 to 60 minutes and disappears nearly completely within six hours, was reported from bovines that acquired such antibodies either actively (Kerr, 1944) or passively (Kerr and Robertson, 1946a). "Tricin" (see p. 522; and Kerr, 1944), ethylene glycol extract (Kerr et al., 1949, 1951), the diethylene glycol-extracted polysaccharide-aminoacid complex (Feinberg and Morgan, 1953), and a soluble polysaccharide fraction (Osaki and Oka, 1962) of T. foetus have been employed as antigens in the skin test. According to Kerr et al. (1949), skin of cattle could be desensitized by intramuscular inoculations of the trichomonad antigen, by absorption of the antigen from the uterus in heavy infections, and by instillation of the freeze-dried antigen into the uteri of nonpregnant cows. Nonspecific desensitization was observed at parturition, as well as after injections of cortisone and of sphingomyelin. Administration of the latter two substances resulted in depression of lymphocytes in the experimental animals (see Kerr et al., 1951, for references), and presumably cortisone-induced lymphopenia coincided with the last stages of parturition in cattle (Kerr et al., 1949, 1951). The changes in the lymphocyte counts, as well as desensitization of skin to T. foetus antigens, were related to the action of cortisone (Kerr et al., 1951).

All the available evidence indicates that the induced humoral antibodies to T. foetus remain for limited time periods, a few weeks to less than six months, in the bloodstream of cattle following natural infection or experimental immunization (Riedmüller, 1932; Witte, 1934; Kerr and Robertson, 1954). These findings are in agreement with those reported for the humoral antibodies induced by other trichomonad species.

The question of the protective value of humoral antibodies induced by T. foetus in cattle deserves some consideration. The early experiments of Kerr (1943) suggested that intravenous inoculations of the parasites might have afforded some protection against infection by a bull carrying the urogenital trichomonads. According to Morgan (1947), a prolonged series (a total of 16 injections in eight weeks) of intramuscular or intravenous injections of T. foetus, which resulted in the appearance of elevated immobilizing antibody titers (up to 1:256), seemed to protect heifers temporarily against infection. The animals were inseminated during the first heat after the last immunizing injection and challenged 24 hours thereafter by the intrauterine introduction of the flagellates—all the heifers calved normally. Groups of heifers receiving fewer intramuscular inoculations prior to insemination appeared not to be protected against subsequent challenge with T. foetus. Regarding active immunity of laboratory animals, Baba's (1958) results indicated that intra-peritoneal injections of heat-killed bovine urogenital trichomonads protected 80 percent of mice against intramuscular challenges with living homologous antigen. However, as indicated previously (see p. 487), these results need not necessarily reflect the activity of circulating humoral antibodies.

As far as passive immunity is concerned, some pertinent earlier experiments are cited by Morgan (1946). According to one of the reports, the prepatent period was prolonged in a heifer injected intravenously with whole blood from immune hosts prior to the introduction of *T. foetus* into the urogenital tract. Another experiment suggested that intravenous inoculations of an immune serum into a heifer protected the animal against subsequent introduction of cultured trichomonads into its vagina. On the other hand, the heifer developed trichomoniasis when bred to an infected bull. The apparent difference in effectiveness of passive immunization against challenge by the flagellates maintained in culture and by those derived from an infected bull was also noted by Garlick et al. (1944). These workers succeeded in protecting two out of three heifers against development of urogenital trichomoniasis by cultured parasites by subjecting them to a series of intravenous injections of defibrinated blood or of sera derived from cows proved immune to natural and experimental infections. Animals receiving the immune blood or sera, however, were not protected when serviced by a bull carrying the urogenital parasite or when infected with prepucial washings of such a bull.

Whereas the above experimental data may suggest some protective value of the humoral antibodies induced by *T. foetus*, the research of Kerr and Robertson (1946b, 1953) throws serious doubts upon any such role of these antibodies in urogenital trichomoniasis of cattle. The experiments reported by these workers (Kerr and Robertson, 1946b) suggested that heifers, which showed high agglutination titers and gave positive skin reactions as a result of intramuscular vaccination with *T. foetus* antigen, were not protected against infection with this parasite. Three out of four heifers aborted when the trichomonads were inoculated into their uteri simultaneously with, or four hours after, artificial insemination. These results did not differ significantly from the ones obtained with the control animals. In the latter group, five out of seven heifers became infected; of these, two aborted, one became sterile, and two showed mild infections which did not interfere with the completion of normal pregnancy. Similar results were reported by Byrne and Nelson (1939) in rabbits whose sera showed a high agglutination titer after intravenous injections of the flagellates, but which were no less susceptible to intravaginally introduced trichomonads than the untreated control animals. Kerr and Robertson (1953) could not demonstrate agglutinating antibodies in uterine washings from cows whose sera showed high antibody titers for weeks or even for months, and similar observations were reported by Florent (1948) with vaginal mucus. Further, no allergic reactions reflecting sensitization of the uterus were noted in such animals upon introduction of the parasites into this organ for the first time. The foregoing findings suggested that the humoral antibodies failed to reach all the body tissues (Pierce, 1959; Robertson, 1963) and that they contributed nothing to the protection of cattle against infection with *T. foetus* (Kerr and Robertson, 1953; Robertson, 1963). Only further investigations of various facets of the host-parasite relationship, including the immunologic aspects, may aid in understanding of the role played by the humoral antibodies in infection with *T. foetus*.

Local Antibodies. The results obtained in the studies of the humoral antibodies to *T. foetus* could not explain the immunologic basis for the numerous findings, according to which urogenital trichomoniasis usually represents a self-limiting infection in cattle (Andrews et al., 1935; Andrews, 1938; Andrews and Miller, 1938; Florent, 1941, 1949, 1957; *see also* Morgan, 1946) and in rabbits (Witte, 1933; Nelson, 1938; Byrne and Nelson, 1939; Byrne, 1942). Further, the evidently low degree of protection against *T. foetus* afforded by the humoral antibodies in natural and experimental infections would hardly be adequate to account for the significant level of resistance to reinfection observed in cattle (Andrews et al., 1935; Andrews, 1938; Andrews and Miller, 1938; Kerr, 1943; Bartlett et al., 1944; Florent, 1949, 1957) and in laboratory animals (Nelson, 1938; Byrne and Nelson, 1939; Byrne, 1943). It seems also that the activity of these antibodies would not explain the results reported from experiments with mice in which 80 percent of animals inoculated intraperitoneally with 5×10^5 living trichomonads were protected against intraperitoneal challenge of 1×10^7 parasites, a dosage found invariably lethal for the controls (Oka and Osaki, 1963).

It is evident from the aforementioned reports that even after a single exposure to *T. foetus*, cattle and laboratory animals show a greater or lesser degree of resistance to subsequent infections with this parasite. Partial resistance is reflected in a shortened course of trichomoniasis, and in many instances immunity appears to be solid after several infections, or less frequently, after a single infection. For reasons that will become evident from the following discussion, the acquired immunity is not permanent. For example, Bartlett et al. (1944) reported that cows which were demonstrated to be refractory to intravaginal infection with *T. foetus* at least once in the course of a prolonged experimental series, developed typical trichomoniasis when serviced by an infected bull two years after immunization.

Perhaps in some instances we may be dealing with resistance to superinfection, for, as pointed out by Morgan (1946), the possibility of continued low grade occult infections cannot be eliminated on the basis of the available information. This type of resistance is common in protozoan infections (*see* Garnham et al., 1963). It appears, however, that the resistance to reinfection with *T. foetus* exhibited by cattle and laboratory animals may depend to a significant degree upon the activity of local antibodies. Indeed, the presence of such antibodies has been demonstrated by many competent investigators.

Florent (1941) noted that the vaginal mucus taken from cattle infected with *T. foetus* agglutinated and immobilized these flagellates. Subsequently, Pierce (1947) was able to demonstrate specificity of the agglutinating antibodies. With the aid of a test in which the mucus was mixed with agar prior to the addition of living trichomonads, this worker showed positive correlation between the time of disappearance of the parasites and that of the appearance of the antibodies. Further, he established that subsequent reappearance of the flagellates in the vagina coincided with the disappearance of these antibodies. The antibodies, shown to be relatively resistant to heating to 60°C, were destroyed rapidly by exposure to 100°C (Pierce, 1947). Inasmuch as the level of agglutination depended to some degree upon the strain employed in the reaction, Pierce (1949b) found it advisable to use both Belfast and Manley strains for demonstrating mucus agglutination in field tests. To avoid false positive readings due to the presence of natural antibodies in the vaginal mucus of normal cattle, all tests were controlled by using 1:10 and 1:20 dilutions of the mucus. A somewhat different method, in which the trichomonads were exposed directly to the vaginal mucus without the use of agar, was devised by Florent (1947). Although in no way quantitative, this latter technique was found to be quite satisfactory in demonstrating the vaginal mucoantibodies which have been said to appear usually six weeks after the first coitus with an infected bull (Florent, 1949).

The complete independence of the local mucoantibodies and the circulating humoral agglutinins was demonstrated by Pierce (1947) and Florent (1948). Sera from many animals whose vaginal mucus reacted strongly with *T. foetus* were devoid of specific agglutinating activity. On the other hand, cattle inoculated with the urogenital trichomonads via subcutaneous or intravenous routes showed high agglutination titers in their sera, but no agglutinating antibodies could be demonstrated in their vaginal mucus (Florent, 1948; Pierce, 1953). Similar results were reported by Kerr and Robertson (1953), who failed to find any antibodies in the uterine washings from cattle whose sera had high agglutinating titers, but were able to show specific antibodies in such washings from animals after infection with the urogenital trichomonad. These workers (Kerr and Robertson, 1947, 1953) demonstrated the presence of agglutinating antibodies in the uterine secretion not only following infection with living trichomonads but also after instillation of dead antigen into the uterus.

As evidenced by the allergic reaction caused by an intrauterine infection of cattle with *T. foetus*, the uterus can be sensitized actively through repeated exposure to the trichomonad antigen, or passively by instillation of bovine antitrichomonad serum (Kerr and Robertson, 1953). Actually, according to Florent (1949), abortion in bovine urogenital trichomoniasis represents an allergic response. No local allergic reactions were observed in cattle whose sera had high agglutinating titers (Kerr and Robertson, 1953). In the light of all the available information, it seems that only antibodies formed as a result of local infection become fixed in the uterine tissues.

According to Pierce (1953) and Florent (1957), the uterine and vaginal agglutinating antibodies are produced independently of each other at the sites of their activity. On the other hand, Kerr (1955), on the basis of experiments reported by Kerr and Robertson (1953), believed that the production of the vaginal mucoantibodies was stimulated by those formed in the uterine cells. Of all sites, the area surrounding the os, which provides the best source of thick mucus rich in the agglutinating antibodies, might represent the principal region of local antibody production. Whatever the relationship may be between the uterine and vaginal mucoantibodies, it has been reported by many workers (Florent, 1948; Kerr and Robertson, 1953; Pierce, 1959) that the uterine antibodies were less persistent than their vaginal counterparts, and it seemed likely to Kerr and Robertson (1953) that this difference might be related to cyclical destruction of the mucosa associated with estrus.

In their extensive discussions, Florent (1949, 1957), Kerr (1955), Pierce (1959), and Robertson (1963) agree that the local mucoantibodies confer a certain protection against reinfection with *T. foetus*. This protection, however, is by no means permanent nor even particularly long-lasting (Bartlett et al., 1944; Kerr and Robertson, 1947; Pierce, 1959). It has been suggested (Pierce, 1959) that the dilution of the vaginal mucoantibodies during the estral mucus flow may represent an important factor in rendering the immunity to urogenital trichomoniasis, as observed in the field, rather short-lived.

According to Robertson (1963), it seems likely that the uterine mucoantibodies have some effect on eliminating *T. foetus* from the uterus in mild infections which do not entail the interruption of pregnancy. They probably play a similar role in cases of temporary sterility in which the parasites diminish in number and finally disappear. Similar, but even stronger statements, regarding the role played by the local mucoantibodies were made by Florent (1949, 1957). Most workers (Kerr and Robertson, 1946b, 1947; Florent, 1949, 1957; Robertson, 1963) assume that the complete and rapid elimination of the trichomonads at the time of abortion is caused by the activity of the uterine antibody, which may also be responsible for the high degree of resistance to reinfection exhibited by cattle for several months after abortion.

As far as the vaginal mucoantibodies are concerned, they might play some role in freeing the vagina from trichomonads found there as a result of their continual passage from the uterus; actually *T. foetus* appears never to settle permanently in the vagina (Robertson, 1963; Pierce, 1949b).

The field tests involving agglutination by the local mucoantibodies appear to give more satisfactory results than those dependent upon serodiagnostic methods (Florent, 1947, 1948, 1949, 1957; Pierce, 1949b, 1959; Robertson, 1963). Still, as indicated by Pierce (1947, 1949b, 1959), only 60 percent of the infected cattle can be expected to give a positive mucoagglutination reaction. Consequently, the reaction seems useful primarily in herd tests.

The understanding of many immunologic aspects of infections with *T. foetus* must await further studies. The introduction of artificial insemination methods by cattle breeders has reduced significantly the dangers associated with urogenital trichomoniasis and rendered the need for finding effective means of diagnosing this infection less urgent. Nonetheless bovine trichomoniasis would seem to provide excellent opportunities for basic studies of immunologic facets of infection involving a pathogenic protozoan parasite.

Tritrichomonas augusta (Alexeieff)

Tritrichomonas augusta is found in the rectum of amphibians, and a morphologically very similar, if not identical, species has been reported in a variety of lizards (Honigberg, 1963). Frogs and toads are the most common hosts of this trichomonad. As far as can be ascertained, *T. augusta* is a harmless commensal.

Using sera from rabbits immunized with one strain of *T. augusta*, Samuels and Chun-Hoon (1964) demonstrated that absorption of such sera with homologous and various intraspecific heterologous antigens resulted in rather significant differences of the agglutination titers of the several strains. It was also evident from the results that some of the strains had very similar antigenic compositions, while others were antigenically quite distinct. By a similar method, *T. augusta* was shown to differ in its antigenic characteristics from one or more strains of *T. foetus*, *T. gallinarum*, and *T. vaginalis*.

Only a relatively small reduction in agglutination by anti-*T. augusta* rabbit sera absorbed with *T. augusta* (especially at lower dilutions) was noted with heterologous antigens, such as *T. foetus* or *T. vaginalis*. The authors interpreted the high residual activity of such sera against heterologous antigens as depending upon the presence of natural antibodies, and this seems a plausible explanation. On the other hand, it is surprising that an equally large part of the activity against *T. augusta* was left in the normal and anti-*T. augusta* sera absorbed with *T. foetus* and *T. vaginalis*. As might be anticipated, at higher dilutions (1:1,024 and 1:2,048), the activity was lower against *T. augusta* in the homologous antisera absorbed with *T. foetus*, which belongs in the same genus with the trichomonad from amphibians, than in those absorbed with *T. vaginalis*. The great variability of their results and of the general trend shown in the cross-absorption experiments may make dubious the conclusion reached by Samuels and Chun-Hoon (1964) that: "The serological relationship of *T. augusta* [strain] 101 to the morphologically closer *foetus* and *suis* (?) did not seem greater than to the morphologically more distant species." A more direct approach to the problem, involving several serologic methods in addition to agglutination, would have to be employed before one would be justified in making any positive statements concerning the evolutionary kinships of trichomonad species based on immunologic considerations. In the light of the presently available morphologic information from both light and electron microscopy (Honigberg, 1963; Mattern et al., 1967) and physiologic evidence (Shorb, 1964), we would anticipate the existence of closer antigenic relationships among the members of a single genus, i.e., *T. augusta* and *T. foetus*, than among *T. augusta* and *T. gallinarum* or *T. vaginalis*, the latter two belonging to genera relatively far removed from *Tritrichomonas*.

The primary object of the investigation reported by Samuels and Chun-Hoon (1964) was the analysis of the natural antibodies, agglutinins and lysins, to *T. augusta* and several other trichomonad genera and species, which are present in sera and various body fluids of a number of vertebrates. The natural agglutinating antibodies could be demonstrated in heat-inactivated sera, whereas only active sera or heated sera supplemented with guinea pig complement had lytic activity. The agglutination titers for *T. augusta* were significantly different in normal sera and other body fluids derived from different animal species. The highest titers (1:128 to 1:512) were recorded with sera from sheep, calves that were six months old or older, and 20-week-old chickens. On the other hand, newborn calves' sera showed no activity. However, the titer observed with the latter sera increased up to six months, at which time comparable agglutination levels could be demonstrated with calf and adult cow sera. Similarly, only very low activity was found in the yolk of fertile hens' eggs and in the yolk sac contents of 12-day-old chick embryos, but good agglutination could be shown in sera from 20-week-old chicks. Agglutination was very low, and sometimes absent, in sera from frogs, rodents (rats, mice, guinea pigs), rabbits, and dogs, as well as in bovine plasma ultrafiltrate and human ascitic fluid. Moderate titers (1:40 to 1:88) were noted with alligator, deer, human, and swine sera. A zone of antibody excess, as revealed by reduced agglutination, was observed at high concentrations of the strongly agglutinating sheep and calf sera. In chemically and electrophoretically fractionated sera, the natural antibodies were localized primarily in the γ-globulins and in the area of their overlap with the β-globulins.

Agglutinating and lytic titers of the same sera were compared by observing percentage of lysis before, and percentage of agglutination after, heat-inactivation. Sheep, cattle, and horse sera had closely parallel agglutinating and lytic activity; however, often a high percentage of lysed organisms with significantly lower agglutination titers were noted in sera derived from 18-day-old chicks, rodents, and rabbits. The authors (Samuels and Chun-Hoon, 1964) suggested that either two distinct antibody types were involved in the agglutinating and lytic reactions, or that the observed differences might be dependent upon the differences in complement content of the various sera or in reactivity of different complements in this system. Since the agglutinating but not the lytic reaction was reduced, they tended to reject the idea of insufficient complement. Possibly, a smaller amount of antibody is required in lysis than in the agglutination reaction, and this antibody requirement is satisfied in sera having higher lytic than agglutinating activity. Also, heat-labile factors other than complement may be involved in lysis in the sera with low agglutinating titers.

No precipitins could be demonstrated by means of gel diffusion in concentrated normal sera or γ-globulins against clarified solutions of lyophilized *T. augusta* antigen. On the other hand, a positive reaction for precipitins was obtained with immune rabbit anti-*T. augusta* serum.

In previous sections of this chapter, ample evidence was presented for the existence of natural antibodies to *T. vaginalis* and *T. foetus*. Such antibodies were shown also in experiments involving *M. colubrorum* and were suggested by the results obtained with *P. hominis* and *T. tenax*. In addition to their study of the natural agglutinins and lysins against *T. augusta* in various vertebrate sera and body fluids, Samuels and Chun-Hoon (1964) demonstrated such antibodies to *T. gallinarum* in normal sera. Results obtained by these investigators in cross-absorption experiments using normal sera and one or more strains of *T. vaginalis*, *T. foetus*, *T. gallinarum*, and *T. augusta* suggested that the natural agglutinins were both species and strain specific. The activity of a normal serum against a given species was virtually eliminated by absorption with the homologous antigen and was reduced to a significantly lesser degree when a heterologous antigen was employed for absorption. As far as strain specificity was concerned, reciprocal absorption tests of normal calf serum with various strains of *T. augusta* indicated the antigenic differences among such strains and, like the results obtained by cross-absorption of immune serum, suggested close kinships among some of the strains. Similar conclusions concerning specificity of natural antibodies were reached by Kerr and Robertson (1954) and Pierce (1955) with regard to *T. Foetus*, but Nigesen (1966) found agglutination titers of normal human sera to be independent of the type of *T. vaginalis* used as antigen.

Studies on the natural antibodies to *T. vaginalis*, *T. foetus*, and *T. augusta* seem to support the contention that antitrichomonad reactions observed in normal vertebrate sera are dependent on antibody activity. However, the question of the origin of these natural, evidently specific, antibodies remains largely unanswered. In this connection, Samuels and Chun-Hoon (1964) considered three general possibilities: (1) occult infections which induced immunization; (2) exposure to heterophil antigens resulting in active immunization; and (3) a genetic predetermination of specific antibodies.

Inasmuch as *T. foetus* was studied with the aid of sera from its normal hosts (Robertson, 1941; Kerr and Robertson, 1954; Pierce, 1955), the appearance of natural antibodies to this species could be explained by a theoretical possibility of previous exposures. Still, even in regard to the bovine urogenital trichomonad, Kerr and Robertson (1954) and Pierce (1955) favored hypotheses involving autogenous origins of the natural antibodies. Samuels and Chun-Hoon (1964) pointed out that it is highly impractical, if not in fact virtually impossible, to expose mammals sufficiently to a series of serologically distinct strains of *T. augusta*, which does not survive at 37°C, to produce specific antibodies against each strain. It should also be noted that each species of serum donors had a rather uniform antibody level; that laboratory-reared chicks never exposed to any trichomonads developed a high natural agglutinin titer; and that normal sera from laboratory rodents, which always harbor large numbers of trichomonads that may be rather closely related to *T. augusta*, had very low agglutinating activity against the latter species. In this connection, the large numbers of organisms needed to induce immunity render the development of immune paralysis unlikely.

The idea of involvement of heterophil antigenic systems would appear most attractive. It could explain the acquisition and progressive increase of activity against *T. augusta* in chicks (Samuels and Chun-Hoon, 1964), and against both *T. augusta* (Samuels and Chun-Hoon, 1964) and *T. foetus* (Kerr and Robertson, 1954; Pierce, 1955) by calves. Still, it was shown (Kerr and Robertson, 1954) that active immunization had no effect on the titer of natural agglutinins against the latter species. To test the role of the heterophil antigen in the production of natural antitrichomonad antibodies, Samuels and Chun-Hoon (1964) employed reciprocal agglutinin-absorption tests of normal calf serum with *T. augusta*, *Aerobacter aerogenes*, *Escher-*

ichia coli, and *Saccharomyces cerevisiae.* The low level of reduction in the agglutinating capacity of *T. augusta* by the bacteria- and yeast-absorbed calf sera could not be interpreted as evidence for the involvement of these three heterophil antigen systems. As pointed out by the authors, the evidence is insufficient at present to draw definite conclusions as to the role of living microorganisms and nonliving materials (such as foodstuffs) in the stimulation of production of the natural antibodies. Still, the ranking of the agglutinating activity of sera derived from various host species agrees closely with that reported by Gibson (1930) for natural antibody levels in such species against certain bacteria, and the heterophil origin of these latter agglutinins could not be excluded (Pierce, 1955).

In view of the foregoing arguments, a third alternative involving the production of natural antibodies as specific hereditary proteins would appear plausible. Indeed, several recent immunologic theories (Lederberg, 1959; Talmage, 1959; Burnet, 1962) consider the hereditary basis of antibody specificity. According to Samuels and Chun-Hoon (1964), "Constancy of level of 'natural' antibody [to trichomonads] in members of a given species could be an expression of their common genetic background. . . ."

It seems that natural antibodies do not play an important role in protecting the animals against infection with trichomonads. In the case of *T. foetus,* all calves develop up to 1:96 (Kerr and Robertson, 1954) or even higher titers (Samuels and Chun-Hoon, 1964), without affording any protection to the hosts. Admittedly, the serum of frogs, the natural hosts of *T. augusta,* seems to have very low agglutinin activity for this species. On the other hand, rodents with low agglutinin activity and sheep or cattle with very high activity are equally insusceptible to infection with this flagellate. Of course, the high body temperature of mammals in itself militates against infection with *T. augusta;* in addition, rodent, cattle, and sheep sera have high lytic activity. It would be interesting to know whether frog sera are capable of lysing their commensal flagellates.

Although, as indicated by Samuels and Chun-Hoon (1964), the so-called natural antibodies against trichomonads are widespread and are susceptible to numerous immunoanalytical methods, it is not likely that their true nature and, especially, their origin will be understood in the near future. Indeed, the nature of the similar antibacterial antibodies is still far from clear, and the latter have been the subject of much investigation.

REFERENCES

Abraham, R., and B. M. Honigberg. 1965. Cytochemistry of chick liver cell cultures infected with *Trichomonas gallinae.* J. Parasit., 51:823-833.
Aburel, E., G. Zervos, V. Titea, and S. Pană. 1963. Immunological and therapeutic investigations in vaginal trichomoniasis. Rumanian Med. Rev., 7: 13-19.

When a Japanese, Polish, or Russian writer included an English translation of the title of his article, it was copied exactly. In the absence of an original translation, the title was transliterated and followed (in parentheses) by my translation into English.

Adler, S., and R. J. V. Pulvertaft. 1944. The use of penicillin for obtaining bacteria-free cultures of Trichomonas vaginalis Donné, 1837. Ann. Trop. Med. Parasit., 38: 188-189.

───── and A. Sadowsky. 1947. Intradermal reaction in trichomonad infection. Lancet, 252: 867-868.

Amino, E. 1958. Biological and immuno-serological studies on Trichomonas vaginalis. J. Jap. Obstet. Gynec. Soc. (Eng.), 5: 77.

Andrews, J. 1938. Self limitation and resistance in Trichomonas foetus infection in cattle. Amer. J. Hyg., 27: 149-154.

───── and F. Miller. 1938. Infection with Trichomonas foetus in heifers. Amer. J. Hyg., 27: 235-249.

───── K. Kerr, and D. Porter. 1935. Cultural and microscopic diagnosis of Trichomonas foetus infection in cattle. J. Parasit., 21: 452.

Anina-Radchenko, N. D. 1959. Opit polucheniia allergena dlia viiavleniia porazhennosti liudei Trichomonas vaginalis (Method of obtaining an allergen for detection of human infection with Trichomonas vaginalis). Desiatoe Soveshchanie po Parazitologicheskim Problemam i Prirodnoochagovim Bolezniam. Moskva-Leningrad, Izdatelstvo Akademii Nauk SSSR, 2: 239-240.

Arai, H. 1959. Studies on Trichomonas vaginalis. 1. Immunological reactions in the experimental and clinical trichomoniasis (In Japanese, English summary). Kiseichugaku Zasshi, 8: 858-867.

Baba, H. 1957. Immunological studies on trichomonads. 1. Comparison of immobilization test and agglomeration reaction (In Japanese, English summary). Nisshin Igaku, 44: 655-664.

───── 1958. Immunological studies on trichomonads. 2. On the protection of mice from trichomonas infection by the immunization with heat-killed trichomonads (In Japanese, English summary). Nisshin Igaku, 45: 16-19.

Bartlett, D., D. M. Hammond, and G. Garlick. 1944. Attempts to develop active immunity to bovine trichomoniasis in breeding females by inoculation prior to breeding age. Amer. J. Vet. Res., 5: 17-21.

Bauer, H. 1962. Besteht Veranlassung und die Möglichkeit zu einer planmäszigen Bekämpfung der urogenitalen Trichomoniasis, der häufigsten venerischen Parasitose des Menschen? Prophylaxe und Therapie, 12: 11-17.

Burnet, F. M. 1962. The Integrity of the Body. Cambridge, Mass., Harvard University Press.

Bushnell, L. D. and N. J. Twiehaus. 1940a. Trichomoniasis in turkeys. Vet. Med., 35: 103-105.

───── and N. J. Twiehaus. 1940b. Poultry disease investigations. Kansas Agric. Exp. Station, 10th Biennial Report (1938-40), pp. 124-125.

Buttrey, B. W. 1956. A morphological description of a Tritichomonas from the nasal cavity of swine. J. Protozool., 3: 8-13.

Byrne, H. 1942. Trichomonas foetus: infection and immunity in rabbits. Thesis (unpubl.), Madison, University of Wisconsin, 35 pp. Cited by Morgan (1946).

───── and P. M. Nelson, 1939. Nature of immunity to Trichomonas foetus infection in rabbits. Arch. Path., 28: 761.

First Canadian Symposium on Non-Gonococcal Urethritis and Human Trichomoniasis, Montreal, Sept., 1959, Parts 3 and 4., 1960. Gynaecologia, 149 (Suppl.): 1-170.

Cavalti, P. A. 1947. The technic of collodion particle agglutination. J. Immun., 57: 141-154.

Cavier, R. and X. Mossion. 1956. Essais d'infestation expérimentale de la ratte par Trichomonas vaginalis (Donné, 1837). C. R. Acad. Sci. [D.] (Paris), 242: 2412-2414.

Combescot, C., M. Pestre, A. Domenech, and A. Verain. 1958. Rôle du terrain endocrinien au cours de l'infestation expérimentale de la ratte albinos par Trichomonas vaginalis (Donné, 1837): Étude de la flore vaginale et du pH vaginal Proc. 15th Int. Congr. Zool., London, July 1958. Hewer, H. R., and Riley, N. D., eds. London, The Congress, Burlington House.

Coutts, W. and E. Silva-Inzunza. 1957. Considérations à propos de certains aspects de l'infestation humaine par Trichomonas vaginalis. (English summary). In Les infestations à Trichomonas, Premier Symposium Européen, Reims, France, May, 1957. Paris, Masson & Cie, pp. 185-188.

Diamond, L. S. 1961. Axenic cultivation of Entamoeba histolytica. Science, 134: 336-337.

───── 1962. Axenic cultivation of Trichomonas Tenax, the oral flagellate of man. I. Establishment of cultures. J. Protozool., 9: 442-444.

────── and I. L. Bartgis. 1965. Axenic cultivation of *Entamoeba histolytica* in a clear liquid medium. *In* Progress in Protozoology, Proc. 2nd Int. Conf. Protozool., London, Aug., 1965. Amsterdam, Excerpta Medica Foundation, Intl. Congr. Ser. No. 91, p. 102.

Doran, D. J. 1957. Studies on trichomonads. I. The metabolism of *Tritrichomonas foetus* and trichomonads from the nasal cavity and cecum of swine. J. Protozool., 4: 182-190.

────── 1959. Studies on trichomonads. III. Inhibitors, acid production, and substrate-utilization by 4 strains of *Tritrichomonas foetus*. J. Protozool., 6: 177-182.

Endress, R. 1939. Verwertbarkeit der Komplementbindungsreaktion, der Agglomeration und der Trichomolyse für die Erkennung der Trichomonadeninfektion des Rindes. Arch. Tierheilk., 75: 65-82.

Farris, V. K. 1965. Comparative pathogenicity of two strains of *Trichomonas vaginalis* Donné in cell cultures. Ph.D. Thesis, Amherst, Mass., University of Mass., 71 pp.

Feinberg, J. G. 1952. A capillary agglutination test for *Trichomonas foetus*. J. Path. Bact., 64: 645-647.

────── and W. T. J. Morgan. 1953. The isolation of a specific substance and a glyco-gen-like polysaccharide from *Trichomonas foetus* (var. Manley). Brit. J. Exp. Path., 34: 104-118.

Fischer, C. 1938. Trichomonadenseuche. Deutsch. Tierärztl. Wschr., 46: 405-406.

Fletcher, S. 1965. Indirect fluorescent antibody technique in the serology of *Toxoplasma gondii*. J. Clin. Path., 18: 193-199.

Florent, A. 1941. La trichomoniase du bétail. Ann. Méd. Vét., 85: 129-142, 165-191.

────── 1947. Pouvoir agglutinant du mucus vaginal vis-à-vis de *Trichomonas foetus* dans la trichomonose du bétail. C. R. Soc. Biol. (Paris), 141: 957-958.

────── 1948. Le pouvoir agglutinant du mucus vaginal vis-à-vis des *Trichomonas*, phéno-mène d'immunité locale dans la trichomoniase du bétail. C. R. Soc. Biol. (Paris), 142: 406-408.

────── 1949. Le phénomène d'agglutination des *Trichomonas* par le mucus vaginal—ou de "muco-agglutination" dans la trichomoniase du bétail. Ann. Méd. Vét., 93: 19-29.

────── 1957. Immunologie dans la trichomonase bovine. (English summary). *In* Les infestations à *Trichomonas*, Premier Symposium Européen, Reims, France, May, 1957. Paris, Masson & Cie, pp. 308-313.

Frost, J. K. 1962. *Trichomonas vaginalis* and cervical epithelial changes. Ann. N. Y. Acad. Sci., 97: 792-799.

────── and B. M. Honigberg. 1962. Comparative pathogenicity of *Trichomonas vaginalis* and *Trichomonas gallinae* for mice. II. Histopathology of subcutaneous lesions. J. Parasit., 48: 898-918.

────── B. M. Honigberg, and M. T. McLure. 1961. Intracellular *Trichomonas vaginalis* and *Trichomonas gallinae* in natural and experimental infections. J. Parasit., 47: 302-303.

Fuller, A. 1938. The formamide method for the extraction of polysaccharides from hae-molytic streptococci. Brit. J. Exp. Path., 19: 130-139.

Garlick, G., D. Bartlett, and D. M. Hammond. 1944. Attempts to demonstrate passive immunity in bovine trichomoniasis. Amer. J. Vet. Res.. 5: 14-16.

Garnham, P. C. C., A. E. Pierce, and I. Roitt, eds. 1963. Immunity to Protozoa. Oxford, Blackwell Scientific Publications.

Gibson, H. J. 1930. Observations on the occurrence, characteristics and specificity of natural agglutinins. J. Hyg. (Camb.), 30: 337-356.

Gierke, A. G. 1933. Trichomoniasis of the upper digestive tract of chickens. California Dept. Agric. Bull., 22: 205-208.

Goldman, M. 1967. An improved microfluorimeter for measuring brightness of fluores-cent antibody reactions. J. Histochem. Cytochem., 15: 38-45.

────── and L. T. Cannon. 1967. Antigenic analysis of *Entamoeba histolytica* by means of fluorescent antibody. V. Comparison of 15 strains of *Entamoeba* with information on their pathogenicity to guinea pigs. Amer. J. Trop. Med. Hyg., 16: 245-254.

────── and N. N. Gleason. 1962. Antigenic analysis of *Entamoeba histolytica* by means of fluorescent antibody. IV. Relationships of two strains of *E. histolytica* and one of *E. hartmanni* demonstrated by cross-absorption techniques. J. Parasit., 48: 778-783.

────── and B. M. Honigberg. 1968. Immunologic analysis by gel diffusion techniques of the effects of prolonged cultivation on *Trichomonas gallinae*. J. Protozool., 15: 350-352.

Gorczyński, M. and M. Józwik. 1966. The serological properties and a chromatographic analysis of haptens obtained from strains of *Trichomonas vaginalis*. (In Polish, English summary). Wiad. Parazyt., 12: 398-403.

Hammond, D. M. and D. E. Bartlett. 1943. The distribution of *Trichomonas foetus* in the preputial cavity of infected bulls. Amer. J. Vet. Res., 4: 143-149.

———— and D. E. Bartlett. 1945. An instance of phagocytosis of *Trichomonas foetus* in bovine vaginal secretions. J. Parasit., 31:82.

———— and W. Leidl. 1957. Experimental infections of the genital tract of swine and goats with *Trichomonas foetus and Trichomonas* species from the cecum or feces of swine. Amer. J. Vet. Res., 18: 461-465.

———— P. R. Fitzgerald, and J. L. Shupe. 1956. Trichomoniasis of the reproductive tract. *In* Yearbook of Agriculture 1956. Washington, D.C., U.S. Department of Agriculture, pp. 277-283.

Hawn, M. C. 1937. Trichomoniasis of turkeys. J. Infect. Dis., 61: 184-197.

Hibler, C. P., D. M. Hammond, F. H. Caskey, A. E. Johnson, and P. R. Fitzgerald. 1960. The morphology and incidence of the trichomonads of swine, *Tritrichomonas suis* (Gruby & Delafond), *Tritrichomonas rotunda*, n. sp. and *Trichomonas buttreyi*, n. sp. J. Protozool., 7: 159-171.

Hinshaw, W. R. 1937. Diseases of turkeys. Univ. Calif., Berkeley, College Agric. Bull. No. 613, 112 pp.

Hoffmann, B. 1966a. Investigations of *Trichomonas vaginalis* serology (In Polish, English summary). Wiad. Parazyt., 12: 349-356.

———— 1966b. An evaluation of the use of the indirect hemagglutination method in the serodiagnostic of trichomonadosis (In Polish, English summary). Wiad. Parazyt., 12: 392-397.

———— and M. Gorczyński. 1964. Serologic types of *T. vaginalis* strains as encountered in the population of Białystok Voivodeship (In Polish, English summary). Wiad. Parazyt., 10: 132-135.

———— W. Kazanowska, W. Kilczewski, and J. Krach. 1963. Serologic diagnosis of *Trichomonas* infection (In Polish, English summary). Med. Dośw. Mikrobiol., 15: 91-99.

Hogue, M. J. 1938. The effect of *Trichomonas foetus* on tissue culture cells. Amer. J. Hyg., 28: 288-298.

———— 1943. The effect of *Trichomonas vaginalis* on tissue-culture cells. Amer. J. Hyg., 37: 142-152.

Holtroff, D. 1957. Einige für die Praxis wichtige Nachweismethoden der Trichomonaden. Abstracts of papers, Wiss. Ges. Geburtsch. Gyn. Med. Akad. Karl Gustav Carus, Dresden, Feb. 2, 1957. Zbl. Gynäk, 79: 1995. (From the *Trichomonas vaginalis* Bulletin, 1958, Eaton Laboratories 1(1): 1.)

Honigberg, B. M. 1961. Comparative pathogenicity of *Trichomonas vaginalis* and *Trichomonas gallinae* for mice. I. Gross pathology, quantitative evaluation of virulence, and some factors affecting pathogenicity. J. Parasit., 47: 545-571.

———— 1963. Evolutionary and systematic relationships in the flagellate order Trichomonadida Kirby. J. Protozool., 10: 20-63.

———— and M. Goldman. 1968. Immunologic analysis by quantitative fluorescent antibody methods of the effects of prolonged cultivation on *Trichomonas gallinae*. J. Protozool., 15: 176-184.

———— R. DiM. Becker, M. C. Livingston, and M. T. McLure. 1964. The behavior and pathogenicity of two strains of *Trichomonas gallinae* in cell cultures. J. Protozool., 11: 447-465.

———— M. C. Livingston, and J. K. Frost. 1966. Pathogenicity of fresh isolates of *Trichomonas vaginalis*: "The mouse assay" versus clinical and pathologic findings. Acta Cytol., 10: 353-361.

———— H. Friedman, and S. Stępkowski. 1969. Effects of immunization methods on agglutination and precipitation reactions involving *Trichomonas gallinae*. (Unpublished.)

Huddleson, I. F., H. W. Johnson, and E. E. Hamann. 1933. A study of the opsonocytophagic power of the blood and allergic skin reaction in *Brucella* infection and immunity in man. Amer. J. Public Health, 23: 917-929.

Hungate, R. E. 1955. Mutualistic intestinal protozoa. *In* Biochemistry and Physiology of Protozoa, 2. Hutner, S. H., and Lwoff, A., eds. New York, Academic Press, Inc., pp. 159-199.

Inoki, S. 1957. Expériences d'immunologie, de biochimie, de génétique sur *Trichomonas vaginalis* (English summary), *In* Les infestations à *Trichomonas*, Premier Symposium Européen, Reims, France, May, 1957. Paris, Masson & Cie, pp. 265-279.

Jaakmees, H. P. 1964a. Vnutrikozhnaia proba pri trichomonoze urogenitalnovo trakta (Intradermal test in urogenital trichomoniasis). Materiali V Konferentsii Tallinskovo Nauchno-Issledovatelskovo Instituta Epidemiologii, Mikrobiologii i Gigieni, Tallinn, pp. 119-121.

—— 1964b. Reaktsia sviazivania komplementa pri trichomonoze urogenitalnovo trakta (Complement-fixation reaction in urogenital trichomoniasis). Materiali V Konferentsii Tallinskovo Nauchno-Issledovatelskovo Instituta Epidemiologii, Mikrobiologii i Gigieni, Tallinn, pp. 121-123.

—— 1964c. Issledovanie komplement-sviazivaiushchikh spetsificheskikh antitel pri trichomonoze urogenitalnovo trakta (Investigation of complement-fixing specific antibodies in urogenital trichomoniasis). Materiali k Tretiemu Nauchno-Koordinatzionnomu Soveshchaniu po Parazitologicheskim Problemam Litovskoi SSR, Latviiskoi SSR i Estonskoi SSR. Vilnius, Gazetno-Zhurnalnoe Izdatelstvo, pp. 116-118.

—— 1965. Reaktsia sviazivania komplementa i vnutrikozhnaia proba pri trichomonoze urogenitalnovo trakta (Complement-fixation reaction and intradermal test in urogenital trichomoniasis). Diss., Cand. Med. Sci., Acad. Sci., Estonian SSR., Inst. Exp. Clin. Med., 29 pp.

—— and J. K. Teras. 1966. Intradermal reaction with specific antigens in cases of genito-urinary trichomonadosis. Wiad. Parazyt., 12: 385-391.

—— J. K. Teras, U. K. Nigesen, H. J. Tompel, and E. M. Rõigas. 1964. Zavisimost reaktsii sviazivania komplementa i reaktsii aggliutinatsii ot serotipa shtamma *Trichomonas vaginalis* u bolnikh trichomonozom (Dependence of the complement-fixation reaction and of the agglutination reaction on the serotype of the strain of *Trichomonas vaginalis* in trichomoniasis patients). Materiali V Konferentsii Tallinskovo Nauchno-Issledovatelskovo Instituta Epidemiologii, Mikrobiologii i Gigieni, Tallinn, pp. 123-125.

—— J. K. Teras, E. M. Rõigas, U. K. Nigesen, and H. J. Tompel. 1966. Complement-fixing antibodies in the blood sera of men infested with *Trichomonas vaginalis*. Wiad. Parazyt., 12: 378-383.

Jeffries, L. and M. Harris. 1967. Observations on the maintenance of *Trichomonas vaginalis* and *Trichomonas foetus*; the effects of cortisone and agar on enhancement of severity of subcutaneous lesions in mice. Parasitology, 57: 321-334.

Johnson, G. and R. E. Trussell. 1943. Experimental basis for the chemotherapy of *Trichomonas vaginalis* infestations. I. Proc. Soc. Exp. Biol. Med., 54: 245-249.

—— M. Trussell, and F. Jahn. 1945. Isolation of *Trichomonas vaginalis* with penicillin. Science, 102: 126-128.

—— A. B. Kupferberg, and C. G. Hartman. 1950. Cyclic changes in vaginal populations of experimentally induced *Trichomonas vaginalis* infections in Rhesus monkeys. Amer. J. Obstet. Gynec., 59: 689-692.

Kelly, D. R. and R. J. Schnitzer. 1952. Experimental studies on trichomoniasis. II. Immunity to reinfection in *T. vaginalis* infections of mice. J. Immun., 69: 337-342.

—— A. Schumacher, and R. J. Schnitzer. 1954. Experimental studies in trichomoniasis. III. Influence of the site of the immunizing infection with *Trichomonas vaginalis* on the immunity of mice to homologous reinfection by different routes. J. Immun., 73: 40-43.

Kerr, W. R. 1943. Trichomoniasis in the bull. II. Vet. J., 99: 4-8.

—— 1944. The intradermal test in bovine trichomoniasis. Vet. Rec., 56: 303-307.

—— 1955. Vaginal and uterine antibodies in cattle with particular reference to *Br. abortus*. Brit. Vet. J., 111: 169-178.

—— 1958. Experiments in cattle with *Trichomonas suis*. Vet. Rec., 70: 613-615.

—— and M. Robertson. 1941. An investigation into the infection of cows with *Trichomonas foetus* by means of the agglutination reaction. Vet. J., 97: 351-365.

—— and M. Robertson. 1943. A study of the antibody response of cattle to *Trichomonas foetus*. J. Comp. Path. Ther., 53: 280-297.

—— and M. Robertson. 1945. A note on the appearance of serological varieties among *T. foetus* strains isolated from infected cattle. Vet. Rec., 57: 221-222.

—— and M. Robertson. 1946a. A study of the passively acquired antibody to *Tr. foetus* in the blood of young calves and its behavior in agglutination tests and intradermal reactions. J. Comp. Path. Ther., 56: 38-48.

—— and M. Robertson. 1946b. Experimental infections in virgin heifers with *Trichomonas foetus* in vaccinated and unvaccinated animals. J. Comp. Path. Ther., 56: 101-113.

—————— and M. Robertson. 1947. A study of the re-exposure to *Tr. foetus* of animals already exposed to the infection as virgin heifers with some observations on the localization of antibody in the genital tract. J. Comp. Path. Ther., 57: 301-313.

—————— and M. Robertson. 1953. Active and passive sensitization of the uterus of the cow *in vivo* against *Trichomonas foetus* antigen, and the evidence for the local production of antibody in that site. J. Hyg. (Camb.), 51: 405-415.

—————— and M. Robertson. 1954. Passively and actively acquired antibodies for *Trichomonas foetus* in very young calves. J. Hyg. (Camb.), 52: 253-263.

—————— J. L. McGirr, and M. Robertson. 1949. Specific and non-specific desensitization of the skin in *Trichomonas* sensitive bovines. J. Comp. Path. Ther., 59: 133-154.

—————— M. Robertson, and J. L. McGirr. 1951. A study of the reaction of the white blood corpuscles in bovines at parturition with a consideration of the evidence of the action of the adrenal cortical hormone (cortisone). J. Hyg. (Camb.), 49: 67-80.

Kirby, H. 1937. Host-parasite relations in the distribution of protozoa in termites. Univ. Calif. Publ. Zool. (Berkeley), 41: 189-212.

—————— 1941. Relationships between certain protozoa and other animals. *In* Protozoa in Biological Research. Calkins, G. N. and Summers, F. M., eds. New York, Columbia University Press, pp. 890-1008.

Korte, W. 1957. Détection de la trichomonase par des méthodes d'immunologie. *In* Les infestations à *Trichomonas*, Premier Symposium Européen, Reims, France, May, 1957. Paris, Masson & Cie, pp. 159-162.

Kott, H. and S. Adler. 1961. A serological study of *Trichomonas* sp. parasitic in men. Trans. Roy. Soc. Trop. Med. Hyg., 55: 333-344.

Kramář, J. and K. Kučera. 1966. Immunofluorescence demonstration of antibodies in urogenital trichomoniasis. J. Hyg. Epidem. (Praha), 10: 85-88.

Kulda, J., and B. M. Honigberg. 1969. Behavior and pathogenicity of *Tritrichomonas foetus* in chick liver cell cultures. J. Protozool., 16: 479-495.

Künstler, J. 1888. Sur quelques infusoires nouveaux ou peu connus. C. R. Acad. Sci. [D] (Paris), 107: 953-955.

Kupferberg, A. B., G. Johnson, and H. Sprince. 1948. Nutritional requirements of *Trichomonas vaginalis*. Proc. Soc. Exp. Biol. Med., 67: 304-308.

Kust, D. 1936a. Die Trichomonadensterilität des Rindes und ihre Bekämpfung. Deutsch. Tierarztl. Wschr., 44: 177-181.

—————— 1936b. Die Diagnose der Trichomonadenseuche des Rindes. Deutsch. Tierarztl. Wschr., 44: 821-825.

Kuvin, S. F., J. E. Tobie, C. B. Evans, G. R. Coatney, and P. G. Contacos. 1962. Fluorescent antibody studies on the course of antibody production and serum gamma globulin levels in normal volunteers infected with human and simian malaria. Amer. J. Trop. Med. Hyg., 11: 429-436.

Laan, I. A. 1965. Ob izmenchivosti patogennosti, aggliutinabilnosti i fermentativnoi aktivnosti *Trichomonas vaginalis* (On changeability of pathogenicity, agglutinability and fermentative activity of *Trichomonas vaginalis*). Diss., Cand. Med. Sci., Acad. Sci., Estonian SSR., Inst. Exp. Clin. Med., 32 pp.

—————— 1966. On the effect of passages in vitro and in vivo on the pathogenicity, agglutinative ability, and fermentative activity of *Trichomonas vaginalis*. Wiad. Parazyt., 12: 173-182.

Lanceley, F. 1958. Serological aspects of *Trichomonas vaginalis*. Brit. J. Vener. Dis., 34: 4-8.

—————— and M. G. McEntegart. 1953. *Trichomonas vaginalis* in the male. The experimental infection of a few volunteers. Lancet, 264: 668-671.

Lederberg, J. 1959. Genes and antibodies. Science, 129: 1649-1653.

Levine, N. D. 1961. Protozoan Parasites of Domestic Animals and of Man. Minneapolis, Burgess Publishing Company.

—————— and C. A. Brandly. 1939. A pathogenic *Trichomonas* from the upper digestive tract of chickens. J. Amer. Vet. Med. Ass., 95: 77-78.

—————— and C. A. Brandly. 1940. Further studies on the pathogenicity of *Trichomonas gallinae* for baby chicks. Poult. Sci., 19: 205-209.

—————— L. E. Boley, and H. R. Hester. 1941. Experimental transmission of *Trichomonas gallinae* from the chicken to other birds. Amer. J. Hyg., 33: 23-32.

MacDonald, E. M. and A. L. Tatum. 1948. The differentiation of species of trichomonads by immunological methods. J. Immun., 59: 309-316.

McEntegart, M. G. 1952. The application of a haemagglutination technique to the study of *Trichomonas vaginalis* infections J. Clin. Path., 5: 275-280.

———— 1956. Serological comparison of a strain of *Trichomonas vaginalis* with the Belfast and Manley strains of *Trichomonas foetus*. J. Path. Bact., 71: 111-115.

———— C. S. Chadwick, and R. C. Nairn. 1958. Fluorescent antisera in the detection of serological varieties of *Trichomonas vaginalis*. Brit. J. Vener. Dis., 34: 1-3.

Magara, M. 1957. Étude des caractères sérologiques et de la pathogénèse expérimentale du *Trichomonas vaginalis* (English summary), *In* Les infestations à *Trichomonas*. Premier Symposium Européen, Reims, France, May, 1957. Paris, Masson & Cie, pp. 197-199.

Mattern, C. F. T., B. M. Honigberg, and W. A. Daniel. 1967. The mastigont system of *Trichomonas gallinae* (Rivolta) as revealed by electron microscopy. J. Protozool., 14: 320-339.

Mazzanti, E. 1900. Due osservazioni zooparassitologiche. G. Soc. Accad. Vet. Ital., 49: 626-631.

Molinaro, G. A., J. C. Jaton, H. C. Isliker, and H. J. Scholer. 1965. Action of papain and pepsin fragments of rabbit immunoglobulin on the motility of *Trichomonas foetus*. Int. Arch. Allerg. 28: 141-149.

Morgan, B. B. 1943. Studies on the immobilization-reaction of *Trichomonas foetus* (Protozoa) in cattle. J. Immun., 47: 453-460.

———— 1944. Normal agglutinins in vertebrate sera for *Trichomonas foetus* (Protozoa). Proc. Helminth Soc. (Washington), 11: 21-23.

———— 1946. Bovine Trichomoniasis. Minneapolis, Burgess Publishing Company, revised ed.

———— 1947. Vaccination studies on bovine trichomoniasis. Amer. J. Vet. Res., 8: 54-56.

———— 1948. Studies on the precipitin and skin reactions of *Trichomonas foetus* (Protozoa) in cattle. J. Cell. Comp. Physiol., 32: 235-246.

Morisita, T. 1939. Studies on the trichomonad, parasitic in the reproductive organs of cattle. Part 3. Serological study, with special reference to agglomeration- and agglutination-phenomena. Jap. J. Exp. Med., 17: 27-41.

Nakabayashi, T. 1952. Immunological studies on the parasitic trichomonads with special reference to the analytical comparison between agglomeration and agglutination. Osaka Daigaku Igaku Zasshi, 4: 11-21.

Nelson, P. 1938. *Trichomonas foetus*. Infection, immunity, and chemotherapy. Sum. Doctoral Dissertations, Madison, University of Wisconsin, 3: 50-51.

Nigesen, U. K. 1963. Importance of the serotypes of *Trichomonas vaginalis* in the agglutination reaction in case of the genito-urinary trichomoniasis (In Russian, English summary). *In* Genito-urinary Trichomoniasis (collection of papers). Teras, J. K., ed. Tallinn, Acad. Sci., Estonian SSR., pp. 51-62.

———— 1964. Issledovania zashchitnovo deistvia sivorotki krovi bolnikh trichomonozom urogenitalnovo trakta (Investigations of protective activity of sera of patients suffering from urogenital trichomoniasis). Materiali k Tretiemu Nauchno-Koordinatzionnomu Soveshchaniu po Parazitologicheskim Problemam Litovskoi SSR, Latviiskoi SSR i Estonskoi SSR. Vilnius, Gazetno-Zhurnalnoe Izdatelstvo, pp. 99-101.

———— 1966. Reaktsia aggliutinatsii i test seroprotektsii pri trichomonoze urogenitalnovo trakta (Agglutination reaction and seroprotection test in urogenital trichomoniasis). Diss., Cand. Med. Sci., Acad. Sci., Estonian SSR, Inst. Exp. Clin. Med., 34 pp.

———— J. K. Teras, H. P. Jaakmees, H. J. Tompel, and E. M. Rõigas. 1964. Reaktsia aggliutinatsii pri trichomonoze urogenitalnovo trakta (Agglutination reaction in urogenital trichomoniasis). Materiali V Konferentsii Tallinskovo Nauchno-Issledovatelskovo Instituta Epidemiologii, Mikrobiologii i Gigieni, Tallinn, pp. 110-112.

Oka, Y. and H. Osaki. 1963. Physiological function of the protozoan cell. VI. Analysis of living and killed parasite immunity to experimental trichomoniasis in mice. Medicine and Biology, 66: 279-282.

Oleinik, G. I. 1964. On the study of antigenic properties of human trichomonads (In Ukrainian, English summary). Mikrobiol. Zh. (Kiev), 26: 50-56.

Osaki, H. and Y. Oka. 1962. Physiological function of the protozoan cell. V. A serological study of ultracentrifugal soluble and insoluble fractions of cell-free extract of *Trichomonas foetus* (In Japanese). Medicine and Biology, 66: 213-215.

Perez-Mesa, C., R. M. Stabler, and M. Berthrong. 1961. Histopathological changes in the domestic pigeon, infected with *Trichomonas gallinae*. Avian Dis., 5: 48-59.

Pierce, A. E. 1947. The demonstration of an agglutinin to *Trichomonas foetus* in the vaginal discharge of infected heifers. J. Comp. Path. Ther., 57: 84-97.

——— 1949a. The agglutination reaction of bovine serum in the diagnosis of trichomoniasis. Brit. Vet. J., 105: 286-294.
——— 1949b. The mucus agglutination test for the diagnosis of bovine trichomoniasis. Vet. Rec., 61: 347-349.
——— 1953. Specific antibodies at mucous surfaces. Proc. Roy. Soc. Med., 46:785-787.
——— 1955. Electrophoretic and immunological studies on sera from calves from birth to weaning. II. Electrophoretic and serological studies with special reference to the normal and induced agglutinins to *Trichomonas foetus*. J. Hyg. (Camb.), 53: 261-275.
——— 1959. Specific antibodies at mucous surfaces. Vet. Rev. Annot., 5: 17-36.
First Polish Symposium on Trichomoniasis, Olsztyn-Kortowo, Sept., 1961, 1962. Wiad. Parazyt., 8 (2): 163-282.
Second Polish Symposium on Trichomoniasis, Lublin, Nov., 1963, 1964. Wiad. Parazyt., 10 (2-3): 103-271.
Third Polish Symposium on Trichomoniasis, Białystok, Nov., 1965. 1966. Wiad. Parazyt. 12 (2-4): 139-508.
Purchase, H. G. and D. T. Clark. 1967. The pathogenicity of two strains of *Tritrichomonas foetus* for mice. J. Protozool., 14: 43-45.
Quisno, R. A. and M. J. Foter. 1946. The use of streptomycin in the purification of cultures of *Trichomonas vaginalis*. J. Bact., 51: 404.
Reardon, L. V., L. L. Ashburn, and L. Jacobs. 1961. Differences in strains of *Trichomonas vaginalis* as revealed by intraperitoneal injections into mice. J. Parasit., 47: 527-532.
Reims Symposium. 1957. Les infestations à *Trichomonas*. Premier Symposium Européen (First European Symposium on Infestations due to *Trichomonas*). Reims, France, May 1957. Paris, Masson et Cie, 381 pp.
Reisenhofer, U. 1963. Über die Beeinflussung von *Trichomonas vaginalis* durch verschiedene Sera. Arch. Hyg., Bakt., 146: 628-635.
Riedmüller, L. 1928. Über die Morphologie, Übertragungsversuche und klinische Bedeutung der beim sporadischen Abortus des Rindes vorkommenden Trichomonaden. Zbl. Bakt. [Orig.], 108: 103-118.
——— 1932. Zur Frage der ätiologischen Bedeutung der bei Pyometra und sporadischen Abortus des Rindes gefundenen Trichomonaden. Schweiz. Arch. Tierheilk., 74: 343-351.
Robertson, M. 1941. Agglutination reactions of certain trichomonads in sera obtained from immunised rabbits, with particular reference to *Trichomonas foetus*. J. Path. Bact., 53: 391-402.
——— 1960. The antigens of *Trichomonas foetus* isolated from cows and pigs. J. Hyg. (Camb.), 58: 207-213.
——— 1963. Antibody response in cattle to infection with *Trichomonas foetus*. *In* Immunity to Protozoa. Garnham, P. C. C., Pierce, A. E., and Roitt, I., eds. Oxford, Blackwell Scientific Publications, pp. 336-345.
Rom, F. de and M. Thiery. 1957. Mise en évidence d'anticorps locaux dans la vaginite à *Trichomonas*. *In* Les infestations à *Trichomonas*, Premier Symposium Européen, Reims, France, May, 1957. Paris, Masson & Cie, pp. 162-163.
Salzer, H. 1938. Infektionsversuche mit Geschlechtstrichomonaden des Rindes. Inaugural Dissertation, Giessen, 44 pp. Cited by Morgan (1946).
Samuels, R. and H. Chun-Hoon. 1964. Serological investigations of trichomonads. I. Comparisons of "natural" and immune antibodies. J. Protozool., 11: 36-45.
Sanborn, W. R. 1955. Microagglutination reactions of *Trichomonas suis*, *Trichomonas* sp., and *T. foetus*. J. Parasit., 41: 295-298.
Schneider, M. 1941. *Trichomonas foetus* in cattle with special reference to diagnosis. Thesis (unpubl.), Madison, University of Wisconsin, 33 pp. Cited by Morgan, (1946) and Pierce (1949).
Schnitzer, R. J. and D. R. Kelly. 1953. Short persistence of *Trichomonas vaginalis* in reinfected immune mice. Proc. Soc. Exp. Biol. Med., 82: 404-406.
——— D. R. Kelly, and B. Leiwant. 1950. Experimental studies on trichomoniasis. 1. The pathogenicity of trichomonad species for mice. J. Parasit., 36: 343-349.
Schoenherr, K. E. 1956. Serologische Untersuchungen über Trichomonaden. Z. Immunitätsforsch, 113: 83-94.
Sharma, N. N. and B. M. Honigberg. 1966. Cytochemical observations on chick liver cell cultures infected with *Trichomonas vaginalis*. I. Nucleic acids, polysaccharides, lipids, and proteins. J. Parasit., 52: 538-555.

———— and B. M. Honigberg. 1967. Cytochemical observations on proteins, alkaline and acid phosphatases, adenosine triphosphatase, and 5'-nucleotidase in chick liver cell cultures infected with *Trichomonas vaginalis*. J. Protozool., 14: 126-140.

Shorb, M. S. 1964. Physiology of trichomonads. *In* Biochemistry and Physiology of Protozoa, 3. Hutner, S. H., ed. New York, Academic Press, Inc., pp. 383-457.

Sinelnikova, N. V. 1961. Kozhno-allergicheskaia reaktsia pri urogenitalnom trichomoniaze cheloveka i eë diagnosticheskoe znachenie (Allergic skin reaction in urogenital trichomoniasis of man and its diagnostic significance). Tr. Odessa Inst. Epidem. Microbiol. Metchnikova, 5: 102-105.

Soszka, S., W. Kazanowska, and K. Kuczyńska. 1962. On injury of the epithelium of the vagina caused by *Trichomonas vaginalis* in experimental animals (In Polish, English summary). Wiad. Parazyt., 8: 209-215.

Stabler, R. M. 1948a. Variations in virulence of strains of *Trichomonas gallinae* in pigeons. J. Parasit., 34: 147-149.

———— 1948b. Protection in pigeons against virulent *Trichomonas gallinae* acquired by infection with milder strains. J. Parasit., 34: 150-153.

———— 1951. Effect of *Trichomonas gallinae* from diseased mourning doves on clean domestic pigeons. J. Parasit., 37: 473-478.

———— 1953. Observations on the passage of virulent *Trichomonas gallinae* through 119 successive domestic pigeons. J. Parasit., 39 (Suppl.): 12.

———— 1954. *Trichomonas gallinae*: A review. Exp. Parasit., 3: 368-402.

———— B. M. Honigberg, and V. M. King. 1964. Effect of certain laboratory procedures on virulence of the Jones' Barn strain of *Trichomonas gallinae* for pigeons. J. Parasit., 50: 36-41.

Stępkowski, S. 1957. Proceedings of discussion of the Biological Veterinary Section of the 5th meeting of the Polish Parasitological Society. Wiad. Parazyt., 3: 345.

———— 1961a. Studies on the properties of trichomonads in swine and cattle. Wiad. Parazyt., 7 (Suppl.): 359-361.

———— 1961b. Collodional phagocytic test in investigation on the antigenic structure of trichomonads. Wiad. Parazyt., 7 (Suppl.): 365-366.

———— 1966. Vergleichende Beobachtungen über die Verwandtschaft zwischen *Trichomonas foetus* and *Trichomonas foetus*-aenlichen Schweine-Trichomonaden. *In* Proceedings of the First International Congress of Parasitology, Rome, Sept., 1964. New York, Pergamon Press, 1: 379-386.

———— and A. Bartoszewski. 1959. The state of investigations of trichomoniasis in people and animals (In Polish). Wiad. Parazyt., 5: 15-19.

———— and B. M. Honigberg. 1969. Relationship between pathogenicity and antigenic structure of *Trichomonas gallinae* strains as revealed by gel diffusion. (MS in preparation.)

Svec, M. H. 1944. Bovine intracutaneous and serological reactions to fractions of *Trichomonas foetus* (protozoon). J. Bact., 47: 505-508.

Talmage, D. W. 1959. Immunological specificity. Science, 129: 1643-1648.

Tatsuki, T. 1957. Studies on *Trichomonas vaginalis*. II. Immunoserological reactions of *Trichomonas vaginalis* by sera and colostra from women infected therewith (In Japanese, English summary). Nagasaki Igakkai Zasshi, 32: 983-993.

Teras, J. K. 1954. Eksperimentalnoe issledovanie patogennosti *Trichomonas vaginalis* (Experimental investigation of pathogenicity of *Trichomonas vaginalis*). Diss., Cand. Med. Sci., Univ. of Tartu, 21 pp.

———— 1959. Nekotorye voprosi izuchenia trichomoniaza urogenitalnovo trakta (Some problems in the study of urogenital trichomoniasis). Desiatoe Soveshchanie po Parazitologicheskim Problemam i Prirodnoochagovim Boleznam. Moskva-Leningrad, Izdatelstvo Akademii Nauk SSSR, 2: 262-263.

———— 1961a. On the protective effect of the blood sera of patients with trichomoniasis of the genito-urinary tract on white mice infected intraperitoneally with cultures of *Trichomonas vaginalis* (In Russian, English summary). Izv. Akad. Nauk Estonskoi SSR., 10 (Biol. Ser. 1961, No. 1): 19-26.

———— 1961b. On the existence of antibodies agglutinating, immobilizing and lysing *Trichomonas vaginalis* in the blood sera of healthy people and rabbits (In Russian, English summary). Akad. Nauk Estonskoi SSR, Inst. Exp. Clin. Med., Issledovania po Mikrobiologii, pp. 43-53.

———— 1961c. On the changes of the agglutinin titre of blood sera in rabbits vaccinated with cultures of *Trichomonas vaginalis* (In Russian, English summary). Akad. Nauk Estonskoi SSR, Inst. Exp. Clin. Med., Issledovania po Mikrobiologii, pp. 55-63.

———— 1962a. Über die agglutinogenen Eigenschaften der *Trichomonas vaginalis* (In Estonian, German summary). Izv. Akad. Nauk Estonskoi SSR, 11 (Biol. Ser. 1962, No. 1): 54-59.

———— 1962b. On the agglutination reaction and complement fixation in trichomoniasis of the genito-urinary tract (In Russian, English summary). Izv. Akad. Nauk Estonskoi SSR, 11 (Biol. Ser. 1962, No. 2): 107-118.

———— 1963a. On the different antigenic structures of the strains of *Trichomonas vaginalis* (In Russian, English summary). *In* Genito-urinary Trichomoniasis (collection of papers), Teras, J. K., ed. Tallinn, Acad. Sci., Estonian SSR., pp. 23-32.

———— 1963b. On the immunogenic properties of *Trichomonas vaginalis* (In Russian, English summary). *In* Genito-urinary Trichomoniasis (collection of papers), Teras, J. K., ed. Tallinn, Acad. Sci., Estonian SSR, pp. 33-42.

———— 1964. Diagnostika, epidemiologiia i lechenie trichomonoza urogenitalnovo trakta (Diagnosis, epidemiology and treatment of urogenital trichomoniasis). Diss., Doct. Med. Sci., Acad. Sci., Estonian SSR, 80 pp.

———— 1965. On the varieties of *Trichomonas vaginalis*. *In* Progress in Protozoology, Proc. 2nd Int. Conf. Protozool., London, Aug., 1955. Amsterdam, Excerpta Medica Foundation, Int. Congr. Ser. No. 91, pp. 197-198.

———— 1966. Differences in the antigenic properties within strains of *Trichomonas vaginalis*. Wiad. Parazyt., 12: 357-363.

———— and H. J. Tompel. 1963. Comparative study of the pathogenicity of monocellular cultures of the serotypes of *Trichomonas vaginalis* TLR and TN (In Russian, English summary). *In* Genito-urinary Trichomoniasis (collection of papers). Teras, J. K., ed. Tallinn, Acad. Sci., Estonian SSR., pp. 43-50.

———— H. P. Jaakmees, U. K. Nigesen, E. M. Rõigas, and H. J. Tompel. 1964. O dinamike komplementzviazivaiushchikh antitel v sivorotke krovi bolnikh trichomonazom zhenshchin i muzhchin posle lechenia metronidazolom (On the dynamics of complement-fixing antibodies in serum of women and men suffering from trichomoniasis after treatment with metronidazole). Materiali V Konferentsii Tallinskovo Nauchno-Issledovatelskovo Instituta Epidemiologii, Mikrobiologii i Gigieni, Tallinn, pp. 114-116.

———— H. P. Jaakmees, U. K. Nigesen, E. M. Rõigas, and H. J. Tompel. 1966a. The dependence of serologic reactions on the serotypes of *Trichomonas vaginalis*. Wiad. Parazyt., 12: 364-369.

———— U. K. Nigesen, H. P. Jaakmees, E. M. Rõigas, and H. J. Tompel. 1966b. The agglutinogenic properties of *Trichomonas vaginalis* in human organism. Wiad. Parazyt., 12: 370-377.

Theokharov, B. A. 1959. Epidemiologiia trichomoniaza mochepolovikh organov i voprosi patogennosti vlagalishchnikh trichomonad (Epidemiology of trichomoniasis of the urogenital organs and problems of pathogenicity of vaginal trichomonads). Diss., Doct. Med. Sci., Leningrad. Cited by Jaakmees and Teras, 1966.

Tobie, J. E. and Coatney, G. R. 1961. Fluorescent antibody staining of human malaria parasites. Exp. Parasit., 11: 128-132.

Tokura, N. 1935. Biologische und immunologische Untersuchungen über die menschenparasitären Trichomonaden. Igaku Kenkyu, 9: 1-13.

Trussell, R. E. 1946. Microagglutination tests with *Trichomonas vaginalis*. J. Parasit., 32: 563-567.

———— 1947. *Trichomonas vaginalis* and trichomoniasis. Springfield, Ill., Charles C Thomas.

———— and S. H. McNutt. 1941. Animal inoculations with pure cultures of *Trichomonas vaginalis* and *Trichomonas foetus*. J. Infect. Dis., 69: 18-28.

———— M. E. Wilson, F. H. Longwell, and K. A. Laughlin. 1942. Vaginal trichomoniasis. Complement fixation, puerperal morbidity, and early infection of newborn infants. Amer. J. Obstet Gynec., 44: 292-295.

Vershinskii, B. V. 1958. O Patogennosti *Trichomonas vaginalis* Donné, 1836 (On pathogenicity of *Trichomonas vaginalis* Donné, 1836). Akush. Ginek., 34: 76.

Volkmar, F. 1930. *Trichomonas diversa* n. sp. and its association with a disease of turkeys. J. Parasit., 17: 85-89.

Wagner, O. and E. Hees. 1937. 156 positive Trichomonasblutbefunde bei Mensch und Tier. Zbl. Bakt. [Orig.], 138: 273-290.

Walton, B. C., B. M. Benchoff, and W. H. Brooks. 1966. Comparison of the indirect fluorescent antibody test and methylene blue dye test for detection of antibodies to *Toxoplasma gondii*. Amer. J. Trop. Med. Hyg., 15: 149-152.

Warren, L. G. and A. C. Chandler. 1958. Host-parasite relations in trichomoniasis. The immune response in mice infected with *Trichomonas gallinae* (Rivolte, 1878) Stabler, 1938. J. Parasit., 44 (Suppl.): 21.

────── W. B. Kitzman, and E. Hake. 1961. Induced resistance of mice to subcutaneous infection with *Trichomonas gallinae* (Rivolta, 1878). J. Parasit., 47: 533-537.

Watkins, W. M. 1959. Enzymes of *Trichomonas foetus*. The action of cell-free extracts on blood-group substances and low-molecular-weight glycosides. Biochem. J., 71: 261-274.

Weld, J. T. and B. H. Kean. 1958. A factor in serum of human beings and animals that destroys *T. vaginalis*. Proc. Soc. Exp. Biol. Med., 98: 494-496.

Wendlberger, J. 1936. Zur Pathogenität der *Trichomonas vaginalis*. Arch. Dermatol. Syph., 174: 583-590.

Wenrich, D. H. and M. A. Emmerson. 1933. Studies on the morphology of *Tritrichomonas foetus* (Riedmüller) (Protozoa, Flagellata) from American cows. J. Morph., 55: 193-205.

Witte, J. 1933a. Bakterienfreie Züchtung von Trichomonaden aus dem Uterus des Rindes in einfachen Nährböden. Zbl. Bakt. [Orig.], 128: 188-195.

────── 1933b. Tierversuche zur Prüfung der Pathogenität der in den Genitalien des Rindes vorkommenden Trichomonaden. Arch. Wiss. Prakt. Tierheilk., 66: 333-343.

────── 1934. Serologische Untersuchungen zum Nachweis der Trichomonadeninfektion der Genitalien des Rindes. Berlin Tierärztl. Wschr., 50: 693-695.

Zeetti, R. 1940, Ricerche sperimentali sul *Trichomonas* "Mazzanti" (German summary). Clin. Vet. Milano, 63: 51-59.

African Trypanosomes

ROBERT S. DESOWITZ
Section of Tropical Medicine and Medical Microbiology, School of Medicine,
University of Hawaii, Honolulu, Hawaii

INTRODUCTION

The foundations of modern immunology were established in the latter part of the 19th century, a time when the Great Powers, Britain, France, and Germany, were embarking upon their colonial adventures in Africa. It soon became apparent to these nations that economic development of their new possessions could not be accomplished unless the debilitating diseases peculiar to that continent could be controlled.

Trypanosomiasis, with its toll of human and domestic animal life, was (and still is) of particular importance in impeding the progress of African development. Immunologic protection was a particularly attractive method of control, and research was soon begun in Europe in this field. Rouget in 1896 recognized that sera of animals infected with *Trypanosoma equiperdum* possessed protective properties. Schilling (1902) demonstrated these antibodies to be trypanolytic, and Levaditi and Muttermilch (1909) showed that in common with other immuno-lytic phenomena, this too required complement.

There is, then, a period of some 60 years during which research on immunity to trypanosomes has been carried out. However, despite the efforts of many scientists in many countries, the goal of immunologic protection of man or his domestic animals against trypanosomiasis has not been achieved. Nor is there available, at present, a reliable serologic test for diagnosis of this disease.

Immunologic protection remains an ideal highly worthy of accomplishment, and the post-World War II years have witnessed a revival of interest in this field. It is, admittedly, a revival that results, to some measure, from an attitude of desperation. During the 10 years after that war, many new chemotherapeutic compounds were developed to cure and control parasitic infections. A chemotherapeutic armamentarium became available for combating trypanosomiasis more effectively than ever before: Antrycide, the dimidiums, and phenanthridiniums for the trypanosomiases of domestic animals, and pentamidine for human trypanosomiasis. But the use of these compounds has not achieved eradication or widespread control of the disease, and in this respect, it has not fulfilled our expectations. The appearance of drug-resistant strains of trypanosomes and the relatively great administrative difficulties in giving the drugs at frequent intervals to large numbers of people or cattle have made it virtually impossible, particularly when dealing with nomadic tribes, to control the disease by chemotherapeutic means. Trypanosomiasis may well disappear when a marked improvement of social conditions and the settlement of nomadic tribes occur, and an increasing amount of land is brought under efficient agriculture. On the other hand, these improvements may depend on the control of the disease in order to allow mixed farming and to provide the protein foods required by an energetic society. The cycle has not yet been broken by chemotherapy, chemoprophylaxis, or tsetse-fly eradication, and in view of this, scientists have again turned to the possibility of immunization, for it is by this method that other infections have been controlled without necessitating drastic change in the socioenvironmental order.

This chapter deals with the immunology of pathogenic trypanosomes. *T. cruzi* is excluded, since it is dealt with in Dr. Goble's chapter for this book. For the most part, the species of trypanosomes with which this review is concerned are of African origin and are cyclically transmitted by tsetse flies. The chapter is not intended to be a comprehensive review of the literature in the sense of being a bibliography. I have attempted to cover the significant developments in the field that have been made during the years since the publication of Taliaferro's *The Immunology of Parasitic Infections* (1929). Older literature is cited in evidencing the evolution of modern concepts and in areas, such as "natural" antibody to trypanosomes, which have been largely neglected by contemporary investigators.

TRYPANOSOME ANTIGENS

Somatic antigens

Prerequisite to any study of immunity is the elucidation of the nature of the stimulating agents—the antigens. The major advances made in the field of biochemistry and immunochemistry during the last 20 years have been applied to trypanosomes by a number of workers. As a result, there is a considerable amount of new information on the chemical composition and the antigens of the parasite.

The percentage of dry matter in fresh weight has been estimated at 8 percent for *T. rhodesiense* (Christophers and Fulton, 1938) and 18 percent for *T. equiperdum*. A good proportion of this is lipoidal material, although the early estimate of 60 percent lipids for *T. evansi* (Kligler and Olitzki, 1936; Kligler et al., 1940) is undoubtedly too high. Later analyses (Ikejiani, 1946; Williamson and Brown, 1964; Godfrey, 1967) generally agree that the total lipid content of pathogenic trypanosomes is about 15 percent. There is, however, no evidence that any of the lipid is in haptenic association with protein so as to constitute an antigen (Williamson and Desowitz, 1961; Williamson and Brown, 1964).

Trypanosomes are almost devoid of any polysaccharide material that could be antigenic. The only detectable carbohydrate present in whole-cell hydrolyzates of *T. rhodesiense*, apart from nucleotide pentose, is a trace of glucosamine (0.2 to 0.3 μg per mg of protein) (Williamson and Desowitz, 1961).

The bulk of trypanosomal antigens consists, then, of protein and is devoid of carbohydrate, lipid, and probably nucleic acid haptenic components. The aminoacid composition of hydrolyzates prepared from nine species and strains of trypanosomes is shown in Table 1 (*see* pp. 554–555). There are relatively few differences in aminoacid composition among the pathogenic trypanosomes. The general aminoacid composition is, rather unexcitingly, not too unlike that of bovine albumin hydrolyzate.

The electrophoretic pattern of trypanosomal extracts has been described by Desowitz (1959a) and Williamson and Desowitz (1961) (*see* Table 2, pp. 556–557). No differences were detectable among the electrophoretic patterns

Table 1

Aminoacid Composition of Nine Different Trypanosomes and a Trypanosomatid Flagellate

Aminoacid composition (moles % ± S.E.)	Hydrolyzate							
	T. cruzi	T. lewisi	T. equinum	T. vivax (i) (ii)	T. brucei	T. rhodesiense (fly)	T. rho-desiense N	T. rho-desiense S
No. of samples	1	1	1	2	2	2	4	3
No. of analyses	3	4	2	6	4	4	8	5
Cysteine + cystine/2	0.1 ± 0.1	1.2 ± 0.8	0.8 ± 0.3	1.1 ± 0.7	0.1 ± 0.1	0.7 ± 0.2	0.7 ± 0.3	0.9 ± 0.5
Histidine	4.1 ± 1.4	5.2 ± 1.2	2.7 ± 0.6	2.9 ± 0.5	—	1.6 ± 0.7	1.3 ± 0.5	2.4 ± 1.6
Lysine	—	5.3	—	5.8	—	—	8.3 ± 1.2	4.8 ± 0.7
Arginine	—	6.8 ± 1.3	—	14.3	—	—	5.9 ± 1.6	19.3 ± 2.1
Lysine + arginine	14.4 ± 0.5	16.8 ± 0.7	13.3 ± 1.1	16.0 ± 1.3	22.5 ± 1.6	18.0 ± 1.2	18.2 ± 0.8	23.2 ± 1.2
Aspartic acid	3.1 ± 1.0	2.1 ± 0.6	5.3 ± 0.7	6.2 ± 0.5	7.4 ± 0.7	5.1 ± 0.5	5.8 ± 0.7	3.5 ± 0.7
Glutamic acid	20.8 ± 6.9	10.2 ± 1.4	12.0 ± 0.7	14.7 ± 1.3	20.0 ± 1.0	20.2 ± 1.5	13.4 ± 0.8	12.1 ± 0.8
Aspartic + glutamic acid	23.9 ± 7.0	12.3 ± 1.5	17.3 ± 1.1	20.9 ± 1.4	27.4 ± 1.2	25.3 ± 1.6	19.2 ± 1.1	15.6 ± 1.1
Glycine	9.1 ± 1.4	8.8 ± 1.0	9.9 ± 1.1	11.8 ± 0.8	14.3 ± 1.3	11.0 ± 1.0	10.3 ± 0.6	7.9 ± 1.4
Serine	8.0 ± 0.3	4.0 ± 0.9	5.6 ± 0.9	5.7 ± 0.6	6.4 ± 0.9	7.3 ± 0.9	5.0 ± 0.6	3.8 ± 0.8
Alanine	19.1 ± 1.2	8.4 ± 1.0	8.9 ± 1.2	14.6 ± 0.9	13.9 ± 1.3	12.6 ± 0.5	13.1 ± 0.7	18.6 ± 1.5
Threonine	3.2 ± 0.4	5.5 ± 0.9	8.3 ± 1.6	5.9 ± 0.3	1.6	4.9 ± 1.4	4.4 ± 0.5	3.3 ± 0.6
Valine	8.7 ± 1.6	6.2 ± 0.9	9.3 ± 0.7	6.8 ± 0.7	4.8 ± 0.8	7.7	8.8 ± 0.5	8.6 ± 0.5
Tyrosine	—	0.5 ± 0.7	1.2 ± 0.3	1.3 ± 0.5	—	—	0.6 ± 0.4	1.3 ± 0.4
Phenylalanine	—	3.4	—	4.2	—	1.8	2.6 ± 0.7	2.6
Leucine/iso-leucine	—	22.2	—	—	—	19.6 ± 1.2	18.8 ± 1.2	19.6
Phenylalanine + leucines	20.6 ± 0.8	29.5 ± 1.9	22.9 ± 1.2	20.9 ± 0.7	16.3 ± 0.7	19.5 ± 0.4	19.6 ± 1.2	20.6 ± 1.0

Table 1 (Continued)

Aminoacid composition (moles % ± S.E.)	T. gambiense*	T. rhodesiense N (supernatant)*	T. rhodesiense N (deposit)*	S. oncopelti	Hydrolyzate Crystalline BPA† (experimental)	BPA‡	Mean: group A§	Mean: group B§
No. of samples	2	1	1	1	2		2	16
No. of analyses	4	2	4	3	7		7	33
Cysteine + cystine/2	0.6 ± 0.3	1.8 ± 0.5	1.6 ± 0.5	tr. —	3.5 ± 0.2	6.1	0.7	0.7
Histidine	3.0	5.0 ± 0.6	7.3 ± 0.9	3.0 ± 0.5	3.1 ± 0.5	3.2	4.7	2.3
Lysine	—	11.0	6.0	—	—	10.8	—	6.3
Arginine	—	13.1	7.9	—	—	4.2	—	13.2
Lysine + arginine	20.5 ± 1.2	17.4 ± 2.2	14.7 ± 0.8	17.0 ± 0.9	18.1 ± 1.8	15.0	15.6	18.9
Aspartic acid	6.0 ± 1.0	2.4 ± 0.4	4.7 ± 0.8	2.9 ± 0.5	5.1 ± 0.6	10.1	2.6	5.6
Glutamic acid	18.2 ± 1.1	13.6 ± 1.7	12.9 ± 0.5	10.1 ± 0.8	19.6 ± 1.5	13.8	15.5	15.8
Aspartic + glutamic acid	24.2 ± 1.5	16.0 ± 1.7	17.6 ± 1.0	13.0 ± 1.0	24.7 ± 1.6	23.9	18.1	21.4
Glycine	11.0 ± 0.6	7.1 ± 1.6	5.4 ± 0.5	8.8 ± 0.7	3.3 ± 0.4	3.0	9.0	10.9
Serine	6.3 ± 0.8	6.3 ± 0.6	5.8 ± 0.5	3.7 ± 0.5	4.0 ± 0.5	4.9	6.0	5.7
Alanine	11.5 ± 1.1	15.9 ± 2.2	9.3 ± 0.8	14.5 ± 0.7	13.6 ± 0.9	8.6	13.8	13.3
Threonine	4.0 ± 0.2	6.6 ± 0.8	5.7 ± 0.8	5.7 ± 0.8	4.9 ± 0.2	6.0	4.4	4.6
Valine	7.8 ± 1.3	8.8 ± 1.7	7.9 ± 0.8	8.6 ± 0.7	7.2 ± 0.7	6.1 (6.7 + Me)	7.5	7.7
Tyrosine	0.7	2.7 ± 0.6	3.0 ± 0.8	2.5 ± 0.7	1.9 ± 0.1	3.4	—	1.0
Phenylalanine	0.8 ± 0.6	—	—	—	—	4.9	—	2.4
Leucine/iso-leucine	22.9	—	—	—	—	14.1	—	20.2
Phenylalanine + leucines	19.9 ± 1.5	23.3 ± 2.0	27.7 ± 1.8	22.4 ± 0.7	20.3 ± 1.5	19.0	25.1	20.0

* Homogenate.
† BPA = bovine plasma albumin (Armour), included as reference standard.
‡ Figures derived from Tristram (1953).
§ Group A = T. cruzi and T. lewisi; Group B = T. equinum, T. vivax, T. brucei, and T. rhodesiense.
From Williamson and Desowitz. 1961. Exp. Parasit. 11:161-175.

Table 2

Summary of Trypanosome Antigens Described by Various Authors

Antigen Designation or Derivation	Technical Description or Method of Fractionation	Authors
Whole trypanosome homogenates 4 fractions	Paper electrophoresis	Desowitz, 1959a; Williamson and Desowitz, 1961
Brucei-group homogenates 9 fractions 11 fractions 22 fractions	Cellulose-acetate electrophoresis Polyacrilamide-gel disc electrophoresis Starch-gel electrophoresis	Njogu and Humphreys, 1967
Brucei-group trypanosomal extracts Variant-specific 4S group (mol. wt. 5 to 16 × 10⁴) Common antigens (uncharacterized nature) Variant-specific 1S group (mol. wt. 1 × 10⁴)	Precipitinogens (gel diffusion); all of unconjugated proteins	Williamson and Brown, 1964
Brucei-group homogenates 11 components 1: Nucleoprotein 2-5: Slow moving components (precipitinogens) 6-11: Components of greater mobility	Starch-gel electrophoresis	Brown, 1963
A antigens (high variant specificity)	Chemical nature of a group of precipitinogens; sensitive to heat, pepsin, sodium metaperiodate	
B antigens (high variant specificity)	Chemical nature of a group of precipitinogens; less heat-sensitive than A antigens, resistant to pepsin, sodium metaperiodate; *Brucei*-group homogenates	
AG-specific antigen	Precipitinogen in *T. rhodesiense*-infected rat serum; strain-specific; not immunogenic	Seed and Weinman, 1963; Seed, 1963

Antigen	Description	Reference
PR-specific antigen	Nonprecipitinogen present as serum exoantigen and somatic antigen; strain-specific; immunogenic; precipitated by ammonium sulfate and adsorbed to calcium phosphate gel	Seed and Gam, 1966a
Common antigens Specific to culture and to blood forms Two antigens common to culture and blood forms	Precipitinogen *Brucei*-group trypanosome homogenates; one common antigen is hexokinase	
Agglutinogen	Produces agglutinin in rabbits infected with *T. gambiense*	Gray, 1965a, b
Protective antigen	Distinct antigen from the agglutinogen; not hexokinase	
Basic antigen	Although classified as a variant-type antigen, it is said to be responsible for antigenic similarity of substrains of tsetse fly-transmitted trypanosome	
Predominant antigen	Variant antigen appearing early in the infection each time a strain is mechanically transmitted to a new host	

of the species examined (*T. vivax*, *T. brucei*, *T. gambiense*, and *T. rhodesiense*). A typical electrophoretogram is illustrated in Figure 1. The extracts are composed of four electrophoretic fractions, although Fraction 4, which appears as a trail, was not present in all samples. Fraction 1 and the closely associated Fraction 2, both of low mobility, constitute 28.8 percent and 28 percent, respectively, of the total protein. Fraction 3 contains 26.7 percent of the protein, and Fraction 4, when present, 16.6 per cent of the total. Fraction 1 shows a faintly positive Feulgen reaction; Fraction 3 gives a positive ferricyanide reaction for thiol groups. No histochemical reaction was given with stains for fats or mucopolysaccharides, which confirmed the chemical analyses. Starch-gel electrophoresis (Brown, 1961, 1963; Williamson and Brown, 1964) of *T. rhodesiense* extract revealed the same four major protein zones, but further resolved them into eleven fractions (*see* Table 2, pp. 556–557). Antigenic constitution seems to expand as a function of technical refinement. The author recalls his personal satisfaction in being able to discern four fractions of trypanosome homogenates by paper electrophoresis (Desowitz, 1959a). Some ten years and several techniques later, Njogu and Humphreys (1967) were able to resolve, by polyacrilamide-gel disc electrophoresis, 11 soluble protein components of *T. rhodesiense* and 22 components by starch-gel electrophoresis of this material (Fig. 2, *see also* Table 2). Some of these complex bands showed multiple enzyme activity, and future work along these lines should allow a correlation between the enzymatic and antigenic properties of these components.

In a series of valuable studies, Brown and Williamson (1962, 1964), Williamson (1961, 1963), and Williamson and Brown (1964) have further characterized the physicochemical nature of the trypansomal antigenic constituents. At pH 8.6, the electrophoretically immobile fraction is a group of antigens composed of ribonucleoprotein, nucleoprotein, or both, with components having a molecular weight range of 1.4×10^6 to 6.0×10^6 (35S, 54S, 72S). The two mobile fractions are of two distinct molecular weights: a "4S" group (molecular weight range of 5 to 16×10^4) of tertiary hydrogen-bonded structures probably involving tyrosine, and a much lighter "1S" group (molecular weight of 1×10^4) which is capable of diffusion through cellophane and is

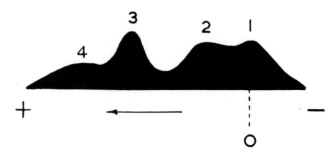

FIG. 1.   Electrophoretic separation of trypanosome protein fractions; a densitometric analysis (Whatman 3MM paper, 130 volts applied for 24 hours, veronal-acetate buffer, pH 8.6; O = origin). (From R. Desowitz, 1959a.)

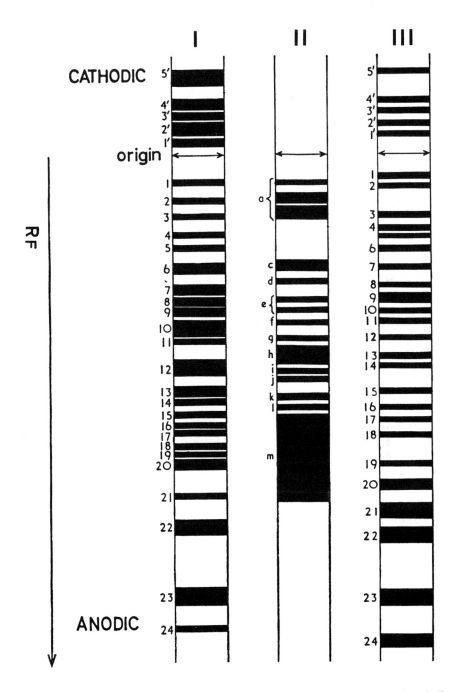

FIG. 2.   Starch-gel electrophoretogram of trypanosomes and rat serum proteins. I. Eatro 691; II. Normal rat serum; III. *T. rhodesiense*. The figure is a combined scale drawing representing several preparations. (After Njogu and Humphreys, 1967. *Nature* (*London*), 216: 280-282.)

incompletely precipitable by trichloroacetic acid. The 1S protein might not
be revealed by conventional paper electrophoresis of the crude homogenate.
An attempt was made by Williamson and Brown to locate the antigens in
subcellular fractions of *Trypanosoma rhodesiense*, but the results were not
particularly distinct. Their tentative conclusion was that the 4S and 1S
groups of antigens were in nuclear, microsomal, and cell-sap fractions. The
authors believe that the 4S antigens in particular are associated with nuclear
structures.

While this is a promising and important area of investigation, the procedures now available seem to be too imprecise to separate the main structural
components of trypanosomes. The complex of antigens undoubtedly elicits
the production of a serologic galaxy of antibodies. The manner in which
these individual antibodies actually function cannot be determined until the
individual antigens are located with reasonable certainty.

Exoantigen

In addition to the somatic antigens there are, in some infections, soluble
trypanosomal products in the circulating plasma. These antigens, which have
been referred to as trypanosomal metabolites or plasma antigens, are now
conventionally designated as exoantigens. Exoantigen of pathogenic trypanosomes was first described by Weitz (1960 a, b), who found that rabbit antisera to *T. brucei* not only agglutinated live trypanosomes but also precipitated infected rat serum. When normal rats were inoculated with trypano-
some-free infected rat serum, they also produced antisera which contained
agglutinin for the living organism and precipitin for exoantigen. The exoantigen has also been detected in the sera of rodents experimentally infected
with *T. vivax* (Gray, 1961; Weitz, 1962a; 1963a), *T. rhodesiense* (Weitz,
1963b; Seed and Weinman, 1963; Seed, 1963), *T. gambiense* (Gray, 1961;
Dodin and Fromentin, 1962; Dodin et al., 1962), and *T. congolense* (Johnson et al., 1963). Exoantigen is usually present in the sera of animals in
which there is a fulminating parasitemia. This relationship, however, is not
consistent, since it may be present in animals, such as goats, with a low parasitemia but absent in animals with a massive infection of *T. vivax*. No soluble antigen is detectable in sheep or cattle with cyclically transmitted *T.
vivax* infections (Gray, 1961).

When a soluble antigen produced *in vitro* by *T. lewisi* was first described
by Thillet and Chandler (1957), it was thought to be a metabolic product
rather than a somatic constituent of the parasite. Research since that time
has revealed a much more complicated picture in that some of the circulating
antigens are derived from the trypanosome cytoplasm. During the course of
infection, there is a constant destruction of parasites, mainly by immuno-
lysis, and the proteins released obviously enter the circulation. For example,
three of the seven precipitin lines developed from *T. vivax*-infected rat serum
and its antisera are of somatic origin, while the other four may be associated

with surface structures of the organism (Gray, 1961). In addition to the precipitins in the infected rat serum, there is an antigen which does not develop in the agar-gel double-diffusion system (Seed, 1963). It has been claimed that it is this nonprecipitating antigen which is immunogenic. (The protective activity of exoantigen will be discussed later—*see* p. 579.) Weitz (1960b) maintained that exoantigen was a distinct entity located on the surface of the trypanosome. In contrast to Seed's findings, Weitz observed a single precipitin band of lower mobility than the γ-globulin component in starch-gel immunoelectrophoresis. It is of interest that in electrophoretic analysis of trypanosome homogenates, the "inert" component has been identified as nucleoprotein. Weitz (1963a) has proposed that exoantigen is not strictly a surface antigen, but occurs naturally on the surface of the organisms and is continuously liberated in the environmental fluids, such as in the serum of the host.

Antigenic alteration

The ability of the pathogenic African trypanosomes to change antigenically during the course of relapsing infections has intrigued (and plagued) research workers since this phenomenon was first described by Franke in 1905. The problem of antigenic variation is of considerable practical importance in that the failure to produce an effective immunity has been attributed to this ability of the parasite to confound its host antigenically.

Almost all the investigations on antigenic variation have employed the *Brucei*-group trypanosomes, which produce a relapsing type of infection in rats, guinea pigs, and rabbits. The normally fulminating course in mice may be aborted by subcurative chemotherapy or inactivated human serum (Inoki et al., 1952). Trypanosomes appearing after such treatment exhibit a pattern of antigenic variation similar to that of trypanosomes in other relapsing infections. A number of serologic methods have been employed to characterize the variants, e.g., neutralization, rechallenge, and agglutination. The great majority of serotype studies have relied on the agglutination reaction, and several modern modifications of the test have been described (Inoki et al., 1952; Soltys, 1957b; Cunningham and Vickerman, 1962). More recently, Brown (1963) has shown that antigenic variation is demonstrable by double-diffusion precipitation of antibody and trypanosome homogenates.

In early experiments on antigenic variation, it was necessary to maintain each variant by "acme" infection in mice. The introduction of deep-frozen strains ("stabilates") by Polge and Soltys (1957) and Lumsden et al. (1963) has greatly simplified experimental procedure.

The question of the extent to which trypanosomes may undergo antigenic variation has not been fully answered as yet. Earlier workers, such as Ritz (1914, 1916), were impressed by the ability of trypanosomes to produce what appeared to be an unlimited number of antigenic types during the course of a relapsing infection. Ritz (1916) recognized 22 antigenic variants of *T. brucei*, Lourie and O'Connor (1937) isolated 13 variants of *T. rhodesiense* from 13 relapses, and Osaki (1959) found 23 variants of *T. gambiense*. Gray (1965a) essentially agreed with the concept that there is no inherent limit to antigenic variation. He has stated that "there seems to be no limit to the number of antigens which can develop in a clone strain of trypanosomes during an untreated infection, other than that imposed by the length of time for which an infected host survives." However, there is some evidence from the work of Inoki and his colleagues (1957, 1960) that the number of relapse serotypes may be limited.

Despite this proliferation of serotypes, there is now a growing body of evidence that the process is not a random one but rather that serotypes develop in a sequence of a well-defined pattern. Gray, in a series of experiments (1962, 1965a, b), noted that after initiating infections with single trypanosomes (clones) derived from the different serologic populations (variants) of a given strain, a discernible pattern of immunologic events usually ensued. First, the variant returned to the serotype of the parent strain (the basic antigen, *see* Table 2). Next, during the first week of infection, a series of similar serotypes (predominant antigens, *see* Table 2) developed. In the later stages of the infection, the appearance of serotypes in ordered sequence was not as apparent as during the first week.

The reversion of a serotype to a basic antigen particularly occurs when new hosts are infected by tsetse-fly cyclical transmission (Broom and Brown, 1940; Gray, 1965b). In these tsetse fly-induced infections of *T. brucei*, the parasites can be detected in the rabbit or goat on the third day following the fly bite, and the sera become serologically positive on the eighth day. The trypanosomes maintain the basic antigenic character, although in some cases there is some carry-over of the parent variant antigen, until the first appearance of antibody on the eighth or ninth day. Thereafter, new serotypes (variants) are produced every three days until the death of the host (Gray, 1965b).

The number, distribution, and relationship of basic antigens found in nature are still unknown, but such information could greatly contribute to a study of the epizootiology of the *Brucei*-group trypanosomiases. Gray (1966), in a limited study of basic antigens in *T. brucei* isolates from cattle from widely separated areas of Nigeria, found little antigenic similarity. However, clones derived from infected cattle in a single herd exhibited considerable antigenic similarity.

How, then, do these antigenic variants arise? There are three obvious hypothetical possibilities: by selection, by mutation, or by adaptation.

The selection theory held primacy among the earlier workers, since it conformed to a Darwinian view of a mixed population being selected via the pressure of some external agency, in this case, antibody. However, the recent work of Gray (1963a, 1965b), who showed that the same pattern of variation occurred after inoculation of a single trypanosome, disproved the mixed-population hypothesis.

While the mutational theory still has a number of advocates, the objec-

tion, as Bray (1967) has pointed out, is in accepting that a series of mutations, normally thought to be a random process, occurs in a predetermined
sequence with reversional mutation to the original type in a new host. Of the
more recent investigators, Watkins (1964) is the chief proponent of the
mutation-selection theory. He argued that his calculated mutation rate of
of 10^{10} trypanosomes per milliliter, his calculated mutation rate of $10^{-5.17}$
trypanosome per division cycle, about 1 in 150,000, would provide sufficient
serologic variants to account for the relative rapidity at which they appear. Furthermore, Watkins was unable to confirm the results of Gray and
others that serologic variants appear in an ordered sequence. Using both
mouse-protection and agglutination tests, he found that: 1. There was always homologous protection, but some sera protected against heterologous
strains more than homologous strains; 2. With nine serologic variants, there
was no consistent pattern of protection; and 3. Absorption tests were erratic
in that sometimes a homologous strain failed to reduce the agglutination
titer. One of the conclusions he drew from these experiments was that "the
cross agglutination reactions were therefore not due to antigenic identity or
even to possession of common major antigens" (Watkins, 1964).

The process by which antigenic variation might arise via adaptation is
not known. One hypothesis, which was proposed by Gray (1967), is that the
antibody enters the trypanosome and alters or chooses the genetic key, causing the new generation to possess an altered antigenic constitution. Bray
(1967) tends to dismiss this theory, since there is no evidence, at present,
to indicate that antibody can directly affect the genetic process in a way
comparable to that of the virus particle.

I espouse an adaptive theory which is based on the possibility that the
tertiary structure of a surface antigen could be altered by the action of antibody. The reasoning for this view is as follows. The major evidence for serologic variation is derived from the agglutination test. The antigen-antibody
reaction leading to this is a surface phenomenon located exterior to the cell
membrane. Indeed, it is questionable whether any form of antibody penetrates the living cell (Coombs and Lachman, 1968). Although the plasma-
lemma itself may be antigenic, exoantigen studies indicate that the serologic
determinant is an antigen elaborated by the trypanosomes which localizes as
an extramembranous deposit. It is tempting to speculate that the exterior
"coat" shown in the electron micrographs of the blood-stream forms of African trypanosomes (Vickerman, 1968) is this antigen or antigen-antibody
complex. A point of departure from the accepted adaptive theory is the proposal that the trypanosome has little or no ability to alter this antigen endo-
genously. This would account for the "basic" or "common" nature of the
antigen during the first few days of an infection. Antibody elaborated would
act by altering the tertiary structure of the "basic" protein antigen and, in
the process, would expose new determinant sites. This would be akin to certain types of drug action which also have been shown to induce antigenic
change of the trypanosome. The altered antigen would induce new antibody
formation, which in turn would further modify the antigen's tertiary struc-

ture, and the seemingly endless succession of serotypes could be accounted for by this continuous feedback mechanism.

Alternatively, the antigenic agent may be an antigen-antibody complex rather than antigen alone.

Furthermore, there probably would be a general, set sequence in which the tertiary structure unfolds. Thus, during the early stages of infection and variation there would remain, in most instances, a sufficiently common structural identity for agglutination by previously formed antibody. This would explain the relatively ordered pattern of antigenic change described by Gray and others. After repeated immunologic attack, the antigen's tertiary structure would have changed to a degree that would cause the lack of ordered sequence which is reported to occur at the later stages of infections (Gray, 1965b). Transmission via the tsetse fly would remove the exterior antigenic coat (Vickerman, 1968), and so the whole process would start again in the new host.

The antigen(s) responsible for antigenic variation has not been localized with any certainty. Brown and Williamson (1964) believe the 4S and 1S somatic antigens to be variant-specific. Miller (1965) has demonstrated exoantigen to be variant-specific. In a brief report, Inoki et al. (1968) claim that an electron microscope study using ferritin-conjugated antibody indicated that the variant-specific antigen has a sedimentation coefficient of 8.2S and is largely located in the flagellum of the parasite.

As is obvious from the foregoing discussion, our present knowledge about antigenic variation is in an almost hopelessly confused state. There is as yet no satisfactory explanation for the mechanism which will fit experimental findings. Indeed, there is considerable disparity in the results obtained by different investigators. Also, there is no agreement as to which is the responsible antigen or antigens. Even more important for practical considerations, it is not known whether the natural hosts, i.e., man, domestic animals, and wild ungulates, respond immunologically in the same highly variant-specific manner as do experimental laboratory animals, or whether they produce a broader-spectrum antibody.

Common antigens

In addition to the complex of species-, variant-, and clone-specific antigens, several workers have revealed the presence of common antigens. Again, however, there is confusion and difficulty in attempting to interpret the results of a serologic method in terms of host immunity. For example, does the satisfactory use of *T. equiperdum* antigen in the complement-fixation reaction for the diagnosis of *T. gambiense* trypanosomiasis (Schoenaers et al., 1953a, b) indicate the presence of a broad-spectrum antibody elicited to a common antigen, or is it only an unknown peculiarity of that serologic technique?

The various immunodiffusion techniques have been favored for determining antigenic relationships. Of the precipitinogenic somatic *Brucei*-group antigens, there are at least two common antigens with a molecular weight greater than 2×10^6. These are probably nucleoproteins. The cell sap also contains common antigens of as yet unknown character (Brown and Williamson, 1962, 1964; Brown, 1963; Williamson and Brown, 1964). Seed (1963) has also identified common antigens among the *Brucei* group, although the number of these common antigens varied from strain to strain. Possibly related to this are the results of a respiratory-inhibition test study (Desowitz, 1961), which suggested that antigenic specificity of *Brucei*-group trypanosomes is associated with their polymorphic character. In old monomorphic strains maintained by prolonged mechanical passage, there was almost complete cross-reactivity among *T. brucei*, *T. gambiense*, and *T. rhodesiense*. Seed (1963) has presented evidence that the common antigen responsible for the respiration-inhibiting antibody is hexokinase, although this antigen-antibody system is not precipitinogenic. Agglutinogenic relationships also indicate common antigens, although these vary from strain to strain and species to species. For example, Taylor (1968) found that rabbits infected with one strain of *T. rhodesiense* usually had high antibody titers to other *T. rhodesiense* strains, as well as to the homologous strain, but there was no cross-reaction with any *T. brucei* strain. The same was true for *T. brucei* in that it cross-reacted with other *T. brucei* strains, but in addition, *T. rhodesiense* was agglutinated, although at low titer.

Precipitin, protection, and immunofluorescent tests have shown exoantigen mainly to be species- or strain-specific (Weitz, 1963a; Seed and Weinman, 1963). However, as noted earlier, exoantigen is an antigenic complex, and Gray (1961) found by double-diffusion analysis, one common antigen band among the exoantigens produced in rats infected with *T. vivax*, *T. brucei*, or *T. gambiense*. A rat-adapted strain and a tsetse fly-transmitted strain of *T. vivax* possessed three common exoantigens, despite their considerably diverse biologic characters and geographic origin.

Investigators studying immunity to trypanosomes have tended to forget that the parasite has a complicated developmental cycle during which profound physiologic and morphologic alterations take place. It is reasonable to conjecture that antigenic changes also are a part of this metamorphosis. Seed has been the only worker who has directed his attention to this problem. Gel-diffusion precipitin patterns revealed the presence of antigens specific to blood and culture forms of *T. rhodesiense* and at least two antigens common to both forms (Seed, 1963; *see also* Table 2). Antibodies formed by rabbits against any one species of *Brucei*-group culture forms will cross-agglutinate culture forms of all three species (*T. brucei*, *T. rhodesiense*, and *T. gambiense*) at nearly the same titers. However, antibody to the *Brucei*-group culture forms did not agglutinate culture forms of *T. cruzi*, *T. conorhini*, or *T. rangeli* (Seed, 1964). Culture techniques which will allow complete invertebrate-phase development to the metacyclic stage are now largely lacking. If and when such "complete" culture methods become available, the comparative characterization of developmental antigens will, undoubtedly, be greatly advanced.

There is, then, ample evidence that common antigens exist among strains and species of the pathogenic trypanosomes. Isolation and characterization of the properties of common antigens have yet to be achieved. Obviously, the determination of their immunogenicity is of great importance if a practical method for protective immunization is to be realized.

IMMUNITY TO TRYPANOSOMES

Natural immunity

In 1902, Laveran observed that normal human sera, when injected into mice infected with *T. brucei*, caused a marked reduction in their parasitemia. During the succeeding thirty years, the natural antibody in normal human sera and some animal sera was the subject of a vast amount of research. However, since that time, work on this phenomenon has been almost entirely neglected. This is indeed regrettable, since modern immunologic techniques could provide answers to many still mysterious facets of natural antibody to trypanosomes.

Earlier workers (Laveran and Mesnil, 1902; Goebel, 1907; Braun and Teichman, 1912) believed that human serum was effective only when inoculated into infected mice and had no activity *in vitro*. Yorke et al. (1929), however, devised an *in vitro* method for the demonstration of natural antibody. Most of the work carried out was concerned with the action of normal human serum on the *Brucei*-group trypanosomes. The members of this group are not equally affected, and moreover, the degree of sensitivity may change after subpassage in the rodent host. Newly isolated strains of *T. rhodesiense* and *T. gambiense* maintained in experimental rodents are not adversely affected by human serum, whereas newly isolated strains of *T. brucei* are susceptible. At some time between the second and eighth rodent-to-rodent subpassage, *T. rhodesiense* becomes susceptible to human serum (Fairbairn, 1933a; Adams, 1933). *T. gambiense*, however, retains a degree of resistance to human serum for many years of mechanical subpassage in rodents. Strains of *T. brucei* maintained in experimental rodents remain highly susceptible.

This difference of trypanocidal action of human serum on *T. rhodesiense*, *T. gambiense*, and *T. brucei* gave rise to the theory that the human trypanosomes have evolved from *T. brucei* and are serum-resistant variants of that organism. Hoare (1948a, b) has proposed that through this process the virulent strains of *T. rhodesiense* arose first, and later a strain of this developed into the better adapted *T. gambiense* which causes a chronic disease. There is, however, no experimental evidence to support this theory. Human serum when inoculated into mice is usually not completely curative, and relapse generally occurs. By successive selection of the relapsing parasites, a strain of *T. brucei* can, by a method similar to isolation of drug-fast strains, be obtained which is totally resistant to the trypanocidal action of human serum. These serum-resistant organisms are still unable to infect man (Collier, 1924). Conversely, a strain of *T. rhodesiense* maintained in rodents becomes serum-susceptible but is still capable of inducing human infections (Corson, 1933). Nor does cyclical transmission of *T. rhodesiense* through the sheep cause it to revert to a *brucei*-like parasite incapable of infecting man (Fairbairn, 1937). Fairbairn (1933b) concluded that:

> If one's whole defence were dependent upon the trypanolytic action of serum, it is extraordinary that *T. gambiense*, which is completely resistant to human serum, should produce a chronic infection in man, while *T. rhodesiense*, which is comparatively susceptible to human serum (even on first isolation) should produce an acute, rapidly fatal disease. There must be some other factor, or lack of one, in unshed blood, which produces these results.

A complete survey of the trypanocidal action of human serum on trypanosomes other than those of the *Brucei* group has not been carried out. Yorke et al. (1930) demonstrated *in vitro* that human serum was lethal for an old laboratory strain of *T. equiperdum* at dilutions up to 1:5,000. Against two recently isolated strains of *T. congolense*, there was activity at dilutions up to 1:10. Human serum is not active against the rat-adapted strain of *T. vivax* (Terry, 1957).

Normal sera from animals other than man may also possess trypanocidal properties, but again no complete survey has been carried out. The most notable is the trypanocidal properties of baboon (*Papio* sp.) serum, which were first reported by Laveran in 1904. Mesnil and Leboeuf (1910) found that when baboon serum was tested against various species of pathogenic trypanosomes, there was a marked variation in response. *T. brucei*, *T. evansi*, and *T. equinum* were highly sensitive, but *T. gambiense* and *T. congolense* were hardly affected. The refractivity of the baboon to infection with the human trypanosomes may, in large part, depend on natural serum antibody, since a low-grade infection of *T. gambiense* confined to the cerebrospinal fluid can be established by direct inoculation into the meningeal space (Regendanz, 1932). Other primate sera also possess trypanocidal properties, but not to the degree of baboon serum. Mesnil and Leboeuf (1910) found that the degree of activity could be arranged in descending order: baboon, mangabey, to mandrill. The sera of *Macacus*, *Cynomologus* and *Cercopithecus* contain no trypanocidal factor. The lack of trypanocidal activity of *Cercopithecus* sera is of interest, since this genus is supposed to be quite closely related to *Papio* spp. Relatively little is known of the trypanocidal action of other animal sera. The only recent work on the subject is the observation by Terry (1957) that normal cotton rat serum contains an antibody active against the rat-adapted strain of *T. vivax*. The antibody is quite specific in that *T. brucei*, *T. equiperdum*, *T. evansi*, *T. rhodesiense*, and *T. cruzi* are unaffected by it. Furthermore, it is not present in the serum of the closely related white rat, nor is it found in the sera of man, horse, sheep, rabbit, guinea pig, or hamster.

The natural antibody in human serum has a number of characteristics that distinguish it from acquired specific antibody. It can be inactivated by heat, but this requires the relatively high temperature of 62° to 64°C for 30 minutes to destroy its trypanocidal action completely. Fresh guinea pig or human sera do not reactivate the trypanolytic power of heated serum, and from this it has been adduced that the mode of action of this system is not complement-mediated. It could be argued that the high temperature of inactivation destroys or denatures the antibody, so reactivation by complement is impossible. There is considerable variation in trypanocidal activity among the sera of different individuals (Laveran and Mesnil, 1912). Age also exerts an influence in that sera from adults have a higher level of the natural antibody than do sera from newborns. Other factors, particularly liver disease, may diminish or entirely ablate the trypanocidal power of the affected individual's serum. The icteric sera from patients with jaundice of diverse etiology have little or no activity, and from this several workers, such as Zeiss (1921) and Rosenthal and Nossen (1921), have concluded that the trypanocidal power of serum is closely related to the function of the liver, and that in all probability the liver is the site of formation of natural trypanocidal antibody. Cancers other than those of the liver are reputed not to affect the trypanocidal properties (Mignoli, 1924). Malnutrition, particularly when aggravated by lack or imbalance of vitamin intake, decreases trypanocidal activity (Grünmandel and Leichtentritt, 1924).

The exact nature of the trypanocidal factor is still not known to any degree of certainty. It appears to be a globulin or associated with that fraction. The only modern attempt at identification is that by Terry (1957), who found that the trypanocidal activity of cotton rat serum for *T. vivax* was present in the β- and faster moving γ-globulin component. The factor certainly is of sufficient size to be antigenic, since antihuman rabbit serum destroys the trypanocidal activity of normal human serum (Handler, 1935). It is relatively nonspecific in that adsorption with bacteria such as *Salmonella typhosa* and *Proteus vulgaris* causes inactivation (Culbertson and Strong, 1935). There is some evidence, however, that the natural antibodies from different animals are not identical. Zimmer (1931) showed that when a strain of trypanosomes was made resistant to normal human serum, it would still be killed by baboon serum.

The precise identification and mode of action of natural trypanocidal antibody has remained enigmatic for over 60 years. There are many obvious parallelisms between this antibody and the antimicrobial factors of normal tissues and fluids. In particular, there is a notable similarity between properdin and the natural trypanocidal antibody. Both are thermolabile and both have certain specific activity; different strains and species of Gram-negative bacteria show a variable sensitivity to properdin (Landy and Pillemer, 1956), and natural trypanocidal antibody, as has been described above, affects only some species and strains of trypanosomes. Skarnes and Watson (1957) consider properdin and natural microbial antibody to be the same substance. Properdin requires the presence of complement and Mg^{++} ions to exhibit bactericidal action. It can be removed from serum by zymosan. It would be of considerable interest to determine whether natural trypanocidal antibody has these same characteristics.

Obviously, factors other than natural antibody are operative in delimiting host-trypanosome relations. As a group, trypanosomes are creatures of remarkable variety with regard to the range of hosts which they can infect. For example, within the morphologically identical *Brucei* group, *T. brucei* will infect a large number of animals ranging from cows to chickens, whereas *T. gambiense* is a reluctant parasite and is not established readily even in common laboratory animals. Some trypanosomes exhibit strange host predilections. *T. simiae* is an example *par excellence of* this phenomenon in that it produces fulminating infections only in the domestic pig and monkeys. Little is known regarding the factors influencing host-trypanosome dependencies. A hypothesis has been advanced by Desowitz and Watson (1954) that trypanosomes become adapted to a host by somehow adsorbing onto their surface a coating of serum protein that protects them, to some extent, against elaborated antibody. The hypothesis was based on the observation that the white rat, which is normally refractive to *T. vivax*, could be infected if sera from hosts normally susceptible to infection, e.g., bovines and sheep, were given as supplement (Desowitz and Watson, 1951, 1952). Sera from refractive hosts, e.g., man, monkey, and rodents, do not facilitate infection. The antibody-protection factor appears to be a serum protein or proteins (Desowitz, 1954), but it has not been definitely identified as yet. It is possible that the extraneous coat seen in electron micrographs (Vickerman, 1968) could be the bound factor.

Other maneuvers can also reduce the defenses of a normally refractory or poorly susceptible host. Splenectomy and reticuloendothelial blockade are two common experimental practices used to induce this effect. For example, splenectomy makes rabbits liable to fatal infections of *T. simiae* (Desowitz and Watson, 1953). The mechanism by which splenectomy and blockade enhances susceptibility to infection is not well understood. The functional efficiency of the macrophage system would be reduced in these animals, although cellular defense has not been generally considered to be significant in trypanosome immunity. The ability to mobilize the immunocompetent cells which elaborate humoral antibody would be impaired, and this is probably an important factor. Kuhn (1938) has presented experimental evidence that splenectomy or blockade acts by interfering with the specific sensitization of the trypanosome to antibody. Biochemical agents, such as cortisone and salicylate, or vitamin deficient diets may also enhance susceptibility. Desowitz (1963) has reviewed the work in this area.

Acquired nonspecific immunity

Despite the high degree of strain- and species-antigenic specificity attributed to trypanosomes, there are a number of nontrypanosomal antigens which will induce a protective or partially protective immunity. The antagonism of bacterial infections on experimental trypanosome infections was demonstrated over 60 years ago by Thomas and Breinl (1905) and by Nissle (1904). An excellent review on the early work on the suppressive effect of intercurrent bacterial infections was given by Laveran and Mesnil in their classic book *Trypanosomes et Trypanosomiases* (1912). In 1907, Trautmann demonstrated that the life of *T. brucei*-infected mice was prolonged when they were concurrently infected with the spirochete of relapsing fever. This phenomenon received little or no further attention until 1951, when Tate found that rats infected with *Spirillum minus* were strongly resistant to *T. equinum*. It was also observed that no protection was engendered when the trypanosomes and spirochetes were inoculated into the rat simultaneously. However, if the trypanosome challenge was administered two to four weeks after the inoculation of *S. minus*, i.e., during the acute phase, there was resistance in that the trypanosome infection was ameliorated to the extent of prolonging the life of the infected animals from the usual 5 to 17 days survival to approximately 49 weeks. There is evidence that not all strains or species of spirochetes induce this protective effect. For example, *S. duttoni*, *S. microti*, and *S. merionesi* give definite protection to mice against Brucei-group trypanosomes, whereas *S. hispanica* and *S. persica* do not (Lapierre et al., 1958; Galliard et al., 1958).

Bacterial endotoxins also exert a protective effect (Singer et al., 1964), although not as pronounced as that induced by spirochetes. Prior administration of endotoxin to mice previously made tolerant to this substance increased their survival time with *T. rhodesiense* and *T. congolense* infections. Simultaneous inoculation of endotoxin and trypanosomes had no effect in influencing the course of infection.

At present, there is no experimental evidence to account for the phenomenon of acquired nonspecific immunity. Singer and his colleagues (1964) have offered the alternative hypotheses of either enhanced natural antibody production or activation of the reticuloendothelial elements engaged in cellular immunity. There is such a paucity of data that one cannot even make a speculative comment on the first hypothesis. Regarding cellular immunity, Taliaferro (1929) described the phagocytosis of trypanosomes by wandering and fixed macrophages. However, cellular immunity does not appear to play an important role in host defense against trypanosomiasis. An important possible consideration, about which nothing is known, is that past or low-grade intercurrent infections with bacteria, spirochetes, or other organisms might influence the course of trypanosomiasis in man and domestic animals.

Acquired specific immunity

As Zuckerman and Ristic (1968) have pointed out, the mystery and uniqueness once attributed to immunity in protozoan infections have gradually given way to the understanding that "immunological phenomena relating to the protozoa are qualitatively similar to those governing other host-parasite combinations." If there is any "uniqueness" of trypanosomal immunity, it is their very broad spectrum of host-parasite relationships, which ranges from fulminating infections to an apparently sterile hyperimmunity. The interplay of inherent parasite virulence and the quantitative and qualitative aspects of the immunologic reaction are the obvious factors governing the nature of the infection. Virtually nothing is known of the mechanisms of virulence in trypanosomiasis or of why a strain or species may be more lethal or produce more disease than another (*see* Desowitz, 1963, for a review). For example, *T. rhodesiense* is presumably more virulent than *T. gambiense*. It may be argued that the antigens of *T. gambiense* are more immunogenic and somehow elicit a more satisfactory immune response; although due to their many basic similarities, it would be difficult to accept this premise.

For the most part, the influence of immunity on limiting trypanosomal infections has not been adequately elucidated. That antibody does occur has been demonstrated by a gamut of serologic reactions, but as in so many other instances, the serologic titer may bear little or no relationship to the degree of immune protection. It has been shown with African breeds of cattle that the nature of the immune response may depend on a complex of factors (Desowitz, 1959b). In West Africa there is a great difference in susceptibility among the various indigenous breeds of cattle to infections produced by *T. vivax* and *T. congolense*. The large, humped Zebu breed may be subject to fatal infections, particularly in areas of heavy exposure. They can, however, survive where the challenge is light and grazing conditions are good. In contrast, the breeds collectively designated by Stewart (1951) as West African Shorthorn possess considerable resistance. These breeds, of which N'Dama and Muturu are two examples, share the common characters of small stature, lack of hump, and relatively short horns. Chandler (1952) has confirmed the ability of N'Dama to survive in tsetse fly-infested areas. The resistance of the shorthorn is not absolute, and under such conditions as nutritional deprivation and intercurrent disease, they may also acquire fatal trypanosomiasis.

Adult Zebu (humped) cattle, born and bred in a tsetse-fly area but uninfected at time of transmission by *T. vivax*-carrying tsetse flies, developed an infection characterized by a series of intense parasitemic attacks during the first 40 days. Thereafter, the animals developed a chronic low-grade parasitemia. The immune response, as measured by the respiratory-inhibition test (Desowitz, 1956, 1959b), was correlative with the parasitemia and obviously influenced the course of infection. The rise in antibody titer was followed by crisis. Recrudescence occurred concomitantly with antibody decrease. Comparable N'Dama, also born and bred in tsetse-fly area, developed only a low-grade transient parasitemia after infection. Their antibody titer was much higher than that in Zebu. The high titer of lytic antibody was sustained for at least 100 days, and antibody was detectable even after 2 years, despite the apparent absence of circulating trypanosomes. However, N'Dama born of hyperimmune dams but raised in a tsetse fly-free area developed only a partial immunity and attendant parasitemia when challenged. Shorthorn cattle from a herd which had not been in contact with trypanosomes for many generations failed to develop any protective immunity, and the experimental infections in these animals ran a fulminating, lethal course. From these observations, it was concluded that the shorthorn breed has a special potential to acquire a hyperimmune protective state. However, the two necessary precursors of hyperimmunity are that: 1. The animal must be born of a hyperimmune dam; and 2. It must be subject to trypanosomal challenge early in life. The exact time when the latter event must take place is not known as yet. When one of these factors is absent, then only partial immunity develops. In the absence of both factors, the animal is virtually incapable of developing any immunity. Fiennes (1950b) provided further evidence that the age at which an animal receives an antigenic stimulus is an important factor in determining the nature of the immune response. He found that in calves infected with *T. congolense* during the first 2 weeks of life, the disease ends in spontaneous recovery with ensuing immunity to the infecting strain of trypanosome. However, there is as yet no direct experimental evidence of maternal transfer of antibodies via the milk or placenta (Werner, 1954).

It is generally believed that humans infected with trypanosomes invariably succumb sooner or later: sooner for those infected with *T. rhodesiense*, and later for those with *T. gambiense*. Ross (1956) argued that this is not necessarily the case. He gave examples from the past literature and from his own case histories of healthy *T. rhodesiense* carriers. The immunologic component in maintaining the "carrier" state in humans is not known, and indeed the existence of this condition requires further documentation.

It has been known for many years that a healthy carrier (reservoir) state exists in wild African ungulates. However, virtually nothing is known about the mechanism whereby an animal can harbor potentially pathogenic trypanosomes such as *T. rhodesiense* without exhibiting any obvious clinical symptoms. It is not known whether or not the immune response participates in establishing this biologically ideal form of host-parasite relationship. Following experimental infection with *T. rhodesiense, T. brucei,* and *T. vivax,* antelopes (*Gazella rufifrons* and *Sylvicapra grimmia*) produce trypanolytic and respiratory-inhibiting antibody(s) during the reservoir state (Desowitz, 1960a). Not all antelopes are resistant to clinical infection, and with some species the animal may succumb (Carmichael, 1934; Ashcroft et al., 1959; Desowitz, 1960a). Comparative studies on antibody elaboration in reservoir species and susceptible species of wild ungulates have not been carried out. The information provided by an investigation of that type would help answer the question of whether immunity is the main determinant in the reservoir state and, if so, whether an antibody is formed which differs from that in susceptible animals. It has already been shown that unlike cattle or experimental laboratory animals, there is, in infected antelopes, a striking elevation of β_2-globulin in addition to the expected elevation of γ-globulin (Desowitz, 1960a). The immunologic properties of this β_2-globulin have not as yet been determined.

SERUM PROTEIN ALTERATIONS

The acquisition of immunity or partial immunity is reflected by characteristic alterations in serum protein fractions. The electrophoretic techniques progressively developed during the past 25 years have been applied by a number of students of trypanosomal immunity.

Early observations, although differing in details, essentially agreed that in trypanosomal infections of man and some experimental animals, the albumin decreased while the γ-globulin increased (Trincao et al., 1953; Petard and Ridet, 1954; Olberg, 1955; Seneca et al., 1958; Pautrizel et al., 1959). Ganzin et al. (1952) found that in guinea pigs infected with *T. brucei*, the α_2 fraction bifurcated on electrophoresis. Both these workers and Gall (1956) found an increase in γ-globulin in humans and monkeys suffering from *T. gambiense*. The γ-globulin not only showed a marked increase, but an extra component also developed which appeared as a shoulder on the γ peak between the β- and γ-globulins (Gall, 1956). It is perhaps significant that Desowitz (1956) also found, by micro-Tiselius electrophoresis, a similar "bump" on the γ-globulin component in sera from N'Dama shorthorn cattle that were hyperimmune to *T. vivax*. Partially immune Zebu cattle, though showing an overall increase in the γ-globulin peak after challenge, did not produce this faster moving γ-globulin component. Isolation and characterization of these faster moving components have not as yet been carried out. At the other end of the host-parasite spectrum, in the fulminating disease in *T. brucei*- and *T. evansi*-infected mice, the γ-globulin and α-globulin levels are lower than those in controls (Hara et al., 1955). The β-globulin fraction increased in these acutely ill animals, but this was attributed to an impaired fat metabolism by the liver rather than to any reaction of immunologic significance. An increase in γ-globulin is sometimes found in the early acute cases of *T. rhodesiense*, but generally, the concentration is unchanged or lowered (Jenkins and Robertson, 1959). Early cases of *T. gambiense* have much higher mean γ-globulin levels than early *T. rhodesiense* infections (Evens and Charles, 1956). This might be due to the more insidious nature of *T. gambiense*. African antelopes, the reservoir hosts of trypanosomes, exhibit unique serum protein alterations following infection with *T. vivax* (Desowitz, 1960a). In bovines and sheep, only γ-globulin shows a significant increase, but in all species of antelope studied there was also a striking increment of increase in the β-globulin as well as in the γ-globulin fraction. The role, if any, that the β-globulin may play in maintaining the immune state associated with a reservoir-type host-parasite relationship is still unknown, but obviously its elucidation would be of great value.

In recent years, interest has centered on the elevation of IgM (β_2-macroglobulin, 19S globulin) which is an early feature of *Brucei*-group infections. The IgM level in human African trypanosomiasis may rise to four times the normal level (Mattern, 1964). In some of the patients, elevated IgM levels were detected prior to the onset of symptomatic disease. The application of measuring macroglobulinemia as a diagnostic aid will be discussed in a succeeding section (*see* pp. 586–587). The IgM level reverts to normal following chemotherapeutic treatment or spontaneous remission (Nicoli et al., 1961; Mattern et al., 1961). There is some evidence that the IgM produced in African trypanosomiasis differs from the macroglobulin of other pathogenic conditions such as Waldenström's disease. The terminal aminoacids of the IgM of trypanosomiasis are glutamic and aspartic acids, whereas the IgM of Waldenström's disease has glutamic acid only (Josselin et al., 1964).

Immunoglobulin changes occur in the cerebrospinal fluid (CSF) of affected individuals. In the cerebrospinal fluids of these patients, there is a rise in γ-globulin, particularly of the γ_2 and γ_3 components. There is also a rise of β_2-globulin, but not of β_1-globulin. The degree of β_2- to β_1-globulin inversion is considered by Janssens et al. (1961) to be a sensitive index of neurologic involvement. IgM and IgA have also been reported in the cerebrospinal fluids of these patients (Bideau and Massayeff, 1964; Mattern et al., 1967).

THE RELATIONSHIP OF CHEMOTHERAPY AND IMMUNITY

Ehrlich and Shiga (1904) were the first to demonstrate that experimental animals chemotherapeutically cured of their trypanosome infections became immunologically refractory to reinfection. In the years following this observation, there has gradually developed an awareness that the relationship of immunity to chemotherapy is an extremely complex bidirectional avenue; not only does chemotherapy induce and influence the immune response, but also the immunologic status of the host affects the activity of the chemotherapeutic agent. Moreover, the mode of action of antibody and some trypanocidal agents may be similar. There may also be a similarity in the process by which trypanosomes become resistant to antibody and to drugs.

The duration of immunity following chemotherapeutic cure of experimental infections has been reported to be anywhere from 8 days (Terry, 1911) to 8 months (Lourie and O'Connor, 1936). The intensity of the parasitemia at the time of drug administration appears to have some effect on the subsequent immunity. Rats given oxophenarsine when the level of parasitemia was 9 trypanosomes per cu mm were immune for at least 87 days, whereas those cured when there were 100,000 parasites per cu mm were refractory to reinfection for at least 110 days (Cantrell, 1957).

Other factors may also contribute to postchemotherapeutic immunity. The species or strain of trypanosome is of importance. Fulton and Lourie (1946) found that mice cured of *T. rhodesiense* had a much higher degree of immunity to superinfection than those cured of *T. congolense*, despite the latter animals' having high titers of trypanolysin. The authors attributed this to a difference in antigenic lability rather than to immunogenic properties. They thought *T. congolense* to be more antigenically labile than *T. rhodesiense* and therefore more capable of emerging through the barrier of homologous immunity. Many studies have shown that in rodents, postchemotherapeutic antibody is highly strain-specific. There is also no cross-immunity between parent and drug-fast strains, although this is not surprising since the latter arise from relapses and thus would be antigenic variants. However, the results obtained by Fulton and Lourie (1946) may be partly attributable to the strain of *T. congolense* they employed, since it has been shown (Browning et al., 1948) that the degree of immunity induced after cure differs markedly with various strains of this trypanosome.

The mechanism by which chemotherapy stimulates antibody production is not known with any certainty. The most likely explanation is that the drug rapidly destroys many parasites and releases their somatic antigens into the circulation, a process which would undoubtedly enhance the immune response. An additional factor may also be contributory. A portion of the trypanosomes' soluble somatic protein, probably a nucleoprotein, readily combines *in vitro* with basic trypanocidal drugs to form a relatively insoluble precipitate (Desowitz, 1960b). Preliminary experiments have indicated the drug-antigen combination affords a higher degree of protection than an equivalent amount of either drug or antigen alone. Possibly, the drug-antigen complexes are protective because their insolubility produces a depot of antigen for continuous stimulus, or the haptenic association of drug and antigen is more immunogenic than the antigen alone, or because of both.

The prophylactic protection afforded by the combined activity of drug and immunity may be of great practical value in the control of trypanosomiasis. Fulton (1944) has shown that the prophylactic action of some aromatic diamidines was considerably enhanced in experimental animals which had received frequent test challenges with trypanosomes. More pertinently, several workers (Fiennes, 1950b; Soltys, 1955; Wilson et al., 1969) have found that cattle given prophylactic compounds, such as Antrycide or Berenil, may be protected for periods of almost a year when exposed to natural challenges by infected tsetse flies. Reinforcing the immunity by a regime of inoculation with virulent organisms followed by drug treatment is also efficacious. Significantly, a sterile immunity is not usually produced by these procedures, but rather a resistance to the clinical disease results. Furthermore, the immunologic coverage may not be of the highly strain-specific type elicited in small laboratory animals. Soltys (1955) reported that the combination of Antrycide and immunity protected cattle from *T. congolense* strains coming from two widely separated areas. Fiennes (1950b) has stated,

> . . . it appears unlikely either drug therapy or immunization alone will prove to be the solution of the problem. So far as can at present be foreseen, immunization will depend on the use of living parasites, and possibly the exposure of very young animals to infection. I believe, therefore, that the final solution may lie in using a combination of drug therapy with the creation of immunity.

It is believed that the immunologic status of the infected host influences the drug dosage required to accomplish cure. There is, however, a disparity between results obtained from experiments in large animals, such as cattle, and those from experimental infections in laboratory rodents. For example, phenanthridium compounds are more effective in curing *T. congolense* infections of cattle when the disease is at the chronic stage (Randall and Laws, 1947). These authors felt that the immunity established during chronicity was essential in assisting drug action. On the other hand, Calver (1945) and Browning et al. (1948) reported that these same trypanocides are more effective in dealing with *T. congolense* of mice when the infection is at "acme." In this instance, too, the difference in drug action has been attributed to an immunologic factor, since it was believed that the relapse strains appearing during chronicity are less sensitive to the drug than are the parasites of the early stages of infection. Soltys (1959) and Soltys and Folkers (1963) have confirmed this hypothesis and have carried out further observations on the problem. Relapse strains of *T. brucei* in rabbits were considered to be antibody-resistant. These relapse trypanosomes were found to be much less sensitive both *in vitro* and *in vivo* to the action of suramin and Antrycide. It was found, for example, that the antibody-resistant strain of trypanosomes required 50 times more drug *in vitro* to render them noninfectious to mice than did the antibody-sensitive trypanosomes. It may be that a common mechanism is operative in the production of antibody resistance and drug resistance. Williamson (1962), in his comprehensive review of chemotherapy and chemoprophylaxis of African trypanosomiasis, states, "The possibility of a relation between virulence, antibody-fastness and drug resistance immediately suggests that in human sleeping sickness, the naturally tryparsamide-fast *T. rhodesiense* developed by a sojourn in an animal reservoir."

THE RELATIONSHIP OF IMMUNITY TO THE PATHOPHYSIOLOGY OF TRYPANOSOMIASIS

There is a rapidly growing body of evidence to indicate that many inappropriate immunologic responses occur which produce a variety of diseases. For example, the sequence of events leading to anoxemia-induced tissue damage in malaria is believed to be as follows: the antigen-antibody complex on a cell-fixed site leads to the release of vascular permeability-increasing factors (e.g., bradykinin), which in turn lead to a "leaky" small vasculature system, then to hypovolemia, to vasoconstriction, and finally to tissue anoxia (Tella and Maegraith, 1962, 1963; Desowitz and Pavanand, 1967; Desowitz et al., 1967; Miller and Chongsuphajaisiddhi, 1968). Very little is known of the mechanisms responsible for the production of clinical disease in trypanosomiasis, nor has the pathophysiology of the infected host been adequately described.

Recent studies implicate an immunologic component in the pathogenesis of trypanosomiasis. Boreham (1968) described the presence of kinins in rabbits, cattle, and man infected with *Brucei*-group organisms. His *in vitro* experiments support the hypothesis that antigen-antibody complexes cause the release of kinins. Boreham hypothetically proposed a pathologic process in trypanosomiasis which is almost identical to that given above for malaria. The possibility that the permeability-increasing factor consists of the pharmacologically active complement components C3a and C5a has not been explored. Alterations in the complementary cascade have been demonstrated in malaria infections (Cooper and Fogel, 1966), and considering the many similarities in the immune response between the two protozoan infections, a defect in the complementary cascade might also occur in trypanosomiasis.

Anemia and other blood abnormalities, such as autoagglutination, are prominent features of experimental and natural trypanosomal infections (see Zuckerman, 1964). Blood loss is a result of hemolysis and erythrophagocytosis, and both processes have been observed in trypanosomal infections. A number of hypotheses have been advanced to account for red-cell destruction. Nissle (1950) and Henderson-Begg (1946) held that trypanosomes and erythrocytes either share common antigens or are sufficiently alike that antibody formed against the parasites would also destroy host erythrocytes. Another mechanism would have trypanosome antigen-antibody complexes form on the surface of the red cell and the lesion so caused lead to the cell's destruction. There is also the possibility of a true autoimmunity. There has been a single report of a positive Coombs' antiglobulin test in a case of human trypanosomiasis (Zoutendyk and Gear, 1951). Additional evidence of autoimmunity is the presence of immunoconglutinin (Ingram et al., 1959), the development of which was considered by Coombs and Coombs (1953) to be "one of the best examples of autoimmunization."

It is likely that autoagglutination is a sign of red-cell alteration or sensitization and is precursive to the cells' destruction by hemolysis or erythrophagocytosis. An agglutinin in the plasma of sleeping-sickness patients was first described by Yorke (1911) and later studied by Gall et al. (1957). This agglutinin is nonspecific in that it is capable of clumping erythrocytes from noninfected individuals, as well as those from the patient. Zuckerman (1964), in reviewing the literature on the erythrocyte autoagglutinin of trypanosomiasis, adduced that it is a cold autoagglutinin. Mattern et al. (1961) found a cryoglobulin that was a β_2-macroglobulin which fixed complement and is therefore presumably an antibody. That trypanosomes adhere to the formed blood elements of infected hosts has been known for many years, and the phenomenon has been the basis for an immunospecific red-cell adhesion test (see review by Zuckerman, 1964). "Adhesin" is a specific antiparasitic antibody that operates in the presence of complement, probably C3. The antibody-coated erythrocyte is presumably more liable to destruction by the host's cellular defenses than is a normal cell. At the time when adhesin appears in the plasma, the surface charge of the host's erythrocytes is significantly lowered (Brown, 1933), an event that would also predispose them to phagocytosis.

Several recent workers have proposed that the organ pathology, particularly the lesions of the central nervous system, in trypanosomiasis is immunologically induced. Gombert et al. (1965) believed that the macroglobulin elaborated in trypanosomiasis becomes fixed to altered nervous tissue, which in turn leads to an altered metabolic behavior of the central nervous system. Similarly, Collomb and Salles (1958) advanced the theory that the multiple mononeuritis often seen in sleeping-sickness patients is caused by a cryoglobulin precipitate on the walls of the vasculature associated with the central nervous system. Seed and Gam (1967) described complement-fixing and precipitating antibodies to normal rabbit-liver antigen in rabbits infected with *T. gambiense*. They believed that host tissue antigens are released by toxin or by hypersensitivity-induced cell destruction. These tissue antigens are not recognized as self-materials by the host, and an autoimmune condition follows.

The relationship of immunity to the pathophysiology of trypanosomiasis is still on the threshold of discovery. Research in this field holds the exciting promise of illuminating the many mysteries surrounding trypanosome-induced disease. Despite this, the pathophysiology of trypanosomiasis has been a neglected field of investigation. It requires no further comment than to note that for the World Health Organization Expert Committee on Trypanosomiasis meeting of 1962, there was not a single working paper on the nature of trypanosomal disease.

IMMUNIZATION

The possibility of producing effective artificial immunization against trypanosomes has occupied the attention of investigators for more than 50 years. Limited success has been achieved in protecting against experimental infections by the inoculation of various trypanosome antigen preparations. However, a practical method of immunizing man or his domestic animals has not as yet been realized, although it is a goal still highly worthy of achievement.

Repeated injections of dead trypanosomes have been found to induce partial protection in that the life of the challenged animal is prolonged (Kligler and Comaroff, 1935). In experimentally infected rodents, the immunity is species- or strain-specific (Kliger and Berman, 1935; Lapierre and Rousset, 1961a), and most reviewers, such as Gray (1967), have attributed the inability to induce effective artificial immunity to the strain specificity of the elaborated protective antibody. Undoubtedly, the relatively low level of protective antibody produced by artificial immunization also contributes to this failure.

The immunogenicity of the antigen is associated with its nature and preparation. Lapierre and Rousset (1961b), for example, noted that immunization with formalin-killed trypanosomes affords a better protection than does immunization with acetic acid-killed organisms. Soltys (1965) reported that *T. brucei* which were inactivated with β-propiolactone induced complete protection in mice, whereas formalin- or phenol-killed trypanosomes did not. Johnson et al. (1963) found that *T. congolense* antigen with saponin or *m*-hexadecylamine adjuvants was highly immunogenic, producing a sterile immunity in a high proportion of their experimental mice. Neither Freund's adjuvant nor potassium aluminum sulfate conferred a similar effect. Chemical enhancement of trypanosome antigens would thus seem to be a promising technique and deserves further investigation.

Most experiments on artificial immunization have employed old laboratory strains of blood-form trypanosomes. The one attempt to immunize rats with a homogenate of a tsetse fly-transmitted strain of *T. brucei* failed (Gray, 1963b). Similarly, immunization with *T. brucei* metacyclics to which saponin or Freund's adjuvant had been added was also unsuccessful (Gray, 1965c). This has been the only attempt to use an antigen from a stage other than the blood form. Invertebrate-stage forms are reputedly less antigenically variable and might conceivably be more effective as immunizing antigens than the blood forms. However, further research in this direction probably must await culture techniques that allow complete test-tube recapitulation of the tsetse-fly cycle of the parasite.

Exoantigen is also immunogenic. Rats and mice can be immunized by repeated injections of exoantigen-containing sera obtained from infected animals. Exoantigen induces only a partial immunity; the life of the immunized animals is prolonged three or four days longer than that of the controls. Exoantigen-induced immunity is strain-specific (Weitz, 1960a, 1963b; Seed and Gam, 1966b; Seed and Weinman, 1963).

Very little experimental work has been carried out on passive immunity. Recently, Seed and Gam (1966b) demonstrated that mice could be completely protected against a monomorphic *T. gambiense* strain, provided that they were given antibody of sufficiently high titer and that the number of trypanosomes in the challenging inoculum was small. It is conceivable that the high-titer antibody in the sera of hyperimmune animals, such as N'Dama cattle (Desowitz, 1959b), could be effective for serum therapy. However, experiments to test this have yet to be carried out.

The foregoing discussion described attempts to confer a protective immunity by the use of nonliving antigens. For many years there has been a school of thought which has held that effective immunologic defense can only be maintained by the continuous presence of living parasites in the host, i.e., a state variously termed latent immunity or premunity. Edmond Sergent (1963), in summarizing his life-long monumental work on premunity, states:

> Premunition keeps the body defences permanently on the alert. It is in continual operation. Therefore in cases where the patient lives in an infected area, one must be careful not to completely disinfect the host by a too active drug, e.g. in trypanosomiasis and malaria. The vaccines used against diseases where premunition occurs, must be, by definition, living vaccines as they must cause a latent infection.

Schilling (1933, 1935) and Van Saceghem (1938) were able to establish premunity in calves, which are reputed to have a higher degree of resistance to trypanosomiasis than older animals, by inoculation of small numbers of trypanosomes. These animals survived longer when exposed to natural infections than did the control calves, provided the challenging trypanosome was antigenically related. Fiennes (1947) also described resistance to superinfection of cattle premunized to *T. congolense*. He noted, however, that these animals were in a poorer state of health than were those which developed a protective immunity following chemotherapeutic cure. Premunity could best be induced by inoculation of nonvirulent organisms in a manner similar to that used for immunization against some viral infections. However, nonvirulent strains with sufficient antigenic similarity to the natural tsetse fly-transmitted strains have not as yet been isolated, nor has a systematic search been made for them.

SEROLOGY AND IMMUNODIAGNOSIS

Antibodies elicited in trypanosomiasis are evidenced by a multiplicity of serologic reactions. Some of these reactions have served as diagnostic aids, others have provided insight into the state of actual immunity, while others remain as immunologic curiosities. The early literature on the subject has been reviewed by Taliaferro (1929), and therefore the present discussion will, for the most part, be confined to more recent investigations.

Complement-fixation test. One of the oldest serologic techniques for trypanosomiasis diagnosis is the complement-fixation test (CFT) introduced by Citron in 1907. There are a number of investigators who still advocate it as the best adjunctive diagnostic method. The antigen reactant has been prepared from disrupted trypanosomes, and it possesses a sufficiently broad spectrum of specificity so that *T. equiperdum* antigen can be used in the serologic diagnosis of *T. gambiense* infections (Schoenaers et al., 1953a, b; Pautrizel et al., 1960, 1962). The reported efficacy of the CFT is indeed impressive; investigations have shown that over 95 percent of proved cases give a positive complement-fixation reaction (Schoenaers et al., 1953; Depaux et al., 1956; Neujean and Evens, 1958; Pautrizel et al., 1960). Moreover, both normal and Wasserman-positive controls were almost invariably negative. Complement-fixing antibodies appear rapidly after infection. For example, *T. equiperdum*-infected rabbits become CFT positive three days after inoculation (Pautrizel et al., 1959), and the sera of experimentally infected human subjects become positive between the seventh and fifteenth day (Neujean and Evens, 1958). In the guinea pig, which generally shows a relapsing infection with *T. equiperdum*, the CF titer falls to approximately one third of its previous level after crisis (Horner, 1939).

The CFT is most applicable in the diagnosis of early cases. As a general rule, the titer diminishes or becomes negative when the infection has progressed to the stage of central nervous system involvement. Following chemotherapy and subsequent clinical cure, the CFT becomes negative. Depaux et al. (1956) observed that in treated early cases, clinical cure precedes the fall in titer, whereas in treated late cases, the opposite occurs.

The CFT is less reliable in detecting relapses. Evens et al. (1953) reported that complement-fixing antibody was detectable in only 80 percent of relapsed patients. Neverthless, even in these cases the CFT is of value since in some instances a positive CFT signalled a relapse in the absence of demonstrable parasites (Evens et al., 1953; Pautrizel et al., 1960).

The difficulties in performing the CFT are well-known, and the test is obviously not suitable for field use. Despite this, its proved reliability recommends its use where facilities are available. The ability to use group-specific antigens is another point in its favor.

Agglutination test. The agglutination test also has a long history, its introduction in pathogenic trypanosome serology being almost contemporaneous with that of the complement-fixation test (Lange, 1911; Laveran and Mesnil, 1912; Mattes, 1912). The killed, formalinized trypanosomes used in the earlier studies did not give sufficient sensitivity for either experimental or diagnostic purposes. A modern modification of the test employs living trypanosomes taken from mice at "acme" (Soltys, 1957b; Cunningham and Vickerman, 1962). Soltys reported the test to be species-specific, while other workers, such as Watkins (1964), Pautrizel et al. (1962), and Gray (1965a,b), have found it to be strain- or clone-specific.

Lumsden (1967) remarked that the direct agglutination test has yielded a great deal of information, but erratic results often make this information difficult to interpret. Lumsden maintained that these inconsistencies result because of a failure to work with a single antigenic type or because the organisms have already been in contact with antibody. He also noted that the direct agglutination test, besides being applicable only to antigens available at high concentrations, is difficult to standardize with respect to the quantities of materials used, and end-point determination is often extremely uncertain.

The agglutination test has been applied to studies on antigenic relationships and variation, a subject which is discussed elsewhere in this chapter (*see* p. 561).

Indirect hemagglutination test. The indirect or passive hemagglutination test (IHA) is also of possible value as a diagnostic tool in trypanosomiasis. The method has already been of considerable value in the serology of such protozoan diseases as amoebiasis, toxoplasmosis, and malaria. The advantages of the IHA are that only small amounts of relatively stable reactants are necessary, and that in experienced hands, it is a highly sensitive and reproducible method of detecting antibody. Gill (1964) has described a passive hemagglutination technique using a cell-free extract prepared from ultrasonicated *T. evansi* as antigen and sera from experimentally immunized rabbits as antibody.

Fluorescent-antibody test. Of the newer immunologic techniques, the fluorescent-antibody (FA) test has undoubtedly excited the most interest, although examination of the literature (Desowitz, 1966) often reveals that the interest is out of proportion to its specificity, ease of performance, and quantitation.

Williams et al. (1963) found that trypanosomes fixed in 5 percent formalin-rhodamine bovine albumin gave optimal results in the presence of immune sera. Rabbits experimentally infected with either *T. rhodesiense* or *T. gambiense* showed a positive FA test as early as one week after inoculation. Intergeneric specificity was not determined in their experiments, but there was an indication of broad-spectrum reaction, since antisera to *T. rhodesiense* and *T. gambiense* gave a strongly positive FA reaction with *T. lewisi* antigen.

In a study with sera from sleeping-sickness patients, Sadun et al. (1963) found that normal human serum controls gave anywhere from 4 percent to 12.5 percent false positive reactions (positive and doubtful reactions). Furthermore, 30 percent and 40 percent of the sera from patients with malaria cross-reacted with *T. rhodesiense* and *T. gambiense*, respectively. In view of the coendemicity of malaria and trypanosomiasis in Africa, this cross-reaction would severely limit the usefulness of the FA test as a diagnostic aid. Bailey et al. (1967) tested the sera of 50 *T. rhodesiense*-infected patients and 130 healthy human controls using the indirect fluorescent-antibody technique. With *T. rhodesiense* antigen, 98 percent of the patients' sera gave a positive reaction and 66 percent of the controls gave a false positive; however, in most instances the degree of fluorescence was much greater with sera from the infected humans.

The cerebrospinal fluid also acquires immunofluorescent antibodies when the infection reaches the stage of central nervous system involvement (Lucasse, 1964; Mattern et al., 1965). All three classes of immunoglobulins, IgG, IgA, and IgM, are reported to participate in the reaction (Mattern et al., 1965).

Cunningham et al. (1967) applied the indirect FA test to immunity in bovine trypanosomiasis. Sera of cattle infected with *T. theileri*, a common nonpathogenic organism, were reactive with *T. brucei*, *T. congolense*, and *T. vivax* antigens, and in view of this these workers recommended that sera to be tested for antibody to the pathogenic trypanosomes should be diluted to 1:40. In confirmation of the findings of Williams et al. (1963), these East African workers concluded that the indirect FA test detects common antibodies. This group also noted that in *T. congolense* infections of Zebu cattle, the antibody detectable by the indirect FA test is usually not continuously present, but it disappears after crisis and reappears at relapse.

Precipitation tests.   Precipitating antibodies are also elaborated in trypanosome infections. Double-diffusion and immunoelectrophoretic techniques have been employed to analyze somatic and exoantigens, as discussed earlier (*see* pp. 553–561). A precipitation test has not, as yet, generally been used for diagnostic purposes. Mattern et al. (1967) detected precipitating antibody in 9 of 59 sleeping-sickness patients. In some cases, antibody was present many years after presumed chemotherapeutic cure. These workers found IgG was a precipitin, but not IgM. Schoenaers (1950) found that sera of bovines infected with *T. vivax* possessed precipitating antibody, although sera from animals infected with *T. congolense* did not. Provided its sensitivity can be improved, the precipitin test has much to recommend it as a potential diagnostic method. It requires small amounts of reactants, nonliving antigen is used, and it is a simple method not requiring elaborate or expensive equipment.

Direct versus indirect immunodiagnostic tests. With the exception of the agglutination test, the serologic methods described above are, in a sense, indirect in that they measure the effect of antibody on the dead trypanosome or extract of the organism. Ideally, a serologic technique should be able to provide information leading to a diagnosis and to give an assessment of the patient's immunologic defense. However, though many of the "indirect" techniques are of diagnostic value, they do not seem to measure functional, protective antibody. For example, Gray (1966) noted that: "Many samples of sera from cattle in enzootic trypanosomiasis areas contained precipitating or agglutinating antibodies to *T. brucei*, but there was little correlation between serum antibody content and infection or species of infecting trypanosome." Because of this deficiency, the application of modern serologic methods has not produced a better fundamental understanding of the mechanisms of immunity to trypanosomiasis. Thus, the tests which actually reflect the action of antibody on the trypanosome's life processes might be of service in this direction.

Neutralization tests. It has been recognized for many years that antibody has a direct deleterious effect upon the trypanosome. In 1911, Leger and Ringenbach demonstrated the presence of specific lytic antibody in the sera of *T. brucei*-infected guinea pigs following parasitic crisis, and this observation led to the development of a neutralization test.

This neutralization test has recently been refined by Soltys (1957a) to yield quantitative, reproducible results. The Soltys neutralization test, essentially, is carried out by mixing trypanosomes and antibody *in vitro* and determining the consequent parasite inactivation by inoculation into mice. In rabbits experimentally infected with *T. brucei*, neutralizing antibody appears within 5 days of inoculation and attains a peak titer on about the 25th day. Following treatment with suramin, the titer gradually declines until it is no longer detectable after 22 weeks. Soltys (1957a) has also demonstrated that rabbits immunized with formalinized trypanosomes produce neutralizing antibody to the same level as do infected rabbits. Neutralizing antibody is species- and, probably, strain-specific. It is also reported to be heat-stable, although in common with other lytic phenomena, it requires complement. However, lysis of the rodent-adapted strain of *T. vivax* differs in that the addition of complement does not appear to be necessary. It has been suggested that this trypanosome produces a complement-like substance itself (Clarkson and Awan, 1969).

A variation of the neutralization test is the mouse-protection test. This technique is carried out by inoculating the serum to be tested into infected mice and then observing if it produces cure or an extension of life in comparison to untreated controls. For many investigative purposes, the neutralization and protection tests have their limitations. They are difficult to quantitate with any precision, it requires several days before results are observable, and they are not particularly instructive as to the mode of antibody action.

Respiratory-inhibition test. Trypanolytic antibody of high titer causes rapid disruption of the parasite. However, at lower levels, it appears to act in a slower, more subtle fashion on the trypanosome's life processes. This phenomenon was exploited in devising an immunorespirometric test in which the oxygen consumption of trypanosomes suspended in normal control serum and in serum which contains antibody is compared (Desowitz, 1956; 1958).

The method provides a quantitative assessment of the effect of antibody directly on the living organism. It has also been shown by sequential study of infected bovines and antelopes that the changes in respiratory-inhibition titers (indices) correlate logically with the course of infection (Desowitz, 1959b, 1960a). Thurston (1958) confirmed the inhibitory effect of antibody on the respiration of *T. brucei*.

The test appears to be species-specific. It has been shown (Desowitz, 1961) that the inhibitory antibody produced by sheep against the three *Brucei*-group trypanosomes was relatively specific against polymorphic strains, while there was almost a complete cross-reactivity between old, laboratory-maintained, monomorphic strains.

The sera of humans infected with *T. gambiense* have been shown to contain respiratory-inhibiting antibody. Desowitz (1958) reported that 17 of 18 patients exhibited respiratory-inhibiting antibody indices ranging from 3.5 to 84.2.* Masseyeff and Gombert (1963) also found that the sera of 16 out of 17 sleeping-sickness patients inhibited the respiration of *T. gambiense*, whereas the sera of normal humans and those from 23 patients with diseases other than trypanosomiasis did not. In another trial, Gombert (1963) found that 59 of 62 sera from sleeping-sickness patients gave a high respiratory-inhibition index. Sera stored at $-20°C$ to $-60°C$ for more than six months had a somewhat lower index. The results of Gombert's experiments are summarized in Table 3.

The respirometric method fulfills two important criteria for a good immunologic technique: it is species-specific and it appears to assess the state of functional immunity. However, the relatively complicated procedure of Warburg respirometry would tend to preclude its use as a standard diagnostic procedure. In our laboratory, we have recently used the polarographic oxygen monitor instead of the Warburg apparatus with highly satisfying results. With this instrument, respirometric determinations are easily performed, and results can be obtained with small amounts of material in a matter of minutes.

Dye test. Molinari (1961) unsuccessfully attempted to adapt the Sabin-Feldman dye test for toxoplasmosis to trypanosomiasis.

---

* Respiratory-inhibition index = $[(A - B)/A] \times 100$.
  A = microliters of O_2 consumption per hour by trypanosomes suspended in normal serum.
  B = microliters of O_2 consumption per hour by trypanosomes suspended in serum tested for antibody.

Table 3
Number of Sera or Cerebrospinal Fluids Giving a Respiratory Inhibition Index

Specimen	Number of Sera or CSF	Respiratory Inhibition Index									
		0–10	11–20	21–30	31–40	41–50	51–60	61–70	71–80	81–90	91–100
T. gambiense patients' sera stored less than six months	62	3	—	—	—	—	—	9	14	27	9
T. gambiense patients' sera stored more than six months	7	3	—	1	1	1	1	—	—	—	—
Patients' sera during the course of treatment	3	—	—	—	—	—	—	2	1	—	—
Sera of treated patients six months after clinical recovery	8	1	2	1	—	—	—	—	—	—	—
Sera of clinically suspect patients but without parasitologic confirmation	3	—	—	—	—	—	—	—	—	3	—
CSF from trypanosomiasis cases	4	—	1	1	—	—	—	—	1	1	—
CSF from uninfected humans	3	2	1	—	—	—	—	—	—	—	—
Sera with a high content of IgM from humans without trypanosomiasis	12	11	—	—	1	—	—	—	—	—	—
Sera with a high content of IgM from humans without sleeping sickness but living in an old endemic area	16	5	4	4	3	—	—	—	—	—	—
Control sera from healthy humans	50	50	—	—	—	—	—	—	—	—	—

From Gombert (1963).

Hyperglobulinemia tests. A number of nonspecific serodiagnostic procedures have been described which do not employ trypanosome antigen. These reactions depend upon alterations in serum protein constituents, chiefly the rise in IgM, occurring in trypanosomal infections. Prior to the modern recognition of the classes of immunoglobulins, it was known that the fractions designated as globulin and euglobulin increased in trypanosomiasis. The elevation of these components in kala-azar and trypanosomiasis produces a positive serum-formalin test, and this reaction has been used as a diagnostic method by various workers since 1925. A history and evaluation of the method has been given by Cookson (1947), who concluded from his study that the serum-formalin reaction was of great value in diagnosing doubtful cases. Its chief virtue is its simplicity of performance which permits its use by the investigator working under primitive conditions.

Griffiths (1958) described a colloidal gum-mastic reaction which depends on the precipitation of mastic from colloidal suspensions of serum in which there is a hyperglobulinemia. Rabbits and sheep experimentally infected with *T. brucei* and *T. rhodesiense* gave a positive reaction, but the test has not been further assessed with sera of sleeping-sickness patients.

A number of investigators have shown that the hypermacroglobulinemia occurring in trypanosomiasis is sufficiently characteristic to be of diagnostic value. However, the condition also occurs in other African diseases, such as malaria, so it is not absolutely pathognomonic of trypanosomiasis. There may be considerable overlap between the results with sera from healthy subjects and those with trypanosomiasis. Furthermore, at least 3 percent of parasitologically positive cases give a negative double-diffusion test (Binz, et al., 1968).

IgM levels in sera and cerebrospinal fluids have been measured by double-diffusion in agar gel or cellulose acetate (Bideau and Masseyeff, 1964) and by immunoelectrophoresis. The "immuno-plate" diffusion method is probably the simplest and most practical technique for diagnostic purposes.

Cunningham et al. (1967) have described the use of dried blood on filter paper from which serum can later be eluted for IgM estimation by immunodiffusion. They consider that the method can be used as a screen test in the diagnosis of human trypanosomiasis. It has the advantage that the blood can be collected in the field and sent by post to a central laboratory. Dutertre and Boisson (1968) compared the results obtained by Cunningham's filter-paper method and the conventional double-diffusion technique. There was a significant correlation between the results of the two methods except when the diameter of the precipitation ring was between 5.1 and 6.0 mm. They suggested that these sera should be re-examined by the conventional double-diffusion technique.

Mattern (1968) has reviewed the measurement of serum IgM increase as a means for presumptive diagnosis. He believes it is of value in a negative way, since the absence of such a rise almost certainly rules out trypanosomal infection. On the other hand, he noted that the rise in cerebrospinal IgM is almost conclusive evidence of late-stage trypanosomal infection with central nervous system involvement. Even in the earlier hemolymphatic stage, 12 out of 60 patients were found to have IgM in their cerebrospinal fluid. On a basis of their own findings, Watson and Chirieleison (1966) generally concur with Mattern, but caution that: "With careful clinical examination of the patient to eliminate other obvious conditions which might cause a rise in IgM titer, the utility of this technique in sleeping sickness diagnosis is considerable. A certain diagnosis is, however, still dependent upon finding trypanosomes."

Immunoconglutination test. Another "nonantigen" serologic method which has been applied to trypanosomiasis is immunoconglutination. The clumping of red blood cells in this reaction is due to a natural antibody to erythrocytes and an aggregating substance termed conglutinin. Ingram et al. (1959) showed that the conglutinin level markedly increased during the acute and chronic phases of *T. brucei* infection in rabbits. In a later study, Ingram and Soltys (1960) found conglutinin to appear 7 days after inoculation of trypanosomes into rabbits or cats, and it reached a peak titer on about the 15th to 30th day, depending upon the virulence of the strain. The conglutinin titer dropped rapidly after effective chemotherapy, whereas the neutralizing-antibody level showed little alteration. Unlike other serologic reactions, the conglutinin titer was elevated only by active infection and not by immunization with dead trypanosomes. Pautrizel et al. (1962) also evaluated the conglutinin test with sera of sleeping-sickness patients and of experimentally infected animals. They felt that it was a more sensitive test than the CFT, but they experienced some difficulty in using it, since some sera had a poor combining affinity and a zone phenomenon also occurred.

Conclusion. It is evident from the foregoing discussion that a number of serologic techniques have potential clinical values. It is also evident that each needs further testing and refinement before it can be confidently accepted as a common diagnostic procedure. The need for a good immunodiagnostic method is very real. Weinman (1963) noted in his review of the literature that based on parasitologic findings alone, the diagnostic failure rate may be as high as 10 percent to 25 percent.

REFERENCES

Adams, A.R.D. 1933. A record of an investigation into the action of sera on the trypanosomes pathogenic to man. Ann. Trop. Med. Parasit., 27:309-326.

Ashcroft, M.T., E. Burtt, and H. Fairbairn. 1959. The experimental infection of some African wild animals with *Trypanosoma rhodesiense, T. brucei,* and *T. congolense.* Ann. Trop. Med. Parasit., 53:147-161.

Bailey, N.M., M.P. Cunningham, and C.D. Kimber. 1967. *In* East African Trypanosomiasis Research Organization Report for 1966. Government Printer, Entebbe, Uganda.

Bideau, J., and R. Masseyeff. 1964. Mise en évidence de la B₂-macroglobuline dans le sérum et dans le L. C. R. des trypanosomes par immuno-diffusion double en acetate de cellulose. Bull. Soc. Path. Exot., 57:1231-1236.

Binz, G., G. Timperman, and M.P. Hutchinson. 1968. Estimation of serum immunoglobulin M as a screening technique for trypanosomiasis. A field trial in the Democratic Republic of the Congo. Bull. W. H. O., 38:523-545.

Boreham, P.F.L. 1968. The possible role of kinins in the pathogenesis of chronic trypanosomiasis. Trans. Roy. Soc. Trop. Med. Hyg., 62:120-121.

Braun, H., and E. Teichmann. 1912. Versuche zur Immunisierung gegen Trypanosomen. Jena, Gustav Fischer.

Bray, R.S. 1967. The question of antigenic variation among parasitic protozoa. J. Fac. Med. Baghdad, 9:102-112.

Broom, J.C., and H.C. Brown. 1940. Studies in trypanosomiasis. IV. Notes on the serological characters of *Trypanosoma brucei* after cyclical development in *Glossina morsitans*. Trans. Roy. Soc. Trop. Med. Hyg., 34:53-64.

Brown, H.C. 1933. Further observations on the electric charge of the erythrocytes in certain protozoal diseases. Brit. J. Exp. Path., 14:413-421.

Brown, K.N. 1961. Studies on the immunology of trypanosomiasis. Ann. Trop. Med. Parasit., 55:143-144.

——— 1963. The antigenic character of the Brucei trypanosomes. *In* Immunity to Protozoa. Garnham, P.C.C., Pierce, A.E., and Roitt, I., eds. Oxford, Blackwell Scientific Publications, pp. 204-212.

——— and J. Williamson. 1962. Antigens of *Brucei* trypanosomes. Nature (London), 194:1253-1255.

——— and J. Williamson. 1964. The chemical composition of trypanosomes. IV. Location of antigens in subcellular fractions of *Trypanosoma rhodesiense*. Exp. Parasit., 15:69-86.

Browning, C.H., K.M. Calver, and H. Adamson. 1948. The chemotherapy of *Trypanosoma congolense* infection with phenanthridinium compounds etc. J. Path. Bact., 60:336-339.

Calver, K.M. 1945. Chemotherapeutic studies on experimental *T. congolense* infections. Ph.D. Thesis, University of Glasgow, Glasgow, Scotland.

Cantrell, W. 1957. Duration of acquired immunity to *Trypanosoma equiperdum* in the rat. J. Infect. Dis., 101:175-180.

Carmichael, J. 1934. Trypanosomes pathogenic to domestic stock and their effect in certain species of wild fauna in Uganda. Ann. Trop. Med. Parasit., 28:41-45.

Chandler, R. L. 1952. Comparative tolerance of West African N'Dama cattle to trypanosomiasis. Ann. Trop. Med. Parasit., 46:127-134.

Christophers, S.R., and J.D. Fulton. 1938. Observations on the respiratory metabolism of malaria parasites and trypanosomes. Ann. Trop. Med. Parasit., 32:43-75.

Citron. 1907. Deutsch. Med. Wschr., 29. Quoted in Laveran and Mesnil, 1912.

Clarkson, M.J., and M.A.Q. Awan. 1969. Complement and immune lysis of trypanosomes. Trans. Roy. Soc. Trop. Med. Hyg., 63:9.

Collier, W. A. 1924. Über einen Versuch, Tsetsetrypanosomen durch Festigung gegen Menschenserum menschenpathogen zu machen. Arch. Schiffs. Trop. Hyg., 28:484-488.

Collomb, H., and P. Salles. 1958. Du rôle possible des facteurs humoraux (cryoglobulines) dans la pathogénie de certaines manifestations nerveuses de la trypanosomiase humaine africaine, des atteintes périphériques en particulier. Bull. Soc. Path. Exot., 51:177-180.

Cookson, L.O.C. 1947. The serum-formalin reaction in *Trypanosoma rhodesiense* sleeping sickness. J. Trop. Med. Hyg., 50:134-140.

Coombs, A.M., and R.R.A. Coombs. 1953. The conglutination phenomenon. IX. The production of immunoconglutinin in rabbit. J. Hyg. (Cambridge), 51:509-531.

Coombs, R.R.A., and P.J. Lachman. 1968. Immunological reactions at the cell surface. Brit. Med. Bull., 24:113-117.

Cooper, N.R., and B.J. Fogel. 1966. Complement in acute experimental malaria. II. Alterations in the components of complement. Milit. Med., 131 (Suppl.):1180-1190.

Corson, J.F. 1933. A note on some experiments on the action *in vitro* of normal human serum on *Trypanosoma brucei* and *T. rhodesiense*. J. Trop. Med. Hyg., 36:53-55.

Culbertson, J.T., and P.S. Strong. 1935. The trypanocidal action of normal human serum. The nature of the substance responsible for the trypanocidal effect and its relationship with the bacteriocidal activity of normal human serum. Amer. J. Hyg., 21:1-17.

Cunningham, M.P. and K. Vickerman. 1962. Antigenic analysis in the *Trypanosoma brucei* group, using the agglutination reaction. Trans. Roy. Soc. Trop. Med. Hyg., 56:48-59.

——— N.M. Bailey, and C.D. Kimber. 1967. East African Trypanosomiasis Research Organization Report of 1966. East African Common Services Organization. Entebbe, Uganda, Government Printers.

Depaux, R., P. Merveille, and J. Ceccaldi. 1956. Étude de la réaction de fixation du complement dans la trypanosomiase humaine. Ann. Inst. Pasteur (Paris), 91:684-692.

Desowitz, R.S. 1954. Studies on *Trypanosoma vivax*. X. The activity of some blood fractions in facilitating infection in the white rat. Ann. Trop. Med. Parasit., 48:142-151.

——— 1956. Effect of antibody on the respiratory rate of *Trypanosoma vivax*. Nature (London), 177:132-133.

——— 1958. The measurement of antibody occurring in human and bovine trypanosomiasis by a respirometric method. Proceedings of the Sixth International Congress on Tropical Medicine and Malaria, Vol. 3, pp. 236-240.

——— 1959a. Paper electrophoresis of trypanosomal extracts. Nature (London), 184:986.

——— 1959b. Studies on immunity and host-parasite relationships. I. The immunological response of resistant and susceptible breeds of cattle to trypanosomal challenge. Ann. Trop. Med. Parasit., 53:293-313.

——— 1960a. Studies on immunity and host-parasite relationships. II. The immune response of antelope to trypanosomal challenge. Ann. Trop. Med. Parasit., 54:281-292.

——— 1960b. Denaturant effect of basic trypanocidal drugs on the protein of cell-free trypanosomal extracts. Exp. Parasit., 9:233-238.

——— 1961. Antigenic relationships between polymorphic and monomorphic strains of the *Brucei* group trypanosomes. J. Immun., 86:69-72.

——— 1963. Adaptation of trypanosomes to abnormal hosts. Ann. N. Y. Acad. Sci., 113:74-87.

——— 1966. Serological techniques in parasitology—Some comments by a devil's advocate. Med. J. Malaya, 21:35-40.

——— and H.J.C. Watson. 1951. Studies on *Trypanosoma vivax*. I. Susceptibility of white rats to infection. Ann. Trop. Med. Parasit., 45:207-219.

——— and H.J.C. Watson. 1952. Studies on *Trypanosoma vivax*. III. Observations on the maintenance of a strain in white rats. Ann. Trop. Med. Parasit., 46:92-100.

——— and H.J.C. Watson. 1953. The maintenance of a strain of *Trypanosoma simiae* in rabbits. The effect of splenectomy on the course of infection. Ann. Trop. Med. Parasit., 47:324-334.

——— and H.J.C. Watson. 1954. Studies on *Trypanosoma vivax*. VI. The occurrence of antibodies in the sera of infected sheep and white rats and their influence on the course of infection in white rats. Ann. Trop. Med. Parasit., 47:247-257.

——— and K. Pavanand. 1967. A vascular-permeability increasing factor in the serum of monkeys infected with primate malarias. Ann. Trop. Med. Parasit., 61:128-133.

——— L.H. Miller, R.D. Buchanan, V. Yuthasastrkosol, and B. Permpanich. 1967. Comparative studies on the pathology and host physiology of malarias. I. *Plasmodium coatneyi*. Ann. Trop. Med. Parasit., 61:365-374.

Dodin, A., and H. Fromentin. 1962. Mise en évidence d'un antigène vaccinant dans le plasma de souris experimentalement infectées par *Trypanosoma gambiense* et par *T. congolense*. Bull. Soc. Path. Exot., 55:128-138.

——— H. Fromentin, and M. Gleyne. 1962. Mise en évidence d'un antigène vaccinant dans le plasma de souris expérimentalement infectées par diverses espèces de Trypanosomes. Bull. Soc. Path. Exot., 55:291-299.

Dutertre, J., and P. Boisson. 1968. La sérologie de la trypanosomiase sur sang desseché. Essai de la methode des confetti de Cunningham. Méd. Trop. (Marseille), 28:649-662.

Ehrlich, P., and K. Shiga. 1904. Farben therapeutische Versuche bei Trypansomenerkrankung. Berlin. Klin. Wschr., 41:329 and 362.

Evens, F., and P. Charles. 1956. Preliminary note on the study of blood proteins in *T. gambiense* sleeping sickness patients. Paper presented at 6th meeting of International Scientific Committee for Trypanosomiasis Research (mimeographed).

——— F. Schoenaers, G. Neujean, A. Kaeckenbeek, and J. Styns. 1953. Valeur practique de la réaction de fixation du complément dans la maladie du sommeil à *T. gambiense*. II. La réaction de fixation du complement lois d'une rechute après traitement medicamenteux. Ann. Soc. Belg. Med. Trop., 33:389-402.

Fairbairn, H. 1933a. Experimental infection of man with a strain of *Trypanosoma rhodesiense*. Ann. Trop. Med. Parasit., 27:185-205.

——— 1933b. The action of human serum *in vitro* on sixty-four recently isolated strains of *T. rhodesiense*. Ann. Trop. Med. Parasit., 27:185-205.

——— 1937. The infectivity to man of a strain of *Trypanosoma rhodesiense* transmitted through sheep by *Glossina morsitans*, and its resistance to human serum *in vitro*. Ann. Trop. Med. Parasit., 31:285-291.

Fiennes, R.N.T.-W.-. 1947. Immunity and premunity in cattle trypanosomiasis. Vet. Rec., 59:292.

——— 1950a. The cattle trypanosomiases: Cryptic trypanosomiases. Ann. Trop. Med. Parasit., 44:222-237.

——— 1950b. The cattle trypanosomiases: Some considerations of pathology and immunity. Ann. Trop. Med. Parasit., 44:42-54.

Franke, E. 1905. Über Trypanosomentherapie. München Med. Wschr., 52:2059-2060.

Fulton, J.D. 1944. The prophylactic action of various aromatic diamidines in trypanosomiasis of mice. Ann. Trop. Med. Parasit., 38:78-84.

——— and E.M. Lourie. 1946. The immunity of mice cured of trypanosome infections. Ann. Trop. Med. Parasit., 40:1-9.

Gall, D. 1956. Blood protein changes in sleeping sickness. J. West Afr. Sci. Ass., 2:152-157.

——— M.P. Hutchinson, and W. Yates. 1957. The erythrocyte sedimentation rate in sleeping sickness. Ann. Trop. Med. Parasit., 51:136-150.

Galliard, H., J. La Pierre, and J. J. Rousset. 1958. Comportement spécifique des différentes espèces de "Borrelia" au cours de l'infection mixte avec "Trypanosoma brucei." Son utilisation comme test d'identification des spirochaetes récurrents. Ann. Parasit. Hum. Comp., 33:177-208.

Ganzin, M., P. Rebeyrotte, M. Macheboeuf, and G. Montezin. 1952. Étude par électrophorese des fractions protéiques du sérum sanguin d'hommes et de cobayes infectés par de trypanosomes. Bull. Soc. Path. Exot., 45:518-524.

Gill, B.S. 1964. A procedure for the indirect haemagglutination test for the study of experimental *Trypanosoma evansi* infections. Ann. Trop. Med. Parasit., 58:473-480.

Godfrey, D.J. 1967. Phospholipids of *Trypanosoma lewisi, T. vivax, T. congolense,* and *T. brucei.* Exp. Parasit., 20:106-118.

Goebel, O. 1907. Pouvoir préventif et pouvoir curatif du sérum humain dans l'infection due au Trypanosome du Nagana. Ann. Inst. Pasteur (Paris), 21:882-910.

Gombert, J. 1963. Contribution à l'etude des anticorps de la trypanosomiase africaine à *T. gambiense.* Thesis. Toulouse, Toulousaine Vve R. Lion.

——— Y. Bresson, and R. Masseyeff. 1965. Comportment métabolique anormal de la macroimmuniglobuline des malades atteints de trypanosome africaine. Bull. Mem. Fac. Mixte Med. Pharm., Dakar, 13:135-144.

Gray, A. R. 1961. Soluble antigens of *Trypanosoma vivax* and of other trypanosomes. Immunology, 4:253-261.

——— 1962. The influence of antibody on serological variation. Ann. Trop. Med. Parasit., 56:4-13.

——— 1963a. Antigenic variation in a fly-transmitted strain of *Trypanosoma brucei*. Seventh Int. Sci. Comm. Tryp. Res., p. 361.

——— 1963b. Cited in the Annual Report on the West African Institute for Trypanosomiasis Research, p. 37.

——— 1965a. Antigenic variation in clones of *Trypanosoma brucei*. I. Immunological relationships of the clones. Ann. Trop. Med. Parasit., 59:27-36.

——— 1965b. Antigenic variation in a strain of *Trypanosoma brucei* transmitted by *Glossina morsitans* and *G. palpalis*. J. Gen. Microbiol., 41:195-214.

——— 1965c. Cited in the Annual Report of the Nigerian Institute for Trypanosomiasis Research, pp. 42-43.

——— 1966. Immunological studies on the epizootiology of *Trypanosoma brucei* in Nigeria. Eleventh Meeting Int. Sci. Comm. Tryp. Res. (Nairobi, 1966). O.A.U./S.T.R.C., Publication No. 100, pp. 57-62.

——— 1967. Some principles of the immunology of trypanosomiasis. Bull. W. H. O., 37:177-193.

Griffiths, B.L. 1958. The colloidal gum mastic reaction in experimental trypanosomiasis. J. Med. Lab. Tech., 15:275-279.

Grünmandel, S., and B. Leichtentritt. 1924. Der Gehalt des kindlichen Serums an trypanozider Substanz. Jahrb. Kinderheilk., 106:203.

Handler, B.J. 1935. Studies on the trypanocidal power of normal human serum. Amer. J. Hyg., 21:18-26.

Hara, K., S. Oka, K. Takagi, K. Nagata, and T. Sawada. 1955. Studies on the variation of serum and liver proteins in mice infected with trypanosome. Gunma J. Med. Sci., 4:295-301.

Henderson-Begg, A. 1946. Heterophile antibodies in trypanosomiasis. Trans. Roy. Soc. Trop. Med. Hyg., 40:331-339.

Hoare, C.A. 1948a. The relationship of the haemoflagellates. *In* Proceedings of the Fourth International Congress of Tropical Medicine and Malaria, pp. 1110-1116.

———— 1948b. Reservoir host of human trypanosomiases. Proc. Roy. Soc. Med., 41:553-558.

Horner, I. 1939. Studies on serum complement of guinea pigs infected with *Trypanosoma equiperdum*. J. Immun., 37:85-89.

Ikejiani, O. 1946. The antigenic composition and the effect of various extracts of *Trypanosoma equiperdum* and *Trypanosoma lewisi* on the leucocyte picture in experimental trypanosomiasis. Amer. J. Hyg., 45:144-149.

Ingram, D. G., and M. A. Soltys. 1960. Immunity in trypanosomiasis. IV. Immunoconglutinin in animals infected with *Trypanosoma brucei*. Parasitology, 50:231-239.

———— H. Barber, D.M. McLean, M.A. Soltys, and R.R.A. Coombs. 1959. The conglutination phenomenon. XII. Immuno-conglutinin in experimental infections of laboratory animals. Immunology, 2:268-282.

Inoki, S. 1960. Studies on the antigenic variation in the Welcome strain of *Trypanosoma gambiense*. II. On the first relapse in mice treated with human plasma. Biken J., 3:223-228.

———— T. Kitaura, T. Nakabayashi and H. Kurogochi. 1952. Studies on the immunological variations in *Trypanosoma gambiense*. I. A new variation system and a new experimental method. Med. J. Osaka Univ., 3:357-371.

———— T. Nakabayashi, H. Osaki, and S. Fukukita. 1957. Studies on the immunological variation in *Trypanosoma gambiense*. III. Process of the antigenic variation in mice. Med. J. Osaka Univ., 7:731-743.

———— Y. Ohno, and T. Takayanagi. 1968. The studies on the antigenic type substance of *Trypanosoma gambiense*. Proceedings of the Twelfth International Congress on Genetics, Vol. 1, p. 72.

Janssens, P. G., D. Karchen, M. Van Sande, A. Lowenthal, and G. Ghysels. 1961. Étude enzymo-électrophoretique du L.C.R. des patients atteints de trypanosomiase africaine *T. gambiense*. Bull. Soc. Path. Exot., 54:322-331.

Jenkins, A.R., and D.H.H. Robertson. 1959. Hepatic dysfunction in human trypanosomiasis. II. Serum proteins in *Trypanosoma rhodesiense* infections and observations found after treatment and during convalescence. Trans. Roy. Soc. Trop. Med. Hyg., 53:524-533.

Johnson, P., R.A. Neal, and D. Gall. 1963. Protective effect of killed trypanosome vaccines with incorporated adjuvants. Nature (London), 200:83.

Josselin, J., J. Gombert, and R. Masseyeff. 1964. Application de la chromatographie en couche mince à la mise en évidence des acides aminés N-terminaux de la macroimmunoglobuline (IgM). Bull. Mem. Fac. Mixte Med. Pharm., Dakar, 12:126-129.

Kligler, I.J., and M. Berman. 1935. Susceptibility and resistance to a trypanosome infection. X. Specific character of the immunity produced in rats by the injection of suspensions of dead trypanosomes. Ann. Trop. Med. Parasit., 29:457-461.

———— and R. Comaroff. 1935. Susceptibility and resistance to a trypanosome infection. IX. Active immunization of rats and guinea pigs and passive immunization of rats to a trypanosome infection. Ann. Trop. Med. Parasit., 29:145-160.

———— and L. Olitzki. 1936. The antigenic composition of *Trypanosoma evansi*. Ann. Trop. Med. Parasit., 30:287-291.

———— L. Olitzki, and H. Kligler. 1940. The antigenic composition and immunizing properties of trypanosomes. J. Immun., 38:317-331.

Kuhn, L.R. 1938. The effect of splenectomy and blockade on the protective titer of antiserum against *Trypanosoma equiperdum*. J. Infect. Dis., 63:217-224.

Landy, M., and L. Pillemer. 1956. Increased resistance to infection and accompanying alteration in properdin levels following administration of bacterial lipopolysaccharides. J. Exp. Med., 104: 383-409.

Lange, E. 1911. Makroskopische Agglutination bei Trypanosomen. Zbl. Bakt. Beiheft, pp. 171-178.

Lapierre, J., and J.J. Rousset. 1961a. Étude de l'immunité dans les infections à *Trypanosoma gambiense* chez la souris blanche. Variations antigéniques au cours des crises trypanolytiques. Bull. Soc. Path. Exot., 54: 332-336.

———— and J.J. Rousset. 1961b. Caractères biologiques d'une souche virulente de *Trypanosoma gambiense*. Immunisation par vaccin tués. Bull. Path. Exot., 54: 336-345.

———— M. Lariviere, and J. J. Rousset. 1958. Protection de la souris contre une souche virulente de *Trypanosoma gambiense* par certaines espèces de *Borrelia*. Bull. Soc. Path. Exot., 51: 173-176.

Laveran, A. 1902. De l'action du sérum humain sur le Trypanosome du Nagana (*Tr. brucei*). C.R. Acad. Sci. (Paris), 134: 735.

———— 1904. Immunité naturelle des Cynocéphales pour les Trypanosomiases—Activité de leur sérum sur les trypanosomes. C.R. Acad. Sci. (Paris), 193: 177.

———— and F. Mesnil. 1902. Recherches morphologiques et expérimentales sur le trypanosome du Nagana ou maladie de la mouche tsé-tsé. Ann. Inst. Pasteur (Paris), 16: 1-55.

———— and F. Mesnil. 1912. Trypanosomes et Trypanosomiases. 2nd Ed., Paris, Masson et Cie.

Leger, A., and J. Ringenbach. 1911. Sur la spécificité de la propriété trypanolytique des sérums des animaux trypanosomies. C.R. Soc. Biol. (Paris), 70: 343.

Levaditi, C., and S. Muttermilch. 1909. Recherches sur la méthode de Bordet et Gengou appliquée à l'étude de trypanosomiases. Z. Immunitätsforsch. Exp. Therap. [Orig.], 2: 702-722.

Lourie, E.M., and R.J. O'Connor. 1936. Trypanolysis *in vitro* by mouse immune serum. Ann. Trop. Med. Parasit., 30: 365-388.

———— and R.J. O'Connor. 1937. A study of *Trypanosoma rhodesiense* relapse strains *in vitro*. Ann. Trop. Med. Parasit., 31: 319-340.

Lucasse, C. 1964. Fluorescent antibody tests as applied to cerebro-spinal fluid in human sleeping sickness. Bull. Soc. Path. Exot., 57: 283-292.

Lumsden, W.H.R. 1967. Trends in research on the immunology of trypanosomiasis. Bull. W. H. O. 37: 167-175.

———— M.P. Cunningham, W.A.F. Webber, K. Van Hoeve, and P.J. Walker. 1963. A method for the measurement of the infectivity of trypanosome suspensions. Exp. Parasit., 14: 269-279.

Masseyeff, R., and J. Gombert. 1963. Inhibition de la respiration de trypanosomes par le sérum de malades atteints de trypanosomiase africaine à *T. gambiense*. Ann. Inst. Pasteur (Paris), 104: 115-122.

Mattern, P. 1964. Techniques et intérêt épidémiologique du diagnostic de la trypanosomiase humaine africaine par la recherche de la β_2-macroglobuline dans le sang et dans L.C.R. Ann. Inst. Pasteur (Paris), 107: 415-421.

———— 1968. État actuel et résultats des techniques immunologiques utilisées à l'Institut Pasteur de Dakar pour le diagnostic et l'étude de la trypanosomiase humaine africaine. Bull. W. H. O., 38: 1-8.

———— M. Bentz, and I.A. McGregor. 1967. Les anticorps précipitants présents dans le sang et dans le liquide cephalo-rachidien des malades atteints de trypanosomiase humaine africaine à *T. gambiense*. Ann. Inst. Pasteur (Paris), 112: 105-112.

———— R. Masseyeff, and P. Peretti. 1961. Étude immunochimique de la B₂-macroglobuline des sérums de malades atteints de trypanosomiase africaine à *T. gambiense*. Ann. Inst. Pasteur (Paris), 101: 382-388.

———— J. Pillot, and R. Bornardot. 1965. Contribution à l'étude des immuno-globulines du liquide cephalo-rachidien responsables du phénomène d'immuno-fluorescence dans la neuro-syphilis et dans la trypanosomiase nerveuse. Med. Afrique Noir, Dakar, 12: 219-221.

Mattes, W. 1912. Agglutinationserscheinungen bei den Trypanosomen der Schlafkrankheit, Nagana, Dourine, Beschälseuche und des Kongoküstenfiebers, unter Berücksichtigung der Färbemethoden der morphologischen und biologischen Verhältnisse der Erreger. Zbl. Bakt. [Orig.], 65: 538-573.

Mesnil, F. and A. Leboeuf. 1910. De l'action comparée de sérums de primates sur les infections à trypanosomes. C.R. Soc. Biol. (Paris), 69: 382.

Mignoli, A. 1924. Del comportamento della tripanocidiasi in diverse forme morbose. Reforma Med., 40:577.

Miller, J.K. 1965. Variation of the soluble antigens of *Trypanosoma brucei*. Immunology, 9:521-528.

Miller, L.H., and T. Chongsuphajaisiddhi. 1968. Comparative studies on the pathology and host physiology of malarias. V. Hypovolaemia in *Plasmodium coatneyi* malaria. Ann. Trop. Med. Parasit., 62:218-232.

Molinari, V. 1961. Considerazioni sulla reazione di agglomerazione. Studio sulla applicazione della tecnicei di Sabin e Feldman alla diagnosi di tripanosomiasi cronica nel coniglio. Acta Med. Ital., 16:205-206.

Neujean, G., and F. Evens. 1958. Diagnostic et traitement de la maladie du sommeil à *T. gambiense*. Acad. Roy. Sci. Coloniales, Classe Sci. Nat. Med., 7:1.

Nicoli, J., J. Bergot, and J. Demarchi. 1961. Études des protéines sériques au cours de la trypanosomiase humaine africaine. Ann. Inst. Pasteur (Paris), 101:596-610.

Nissle, A. 1904. Hygiene Rundschau, 14:1039 (quoted in Laveran and Mesmil, 1912.)

——— 1950. Eine Theorie zur Erklärung der Pathogenese von Infektions-krankheiten. Z. Immunitätsforsch., 107:84-89.

Njogu, A.R., and K.C. Humphreys. 1967. Electrophoretic separation of the soluble proteins of *Brucei* sub-group trypanosomes. Nature (London), 216:280-282.

Olberg, H. 1955. Über die Blutweissveranderungen bei experimenteller Infektion von Mäusen mit *T. brucei*. Zbl. Bakt. [Orig.], 162:120-135.

Osaki, H. 1959. Studies on the immunological variation in *Trypanosoma gambiense* (serotypes and the mode of relapse). Biken J., 2:113-127.

Pautrizel, R., A. Lafaye, and J. Duret. 1959. Anticorps et modifications plasmatiques au cours de la trypanosomose expérimentale du lapin par *Trypanosoma equiperdum*. Rev. Immun. (Paris), 23:323-335.

——— P. Mattern, and J. Duret. 1960. Diagnostic sérologique de la maladie du sommeil. II. Les anticorps fixant le complément au cours de l'infection. Bull. Soc. Path. Exot., 53:878-885.

——— J. Duret, J. Tribouley, and C. Ripert. 1962. Étude de la spécificité de la réaction d'agglutination des trypanosomes au cours des trypanosomiases. Bull. Soc. Path. Exot., 55:383-390.

Petard, P. H., and H. Ridet. 1954. Serological studies of African trypanosomiasis in man. Med. Trop. (Marseilles), 14:78-94.

Polge, C., and M.A. Soltys. 1957. Preservation of trypanosomes in the frozen state. Trans. Roy. Soc. Trop. Med. Hyg., 51:519-526.

Randall, J.B., and S.G. Laws. 1947. The effect of the stage of infection on the response of *T. congolense* in cattle to phenanthridinium 1553. Vet. Rec., 59:1-3.

Regendanz, P. 1932. Die experimentelle Erzeugung von Schlafkrankheit beim natürlich immunen Pavian durch Infektion des Liquor cerebrospinalis. Arch. Schiffs. Trop. Hyg., 36:409-425.

Ritz, H. 1914. Über Rezidive bei experimenteller Trypanosomiasis. Deutsch. Med. Wschr., 40:1355.

——— 1916. Über Rezidive bei experimenteller Trypanosomiasis. II. Mitteilung. Arch. Schiffs. Trop. Hyg., 20:397-420.

Rosenthal, F., and H. Nossen. 1921. Serologische Trypanosomenstudien. II. Mitteilung. Eine Serodiagnose verschiedener menschlicher Ikterusformen. Berlin. Klin. Wschr., 58:1093.

Ross, R. 1956. "Healthy carrier" cases of human trypanosomiasis in Southern Rhodesia. Int. Sci. Comm. Tryp. Res. (6) 2, (mimeographed report).

Rouget, J. 1896. Contribution à l'étude du trypanosome des mammifères. Ann. Inst. Pasteur (Paris), 10:716-728.

Sadun, E.H., R.E. Duxbury, J.S. Williams, and R.I. Anderson. 1963. Fluorescent antibody test for the serodiagnosis of African and American trypanosomiasis in man J. Parasit., 49:385-388.

Schilling, C. 1902. Bericht über die Surra-Krankheit der Pferden und Rinder im Schutzgebiete Togo. Zbl. Bakt. [Orig.] 31:452-459.

——— 1933. The immunization of cattle against trypanosomiasis. Bull. Soc. Path. Exot., 27:170-173.

——— 1935. Immunization against trypanosomiasis. J. Trop. Med. Hyg., 36:106-108.

Schoenaers, F. 1950. Voyage d'études vétérinaires au Congo Belge. Bull. Agric. Congo Belge, 41:1007-1036.

———— G. Neujean, and F. Evens. 1953a. Valeur pratique de la réaction de fixation du complement dans la maladie du sommeil à *T. gambiense*. Première Partie: Le diagnostic de la maladie. Ann. Soc. Belge Med. Trop., 33:141-169.

———— G. Neujean, and F. Evens. 1953b. Valeur pratique de la réaction de fixation du complement dans la maladie du sommeil à *T. gambiense*. Deuxième Partie: La réaction de fixation du complement lors d'une rechute après traitement medicamenteux. Ann. Soc. Belge Med. Trop., 33:389-402.

Seed, J.R. 1963. The characterization of antigens isolated from *Trypanosoma rhodesiense*. J. Protozool., 10:380-389.

———— 1964. Antigenic similarity among culture forms of the *"brucei"* group of trypanosomes. Parasitology, 54:593-596.

———— and A.A. Gam. 1966a. The properties of antigens from *Trypanosoma gambiense*. J. Parasit., 52:395-398.

———— and A.A. Gam. 1966b. Passive immunity to experimental trypanosomiasis. J. Parasit., 52:1134-1140.

———— and A.A. Gam. 1967. The presence of antibody to a normal rabbit liver antigen in rabbits infected with *Trypanosoma gambiense*. J. Parasit., 53:946-950.

———— and D. Weinman. 1963. Characterization of antigens isolated from *Trypanosoma rhodesiense*. Nature (London), 198:197-198.

Seneca, H., J.B. Sang, and O.K. Truc. 1958. The electrophoretic pattern of the serum proteins in experimental haemoflagellate infections. Trans. Roy. Soc. Trop. Med. Hyg., 52:230-234.

Sergent, E. 1963. Latent infections and premunition. Some definitions of microbiology and immunology. *In* Immunity to Protozoa. Garnham, P.C.C., Pierce, A.E., and Roitt, I., eds. Oxford, Blackwell Scientific Publications, pp. 39-47.

Singer, I., E.T. Kimble, III, and R.E. Ritts. 1964. Alterations of the host-parasite relationship by administration of endotoxin to mice with infections of trypansomes. J. Infect. Dis., 114:243-248.

Skarnes, R.C., and D.W. Watson. 1957. Antimicrobial factors of normal tissues and fluids. Bact. Rev., 21:273-294.

Soltys, M.A. 1955. Studies on resistance to *Trypanosoma congolense* developed by Zebu cattle treated prophylactically with Antrycide pro-salt in an enzootic area of East Africa. Ann. Trop. Med. Parasit., 49:1-8.

———— 1957a. Immunity in trypanosomiasis. I. Neutralization reaction. Parasitology, 47:375-389.

———— 1957b. Immunity in trypanosomiasis. II. Agglutination reaction with African trypanosomes. Parasitology, 47:391-395.

———— 1959. Immunity in trypanosomiasis. III. Sensitivity of antibody-resistant strains to chemotherapeutic drugs. Parasitology, 49:143-152.

———— 1965. Immunogenic properties of *Trypanosoma brucei* inactivated by ß-propiolactone. *In* Progress in Protozoology, Second International Conference on Protozoology. Amsterdam, Excerpta Medica Foundation, p. 138.

———— and C. Folkers. 1963. The effect of immunity on chemotherapy in trypanosomiasis. *In* Immunity to Protozoa. Garnham, P.C.C., Pierce, A.E., and Roitt, I., eds. Oxford, Blackwell Scientific Publications.

Stewart, J.L. 1951. The West African shorthorn cattle: Their value to Africa as trypanosomiasis-resistant animals. Vet. Rec., 63:454-457.

Taliaferro, W.H. 1929. The Immunology of Parasitic Infections. New York, The Century Co.

Tate, P. 1951. Antagonism of *Spirillum minus* infections in rats towards *Trypanosoma lewisi* and *T. equinum*. Parasitology, 41:117-127.

Taylor, A. 1968. Immunological studies on the subgenus *Trypanozoon* and *Trypanosoma lewisi*. Trans. Roy. Soc. Trop. Med. Hyg., 62:128-129.

Tella, A., and B.G. Maegraith. 1962. Bradykinin in *P. knowlesi* infection (Laboratory demonstration). Trans. Roy. Soc. Trop. Med. Hyg., 56:6.

———— and B.G. Maegraith. 1963. Further studies on bradykinin involvement in *P. knowlesi* infection (Laboratory demonstration). Trans. Roy. Soc. Trop. Med. Hyg., 57:1-2.

Terry, B.T. 1911. Chemotherapeutic trypanosome studies with special reference to the immunity following cure. Rockefeller Institute for Medical Research, Monograph No. 3.

Terry, R.J. 1957. Antibody against *Trypanosoma vivax* present in normal cotton rat serum. Exp. Parasit., 6:404-411.

Thillet, C.J., and A.C. Chandler. 1957. Immunization against *T. lewisi* in rats by injections of metabolic products. Science, 125:346-347.

Thomas and Breinl. 1905. Liverpool School of Tropical Medicine Memoirs, 15:1. (Quoted in Laveran and Mesnil, 1912).

Thurston, J.P. 1958. The effect of immune sera on the respiration of *Trypanosoma brucei in vitro*. Parasitology, 48:463-467.

Trautmann, R. 1907. Étude expérimentale sur l'association du spirille de la tick-fever et de divers trypanosomes. Ann. Inst. Pasteur (Paris), 21:803-824.

Trincao, C., E. Gouveia, A. Franco, and F. Perreira. 1953. Disturbance of blood protein in sleeping sickness. Bull. Soc. Path. Exot., 46:680-685.

Tristram, G.R. 1953. The amino acid composition of proteins. *In* The Proteins, Vol. 1. Neurath, H., and Bailey, K., eds. New York, Academic Press, Inc.

Van Saceghem, R. 1938. The immunization of cattle against trypanosomiasis. Bull. Soc. Path. Exot., 31:296-298.

Vickerman, K. 1968. Cyclical changes in surface structure in pathogenic trypanosomes. Abstracts and Reviews, Eighth International Congress of Tropical Medicine and Malaria, p. 304.

Watkins, J.F. 1964. Observations on antigenic variation in a strain of *Trypanosoma brucei* growing in mice. J. Hyg. (Cambridge), 62:69-80.

Watson, H.J.C., and G. Chirieleison. 1966. Titres of the IgM class of immunoglobulins in Gambian sleeping sickness and other disease conditions. Eleventh Meeting Int. Sci. Comm. Tryp. Res. (Nairobi, 1966). O.A.U./S.T.R.C. Publication No. 100, pp. 183-185.

Weinman, D. 1963. Problems of diagnosis of trypanosomiasis. Bull. W.H.O., 28:731-743.

Weitz, B. 1960a. A soluble protective antigen of *Trypanosoma brucei*. Nature (London), 185:788-799.

———— 1960b. The properties of some antigens of *Trypanosoma brucei*. J. Gen. Microbiol., 23:589-600.

———— 1962a. Immunity in trypanosomiasis. *In* Drugs, Parasites and Hosts. Biological Council Symposium. London, J.A. Churchill, Ltd., p. 180.

———— 1963a. Immunological relationships between African trypanosomes and their hosts. Ann N.Y. Acad. Sci., 113:400-408.

———— 1963b. The antigenicity of some African trypanosomes. *In* Immunity to Protozoa. Garnham, P.C.C., Pierce, A.E., and Roitt, I., eds. Oxford, Blackwell Scientific Publications, p. 196.

Werner, H. 1954. Über die Frage der placentaren Trypanosomen-Infektion und Übertragung von Trypanosomen und Antikörpen durch die Milch auf das Neugeborene. Z. Tropenmed. Parasit., 5:422-442.

Williams, J.S., R.E. Duxbury, R.I. Anderson, and E.H. Sadun. 1963. Fluorescent antibody reactions in *Trypanosoma rhodesiense* and *T. gambiense* in experimental animals. J. Parasit., 49:380-384.

Williamson, J. 1961. Chemical composition of trypanosomes. Ann. Trop. Med. Parasit., 55:146-147.

———— 1962. Chemotherapy and chemoprophylaxis of African trypanosomiasis. Exp. Parasit., 12:323-367.

———— 1963. The chemical composition of trypanosomes. Proceedings of the 16th International Congress of Zoology, Vol. 4. pp. 189-195.

———— and R.S. Desowitz. 1961. The chemical composition of trypanosomes. I. Protein, amino acid and sugar analysis. Exp. Parasit., 11:161-175.

———— and K.N. Brown. 1964. The chemical composition of trypanosomes. III. Antigenic constituents of *Brucei* trypanosomes. Exp. Parasit., 15:44-68.

Wilson, A.J., M.P. Cunningham, J.M.B. Harley. 1969. The use of Berenil to stimulate the protective immune response of cattle to pathogenic trypanosomes. Trans. Roy. Soc. Trop. Med. Hyg., 63:124.

World Health Organization Expert Committee on Trypanosomiasis. 1962. WHO/Tryp/ 1-35.

Yorke, W. 1911. Autoagglutination of red blood cells in trypanosomiasis. Proc. Roy. Soc. [Biol.], 83:238-258.

———— A.R.D. Adams, and F. Murgatroyd. 1929. Studies in chemotherapy. I. A method for maintaining pathogenic trypanosomes alive *in vitro* at 37°C for 24 hours. Ann. Trop. Med. Parasit., 23: 501-518.

———— A.R.D. Adams, and F. Murgatroyd. 1930. Studies in chemotherapy. II. The action *in vitro* of normal human serum on the pathogenic trypanosomes, and its significance. Ann. Trop. Med. Parasit., 24: 115-163.

Zeiss, H. 1921. Die Einwirkung menschlichen Serums auf menschenpathogene Trypanosomen. Arch. Schiffs. Trop. Hyg., 24: 73-92.

Zimmer, G. 1931. Zbl. Bakt. [Orig.], 120: 422.

Zoutendyk, A., and J. Gear. 1951. Autoantibodies in the pathogenesis of disease. S. Afr. Med. J., 25: 665-668.

Zuckerman, A. 1964. Autoimmunization and other types of indirect damage to host cells as factors in certain protozoan diseases. Exp. Parasit., 15: 138-183.

———— and M. Ristic. 1968. Blood parasite antigens and antibodies. *In* Infectious Blood Diseases of Man and Animals. Weinman, D., and Ristic, M., eds. New York, Academic Press, Inc., pp. 80-115.

South American Trypanosomes

FRANS C. GOBLE
Smith, Miller, and Patch, Inc., New Brunswick, New Jersey

INTRODUCTION

Systematic position of South American trypanosomes

The terms "pathogenic," "South American," and "nonpathogenic," as
applied to trypanosomes in this chapter will be meaningful to most parasitol-

Table 1
Classification of Mammalian Trypanosomes

A. Section Stercoraria	Normal Host
Subgenus *Megatrypanum* Hoare, 1964	
Trypanosoma (Megatrypanum) theileri Laveran, 1902	bovines, antelopes
T. (M.) tragelaphi Kinghorn et al., 1913	antelopes
T. (M.) melophagium Flu, 1908	sheep
T. (M.) mazamarum Mazza et al., 1932	deer
T. (M.) cephalophi Bruce et al., 1913	antelopes
T. (M.) ingens Bruce et al., 1910	cattle, antelopes, chevrotains
Subgenus *Herpetosoma* Doflein, 1901	
Trypanosoma (Herpetosoma) lewisi (Kent, 1880) Laveran & Mesnil, 1901	rats
T. (H.) duttoni Thiroux, 1900	mice
T. (H.) grosi Laveran & Pettit, 1909	wood mice
T. (H.) rabinowitschae Brumpt, 1906	hamsters
T. (H.) primatum Reichenow, 1917	anthropoid apes
T. (H.) nabiasi Railliet, 1895	rabbits
T. (H.) zapi Davis, 1952	jumping mice
T. (H.) rangeli Tejera, 1920	man, dogs, opossums, monkeys
T. (H.) otospermophili Wellman & Wherry, 1910	ground squirrels
Subgenus *Schizotrypanum* Chagas, 1909; emend. Nöller, 1931	
Trypanosoma (Schizotrypanum) cruzi Chagas, 1909	man, dogs, cats, armadillos, opossums, etc.
T. (S.) vespertilionis Battaglia, 1904	bats
T. (S.) pipistrelli Chatton & Courrier, 1921	bats
T. (S.) phyllostomae Cartaya, 1910	bats
T. (S.) hipposideri Mackerras, 1959	bats
T. (S.) prowazeki Berenberg-Gossler, 1908	uakari monkeys
T. (S.) lesourdi Leger & Porry, 1918	spider monkeys
T. (S.) sanmartini Garnham & Gonzalez-Mugaburu, 1962	squirrel monkeys
Genus *Endotrypanum* Mesnil & Brimont, 1908	
E. schaudinni M. & B., 1908	sloths

ogists, although they are not entirely accurate, descriptive, or satisfactorily inclusive or exclusive. In some hosts (e.g., *Peromyscus*), the "pathogenic" types do not produce disease (Packchanian, 1950). One of the "South American" types is a classical pathogen. Under certain conditions, members of the "nonpathogenic" group may be lethal.

Classification of trypanosomes of mammals has been developing during the past 30 years through the efforts of Hoare, and this generally accepted system will be reviewed in pointing out the taxonomic position of the organisms designated "South American trypanosomes" (Table 1). Hoare (1966) divided the mammalian trypanosomes into two sections, designated Stercoraria and Salivaria. The Salivaria include the species to which the term "pathogenic" is applied (*see* chapter by Desowitz, pp. 551–596). They are trypano-

Table 1 (Continued)

B. Section Salivaria	
Subgenus *Duttonella* Chalmers, 1918	
Trypanosoma (Duttonella) vivax Ziemann, 1905	ruminants, equines
T. (D.) uniforme Bruce et al., 1911	ruminants
Subgenus *Nannomonas* Hoare, 1964	
Trypanosoma (Nannomonas) congolense Broden, 1904	ruminants, equines, pigs, dogs
T. (N.) dimorphon Laveran & Mesnil, 1904	equines, ruminants, pigs
T. (N.) simiae Bruce et al., 1911	pigs, warthogs
Subgenus *Pycnomonas* Hoare, 1964	
Trypanosoma (Pycnomonas) suis Ochmann, 1905	pigs
Subgenus *Trypanozoon* Lühe, 1906	
Trypanosoma (Trypanozoon) brucei Plimmer & Bradford, 1899	all domestic mammals, antelopes
T. (T.) rhodesiense Stephens & Fantham, 1910	man, antelopes
T. (T.) gambiense Dutton, 1902	man
T. (T.) evansi Steel, 1885	camels, equines, bovines, dogs
T. (T.) equinum Voges, 1901	equines, bovines
T. (T.) equiperdum Doflein, 1901	equines

The first species in each subgenus is the type species.

Classification from Hoare. 1966. *Ergebn. Mikrobiol. Immunitätsforsch. Exp. Therap.*, 39:43-57.

somes in which a free flagellum may be present or absent, the kinetoplast is terminal or subterminal, and the posterior end of the body is usually blunt. Multiplication in the mammalian host is continuous and takes place in the trypanosomal (trypomastigote) stage. Development in the vector is completed in the anterior station (except in mechanical vectors) and transmission is inoculative (except in *T. equiperdum*). Most of the species occur in tropical Africa and cause debilitating and often fatal disease in man and domestic stock, while some of the species afflicting equine hosts are more wide-spread in both hemispheres. Those Salivaria which occur in South America (*T. equinum* and *T. evansi*), however, are not to be considered in this chapter.

The section Stercoraria comprises those trypanosomes in which the free flagellum is always present, the kinetoplast is large and not terminal, and the posterior end of the body is pointed. Multiplication in the mammalian host is discontinuous and typically takes place in the crithidial (epimastigote) or leishmanial (amastigote) stages. Development in the vector is completed in the posterior station and transmission is contaminative (although in *T. rangeli*, it also occurs in the anterior station, with inoculative transmission). Although members of this section are typically not pathogenic, one species (*T. cruzi*) is a well-known exception, causing the pantropic pathosis of man and certain animals known as Chagas' disease.

The Stercoraria includes one subgenus, *Megatrypanum*, which has not been extensively studied, and very little is known concerning the immunology of it. These are parasites of cloven-hoofed animals and are transmitted by flies. Also included is a taxon, *Endotrypanum*, which Hoare recognized as a genus, the only species of which is a parasite of sloths and is presumably transmitted by *Phlebotomus* flies. Stercoraria also includes the members of the subgenus *Herpetosoma*, which may be considered "the nonpathogenic rodent trypanosomes" (*see* chapter by D'Alesandro, pp. 691–738), although some of the species have primates, lagomorphs, carnivores, or marsupials as hosts. They are typically transmitted by fleas. However, *T. rangeli* has a triatome bug as its intermediate host, and other vectors may be represented in those life-cycles which are unknown.

The subgenus *Schizotrypanum* includes species chiefly infesting bats and monkeys, but its most important member, *T. (Schizotrypanum) cruzi*, the causative agent of Chagas' disease, has been found in a wide variety of natural hosts—well over 75 species and/or subspecies in over 40 genera in nine orders of mammals.

What, then, are the South American "trypanosomes"? Although *T. mazamarum*, *Endotrypanum schaudinni*, and several species of bat and monkey trypanosomes of the subgenus *Schizotrypanum* were described from South America, it is probable that none of these comes to mind as readily as the two species which are found in man, are transmitted by triatome bugs, and are more abundant in South America than in any other continent. One of these is *T. rangeli*, which is nonpathogenic and occurs in dogs, opossums, and monkeys. The other is *T. cruzi*, a zoonotic species, the original sylvatic hosts of which were probably armadillos and opossums. Most of this chapter will be devoted to this species and to the immunology of Chagas' disease. Only minor and incidental reference will be made to *T. rangeli*, which has not been studied from an immunologic point of view.

Vectors, life cycle, and pathogenesis

Both *T. cruzi* and *T. rangeli* have as vectors species of reduviid bugs of the subfamily Triatominae. These bugs ingest trypanosomes when feeding on infective vertebrate hosts, and they harbor the parasites in their intestinal tracts during a period of multiplication and development. There the similarity in behavior of the two species ends.

T. rangeli passes from the intestine into the hemocoel of its intermediate host (usually *Rhodnius prolixus*), and after a few days of growth in the hemolymph, it invades the salivary glands, where metacyclic trypanosomes are found which may infect the vertebrates on which the insects feed. The infections which result are low in intensity, and although they may persist for some time, they do not appear to be pathogenic. The cycle is completed when suitable triatomes feed on infected vertebrates and the parasites are returned to the intermediate host (*see* Tobie, 1964, for references).

T. *cruzi*, on the other hand, remains in the intestine of the bug. There metacyclic trypanosomes eventually develop which infect definitive hosts by the contaminative route. While they are feeding on vertebrates, the bugs defecate, and the parasites in the triatome feces penetrate either the wound resulting from the bite or another site of access, such as the conjunctiva or the oral mucosa. The organisms which thus effect entry into the body attack a variety of organs and tissues, setting up intracellular foci in which multiplication takes place by binary fission. This results in the production of new parasites. The new parasites eventually leave the intracellular sites, destroy the cells in which they developed, and reinvade new tissues in which the cycle is repeated.

Although striated-muscle (including cardiac), reticuloendothelial, and nervous tissues are the most commonly invaded, the parasites may attack almost any organ, and the manifestations of the disease, in some hosts, may be protean. It is probable that no spontaneous cures occur, and that individuals once infected will harbor parasites for the rest of their lives, sometimes without apparent effects, but often with progressive debilitating processes leading to irreversible damage and multiple malfunctions.

Feeding of triatomes on infected humans or other animals completes the cycle. This may occur under domiciliary conditions in which bugs transmit the disease from man to man, from man to domestic animal (dog, cat, or guinea pig), or from animal to man. Under sylvatic conditions, other species of triatomes transmit the disease from wild animal to wild animal, to domestic animal, or to man, in one or another of a variety of passages. In contrast to *T. rangeli*, which has as its normal vector only one species (*Rhodnius prolixus*), *T. cruzi* can be transmitted by a number of genera and species of triatomes. The most important transmitting species belong to the genera which have the greatest number of species—*Triatoma* (with about 30 species in the neotropical region), *Panstrongylus* (with about 10 species), and *Rhodnius* (with 10 species).

NATURAL RESISTANCE

Factors affecting susceptibility

Host factors—*Species.* In contrast to many other members of the section Stercoraria, *Trypanosoma cruzi* has remarkably little host specificity, although quantitative differences in susceptibility among the various species are notable. Mammals are the typical hosts, and, if we can exclude bats (which harbor a number of related nonpathogenic species and which are of doubtful importance as reservoirs of *T. cruzi*), susceptible mammals fall into eight orders, seven of which are found to be infected in nature (Table 2) and one of which (Monotremata) has been found only experimentally (Table 3). The degrees of infection range from those in which only low and transient parasitemias are observed and tissue stages are difficult or impossible to find

Table 2

Natural Hosts of *Trypanosoma cruzi*

Host	Author*	North America	Middle America	South America	Asia†
Marsupialia					
Didelphis azarae (=*paraguayensis*)	D			+	
Didelphis marsupialis	D	+	+	+	
Didelphis marsupialis aurita	P			+	
Didelphis marsupialis mesamericanus	D	+			
Didelphis marsupialis etensis	D		+	+	
Didelphis virginianus	P	+			
Lutreolina crassicaudata crassicaudata	D			+	
Lutreolina crassicaudata paranalis	D			+	
Marmosa mitis certa	D			+	
Marmosa agilis agilis	B			+	
Marmosa cinerea	D			+	
Marmosa pallidior	B			+	
Metachirus nudicaudatus	D			+	
Monodelphis domestica	B			+	
Philander opossum	P			+	
Philander philander	B			+	
Carnivora					
Canis familiaris	D	+	+	+	
Felis domesticus	D			+	
Grison vittatus	D			+	
Grison cuja	D			+	
Mephitis mephitis nigra	D			+	
Procyon lotor	P,B	+	+		
Dusicyon calpaeus c.	D			+	
Dusicyon gracilis gracilis (=*griseus griseus*)	D			+	
Dusicyon griseus graislis (=*culpaeus andinus*)	D			+	
Tarya barbara	D			+	
Urocyon cinereoargenteus	P	+			
Nasua narica	L		+		
Cerdocyon thous	B			+	
Rodentia					
Akodon arviculoides cursor	B			+	
Cavia porcellus	D			+	
Cercomys cunnicularius laurentius	B			+	
Citellus leucurus cinnamoneus	B	+			
Coelogenus subniger	D			+	
Coendous mexicanus laenatus	B		+		
Coendous prehensilis	D			+	
Cuniculus paca paca (=*subniger*)	B			+	
Dasyprocta agouti	D			+	
Dasyprocta rubrata	D			+	
Galea spixii spixii	B			+	
Guerlinguetus gilirgularis	B			+	
Leptosciurus argentinus	D			+	
Mus musculus	D	+			
Mus musculus brevirostris	F			+	
Nectomys squamipes amazonicus	P			+	
Neotoma albigula albigula	D	+			

The nomenclature of Walker (1964) has been followed whenever possible in this table.

* D = Dias, 1956; P = Pessoa, 1963; B = Barretto, 1964; L = Lainson, 1965; F = Ferriolli and Barretto, 1965.

† These are considered by Hoare (1963) to be accidental infections.

Table 2

Natural Hosts of *Trypanosoma cruzi*

Host	Author*	North America	Middle America	South America	Asia†
Rodentia (cont.)					
Neotoma alleni	B	+			
Neotoma fuscipes macrotis	D	+			
Neotoma micropus canescens	B	+			
Neotoma micropus micropus	D	+			
Octodon degus degus	D			+	
Oryzomys subflavus subflavus	B			+	
Peramys domesticus	B			+	
Peromyscus boylii rowlei	D	+			
Peromyscus truei gilberti	D	+			
Rattus rattus rattus	B			+	
Rattus rattus alexandrinus	B			+	
Rattus rattus frugivorus	F			+	
Rattus norvegicus	D	+		+	
Sciurus gerrardi morulus	D		+		
Sciurus (guerlinguetus) sp.	D			+	
Zygodontomys pixuna	A			+	
Lagomorpha					
"Wild rabbit" (probably *Sylvilagus orinoci*)	D			+	
Oryctolagus cuniculus	B			+	
Edentata					
Cabassous tatouya	D			+	
Cabassous unicinctus	P			+	
Chaetophractus vellerosus vellerosus	D			+	
Chaetophractus vellerosus pannosus	D			+	
Chaetophractus villosus	D			+	
Dasypus hybridus	P			+	
Dasypus novemcinctus	D			+	
Dasypus novemcinctus fenestratus	D		+		
Dasypus novemcinctus mexicanus	D	+			
Dasypus novemcinctus texanus	D	+			
Dasypus paraguayensis	P			+	
Dasypus pentadactylus	P			+	
Euphractus sexcinctus	D			+	
Tamandua tetradactyla	D			+	
Tolypeutes matacus	D			+	
Zaedyus pichi caurinus	D			+	
Primata					
Aloutta senicola	D			+	
Callithrix jacchus	B			+	
Cebus apella	B			+	
Cebus capucinus	D			+	
Cebus (probably *fulvus*)	B			+	
Cebus sp.	D			+	
Macaca irus	D				+
Macaca mulatta	B				+
Saimiri sciureus	D			+	
Saimiri boliviensis	B			+	
Artiodactyla					
Sus scrofa domesticus	D			+	
Capra hircus	B			+	

The nomenclature of Walker (1964) has been followed whenever possible in this table.

* D = Dias, 1956; P = Pessoa, 1963; B = Barretto, 1964; F = Ferriolli and Barretto, 1965; A = Alencar et al., 1962.

† These are considered by Hoare (1963) to be accidental infections.

Table 3

Experimental Hosts of *Trypanosoma cruzi*

Host	Author
Monotremata	
Tachyglossus aculeatus	Backhouse and Bolliger, 1951
Marsupialia	
Trichosurus vulpecula	Backhouse and Bolliger, 1951
Rodentia	
Cavia porcellus	Chagas, 1909
Mesocricetus auratus	Cariola et al., 1950
Mus musculus	Blanchard 1912, Mayer and daRocha-Lima, 1912
Octodon degus degus	Christen and Neghme, 1950
Peromyscus californicus insignis	Wood, 1951
Peromyscus maniculatus gambeli	Cariola et al., 1950
Rattus rattus	Blanchard 1912, Mayer and daRocha-Lima, 1912
Lagomorpha	
Rabbit (probably *Oryctolagus cuniculus*)	Chagas, 1909, Agosin and Badinez, 1949
Primata	
Callithrix jacchus	Blanchard, 1912
Callithrix penicillata	Chagas, 1909
Erythrocebus patas	Blanchard, 1912
Macaca mulatta	Mayer and daRocha-Lima, 1912
Artiodactyla	
Bos taurus	Diamond and Rubin, 1958
Capra hircus	Diamond and Rubin, 1958
Ovis aries	Brumpt, 1913
Sus scrofa domestica	Brumpt et al., 1939, Mazza, 1940
Carnivora	
Canis familiaris	Chagas, 1909
Felis domestica	Blanchard, 1912

(as occurs in most of the wild reservoir hosts) to those with severe intracellular involvement, resultant extensive tissue damage, and parasitemias (as occurs in certain domestic hosts and experimental animals, e.g., in dogs, cats, and inbred mice). Within each of these host species, there are also variations in susceptibility (depending on strain or breed, age, and sex) which have not been well-studied except in mice.

Dias (1956) pointed out that the only animals other than man which become sick as a result of infection are dogs and cats, and that dogs sometimes die of natural infections. There seems to be no evidence that infection is lethal to the other reservoir hosts in nature. Artificially infected mice (certain strains), rats (usually young), hamsters, phalangers (*Trichosurus vulpecula*), and dogs succumb to the disease, often showing lesions typical of the acute disease in man and occasionally showing signs simulating certain phases of the chronic disease. About 75 percent of experimentally inoculated *Octodon degus* survived the infection, and the other species of rodents (guinea pig and *Peromyscus* sp.), monotremes, primates, and artiodactyls (*see* Table 3) are generally tolerant to artificial infections, developing low and transient parasitemias without other signs of disease.

Muniz and Borriello (1945) observed that normal human or guinea pig sera lysed the crithidial forms of *T. cruzi* from cultures, leaving the meta-cyclic trypanosomal forms unharmed. The fresh sera of a number of mammals have been tested for lytic effect against culture and blood forms of *T. cruzi* (Rubio, 1956b). Normal sheep and rat sera also produced a rapid destruction of crithidial stages from cultures over a range of temperatures. Only mouse serum did not show this property. The lytic activity was destroyed by heating at 56°C for 10 minutes or by standing a long time at room temperatures, but the lack of the C2 and C4 components of complement did not influence the lytic activity since sheep serum was effective without these components. Sheep, rat, and guinea pig sera which had been inactivated could be reactivated by the addition of mouse serum, which, by itself, was not lytic for crithidia. The blood forms were not lysed by the undiluted serum of any of the mammals tested. However, undiluted chicken serum lysed both crithidial and blood forms. Warren and Borsos (1959) point out that fowl sera contain at least two factors active against the crithidial forms: a heat-stable one, which is probably an agglutinating and sensitizing antibody, and a heat-labile factor, which they believe to be complement. The antibody which is present in mature chickens is transmitted to the yolk and thence to the embryo. It is greatly reduced or lost after hatching, but it is regained with immunologic maturation. Germ-free birds had antibody in their sera shortly after hatching, but on losing it, did not regain it. It was felt that the agglutinating antibody resulted from a response to cross-reacting antigen present in a common contaminant of fowls.

Although chick embryos have been used in the cultivation of *T. cruzi* by a number of investigators, embryo-to-embryo passage of the infection has not been generally reported, and it has been felt that the limited success of this system does not justify the use of the technique on a large scale (Pipkin, 1960). Under certain circumstances, embryonic chicken tissues are susceptible to infection by *T. cruzi* in tissue culture, as demonstrated by Romaña and Meyer (1942) and Meyer and de Oliviera (1948). Chicken macrophages also supported the growth of *T. cruzi* in roller-tube cultures provided the chicken serum used in the medium was heat-inactivated (Warren 1958). The chicken may not be typical of all birds, however, since Rubio (1956b) observed that the trypanosome forms of *T. cruzi* are not lysed by pigeon serum as they are by fowl serum.

Rubio's (1956a) study included sera from a toad (*Bufo chilensis*) and from a frog (*Pleurodema dibronii*), both of which possessed lytic properties for crithidial forms. There was, however, a differential activity against the blood (trypanosome) forms, the frog serum being more active. Despite the earlier report (Niño, 1925) that the toad (*Bufo marinus*) was susceptible to inoculation with *T. cruzi*, later authors agree that cold-blooded animals are not susceptible (Bruni, 1926; Brumpt, 1927; Dios et al., 1929; Dias, 1933,

1944; Dios and Bonacci, 1943), with the possible exception of certain lizards (*Gerrhonotus multicarinatus webbii*) which Ryckman (1954) infected by feeding them *Triatoma protracta*. Another species of lizard (*Sceloporus occidentalis biseriatus*) did not become infected.

Not noted in the above lists (*see* Tables 2 and 3) are the numerous species of bats which have been found to harbor *T. cruzi*-like organisms and various species of the subgenus *Schizotrypanum*. These parasites are indistinguishable morphologically from *T. cruzi* and are also transmitted by reduviid bugs. Some authors (e.g., Dias, 1956) do not consider them to be *T. cruzi*, while others (e.g., Marinkelle, 1966) stress the role of bats as reservoirs of Chagas' disease. A full discussion of this controversial point would probably not be useful here.

Host strain.   Systematic studies on differences in susceptibility among strains of mice were begun by Hauschka (1947a). He used several inbred strains (A, C, C$_3$H, and DBA) and found A mice to be most susceptible, C mice to be most refractory, and the others intermediate in their response to the infection. Pizzi et al. (1949) studied a number of strains and found A, C57, DBA, and C$_3$H strains to be relatively susceptible, whereas Ay, Ak, Daab, and Rockefeller strains were more resistant. Goble (1951) compared inbred A mice with random-bred Webster mice and also found the former to be less resistant, but he did not feel that this difference, although significant and reproducible, warranted special procurement of the more susceptible A mice for most experiments. Seneca and Peer (1963a, b) made a point of using a hybrid from A male and C57 females, but the advantages thereof are not apparent. Marcuse et al. (1964) reported no significant differences among the five strains they studied (CFW, NMRI, CBH/He, DBH/2, C57/B/6).

Many competent investigators have not designated the strains of mice used. Although certain highly inbred strains are more susceptible than others and might therefore be more useful in establishing a laboratory infection in mouse-to-mouse passage, it may be that once this continuous passage has been attained, factors related to the parasite (such as the strain of *T. cruzi* or the size of inoculum) rather than to the host are more important. Kagan and Norman (1960) and Hewett et al. (1963) have used random-bred, general purpose mice successfully in immunologic and chemotherapeutic studies, respectively.

Little is known about possible strain differences in animals other than mice; in most instances, the strains of rats, guinea pigs, hamsters, rabbits, and dogs have not been recorded in work dealing with these hosts.

Age.   Since Chagas' first investigations (1909), it has been recognized that the course of *T. cruzi* infections is more severe in younger individuals than in older. Experimental confirmation of this was provided by Regendanz (1930) and Niimi (1935), who found that young mice, rats, and rabbits suffered more intense infections than did older ones. On the other hand, Zuccarini (1930) found that guinea pigs were equally susceptible at all ages. Kolodny (1939a, b, c) found in a series of studies that suckling rats up to 20 days of age could not respond to the infections with production of sufficient protective antibody to be demonstrable in a protection test. Rats infected at 30 days of age produced antibody which could be detected about 15 days after infection and which attained a maximum (which was lower than that in older animals) at about 35 days. Rats 60 days of age and older produced antibody which was demonstrable 8 days after infection, and the titer was somewhat higher at 35 days after infection than that of the 30-day-old animals (Kolodny, 1940a).

Kolodny, in his work with rats, and Culbertson and Kessler (1942), in their work with mice, used both intraperitoneal and oral routes of inoculation. They found age resistance in either case, but less intense and less frequently fatal infections occurred when the inoculum was given *per os*. Pizzi (1957) pointed out that the maximum susceptibility to the virulent Tulahuén strain was in mice less than 75 days old, and Galliard et al. (1962b) noted longer survival times in adult mice as compared with young mice infected with this strain. Marcuse et al. (1964) reported that newborn mice died 2 to 3 days after infection, but the average time between the appearance of parasitemia and death in other than newborn mice was 7 to 9 days, regardless of age. With a strain of parasite which killed all mice less than a month old, there were some survivors among more mature (70-day-old) animals. Goble (1952a) found that in untreated infections with strains which were uniformly fatal to puppies, adult dogs sometimes showed resistance with ensuing spontaneous recovery.

Sex. Although there are a number of clinical references indicating that Chagas' disease has greater incidence and severity in males, these data might be interpreted as resulting from a greater risk of exposure for males. Experimental studies, however, have shown that there is a fundamental difference in the response of each sex to the disease. Hauschka (1947a) pointed out that a consistent difference was present in four different strains of mice (A, C, C₃H, and DBA) when infected with three strains of *T. cruzi* (Brasil, Culbertson, and WBH). The greater susceptibility of males was manifested in terms of parasitemia, degree of tissue invasion, and survival rate.

Goble (1951) also found a greater susceptibility in male mice infected with two strains (Brasil and A), but Streber (1950), working with another strain (Izurcar, from Mexico), found, to the contrary, that females showed higher parasitemias than did males in tests with both mice and rats. He reported that the myocardial invasion by parasites was greater in females and considered his observations to be evidence that different strains of *T. cruzi* might react differently to the hormones of the host. No other findings similar to Streber's have been reported, and numerous subsequent studies (Galliard et al., 1962b; Goble, unpublished) with additional strains of parasites (Tulahuén, Peru, and Y) have consistently confirmed Hauschka's observations that males are more susceptible than females. This is true not only in the untreated disease but also in chemotherapeutic experiments. The females responded more readily to chemotherapy, presumably because some immune mechanisms were concurrently in operation (Konopka et al., 1965, 1966).

That substances other than the steroids of the adult gonads are involved seems to be indicated by the prepuberal occurrence of the sex difference in susceptibility and by the fact that the course of the disease is not influenced by the administration of hormones characteristic of the opposite sex to males or females during infection (Goble, 1952b, 1966).

Wood (1934) attempted to augment the pathogenicity of an avirulent strain in rats by administration of aqueous testicular extracts. Krampitz and Disko (1966) made some interesting ancillary observations which require clarification. They found that mice infected with *T. cruzi* show a slight increase in the number of parasites during pregnancy. During lactation, however, the development of parasites is retarded. Lactating infected mice live longer than nonlactating controls and often may survive. With infections which are uniformly fatal to normal mice, up to 50 percent survival may be found in lactating mice. This has been noted with two different strains of parasite (NMRI/Tubingen and WBH).

Goble (1952a) found that in dogs the prepatent periods and survival times did not differ between the sexes, but parasitemias in males were higher than in females. This sex difference was also prepuberal. In juvenile dogs which succumbed to acute experimental Chagas' disease and died from myocarditis and cardiac insufficiency between 25 and 49 days after infection, their thyroid glands showed striking differences which were dependent on sex. The glands from all but one of 17 males were normal compared to material from uninfected controls, whereas those from females showed diffuse parenchymatous changes in 12 of the 17 examined (Goble, 1954). These observations were made with the Brasil strain of *T. cruzi*, but have not been noted in infections with other strains.

Environmental factors—*Endocrine state.* Non-sex-dependent endocrine factors are perhaps more susceptible to the influence of environment than are the fundamental differences associated with maleness and femaleness. The environment can influence hormonal systems by stress, which involves changes in the adrenal-pituitary axis and the concomitant effects of varying levels of adrenocorticotropic hormones and cortisone.

The effects of cortisone began to be studied in 1951. There were planned tests in mice by Chilean workers who decided to investigate the possibility that cortisone might alter the course of experimental Chagas' disease (Jarpa et al., 1951). On the other hand, there were fortuitous observations of certain North American neurologists who were using cortisone along with the administration of monkey brain and adjuvants in the study of experimental disseminated encephalomyelitis in Rhesus monkeys (Wolf et al., 1951, 1953). The first group found that cortisone had a marked unfavorable effect on the course of experimental Chagas' disease in DBA mice, which could not be controlled by usually favorable chemotherapeutic doses of pentaquine. The latter group found that cortisone exacerbated latent *T. cruzi* infections in monkeys (Seneca and Wolf, 1955).

The Chilean workers conducted a series of studies on the action of cortisone in C_3H and DBA mice with Chagas' disease, and found that the steroid not only effected a greater degree of tissue parasitism but also caused a shift in the sites of predilection from the heart and skeletal muscle (where most parasites were found in untreated animals) to the liver (Neghme et al., 1951). They also found that cortisone enhances the antitumor effect of *T. cruzi* infections in C_3H mice (Christen et al., 1951). It enhances uncomplicated, untreated *T. cruzi* infections in Rockefeller mice (Pizzi et al., 1952) and in normal DBA mice (Thierman and Christen, 1952), as well as in adrenalectomized DBA mice in which even more pronounced effects were observed (Neghme et al., 1952). It was also reported to enhance the aggravating effect of chlortetracycline on the infection in DBA mice (Thierman and Christen, 1952). Additional articles by Agosin, Jarpa, Pizzi, Prager, Rubio and their colleagues have been reviewed by Pizzi (1952, 1957).

Chronic and mild infections in rats of the A/c strain were reported to be unaffected by administration of high doses of cortisone (Pizzi et al., 1952), but Seneca and Rockenbach (1952) found that acute fatal infections could be induced in baby rats by the use of cortisone. At about the same time, Friebel (1952) reported that cortisone abolished the temporary inhibitory effect of trypan blue on *T. cruzi* infections. Later, Seneca and Ides (1955) found that hydroxycortisone exerted a lesser effect than cortisone in DBA mice and that with certain regimens, compound S (17-hydroxydesoxycorticosterone) partially protected the animals against the resistance-lowering effects of cortisone. Galliard et al. (1962b) also found cortisone to aggravate *T. cruzi* infections, as well as to abolish the cross-resistance which results from prior infections with heterologous strains (Galliard et al., 1962a, c).

In experimental animals, cortisone has usually been shown to exert an infection-enhancing effect which nullifies the chemotherapeutic action of agents which are effective in mice not receiving steroids. In man, however, Espinosa (1959) has reported a salutary effect of cortisone administration concurrent with primaquine therapy, allowing prolonged treatment regimens without untoward side-effects.

Adrenocorticotropic hormone (ACTH) is reported to have an opposite effect to that of cortisone when given to dogs with acute experimental Chagas' disease. The animals showed marked improvement with ACTH administration and survived infections which caused death in untreated animals (Robles Gil et al., 1950, 1951). Philocreon (1951), on the other hand, found it to be ineffective in two human patients with cardiopathy of Chagas' disease.

Somatropic hormone (STH) was found by Sommer (1955) to shorten the survival time of mice (GN strain) infected with *T. cruzi*, although to a lesser extent than did cortisone. However, Galliard et al. (1962b) found STH to be without effect. Although the spleen-shrinking and body-weight depressing effects of cortisone were partially antagonized by STH, there was no effect of STH on the course of the infection in cortisone-treated animals.

The coincidental occurrence of goiter in areas in which there was a high incidence of *T. cruzi* infection led Chagas to consider that thyroid abnormality was one of the signs of Chagas' disease. Later workers have indicated, however, that *T. cruzi* infection is not involved in the etiology of goiter, and that the thyroid functions in Chagas' disease patients and in non-Chagas' disease controls, living in a region where there is high prevalence of both Chagas' disease and goiter, did not differ significantly (Lobo et al., 1962). Since the incidence of goiter in the region studied was the same in patients with Chagas' disease as in those uninfected, it also appears that hypothyroidism does not predispose to *T. cruzi* infection. Hyperthyroidism, however, when induced in rats by feeding them iodinated casein, was accompanied in some *T. cruzi*-infected animals by cardiac damage which did not appear in infected rats on control diets (Yaeger and Miller, 1966).

Nutrition. Although caloric restriction has little effect on the susceptibility of rats to experimental Chagas' disease (Yaeger and Miller, 1966), rats fed a purified diet containing a low quality protein (gluten) were more susceptible than those receiving a high quality protein (casein). Supplementing the caloric diet with lysine markedly reduced the susceptibility of the rats on that diet, although the parasitemia and cardiac damage could not be reduced to the level of those in the control animals (Yaeger and Miller, 1963b, c). Riboflavin deficiency did not effect a significant increase in susceptibility (Yaeger and Miller, 1960b), but thiamine deficiency resulted in higher parasitemias and greater cardiac damage (Yaeger and Miller, 1960a). Similar increases in susceptibility resulted with pantothenate deficiency and pyridoxine deficiency, as well as with vitamin A deficiency (Yaeger and Miller, 1960c, d, 1963a). Ofman (1944) and Pizzi (1944), however, found that scorbutic guinea pigs are less susceptible to *T. cruzi* infection than are normal animals. It has been suggested that this may be attributable to the ascorbate requirement of the parasite (Lwoff, 1938).

Environmental temperature. After having observed that the parasitemia in rats inoculated with *T. cruzi* varied according to the season of the year (being more benign in the summer), Kolodny (1939b, 1940b) studied infected rats which were kept at different temperatures. He found that those kept at near body temperature (90° to 95°F) had lower parasitemias than those kept at room temperature (70° to 74°F), and that animals kept in the cold (40° to 45°F) had severe parasitemias and died.

Hauschka (1949b) observed seasonal variation in parasitemias in mice infected with *T. cruzi*, as did Galliard et al. (1962b). The severity of the infection was inversely correlated with the ambient temperature. Franca-Rodriguez and MacKinnon (1962) found that *T. cruzi* infections in mice were less intense in animals kept at body temperature than in those kept at room temperature. These results were confirmed by the studies of Trejos et al. (1965), who not only kept mice at different temperatures but changed the ambient temperature of some of the mice during the course of the experiment. Animals started at 37°C with low parasitemias had rapid increases in their parasitemias when changed to 18°C, and animals at the lower temperature with high parasitemias showed a reversal in parasitemias when transferred to the high temperature.

Amrein (1967) studied male Swiss mice infected with *T. cruzi* (Yucatan strain) after one week at temperatures of 10°C and 35°C. All of the animals kept at 35° survived, while those kept at 10° died in 21 to 26 days. Surprisingly, however, if the mice were treated with a steroid (dexamethasone), the results were reversed. Those kept at 10° survived and those kept at 35° suffered a 60 percent mortality. Reduction of the body temperature of mice with chlorpromazine was reported by Friebel and Kastner (1955) to aggravate *T. cruzi* infection, effecting increases in parasitemias and earlier deaths in treated mice than in untreated animals, but this could not be confirmed by Neva et al. (1961).

Victoria (1954), Victoria and Dalma (1956), and Dalma (1956, 1961) attempted pyretotherapy in human patients with Chagas' disease. They induced fever by the intravenous injection of bacterial vaccines or by intramuscular injection of sterile milk. Some of their patients, however, were also treated with spirotrypan or with 8-aminoquinolines (pentaquine, isopentaquine, and primaquine), so the salutary effects that they observed could not be entirely attributable to the fever treatment and, in any case, were not statistically significant.

Intercurrent infection. As early as 1907, Trautmann observed that intercurrent infections with *Borrelia duttoni* had a protective effect on infections with the African pathogenic trypanosomes. Galliard (1930a) extended these studies to a number of other species of *Borrelia*. He observed a relative attenuation of acute *T. cruzi* infections in mice when *Borrelia crocidurae* was the concurrent agent. Later, he and his colleagues studied *Borrelia duttoni* and *B. persica* and confirmed the antagonistic effect of these spirochetes on experimental Chagas' disease in mice (Galliard et al., 1959). It has been suggested that damage to the reticuloendothelial system is involved in spirochete infections, and that compensatory hyperactivity of that system in response to the injury may be the basis of the attenuating effect on trypanosome infections (Hassko, 1931; Schlossberger and Grillo, 1935). This view seems to be supported by Galliard's observation (1930b) that the effect is reduced in animals which are splenectomized.

Zeledon and Lizano (1962) infected guinea pigs with *T. cruzi* (PE strain, from cardiac blood) given intraperitoneally, and after 60 days, they superimposed an infection with *Leishmania enriettii* from a nasal nodule, also given intraperitoneally. A month after inoculation with *Leishmania*, the guinea pigs with the concurrent *T. cruzi* infection showed a slight, soft orchitis, while most animals with leishmaniasis alone had some nodular periorchitic lesions, which did not appear until later in the *T. cruzi*-infected group. Deaths, attributable to secondary infection, began to occur earlier in the animals infected with only *Leishmania* than in those with concurrent *T. cruzi* infection. The electrophoretic picture will be referred to later (*see* pp. 631–632).

In combined infections with *T. cruzi* and *Schistosoma mansoni* in mice (Abath et al., 1966), the concurrent schistosome infection did not effect any change in the histopathologic picture of Chagasic polymyositis, but the death rates in groups with intercurrent infection with both parasites suggested that the experimental Chagas' disease had a protective effect against the schistosome infection. The mortality rates in the dual infections (11 and 17 percent) were significantly different (p<0.01) from that in the schistosome infection alone (61 percent). On the clinical side, there is a suggestion (Torres Pereyra, 1967) that a paratyphoid A infection may have reactivated a chronic *T. cruzi* infection in a child, resulting in acute myocarditis.

Irradiation. Unpublished experiments of Pizzi indicate that x-irradiation of rats results in high tissue invasion and parasitemia following infection with a *T. cruzi* strain which normally produces a low level of infection in this host (Goble and Singer, 1960).

Parasite factors—*Strain.* Differences in the behavior of strains of *T. cruzi* were recognized by Brumpt (1913a), who studied two strains which differed in virulence and found that infection with the avirulent one (Bahia) induced resistance to the virulent one (Chagas). Characteristics other than virulence (as measured by mortality), which have been reported to differ among strains, are morphology (Brener and Chiari, 1963b), aspects of early growth (Brener and Chiari, 1966), tissue affinity and course of parasitemia (von Brand et al., 1949; Goble, 1958; Biagi et al., 1965; Galliard, 1965; Watkins, 1966), drug susceptibility and response to seasonal temperature (Hauschka, 1949b), prepatent period (Brener, 1965), and elaboration of various antigens (Moore, 1957; Nussenzweig et al., 1962, 1963; Nussenzweig, 1963; Nussenzweig and Goble, 1964, 1966).

The virulence of some strains can be influenced by the size of the inoculum used; smaller numbers of infective organisms give rise to less acute infections and lower mortality (Phillips, 1960). Other strains, however, are intrinsically different, and reduction in inoculum size may delay the fatal outcome of the infection but not prevent it.

Virulence does not seem to be directly associated with immunogenicity. Strains attenuated by long passage in culture (Pizzi and Prager, 1952; Menezes, 1968) or strains of naturally low virulence (Hauschka et al., 1950; Norman and Kagan, 1960) are able to induce protective immunity to challenge with highly virulent strains.

Passage. In a number of microorganisms, the way in which a strain is maintained is known to affect their virulence. The general observations are that prolonged maintenance in culture media may decrease virulence, and that passage through susceptible animals may result in greater pathogenicity. These generalizations are, however, not without exception and may be conditioned by many factors. Although Goble (1951) and Pizzi and Prager (1952) observed diminution in virulence in some *T. cruzi* strains following prolonged *in vitro* passage, Goble found that one strain, which was maintained under the same conditions as one which became avirulent, did not change its infectivity or pathogenicity during several years in culture. Packchanian and Sweets (1947) reported that infectivity was retained by a strain maintained in culture for 13 years without any intervening animal passage. Norman and Kagan (1960) have reported an increase in virulence in weanling mice of several strains of relatively low virulence maintained in culture without animal passage. So it appears that passage in culture media may reduce infectivity, enhance it, or effect no change, depending on factors which have not been defined. Inasmuch as protective immunity can be induced by both virulent and avirulent strains, these variations in pathogenicity, uncorrelated with immunogenicity, emphasize that the importance of the method of culture cannot be stated with certainty.

The effects of animal passage are likewise unpredictable. Although it is not well-documented, it seems probable that most of the virulent strains which have been maintained for some time in mouse-to-mouse passage were isolated from human cases of Chagas' disease or from bugs in areas where human cases are frequent. It appears that most animal isolates are less virulent than human strains (Norman et al., 1959; Nussenzweig et al., 1963). The latter apparently show an inherent trait of virulence which does not occur in most animal isolates. There is no report to date indicating that a strain of originally low virulence has ever been established in animal passage with a resulting increase in virulence. A strain of inherent virulence which has lost it by prolonged passage in culture or passage through bugs has, however, the potential of having its virulence restored by repeated animal passage (Goble, 1951; Phillips, 1960).

Size of inoculum.   As early as 1921, Nattan-Larrier, using blood forms of *T. cruzi* as inocula, found that reducing the number of parasites given resulted in attenuated infections. Dias (1934) also noted the correlation between the number of organisms inoculated and the severity of the disease. Although Kolodny (1939a) did not obtain similar correlation in rats, Mazotti (1940a), and Pizzi and Prager (1952) found partial correlation. Romaña and Terracini (1945), Da Silva and Nussenzweig (1953), Ghelelovich and Chassignet (1957), and Hewitt et al. (1963) reported complete correlation. The last authors found that infections resulting from intraperitoneal inoculations were more erratic than those initiated by the subcutaneous route, and that the gradation among the infections resulting from dilution of inocula was far more uniform when the infections were given subcutaneously. Phillips (1960) pointed out that there are two types of experimental *T. cruzi* infections, each depending on the strain characteristics. In one type, the intensity and course of infection is associated with the number of parasites inoculated. In the other type, reducing the size of the inoculum does not reduce the virulence or pathogenicity; the prepatent period or survival time may be prolonged, but the eventual mortality cannot be influenced by reduction of the inoculum. Mazzoti (1940) found that inoculation into mice of varying numbers (from 800 to 8,000) of parasites from the intestinal contents of *Triatoma* did not result in measureable differences in the course of the parasitemia. It should be pointed out that this was a nonfatal strain of *T. cruzi* and that the numbers of organisms inoculated were relatively low. Goble (1951) found that increasing the size of the inoculum from 10 million to 30 million culture organisms resulted in an increase in mouse mortality from 10 percent to 98 percent.

Stage of parasite inoculated.   Marsden (1968), using the Peru strain, compared infectivity and virulence of the forms from mouse blood (after numerous passages) and from bug (*Rhodnius prolixus*) feces. He found that the fecal flagellates were more infectious but caused fewer deaths. The fecal forms also induced infections by the conjunctival route more often than did the blood forms.

Mechanisms of natural resistance

Although normal sera of various animals contain substances which are lytic to the crithidial forms of *T. cruzi*, the main defense against the parasite seems to be phagocytosis by inflammatory macrophages, perhaps assisted by non-lytic or opsonin-like factors (Pizzi, 1957, 1963; Pizzi et al., 1953). The cellular aspects, therefore, will be discussed first.

Cellular factors. Although Souza Campos (1929a, b, 1934), Souza Campos and Artigas (1932), Dias (1932, 1934), and Mazza et al. (1935a, b, 1943) recognized the close relation of *T. cruzi* to certain cells of the reticuloendothelial system, they were particularly impressed by the role of macrophages as host cells for the parasite. Pizzi (1954) and his collaborators (Pizzi et al., 1953, 1954; Pizzi and Rubio, 1955; Taliaferro and Pizzi, 1955) pointed out the functions of the lymphoid-macrophage system in relation to natural resistance to experimental Chagas' disease. When culture forms of low virulence are injected into nonimmune (as well as immune) mice, they are rapidly destroyed, especially by the inflammatory macrophages. When virulent blood forms are injected into nonimmune mice, only a relatively small number are digested in the macrophages and most develop normally into intracellular fission forms in free and fixed macrophages (reticular cells, littoral cells, and histiocytes) which are eventually destroyed. In rats infected with virulent blood forms, the rate of intracellular reproduction of the parasites is less than it is in mice, and the inflammation at the site of inoculation is accelerated, with abundant macrophages appearing early. Pizzi et al. (1954) pointed out that the higher degree of innate immunity in rats is associated with a marked ability to develop acquired immunity, and that the cellular immunity is probably assisted by non-lytic antibodies. Even in lower animals, such as frogs and toads, the sera of which are lytic for crithidial forms of *T. cruzi* at 1:10 dilution *in vitro*, defense seems to be effected by rapid phagocytosis and digestion of the parasites at the point of inoculation. Some trypanosomes are able to reach the blood stream, and these are destroyed mainly in the liver and kidney by macrophages, polyblasts, and heterophils (Rubio, 1956).

Some attempts have been made to elucidate the importance of the cellular aspects of resistance to *T. cruzi* by manipulations calculated to alter the function of the reticuloendothelial system. Splenectomy has consistently been reported to have no influence on the infection in mice, rats, guinea pigs, or dogs (Kritschewski and Schwartzman, 1928; Nieschulz and Wawo-Roentoe, 1930; Galliard, 1930; Regendanz, 1930; Wood, 1934; Kelser, 1936; Galliard et al., 1962b; Dias, 1934; Kofoid and Donat, 1933; Ofman, 1944;

Pizzi, 1957). However, Pizzi and Knierman (1955) found antibody titers to be reduced in splenectomized mice. Similarly, attempts at reticuloendothelial blockade (Friebel, 1952; Pizzi, 1954; Dias, 1934) have not resulted in alterations in the course of infection, although antibody titers were reduced (Denison, 1943a, b). Goble and Boyd (1962), however, were able to lower the resistance of mice to strains of *T. cruzi* of low infectivity by intravenous injection of colloidal thorium dioxide on five consecutive days starting on the fourth day before infection. They were not able to affect the course of the infection by the administration of rabbit antimouse-spleen serum, which when administered in murine *T. congolense* infections results in acceleration of the disease.

Humoral factors. Muniz and Borriello (1945) reported that normal human and guinea pig sera lysed the crithidial forms in culture, but not the metacyclic trypanosome forms (which are the stages which are infective to the vertebrate host). It is possible that the latter are not affected because they have an ability not found in the crithidial forms to survive the humoral defenses of the host on inoculation and to invade cells and transform into intracellular stages. Rubio (1956b) found that sera from sheep, rats, hamsters, fowl, chickens, frogs, and toads behaved similarly when undiluted, and that certain sera were lytic for crithidial forms within one hour, even when diluted 1:10. These were the sera from sheep, rats, guinea pigs, frogs, and toads, diluted hamster and chicken sera were not lytic for crithidial forms within one hour but were in 24 hours. Only the sera (undiluted) from the fowl, frogs, and toads were lytic for the metacyclic trypanosome forms in culture, and only the frog sera showed this activity in the 1:10 dilution in one hour; diluted fowl and toad sera were, however, lytic in 24 hours. Warren and Borsos (1959) studied fowl serum more extensively and concluded that two factors active against crithidial forms were present: (1) a heat-stable factor, which is probably an agglutinating and sensitizing antibody, and (2) a heat-labile factor, complement.

ACQUIRED RESISTANCE

That an initial infection with *T. cruzi* confers resistance to subsequent infection has been known since the time of Blanchard (1912a, b). His reports were soon followed by that of Brumpt (1913b), who found that infection of mice with a strain of low virulence led to cross-resistance to challenge with a virulent strain. The humoral aspect of this acquired immunity was demonstrated by Guerrero and Machado (1913), who adapted the Bordet-Gengou reaction for the detection of complement-fixing antibody in Chagas' disease. Mayer and Rocha Lima (1914) also recognized that rats which acquired immunity during the course of the acute infection remained thereafter resistant to superinfection. They were not, however, able to demonstrate protective or curative effects with sera from immune animals.

Collier (1931) attenuated a strain of *T. cruzi* (by subjecting it to trypaflavine) and used it to produce mild infections in mice, which were thereafter resistant to superinfection with a virulent nonattenuated strain. He pointed out that this was not a sterile immunity, but it was a resistance that depended on the presence of residual infection with the avirulent organism.

Dias (1934) and Wood (1934) confirmed the existence of strong immunity in animals which survived infection. The former attempted (but was unable) to demonstrate passive immunity by transfer of sera from immune animals to infected nonimmune animals.

Packchanian (1935) studied agglutination and precipitin production in rabbits injected with *T. cruzi*. Kelser (1936) made a significant breakthrough in the practice of the complement-fixation test by introducing the use of antigen made from culture organisms rather than from organs of infected animals.

The most systematic early experimental work in acquired immunity was begun by Culbertson and Kolodny (1938). They studied Chagas' disease in rats, which have greater natural immunity than do mice, and which do not ordinarily succumb to the disease after they have reached young adulthood. Rats which recovered from initial infections were completely resistant to reinfection, and their sera conferred passive protection to nonimmune rats on subcutaneous injection. Kolodny (1939a) continued these studies, defining the influence of age on the development of the immune response and recording the rate of antibody production in various age groups as determined by protection tests.

Darman (1941) made additional observations of cross-immunity between strains of *T. cruzi* in mice. Culbertson and Kessler (1942) studied age immunity in mice, which had been noted in rats by Regandanz (1930). Denison (1943a, b) pointed out that sera from immune rats lysed the culture forms of *T. cruzi*, and the titer of these antibodies diminished in animals which were splenectomized or subjected to reticuloendothelial blockade.

The modern period in the experimental study of acquired immunity may be said to have started in the late 1940's with the work of Hauschka et al. (1950) and Pizzi et al. (reviewed by Pizzi, 1957), whose findings will be discussed under the appropriate topics below, along with observations of later authors.

Factors affecting immune response

It may be presumed that all of the factors, such as those of the host, environment, and parasite, which condition natural resistance may also be involved in acquired resistance, although specific documentation may be difficult to adduce. Some examples, however, may be cited. Host species differences in response to trypanosome infection are generally recognized, and it appears that rats demonstrate an immune response to infection more promptly than mice (Pizzi et al., 1954). Strain differences in reticuloendothelial structure and function have been reported for mice (Stern, 1948; Duque, 1965), but have not specifically been correlated with response to *T. cruzi* infection. Marr and Pike (1967), however, found differences in the degree of protection developed by different strains of mice in response to injection with an avirulent strain (Corpus Christi) of *T. cruzi*. In four strains of mice (DBA-2J, C57BL-6J, LAF₁, and SWR-J), the response was enough to protect 100 percent of the previously inoculated mice against subsequent challenge with the virulent Brasil strain. In two other strains (C3H-HeJ and C57BR-cdJ), only partial protection was effected (29 percent and 57 percent, respectively). Immunization has been found to differ as much as ten-fold between different strains of mice in response to tetanus toxoid (Ipsen, 1959), and genetic control of combining sites of antibodies and of immunoglobulin synthesis has been demonstrated in various species with various antigens (Lennox, 1966; Oudin, 1966). The ability of rats to produce antibodies in experimental Chagas' disease has been shown to be definitely dependent on age (Kolodny, 1939a). There is ample evidence from other systems that the immune response is different in the two sexes (Galton, 1967), and that both cellular (Hartveit, 1966; Halberg et al., 1957) and humoral (Lawford and White, 1964; Reuter and Kennes, 1966; Butterworth et al., 1967) elements are sex-dependent.

Mechanisms of acquired resistance

Pizzi et al. (1954) and Taliaferro and Pizzi (1955) have pointed out that the main defensive mechanism in acquired resistance to Chagas' disease is, as in natural resistance, cellular immunity, and that the role of humoral factors is not clear.

Cellular factors. The manner in which cellular elements are mobilized following infection with Chagas' disease in the nonimmune animal has been noted (*see* pp. 614–615). It has been pointed out that the difference between the defensive reactivity in nonimmune animals and that in immune ones is quantitative. Those with acquired immunity mobilize inflammatory macrophages as do nonimmune animals, but they do so more rapidly and more intensively, and the response is possibly assisted by non-lytic humoral factors (Pizzi et al., 1954; Taliaferro and Pizzi, 1955). These authors note the similarity between the immune mechanisms in Chagas' disease and those in malaria, i.e., the involvement of macrophage defense with probable opsonin cooperation. However, they emphasize the difference in the sites of parasite distribution; in Chagas' disease the macrophages in the connective tissue of various organs are primarily involved, whereas in malaria the spleen is the outstanding site of predilection.

Humoral factors and passive transfer. Muniz and de Freitas (1946) noted that the effects of immune serum on culture forms of the parasite *in vitro* may not be at all indicative of the role which humoral factors play in the body. Although not reported in detail, it seems likely that they observed some of the phenomena more comprehensively described later by Adler (1958), who grew *T. cruzi* in media containing various dilutions of specific antisera prepared in rabbits. Adler noted agglutination, such as that observed by Muniz and de Freitas with sera from patients with Chagas' disease, as well as the development of colonies and multinucleated masses from flagellates which survived the effects of the antiserum. These papers, which should be consulted in the original, do not, however, elucidate the possible mode of action of humoral factors *in vivo*. It seems likely that whatever effects are exerted against the parasite during the course of the disease are mediated through synergism with cellular factors. Since immune sera are ineffective against the trypanosomal (blood) forms *in vitro*, experiments indicating their activity *in vivo* are of interest.

Culbertson and Kolodny (1938) found that the sera of rats which had recovered from *T. cruzi* infection conferred protection to normal rats (10 to 15 days old) when injected into these animals. Prophylactic administration did not completely prevent infection, but permitted only a low-grade infection. Therapeutic administration caused an incomplete crisis in which the parasitemia fell temporarily, with relapses occurring soon after the serum injections were suspended. The authors presumed that the action was against only the blood forms, and that the serum did not reach the intracellular stages.

Hauschka et al. (1950) were unable to protect mice against lethal infections by passive transfer of large amounts of antiserum administered either prophylactically or therapeutically. Kagan and Norman (1961), however, prophylactically protected mice by intraperitoneal administration of immune mouse serum, but Voller and Shaw (1965) were unable to alter the course of the infection by the injection of antiserum on the 15th day after infection. Ryckman (1965) studied passive transfer of resistance to young rats (7 days old) which were given sera from recovered rats prior to infection. He also reported that milk from chronically infected females was protective for baby rats.

Antigens and other cell products

Antigenic analyses. Earlier studies on antigens of *T. cruzi* were mainly concerned with the specificity of serologic reactions, usually agglutination, and with the presence of common antigens with other species of trypanosomes or other genera of hemoflagellates (Packchanian, 1935, 1940; Chang and Negherbon, 1947; Menolasino and Hartman, 1954). In many studies, only one strain of *T. cruzi* was used. When a number of strains were tested simultaneously, it was found that some variations in titer might occur between different strains, but that strains could not be distinguished by simple agglutination tests (Senekjie, 1943; Hauschka et al., 1950).

With the advent of gel-diffusion techniques (Ouchterlony, 1949), a new tool became available. This method was first applied to *T. cruzi* antigens by Moore (1957), who studied two strains of *T. cruzi* from Texas (Corpus Christi and Houston) in comparison with one from Brazil (Brasil), as well as two species of *Leishmania*. He prepared antigens both from washed organisms and from the parasite-free liquid phase of the diphasic medium in which the organisms were grown. Antisera were prepared in rabbits. In the gel-diffusion tests, there were apparently common antigens between *T. cruzi* (Brasil) and *Leishmania tropica* (Teheran) which were not found in the Corpus Christi or Houston strains of *T. cruzi*. There were no common lines between *L. donovani* and the *T. cruzi* strains. The Brasil strain of *T. cruzi* appeared to have more antigenic components than the North American strains.

Nussenzweig et al. (1962, 1963a) used rabbit sera for agglutination tests, which they performed both before and after absorption of the antisera. In gel-precipitation tests, they reported that rabbit sera reacted with several components of the antigens used, giving rise to at least ten different precipitation lines in double-diffusion plates and immunoelectrophoresis. These lines were not sharp and their number depended on the concentration of the antigen extracts used. Absorption of the antisera did not clarify the results. Seneca and Peer (1963a, b) reported nine different lines when rabbit sera were used, but only three appeared with horse serum.

Nussenzweig and his coworkers found that horse serum with its fewer reactive components could be used in double-diffusion tests and electrophoretic studies to demonstrate two immunologic types of *T. cruzi*: one, type A, included strains which could completely absorb agglutinins from anti-A sera; the other, type B, included strains which can absorb only part of the agglutinins from anti-A sera. Subsequent studies (Nussenzweig, 1963; Nussenzweig and Goble, 1964, 1966) categorized an additional number of strains, bringing the total examined to 36. In addition to the original two types, A and B, a third (designated C), differing from both A and B but probably closer to A, was found in only one host species, *Tayra barbara*, a carnivore from Brazil. These immunologic types were not clearly associated with either the species of host (both A and B types were found among isolates from both man and raccoons), geographic distribution (both A and B types were found in North and South America), or pathogenicity.

Vaccines. As has been pointed out elsewhere (p. 627), the inability to predict the virulence for man of so-called avirulent strains precluded the suggestion that strains of naturally low virulence or live attenuated strains (Collier, 1931) be used for the induction of active immunity by vaccination. Some attention has been given to preparations of killed *T. cruzi* material as vaccines. In 1946, Muniz et al. prepared vaccine from culture organisms killed with thimerosal and attempted to immunize monkeys against subsequent challenge with parasites from the feces of triatomes. They obtained serum agglutinin titers but no protection. Subsequently, Hauschka et al. (1950) treated blood and culture forms with formalin. These were ineffective in protecting mice from challenge with virulent blood forms. Hauschka suggested that effective protection was dependent on antibodies which are produced only as a result of active infection.

The work of Hauschka et al. (1950) provided a hint that killed *T. cruzi* materials might have some protective antigenicity. They ground freshly lyophilized spleens from infected mice into a powder which was then suspended in Ringer-Locke solution and injected subcutaneously into mice. Following subsequent challenge with the homologous parasite, there was an insignificantly lower parasitemia in the spleen-treated mice as compared with untreated controls, and their survival time was slightly greater.

In a study which was designed to document the histopathologic changes in mice infected with *T. cruzi* under different conditions of resistance, Rego (1956) gave repeated subcutaneous injections ("sensitizing doses") of triturated freeze-dried culture organisms to mice, and then followed this series with a large "shocking" dose (intraperitoneally) 9 to 15 days after the original series. About three weeks later, these animals were infected by intraperitoneal injection of virulent blood forms (Y strain). All of the mice contracted the infection and showed parasitemia and mild signs of disease at about 10 days after infection, but were normal at 15 days. All survived for 53 days, at which time they were sacrificed. However, six out of seven control mice died in 10 to 12 days. Although Rego pointed out in his summary that the series of "sensitizing" doses followed by the "shocking" dose conferred resistance to subsequent infection, he did not seem to appreciate his breakthrough in demonstrating that protection could be conferred by nonliving material, nor did he refer to the earlier observations of Collier (1931), Muniz et al. (1946), or Hauschka et al. (1950).

In 1959, Goble and co-workers began an investigation on preparations of *T. cruzi* killed by various physical means, having ascertained that a variety of chemical methods of killing the parasites resulted in nonprotective materials. Culture organisms disrupted by ultrasonication, by pressure, or by shaking with glass beads were used as experimental vaccines and were found to be protective in mice. Inasmuch as only an abstract was published referring to this work (Goble et al., 1964), a more detailed description of these investigations will be given: The Brasil strain of *T. cruzi* was cultured at room temperature in a modification of Johnson's diphasic medium (Goble, 1952a) or in Warren's HM liquid medium (Warren, 1960). Ten-day-old cultures were centrifuged to concentrate the cells. The cells were then washed with Locke's solution and resuspended in one-tenth of the original volume. The resulting suspensions, containing about 300 million cells per milliliter, were placed in the chamber of a magneto-restrictive oscillator (Ratheon Model DF-101) and subjected to vibration at a frequency of 10 kilocycles per second, for periods ranging from 15 minutes to 1 hour, until no intact cells could be found on microscopic examination of samples of the fluid. Samples were also cultured to confirm the sterility of the preparations.

In the first test (Fig. 1), DBA mice were injected subcutaneously with virulent blood forms of *T. cruzi* (over one million parasites per mouse). A

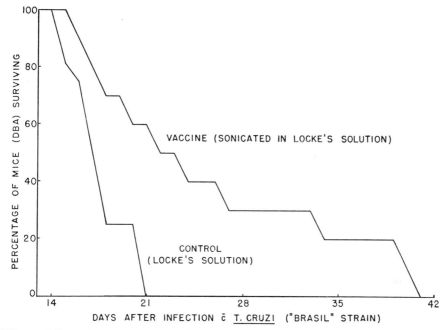

FIG. 1. Effect of vaccination with homogenate of *T. cruzi* prepared by sonication on survival rate of mice challenged with Chagas' disease.

severe infection ensued, killing all of the control mice in 21 days. Although all of the vaccinated mice died within 41 days, there was an increase in the survival time of the immunized group, which although significant only at the 2.5 percent level, encouraged the pursuit of the problem. Later experiments were done with CF1 mice, and a challenge time (21 days after vaccination) and challenge dose (20,000 trypanosomes per mouse) were established for assay purposes. In addition to microscopic examinations and culturing of homogenates to be sure no live organisms were present in the vaccines, blood samples were taken on a number of tests from the mice before challenge and cultured to secure that there were no subpatent infections.

On the supposition that oxidation might accompany sonication, various thiol compounds were added to the suspensions, and more effective preparations resulted. Although cystine gave better results than mercaptoethanol, it was eventually abandoned because of the formation of insoluble precipitates of cystine as it was oxidized, and eventually glutathione was used as the material of choice.

Although it was also possible to get some effective preparations by the use of the French pressure cell, the best results were obtained with the products of disintegration resulting from shaking the organisms with ballotini in the Shockman (1957) apparatus in a refrigerated centrifuge. These preparations were less labile, and eventually good preparations were made without the use of thiol compounds. One preparation in this series was stored at 70°C for over 3 months and was still effective. At temperatures above freezing, however, the ability of the homogenates to induce protective immunity decreased rapidly (Fig. 2).

The increase in the immune response with an increase in time between vaccination and challenge is shown in Table 4. The highest values were observed when the interval was 3 weeks or more. These levels of protection were maintained up to 7 weeks, after which time there was some decline. However, protection was demonstrable for at least 4 months, the longest interval tested.

Kagan and Norman (1961) prepared a vaccine of culture organisms with thimerosal. Their material did not give any protection, either immediately (within a few days) after the vaccine dose or 10 weeks later.

Johnson et al. (1963) reported successful immunization of mice against experimental Chagas' disease by the use of *T. cruzi* killed by alternate freezing and thawing, but their preparations were only active when given in combination with adjuvants, the most effective of which was a saponin from the Chilean soap tree. In their experiments, the parasitemias were decreased and survival times increased, but sterile immunity was not achieved.

Subsequently, other studies have been done using ultrasonication (Garcia, 1967), pressure (Gonzalez et al., 1966a, b), and lyophilization (Menezes, 1965) in the preparation of vaccine material. The physical methods of killing the parasites have been almost universally more effective than chemical means in the production of protective antigens, but Seneca et al. (1966) reported that lipopolysaccharide material from *T. cruzi*, prepared by

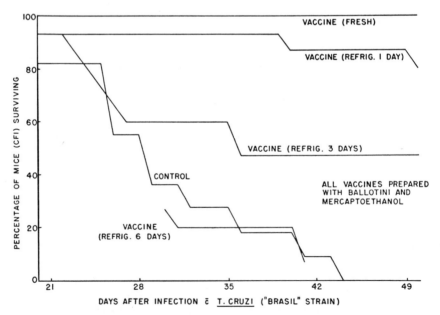

FIG. 2. Effect of vaccination with homogenate of *T. cruzi* prepared by shaking with ballotini on survival rate of mice challenged with Chagas' disease.

Table 4

Influence of Interval between Vaccination and
Challenge on the Effectiveness of Acquired
Immunity Induced by Subcutaneous Injection
of Homogenates of Culture Organisms

No. of Mice in Test Group	Interval between Vaccination and Challenge (Days)	Median Survival Time of Controls (Days)	Percent Vaccinated Survivors at 60 Days (All controls dead except as noted)
18	9	24	22
17	14	23	65
22	14	19	73
22	17	21	82
19	17	26	89
15	21	23	93
15	21	28	93
15	21	31	100
18	28	23	94
15	28	40	100
22	35	27	90
21	45	26	90
15	49	41	100
15	70	35	83
15	91	32	86*
15	112	33	73†

* 7% of controls surviving.
† 13% of controls surviving.

a method modified from Westphal et al. (1952) and involving the use of phenol, has a protective effect.

Another approach to the idea of vaccination against *T. cruzi* is that set forth in the studies of Fernandes (1965) and his colleagues (1965, 1966), who found that actinomycin D, when added to cultures of *T. cruzi*, blocks RNA synthesis, which is followed by inhibition of DNA and protein synthesis. Culture forms so affected remain motile but cannot multiply. They cannot infect mice or tissue cultures, but they are antigenic when injected into mice, stimulating resistance to subsequent challenge with virulent parasites.

Toxins. Since the early work of Chagas (1916) and Chagas and Villela (1922), there have been allusions to toxins from the parasite as possible factors in the pathogenesis of lesions in *T. cruzi* infection. Damage to tissues which are not actually invaded by the parasite could be explained by hypothesizing the presence of such substances. Such an explanation was suggested by Goble (1954) as a result of studies on thyroid changes in experimental Chagas' disease in dogs. Similarly, Köberle (1956) proposed that a "neurotoxin" was liberated by the disintegration of the amastigote tissue forms of the parasite, and caused destruction to the ganglion cells of the muscular hollow organs, the denervation of which results in dilatations (cardiomegaly, megacolon, and megaesophagus). Köberle amplified his views in subsequent articles (1957, 1958, 1959) which inspired attempts to isolate substances with such action from preparations of *T. cruzi* grown in liquid culture (Eichbaum, 1961; Jörg, 1964) or in tissue culture (Musacchio and Meyer, 1959). Failure to find such activity in preparations of epimastigote and trypomastigote forms from such cultures does not, of course, affect the hypothesis if it is based on *in vivo* disintegration of amastigote forms. It is the opinion of Andrade and Andrade (1966) that the Auerbach plexus is damaged by inflammation, and that neither toxins nor enzymes noxious to the nerve cells are involved.

As early as 1931, Roskin and Ekzemplarskaya noted that in mice infected with *T. cruzi*, there was inhibition or even destruction of certain tumors. This action was later (Roskin and Romanova, 1935) attributed to substances designated "endotoxins." These were purportedly present in the blood forms of trypanosomes which were killed by heating the plasma containing them in a water bath at 40°C to 50°C for 20 minutes. When plasma containing the killed trypanosomes was injected into mice following tumor inoculation, carcinolytic action could be demonstrated. They reported that the material lost its potency on storage (Roskin, 1946). Because reticuloendothelial blockade interfered with the antitumor activity of the "endotoxin," they suggested that in addition to a direct action on tumor cells, there was an indirect effect resulting from reticuloendothelial stimulation. Subsequent studies by the Russian workers led to the preparation of "endotoxin" from culture forms of *T. cruzi*. The earlier works of Roskin and his colleagues were reviewed by Hauschka (1947b) and Hauschka et al. (1947), who confirmed the antagonism of *T. cruzi* infections for experimental murine tumors (carcinoma 119, mammary adenocarcinoma of C₃H mice, and sarcoma 37). They concluded that the retardation of tumor growth in mice injected with *T. cruzi* was attributable to nonspecific effects, such as nutritional depletion and weight loss, impairment of circulation and interference with tumor vascularization, toxic metabolites, or competition for growth factors required by tumor cells.

Knop et al. (1949) reported a similar effect of *T. cruzi* infection on mouse leukemias, Bch and Ech, as well as on a transplanted mammary tumor. Brncic and Hoecker (1949), however, found no such action in chicks with fibrochondrioangiosarcoma IB₃, although a large number of parasites were inoculated. They concluded that *T. cruzi* could not be expected to influence the growth of tumors in hosts which are refractory to the parasite.

Using lysates of culture forms according to methods proposed by Klyueva and Roskin (1946), Malisoff (1947) confirmed the activity of such preparations in two mouse tumors. Hauschka et al. (1947, 1948), however, were unable to get any active preparations from a number of strains of *T. cruzi*, including one used by Malisoff and one which Roskin and Klyueva claimed to be a source of tumor-destroying material. Cohen et al. (1947), Gruhzit and Fisken (1948), Spain et al. (1948), and Jedeloo et al. (1949, 1950) were likewise unable to demonstrate antitumor effects.

Interest continued, however, in continental Europe with studies by Klyueva (1947), Galliard et al. (1950), Lob (1949, 1950), Coudert and Juttin (1950), Coudert (1956a,b, 1961a,b), Klyueva and Roskin (1957), Coudert et al. (1960), Trufanov and Palkina (1960), Mounier-Kuhn et al. (1961), and Krause (1964). Coudert points out the lability of the active material to heat and freezing, and he emphasizes that strains differ in antitumor activity so that a proper one must be selected. His preparations are preserved by lyophilization, and a commercial product (Trypanosa) is available from a firm in Lyon, France.

The designation "endotoxin" as used by Roskin was an unfortunate one, and is particularly misleading at the present, now that the term is almost universally applied to high molecular-weight polysaccharide complexes (Landy, 1962), some of which are undoubtedly present in the various preparations of intracellular materials from *T. cruzi*. There is, however, no evidence that these materials are the antitumor agents, and Coudert, who employs the less specific description "extracts," believes the active material is proteinaceous or enzymatic in nature. Later Russian authors refer to the material as "the antibiotic Krutsin" (Trufanof and Palkina, 1960; Krause, 1964).

A preparation which has been more specifically defined as a lipopolysaccharide is one which Seneca et al. (1966) call "Chagastoxin." It is prepared by a modification of the method of Westphal et al. (1952) for the extraction of endotoxin from cell walls of Gram-negative bacteria. This material is toxic and pyrogenic, produces leukocytosis, gives a reaction in intradermal tests suggestive of endotoxin, and is reported by Seneca et al. to induce protective immunity in mice. It is also stated to have a cortisone-like effect, exacerbating chronic latent *T. cruzi* infections into an acute fatal stage. This material is the product of a series of studies by Seneca that began with the preparation of trypanosome extracts which were intended to stimulate nonspecifically the resistance of patients to various infections but which revealed skin reactions in patients with cancer (Columbia Univ. Rep., 1959).

Cross-immunity between strains

Cross-immunity between strains of *T. cruzi* was observed as early as 1913 by Brumpt, who infected mice with *T. cruzi* from the feces of bugs by using a strain of low virulence (designated Bahia) and subsequently challenging them with a virulent strain (designated Chagas). In these studies, he found that the incubation period and the survival time was prolonged in the animals which had been infected earlier with the strain of low virulence.

Darman (1941) challenged mice which had recovered from infections with the Tehuantepic strain by inoculation with the "vickersae" strain (which he had obtained from Mayer at Hamburg and which was probably the strain isolated by Malamos from a cynomolgus monkey from Java). He reported that there was resistance to "vickersae" strain, but that it was less than the resistance to challenge with the homologous Tehuantepic strain.

Subsequently, Hauschka et al. (1950) showed that seven heterogeneous strains were immunologically related, and that after spontaneous or drug-induced recovery from infections with any of these strains, mice were resistant to challenge with a lethal mouse-to-mouse passage strain.

Norman and Kagan (1960a, b) infected mice with seven strains of low virulence isolated from wild animals from Georgia and Florida and challenged the mice 30 days later with the virulent mouse-passage strain Tulahuén. All of the animal strains gave some protection against challenge with the virulent strain. Goble (unpublished studies) used these same strains and an additional one from Louisiana (Lafitte) in dogs and challenged some of the animals with the Tulahuén strain and the others with the Brasil strain. The results are shown in Table 5. In these experiments, protection against the Tulahuén strain was not effected except in those animals which received an inoculation with the Brasil strain between the time of infection with the avirulent strains and the time of challenge with Tulahuén.

Deane (1960) found that previous infection with a strain from a wild rat (*Nectomys*) protected mice against challenge with a virulent human strain (Y). Goble (1961) reported that the Houston strain gave protection against both the Brasil strain and the Corpus Christi strain in dogs, and that the Corpus Christi strain (a human isolate) and the Patuxent strain (from raccoons) protected against infection with the Brasil strain. Protection of mice against the Brasil strain by previous inoculation with the Corpus Christi strain was accomplished somewhat later by Marr and Pike (1967). Galliard et al. (1962a, c) studied the protection conferred by certain avirulent strains, Cura (from Uruguay) and Romero (from Venezuela), against the virulent Tulahuén (from Chile) and showed that the resistance to challenge with the virulent strain could be abolished by the use of cortisone.

Nussenzweig et al. (1963b) tested five strains of two different immuno-

Table 5

Results of Cross-Protection Experiments in Nine Dogs,
each Infected with a Different Strain of *T. cruzi* and each
Subsequently Challenged with Heterologous Trypanosomes

	Primary Infection		2 months		5 months		8 months	
Strain	Positive from Day	Negative from Day	Strain*	Result†	Strain*	Result†	Strain*	Result†
Lafitte	19	29	T	d				
FR₄	—	—	T	d				
OR₂₁	19	34	B	s	G	d		
Skunk	26	34	B	s	G	d		
FH₄	21	29	B	s	G	m	T	s
FH₅	18	28	B	s	G	m	T	s
FH₆	18	30	B	s	G	m	T	s
FR₄	—	—	B	s	G	m	T	s
Raccoon	18	62	—	—	B	s	T	d

* B = *T. cruzi* Brasil; T = *T. cruzi* Tulahuén; G = *T. gambiense*.

† d = died; m = treated and survived; s = survived.

logic types (A and B) for cross-resistance as evidenced by protection of mice against challenge, and found that infection with either immunologic type gave protection against challenge with the lethal Y strain. This result suggested that the antigens responsible for the *"in vitro"* typing were not necessarily those involved in protective immunity. Although these demonstrations of protection against virulent *T. cruzi* infections by prior inoculations with strains of low virulence might suggest that living vaccines could be useful, the fact that there is no animal test which is predictive of the virulence for man of a so-called avirulent strain precludes the possibility of developing such procedures at this time.

Immunity in relation to therapy

Chemotherapeutic agents. Collier (1931) used acriflavine to modify the virulence of *T. cruzi* so that nonlethal infections could be produced which would lead to the development of resistance, which laid the basis for subsequent studies with drugs as tools in immunology. These, however, came much later, in part due to the paucity of compounds with activity against *T. cruzi*.

Hauschka et al. (1950) used Bayer 7602 to control the highly virulent WBH and Brasil strains so that mice could be saved from otherwise fatal infection and could later be challenged with either homologous or heterologous strains. In no case did they begin treatment before the second day after infection, and when the WBH-infected animals were challenged from 6 to 25 weeks later with the same strain, there was 100 percent protection. In mice infected with the Brasil strain, treated, and then challenged 2 to 34 weeks later, only 62.5 percent survived. Two weeks, however, does not allow for the development of peak resistance, and it may be that the animals that succumbed were those with the shortest period between immunization and challenge, although this is not noted in their paper.

Pizzi et al. (1954) used primaquine to suppress virulent infections with the Tulahuén strain in mice. They found that along with retardation of the development of the parasites, there was more inflammation and more marked phagocytic activity. A low-grade infection resulted, which led to strong immunity against superinfection. They pointed out, however, that antibodies (which were demonstrable in mice immunized with culture forms of low virulence) were not observed. Pizzi (1957) subsequently noted that immunization by treatment of an infection with virulent organisms was not as regular or sure as that effected by inoculation of attenuated culture material. This could possibly be attributed to early medication with primaquine which, according to his graphs, seems to have been begun on the day after infection.

Browning et al. (1946) found that mice which had been given certain phenanthridinium compounds, which suppressed or cured their *T. cruzi* infections, were refractory to subsequent inoculations with the homologous parasite, even many months after the primary infection. Brener (1961, 1962), using nitrofurazone and furadantin, found that if medication was begun on the day after infection by the Y strain, the suppression of the parasite was so complete that no immunity to challenge developed and reinfection after 10 weeks resulted in 100 percent mortality. When treatment was begun on the fourth day after infection, resistance developed (as evidenced by low parasitemias compared with controls) and persisted at about the same level for 1 to 3 months, eventually showing a decrease in animals challenged at 5 to 7 months. Brener and Chiari (1963a) found that a strong immunity developed in mice in which the infection had been driven into the chronic stage by furaltadone treatment, and that the resistance was not diminished by cortisone, as was observed in acute infections.

Another aspect of immunology in relation to therapy is that which Seneca and Peer (1963a, b) have termed "immunochemotherapy." By the use of hyperimmune rabbit serum in combination with furaltadone, they were able to effect 100 percent survival of mice infected with a lethal strain (Tulahuén) of *T. cruzi*. Animals treated with furaltadone alone had a survival rate of 86.7 percent. With the number of animals used in this experiment, the 95 percent confidence limits for 86.7 percent is 69 to 96, and for 100 percent is 90 to 100. It seems clear, therefore, that no definite conclusion as to the superiority of the combined treatment can be made.

Effects of tetracyclines.   Still another type of therapy-immunity relation is that in which a drug may alter the immune responses. Although there are substances which can stimulate bodily defenses (usually by their effects on the reticuloendothelial system), they are not materials which are generally regarded as chemotherapeutic agents. The question has been raised, however, in connection with Chagas' disease concerning the possibility that the tetracyclines may depress the host's resistance mechanisms and cause an enhancement of the infection.

Soon after the introduction of the antibiotic, chlortetracycline, it was tested in experimental Chagas' disease by Jarpa et al. (1949), who reported that it increased the severity of the disease when administered to mice infected with the Tulahuén strain of *T. cruzi*. They indicated that the mean levels of parasitemia in the treated group (8 males and 7 females) was more than four times that of the control group (11 males and 3 females), and that the mean survival time of the medicated animals was less than half that of the controls.

Chlortetracycline was subsequently reported by Galliard and Boutet (1951) to enhance the virulence of *T. cruzi* (Cura strain) in a nonfatal murine infection. The control parasitemias increased linearly from the tenth day to the peak at 30 days and then showed a similar decrease, so that the curve of parasitemia resembled an isosceles triangle. One mouse was treated with chlortetracycline and its parasitemia was compared with that of one control mouse which was not medicated. The peak of parasitemia in the treated mouse was about two times higher and occurred about five days later than that in the control mouse. It was also reported that the mouse which received chlortetracycline became anemic.

The above two articles were referred to by Guzman et al. (1952), who reported that chlortetracycline appeared to aggravate the infection in a fatal case of Chagas' disease they had treated in a Chilean infant. Later, Thiermann and Christen (1952) noted higher parasitemais and greater mortality in mice receiving chlortetracycline than those in untreated controls. Treatment with cortisone effected much higher parasitemias, however, and when chlortetracycline was used with cortisone, this effect of cortisone was partially reversed.

Packchanian (1953) did not report an infection-enhancing effect for chlortetracycline, but Woody and Woody (1961) stated that "definite clinical and experimental evidence exists to show that steroids and chlortetracyclines exacerbate the infection and should not be used." They had previously (1955) used tetracycline in treating a child with Chagas' disease, and had reported that within 48 hours after therapy was initiated, the patient became afebrile. Goble (1956) expressed doubt that the elimination of the fever was effected by the tetracycline, and quoted Hewitt et al. (1954, 1955), who reported that it was "not effective against trypanosomes." Agosin et al. (1951) and Packchanian (1953) had indicated that oxytetracycline was also ineffective in experimental Chagas' disease. Ribeiro (1957), however, used oxytetracycline in three cases of acute Chagas' disease and reported amelioration of the symptoms in all three, though without effecting cures. He also used oxytetracycline and tetracycline in combination with spirotrypan in two cases.

In view of the possibility that medication with one or another of the tetracyclines might be indicated in some infections which might occur concurrently with Chagas' disease in patients from Latin American countries, Goble et al. (1964) decided to reinvestigate the effects of these compounds to establish more clearly whether admonitions against tetracycline treatment in patients possibly infected with *T. cruzi* were indeed warranted. Blood forms of the Brasil strain of *T. cruzi* were used to infect CF1 mice, and commercial samples of three tetracyclines were used: chlortetracycline (Aureomycin), oxytetracycline (Terramycin), and tetracyline (Achromycin). The compounds were given in the diet, *per os* by stomach tube, or subcutaneously. At least ten mice were used in each group, and mortality was recorded during a period of 7 weeks after infection. The survival data were analyzed for significance by the nonparametric Mann-Whitney test and by the test on square-root transformation.

When chlortetracycline was given *per os* at a level of 1,000 mg per kg of body weight per day starting on the day of infection, there was no enhancement of the disease and the mortality. There was also no enhancement of the infection when the same doses were given beginning 3 days and 6 days before infection on different regimens varying from 4 to 13 doses.

When oxytetracycline was given subcutaneously at 125 mg per kg of body weight per day on 13 consecutive days beginning either on the day of infection, 3 days before, or 3 days after, significant delays in deaths were observed in the treated animals. *Per os* doses of 250 mg per kg of body weight per day according to the same regimens had no effect on the course of the disease. At 200 mg per kg of body weight per day given for 15 days by stomach tube, none of the three tetracyclines caused an enhancement of the infection and chlortetracycline had a slight tendency to delay deaths.

When given in the diet at 0.1 percent, which may be assumed to have effected the maintenance of more substantial blood levels, there was delay in deaths in all of the treated groups, the median survival time being about one week later than that of the controls. The effects on the parasitemia in two different tests is shown in Figure 3.

The findings were the same whether the medication was commenced 4 days before or 6 days after infection, and in another test in which medication (also in the diet) was begun on the day after infection and continued for three different periods (14 days, 21 days, and 28 days), the results were the same for all regimens.

An experiment was also done in which the amount of the drugs in the diet was increased from 0.1 percent to 0.2 percent and later to 0.3 percent, at which level the food intake dropped and the animals began to lose weight. Even under these conditions of exposure to toxicity, the course of the disease was not accelerated; in fact, the median survival time for each group was at least 3 days longer than that of the controls.

Although it is possible that the findings of earlier workers are attributable to the use of dosages more toxic than those obtained in these experiments, it is believed that the contradictions might also be accounted for in terms of the use of limited numbers of animals in a system in which there is

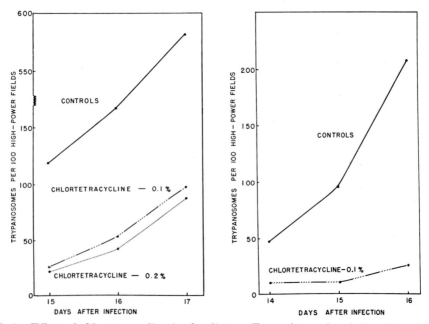

FIG. 3.   Effect of chlortetracycline in the diet on *T. cruzi* parasitemia in mice.

sometimes considerable variation in the values which were used as criteria of enhanced infection, i.e., parasitemic levels and survival times.

On the basis of the tests of Goble et al. (1964), which involved more than 800 animals and which did not furnish any evidence indicating that chlortetracycline, oxytetracycline, or tetracycline aggravate or enhance experimental Chagas' disease when administered in tolerated or therapeutic doses, it is believed that there is no reason for avoiding the use of these agents in patients with Chagas' disease, if this use is indicated for the treatment of some concurrent infection.

In spite of the above evidence, however, the question continues to arise when tetracycline is used in patients with Chagas' disease (Pizzi et al., 1963; Rubio et al., 1967).

Monitoring by serologic tests. The use of serologic tests to monitor the efficacy of chemotherapeutic treatment has been discussed by Pedreira de Freitas (1963), who pointed out the necessity of distinguishing between the acute and chronic forms of the disease, and of using the precipitin reaction in the former, and complement fixation for the latter. He emphasized the fact that the precipitin titers during the acute phase may drop rapidly even in the absence of therapy, and that quantitation of therapeutic effects by complement-fixation tests in the chronic disease is difficult because of the low titers of antibody.

Electrophoretic studies

Gotta (1946) noted hypoproteinemia in an acute case of Chagas' disease, with lowered albumin and inversion of the albumin:globulin quotient. As the case progressed into the chronic stage, there was a recovery but without the serum protein values becoming completely normal. Benning (1953) studied cases of so-called tropical myocarditis in Venezuela and noted high levels of γ-globulin with a drop in albumin. Taquini et al. (1956) carried out protein determinations on sera from 22 cases of uncomplicated Chagas' myocarditis and found normal values for protein, with an increase in α-globulin, a reduction in albumin, and a consequent reduction in the albumin:globulin ratio.

Lacaz et al. (1957) concluded from the examination of 10 sera from acute cases that there was a reduction in albumin and an increase in α_2- and γ-globulins. Later (Salum et al., 1959), these cases were reviewed, and five more cases were added in which it was noted that early determinations showed hypoproteinemia, hypoalbuminemia, and hyperglobulinemia with the α_1- and β-globulin fractions within normal limits. As the disease evolved, there was an increase in total protein and a reversion of the α_2- and γ-globulin values toward the normal. Pinto and Falcao (1958) studied seven chronic patients and noted low protein values and high α_2- and γ-globulin, with the albumin:globulin quotient below normal. They pointed out that the patterns differed enough from those in leishmaniasis to be useful in diagnosis.

Chattas et al. (1958, 1959) examined the sera of 16 children with the acute disease and found dysproteinemia in all cases, with increased α_2- and γ-globulin. Similar changes were observed in 10 acute cases by Minoprio et al. (1962), who also reported a tendency for the profile to return toward normal as the acute stage ends. These authors also reported that the serum protein pattern was different from that in leishmaniasis, which would allow for differential diagnosis. Ferreira and Elejalde (1960) found hypoalbuminemia in 10 of 11 chronic cases and elevated α_2-globulin in all 11, with no other important changes. Howard et al. (1962) also reported on 10 cases in children. They found no typical differences between acute and chronic stages and, in general, no unusual values in albumin, α_1-, α_2-, or β-globulins, although the γ-globulin fractions were high.

There are few such studies in experimental animals. Seneca et al. (1958) reported that in DBA mice infected with *T. cruzi* for 2 weeks, albumin was reduced, γ-globulin was markedly increased, while α- and β-globulins were moderately increased. Total serum protein was moderately lowered. Zeledon and Lizano (1962) studied sera of guinea pigs in which leishmanial infections (*L. enriettii*) were superimposed on *T. cruzi* infections. Total serum proteins showed a tendency to decrease in the animal infections with both species of parasite, though in animals with only leishmanial infections there was no decided change. The *T. cruzi* infection produced an increase in γ-globulin, and when leishmaniasis was superimposed, there was also an increase in the β-globulin fraction.

IMMUNODIAGNOSTIC TESTS

Immunologic tests are of great importance in the diagnosis of Chagas' disease. Isolation and identification of the parasite from the blood or tissues is difficult or impossible except during the acute phase of the disease, which obtains for only a relatively short time compared with the duration of the chronic stages. Notable reviews concerning immunologic tests are those of Barreto (1946), Pedreira de Freitas (1947), Pifano (1960), Muniz and Moraes (1962), and Maekelt (1964).

Serologic tests

The serologic tests which have been devised are discussed below in the chronologic order of their development.

Complement-fixation tests. The complement-fixation (CF) test is not only the oldest method for the serodiagnosis of Chagas' disease, but it is now the most widely used and best evaluated technique. The early history of its development is largely a story of the search for and modification of suitable antigenic materials, a process which still continues. The later history involves the extension of its use to wide epidemiologic investigation and the perfection of quantitative techniques and sophisticated analyses.

The variations in antigens and methods used in different laboratories have made various studies difficult to compare with each other. The need for standardization at last became so apparent that a study group was organized in 1966 under the auspices of the Pan American Health Organization (PAHO) to attempt to resolve some of the problems and to establish a quantitatively standardized complement-fixation procedure by which a number of types of antigens could be evaluated.*

Because of the importance of antigen in the test, this aspect will be discussed first. This will be followed by remarks on specificity and sensitivity, after which modifications of methods and the results of epidemiologic studies using the CF test will be reviewed.

Antigens. Four years after the discovery of *T. cruzi*, Guerreiro and Machado (1913) adapted the Bordet-Gengou reaction to use for the diagnosis of Chagas' disease, and although the procedure has subsequently been modified in a number of ways, it is still commonly called the Machado-Guerreiro test. These authors found that the use of aqueous extracts of spleens from infected puppies as antigen was superior to the use of various aqueous and alcoholic extracts of trypanosomes collected from the blood of infected dogs by differential centrifugation. They also tested antigens made from infected livers, and in addition to their examinations of sera of various infected animals, sera from patients with Chagas' disease were studied (Villela and Bicalho, 1923). Other early investigators (Mayer and da Rocha Lima, 1914; Villela and Da Cunha, 1919, 1920; Leao, 1923; La Corte, 1926, 1927; Patto, 1931; Minning, 1935) also used organs of infected animals for the preparation of antigen.

In 1930, Muniz experimented with the so-called Watson antigen (prepared from *Trypanosoma equiperdum*) in the complement-fixation test for Chagas' disease, but the breakthrough came in 1936 when Kelser introduced antigen made from culture forms of *T. cruzi*. This opened the way for the preparation of large quantities of parasite material uncomplicated by the presence of host tissues. This type of antigen was quickly accepted and used either according to Kelser's method (Cardoso, 1940a, b, 1941, 1943) or with modifications, such as desiccation (Liem, 1938; Liem and Van Thiel, 1941) or rupture of the cells by freezing and thawing (Davis, 1943a). Only a few workers continued to use organ extracts as antigen after the introduction of culture preparations (Iriarte, 1941). Antigens prepared from whole culture organisms of *T. cruzi* continued to be used (Dias, 1946; Muniz and Freitas, 1946; Knierim, 1959) throughout the period when extraction and fractionation of various cellular components were being increasingly employed.

Although the introduction of antigens made from culture organisms

* The original composition of this study group consisted of Jose Oliveira de Almeida, Antonio D'Alessandro, Fernando Beltran, Earl H. Fife, Jr., Irving G. Kagan, Feliza Knierim, G. A. Maekelt, Franklin A. Neva, Aluizio Prata, Bryce C. Walton, and Louis J. Olivier (Secretary). Other individuals collaborated in the preparation of antigens and the conduct of the tests, and will be mentioned later.

reduced the incidence of nonspecific reactions observed with syphilitic sera or even with some sera from healthy individuals, nonspecific reactions were still encountered (Liem and Van Thiel, 1941). Romaña and Dias (1942) tried to overcome this by acetone extraction of certain lipid components from antigen preparations, but Muniz and Freitas (1944b) considered antigens so treated to be less satisfactory than aqueous extracts. The latter authors prepared a highly purified polysaccharide antigen. Romaña and Cossio (1944) used alcohol to extract desiccated, triturated organisms. Later Romaña and Gil (1946) prepared antigen from a 10 percent suspension of culture forms in physiologic saline with 5 percent phenol, which was then shaken with fractured glass to rupture the cells. The resulting homogenate was used as antigen. Pedreira de Freitas (1950) used desiccated organisms, chloroform as a preservative, and benzene for extraction. Chaffee et al. (1956) prepared an improved antigen by extracting desiccated culture forms of *T. cruzi* with anhydrous ether in the cold prior to final extraction with alkaline buffer. Maekelt (1962) extracted freeze-dried organisms with benzene and prepared a water-soluble antigen. Gaikhorst (1960) used ether extraction and also obtained a water-soluble product.

In the meantime, others had fractionated culture preparations in order to isolate certain antigenic carbohydrate and protein components. Pellegrino and Brener (1952) distinguished a protein complex, a protein fraction, and a polysaccharide complex. Gonçalves and Yamaha (1959) obtained a polysaccharide-polypeptide complex. Fife and Kent (1960) found separate protein and carbohydrate fractions, each of which showed high reactivity in CF tests. They found the protein fraction to be the antigen of choice. In 1962, Maekelt described the chemical methods (saline precipitation of proteins and extractions of lipids with acetone, ether, and benzol) used to fractionate the lyophilized culture forms of *T. cruzi*. He determined the antigenic properties of each fraction in CF tests by block titration. The preparations he tested were: (1) extracts of aqueous solutions from organisms, (2) suspensions of homogenized organisms, (3) water-soluble protein fractions without benzol-, ether-, and acetone-soluble substances, (4) water-soluble fractions of globulin character, subfractions of these, and fractions of albumin character, and (5) lipid extracts. Specific antigenic substances were found in different fractions. There were some thermostable substances with highly specific antigenic properties. There was no marked difference among the specific antigenic properties of the different protein fractions from which the lipid material had been removed. Specific antigenic substances were also found in the lipid fractions.

Methods for the comparative study of antigens prepared either simultaneously or at different times from the same culture material have been described by Siqueira (1964a, b), which use isofixation curves (after the method of Almeida, 1956) and sequential analysis.

When the PAHO Study Group (*see* p. 633) on the serology of Chagas' disease met in 1966, the consensus was that the following antigens are the most commonly used:

1. Chloroform-jelly antigen (Pedreira de Freitas and Almeida, 1949; Almeida et al., 1959). *T. cruzi*, cultured in diphasic blood medium, are washed several times in saline until the supernatant is colorless and free of blood elements. They are then frozen (−20°C) and dried under vacuum over calcium chloride. The dried organisms are extracted with benzene in a glass homogenizer and redried. The material is extracted again in nine volumes of distilled water plus three volumes of chloroform and shaken thoroughly with glass beads. The antigen is stored frozen.

2. Delipidized (benzene) antigen (Maekelt, 1960). The organisms are grown on a sterile diphasic medium consisting of Difco brain-heart infusion agar (37 g), dextrose (10 g), agar (20 g), and distilled water (1,000 ml) in 125-ml Erlenmeyer flasks. Stock cultures are also grown on the above medium, but 2.5 ml of defibrinated rabbit blood is added to each flask along with antibiotics. The organisms harvested from the medium without blood are disrupted by alternate freezing and thawing in a dry-ice and alcohol bath ten times and then are lyophilized. The lyophilized organisms are extracted with benzene, dried under vacuum, extracted again with benzene, dried under vacuum, extracted with distilled water, brought to isotonicity with 1.7 percent NaCl with thimerosal (1:5,000), and then centrifuged. The opalescent supernatant is tubed in small amounts and stored at −20° C.

3. Delipidized (benzene) antigen (Maekelt, 1964). This antigen is prepared from *T. cruzi* grown in cellulose sacs containing saline and suspended in a medium containing Bacto brain-heart infusion (37 g), dextrose (19 g), hemoglobin (200 ml), and distilled water (1,000 ml). After 21 days of incubation with continuous agitation at 27°C, the organisms are harvested, sonicated,* and lyophilized. The lyophilized powder is extracted as in delipidized antigen preparation 2 (above). The antigen is lyophilized and stored at −20°C.

4. Crude water-soluble antigen (Knierim and Saavedra, 1966). The antigen is prepared from trypanosomes cultivated in a diphasic medium. Freshly harvested organisms are diluted with distilled water and subjected to six alternate freeze-thaw treatments. After centrifugation, the soluble product (antigen) is made isotonic with NaCl solution and stored at −20°C.

5. Somatic protein antigen (Fife and Kent, 1960). This is a protein fraction isolated from cultures cultivated in cellulose sacs, the dried blood-clot component of the Little and Subbarow (1948) medium being placed outside the sacs. Lyophilized harvests are first treated with anhydrous ether and then are extracted with buffered salt solution. The protein fraction obtained by chloroform-gel fractionation is used as antigen. The antigen is lyophilized for storage.

6. Exoantigen (Tarrant et al., 1965). This antigen is a culture-filtrate product obtained from *T. cruzi* cultivated in cellulose sacs in the medium uti-

---

* Sonication had previously been used by Correa et al. (1959), who placed culture forms suspended in saline (with 1:10,000 thimerosal) in a Siemens apparatus; the cells were first subjected to sonication at 800 kilocycles for 10 minutes with air energy consuming 30 watts, and then subjected to 2,400 kilocycles for an additional 10 minutes with an energy consumption of 38 watts.

lized for somatic protein antigen (above). The trypanosomes are removed, the supernatant antigen is dialyzed against saline, and certain nonantigen components are removed by isoelectric precipitation at pH 4.6. The soluble components comprise the exoantigen and are preserved by lyophilization.

7. Methylic antigen (Batista and Santos, 1959). This antigen is prepared from *T. cruzi* cultures grown on diphasic or liquid medium. The harvested organisms are dried and treated with benzene. The material is then extracted with pure anhydrous methanol and autoclaved for 15 minutes at 30 psi pressure (120°C). The antigen is stable at warm temperatures.

Seven types of antigen were selected by the PAHO group for comparative study in quantitative tests. These were:

1. Benzene-chloroform
2. Methanol extract (two sources)
3. Delipidized aqueous extract (three sources)
4. Aqueous extract (two sources)
5. Amastigote exoantigen from tissue culture
6. Somatic protein antigen
7. Epimastigote exoantigen.

The evaluation of the antigens* will be accomplished in two general steps, first an initial critical evaluation for nonspecific reactivity, and finally an evaluation for specific reactivity (sensitivity). This will be done according to a quantitatively standardized procedure devised in accordance with current knowledge of immunohemolysis and complement fixation.

Gonzalez et al. (1966) prepared antigens at different pressures in the refrigerated Ribi cell fractionator (Duerr and Ribi, 1963) and studied their ability to fix complement. Very high titers were obtained compared with those prepared by the method of Davis (1943); the antigen preparations obtained at pressures of 20,000 to 25,000 psi were the most potent. Antigens with lower activities resulted from the use of pressures above and below those values. Complement-fixing ability was greatly lowered when antigens were stored at 40°C for 30 days, and preservation with phenol, sodium azide, or thimerosal did not improve the stability, although the final potencies were still greater than were those obtained by use of Davis' techniques.

In addition to the antigen prepared from *T. equiperdum* by Muniz (1930) mentioned earlier (*see* p. 633), a few other species of flagellates have been used as sources for antigens which were tested against sera from Chagas' disease patients. Muniz and de Freitas (1944a, b) found that antigens prepared from *Leishmania brasiliensis* and *T. equinum* fixed complement in the presence of chagasic sera. Berrios and Zeledon (1960) made antigen from *Strigomonas oncopelti*, a parasite of insects, which can be grown in very such simpler media than those for *T. cruzi*. They found that

---

* These eleven antigens were prepared in nine different laboratories, some by members of the original group (listed above on p. 633) and some by additional collaborators, O. Baracchini and J. A. Cerisola. The seven laboratories selected to participate in the antigen evaluation were those of J. O. Almeida, Ribeirao Preto; G. A. Maekelt, Caracas; J. A. Cerisola, Buenos Aires; R. Zeledon, San Jose; F. Knierim, Santiago; I. G. Kagan, Atlanta; and E. H. Fife, Jr., Washington, D.C.

it did not fix complement in the qualitative (Kolmér) test, although in the quantitative (Pedreira de Freitas) test, low titers were observed. This antigen was less specific than *T. cruzi* antigen in that it reacted more strongly against sera from cases of cutaneous leishmaniasis than did *T. cruzi* antigen.

Specificity.   Rosenbaum and Cerisola (1958) have reviewed the observations on the specificity of the complement-fixation reaction in Chagas' disease, and they discussed the possible false positives which may result in the testing of sera from patients with other diseases. They noted that the report of Liem and Van Thiel (1941), who recorded weak CF reactions for Chagas' disease in 4 out of 146 Wasserman-positive sera in Holland, was the only reference to nonspecificity with syphilitic sera in which the presence of Chagas' disease could be excluded with certainty.

The specificity and independence of the reactions of *T. cruzi* antigen, cardiolipin, and tubercle bacillus antigen were emphasized in the test devised by Almeida et al. (1954) in which a triple antigen was used with sera of blood donors in simultaneous testing for syphilis, tuberculosis, leprosy, and Chagas' disease. Chaffee et al. (1956), however, recorded a number of false positives with sera of healthy individuals who had never resided in a Chagas' disease zone, and of syphilitic patients, also from a nonendemic area. In these tests, nonspecific ether-soluble components were not removed from the antigen. With ether extraction, the incidence of false positives was reduced, and some preparations showed no nonspecific reactions with either healthy or syphilitic sera. Subsequent preparations by Maekelt (1960, 1962) and others have given no cross-reactions with syphilitic or normal sera in thousands of tests (Mora Marquez et al., 1960).

In studying the CF test for Chagas' disease in patients with leprosy, Pedreira de Freitas (1947), Dinis and Pellegrino (1948), and Dinis (1949) reported in the neighborhood of 5 percent false positives, but later Pedreira de Freitas (1951), using an improved antigen in the quantitative CF test, reported no false positives in a series of 31 additional cases of leprosy. Maekelt (1960) also had no false positives with antigen prepared by his method.

Cutaneous leishmaniasis, as might be expected, can probably cause the greatest confusion in connection with CF tests for Chagas' disease. This is because of the presence of common antigens among the various genera of hemoflagellates and because of the presence of concurrent infections with leishmaniasis and Chagas' disease in a number of areas in Latin America. Some of the purified antigens, such as those of Chaffee et al. (1956) and Fife and Kent (1960), react strongly with sera from cases of leishmaniasis, even after cross-reactions with syphilitic and helminthic infections have been eliminated. Maekelt (1962), however, reported that his antigen preparation (Maekelt, 1960) gave no false positives in leishmaniasis.

Rosenbaum and Cerisola (1958b) concluded on the basis of findings by Manso Soto and Loretti (1953) and Bettinotti et al. (1953b) that brucellosis does not cause false positives in the CF test for Chagas' disease. They also referred to the observations of Pedreira de Freitas (1947) that the CF test for Chagas' disease was negative in 14 cases of rheumatic fever, 4 of malaria, 3 of paracoccidioidomycosis, 3 of lymphogranuloma venereum, and 1 of infectious mononucleosis. One of two cases of soft chancre (*Hemophilus ducreyi*) which gave positive CF tests was found to be positive by xenodiagnosis, and the other was from an endemic area. This is at variance with earlier reports of Liem (1938) and Liem and Van Thiel (1941), who found that three of six cases of soft chancre in Holland reacted positively, and noted that serum from a rabbit which had been injected with Dmelocos vaccine became positive in the CF test for Chagas' disease. Another study of Pedreira de Freitas (1951) indicated that smallpox vaccination did not cause false positives and that cases of pemphigus which were positive came from endemic areas.

Maekelt (1960) checked the sensitivity of his antigen against sera from cases of histoplasmosis, coccidioidomycosis, and cancer, in addition to a number of the conditions noted above, and found no false positives in these conditions. He also believes (along with Tejera and Pifano, 1959) that there is no cross-reaction with sera from persons with *T. rangeli*, if *T. cruzi* culture antigen is used in the test.

Rosenbaum and Cerisola (1958b) estimated that the incidence of non-specificity in the CF test for Chagas' disease is less than 1 percent. It is probable that most of the false positives are attributable to cross-reactions with antileishmanial antibodies when unrefined preparations from *T. cruzi* culture organisms are used as antigen.

Sensitivity.   Rosenbaum and Cerisola (1958) have estimated the sensitivity of the CF test in Chagas' disease to be between 90 and 95 percent in the chronic stage and 99 percent in the presence of chronic myocarditis, which is comparable to the sensitivity of the Wasserman reaction. Although positive reactions have been observed as early as one week after infection (Pellegrino and Brener, 1952), it appears that complement-fixing antibodies do not generally become detectable until 20 to 45 days after infection, so during the acute stage only 40 to 50 percent of sera are positive. Chagas (1936) found positives as early as 10 to 26 days after infection in experimentally infected cases, Mazza (1938) noted positives at 17 and 20 days, and Osimani (1947c) at 18 and 21 days. Pellegrino and Brener (1952) found positives at 7, 17, 18, 19, 28, and 30 days after infection, but they also found negatives at 5, 10, 15, 26, 27, and 30 days with a doubtful case at 17 days. Pedreira de Freitas (1951), using the quantitative teachnique, found positives at 30, 60, and 90 days, negatives from a few days to 20, 40, and 90, and doubtfuls at 15 and 18 days after infection. In monkeys inoculated through the conjunctiva, Davis (1943b) found positives in 4 to 6 weeks. In dogs, Pellegrino and Brener (1953) found positives in 6 to 8 days in six animals, in 9 to 11 days in four, and two others remained negative. Later in the acute stage, the sensitivity greatly increases; Dias (1955) found almost 95 percent of the patients positive in a series of 300 patients diagnosed as positive by other methods.

Methods and modifications.   A comprehensive review of the history of procedures used in the complement-fixation reaction for Chagas' disease was made by Maekelt in 1960. The earlier investigators employed only qualitative tests modeled on the lines of the Wasserman or Kolmér reactions. As early as 1927, Wadsworth had described quantitative CF procedures which were subsequently elaborated by Wadsworth et al. (1931, 1938), but it was not until 1946 that the 50 percent hemolysis endpoint for complement-fixation determinations was suggested for parasitic diseases (Bozicevich et al., 1946). By 1949, Pedreira de Freitas and Almeida had worked out a quantitative method which they developed extensively during the following years (Pedreira de Freitas, 1951, 1952; Almeida and Pedreira de Freitas, 1953; Almeida et al., 1953, 1954). Uvo et al. (1954) attempted to compare qualitative with quantitative techniques. Chaffee et al. (1956) used a quantitative test based on the earlier work of Kent et al. (1946) to which Bozicevich et al. (1946) referred; Rassi et al. (1958) used a similar method, as did Knierim (1958, 1959).

Two methods were developed independently and almost simultaneously in which the complement-fixation reaction was adapted for use with small amounts of reagents. In these methods, drops of the various reactants are mixed either in wells of a Plexiglas plate (Lobo and da Silva, 1962, based on a technique of Roitt and Doniach, 1958) or on a flat plate (Almeida, 1963a, based on a technique of Fulton, 1949). Both methods are applicable to quantitative testing, the latter having been used in the isohemolytic curves methods (Almeida, 1963b). The plate method has also been used to test pericardial fluid taken at autopsy of suspected cases of Chagas' disease (Lopes et al., 1966).

Cerisola et al. (1967) tested the specificity of the complement-fixation test, performed by two different methods, in comparison with hemagglutination test and the immunofluorescence technique. They found no false positives in a series of 331 sera from residents of Germany, but anticomplementary results in the two different CF tests lowered the index of specificity for those methods to 99.6 and 97.5 percent.

Villela and Bacalho (1923) first used the complement-fixation test with cerebrospinal fluids (CSF) from patients with Chagas' disease. Four of the cerebrospinal fluids were positive. The test was mentioned again shortly thereafter (Villela, 1924), but then 25 years passed before the test was used again (Dias, 1950). Dalma (1953, 1954) studied 12 cases of Chagas' disease with neurologic complications and found the spinal fluid to be positive in four. Elejalde (1959, 1961), however, found no positive CF reactions with the spinal fluids of seven patients whose sera gave positive reactions.

In order to facilitate the storage and shipment of serum samples from rural areas for serologic testing, the possibility of using preparations dried on various cellulose-containing materials was investigated by Maekelt and Colmenares de Alayon (1960). Various types of filter paper, cotton, paper towels, gauze, and toilet paper were tested. In each test, 0.2 ml of serum was placed in the center of the paper and allowed to dry, having been suitably covered to protect it from flies and other contamination. After transportation to the laboratory, the samples were rehydrated, inactivated, and used in the complement-fixation test. Toilet paper proved to be the most useful and practical, and it is recommended for field use. Tests were made with 218 sera to compare dried sera with sera tubes, and agreement was found in 86 percent of the tests. The main discrepancies resulted from the development of anticomplementary effects from absorption and drying on paper. The usefulness of the method, in spite of this drawback, was emphasized.

Use of CF test in epidemiologic surveys.   Tables 6 to 12 list most of the publications in which large numbers of sera were reported to have been examined in the complement-fixation test for Chagas' disease. These show the extent of experience with the test in various countries and the variations in infection rate by area, as well as furnish references for more detailed study of techniques.

Agglutination.   Agglutination titers in rabbits immunized with living and killed cultures forms of *T. cruzi* were measured by Packchanian (1940), Senekjie (1943a), and Chang and Negherbon (1947). Senekjie (1943b) proposed the use of a slide agglutination test in experimental studies as well as in clinical diagnosis. Although the highest titers were observed with homologous *T. cruzi* organisms, cross-reactions at lower dilutions occurred with other hemoflagellates, *L. brasiliensis*, *L. donovani*, and *L. tropica* (Senekjie and Lewis, 1944). Muniz and Freitas (1944a) studied agglutination in comparison with complement fixation and pointed out that agglutination titers in acute cases were greater than those in chronic cases. These authors later (1946) reported on the difficulties involved in interpretation of low agglutination titers.

Hauschka et al. (1950) also used a slide agglutination test with both experimental mouse sera and clinically obtained human sera. They pointed out that certain strains of *T. cruzi* were unsatisfactory for use as antigen in such tests. The Culbertson strain was peculiarly refractory to the nonspecific agglutinins in normal human sera, yet it was highly responsive to agglutinating antibody in sera from patients with Chagas' disease.

Goble (1952a), using Hauschka's method, found that nonspecific agglutinations occurred with sera of uninfected dogs, sometimes causing positive reactions at 1:200 dilutions, so that dog sera had to be tested at 1:400 dilution. However, the results were not consistent during any of the periods of the disease.

The consensus at present seems to be that agglutination tests are difficult to interpret (Muniz and Moraes, 1962; Pedreira de Freitas, 1963; Pifano, 1960; Maekelt, 1964), and that although they are of some value in scientific investigation, they offer little as routine diagnostic methods.

Precipitin reactions.   Packchanian (1935) was the first to use the precipitin reaction in the diagnosis of Chagas' disease. He used antigens prepared by extracting *T. cruzi* with alcohol, ether, or water. He reported the reaction to be specific but with very low titers.

The importance of the precipitation reaction in the early stages of Chagas' disease was recognized by Muniz and de Freitas (1944b). They isolated a polysaccharide from culture forms and developed the precipitation test into a simple technique which used small quantities of serum and gave

Table 6

Incidence of Positive Reactions in Complement-Fixation Tests
in Various Localities of North and Central America

Country (State)	Date	Authors	Population Sample	Number Examined	Percent Positive*
U.S.A.					
Texas	1946	Davis and Sullivan	unselected	1,909	0.05
Texas	1961	Woody et al.	unselected	500	1.5
Georgia	1963	Ferrar et al.	hospital patients	474	0.5
			unselected rural	449	0.5
			diffuse myocardial disease	28	7
Texas	1965	Woody et al.	persons bitten by triatomes	117	2.5† 3.4‡
Mexico		Perrin et al.,	unselected	48	8
Michoacan	1947	Dias et al.			
	1966	Tay et al.	unselected	165	7
Guatemala	1966	Walton	unselected	3,187	2
	1959	de Leon	unselected	6,126	14
El Salvador	1966	Walton	unselected	2,508	5
	1957	Penalver et al.	hospital patients	309	44
			cardiac patients	47	47
			children (urban)	200	1.5
			children (rural)	176	20
Nicaragua	1966	Walton	unselected	2,511	9
Costa Rica	1952	Zeledon	endemic zone	317	6
			nonendemic zone	90	1
	1960	Berrios	hospital patients	706	6
			blood donors	221	8
			insane asylum	73	8
Panama	1936	Kelser	unselected	1,626	4
	1937	Johnson and Kelser	unselected	1,251	4

* Percentages greater than five have been rounded to the nearest one percent, those under five to the nearest half percent, with one exception.
† strong
‡ weak

Table 7

Incidence of Positive Reactions in Complement-Fixation Tests
in Various Localities of Northern South America

Country (Locality)	Date	Authors	Population Sample	Number Examined	Percent Positive*
Netherlands W. Indies					
Aruba	1961	Gaikhorst	unselected	2,243	0
Curaçao	1965	Van der Sar and Vincke	blood donors and cardiac patients	396	1.5
Colombia					
Tibu	1962	Gutierrez	———	93	67
Venezuela					
Valencia	1959	Maekelt	unselected patients	200	34
			blood donors	449	12
Guarico	1959	Maekelt	unselected	83	28
Caracas	1960	Maekelt and Alcaniz	hospital patients	1,374	25
			outpatient, police	858	10
			outpatient, cardiology	176	40
	1961	Maekelt	———	2,699	21
	1962	Salazar et al.	blood donors	—	5
	1962	Figallo	maternity cases	500	11
	1964	Mora-Marques	healthy soldiers	17,000	7
Belen, Eneal	1966	Puigbo et al.	endemic area	1,110	47
Ecuador					
Guayaquil	1950	Montalvan	hospital patients	560	10
	1950	Montalvan	hospital patients	683	9
	1950	Rodriguez	mostly hospital patients	553	8
	1955	Espinoza	unselected	557	24
various	1955	Espinoza	students	443	2.5
Guyas	1955	Espinoza	hospital patients	223	10
various	1959	Rodriguez	various	3,587	14
Peru					
Tarata (Tacna)	1955	Naquira and Naquira	unselected	66	77
	1957	Naquira and Naquira	unselected	284	29
Lima	1962	Cornejo Donayre et al.	———	199	4
San Martin	1965	Larrain	unselected (over 10 years old)	237	13

* Percentages greater than five have been rounded to the nearest one percent, those under five to the nearest half percent.

Table 8

Incidence of Positive Reactions in Complement-Fixation Tests
in Various Localities in Northern Brazil

State (Locality)	Date	Authors	Population Sample	Number Examined	Percent Positive*
Goias					
Montevidiu	1951	Pedreira de Freitas and Mendonca	from infested homes	26	35
			others	42	36
Rio Verde	1951	Pedreira de Freitas and Mendonca	adults	26	12
			school children	115	2.5
Goiania	1951	Pedreira de Freitas and Figueiredo	suspected of cardiac Chagas' disease	148	53
Trindade	1951	Pedreira de Freitas and Figueiredo	students and professors	43	0
			unselected	40	27
Hidrolandia			unselected	60	13
Paraiba				3,598	20
Inga and Itabaiana	1956	Da Silva et al.	unselected	—	0.5
Bananeiras and Solanea			unselected	—	1
Taperoa			unselected	—	11
Patos and Cajazeiras			unselected	—	12
Mata	1957	Lucena and Costa	unselected	—	19
Agreste			unselected	—	18
Sertao			unselected	—	23
Pernambuco					
Timbauba	1957	Lucena	unselected dogs	60	12
			unselected humans	228	10
	1958	Lucena	unselected	3,267	15
Recife	1959	Lucena	unselected	97	26
Timbuaba	1959	Lucena	unselected	1,062	13
Alagoas	1961	Lucena et al.	unselected	3,015	25
Ceara					
Russas	1959	Alencar	unselected	146	12
Limeiro do Norte	1965	Alencar	unselected	114	17
Monte Claro	1962	Alencar et al.	unselected	18	28
Boa Vista			unselected	38	18
Cairiri	1963	Alencar et al.	unselected	370	37
Baturite			unselected	200	12
Rio Grande do Norte	1962	Lucena	unselected	2,280	12

* Percentages greater than five have been rounded to the nearest one percent, those
under five to the nearest half percent.

Table 9

Incidence of Positive Reactions in Complement-Fixation Tests
in Various Localities in Minas Gerais, Brazil

Locality	Date	Authors	Population Sample	Number Examined	Percent Positive*
Belo Horizonte	1948	Pellegrino and Borrotchin	hospital patients	181	20
	1949	Pellegrino	blood donors	179	1.5
Iguatama and Campos Altos	1949	Dias et al.	Railway workers and their families	213	39
Bambui	1950	Dias	———	1,290	60
Belo Horizonte	1951	Pellegrino et al.	blood donors	576	25
Ibiraci	1951	Brant et al.	———	125	59
Pirapora	1952	Pellegrino et al.	school children	207	10
Belo Horizonte	1952	Rezende et al.	hospitalized children (6–15 years)	200	7
Campo Florida	1952a	Pedreira de Freitas et al.	dogs	143	11
Araguari	1953	Biancalana et al.	———	225	19
Uberaba	1959	Jatene and Jacomo	blood donors	640	15
			upper class	219	7
			rural	112	25
Jacui	1963	Brant	unselected	1,222	33
			in city	—	28
			in country	—	36
Uberaba	1963	Sabino de Freitas	not stated	—	64
			blood donors	—	22
Triangulo Minero	1966	Oliveira et al.	pregnant women	200	33
Bambui	1967	Dias	children: 1–6 yrs.	225	1.5
			children: 7–12 yrs.	354	11

* Percentages greater than five have been rounded to the nearest one percent, those under five to the nearest half percent.

Table 10

Incidence of Positive Reactions in Complement-Fixation Tests
in Various Localities in São Paulo State, Brazil

Locality	Date	Authors	Population Sample	Number Examined	Percent Positive*
Sorocaba	1948	Pedreira de Freitas	hospital patients	58	33
			school children (7–13 yrs.)	105	8
São Carlos	1950	Pedreira de Freitas et al.	blood donors	786	5
Echaporã	1951	Pedreira de Freitas and Almeida	children (7–14 yrs.)	—	—
			rural	165	20
			urban	246	8
			adults		
			rural	49	39
			urban	50	6
Paraiba (Queluz)	1951	Unti and da Silva	unselected	136	8
Santo Rita do Passa Quatro	1952	Ramos	unselected	190	15
	1952	Unti and da Silva	unselected	3,737	17
			under 10 years old	2,210	14
Mococo	1952	Dias et al.	————	16	38
Various	1952b	Pedreira de Freitas et al.	————	1,623	2
Riberão Preto	1953	Biancalana et al.	————	19	21
São Paulo	1953	Passalcqua et al.	blood donors	536	4
Rio Preto	1953	Biancalana et al.	————	134	15
Various	1954	da Silva	————	40,815	12
Itaporanga	1954	Portugal et al.	ambulatory patients	204	41
S. Caetano do Sul	1954 a, b, c	Carvalhal et al.	non-endemic zone	211	6
			suspicious zone	624	10
			endemic zone	626	12
São Paulo	1958	Passos	pregnant women	2,632	3
São Paulo	1959	Passos	pregnant women	2,688	3
	1965	Mellone and Pagenotto	blood donors	62,575	1.5
	1965	Amato Neto et al.	pregnant women	750	4
Riberào Prego	1967	Haddad	unselected	1,362	5
São Paulo	1968	Amato Neto et al.	mothers of prematures	402	7

* Percentages greater than five have been rounded to the nearest one percent, those under five to the nearest half percent.

Table 11

Incidence of Positive Reactions in Complement-Fixation Tests
in Various Localities in Chile

Province (Locality)	Date	Authors	Population Sample	Number Examined	Percent Positive*
Various	1940	Bertin-Soto	not stated	600	31
	1942	Dussert and Faiguenbaum	not stated	246	39
	1948	Neghme and Roman	unselected (from endemic zones)	8,142	17
	1949	Neghme et al.	unselected	10,666	14
Tarapaca Arica	1957	Naquira and Neghme	unselected (over 12 yrs.)	20	46
	1959	Knierim	endemic zone	145	47
			non-endemic zone	100	2
	1959	Neghme and Schenone	xenodiagnosis positive	129	77†
			xenodiagnosis positive	57	91‡
Various	1960, 1962	Neghme and Schenone	endemic zones	14,902	15
Tarapaca			endemic zones	263	27
Antofagasta			endemic zones	285	8
Antacama			endemic zones	892	24
Coquimbo			endemic zones	237	37
Valparaiso and Aconcagua			endemic zones	838	20
Santiago			endemic zones	1,494	11
O'Higgins and Colchagua			endemic zones	31	3
Coquimbo Elqui	1960	Apt et al.	unselected	186	35
Isla de Pascua	1961	Morales et al.	unselected	61	0
Santiago	1962	Howard	mothers of prematures	100	4
	1964	Apt and Niedmann	pregnant women	55	24
Colchagua Santa Cruz	1966	Schenone et al.	unselected	50	42

* Percentages greater than five have been rounded to the nearest one percent, those under five to the nearest half percent.
† Using 100% endpoint.
‡ Using 50% endpoint.

Table 12

Incidence of Positive Reactions in Complement-Fixation Tests
in Various Localities of Argentina

Province (Locality)	Date	Authors	Population Sample	Number Examined	Percent Positive*
San Luis	1936	Miyara	asylum inmates	39	20
	1946	Romaña and Gil	unselected	500	49
	1946	Romaña and de Romaña	children (7–14 yrs.)	72	42
	1949	Romaña	———	1,263	48
	1950	Manso Soto et al.	———	83	35
Rosario	1951	Manso Soto and de Rosa	———	150	9
Catamarca Andalgalá	1951	Romaña and Kirschbaum	unselected	94	36
Federal District	1951	Manso Soto et al.	patients (majority, cardiac)	1,080	59
			healthy persons	1,280	12
Cordoba	1951	Bettinotti	———	493	32
Mendoza	1952	Manso Soto and Rispoli	unselected	1,548	21
Federal District	1953	Rispoli	unselected	5,000	3.5
Catamarca	1953a	Bettinotti et al.	———	24	44
Corrientes	1953	Romaña	———	257	24
Cordoba	1953b	Bettinotti et al.	———	72	17
Villa del Rosario			———	22	36
Tucuman	1954	Romaña and Abalos	———	—	—
Amaicha	1954	Romaña and Abalos	unselected	41	34
Colalao del Valle	1954	Romaña and Abalos	———	32	12
Valle del Ris Santa Maria	1954	Romaña and Abalos	———	72	48
Cordoba	1954	Bettinotti	———	493	32
Cordoba and Santiago del Estero	1957a	Rosenbaum and Cerisola	unselected	—	69
Pampa	1957b	Rosenbaum and Cerisola	unselected	352	19
Chaco Resistencia	1959	Torrico	patients (majority chronic cardiac)	575	27
Salta Cafoyate	1960	Romaña	———	80	21
Federal District Buenos Aires	1965	Lausi	healthy children	197	15

* Percentages greater than five have been rounded to the nearest one percent, those under five to the nearest half percent.

immediate (1- to 2-minute) results (Muniz and de Freitas, 1946; Muniz, 1947).

Chang and Negherbon (1947) used a quantitative precipitation reaction with four different aqueous extracts of *T. cruzi* obtained by lyophilization, freezing, lysis by distilled water, and trituration with sand. They evaluated the test with sera of guinea pigs and dogs immunized with *T. cruzi* and three species of *Leishmania*. Positive reactions were obtained in ring tests only at low dilutions, and there were cross-reactions between *T. cruzi* antigens and heterologous sera from animals with *L. tropica* and *L. brasiliensis* infections.

Packchanian (1949) reported greater sensitivity with polysaccharide antigen than with crude aqueous extracts. Knierim (1954) studied precipitins in the sera of rats, guinea pigs, and mice.

Pellegrino and Rezende (1953) introduced a simplified procedure for the use of capillary blood from babies; they found a high sensitivity (more than 97 percent) in the precipitin reaction in 48 acute cases of Chagas' disease and a high specificity when tested in 18 cases of leishmaniasis. Brener and Pellegrino (1957, 1958), however, noted cross-reactions in cases of human and canine kala-azar. Pifano (1960) reaffirmed the high sensitivity of the precipitin reaction in 36 acute cases, but only 9 percent of 52 chronic cases were positive.

Heterophile antibody reactions.   Although it is not specific, heterophile antibody occurs in the earlier stages of Chagas' disease with great regularity, and it is usually found in relatively high levels. Graña (1944) reported heterophile antibody reactions, at the same time, Muniz and de Freitas (1944a) noted them in the course of some work on agglutination. The phenomenon must be taken into account in the practice of hemagglutination tests (Muniz and Santos, 1950a, b, c), as will be mentioned below. Enos and Elton (1950) reported a heterophile antibody reaction to be the only significant laboratory finding in a case of Chagas' disease in Panama which was not diagnosed until autopsy. Only small numbers of patients have been studied (five by Goes, 1947; ten by Goes and Bruno Lobo, 1951), but the reaction is considered to be an auxilliary method of diagnostic testing in acute and subacute cases. Goble (1952) found it to be positive in dogs in the acute stage of infection.

Amato Neto (1958) found considerable variation in the titers of heterophile antibody in acute cases of Chagas' disease. In only a few, however, were the titers insignificant. From absorption studies with guinea-pig kidney and ox red cells, he concluded, in concurrence with Goes and Bruno Lobo (1959), that the heterophile antibodies in Chagas' disease were different from those found in normal individuals and in patients with mononucleosis, and that they were similar to those found in serum sickness. He pointed out that such absorption tests were indispensible in making the heterophile antibody test more than presumptive, so that confirmation of Chagas' disease can be sought by other, specific laboratory tests.

Indirect hemagglutination tests.   As Maekelt (1964) has pointed out, there are several types of indirect hemagglutination tests for Chagas' disease. The first to be introduced was the method of Muniz (1949, 1950a, b, c) in which unmodified red cells were used with a polysaccharide fraction of *T. cruzi* as antigen. In ten subacute and chronic cases, he observed titers of from 1:8 to 1:256. It had already been established that the sera had to be previously adsorbed with sheep red cells and guinea pig kidney in order to eliminate the heterophile antibodies which are usually present in sera of acute cases of Chagas' disease and which give titers up to 1:1,280. In chronic cases, the heterophile antibody titers were much lower (1:128). Heterophile antibodies may produce false positives with sera of healthy persons or of patients with other diseases.

Muniz (1950a) introduced a modification in which complement was added to the antigen-antibody complex (red cells were sensitized with trypanosome polysaccharide and placed in contact with the patient's serum), effecting a specific hemolysis which he termed "conditioned hemolysis." The sera were previously adsorbed with guinea-pig kidney and sheep red cells to eliminate heterophile antibody. Bettinotti (1952) believed that this system was as good as, if not better than, the complement-fixation reaction.

Bouisset et al. (1960) were the first to use red cells, modified at their surface with tannic acid, to adsorb a soluble antigen of *T. cruzi*. Their studies were conducted in laboratory animals, but Cerisola et al. (1962) introduced this reaction for use in routine examination of human sera and compared the results with those obtained by complement fixation. They used a fresh isotonic lysate as antigen, which was prepared daily and absorbed on human red cells of group O previously treated with tannic acid. The test is qualitative, performed in welled plates of the Kline type, and read macroscopically. In a series of nearly 800 sera tested by this method, there was 99 percent agreement with the results obtained in the CF test, using the 50 percent hemolysis endpoint (Knierim, 1959). Later, Cerisola and Lazzari (1963) reported on 7,308 sera tested by hemagglutination in comparison with tests by complement fixation (modified Eagle-Deffis and Bozicevich-Knierim methods). Of 508 CF-positive sera, 27 were doubtful or negative by hemagglutination; of 6,688 CF-negative sera, 26 were positive by hemagglutination, and many of these patients from whom the sera were obtained, when studied clinically, showed electrocardiographic pictures suggestive of the chronic myocardiopathy of Chagas' disease. The test is regarded by Cerisola et al. (1964) to be an excellent diagnostic method of notable simplicity and speed.

Maekelt (1963) independently began to use an indirect hemagglutination technique employing as antigen either a water-soluble whole-trypanosome extract or a water-soluble protein extract of *T. cruzi* prepared from lyophilized material and adsorbed on sheep red cells. The technique is quantitative; it is carried out in tubes according to the method used by Jacobs and Lunde (1960) in toxoplasmosis and is read macroscopically. In 100 sera evaluated with both antigens in the hemagglutination test, there was high correlation with the results in complement-fixation tests. The water-soluble protein antigen from which benzene-soluble substances had been extracted was preferable to the water-soluble whole extract of the parasite.

Serravalle (1963) reported the use of a hemagglutination test with sera of dogs from São Amaro, Bahia. Of 22 sera examined, 2 were positive (9 percent), whereas 24 percent were positive by the complement-fixation test.

Montano and Ucros (1965) made a comparison of hemagglutination (technique of Stavitsky, 1954) and complement-fixation (method of Knierim, 1958) reactions with 8,124 sera from Colombia, conducting the tests simultaneously. In the CF test, 538 sera were positive (6.6 percent) and 72 were anticomplementary (0.86 percent). In the hemagglutination test, 707 were positive (8.7 percent) and 29 were doubtful (0.35 percent). Of the 72 anticomplementary sera, 16 (22.2 percent) were positive and 5 (6.9 percent) doubtful in the hemagglutination test. Of the 29 sera doubtful by the hemagglutination test, 5 were CF-positive. The 2.1 percent difference between the number of positive reactions in the two techniques was of statistical significance ($p < 0.001$). Of the 538 CF-positive sera, only 6 (1.1 percent) were negative by hemagglutination. Of the 707 hemagglutination-positive sera, only 1.1 percent were negative by complement fixation. The intensity of the positive reactions also was correlated in the two types of test.

The sensitivity of the reactions were studied further in 51 persons with confirmed Chagas' disease (positive by xenodiagnosis or blood inoculation) and in 50 artificially infected guinea pigs. Of the 51 human sera, 50 (98 percent) were positive by hemagglutination and 48 (94.4 percent) were positive by complement fixation. The sera of 20 guinea pigs with chronic infection were positive with both techniques. Of the 30 guinea pigs tested in the acute state, 16 (53.3 percent) were positive by hemagglutination and 9 (30 percent) by complement-fixation tests. These results had little statistical significance ($p < 0.01$), but they suggest that antibodies detected by hemagglutination appear earlier than those found by complement fixation. The specificity of the hemagglutination reaction was considered to be similar to that of the complement-fixation reaction, and, in view of its sensitivity and the advantage of being able to evaluate sera which are anticomplementary, the hemagglutination test was recommended as a preferred laboratory procedure.

Neal and Miles (1968) employed a technique adapted from that of Gill (1964). They found no cross-reactions with sera from patients with malaria, tuberculosis, syphilis, or amoebiasis. Titers of sera from patients with Chagas' disease varied from 1:1,000 to 1:512,000. At a dilution of 1:100, there were reactions with one serum from a case of kala-azar and with two sera from cutaneous leishmaniasis, but these patients were from Brazil and Costa Rica, respectively, so concurrent Chagas' disease could not be excluded.

Immobilization tests. Based on the treponema immobilization test (Nelson and Meyer, 1949), Rodriguez (1952) devised an immobilization reaction for use in Chagas' disease. The test is conducted with live culture organisms suspended in saline. These are mixed on a plate with the patient's serum (inactivated) and complement (guinea pig). The percentage of mobile and immobile organisms was recorded at various intervals; the most common interval was 16 hours. Although the test was applied to only a few human sera, the results suggested that further studies might be of interest. Apparently this approach has not been followed up.

Another type of immobilization test was mentioned by Gonzalez-Angulo and Ryckman (1967) in which the patient's serum was mixed, in various proportions, with a mixture of live *T. cruzi* organisms and rat blood. They reported that serum from a patient suspected of Chagas' disease immobilized the parasites to the rat red blood cells in greater proportion than that observed with normal human serum.

Antiglobulin (Coombs) test. In 1955, Nussenzweig and Faria reported on the application of the antiglobulin (Coombs) test to the diagnosis of Chagas' disease in the chronic phase. Inactivated sera were adsorbed with sheep red blood cells for 12 hours in the cold to eliminate heterophile antibody. The antigen was a 2 percent suspension of washed culture forms of *T. cruzi*. Antiglobulin serum agglutinated the parasites and therefore had to be adsorbed three times (4 hours each) with an excess of flagellates. After this treatment, the Coombs serum was titrated with human serum from known cases of Chagas' disease. The titer of antiglobulin serum for the Chagas system was much lower than that for the Rh system. The authors recommended that commercial antiglobulin-diluted serum for hemagglutination tests should not be used without previous titration. Serum to be tested (0.1 ml) was mixed with antigen suspension (0.4 ml) and incubated at 37°C for one hour. After three subsequent washings, one drop of the mass of trypanosomes was mixed on a slide with one drop of previously adsorbed and titrated antiglobulin serum. Intense immediate reactions with large aggregates were considered positive. Of 61 sera positive by complement-fixation tests, 60 had a positive Coombs test. Among 6 with doubtful CF reactions, 4 had a positive Coombs test. Optical results were obtained only with living organisms as antigen; chemically killed organisms were less agglutinable and could only be stored for a short period of time.

Fluorescent-antibody tests. As Essenfeld and Fennell (1964) have pointed out, the fluorescent-antibody technique introduced by Coons et al. (1941) may be employed as either a direct or indirect method. The direct technique involved application of a conjugate containing the antibody to a smear or section. The indirect technique involved application of the specific antibody which, when bound to the antigens, is identified by staining with a conjugate containing an antibody against the specific antibody.

The indirect method was first adapted for use in *T. cruzi* infections by Fife and Muschel (1959), who gave an improved method for purifying antibody, prior to conjugation with fluorescein. They evaluated their procedure with homologous and heterologous sera by comparing their results with human sera to those obtained in complement-fixation tests. They found that nonspecific staining occurred in tests using dried smears of trypanosomes, but the specificity was excellent when the reactions were conducted in test tubes where drying was prevented. Sadun et al. (1963), however, were able to use the indirect technique on slides, and Toussaint et al. (1965a, b) employed soluble antigens, which they found to be as specific and sensitive as somatic protein antigens.

Biagi et al. (1964) prepared antigen for immunofluorescence studies from the amastigote forms from the myocardium of infected mice, and they reported good correlation with the results of complement-fixation tests in 236 sera. Essenfeld and Fennell (1964) and Voller and Shaw (1965) reported using the direct technique; the former authors also used the indirect technique, and the latter employed a one-step inhibition procedure adapted from Goldman's *Toxoplasma* test (1957) based on the inhibition of specific staining. Voller and Shaw did not, however, test the specificity of the inhibition method, and they felt it was less suitable than the indirect technique for quantitative studies.

Girola et al. (1965) found a 96 percent correlation between the fluorescent-antibody test, performed on slides with antigen from culture forms and the complement-fixation test. Camargo (1966) used the fluorescent-antibody test with eluates of blood smears on filter papers, as well as with sera, and observed close agreement between this test and the CF test.

Alvarez et al. (1967) evaluated the immunofluorescence method in comparison with the complement-fixation and the indirect hemagglutination techniques with 1,083 sera, and they concluded that in the chronic stage, the fluorescence technique was as sensitive as the hemagglutination method and slightly superior to the complement-fixation reaction. In the acute stage, the fluorescence method was far more sensitive than either of the other two methods.

In the tube test of Fife and Muschel (1959), two of 20 syphilitic sera gave weak reactions. In the slide test of Sadun et al. (1963), cross-reactions occurred with some frequency with sera from patients with African trypanosomiasis, which, of course, would almost never be a diagnostic problem. There were positive reactions with one out of four sera from patients with leishmaniasis (type not specified) and with one of 13 syphilitic sera, and there were three doubtful reactions among the latter group.

In fluorescent-antibody tests performed with the soluble antigen of Toussaint et al. (1965a, b), there were no cross-reactions with sera either from syphilitics or patients with a number of diverse parasitic infections.

Shaw and Voller (1963), in fluorescent-antibody studies with *Endotrypanum schaudinni*, reported no cross-reactions with *T. cruzi*, although they found positive reactions with culture forms of *Leishmania mexicana* and *L. tropica*.

Camargo (1966) found cross-reactions with sera or with filter-paper eluates in about 50 percent of cases of kala-azar, in 100 percent of cases of mucocutaneous leishmaniasis, in about 10 percent with tuberculosis, and in about 7 percent with lepromatous leprosy.

Dye test. Scorza et al. (1958, 1959) applied the principle of the Sabin-Feldman dye test (1948) for toxoplasmosis to the study of sera from normal persons and patients with Chagas' disease, using methylene blue and toluidine blue as vital stains at pH 11.0. In their method, inactivated test serum is mixed in a tube with fresh guinea pig serum and a suspension of washed culture organisms of *T. cruzi*, incubated one hour, and then mixed (on a slide) with a solution of glucose, sodium hydroxide, and dye. The preparation is examined under the microscope to ascertain whether the cells take up the dye. In a series of 12 patients with positive complement fixation and xenodiagnosis, the percentage of culture forms which did not take up the dye was from 78 to 100 percent. In a group of 19 individuals with negative complement fixation and xenodiagnosis, the "anticrithidial" reaction was from 0 to 6 percent. In another group of 12 patients with positive xenodiagnosis, all were positive in the dye test; although by complement fixation, only 2 were strongly positive, 5 were doubtful, and 5 were negative. Other tests also confirmed the sensitivity of the dye test. It has not, however, apparently been critically examined by other workers.

As Scorza et al. (1958, 1959) pointed out, the adaptation of the dye test to *T. cruzi* diagnosis is an extension of the observations of Muniz and Boriello (1945), Lopez and Franca (1954), and Silva (1955). These workers observed the differential action of sera from normal and immune persons on the survival of culture organisms of *T. cruzi*. The addition of dye furnishes an indicator of the cytologic condition of the cell in the presence of serum, since the uptake of the vital stains is inhibited in cells which are affected by antibody in the presence of certain other essential reagents, sometimes designated "accessory factor." Feldman (1956) has suggested that this accessory factor is similar to if not identical with the properdin system (Pillemer et al., 1954).

Card test. In 1966, Fife et al. reported on the adaptation, for use in Chagas' disease, of a card test based on a procedure used in surveys for syphilis, schistosomiasis, and trichinosis (*see* Schulz et al., 1967, for references). *T. cruzi* soluble antigen (the exoantigen of Tarrant et al.; *see* p. 635) is adsorbed on cholesterol-lecithin crystals. The sensitized crystals are then sedimented and resuspended in a diluting medium containing EDTA, choline chloride, and activated charcoal. The EDTA and choline chloride stabilize the antigen emulsion and permit the testing of unheated serum or plasma; the charcoal is incorporated to facilitate reading of the tests visually without magnification. Tests are performed by mixing a drop of the antigen emulsion with 0.03 ml of unheated serum or plasma on a specially designed disposable test card and rotating for 8 minutes. A reaction is evidenced by an easily recognized clumping of the charcoal particles. A drop of blood obtained by finger puncture and drawn into an heparinized capillary tube will provide sufficient plasma for the test.

In tests with sera from 27 individuals with clinically diagnosed Chagas' disease, 23 (85 percent) reacted positively in the card test. The four sera which did not react were also nonreactive in the standard complement-fixation test. There were five (3 percent) false positives among 176 sera from syphilitic individuals, and 32 (3 percent) false positives among 1,168 sera from healthy individuals. In subsequent studies on sera from individuals residing in a highly endemic Chagas' disease area, it was found that sensitivity and specificity were profoundly influenced by the relative concentrations of antigen and lecithin. Experiments to determine the optimum concentrations and ratios of these are still underway so that, hopefully, this test can be soon made available for epidemiologic surveys and blood-bank monitoring.

Intradermal reactions

In 1941, Mayer and Pifano prepared a phenolized antigen (which they called "cruzin") from culture forms of *T. cruzi*, and they tested it in six confirmed cases of Chagas' disease which gave strongly positive intradermal reactions and in six apparently healthy individuals from an endemic area, five of whom were negative. The one in the latter group who was positive also had positive xenodiagnosis. Twelve individuals with diverse other diseases were negative, and the authors concluded that the intradermal reaction with "cruzin" was of great practical value, more certain than the CF test, and at least as valuable as xenodiagnosis, which took more time.

Pessoa and Cardoso (1942) tried an intradermal reaction in three patients with Chagas' disease (one was acute, two were chronic) and had negative results. In guinea pigs sensitized by intracardial inoculation of large doses of culture forms, they also obtained negative results 10 days after the last sensitizing dose. Senekjie (1943b) obtained positive intradermal reactions in rabbits immunized against *T. cruzi*. At 12 hours, there was an erythematous papule which attained its maximum size at 24 hours and disappeared after 3 days.

Mazza et al. (1943) tested an intradermal antigen prepared by lysis-filtration-dialysis. This was highly reactive in 14 Chagas' disease patients and positive in 3 out of 7 patients from an endemic zone who had not been diagnosed as having Chagas' disease. Later, the antigen was tested in three foreigners and in three individuals born and raised in Buenos Aires, and the results were completely negative. This, however, was after the material had been stored for one year.

Muniz and de Freitas (1944b) prepared several different types of antigens for intradermal testing and used them in six patients with Chagas' disease; two were in the chronic phase with positive xenodiagnosis, and four were in the acute phase of the disease. The following antigens were tested:
1. Autolysate of culture forms
2. Suspension of culture forms in serum containing thimerosal (1:10,000)
3. Suspension of culture forms in serum with 0.5 percent phenol
4. Suspension of culture forms in serum with 0.2 percent formalin
5. Polysaccharide fraction of culture forms.

The intradermal results were completely negative with all of the antigens used.

Pellegrino (1946) prepared two kinds of antigens for testing in dogs. One, used in the testing of acute (six dogs) and transitional (eight dogs) stages of the disease, was prepared from blood forms of *T. cruzi*. The other, used in the testing of chronic (five dogs) stages, was prepared from culture forms. In all cases, the intradermal reactions were negative.

These discouraging results, summarized by Pedreira de Freitas (1947), probably account for the long delay in further studies. It was not until 1964 that Amato Neto et al. tried a new approach, using tissue culture antigen, which they tested in normal individuals (with one false positive among three persons tested) and in cases of Chagas' disease (12) and cutaneous leishmaniasis (7). In the patients with leishmaniasis, the results were all positive and intense. In the patients with Chagas' disease (all chronic), 8 out of 12 were positive and all were mild reactions. These authors did not advise the use of this antigen in diagnosis, but recommended its further study.

Intradermal cross-reactions are of interest because of the use, in some areas where Chagas' disease may occur concurrently with cutaneous leishmaniasis, of a test devised by Montenegro (1926) involving the intradermal injection of a suspension of *Leishmania brasiliensis* organisms which provokes a local reaction in individuals sensitized by the infection. Sales Gomes (1939) modified the Montenegro reaction by introducing an antigen prepared from *T. cruzi* rather than *Leishmania*, but he did not obtain the characteristic local reaction in ten patients who were Montenegro-positive, possibly because an inadequate amount of antigen was used. Pessoa and Pestana (1941) reported that when they prepared antigen from *T. cruzi* under conditions identical to those used in preparing Montenegro antigen, they obtained positive reactions in patients with cutaneous leishmaniasis. These results were later confirmed by Mayer and Pifano (1940), Pessoa and Cardoso (1942), Romaña and Conejos (1946, 1947), and Navarrete and Biagi (1960).

Pessoa and Cardoso (1942) found that although patients with cutaneous leishmaniasis showed positive reactions when tested with antigen from either *L. brasiliensis* or *T. cruzi*, patients (and guinea pigs) with Chagas' disease reacted to neither of the antigens. Pellegrino and Guimaraes (1953) tested six patients with Chagas' disease with antigens prepared from both *T. rangeli* and *L. brasiliensis* culture forms, and they found that none of them gave an intradermal reaction with either antigen.

Effects of *T. cruzi* infection on diagnostic tests for other diseases

Infectious mononucleosis. It has been implied in the discussion of the heterophile antibody reaction (*see* p. 648) that there is a possibility of nonspecific cross-reactions between *T. cruzi* and infectious mononucleosis which might make presumptive tests misleading. It was noted that the heterophile antibodies in Chagas' disease, however, are similar to those in serum sickness and should therefore be adsorbable by guinea-pig or horse kidney.

These antibodies should thus be distinguishable from the non-Forssman types in infectious mononucleosis.

Syphilis. According to La Corte (1942), false positive Wassermann reactions occur in about 14 percent of sera with positive complement fixation for Chagas' disease. A few other authors have suggested, without extensive documentation, that Wassermann and flocculation tests (Kahn and Meinicke) might be affected in Chagas' disease (Vianna Martins et al., 1941; Manso Soto and Rispoli, 1952; Dias, 1955; Gotta, 1946). However, Almeida et al. (1954) did not regard this as a problem, and Amato Neto (1958) strongly emphasized that no false positives are seen in Wassermann, Kahn, and Kline tests as a result of *T. cruzi* infection.

Toxoplasmosis. Awad (1954) reported that mice convalescing from *T. cruzi* infections cross-reacted in the Sabin-Feldman dye test for toxoplasmosis, and Westphal (1954) reported positive complement fixation for *Toxoplasma* in rats and hamsters with *T. cruzi*. Jacobs (1956), however, did not find antibodies for *Toxoplasma* in rats with Chagas' disease. Groenroos and Salminen (1955) also found no false reactions in rats with *T. cruzi* in either CF or dye tests.

Cathie (1957) found that in 15 sera from Chagas' disease patients in Brazil, 6 were positive at low titers in the dye test, and, assuming that the incidence of toxoplasmosis was the same in Brazil as in Britain, they concluded that *T. cruzi* infection would not interfere with the dye test for toxoplasmosis in man, in spite of the observations in animals.

Thiermann et al. (1958) studied 169 sera with positive complement-fixation tests for Chagas' disease in both the dye test and the complement-fixation test for toxoplasmosis. They found that the incidence of positives in the dye test (titers of 1:16 to 1:512) obtained in the Chagas' disease group was not higher than that in 131 normal blood donors of similar age, but the complement-fixation test for toxoplasmosis revealed a higher percentage (22.8 percent) of positive results in the Chagas' disease group than in the controls (2.3 percent). It was suggested that either the *T. cruzi* infection may have stimulated the development of specific *Toxoplasma* antibodies, or the one infection might have furthered the spread of the other. Maekelt and Gomez (1962) reported that no cross-reactions were observed in dye tests with sera from 78 persons with Chagas' disease. Mas Bakal (1962) tested the blood of rabbits infected with *T. cruzi* with negative results.

Leishmaniasis. Marques da Cunha and Dias (1939), using a complement-fixation test for leishmaniasis with an antigen prepared from culture forms of *Leishmania*, found positive cross-reactions with sera from three cases of Chagas' disease. Brener (1952) also used culture material of *L. brasiliensis* to prepare antigen according to Davis' method (1943). Of 11 cases of cutaneous leishmaniasis, 10 reacted positively, and of 15 cases of Chagas' disease, 14 were positive. Pessoa and Cardoso (1942) used material prepared from culture forms of *T. cruzi* according to the method of Kelser (1936) as antigen in complement-fixation tests for cutaneous leishmaniasis. Of 26 cases of cutaneous leishmaniasis, 19 were positive. Two out of three cases of Chagas' disease were positive.

Brener and Pellegrino (1957) prepared polysaccharide fractions of culture forms of both *T. cruzi* and *L. brasiliensis* which they used as antigens in precipitin tests with sera of humans and dogs with visceral leishmaniasis. Positive ring tests were observed in all of six human sera with the *T. cruzi* antigen, and in five out of six with the leishmanial antigen. Two out of four dog sera reacted with both antigens. The same authors (1958) performed complement-fixation tests in eight dogs using antigen prepared from *Mycobacterium*, which is commonly used in tests for visceral leishmaniasis. All of the sera from these dogs (which were shown to be infected with *T. cruzi* by complement-fixation tests with homologous antigen, by precipitin test, or by xenodiagnosis) reacted positively in the complement-fixation test for leishmaniasis.

ALLERGIC PHENOMENA

The presence of numerous inflammatory foci in the myocardium, associated more with necrotic cardiac muscle cells than with living parasitized cells, has been regarded as evidence that myocarditis of Chagas' disease is indirectly induced by an autoimmune reaction. This was suggested by Torres (1929) and Mazza and Jörg (1939). Based on a comparative histologic study, Jaffe (1946) also hypothesized that myocardial changes could result from autoallergic processes, which could explain the heart lesions in Chagas' disease.

Muniz and de Azevedo (1947) reported experiments in which they sensitized monkeys by five injections of killed culture organisms or lysates, and later gave "shocking" doses which provoked inflammatory reactions resembling those found in Chagas' disease. They also reported passive transfer of hypersensitivity. During the same period, Cavelti (1947) and Jaffe and Holz (1948) injected cardiac extracts into animals, which produced cardiac antibodies as well as myocardial lesions.

Pizzi (1951) and Taliaferro and Pizzi (1955) also remarked on the lack of correlation between invasion by parasites and the inflammatory response, and they expressed the view that most inflammation in immune animals is probably allergic and is associated with the production of antibodies against *T. cruzi*, or a tuberculin-type of cellular hypersensitivity.

Continuing earlier studies, Jaffe et al. (1961) and Kozma (1962) carried out serologic tests by gel-precipitation, as well as histologic examinations, with animals sensitized with homologous cardiac extracts. Kozma (1962) found that guinea pig sera from *T. cruzi*-infected animals reacted positively with purified cardiac extracts in Ouchterlony tests, and the percentage of reactions increased from 56 percent at 3 months after infection to 80 percent after 10 months. He also tested sera of 32 patients with positive CF tests for Chagas' disease, and found that 27 (84 percent) reacted positively with homologous cardiac extract. Jaffe and Kozma (1960) reported that Tejada and Castro (1958) also made similar observations.

De Brito et al. (1963) sensitized guinea pigs to cardiac muscle (using

Freund's adjuvant). In their view, the "autoallergic" myocarditis thus produced did not immunoallergically or histopathologically resemble that seen in guinea pigs during the course of experimental Chagas' disease.

REFERENCES

Abath, G. M., E. Coutinho-Abath, and J. M. Barbosa. 1966. Histopathology of skeletal muscle in experimental Chagas' disease. II. Alterations in late phase and in combined infection with *Schistosoma mansoni*. Amer. J. Trop. Med. Hyg., 15:141-145.

Adler, S. 1958. The action of specific serum on a strain of *Trypanosoma cruzi*. Ann. Trop. Med. Parasit., 52:282-301.

Agosin, M., and O. Badinez. 1949. Algunas caracteristicas de la infestacion experimental con *T. cruzi* en el conejo. Bol. Inform. Parasit. Chile., 4:6-7.

—— R. Christen, A. Jarpa, and W. Atias. 1952. Ensayos de quimoterapia en la enfermedad de Chagas experimental. V. Terramicina. Bol. Inform. Parasit. Chile., 6:5-6.

Alencar, J. E. de. 1959. A moléstia de Chagas no Ceará. An. Congr. Internac. Doença de Chagas, 1:35-50.

—— 1965. Estudos sôbre a epidemiologia da doença de Chagas no Ceará, III. Região do Baixo Jaguaribe. Rev. Brasil. Malar., 17:149-158.

—— J. O. de Almeida, V. Sherlock, A. Pereira de Franca, and L. Leite. 1963. Estudos sôbre a epidemiologia da doença de Chagas no Ceará. II. Novos dados. Rev. Brasil. Malar., 15:551-565.

—— E. P. Pessoa, V. R. A. Sherlock, G. S. Tome, and R. V. Cunha. 1962. Estudos sôbre a epidemiologia da doença de Chagas no Ceará. I. Dados preliminares. Rev. Brasil. Malar., 14:201-220.

Almeida, J. O. 1956. Isofixation curves as a method of standardizing quantitative complement-fixation tests. J. Immun., 7:259-263.

—— 1963a. Reação quantitativa de fixação de complemento em gotas sôbre placas, pelo método das curvas iso-hemolíticas. Rev. Inst. Med. Trop. S. Paulo, 5:176-189.

—— 1963b. Tecnica de la reacción de fijación del complemento en gotas para excluir donadores de sangre chagasicos. Bol. Ofic. Sanit. Panamer., 55:133-145.

—— and J. L. Pedreira de Freitas. 1953. Reações atípicas em fixação de complemento nos sistemas sífilis e doença de Chagas, pelo método quantitativo, interpretação e determinação de títulos. Rev. Brasil. Biol., 13:1-12.

—— L. G. Saraiva, and V. Nussenzweig. 1953. Estudos sôbre as reações quantitativas de fixação do complemento. I. Alteração de títulos em reações de fixação do complemento pela inactivação e manutenção dos soros em geladeira, nos sistemas sífilis, doença de Chagas, tuberculose e lepra. Rev. Paulista Med., 43:446.

—— J. L. Pedreira de Freitas, and H. Brandao. 1954. Complement fixation test with a triple antigen for syphilis, tuberculosis, leprosy or Chagas' disease in blood banks. Amer. J. Trop. Med. Hyg., 3:490-494.

—— J. L. Pedreira de Freitas, and A. F. Siqueira. 1959. Capacidade reativa específica do antigeno com anticorpo em reações de fixação de complemento para moléstia de Chagas. Rev. Inst. Med. Trop. S. Paulo, 1:266-272.

Alvarez, M., J. A. Cerisola, and R. W. Rohwedder. 1967. Test de immunofluorescencia para el diagnostico de la enfermedad de Chagas. Primer Congreso Latinoamericano de Parasitologia, Santiago de Chile, Resumenes, p. 32.

Amato Neto, V. 1958. Contribuição ao conhecimento da forma aguda da doença de Chagas. Thesis, Faculdade de Medicina da Universidade de São Paulo, Brasil, 332 pp.

—— C. Magaldi, and S. B. Pessoa. 1964. Intradermoreação para o diagnóstico da doença de Chagas com antigeno de *Trypanosoma cruzi* obtido de cultura de tecido. Rev. Goiana Med., 10:121-126.

—— J. E. C. Martins, L. de Oliveira, and E. Tsuzuki. 1965. Incidência da doença de Chagas entre gestantes, no Hospital das Clínicas de São Paulo. Rev. Inst. Med. Trop. S. Paulo, 7:156-159.

—— J. E. C. Martins, L. de Oliveira, and E. Tsuzuki. 1968. Incidência da doença de Chagas entre mães de prematuros, no Hospital das Clínicas de São Paulo. Rev. Inst. Med. Trop. S. Paulo, 10:192-195.

Amrein, Y. U. 1967. Effects of environmental temperature on *Trypanosoma cruzi* infection in mice. Parasitology, 53:1160.

Andrade, S. G., and Z. A. Andrade. 1966. Doença de Chagas e alteracões neuronais no plexo de Auerbach. Rev. Inst. Med. Trop. S. Paulo, 8:219-224.

Apt, W., and G. Neidmann. 1964. Serologia de la toxoplasmosis y enfermedad de Chagas en el embarazo. Bol. Chile. Parasit., 19:55-59.

———— O. Diaz, and C. Ramos. 1960. Algunos indices epidemiologicos sobre enfermedad de Chagas en el Departamento de Elqui (Provincia de Coquimbo). Bol. Chile. Parasit., 15:23-28.

Awad, F. I. 1954. The diagnosis of toxoplasmosis. Lack of specificity of Sabin-Feldman dye test. Lancet, 2:1055-1056.

Backhouse, T. C., and A. Bolliger. 1951. Transmission of Chagas' disease to the Australian marsupial *Trichosurus vulpecula*. Trans. Roy. Soc. Trop. Med. Hyg., 44:521-533.

Barreto, A. L. de B. 1946. Provas subsidiárias no diagnóstico da doença de Chagas. Arq. Univ. Bahia Fac. Med., 1:285-320.

Barretto, M. P. 1964. Reservatórios do *Trypanosoma cruzi* nas Américas. Rev. Brasil. Malar., 16:527-552.

Batista, S. M., and U. M. Santos. 1959. Methyl antigen from a *"Schizotrypanum cruzi"* culture. Hospital (Rio de Janeiro), 56:1045-1051.

Berrios, A. 1960. Investigaciones sobre enfermedad de Chagas en Costa Rica por la reacción de fijación del complemento. Rev. Biol. Trop., 8:203-217.

———— and R. Zeledon. 1960. Estudio comparativo entre los antigenos de *Schizotrypanum cruzi* y de *Strigomonas oncopelti* en la reacción de fijación del complemento para enfermedad de Chagas. Rev. Biol. Trop., 8:225-231.

Bertin Soto, V. 1940. Consideraciones sobre la epidemiologia de la enfermedad de Chagas en Chile y su profilaxis. Bol. Med. Soc., 7:565-634.

Bettinotti, C. M. 1951. *Trypanosoma cruzi* in Cordoba. Acta Argent. Fisiol. Fisiopatol., 1:691-703.

———— 1952. Las cardiopatias y la enfermedad de Chagas. Estudio serologico—nota previa. Semana Med., 101:675-680.

———— 1953. Difusion de la enfermedad de Chagas en Cordoba. Primera Conferencia Nacional de la Enfermedad de Chagas, Argentina, pp. 153-158.

———— 1954. Difusion de la enfermedad de Chagas en Cordoba (R.A.) (Y distribucion de casos observados en la Provincia). Semana Med., 104:98-107.

———— M. A. Nores, and J. A. Restanio. 1953a. La prueba de fijación de complemento en el diagnostico de casos inaparentes de enfermedad de Chagas. Comunicación previa. Semana Med., 103:196-200.

Biagi, F., J. Tay, and R. M. Murray. 1964. La reacción de immunofluorescencia en el diagnostico de la enfermedad de Chagas. Bol. Ofic. Sanit. Panamer., 57:234-240.

———— J. Tay, and M. Gutierrez. 1965. Behavior of different Mexican strains of *Trypanosoma cruzi* in the white mouse (*Mus musculus*). *In* Progress in Protozoology, Abstracts. Second International Congress on Protozoology, London, 1965. Amsterdam, Excerpta Medica Foundation, International Congress Series No. 91, p. 142.

Biancalana, A., J. O. Pedreira de Freitas, V. Amato Neto, V. Nussenzweig, and R. Sonntag. 1953. Investigações sorológicas sôbre doença de Chagas entre candidatos a doadores em Bancos de Sangue nos Estados de São Paulo e Minas Gerais. Hospital (Rio de Janeiro), 44:745-749.

Blanchard, M. 1912a. Marche de l'infection à *"Schizotrypanum cruzi"* chez le cobaye et la souris. Bull. Soc. Path. Exot., 5:598-599.

———— 1912b. Sur un travail de M. le Dr. E. Brumpt intitulé: Étude experimentale de la trypanosomose americaine de C. Chagas. Bull. Acad. Med. Paris, 67:428-433.

Bozecevich, J., H. M. Hoyem, and V. M. Walston. 1946. A method of conducting the 50 per cent hemolysis end point complement fixation test for parasitic diseases. Public Health Rep., 61:529-534.

Bouisset, L., J. Ducos, and J. Ruffie. 1960. Technique d'hemagglutination passive dans la recherche de l'immunisation trypanosomienne. Path. Biol. (Paris), 8:91-98.

Brant, C. T., T. Caldeira, A. Moraes, E. Dias, and F. S. Laranja. 1951. Reference in Brant, 1962, Rev. Brasil. Malar., 14:3.

Brener, Z. 1952. A reação de fixação do complemento com antigeno de *L. brasiliensis* na leishmaniose tegumentar americana e na doença de Chagas. Hospital (Rio de Janeiro), 41:269-275.

———— 1961. Atividade terapêutica do 5-nitro-furaldeido-semicarbazona (Nitrofurazona) em esquemas de duração prolongada na infecção experimental do camundongo pelo *Trypanosoma cruzi*. Rev. Inst. Med. Trop. S. Paulo, 3:43-49.

———— 1962. Observações sôbre a imunidade à superinfecções em camundongos experimentalmente inoculados com *Trypanosoma cruzi* e submetidos a tratamento. Rev. Inst. Med. Trop. S. Paulo, 4:119-123.

———— 1965. Comparative studies of different strains of *Trypanosoma cruzi*. Ann. Trop. Med. Parasit., 59:19-26.

———— and J. Pellegrino. 1957. Reação de precipitina cruzada, no calazar, com fração polissacaridea isolada de formas de cultura do *Schizotrypanum cruzi* e *Leishmania brasiliensis*. Rev. Brasil. Malar., 9:501-502.

———— and J. Pellegrino. 1958. Reações imunológicas cruzadas em cães com doença de Chagas e leishmaniose visceral, naturalmente infectados. Rev. Brasil. Malar., 10:45-49.

———— and E. Chiari. 1963a. Observações sôbre a fase crônica da doença de Chagas experimental no camundongo. Rev. Inst. Med. Trop. S. Paulo, 5:128-132.

———— and E. Chiari. 1963b. Variações morfológicas observadas em diferentes amostras de *Trypanosoma cruzi*. Rev. Inst. Med. Trop. S. Paulo, 5:220-224.

———— and E. Chiari. 1966. Aspects of early growth of different *Trypanosoma cruzi* strains in culture medium. J. Parasit., 51:922-926.

Brito, T. de, D. Penna, S. Almeida, P. A. Galvao, and A. A. Pryso. 1963. Auto-agressão na cárdite chagárica experimental do cobaia. Proceedings of the Seventh International Congress of Tropical Medicine and Malaria (Rio de Janeiro), Vol. 2, p. 256.

Brncic, D., and G. Hoecker. 1949. Acción del *Trypanosoma cruzi* sobre un sarcoma aviario transmisible. Bol. Chile. Parasit., 4:42-43.

Browning, C. H., K. M. Calver, M. W. Leckie, and L. P. Walls. 1946. Phenanthridine compounds as chemotherapeutic agents in experimental *T. cruzi* infections. Nature (London), 157:263-264.

Brumpt, E. 1913a. Immunité partielle dans les infections à *Trypanosoma cruzi*; transmission de ce trypanosome par *Cimex rotundatus*; rôle régulateur des hôtes intermediaires; passage à travers la peau. Bull. Soc. Path. Exot., 6:172-176.

———— 1913b. Précis de Parasitologie. 2nd Ed. Paris., p. 186.

———— 1927. Eclectisme alimentaire des reduvides vecteurs du *Trypanosoma cruzi*. Presse Med., 35:1161-1162.

———— L. Mazzotti, and L. C. Brumpt. 1939. Enquêtes épidémiologiques sur la maladie de C. Chagas au mexique. Reduvides vecteurs. Animaux reservoirs de virus. Cas humains. Ann. Parasit. Hum. Comp., 17:299-312.

Bruni, N. 1926. Observations et recherches sur *Trypanosoma lewisi* et *Schizotrypanum cruzi*. Bull. Soc. Path. Exot., 19:791-794.

Butterworth, M., B. McClellan, and M. Allansmith. 1967. Influence of sex on immunoglobulin levels. Nature (London), 214:1224-1225.

Camargo, M. E. 1966. Fluorescent antibody test for the serodiagnosis of American trypanosomiasis. Technical modification employing preserved culture forms of *Trypanosoma cruzi* in a slide test. Rev. Inst. Med. Trop. S. Paulo, 8:227-234.

Cardoso, F. A. 1940a. A reação de fixação do complemento na trypanosomose experimental americana, com antigens de cultura. Rev. Asoc. Paulista Med., 17:88-89.

———— 1940b. A reação de fixação de complemento na trypanosomose experimental americana com antigeno de cultura. An. Paulistas Med. Cirurg., 40:404-405.

———— 1941. Tripanosomiasis—Reação de fixação do complemento. Bol. Ofic. Sanit. Panamer., 20:621.

———— 1943. Reação de fixação do complemento na tripanossomose americana experimental da cobaia, feita com antigeno de cultura de *Trypanosoma cruzi* Chagas, 1909 (Tipo Kelser). Bol. Inst. Hig. S. Paulo, 79:3-12.

Cariola, J., R. Prado, M. Agosin, and R. Christen. 1950. Susceptibilidad del Hamster (*Cricetus auratus*) y Peromyscus (*Peromyscus maniculatus gambeli*) a la infección experimental por *Trypanosoma cruzi*, cepa Tulahuén. Bol. Inform. Parasit. Chile., 5:44-45.

Carvalhal, S., A. Ferracci, A. Younes, O. Pilagallo, D. Uvo, and A. A. Aguiar. 1954a. Estudos sôbre a moléstia de Chagas numa coletividade operária no município de S. Caetano do Sul, Estado de São Paulo (Considerações clínicas epidemiológicas). Folia Clin. Biol. S. Paulo, 22:9-22.

———— A. A. Aguiar, O. Pilagallo, and A. Ferracci. 1945b. Considerações sôbre o comportamento da R.F.C. (técnica qualitativa) num grupo de indivíduos seguramente não portadores de infecção chagásica. Folia Clin. Biol. S. Paulo, 22:65-68.

———— O. P. Portugal, T. L. Da Silva, O. Ramos, N. Paladino, and A. A. Aguiar. 1954c. Considerações sôbre os resultados da RFC relacionados com os dados epidemiológicos relativos a endemia chagásica. Estudos sôbre indivíduos examinados serológica, clínica e epidemiològicamente. Folia Clin. Biol. S. Paulo, 22:97-104.

Cathie, I. A. B. 1957. An appraisal of the diagnostic value of the serological tests for toxoplasmosis. Trans. Roy. Soc. Trop. Med. Hyg., 51:104-110.

Cavelti, P. A. 1947. Studies on pathogenesis of rheumatic fever; cardiac lesions produced in rats by means of autoantibodies to heart and connective tissue. Arch. Path. (Chicago), 44:13-27.

Cerisola, J. A., and O. Lazzari. 1963. Resultados obtenidos con el test de hemaglutinación para diagnostico de la enfermedad de Chagas. Proceedings of the Seventh International Congress of Tropical Medicine and Malaria (Rio de Janeiro), Vol. 2, pp. 252-253.

———— M. Fatala Chaben, and J. O. Lazzari. 1962. "Test" de hemaglutinacion para el diagnostico de la enfermedad de Chagas. Prensa Med. Argent., 49:1761-1767.

———— J. Lazzari, and C. A. Dioorleto. 1964. Nuestra experiencia con el test de hemaglutinación para el diagnostico de la enfermedad de Chagas. Primeras Journadas Enf. Trans. Carlos Paz (Cordoba).

———— R. W. Rohwedder, and C. Di Corletto. 1967. Estimación de la especificidad de reacciones serologicas para enfermedad de Chagas. I. Sueros de zona libre de tripanosomiasis. Primer Congreso Latinoamericano de Parasitologia, Santiago de Chile, Resumenes, p. 30.

Chaffee, E. F., E. H. Fife, Jr., and J. F. Kent. 1956. Diagnosis of *Trypanosoma cruzi* infection by complement fixation. Amer. J. Trop. Med. Hyg., 5:763-771.

Chagas, C. 1909. Nova tripanosomiase humana. Estudos sôbre a morfologia e o ciclo evolutivo do *Schizotrypanum cruzi* n. gen., n. sp., agente etiológico de nova entidade mórbida do homen. Mem. Inst. Oswaldo Cruz, 1:159.

———— 1916. Processos patogênicos da tripanosomiase americana. Mem. Inst. Oswaldo Cruz, 8(Part 2):5-36.

———— 1936. Infecção experimental do homen pelo *Schizotrypanum cruzi*. Novena Reunion Sociedad Argentina de Patologia Regional, 1:136-159.

———— and E. Villela. 1922. Forma cardiaca da tripanosomiase americana. Mem. Inst. Oswaldo Cruz, 14:5-61.

Chang, S. L., and W. O. Negherbon. 1947. III. Studies on hemoflagellates. The specificity of serological reactions of *Leishmania donovani, L. brasiliensis, L. tropica,* and *Trypanosoma cruzi.* J. Infect. Dis., 81:209-227.

Chattas, A., R. Zamar, and H. H. Machado. 1958. Estudio electroforetico de las proteinas del suero en niños afectados de enfermedad de Chagas. Rev. Med. Cordoba, 46:293-297.

———— R. Zamar, and H. H. Machado. 1959. Estudio electroforetico de las proteinas del suero en niños afectados de enfermedad de Chagas. Rev. Med. Cordoba, 47:190-193.

Christen, R., and A. Neghme. 1950. Susceptibilidad del *Octodon d. degus* (Molina) a la infección experimental por el *Trypanosoma cruzi*. Bol. Inform. Parasit. Chile., 5:6-7.

———— M. Agosin, O. Badinez, O. Pizarro, A. Neghme, A. Jarpa, G. Gasic, and G. Hoecker. 1951. Cortisona, *Trypanosoma cruzi* y tumores. I. Acción del *Trypanosoma cruzi* y del acetato de cortisona sobre un adenocarcinoma mamario transplantable del raton. Bol. Chile. Parasit., 6:52-54.

Cohen, A. L., H. Borsook, and J. W. Dubnoff. 1947. The effect of a *Sporosarcina ureae* preparation on tumor cells *in vitro*. Proc. Soc. Exp. Biol. Med., 66:440-444.

Collier, W. A. 1931. Über Immunität bei der Chagas Krankheit der weissen Maus. Z. Hyg. Infekt. Krankh., 112:88-92.

Columbia Univ. Rep. 1959. Excerpt from the Combined Annual Report, Columbia University and Presbyterian Medical Center, p. 197.

Coons, A. H., H. J. Creech, R. N. Jones, and E. Berliner. 1942. The demonstration of pneumococcal antigen in tissues by the use of fluorescent antibody. J. Immun., 45:159-170.

Cornejo Donayre, A., A. Berrocal, and E. Cubas. 1962. Chagas' disease in Lima, Peru. Amer. J. Trop. Med. Hyg., 11:610-612.

Correa, M. O. A., M. de Britto e Silva, and V. Amato Neto. 1959. Emprêgo de ondas ultra-sônicas no preparo do antigeno para diagnóstico da moléstia de Chagas mediante fixação do complemento. Nota prévia. Rev. Inst. Adolfo Lutz, S. Paulo, 19:5-8.

Coudert, J. 1956a. Intérêt des antigenes lyophilisés en parasitologie. Maroc. Med., 35:1257-1259.

—— 1956b. Recherches expérimentales et cliniques sur l'action d'un extrait lyophilisé de *Trypanosoma cruzi* vis-à-vis de quelques neoplasies. Sem. Hôp. Paris, 32:3947-3954.
—— 1958. Que peut-on attendre de l'utilisation des extraits de *Trypanosoma cruzi* dans le traitement des neoplasmes. Sem. Med. Prof. (Paris), 34:1290-1294.
—— 1961a. Clinical and experimental investigations into the effect of *Trypanosoma cruzi* lyophilized extract on some forms of cancer (In Russian). Antibiotiki, 6:99-105.
—— 1961b. Recherches sur quelques actions d'un extrait de *T. cruzi* sur les cellules cancereuses. An. Congr. Internac. Doença de Chagas, Rio de Janeiro, 2:447-457.
—— and P. Juttin. 1950. Note sur l'action d'un lysat de *Trypanosoma cruzi* vis-à-vis d'un cancer greffe du rat. C. R. Soc. Biol. (Paris), 144:847-849.
—— M. R. Battesti, and C. Papageorgiou. 1960. Modifications de l'indice mitotique des cellules neoplasiques en culture (souche KB) sous l'influence d'un extrait de *Trypanosoma cruzi*. C.R. Soc. Biol. (Paris), 154:612-615.
—— and W. R. Kessler. 1942. Age resistance of mice to *Trypanosoma cruzi*. J. Parasit., 28:155-158.
Culbertson, J. T., and M. H. Kolodny. 1938. Acquired immunity in rats against *Trypanosoma cruzi*. J. Parasit., 24:83-90.
Dalma, J. 1953. Nota sobre el liquido cefalorraquideo en la enfermedad de Chagas. Primera Conferencia Nacional de la Enfermedad de Chagas, Argentina, pp. 129-133.
—— 1954. Nota sobre el liquido cefalorraquideo en la enfermedad de Chagas. An. Inst. Med. Regional (Tucuman), 4:47-55.
—— 1956. Primeros ensayos de piretoterapia en la enfermedad de Chagas (Resumen de observaciones parciales en 43 casos tratodos). Rev. Med. del Norte, 3:187-193.
—— 1961. Piretoterapia en la enfermedad de Chagas. Rev. Fac. Med. Tucuman, 3:301-304.
Darman, M. 1941. Multiplication du *Trypanosoma cruzi* dans le sang peripherique de la souris par passages successifs. Recherche de la prémunition vis-à-vis des souches homologues et heterologues. Ann. Parasit. Hum. Comp., 18:166-179.
Davis, D. J. 1943a. An improved antigen for complement fixation in American trypanosomiasis. Public Health Rep., 58:775-777.
—— 1943b. Infection in monkeys with strains of *Trypanosoma cruzi* isolated in the United States. U.S. Public Health Dept., No. 58, pp. 1006-1010.
—— and T. de S. Sullivan. 1946. Complement fixation tests for American trypanosomiasis in Texas. Public Health Rep., 61:1083-1084.
Deane, L. de M. 1960. Sôbre um tripanossomo do tipo cruzi encontrado num rato silvestre, no Estado do Pará. Rev. Brasil. Malar., 12:87-102.
De Leon, J. R. 1959. Estado actual de la enfermedad de Chagas en Guatemala. Resumen epidemiologico. Rev. Goiana Med., 5:445-455.
Denison, N. 1943a. Immunological studies on experimental *Trypanosoma cruzi* infections I. Lysins in blood of infected rats. Proc. Soc. Exp. Biol. Med., 52:26-27.
—— 1943b. Experimental studies on *Trypanosoma cruzi* infections and reticuloendothelial blockade in rats. Amer. J. Hyg., 38:178-184.
Diamond, L. S., and R. Rubin. 1958. Experimental infection of certain farm mammals with a North American strain of *Trypanosoma cruzi* from the raccoon. Exp. Parasit., 7:383-390.
Dias, E. 1932. Le *Trypanosoma cruzi* et ses rapports avec le systeme reticuloendothelial. C. R. Soc. Biol. (Paris), 110:206-210.
—— 1933. Immunité naturelle des animaux à sang froid vis-à-vis de l'infection par le *Trypanosoma cruzi*. C. R. Soc. Biol. (Paris), 112:1474-1475.
—— 1934. Estudos sôbre o *Schizotrypanum cruzi*. Mem. Inst. Oswaldo Cruz, 28:1-110.
—— 1944. Não receptividade do pombo doméstico à infecção por *Schizotrypanum*. Mem. Inst. Oswaldo Cruz, 40:191-193.
—— 1946. Acerca de 254 casos de doença de Chagas comprovados em Minas Gerais. Brasil-Med., 60:41-44.
—— 1950. Considerações sôbre a doença de Chagas. Hospital (Rio de Janeiro), 21:921-926.
—— 1955. Informações acerca de 300 casos de doença de Chagas com período inicial conhecido, fichados no Centro de Estudos de Bambui. Hospital (Rio de Janeiro), 47:9-17.
—— 1956. Chagas-Krankheit. Chagas' disease. *In* E. Rodenwaldt's Welt-Seuchen Atlas, 2:135-140.
—— T. G. Perrin, and M. Brenes. 1947a. Nota previa sobre las primeras comprobac-

iones suorologicas de la enfermedad de Chagas en Mexico. Gac. Med. Mex., 77:180-183.
———— T. G. Perrin, and M. Brenes. 1947b. Nota previa sobre las primeras comprobaciones suerologicas de la enfermedad de Chagas en Mexico. Arch. Inst. Cardiol. Mex., 17:20-24.
———— F. Laranja, and J. Pellegrino. 1949. Inquérito clínico-epidemiológico sôbre doença de Chagas feito entre as Estações de Iguatama e Campos Altos, oeste de Minas Gerais. Primer Reunion Panamericano Enfermedad de Chagas, pp. 33-34.
———— T. Caldeira Brant, and R. M. Santos. 1952. Casos de cardiopatia chagásica crônica no município de Mococa, Estado de São Paulo. Rev. Brasil. Malar., 4:184-186.
Dias, J. C. 1950. A cardiopatia crônica da moléstia de Chagas. Res. Clin. Cient., 19:9-17, 53-61.
———— 1967. Prevalência da doença de Chagas entre crianças da zona rural de Bambui, MG, após ensaio profilático. Rev. Brasil. Malar., 19:135-159.
Diniz, O. 1949. Lepra e doença de Chagas. Arq. Mineiros Leprologia, 9:155-171.
———— and J. Pellegrino. 1948. A reação de fixação do complemento com antigeno de cultura de "Schizotrypanum cruzi" em soros de leprosos. Arq. Mineiros Leprologia, 8:111-120.
Dios, R. L., and H. Bonacci. 1943. Sensibilidad de los sapos (Bufo arenarum) a la inoculación experimental del Trypanosoma cruzi. Segunda comunicación. Rev. Inst. Bact. Carlos Malbran, Buenos Aires, 12:27-36.
———— E. T. Werngren, and P. Perez. 1929. Sensibilité du crapaud a l'infection experimentale par Trypanosoma cruzi. C. R. Soc. Biol. (Paris), 102:1100-1101.
Duque, O. 1965. Histology of the reticuloendothial system of the spleen in mice of inbred strains. J. Nat. Cancer Inst., 35:15-27.
Dussert, E., and J. Faiguenbaum. 1942. La reacción de desviación del complemento de Machado-Guerrero en Chile. Proceedings of the Eighth American Scientific Congress, 6:241.
Eichbaum, F. W. 1961. Pesquisas sôbre a presença substâncias tóxicas em culturas de Trypanosoma cruzi. An. Congr. Internac. Doença de Chagas, 2:479-489.
Elejalde, P. 1961. Alguns achados no líquido cefaloraquidiano na forma aguda da doença de Chagas. An. Congr. Internac. Doença de Chagas, 2:491-502.
Enos, F. L., and N. W. Elton, 1950. Fatal acute Chagas' disease in a North American in the Canal Zone. Amer. J. Trop. Med., 30:829-833.
Espinoza, L. 1955. Epidemiologia de la enfermedad de Chagas en la Republica del Ecuador. Rev. Ecuator. Hig. Med. Trop., 12:25-105.
———— 1959. Ensayos de terapia en la enfermedad de Chagas aguda con la asociación del 8-(4-amino-1-metilbutilamino)-6-metoxiquinolina difosfato o difosfato de primaquina y acetato de cortisona. Proceedings of the Sixth International Congress of Tropical Medicine and Malaria, Vol. 6, pp. 885-907.
Essenfield, E., and R. H. Fennell, Jr. 1964. Immunofluorescent study of experimental Trypanosoma cruzi infection. Proc. Soc. Exp. Biol. Med., 116:728-730.
Farrar, W. E., I. G. Kagan, F. D. Everton, and T. F. Sellers. 1963. Serologic evidence of human infection with Trypanosoma cruzi in Georgia. Amer. J. Hyg., 78:166-172.
Feldman, H. A. 1956. The relationship of Toxoplasma antibody activator to the serum-properdin system. Ann. N. Y. Acad. Sci., 66:263-267.
Fernandes, J. F. 1965. The effect of drugs on protein and nucleic acid metabolism in Trypanosoma cruzi. In Progress in Protozoology. Amsterdam, Excerpta Medica Foundation, International Congress Series No. 91, pp. 79-80.
———— M. Halsman, and O. Castellani. 1965. Effect of actinomycin D on the infectivity of Trypanosoma cruzi. Nature (London), 207:1004-1005.
———— M. Halsman, and O. Castellani. 1966. Effect of mitomycin C, actinomycin D, and pyrimidine analogs on the growth rate, protein and nucleic acid synthesis, and on the viability of Trypanosoma cruzi. Exp. Parasit., 18:203-210.
Ferreira, M. P., and P. Elejalde. 1960. Estudo eletroforético das proteinas séricas na forma crônica da doença de Chagas. Brasil-Med., 74:108-116.
Ferriolli, F., and M. P. Barretto. 1965. Estudos sôbre reservatórios e vectores silvestres do Trypanosoma cruzi. Rev. Inst. Med. Trop. S. Paulo, 7:169-179.
Fife, E. H., Jr., and L. H. Muschel. 1959. Fluorescent-antibody technic for serodiagnosis of Trypanosoma cruzi infection. Proc. Soc. Exp. Biol. Med., 101:540-543.
———— and J. F. Kent. 1960. Protein and carbohydrate complement fixing antigens of Trypanosoma cruzi. Amer. J. Trop. Med. Hyg., 9:512-517.

——— G. S. Warner, and C. J. Tarrant. 1966. Development and evaluation of a rapid card test for the diagnosis of Chagas' disease. Presented at the 15th Annual Meeting Amer. Soc. Trop. Med. Hyg., San Juan, Puerto Rico.

Figallo, L. E. 1962. La enfermedad de Chagas congenita. Arch. Venez. Med. Trop. Parasit. Med., 4:243-264.

Franca-Rodriguez, M. E., and J. E. Mackinnon. 1962. Efecto de la temperatura ambiental sobre la infección por *Trypanosoma cruzi*. An. Fac. Med. Univ. Repub., Montevideo, 47:310-313.

Friebel, H. 1952. Über den Einfluss des Cortisons auf die Behandlung der experimentellen Trypanosomen-Infektion mit Trypanblau. Arch. Exp. Path. Pharmakol., 216:536-540.

——— and H. Kästner. 1955. Der Einfluss von Megaphen auf den Verlauf von experimentellen Trypanosomenerkrankungen von Mäusen (*Tr. cruzi* und *evansi*). Arch. Exp. Path. Pharmakol., 225:210-236.

Fulton, F. 1949. The measurement of complement fixation by virus. Advances Virus Res., 5:247-287.

Gaikhorst, G. 1960. The presence of *Trypanosoma cruzi* on the island of Aruba and its importance to man. Trop. Geogr. Med., 12:59-61.

Galliard, H. 1930a. Localisation peritoneale exclusive au cours de l'infection a *Trypanosoma cruzi*. Ann. Parasit. Hum. Comp., 8:140.

——— 1930b. Infections à *Trypanosoma cruzi* chez les animaux splenectomisés. Bull. Soc. Path. Exot., 23:188-192.

——— 1965. Variété des tropismes de différentes souches de *Trypanosoma cruzi* chez la souris. *In* Progress in Protozoology. Second International Congress on Protozoology, London, 1965. Amsterdam, Excerpta Medica Foundation, International Congress Series No. 91, pp. 143-144.

——— and R. Boutet. 1951. Modifications de l'évolution et de la virulence d'une souche de *Trypanosoma cruzi* Chagas sous l'action de divers produits chimiotherapiques et antibiotiques. Ann. Parasit. Hum. Comp., 26:5-18.

——— L. Brumpt, and R. Martinez. 1950. Infections expérimentales à *Trypanosoma cruzi* Chagas chez l'homme à propos de la biotherapie du cancer. Bull. Soc. Path. Exot., 43:204-216.

——— J. Lapierre, and J. J. Rousset. 1959. Attenuation de l'infection à *Trypanosoma cruzi* chez la souris blanche par différentes souches de *Borrelia*. Bull. Soc. Path. Exot., 52:272-276.

——— J. Lapierre, and M. Coste. 1962a. Protection croisée entre souches heterologues de *Trypanosoma cruzi* chez la souris. Son inhibition par la cortisone. C. R. Soc. Biol. (Paris), 156:1267-1270.

——— J. Lapierre, and M. Coste. 1962b. Contribution à l'étude d'une souche pathogène de *Trypanosoma cruzi*. (Souche Tulahuén, Chile). Effets de la splenectomie, des traitements par la cortisone et l'hormone somatotrope. Ann. Parasit. Hum. Comp., 37:495-503.

——— J. Lapierre, and M. Coste. 1962c. Contribution à l'étude d'une souche pathogène de *Trypanosoma cruzi*. (Souche Tulahuén, Chile). II. Premunition croisée entre souches heterologues. Reveil de l'infection chronique par la cortisone. Ann. Parasit. Hum. Comp., 37:504-513.

Galton, M. 1967. Factors involved in the rejection of skin transplanted across a weak histocompatibility barrier: Gene dosage, sex of recipient, and nature of expression of histocompatibility genes. Transplantation, 5:154-168.

Garcia, A. 1967. Estudios sobre la duración de la inmunidad y riesgo de lesiones en la vacunación contra la enfermedad de Chagas. Primer Congreso Latinoamericano de Parasitologia, Santiago de Chile, Resumenes, p. 35.

Ghelelovitch, S., and R. Chassignet. 1957. Évolution de la parasitemie chez les souris infectées de *Trypanosoma cruzi*. Rôle de l'inoculat. Bull. Soc. Path. Exot., 40:135-143.

Gill, B. S. 1964. A procedure for the indirect haemagglutination test for the study of experimental *Trypanosoma evansi* infections. Ann. Trop. Med. Parasit., 58:473-480.

Girola, R., G. J. W. Martini, and A. Milic. 1965. La reacción de inmuno-fluorescencia en el diagnostico de la enfermedad de Chagas. Segundas Jornadas Entomoepidem. Argent., Salta.

Goble, F. C. 1951. Studies on experimental Chagas' disease in mice in relation to chemotherapeutic testing. J. Parasit., 37:408-414.

————— 1952a. Observations on experimental Chagas' disease in dogs. Amer. J. Trop. Med. Hyg., 1:189-204.
————— 1952b. Lack of effect of sex hormones on the course of experimental Chagas' disease in mice. J. Parasit., 38 (Suppl.):15.
————— 1954. Thyroid changes in acute experimental Chagas' disease in dogs. Amer. J. Path., 30:599-607.
————— 1956. American trypanosomiasis. J.A.M.A., 161:269-270.
————— 1958. A comparison of strains of Trypanosoma cruzi indigenous to the United States with certain strains from South America. Proceedings of the Sixth International Congress of Tropical Medicine and Malaria, Vol. 3, pp. 158-166.
————— 1961. Observations on cross-immunity in experimental Chagas' disease in dogs. An. Congr. Internac. Doença de Chagas, 2:603-611.
————— 1966. Pathogenesis of blood protozoa. Soulsby, E. J. L., ed., In Biology of Parasites. New York, Academic Press, Inc., pp. 237-254.
————— and I. Singer. 1960. The reticuloendothelial system in experimental malaria and trypanosomiasis. Ann. N. Y. Acad. Sci., 88:149-171.
————— and J. L. Boyd, 1962. Reticulo-endothelial blockade in experimental Chagas' disease. J. Parasit., 48:223-228.
————— J. L. Boyd, M. Grimm-Wehner, and M. Konrath. 1964. Vaccination against experimental Chagas' disease with homogenates of culture forms of Trypanosoma cruzi. J. Parasit., 50 (Suppl.):19.
————— E. A. Konopka, and J. L. Boyd. 1964. Tetracyclines in experimental Chagas' disease (unpublished). Presented at the 13th Annual Meeting Amer. Soc. Trop. Med. Hyg., New York, N.Y., 1964.
Goes, P. de. 1947. Estudos sôbre a imunidade cruzada. Thesis. Fac. Nac. Farmácia, Rio de Janeiro, 352 pp.
————— and M. Bruno Lobo. 1950. Sôbre o comportamento do anticorpo heterologo ocorrente na doença de Chagas. Arq. Brasil. Med., 40:307-318.
————— and M. Bruno Lobo. 1951. Sôbre o comportamento do anticorpo heterólogo ocorrente na doença de Chagas. An. Microbiol., Rio de Janeiro, 1:69-77.
Goldman, M. 1957. Staining Toxoplasma gondii fluorescein-labeled antibody. J. Exp. Med., 105:557-573.
Gomes, L. Salles. 1939. (teste Romaña, C. and M. Conejos, 1946).
Gonzalez-Angelo, W., and R. E. Ryckman. 1967. Epizootiology of Trypanosoma cruzi in southwestern North America. IX. An investigation to determine the incidence of Trypanosoma cruzi infections in triatominae and men on the Yucatan peninsula of Mexico. J. Med. Entom., 4:44-47.
Gonzalez-Cappa, S. M., G. A. Schmuñis, O. C. Traversa, J. F. Yanovsky, M. E. Etcheverry, and H. J. Garavelli. 1966. Nueva tecnica para la preparación de antigenos del Tripanosoma cruzi. I. Efecto de la presion sobre el antigeno fijador del complemento. Rev. Soc. Argent. Biol., 42:78-84.
————— A. S. Parodi, G. Schmuñis, O. Traversa, and J. F. Yanovsky. 1967a. Efectos de la presion sobre el valor de los antigenos de Trypanosoma cruzi. 1967. Primer Congreso Latinoamericano de Parasitologia, Santiago de Chile, Resumenes, p. 37.
————— A. S. Parodi, G. Schmuñis, O. Traversa, and J. F. Yanovsky. 1967b. Vacunación para la enfermedad de Chagas experimental en el ratón. Primer Congreso Latinoamericano de Parasitologia, Santiago de Chile, Resumenes, pp. 35-36.
Gonçalves, J. Moura, and T. Yamaha. 1959. Immunopolissacarideo de Trypanosoma cruzi. Resumos Congreso Internacional sobre la Enfermedad de Chagas, pp. 71-72.
Gotta, H. 1946. Enfermedad de Chagas. Medicina (Buenos Aires), 6:627-642.
Graña, A. 1944. Anticuerpos heterofilos. Clinica e inmunologia. Buenos Aires, Espasa-Calpe Argentina S.A., 106pp.
Groenroos, P., and A. Salminen. 1955. Studies on Toxoplasma and the serology of toxoplasmosis. Ann. Med. Exp. Biol. Fenn., 33 (Suppl. 2):1-113.
Gruhzit, D. M., and R. A. Fisken. 1948. Failure of Trypanosoma cruzi lysate in treatment of Brown-Pierce carcinoma of rabbit. Fed. Proc., 7:271.
Guerreiro, C., and A. Machado. 1913. Da reação de Bordet e Gengou na moléstia de Carlos Chagas como elemento diagnóstico. Brasil-Med., 27:225-226.
Guzman, A. F., W. C. Leiva, and R. B. Monreal. 1952. Caso agudo mortal de enfermedad de Chagas en un lactante. Bol. Inform. Parasit. Chile., 7:28.
Haddad, N. 1967. Inquérito epidemiológico sôbre moléstia de Chagas e sífilis em um bairro de Ribeirão Prêto. Rev. Inst. Med. Trop. S. Paulo, 9:333-342.

Halberg, F., O. Hamerston, and J. J. Bittner. 1957. Sex difference in eosinophil counts in tail blood of mature B₁ mice. Science, 125:73.

Hartveit, F. 1966. Peritoneal exudate formation in C₃H mice and in mice of an unrelated closed colony. Acta Path. Microbiol. Scand., 68:194-196.

Hassko, A. 1931. Experimentelle Untersuchungen über Misch- und Sekundarinfektion. II. Zbl. Bakt. [Orig.], 123:140-150.

Hauschka, T. S. 1947a. Sex of host as a factor in Chagas' disease. J. Parasit., 33:399-404.

———— 1947b. Protozoa and cancer. In Approaches to Tumor Chemotherapy. Moulton, F. R., ed. Washington, D. C., American Association for the Advancement of Science, pp. 250-257.

———— 1949. Persistence of strain specific behavior in two strains of Trypanosoma cruzi after prolonged transfer through inbred mice. J. Parasit.. 35:593-599.

———— L. H. Saxe, and M. Blair. 1947. Trypanosoma cruzi in the treatment of mouse tumors. J. Nat. Cancer Inst., 7:189-197.

———— and M. B. Goodwin. 1948. Trypanosoma cruzi endotoxin (KR) in treatment of malignant mouse tumors. Science, 107:600-607.

———— M. B. Goodwin, J. Palmquist, and E. Brown. 1950. Immunological relationship between seven strains of Trypanosoma cruzi and its application in the diagnosis of Chagas' disease. Amer. J. Trop. Med., 30:1-16.

Hewitt, R. I., A. R. Gumble, W. S. Wallace, and J. H. Williams. 1954. Experimental chemotherapy of trypanosomiasis. IV. Reversal by purines of the in vivo activity of puromycin, and an amino nucleoside analog, against Trypanosoma equiperdum. Antibiotics and Chemotherapy, 4:1222-1227.

———— A. R. Gumble, W. S. Wallace, and J. H. Williams. 1955. Experimental chemotherapy of trypanosomiasis. V. Effects of puromycin analogues against Trypanosoma equiperdum in mice. Antibiotics and Chemotherapy, 5:139-144.

———— J. Entwistle, and E. Gill. 1963. Quantitative determinations of critical mortality periods in untreated and treated infections with the B strain of Trypanosoma cruzi in mice. J. Parasit., 49:22-30.

Hoare, A., 1963. Does Chagas' disease exist in Asia? J. Trop. Med. Hyg., 66:297-299.

———— 1966. The classification of mammalian trypanosomes. Ergebn. Mikrobiol. Immunitätsforsch. Exp. Therap., 39:43-57.

Howard, J. E. 1962. La enfermedad de Chagas congenita. Thesis. Universidad de Chile.

———— J. Martner, and M. Rubio. 1962. Estudio de las proteinas sanguineas en 10 niños con enfermedad de Chagas en diferentes periodos de evolución. Comunicación preliminar. Bol. Chile. Parasit., 17:36-39.

Ipsen, J. 1959. Differences in primary and secondary immunizability of inbred mice strains. Immunology, 83:448-457.

Iriarte, D. R. 1941. Xenodiagnostico y reacción de Machado-Guerreiro en la enfermedad de Chagas. Bol. Lab. Clin. Luis Razetti, 2:102-107.

Jacobs, L. 1956. Discussion of paper no. 395. International Congress of Pediatrics, Copenhagen.

———— and M. N. Lunde. 1957. A hemagglutination test for toxoplasmosis. J. Parasit., 43:308,

Jaffe, R. 1946. Myocarditis chronica als selbstandiges Krankheitsbild. Cardiologia, 10:402-412.

———— and E. Holz. 1948. Experimental allergic myocarditis. Exp. Med. Surg., 6:189-202.

———— and C. Kozma. 1960. Über die Myocarditis venezolana und die Bedeutung autoallergischer Prozesse fur ihre Pathogenese. Jubilee Volume, 100th Anniversary of the Rudolf Virchow Medical Society, pp. 199-218.

———— A. Dominguez, C. Kozma, and B. von Gavaller. 1961. Bemerkungen zur Pathogenese der Chagas Krankheit. Z. Tropenmed. Parasit., 21:137-146.

Jarpa, A., R. Christen, M. Agosin, and T. Pizzi. 1949. Ensayos de quimioterapia en enfermedad de Chagas experimental I. Aureomicina. Bol. Inform. Parasit. Chile., 4:49-51.

———— M. Agosin, R. Christen, and A. V. Atias. 1951. Ensayos de quimioterapia de la enfermedad de Chagas experimental. VII. Cortisona y fosfato de Pentaquina. Bol. Inform. Parasit. Chile., 6:25-27.

Jatene, A. D., and R. Jacomo. 1959. Doença de Chagas e transfusão de sangue. Rev. Goiana Med., 5:23-30.

Jedeloo, G. C., G. O. E. Lignac, A. J. Ligtenberg, and P. H. van Thiel. 1949. Onderzock naar de biotherapeutische werking van *Trypanosoma cruzi* op munizentcerkanker. Nederl. T. Geneesk., 93:3147-3153.

———— G. O. E. Lignac, A. J. Ligtenberg, and P. H. van Thiel. 1950. Biotherapeutic action of *Trypanosoma cruzi* on tar carcinoma in mice. J. Nat. Cancer Inst., 10:809-813.

Johnson, C. M., and R. A. Kelser. 1937. The incidence of Chagas' disease in Panama as determined by the complement fixation test. Amer. J. Trop. Med., 17:385-392.

Johnson, P., R. A. Neal, and D. Gall. 1963. Protective effect of killed trypanosome vaccines with incorporated adjuvants. Nature (London), 200:83-84.

Jörg, M. E. 1964. Imposibilidad de demostrar toxinas en *Trypanosoma cruzi* de cultivos. Bol. Chile. Parasit., 19:84-87.

Kagan, I. G., and L. Norman. 1960. Immunologic studies of *Trypanosoma cruzi*. I. Susceptibility of CFW stock mice for the "Tulahuén" strain of *T. cruzi*. J. Infect. Dis., 107:165-167.

———— and L. Norman. 1961. Immunologic studies of *Trypanosoma cruzi*. III. Duration of acquired immunity in mice initially infected with a North American strain of *T. cruzi*. J. Infect. Dis., 108:213-217.

Kelser, R. A. 1936. A complement fixation test for Chagas' disease employing an artificial culture antigen. Amer. J. Trop. Med., 16:405-415.

Kent, J. F., S. C. Bukantz, and C. R. Rein. 1946. Studies in complement-fixation. I. Spectrophotometric titration of complement; construction of graphs for direct determination of the 50 per cent hemolytic unit. J. Immun., 53:37-50.

Klyueva, N. G. 1947. Paths of cancer biotherapy. Amer. Rev. Soviet Med., 4:408-414.

———— and G. Roskin. 1946. Cancerolytic substance of *Schizotrypanum cruzi*. Amer. Rev. Soviet. Med., 4:127-129.

———— and G. Roskin. 1957. Le problème des antibiotiques anticancereux. Moscow, 247pp.

Knierim, F., 1954. Estudio serologico en animales experimentalmente infectados por *Trypanosoma cruzi*. Bol. Chile. Parasit., 9:2-6.

———— 1958. Tecnica de la reacción de fijación del complemento segun el metodo del 50% de hemolise de Bozicevich aplicada al diagnostico de la enfermedad de Chagas. Bol. Chile. Parasit., 13:75-78.

———— 1959. Resultados obtenidos con la reacción de fijación del complemento segun el 50% de hemolisis en el diagnostico de la enfermedad de Chagas. Bol. Chile. Parasit., 14:5-6.

———— and P. Saavedra. 1966. Technica de la reacción de hemaglutinación aplicada al diagnostico serologico de las parasitoses. Bol. Chile. Parasit., 21:29-44.

Knop, K., G. Hoecker, D. Brncic, and G. Gasic. 1949. Acción del *Trypanosoma cruzi* sobre tumores transplantados del ratón. Bol. Chile. Parasit., 4:5-6.

Köberle, F. 1956. Über das Neurotoxin des *Trypanosoma cruzi*. Zbl. Allg. Path., 95:458-475.

———— 1957. Patogenia da molestia de Chagas; estudo dos orgãos musculares ocos. Rev. Goiana Med., 3:155-180.

———— 1958. Cardiopathia chagasica. An. Brasil. Ginecol., 53:311-346.

———— 1959. Die Chagaskrankheit—ihre Pathogenese und ihre Bedeutung als Volksseuche. Z. Tropenmed. Parasit., 3:236-268.

Kofoid, C. A., and F. Donat. 1933. The experimental transfer of *Trypanosoma cruzi* from naturally infected *Triatoma protracta* to mammals in California. Bull. Soc. Path. Exot., 26:257-259.

Kolodny, M. 1939a. Studies on age resistance against trypanosome infections. I. The resistance of rats of different ages to infection with *Trypanosoma cruzi*. Amer. J. Hyg., 29c:13-24.

———— 1939b. Seasonal variations in the intensity of experimental infection with *Trypanosoma cruzi* in young rats. Amer. J. Hyg., 29c:131-133.

———— 1939c. Studies on age resistance against trypanosome infections. V. The influence of the age of the rat upon experimental infection with *Trypanosoma cruzi* per os. Amer. J. Hyg., 29c:155-161.

———— 1940a. Studies on age resistance against trypanosomose infections. VII. The influence of age upon the immunological response of rats to infection with *Trypanosoma cruzi*. Amer. J. Hyg., 31c:1-8.

———— 1940b. The effect of environmental temperature upon experimental trypanosomiasis (*T. cruzi* of rats). Amer. J. Hyg., 32c:21-23.

Konopka, E. A., F. C. Goble, and J. S. Donovan. 1965. Sex of host as a factor in chemotherapy of protozoal infections. Abstracts, Fifth Interscience Conference on Antimicrobial Agents and Chemotherapy, Fourth International Congress of Chemotherapy. Washington, D. C., p. 122.

―――― F. C. Goble, and J. S. Donovan. 1966. Sex of host as a factor in protozoal chemotherapy. Abstracts, Third International Pharmacological Congress, São Paulo, Brasil, pp. 212-213.

Kozma, C. 1962. Über den Nachweis spezifischer Herz-Autoantikörper bei der Chagas-Myokarditis. Z. Tropenmed. Parasit., 13:175-180.

Krampitz, H. E., and R. Disko. 1966. Retardation of parasitemia, prolongation of life or survival of lactating mice in infections with Trypanosoma cruzi. Nature (London), 209:526.

Krause, W. S. 1964. Symposium über das Problem: Kruzin als Krebtherapeutikum. Arch. Geschwulstforsch., 24:51-52.

Kritchewski, I. L., and L. Schwartzmann. 1928. Die Bedeutung des retikulo-endothelialen Apparatus bei Infektionskrankheiten. Z. Immunitätsforsch., 56:322-329.

Lacorte, J. G. 1926. A reação de desvio de complemento na moléstia de Chagas. Thesis. Tip. do Inst. Oswaldo Cruz, 49pp.

―――― 1927. A reação de desvio de complemento na moléstia de Chagas. Mem. Inst. Oswaldo Cruz, 20:197-224.

―――― 1942. A reação de fixação do complemento aplicado à moléstia de Chagas (reação de Machado ou Machado Guerreiro). Acta Med., 10:87-94.

Lacaz, P. S., J. Salum, C. Borges, A. Rassi, and J. M. Rezende. 1957. Electroforese das proteínas séricas na fase aguda da doença de Chagas. Estudo de 10 casos. Simpósio sôbre doença de Chagas. Fac. Nac. Med. Univ. Brasil.

Lainson, R. 1965. Parasitological studies in British Honduras. I. A parasite resembling Trypanosoma (Schizotrypanum) cruzi in the coati, (Carnivora, Procyonidae), and a note on Trypanosoma legeri from the ant-eater Tamandua tetradactyla (Edentata). Ann. Trop. Med. Parasit., 59:37-42.

Landy, M. 1962. Bacterial endotoxins. Texas Rep. Biol. Med., 20:1-11.

Larrain, P., Jr. 1956. Enfermedad de Chagas en el departamento de San Martin. Rev. Sanid. Polic., 25:256-261.

Lausi, L. 1965. Encuesta sobre enfermedad de Chagas-Mazza en escolares de Villa Soldati, Buenos Aires, Argentina. Rev. Asoc. Med. Argent., 79:123-127.

Lawford, D. J., and R. G. White. 1964. Abnormal serum components after Escherichia coli endotoxin administration to male and female rats. Nature (London), 201:705-706.

Leão, A. E. de Area. 1923. Do diagnóstico das trypanosomoses pela reação de desvio do complemento. Cienc. Med., 1:126-134.

Lennox, E. S. 1966. The genetics of the immune response. Proc. Roy. Soc. (Biol.), 166:222-231.

Liem, S. D. 1938. Onderzoeckingen over Triatoma infestans als overbrenger van de pathogene organismen en over de complement bindingreactie bij de zeikte van Chagas. Thesis, University of Leiden. Trop. Dis. Bull., 35:719-720.

―――― and P. H. Van Thiel. 1940-1941. The complement fixation test for Chagas' disease employing a dried culture antigen. Acta Leiden. Schol. Med. Trop., 15-16:259-274.

Lob, M. 1949. L'action de Trypanosoma cruzi sur le cancer expérimental de la souris. Schweiz. Med. Wschr., 79:554-556.

―――― 1950. L'action du Schizotrypanum cruzi sur l'adenocarcinome provoqué de la mamelle chez la souris. Schweiz. Z. Allg. Path. Bakt., 13:279-296.

Lobo, L. C. Calvao, and M. M. da Silva. 1962. Técnica simplificada de reação de Guerreiro e Machado para o diagnóstico da doença de Chagas. Hospital (Rio de Janeiro), 61:751-758.

―――― J. Friedman, D. Rosenthal, R. Ulysses, and S. Franco. 1962. Interrelationship of endemic goiter and Chagas' disease. J. Clin. Endocr., 22:1182-1186.

Lopes, E. R., E. Chapadeiro, J. H. M. Furtado, W. Hial, J. R. M. Cintra, E. L. Pereira, and A. Compos Netto. 1966. Reação de Guerreiro e Machado no líquido pericárdico de portadores da cardite Chagásica crônica. Rev. Inst. Med. Trop. S. Paulo, 8:60-61.

Lopez Fernandez, J. R., and M. E. Franca Rodriguez. 1954. Las modificaciónes cinetomorfologicas de las formas sanguicolas de Trypanosoma cruzi, "in vitro" (adherencia de los tripanosomas, transformacion leishmanioide e inmovilizacion) y su aplicación para el diagnostico de la enfermedad de Chagas. (nota previa) An. Fac. Med. Univ. Repub., Montevideo, 39:233-240.

Lucena, D. T., de. 1957. Reação de Guerreiro-Machado em cães do município de Timbauba. Rev. Brasil. Malar., 9:447-450.

———— 1958. A doença de Chagas em Pernambuco, Brasil. Rev. Brasil. Malar., 10:405-416.

———— 1959. Epidemiologia da doença de Chagas em Pernambuco. A reação de Guerreiro-Machado na determinação do nível endêmico. Rev. Brasil. Med., 16:864-866.

———— and L. Costa. 1957. Inquérito sorológico sôbre a doença de Chagas na Paraíba. Rev. Brasil. Med., 14:325-327.

———— and O. T. de Lima. 1962. Epidemiologia da doença de Chagas no Rio Grande do Norte. III. A. infecção humana determinada pela reação de Guerreiro-Machado. Rev. Brasil. Malar., 14:361-366.

———— D. Da Rosa, and J. N. Calheiros. 1961. Epidemiologia da doença de Chagas em Alagoas. II. A endemicidade avaliada pela reação de Guerreiro-Machado. Rev. Brasil. Med., 18:258-261.

Lwoff, M. 1938. L'hematine et l'acide ascorbique, facteur de croissance pour le flagelle Schizotrypanum cruzi. C. R. Acad. Sci. [D] (Paris), 206:540-542.

Maekelt, G. A. 1959. Contribución para el estudio de la enfermedad de Chagas en Venzuela. Investigaciones serologicas de la enfermedad de Chagas mediante la reacción de fijación del complemento. Arch. Venez. Patol. Trop. Parasit. Med., 3:252-271.

———— 1960. Die Komplementbindungsreaktion der Changaskrankheit. Z. Tropenmed. Parasit., 2:152-186.

———— 1961. Encuesta serologica-estadistica sobre la prevalencia de la infección chagasica en el Hospital Vargas. Arch. Hosp. Vargas, Caracas, 3:381-391.

———— 1962. Fracciones antigenicas del Schizotrypanum cruzi como fijador del complemento. Arch. Venez. Med. Trop. Parasit. Med., 4:213-242.

———— 1963. Diagnostico de laboratorio de las trypanosomiasis Americanas. Proceedings of the Seventh International Congress of Tropical Medicine and Malaria (Rio de Janeiro), Vol. 2, pp. 227-228.

———— 1964. Diagnostico de laboratorio de las tripanosomiasis Americanas. Rev. Venez. Sanid. Asist. Soc., 29:1-18.

———— and M. P. Alcaniz. 1960. Estudio seriologico sobre la incidencia de la infección Chagasica en pacientes no seleccionados del hospital Vargas. Arch. Hosp. Vargas, Caracas, 2:249-259.

———— and C. Colmenares de Alayon. 1960. Metodo sencillo para el envio de sueros Chagasicos desde la zonas rurales. Arch. Venez. Med. Trop. Parasit. Med., 3:133-142.

———— and Z. Gomez. 1962. Primeras experiencias co la prueba de Sabin-Feldman para el diagnostico de la toxoplasmosis. Arch. Venez. Med. Trop. Parasit. Med., 4:265-275.

Malisoff, W. M. 1947. The action of the endotoxin of Trypanosoma cruzi (KR) on malignant mouse tumors. Science, 106:591-594.

Manso Soto, A. E., and J. de Rosa. 1951. Enfermedad de Chagas en la ciudad de Rosario. Misión de Estudios de Patologia Regional Argentina, 22:9-12.

———— and J. A. Rispoli. 1952. Enfermedad de Chagas en Mendoza. Su importancia como problema sanitario. Misión de Estudios de Patologia Regional Argentina, 81-82:13-19.

———— and G. A. Loretti. 1953. Enfermedad de Chagas y brucelosis. Misión de Estudios de Patologia Regional Argentina, 24:9-12.

———— G. A. Loretti, and J. A. Rispoli. 1950. Diagnostico de enfermedad de Chagas reacción de fijación del complemento. Misión de Estudios de Patologia Regional Argentina, 21:5-35.

———— G. A. Loretti, and J. A. Rispoli. 1951. La enfermedad de Chagas en la Capital Federal. Reacción de fijación de complemento. Misión de Estudios de Patologia Regional Argentina, 22:5-11.

Marcuse, M., R. Wigand, and M. Piroth. 1964. Über die Resistenz von Mäusen gegenüber Trypanosoma cruzi. Z. Tropenmed. Parasit., 15:279-288.

Marinkelle, C. J. 1966. Observations on human, monkey and bat trypanosomes and their vectors in Colombia. Trans. Roy. Soc. Trop. Med. Hyg., 60:109-116.

Marques da Cunha, A., and E. Dias. 1939. Reação de fixado do complemento nas leishmanioses. Brasil-Med., 53:89-92.

Marr, J. S., and H. Pike. 1967. The protection of mice by "Corpus Christi" strain of Trypanosoma cruzi when challenged with "Brasil" strain. J. Parasit., 53:657-659.

Marsden, P. D. 1968. Infectivity of white mice of a Peru strain of *Trypanosoma cruzi* obtained from two sources: bug faeces and mouse blood. Trans. Roy. Soc. Trop. Med. Hyg., 62:139.

Mas Bakal, P. 1962. The specificity of Sabin and Feldman's dye test in the diagnosis of toxoplasmosis. Trop. Geogr. Med., 14:56-66.

Mayer, M., and H. da Rocha-Lima. 1912. Zur Entwicklung von *Schizotrypanum cruzi* in Säugetieren. Arch. Schiffs. Tropen. Hyg., 16:90-94.

——— and H. da Rocha-Lima. 1914. Zum Verhalten vom *Schizotrypanum cruzi* in Warmblutern und Artropoden. Arch. Schiffs. Tropen. Hyg., 18:101-136.

——— and C. F. Pifano. 1941a. Neuvos metodos para el diagnostico de la enfermedad de Chagas. Rev. Venez. Sanid. Asist. Soc., 6:311-316.

——— and C. F. Pifano. 1941b. O diagnóstico da moléstia de Chagas por intradermo-reação com cultivo de *Schizotrypanum cruzi*. Brasil-Med., 55:317-319.

Mazza, S. 1938. Metodos diagnosticos de la enfermedad de Chagas. Valor y oportunidad de cada uno. Actas y Trabajos, Sexto Congreso Nacional de Medicina, Cordoba, 3:155.

——— 1940. Otros mamiferos infectados naturalmente por *Schizotrypanum cruzi*, o cruzi similes en provincias de Jujuy y Salta. Misión de Estudios de Patologia Regional Argentina, 45:119-134.

——— and M. E. Jörg. 1935a. Consideraciones sobre la patogenia de la enfermedad de Chagas. (Los periodos anatomo-clinicos de la tripanosomiasis.) Novena Reunion Sociedad Argentina de Patologia Regional, 1:221-231.

——— and M. E. Jörg. 1935b. Infección natural mortal por *S. cruzi* en cachorro de Perro "Pila" de Jujuy. Novena Reunion Sociedad Argentina de Patologia Regional, 1:365-411.

——— and M. E. Jörg. 1939. Diferencias entre anatomia patologica de carditis de enfermedad de Chagas. Misión de Estudios de Patologia Regional Argentina, 42:74-97.

——— G. Basso, R. Basso, M. E. Jörg, and S. Miyara. 1943. Investigaciones sobre enfermedad de Chagas. Naturaleza histopatologica de reacciones alergicas cutaneas provocadas en chagasicos con lisados de cultivos de *S. cruzi*. Misión de Estudios de Patologia Regional Argentina, 64:3-143.

Mazzotti, L. 1940a. Effects of inoculating small and large numbers of *Trypanosoma cruzi* in mice. Amer. J. Hyg., 31(c):86.

——— 1940b. Variations in virulence for mice and guinea pigs in strains of *Trypanosoma cruzi* Chagas from different species of bugs (Triatomidae) from different localities in Mexico. Amer. J. Hyg., 31(c):67.

Mellone, O., and J. Pagenotto. 1965. Incidência de sorologia positiva para sífilis e doença de Chagas em 62.575 doadores de sangue. Rev. Hosp. Clin. Fac. Med. Univ. S. Paulo, 20:165-167.

Menezes, H. 1965. O emprêgo de adjuvantes na vacinação de camundongos com *Trypanosoma cruzi* II. Rev. Brasil. Med., 22:536-538.

——— 1968. Protective effect of an avirulent (cultivated) strain of *Trypanosoma cruzi* against experimental infection in mice. Rev. Inst. Med. Trop. S. Paulo, 10:1-4.

Menolasino, N. J., and E. Hartman. 1954. Immunology and serology of some parasitic protozoan flagellates. II. The hemoflagellate protozoa, *Leishmania donovani* and *Trypanosoma cruzi*. J. Protozool., 1:111-113.

Meyer, H., and M. X. De Oliveira. 1948. Cultivation of *Trypanosoma cruzi* in tissue culture: A 4-year study. J. Parasit., 39:91.

Minning, W. 1935. Zur Spezifität der Komplement-Bindungs-Reaktion bei der amerikanischen Trypanosomiasis (Chagas-Krankheit). Arch. Schiffs. Tropen. Hyg., 39:315-328.

Minoprio, J. L., M. Pirinoli, R. S. Perez, and E. Lemos. 1962. La electroforesis en la enfermedad de Chagas aguda. An. Congr. Internac. Doença de Chagas, 2:899-910.

Miyara, S. 1936. Enfermos con reacción de Machado positiva determinados en la provincia de San Luis. Novena Reunion Sociedad Argentina de Patologia Regional, 1:422-438.

Montalvan, C. J. A. 1950. Algunas consideraciones sobre el problema de la enfermedad de Chagas en el Ecuador. Rev. Ecuator. Hig. Med. Trop., 7:1-6.

Montano, G., and H. Ucros. 1965. Comparación entre las reacciones de hemaglutinación y fijación del complemento en el diagnostico serologico de la enfermedad de Chagas. Bol. Chile. Parasit., 20:62-67.

Montenegro, J. 1926. Cutaneous reaction in leishmaniasis. Arch. Derm. Syph., 13:187-194.

Moore, D. V. 1957. Antigenic relationships of certain hemoflagellates as determined by the Ouchterlony gel diffusion technique. J. Parasit., 43(Suppl.):16.

Mora-Marques, R. 1964. Estudio epidemiologico sobre la infección chagasica en miembros de las Fuerzas Armadas de Venezuela. Aspecto serologico. Rev. Venez. Sanid. Asist. Soc., 29:457-464.

———— I. Arape Crespo, and G. A. Maekelt. 1960. Estudio sobre la incidencia de la infección chagasica entre los donantes de sangre de las Fuerzas Armadas de Venezuela. Arch. Venez. Med. Trop. Parasit. Med., 3:125-131.

Morales, A., A. Mosca, S. Silva, A. Sims, E. Thiermann, F. Knierim, and A. Atias. 1961. Estudio serologico sobre toxoplasmosis y otras parasitosis en Isla de Pascua. Bol. Chile. Parasit., 16:82-87.

Mounier-Kuhn, P., J. Gaillard, J. Fontvielle, and L. Gaillard. 1961. Utilizzazione di estratti di Trypanosoma cruzi nel trattamento di alcune neoplasie di competenza ORL. Minerva Med., 52:2254-2257.

Muniz, J. 1930. Del uso del antigeno Watson (Trypanosoma equiperdum) en la reacción de desviación del complemento en la enfermedad de Chagas. Sociedad Argentina Patologia Regional Norte, Quinta Reunion, 2:897-901.

———— 1947. Do valor da reação de precipitina no diagnóstico das formas agudas e subagudas de "Doença de Chagas" ("Trypanosomiasis Americana"). Brasil-Med., 61:261-267.

———— 1949. Action of red cells sensitized with the polysaccharide fraction of the Schizotrypanum cruzi in the presence of specific sera. Conditioned hemolysis as a phenomenon of a more general character. Secção do Rio de Janeiro da "Society of American Bacteriologists, Newsletter" (1 Jan.), p. 9.

———— 1950a. A hemolise condicionada como um fenomeno de ordem mais geral. Quinto Congresso Internacional Microbiologia, Abstracts, pp. 144-145.

———— 1950b. Comportamento de hematias sensibilizadas com a fração polissacarídea do Schizotrypanum cruzi quando em presença de soros específicos. "Hemolise condicionada", um caso particular dentro das reações de imunidade. Hospital (Rio de Janeiro), 37:199-205.

———— 1950c. On the value of "conditioned hemolysis" for the diagnosis of American Trypanosomiasis. A comparative study with complement fixation and sensitized erythrocytes agglutination tests. Hospital (Rio de Janeiro), 38:685-691.

———— and G. de Freitas. 1944a. Contribuição para o diagnóstico da doença de Chagas pelas reações de imunidade. I. Estudo comparativo entre as reações de aglutinação e de fixação do complemento. Mem. Inst. Oswaldo Cruz., 41:303-333.

———— and G. de Freitas. 1944b. Contribuição para o diagnóstico da doença de Chagas pelas reações de imunidade. II. Isolamento de polisacarídeos de Schizotrypanum cruzi e de outros tripanosomídeos, seu comportamento nas reações de precipitação de fixação de complemento e de hiper-sensibilidade. Os testes de floculação (sublimado e formol-gel). Rev. Brasil. Biol., 4:421-438.

———— and A. Boriello. 1945. Estudo sôbre a ação lítica de diferentes soros sôbre as formas de cultura e sanguícolas do Schizotrypanum cruzi. Rev. Brasil. Biol., 5:563-576.

———— and G. de Freitas. 1946. Estudos sôbre a imunidade humoral na doença de Chagas. Brasil-Med., 60:337-341.

———— and A. P. de Azevedo. 1947. Novo conceito da patogenia da doença de Chagas (Trypanosomiasis americana). Hospital (Rio de Janeiro), 32:165-183.

———— and M. C. F. dos Santos. 1950a. Anticorpos heterófilos na trypanosomiasis Americana. Quinto Congresso Internacional Microbiologia, Resumo dos Trabalhos, pp. 142-143.

———— and M. C. F. dos Santos. 1950. Heterophile antibodies in American trypanosomiasis. The presence of heterogenetic component(s) in the antigenic structure of the Schizotrypanum cruzi shown by "conditioned hemolysis" reaction. Hospital (Rio de Janeiro), 38:601-616.

———— and M. C. F. dos Santos. 1950c. Technic of "conditioned hemolysis" applied in the diagnosis of American trypanosomiasis. Hospital (Rio de Janeiro), 38:617-620.

———— and J. A. C. Moraes. 1962. Das reações de imunidade no diagnóstico da doença de Chagas. Rev. Inst. Med. Trop. S. Paulo, 4:112-118.

————— G. Nobrega, and M. da Cunha. 1946. Ensaios de vacinação preventiva e curativa nas infecções pelo *Schizotrypanum cruzi*. Mem. Inst. Oswaldo Cruz, 44:529-541.

Musacchio, M. de Oliveira, and H. Meyer. 1962. Ação do *Schizotrypanum cruzi*, degenerado ou em suspensão de Tripanosomas mortos, sôbre células nervosas em culturas de tecido de embrião de galinha. An. Congr. Internac. Doença de Chagas, 2:1065-1068.

Naquira, F., and N. Naquira. 1955. Contribución al estudio de la enfermedad de Chagas. Encuesta epidemiologica en el sur del Peru. (Provincia de Tarata, Departamento de Tacna). Bol. Chile. Parasit., 10:29-31.

————— and N. Naquira. 1957. Contribución al estudio de la enfermedad de Chagas. II. Nuevas invesigaciones epidemiologicas en el sur del Peru. Bol. Chile. Parasit., 12:46-50.

————— and A. Neghme. 1957. Contribución al estudio de la enfermedad de Chagas. III. Encuesta epidemiologica en algunas localidades del Departamento de Arica (Provincia de Tarapaca, Chile). Bol. Chile. Parasit., 12:22-23.

Nattan-Larrier, L. 1921. Infections à trypanosomes et voies de pénétration des virus. Bull. Soc. Path. Exot., 14:537-542.

Navarrete, F., and F. Biagi. 1960. Leishmaniasis cutanea. Espicificidad de la reacción intradermica de Montenegro. Prensa Med. Mex., 25:2-3.

Neal, R. A., and R. A. Miles. 1968. An indirect haemagglutination test for *Trypanosoma cruzi* (Chagas' disease). Trans. Roy. Soc. Trop. Med. Hyg., 62:7.

Neghme, A., and J. Roman. 1948. Present state of Chagas' disease surveys in Chile. Amer. J. Trop. Med., 28:835-839.

————— and H. Schenone. 1960. Resumen de veinte anos de investigación sobre la enfermedad de Chagas de Chile. Rev. Med. Chile., 88:82-93.

————— and F. H. Schenone. 1962. Enfermedad de Chagas en Chile. Veinte anos de investigacion. An. Congr. Intnac. Doença de Chagas, 3:1069-1105.

————— J. Roman, and R. Sotomayor. 1949. Nuevos datos sobre la enfermedad de Chagas en Chile. Bol. Ofic. Sanit. Panamer., 28:808-816.

————— M. Agosin, R. Christen, A. Jarpa, and A. V. Atias. 1951. Ensayos de quimioterapia de la enfermedad de Chagas experimental. VIII. Acción de cortisona sola y asociada al fosfato de pentaquina o al compuesto de sulfato de quinina-fosfato de penaquina. Estudio histopathologico (Resumen). Bol. Inform. Parasit. Chile. 6:36.

————— O. Badinez, A. Jarpa, E. Thiermann, M. Agosin, and R. Christen. 1952. Acción de la cortisona sobre la trypanosomosis chagasica experimental del ratón suprarreno-privo y total. (Comunicación preliminar). Bol. Inform. Parasit. Chile., 7:4-6.

Nelson, R. A., and M. M. Mayer. 1949. Immobilization of *Treponema pallidum in vitro* by antibody produced in syphilitic infection. J. Exp. Med., 89:369-393.

Nieschulz, O., and F. K. Wawo Roentoe. 1930. Über den Einfluss der Milz-extirpation bei Infektionen mit *Trypanosoma gambiense* und *Schizotrypanum cruzi*. Z. Immunitätsforschung., 65:312-317.

Niimi, S. 1935. Studies on experimental Chagas' disease. Jap. J. Exp. Med., 13:543-564.

Niño, F. 1925. Ensayos de infección experimental del *Bufo marinus* (sapo) con *Schizotrypanum cruzi*. Prensa Med. Argent., 11:1154.

Norman, L., and I. G. Kagan. 1960a. Studies on the immunology of experimental Chagas' disease. J. Parasit., 46 (suppl.):44.

————— and I. G. Kagan. 1960b. Immunologic studies on *Trypanosoma cruzi*. II. Acquired immunity in mice infected with avirulent American strains of *T. cruzi*. J. Infect. Dis., 107:168-174.

Nussenzweig, V. 1963. Immunological types of *Trypanosoma cruzi*. Abstracts, Seventh International Congress of Tropical Medicine and Malaria (Rio de Janeiro), p. 131.

————— and R. Faria. 1955. Prova da antiglobulina no diagnostico da doença de Chagas na fase cronica. Hospital (Rio de Janeiro), 47:81-92.

————— and F. C. Goble. 1964. Further studies on the antigenic constitution of strains of *Trypanosoma (Schizotrypanum) cruzi*. J. Protozool., 11: (Suppl.):16.

————— and F. C. Goble. 1966. Further studies on the antigenic constitution of strains of *Trypanosoma (Schizotrypanum) cruzi*. Exp. Parasit., 18:224-230.

————— L. M. Deane, and J. Kloetzel. 1962. Diversidade na constituição antigênica de amostras de *Trypanosoma cruzi* isoladas do homeme de gambas. Rev. Inst. Trop. Med. S. Paulo, 4:409-410.

————— L. M. Deane, and J. Kloetzel. 1963a. Differences in antigenic constitution of strains of *Trypanosoma cruzi*. Exp. Parasit., 14:221-232.

—————— J. Kloetzel, and L. M. Deane. 1963b. Acquired immunity in mice infected with strains of immunological Types A and B of *Trypanosoma cruzi*. Exp. Parasit., 14:233-239.

Ofman, J. 1944. Contribuciones al estudio experimental de la enfermedad de Chagas. I. Acción de la esplenectomia y Vitamin C sobre la virulencia del *Trypanosoma cruzi* en el cuy. Thesis. Facultad de Medicina, Universidad de Chile.

Oliveira, F. da C., E. Chapadeiro, M. T. Alonso, E. R. Lopes, and F. E. L. Pereira. 1966. Doença de Chagas e gravidez. I. Incidência da tripanosomiase e abortamento espontaneo em gestantes chagásicas crônicas. Rev. Inst. Med. Trop. S. Paulo, 8:184-185.

Osimani, J. J. 1947a. Los antigenos en la reacción de fijación del complemento para el diagnostico de la enfermedad de Chagas. Arch. Soc. Biol. Montevideo, 14:19-27.

—————— 1947b. Tecnica usada en la reacción de fijación del complemento para el diagnostico de la enfermedad de Chagas. Arch. Soc. Biol. Montevideo, 14:28-35.

—————— 1947c. Resultados obtenidos co el uso de la fijacion del complemento en el diagnostico de la enfermedad de Chagas. Arch. Uruguay. Med. Cirug. Especial., 31:125-156.

Ouchterlony, O. 1949. Antigen-antibody reactions in gels. Acta Path. Microbiol. Scand., 26:507-515.

Oudin, J. 1966. The genetic control of immunoglobulin synthesis. Proc. Roy. Soc. (Biol.), 166:207-219.

Packchanian, A. 1935. Agglutination and precipitation tests for the diagnosis of *Trypanosoma cruzi* (Chagas disease). J. Immun., 29:84-85.

—————— 1940. Experimental production of agglutinins for *Trypanosoma cruzi*. Public Health Rep., 55:2116-2124.

—————— 1949. Precipitin test for the diagnosis of Chagas' disease with special reference to the specificity of polysaccharides. Fed. Proc., 8:408.

—————— 1950. Relative immunity of the American forest deer mouse, *Peromyscus leucopus noveboracensis*, against hyperinfection and reinoculations with *Trypanosoma brucei*. Amer. J. Trop. Med., 30:17-26.

—————— 1953. Chemotherapy of experimental Chagas' disease with thirty antibiotics. Amer. J. Trop. Med. Hyg., 2:243-253.

—————— and H. H. Sweets, Jr. 1947. Infectivity of *Trypanosoma cruzi* after cultivation for thirteen years in vitro without animal passage. Proc. Soc. Exp. Biol. Med., 64:169.

Passos, E. M. C. 1958. Moléstia de Chagas na clínica obstétrica. Thesis. Faculdade de Medicina, Universidade do Brasil.

Patto, J. Ortiz. 1931. Fixação do complemento no bócio endêmico. An. Fac. Med. Univ. Minas Gerais (Belo Horizonte), 1:95-103.

Pedreira de Freitas, J. L. 1947. Contribuição para o estudo do diagnóstico da moléstia de Chagas por processos de laboratório. Thesis. Faculdade de Medicina, Universidade de São Paulo, 160 pp.

—————— 1950. Observações sôbre a estabilidade de antigenos de culturas de *Trypanosoma cruzi* para reações de fixação do complemento. Hospital (Rio de Janeiro), 38:513-519.

—————— 1951. Reação de fixação de complemento para diagnóstico da moléstia de Chagas pela técnica quantitativa. Arq. Hig. Saúde Pública (S. Paulo), 16:55-94.

—————— 1952. O diagnóstico de laboratório da moléstia de Chagas. Rev. Clin. S. Paulo, 28:1-10.

—————— . 1958. Processos de laboratório para diagnóstico da moléstia de Chagas. Rev. Goiana Med., 4:135-147.

—————— 1963. Aspectos sorológicos na padronização dos métodos para avaliação dos efeitos da terapêutica na doença de Chagas. Rev. Inst. Med. Trop. S. Paulo, 5:207-215.

—————— and W. Mendonça. 1951. Inquérito sôbre moléstia de Chagas no muincípio de Rio Verde (Estado de Goiás). Hospital (Rio de Janeiro), 39:251-261.

—————— and C. Figueiredo, 1951. Resultados de investigações sorológica sôbre moléstia de Chagas realizadas no Estado de Goiás. Arq. Hig. Saúde Pública (S. Paulo), 16:277-230.

—————— and J. O. de Almeida. 1949. Nova técnica de fixação do complemento para moléstia de Chagas. (Reação quantitativa com antigeno gelificado de culturas de *Trypanosoma cruzi*.) Hospital (Rio de Janeiro), 35:787-800.

—————— U. F. Rocha, J. A. Z. Vasquez, and T. N. Aftimus. 1952a. Inquérito preliminar sôbre a infecção pelo *Trypanosoma cruzi* (Chagas, 1909) entre cães e gatos domésticos no município de Campo Florida (Triângulo Mineiro) Minas Gerais, Brasil. Rev. Fac. Med. Vet. Univ. S. Paulo, 4:545-551.

―――― A. Biancalana, V. Amato Neto, V. Nussenzweig, R. Sonntag, and J. G. Barreto. 1952b. Primeras verificações de transmissão acidental da moléstia de Chagas a homem por transfusão de sangue. Rev. Paulista Med., 40:36-40.

―――― and J. P. de Almeida. 1951. Inquérito sorológico sôbre moléstia de Chagas realizado no município de Echapora (Estado de São Paulo). Arq. Hig. Saúde Pública (S. Paulo), 16:231-236.

Pellegrino, J. 1946. A reação intradérmica com antigeno do *Schizotrypanum cruzi* na doença de Chagas experimental do cão. Rev. Brasil. Biol., 6:443-450.

―――― 1949. Trasmisão de doença de Chagas pela transfusão de sangue. Primeiras comprovações serológicas em doadores e em candidatos a doadores de sangue. Rev. Brasil. Med., 6:297-301.

―――― and M. Borrotchin. 1948. Inquerito sôbre a doença de Chagas no Hospital da Santa Casa de Belo Horizonte (Minas Gerais, Brasil). Mem. Inst. Oswaldo Cruz, 46:419-457.

―――― and Z. Brener. 1952. A reação de fixação do complemento na doença de Chagas. IV. Observações feitas em casos agudos de esquizotripanose. Hospital (Rio de Janeiro), 42:755-761.

―――― and Z. Brener. 1953. A reação de fixação do complemento com antigeno de formas de cultura do *Schizotrypanum cruzi* na doença de Chagas experimental no cão. Hospital (Rio de Janeiro), 43:481-483.

―――― and F. Nery Guimaraes. 1953. A reação intradérmica com antigeno de *Tr. rangeli* em pacientes com leishmaniose tegumentar ou com doença de Chagas. Sexto Congresso Internacional Microbiologia, Resumo dos Trabalhos 2, pp. 531-532.

―――― and C. L. de Rezende. 1953. Técnica para a reação de precipitina no diagnóstico da doença de Chagas com sangue colhido na polpa digital. Hospital (Rio de Janeiro), 51:895.

―――― J. M. Borrotchin, G. Leite, and Z. Brener. 1951. Inquérito sôbre a doença de Chagas em candidatos a doadores de sangue. Mem. Inst. Oswaldo Cruz, 49:555-564.

―――― C. L. Rezende, and A. Canelas. 1952. A doença de Chagas em crianças de idade escolar. II. Inquérito realizado em Varzea de Palma (Municipio de Pirapora, Minas Gerais). VI. Jornada Brasil. Pediat. Puericult., Belo Horizonte.

Peñalver, L. M., M. I. Rodriguez, and G. Sancho. 1957. Nuevos datos sobre trypanosomiasis en El Salvador. Arch. Coleg. Med. El Salvador, 10(1):14-21.

Perrin, T. G., E. Dias, and M. Brenes. 1947. Nota prévia sôbre as primeiras comprovações sorológicas da doença de Chagas no México. Mem. Inst. Oswaldo Cruz, 45:395-400.

Pessoa, S. B. 1963. Reservatórios animais do *Trypanosoma cruzi*. A doença de Chagas e uma zoonose. An. Congr. Internac. Doença de Chagas, 4:1155-1180.

―――― and B. R. Pestana. 1941. A intradermo reação de Montenegro nas companhas sanitárias contra a leishmaniose. Arq. Hig. Saúde Pública (S. Paulo), 6:125-137.

―――― and A. F. Cardosa. 1942. Nota sôbre a imunologia cruzada na *leishmaniose* e na moléstia de Chagas. Hospital (Rio de Janeiro), 21:187-193.

Phillips, N. R. 1960. Experimental studies on the quantitative transmission of *Trypanosoma cruzi*: Considerations regarding the standardization of materials. Ann. Trop. Med. Parasit., 54:60-70.

Philocreon, D. R. 1951. Do emprêgo do ACTH na moléstia de Chagas. Arq. Univ. Bahia Fac. Med., 6:107-115.

Pifano, C. F. 1960. Evaluacion de los procedimientos de laboratorio empleados en el diagnostico de la enfermedad de Chagas. Bol. Ofic. Sanit. Panamer., 49:563-571.

Pillemer, L., L. Blum, J. H. Lepow, O. A. Ross, E. W. Todd, and A. C. Wardlaw. 1954. The properdin system and immunity. I. Demonstration and isolation of a new serum protein, properdin, and its role in immune phenomena. Science, 120:279.

Pinto, C., and P. Falcão. 1958. Electroforese na doença de Chagas. Rev. Brasil. Med., 15:536-539.

Pipkin, A. C. 1960. Avian embryos and tissue culture in the study of parasitic protozoa. II. Protozoa other than *Plasmodium*. Exp. Parasit., 9:167-203.

Pizzi, T. 1944. Contribuciones al estudio experimental de la enfermedad de Chagas. II. Estudio histopatologico en el cuy. Thesis. Facultad de Medicina, Universidad de Chile.

———— 1952. Cortisona en las enfermedades protozoaias (revision critica). Bol. Inform. Parasit. Chile., 7:25-27.

———— 1954. Inflamacion en las enfermedades parasitarias. Bol. Chile. Parasit., 9:54-59.

———— 1957. Inmunologia de la enfermedad de Chagas. Monogr. Biol. Univ. Chile, No. 7, 183 pp.

———— 1961. Inmunologia de la enfermedad de Chagas: Estado actual del problema. Bol. Ofic. Sanit. Panamer., 51:450-464.

———— 1963. Aspectos celulares de la inmunidad en la enfermedad de Chagas. An. Congr. Internac. Doença de Chagas, 4:1217-1229.

———— R. Prager. 1952. Inmunidad a la sobreinfección inducida mediante cultivos de *Trypanosoma cruzi* de virulencia atenuada. (Communicación preliminar). Bol. Inform. Parasit. Chile., 7:20-21.

———— and M. Rubio. 1955. Aspectos celulares de la inmunidad en la enfermedad de Chagas. Bol. Chile. Parasit., 10:4-9.

———— M. Agosin, R. Christen, G. Hoecker, and A. Neghme. 1949. Estudios sobre inmunobiologia de las enfermedades parasitarias: I. Influencia de la constitución genética en la resistencia de las luchas a la infección experimental por *Trypanosoma cruzi*. Bol. Inform. Parasit. Chile., 4:48-49.

———— G. Niedman, and A. Jarpa. 1963. Report of three cases of acute Chagas' disease due to accidental infection in the laboratory. Bol. Chile. Parasit., 18:32-36.

———— M. Rubio, R. Prager, and R. Silva. 1952. Acción de la cortisona en la infección experimental por *Trypanosoma cruzi* (Communicación preliminar). Bol. Inform. Parasit. Chile., 7:22-24.

———— M. Rubio, and F. Knierim. 1953. Contribución al conocimiento de los mecanismos inmunitarios en la enfermedad de Chagas experimental de la rata. Bol. Inform. Parasit. Chile., 8:66-72.

———— and F. Knierim. 1955. Modificaciónes del bazo en relacion con la tasa de anticuerpos circulantes en ratones experimentalmente infectados con *Trypanosoma cruzi*. Bol. Chile. Parasit., 10:42-49.

———— M. Rubio, and F. Knierim. 1954. The immunology of Chagas' disease. Bol. Chile. Parasit., 9:35-47.

Portugal, O. P., S. Carvalhal, N. Paladino, O. L. Ramos, T. L. Da Silva, and H. Mafra. 1954. Inquérito clínico epidemiológico e sorológico sôbre a moléstia de Chagas no município de Itaporanga, Estado de S. Paulo. Folia Clin. Biol. S. Paulo, 22:69-78.

Puigbó, J. J., J. R. Nava Rhode, H. Garcia Barrios, J. A. Suarez, and C. Gil Yepez. 1966. Clinical and epidemiological study of chronic heart involvement in Chagas' disease. Bull. W. H. O., 34:655-669.

Ramos, A. da S. 1952. Inquérito epidemiológico sôbre a moléstia de Chagas em Santa Rita do Passa (Estado de São Paulo). Folia Clin. Biol. S. Paulo, 18:99-108.

Rassi, A., C. Borges, J. M. Rezende, O. Carneiro, J. Salum, I. B. Ribeiro, and H. O. Paula. 1958. Fase aguda da doença de Chagas. Aspectos clínicos observados em 18 casos. Rev. Goiana Med., 4:161-189.

Regendanz, P. 1930. Der Verlauf der Infektion mit *Schizotrypanum cruzi* (Chagas) bei jungen Ratten und über die Unempfänglichkeit erwachsener Ratten für *Schizotrypanum*. Zbl. Bakt. [Orig.], 116:256-264.

Rego, S. Ferreira de Morais. 1956. Estudo das lesões provacadas pelo "*Trypanosoma Cruzi*" Chagas, 1909, no baço e no fígado do camundongo branco ("*Mus musculus*") com diversos graus de resistência. J. Brasil. Med. 1:23-98(599-674).

Reuter, A. M., and F. Kennes. 1966. Strain and sex dependency of pre-albumin in mice. Nature (London), 210:745.

Rezende, C. L., J. Pellegrino, and A. Canelas. 1952. Inquerito sôbre a doença de Chagas em crianças internadas em hospitais de Belo Horizonte (Minas Gerais, Brasil). Hospital (Rio de Janeiro), 18:241-250.

Ribeiro, I. B. 1957. Forma aguda da doença de Chagas em Ceres. Resultados de diversos tratamentos empregados. Rev. Goiana Med., 3:3-20.

Rispoli, J. A. 1953. La enfermedad de Chagas en la Capital Federal. Asoc. Med. Cienc. Hosp. Rawson, Buenos Aires, Aug. 28.

Robles Gil, J., and M. Perrin. 1950. Nota preliminar del estudio experimental sobre la acción de la hormona adrenocotropica de la hipofisis en la enfermedad de Chagas. Arch. Inst. Cardiol. Mexico, 20:314-326.

———— M. Perrin, and J. Balcazar. 1951. Action of adrenocorticotrophic hormone in

Chagas' disease. An experimental study. Proceedings of the Second Clinical ACTH Conference, 1:468-477.

Rodriguez, J. D. 1950. Inmunidad en la enfermedad de Chagas. La reacción de fijación del complemento. Rev. Ecuator. Hig. Med. Trop., 7:65-74.

——— 1952. Inmunidad en la tripanosomiasis Americana. Presencia de "inmovilisimas." Rev. Ecuator. Hig. Med. Trop., 8/9:107-112.

——— 1959. Epidomiologie de la enfermedad de Chagas en la Republica del Ecuador. Rev. Goiana Med., 5:411-438.

Roitt, I. M., and D. Doniach. 1958. Human auto-immune thyroiditis. Lancet, 2:1027.

Romaña, C. 1949. Informe sobre la enfermedad de Chagas en la Argentina: situacion actual del problema. Bol. Ofic. Sanit. Panamer., 28:993-1004.

——— 1953. Panorama epidemiologico de la enfermedad de Chagas en la Argentina a traves de investigaciones sistematicas. Primera Conferencia Nacional de la Enfermedad de Chagas, Argentina, pp. 199-204.

——— 1960. Aplicacion de la tecnica de Kolmer-Boerner modificada a la reacción de fijación de complemento para el diagnostico de la enfermedad de Chagas. An. Inst. Med. Regional (Tucuman), 5:47-54.

——— and E. Dias. 1942. Reação de fixação do complemento na doença de Chagas, com antigeno alcoólico de cultura do Schizotrypanum cruzi. Mem. Inst. Oswaldo Cruz, 37:1-10.

——— and H. Mayer. 1942. Estudos do ciclo evolutivo do Schizotrypanum cruzi em cultura de tecidos de embrião de galinha. Mem. Inst. Oswaldo Cruz, 37:19-27.

——— and F. Cossio. 1944. Formas cronicas cardiacas de la enfermedad de Chagas. An. Inst. Med. Regional (Tucuman), 1:9-91.

——— and E. Terracini. 1945. Comportamiento de las infecciones de lauchas por S. cruzi segun la concentración de parasitos inoculados (infecciones cronicas iniciales). An. Inst. Med. Regional (Tucuman), 1:141-164.

——— and M. Conejos. 1946. Intradermo-reacción con antigeno de S. cruzi en la leishmania tegumentaria americana. An. Inst. Med. Regional (Tucuman), 1:289-296.

——— and J. Gil. 1946. Reacción de fijación de complemento con antigeno de cultura de S. cruzi en 500 sueros humanos. An. Inst. Med. Regional (Tucuman), 1:297-304.

——— and M. S. de Romaña. 1946. Indices de infección de niños por S. cruzi en escuelas de Tucuman, Santiago del Estero y Catamarca. An. Inst. Med. Regional (Tucuman), 1:317-332.

——— and M. Conejos. 1947. Intradermoreacción de Montenegro con antigeno de S. cruzi. Semana Med., 54:88.

——— and M. Kirschbaum. 1951. Encuesta sobre enfermedad de Chagas en las vecindades de Andalgala (Catamarca). An. Inst. Med. Regional (Tucuman), 3:123-128.

——— and J. W. Abalos. 1954. La enfermedad de Chagas en el Provincia de Tucuman. An. Inst. Med. Regional (Tucuman), 4:57-60.

Rosenbaum, M. B., and J. A. Cerisola. 1957a. Encuesta sobre enfermedad de Chagas en el Norte de Cordoba y Sur de Santiago de Estero. Prensa Med. Argent., 44:2713.

——— and J. A. Cerisola. 1957b. Encuesta sobre enfermadad de Chagas en la provincia de la Pampa. Prensa Med. Argen., 44:3485-3493.

——— and J. A. Cerisola. 1958. La reacción de fijación de complemento para el diagnostico de la enfermedad de Chagas. II. Valoración clinica. Prensa Med. Argent., 45:1551-1560.

Roskin, G. 1946. Toxin therapy of experimental cancer. The influence of protozoan infections upon transplanted cancer. Cancer Res., 6:363-365.

——— and E. Ekzemplarskaya. 1931. Protozoeninfektion and experimenteller Krebs. Z. Krebsforschung., 34:628-645.

——— and K. Romanowa. 1935. Action des toxines sur le cancer experimental. Acta Cancrologica, 1:323-334.

Rubio, M. 1956a. Estudio de la enfermedad de Chagas experimental del batracio. I. Factores que intervienen en la inmunidad natural. Bol. Chile. Parasit., 11:28-32.

——— 1956b. Activadad litica de sueros normales sobre formas de cultivo y sanguineas de Trypanosoma cruzi. Bol. Chile. Parasit., 11:62-69.

——— N. Allende, C. Roman, I. Ebensperger, and L. Moreno. 1967. Compromiso del sistema nervioso central en un caso de enfermedad de Chagas congenita. Bol. Chile. Parasit., 22:119-122.

Ryckman, R. E. 1954. Lizards: a laboratory host for triatominae and Trypanosoma cruzi Chagas (Hemiptera: Reduvidae. Protomonadina: Trypanosomidae). Trans. Amer. Micr. Soc., 73:215-218.

―――― 1965. Epizootiology of *Trypanosoma cruzi* in southwestern North America. VII. Experimental control of *Trypanosoma* by immunological methods. J. Med. Entom., 2:105-108.

Sabin, A., and H. A. Feldman. 1948. Dyes as microchemical indicators of a new immunity phenomenon affecting a protozoan parasite (*Toxoplasma*). Science, 108:660-663.

Sabino de Freitas, A. 1963. Parasitoses endêmicas no Brasil Central. Proceedings of the Seventh International Congress of Tropical Medicine and Malaria (Rio de Janeiro), Vol. 2, pp. 204-205.

Sadun, E. H., R. E. Duxbury, J. S. Williams, and R. I. Anderson. 1963. Fluorescent antibody test for the serodiagnosis of African and American trypanosomiasis in man. J. Parasit., 49:385-388.

Salazar, H. T. Arends, and G. A. Maekelt. 1962. Comprobación en Venezuela de la transmisión del *Schizotrypanum cruzi* por transfusión de sangre. Arch. Venez. Med. Trop. Parasit. Med., 4:355-363.

Salum, J., P. S. da Lacaz, C. Borges, A. Rassi, and J. M. Rezende. 1959. Eletroforese das proteínas séricas na fase aguda da doença de Chagas. Comportamento evolutivo observado em 15 casos. Rev. Goiana Med., 5:13-21.

Schenone, H., M. Ramirez, H. Reyes, A. Rojas, and L. Diaz. 1966. Contribución a la epidemiologia de la enfermedad de Chagas en Chile. Estudo epidemiologico en la Provincia de Colchagua. Bol. Chile. Parasit., 21:66-69.

Schlossberger, H., and J. Grillo. 1935. Experimentelle Untersuchungen über Misch und Sekundarinfektion. VI. Zbl. Bakt. [Orig.], 135:203-215.

Schultz, M. G., I. G. Kagan, and G. S. Warner. 1967. Card flocculation in the field diagnosis of trichinosis. Amer. J. Clin. Path., 47:26-29.

Scorza, J. V., A. Alvarez, I. Ramos, C. Dagert, A. Diaz Vasquez, and J. F. Torrealba. 1958. Estudio comparativo de las alteraciones citoplasmicas del *Trypanosoma cruzi* de cultivo cuando se le incuba con sueros de pacientes chagoso y de personas normales. Gac. Med. Caracas, 64:435-438.

―――― A. Alvarez, I. Ramos, C. Dagert, A. Diaz Vasquez, and J. F. Torrealba. 1959. Nuevo metodo rapido para el diagnostico de la enfermedad de Chagas en su fase cronica. Arch. Venez. Patol. Trop. Parasit. Med., 3:121-135.

Seneca, H., and J. Rockenbach. 1952. Fatal *Trypanosoma cruzi* infection in the white rat. Science, 116:14-15.

―――― and D. Ides. 1955. The effect of oxysteroids on *Trypanosoma cruzi* infection in mice. Amer. J. Trop. Med. Hyg. 4:833-836.

―――― and A. Wolf. 1955. *Trypanosoma cruzi* infection in the Indian Monkey. Amer. J. Trop. Med. Hyg., 4:1009-1014.

―――― and P. Peer. 1963a. Immunology and immunochoemotherapy of *Trypanosoma cruzi* infections. Proceedings of the Seventh International Congress of Tropical Medicine and Malaria (Rio de Janeiro), Vol. 2, p. 239.

―――― and P. Peer, 1963b. Immunochemistry of *Trypanosoma cruzi* and immunochemotherapy of experimental Chagas disease. Antimicrobial Agents and Chemotherapy, pp. 560-565.

―――― J. B. Sang, and A. K. Troc. 1958. The electrophoretic pattern of the serum proteins in experimental hemoflagellatic infections. Trans. Roy. Soc. Trop. Med. Hyg., 52:230-234.

―――― P. Peer, and B. Hampar. 1966. Active immunization of mice with chagastoxin. Nature (London) 209:309-310.

Senekjie, H. A. 1943a. Flagellar and somatic agglutinogens of *Trypanosoma cruzi*. Proc. Amer. Fed. Clin. Res., 1:33.

―――― 1943b. Immunologic studies in experimental *Trypanosoma cruzi* infections. 2. Slide agglutination and intradermal tests. Proc. Soc. Exp. Biol. Med., 52:56-69.

―――― and R. A. Lewis. 1944. Diagnosis of leishmaniasis by slide agglutination. Proc. Soc. Exp. Biol. Med., 57:17.

Serravalle, A. 1963. Reações de Guerreiro e Machado e de hemoglutinação em cães. An. Congr. Internac. Doença de Chagas, 4:1499-1503.

Shockman, G. D., J. J. Kolb, and G. Toennies. 1957. Highspeed shaker for the disruption of cells at low temperatures. Biochim. Biophys. Acta, 24:203-204.

Silva, L. H. P. da, and V. Nussenzweig. 1953. Sôbre uma cepa de *Trypanosoma cruzi* altamente virulenta para o camundongo branco. Folia. Clin. Biol. S. Paulo, 20:191-207.

―――― S. B. Carvalho, and N. R. Carneiro. 1956. Doença de Chagas na Paraíba. Inquérito sorológico preliminar. Rev. Brasil. Malar., 8:281-288.

Silva, T. L. da. 1954. Aspectos da epidemiologia e profilaxia da moléstia de Chagas no Estado de São Paulo. Arq. Hig. Saúde Pública (S. Paulo), 19:3-6.

Silva, I. I. 1955. Acerca de la acción tripanolitica de las sangres sobre los cultivos de *Trypanosoma* (*S.*) *cruzi* y observaciones sobre el desarrolo del mismo en un nuevo medio de cultivo. Universidad Nacional de Tucuman: Instituto de Medicina Regional, Publicacion No. 706, Monogr. 3, pp. 1-69.

Siqueira, A. F. 1964a. Comparação de antigenos de *Trypanosoma cruzi* para reações quantitativas de fixação do complemento. I. Linearidade entre complexo imune e complemento. Rev. Inst. Med. Trop. S. Paulo, 6:101-110.

————— 1964b. Comparação de antigenos de *Trypanosoma cruzi* para reações quantitativas de fixação do complemento. II. Análise sequential de probabilidade direta aplicada ao sistema moléstia de Chagas. Rev. Inst. Med. Trop. S. Paulo, 6:268-276.

Sommer, S. 1955. Zum Einfluss von somatropen Hormon und Cortison auf den Verlauf einer experimentellen Trypanosomen-Infektion (*Trypanosoma cruzi*). Arch. Exp. Pathol. Pharmakol., 226:527-531.

Souza Campos, E. de. 1929a. Corpos intranucleares nas células do retículo endothelial do ganglio lymphatico parasitado pelo *Trypanosoma cruzi*. Nota prévia. Bol. Biol. S. Paulo, 16:99-102.

————— 1929b. Estudo sôbre a anatomia patológica do ganglio lymphatico na trypanosomiase do ganglio lymphatico na trypanosomiase americana experimental. Alterações do sistema reticulo-endothelial. Corpos intranucleares. Myelopoese. An. Fac. Med. Univ. S. Paulo, 4:75-90.

————— 1934. Função do retículo endothelio na trypanosomiase americana experimental. Rev. Biol. Hig. S. Paulo, 5:48-49.

————— and P. de Toledo Artigas. 1932. Alterações do pulmão na trypanosomiase americana experimental e contribução para o estudo da natureza das células phagocytasias do pulmão. An. Fac. Med. Univ. S. Paulo, 7:95-115.

Spain, D. M., N. Molout, and L. J. Warshaw. 1948. Preparations of lysates from cultures of *T. cruzi* and their effects on normal and tumor-bearing mice. Proc. Soc. Exp. Biol. Med., 69:134-136.

Stavitsky, A. B. 1954. Procedure and general applications of hemagglutination and hemagglutination-inhibition reactions with tannic acid and protein-treated red blood cells. J. Immun., 72:360-367.

Stern, L. 1948. Storage of carmine in mice of inbred strains. Proc. Soc. Exp. Biol. Med., 67:315-317.

Streber, F. 1950. Influencia del sexo en infecciónes experimentales por *Schizotrypanum cruzi* 1909. Rev. Palud. Med. Trop. Mexico, 2:73-78.

Taliaferro, W. H., and T. Pizzi. 1959. Connective tissue reactions in normal and immunized mice to a reticulotropic strain of *Trypanosoma cruzi*. J. Infect. Dis., 96:199-226.

Taquini, A. C., S. A. Plesch, B. A. Noir, and B. N. Badano. 1956. Über die Plasmaeiweisskörper bei der chronischen Chagas-Myocarditis. Cardiologia, 28:306-318.

Tarrant, C. J., E. H. Fifer, and R. I. Anderson. 1965. Serological characteristics and general chemical nature of the "in vitro" exoantigens of *T. cruzi*. J. Parasit., 51:277-285.

Tay, J., E. Navarrete, E. R. Corominas and F. Biagi. 1966. La enfermedad de Chagas en el municipio de Tuxpan, Estado de Michoacan, Mexico. Rev. Fac. Med. Mex., 8:263-270.

Tejada Valencuela, C., and F. Castro. 1958. Miocarditis cronica en Guatemala. Rev. Coleg. Med. Guatemala, p. 9.

Tejera, E., and C. F. Pifano. 1959. La trypanosomiasis rangeli en Venezuela. Congr. Internac. Doença de Chagas, Resumos Trabalhos, pp. 78-81.

Thiermann, E., and R. Christen. 1952. Influencia del acetato de cortisona y de la aureomicina como agent agravador de la infección chagasica atenuada. Bol. Inform. Parasit. Chile., 7:53-55.

————— G. Niedmann, and F. Naquira. 1958. Contribution to toxoplasma serology. III. Toxoplasma dye test and complement fixation test in 169 blood samples from individuals with Chagas infection. Biologica, pp. 36-51.

Tobie, E. J. 1964. Increased infectivity of a cyclically maintained strain of *Trypanosoma rangeli* to *Rhodnius prolixus* and mode of transmission by intermediate host. J. Parasit., 50:593-598.

Torres, C. Magarinos. 1929. Patogenia de la miocardite cronica en la enfermedad de Chagas. Sociedad Argentina Patologia Regional del Norte, Quinta Reunion, 2:902-916.

Torres Pereya, J. 1967. Asociacion de paratifus A con probable miocardiopatia chagasica. Bol. Chile. Parasit., 22:165-167.

Torrico, R. A. 1959. Casuistica de la enfermedad de Chagas por la reacción de fijación de complemento en cardiacos del Chaco (Argentina). An. Inst. Med. Regional (Resistencia), 5:79-81.

Toussaint, A. J., C. J. Tarrant, and R. I. Anderson. 1965a. Soluble antigen fluorescent antibody (SAFA) test for the serorecognition of infection with Trypanosoma cruzi. J. Parasit., 51:29.

—— C. J. Tarrant, and R. I. Anderson. 1965b. An indirect fluorescent antibody technique using soluble antigens for serodiagnosis of Trypanosoma cruzi. Proc. Soc. Exp. Biol. Med., 120:783-785.

Trautmann, R. 1907. Étude expérimentale sur l'association du spirille de la tick-fever et de divers trypanosomes. Ann. Inst. Pasteur (Paris), 21:803-824.

Trejos, A., M. A. De Urquilla, and A. R. Paredes. 1965. Influence of environmental temperature on the evolution of experimental Chagas' disease in mice. In Progress in Protozoology. Second International Congress on Protozoology, London, 1965. Amsterdam, Excerpta Medica Foundation, International Congress Series No. 91, p. 144.

Trufanov, A. V., and N. A. Palkina. 1960. Deistvie antibiotika krutsina na suktsindegidrazy i tsitokhromoksidazy opukholevoi tkani. Biokhimiia, 25:787-789.

Unti, O., and T. L. da Silva. 1951. Moléstia de Chagas no vale do Paraíba Estado de São Paulo. Nota sôbre profilaxia e epidemiologia. Arq. Hig. Saúde Pública (S. Paulo), 16:131-138.

—— and T. L. da Silva. 1952. Levantamento da moléstia de Chagas no Estado de São Paulo pela reação sorológica. Arq. Hig. Saúde Pública (S. Paulo), 17:123-132.

Uvo, D., A. A. Aguiar, S. Carvalhal, N. Paladino, and N. V. Soubihe. 1954. Estudo comparativo dos resultados da R.F.C. para diagnóstico da moléstia de Chagas, obtidos com a realização das técnicas qualitativa e quantitativa. Folia Clin. Biol. S. Paulo, 22:85-96.

Van der Sar, A., and B. Vinke. 1965. Investigation into the occurrence of Trypanosoma cruzi in Curação. Trop. Geogr. Med., 17:225-28.

Vianna Martins, A., V. Versiani, A. Tupinamba, A. Torres Sobrinho, J. E. Lasmar, and A. A. Teixeira. 1941. Sôbre 24 casos agudos de moléstia de Chagas observados em Minas Gerais. Mem. Inst. Biol. Ezequiel Dias, 3/4:5-70.

Victoria, V. 1954. Communicacion previa sobre tratamiento del sindrome oculoganglionar chagasico con la piretoterapia controlada. Rev. Med. del Norte, 1:10.

—— and J. Dalma. 1956. La piretoterapia en la enfermedad de Chagas. Acta 5 Congreso Panamericano Optalmologia, Santiago de Chile.

Villela, E. 1924. Paralysie expérimentale chez le chien pour le Trypanosoma cruzi. C. R. Soc. Biol. (Paris), 9:979.

—— and J. C. Bacalho. 1923. As pesquisas de laboratório no diagnóstico da moléstia de Chagas. Mem. Inst. Oswaldo Cruz, 16:13-29.

—— and A. M. da Cunha. 1919 and 1920. In Villela and Bacalho, 1923.

Voller, A., and J. J. Shaw. 1965. Immunological observations on an antiserum to Trypanosoma cruzi. Z. Tropenmed. Parasit., 16:181-187.

Von Brand, T., E. J. Tobie, R. E. Kissling, and G. Adams. 1949. Physiological and pathological observations on four strains of Trypanosoma cruzi. J. Infect. Dis., 85:5-16.

Wadsworth, A. 1927. Standard Methods of the Division of Laboratories and Research of the New York Department of Health. Baltimore, Williams and Wilkins Co.

—— E. Maltaner, and F. Maltaner. 1931. The quantitative determination of the fixation of complements by immune serum and antigen. J. Immun., 21:313-339.

—— E. Maltaner, and F. Maltaner. 1938. Quantitative studies of the reaction of complement fixation with tuberculous immune serum and antigen. J. Immun., 35:93-103.

Walker, E. P. 1964. Mammals of the World. Vols. 1 and 2. Baltimore, John Hopkins Press, 1500 pp.

Walton, B. C. 1966. Prevalence of antibodies to T. cruzi in a statistically representative survey of Guatemala, El Salvador and Nicaragua. Presented at the Annual Meeting Amer. Soc. Trop. Med. Hyg., San Juan, Puerto Rico.

Warren, L. G. 1958. Biochemical studies on chicken macrophages infected in vitro with Trypanosoma cruzi. Exp. Parasit., 7:82-91.

—— 1960. Metabolism of Schizotrypanum cruzi Chagas. I. Effect of culture agent substrate concentration on respiratory rate. J. Parasit., 46:529.

—— and T. Borsos. 1959. Studies on immune factors occurring in sera of chickens against the crithidia stage of Trypanosoma cruzi. J. Immun., 82:585-590.

Watkins, R. 1966. Comparison of infections produced by two strains of *Trypanosoma cruzi* in mice. J. Parasit., 52:958-961.

Westphal, A. 1954. Zur Systematik von *Toxoplasma gondii*. Die Toxoplasmen als Trypanosomidae. Z. Tropenmed. Parasit., 5:3-40.

Westphal, O., O. Luderitz, and F. Bister. 1952. Über die Extraktion von Bakterien mit Phenol/Wasser. Z. Naturforschung., 7b:148-155.

Wolf, A., E. A. Kabat, A. E. Bezer, and J. R. C. Fonseca. 1951. Activation of trypanosomiasis in rhesus monkeys by cortisone. Fed. Proc., 10:375.

———— A., E. A. Kabat, A. E. Bezer, and J. R. C. Fonseca. 1953. The effect of cortisone in activating latent trypanosomiasis in rhesus monkeys. *In* Symposium on the Effect of ACTH and Cortisone upon Infection and Resistance, Chapter 10. Schwartzmen, G., ed. New York, Columbia University Press, pp. 122-139.

Wood, F. D. 1934. Experimental studies on *Trypanosoma cruzi* in California. Proc. Soc. Exp. Biol. Med., 32:61-62.

Wood, S. W. 1951. Development of Arizona *Trypanosoma cruzi* in mouse muscle. Amer. J. Trop. Med., 31:1-11.

Woody, N. C., and H. B. Woody. 1955. American trypanosomiasis (Chagas' disease). First indigenous case in the United States. J. A. M. A., 159:676-677.

———— and H. B. Woody. 1961. American trypanosomiasis. I. Clinical and epidemiologic background of Chagas' disease in the United States. J. Pediat., 58:568-580.

———— N. DeDianous, and H. B. Woody. 1961. American trypanosomiasis. II. Current serologic studies in Chagas' disease. J. Pediat., 58:738-745.

———— A. Hernandez, and B. Suchow. 1965. American trypanosomiasis. III. The incidence of serologically diagnosed Chagas' disease among persons bitten by the insect vector. J. Pediat., 66:107-109.

Yaeger, R. G., and O. N. Miller. 1960a. Effect of malnutrition on susceptibility of rats to *Trypanosoma cruzi*. I. Thiamin deficiency. Exp. Parasit., 9:215-222.

———— and O. N. Miller. 1960b. Effect of malnutrition on susceptibility of rats to *Trypanosoma cruzi*. II. Riboflavin deficiency. Exp. Parasit., 10:227-231.

———— and O. N. Miller. 1960c. Effect of malnutrition on susceptibility of rats to *Trypanosoma cruzi*. III. Pantothenate deficiency. Exp. Parasit., 10:232-237.

———— and O. N. Miller. 1960d. Effect of malnutrition on susceptibility of rats to *Trypanosoma cruzi*. IV. Pyridoxine deficiency. Exp. Parasit., 10:238-244.

———— and O. N. Miller. 1963a. Effect of malnutrition on susceptibility of rats to *Trypanosoma cruzi*. Vitamin A deficiency. Exp. Parasit., 14:9-14.

———— and O. N. Miller. 1963b. The influence of quality of dietary protein on susceptibility of rats to infections with *Trypanosoma cruzi* and *Trypansoma gambiense*. Proceedings of the Fifth International Congress of Tropical Medicine and Malaria, Vol. 2, p. 235.

———— and O. N. Miller. 1963c. Effect of lysine deficiency on Chagas' disease in laboratory rats. J. Nutrition, 81:169-174.

———— and O. N. Miller. 1966. The effect of certain dietary stresses on susceptibility of the rat to infection with *Trypansoma cruzi*. Bull. Tulane Univ. Med. Fac., 25:13-20.

Zeledon, R. 1952. El problema de la tripanosomiasis americana o enfermedad de Chagas en Costa Rica. Thesis. Ministerio Salubridad Publica, San Jose, Costa Rica. 109 pp.

———— and C. Lizano. 1962. Experimental infection of the guinea pig with Chagas' disease and superimposed leishmaniasis and electrophoretic analysis of the serum. Rev. Inst. Med. Trop. S. Paulo, 4:124-129.

Zuccarini, J. A. 1930. Estudio experimental sobre el *Trypanosoma cruzi*. Rev. Soc. Argent. Biol., 6:217-224.

Supplementary Bibliography

The following articles have not been referred to specifically in the text for a variety of reasons but contain pertinent information which should be consulted by those interested in further details:

Agosín, M. 1951. Cortisona y enfermedad de Chagas experimental. Biologica (Santiago), 14-15:29-54.

———— R. Christen, and A. Jarpa. 1951. Action of cortisone alone or associated to pentaquine phosphate or to the compound pentaquine phosphate-quinine sulfate on experimental trypanosomiasis (*T. cruzi*) in mice. Parasitology, 37 (No. 5, Suppl.):31.

———— R. Christen, A. Jarpa, and A. Atias. 1951. Cortisona y enfermedad de Chagas experimental. Biologica (Santiago), 14-15:29-54.

———— R. Christen, A. Jarpa, V. A. Atias, and A. Neghme. 1952. Cortisona y enfermedad de Chagas experimental. Rev. Med. Chile, 80:34-37.

Aguilar, F. J. 1956. Diagnóstico de laboratorio en la enfermedad de Chagas o tripanosomiasis americana. Rev. Med. Trop. Parasit. (Habana), 12:58-60.

Almeida, J. O. De, and A. F. Siqueira. 1960. Estudo da discrepancia relativa entre pares de reações simultaneas de fixação de complemento no sistema moléstia de Chagas. Rev. Inst. Med. Trop. S. Paulo, 2:204-212.

Amato Neto, V., and L. H. P. da Silva. 1954. Anticorpos heterofilos na doença de Chagas. Resultados obtidos e casos agudos e cronicos. Hospital (Rio de Janeiro), 45:159-169.

Andrade, Z. A., and A. Paiva. 1962. Reações imuno-celulares na tripanosomiase cruzi experimental. Rev. Med. Bahia, 18(1):27-33.

Baracchini, O., A. Costa, and J. Carloni. 1965. Emprêgo do calor e do metanol no preparo de antigeno de *Trypanosoma cruzi*. Hospital (Rio de Janeiro), 67:1313-1319.

———— A. Costa, and J. Carloni. 1966. Emprêgo do calor a temperatura de 120° C. e do metanol no preparo de antigeno de *Trypanosoma cruzi*. Hospital (Rio de Janeiro), 70:81-84.

Beck, J.S., and P. J. Walker. 1964. Antigenicity of trypanosome nuclei: Evidence that DNA is not coupled to histone in these protozoa. Nature (London), 204:194-195.

Benavides, R. M. 1953. Estudio comparativo de tres cepas de *Schizotrypanum cruzi* Chagas 1909. Thesis. Instituto Politecnico Nacional, Mexico.

Bettinotti, C. M., M. A. Nores, and J. A. Restanio. 1953. La prueba de fijación de complemento en el diagnostico de casos inaparentes de la enfermedad de Chagas. Primera Conferencia Nacional de la Enfermedad de Chagas, Argentina, pp. 123-127.

Borrotchin, M., and J. Pellegrino. 1954. Provas de laboratório para o diagnóstico na doença de Chagas e estudo electrocardiográfico em 38 casos de megaesôfago e megacolon. Rev. Assoc. Med. Minas Gerais, 5:37-38.

Brant, C. T. 1962. Importância médico-social da doença de Chagas. Rev. Brasil. Malar., 14:13-19.

———— 1963. Alterações electrocardiográficas em áreas de triatomineos—município de Jacui, Estado de Minas Gerais. Rev. Brasil. Malar., 15:251-254.

———— F. M. De Bustamante, A. L. De Mello, and S. M. Batista. 1955. Doença de Chagas no município de Itaqui, Estado do Rio Grande do Sul. Rev. Brasil. Malar., 7:177-180.

———— F. S. Laranja, F. M. De Bustamente, and A. L. De Mello. 1957. Dados sorológicos e electrocardiográficos obtidos em populações não selecionadas de zonas endêmicas de doença de Chagas no Estado do Rio Grande do Sul. Rev. Brasil. Malar., 9:141-148.

Brener, Z. 1952. A reação de fixação do complemento com antigeno de *L. brasiliensis* na Leishmaniose tegumentar americana e na doença de Chagas. Hospital (Rio de Janeiro), 41:269-275.

Bustamante, F. M. de, and J. B. Gusmão. 1953. Sôbre um foco de *Triatoma* infestam os Municipios de Resende e Itavera, Estado do Rio de Janeiro. Rev. Brasil. Malar., 50:1129.

———— 1953. Dados sôbre a reação de fixação do complemento do diagnóstico da doença de Chagas. Hospital (Rio de Janeiro), 43:777-780.

Cabral, H. R., C. Montenegro Iniguez, and R. W. De Paolasso. 1966. Acerca del poder aglutinante del suero de pacientes chagasicos agudos sobre eritrocitos de carnero sensibilizados y no sensibilizados. Rev. Fac. Cienc. Med. Cordoba, 24:395-400.

Cerisola, J. A., and M. B. Rosenbaum. 1958. La reacción de fijación de complemento para el diagnostico de la enfermedad de Chagas. I. Tecnica. Prensa Med. Argent., 45:1454-1463.

Chapadeiro, E., J. H. Furtado, and E. R. Lopes. 1968. The complement fixation test of Guerreiro and Machado in the pericardial fluid in chronic Chagas heart disease. J. Trop. Med. Hyg., 71:81-82.

Chatard, H. 1957. À propos de l'extrait de trypanosomes utilisé dans le traitment des affections malignes; possibilité de contre-indications. Lyon Med., 89:171-174.

Chiari, E., E. Neto Mansur, and Z. Brener. 1968. Some effects of gamma-radiation on *Trypanosoma cruzi*, culture and blood forms. Rev. Inst. Med. Trop. S. Paulo, 10:131-137.

Costa, J. Ferreira da, and A. Costa. 1960. Verificações experimentais sôbre imunidade humoral na moléstia de Chagas. Publicações Med., 31:29-31; 33-37.

Coudert, J., and J. Michel-Brun. 1963. Extrait de *Trypanosoma cruzi* et metabolisme de la cellule sarcomateuse. Proceedings of the Seventh International Congress of Tropical Medicine and Malaria (Rio de Janeiro), Vol. 2, p. 240.

―――― and J. Michel-Brun. 1963. Cancerologie. Modifications des processus glycolytiques de la cellule sarcomateuse sous l'influence de extrait de *Trypansoma cruzi*. Soc. Biol. Lyon, 68:71.

―――― J. Michel-Brun, and P. Ambroise-Thomas. 1963. Cancerologie. Influence des extraits de *T. cruzi* sur les acides nucléiques de la cellule du sarcoma d'Ehrlich de la souris. Societe de Biologie de Lyon, 68:72-75.

―――― J. Michel-Brun, and P. Thomas-Ambroise. 1964. Influence des extraits de *T. cruzi* sur les acides nucléiques de la cellule du sarcome d'Ehrlich de la souris. C. R. Soc. Biol. (Paris), 158:72-75.

Coura, R. 1966. Contribuição ao estudo da doença no estado da Guanabara. Rev. Brasil. Malar., 18:9-98.

―――― E. S. Nogueira, and J. Rodrigues da Silva. 1966. Índices de transmissão da doença de Chagas por transfusão de sangue de doadores na fase crônica da doença. Hospital (Rio de Janeiro), 69:991-998.

Coutinho, J. O. 1941. Dados epidemiológicos sôbre a doença de Chagas em uma zona restrita do Estado de S. Paulo. Rev. Inst. Adolfo Lutz, S. Paulo, 1:381-388.

Cox, H. W. 1964. Immune response of rats and mice to trypanosome infections. J. Parasit., 50:15-22.

Culbertson, J. T. 1935. Trypanocidal action of normal human serum. Arch. Path. (Chicago), 20:767-790.

Cunha, A. N. da. 1931. Diagnóstico da leishmaniose tegumentar pelo desvio de complemento e intradermoreação. Rev. Med. Cirurg. Brasil, 29:37.

Davidsohn, I., and K. Stern. 1949. Natural and immune antibodies in mice of low and high tumor strains. Cancer Res., 9:426-435.

Del Rey, C. J., I. G. Kagan, and A. J. Sulzer. 1966. Prueba sencilla de inmunofluorescencia aplicable a la enfermdad de Chagas (estudio de las fracciones de anticuerpos detectables por los tests empleados en la valoracion diagnostica). Med. Trop. (Madrid), 42:211-219.

Depouey, P., and J. Marechal. 1966. Structure antigenique des trypanosomes. I. Étude des antigènes de trois espèces de trypanosomes (*T. mega, T. cruzi, T. gambiense*) par la fixation du complement, la précipitation en gel et l'immuno-fluorescence. Ann. Inst. Pasteur (Paris), 110:889-911.

Diamond, L. S., and R. Rubin. 1956. Susceptibility of domestic animals to infection with *Trypanosoma cruzi* from the raccoon. J. Parasit., 42 (Suppl.):21.

Dias, E. 1946. Acerca de 254 casos de doença de Chagas comprovadas em Minas Gerais. Brasil-Med., 60:41-44.

―――― and T. Caldeira Brant. 1952. Inquérito sôbre doença de Chagas realizado nas localidades de Pedra Branca e Sertãozinho, Município de Bambui, Minas Gerais. Rev. Brasil. Malar., 4:227-230.

―――― F. S. Laranja, F. Nery-Guimarães, and T. Caldeira Brant. 1953. Estudo preliminar de inquéritos serológico-electrocardiográficos em populações não selecionadas de zonas não endêmicas e de zonas endêmicas de doença de Chagas. Rev. Brasil. Malar., 5:205-210.

Dios, R. L., and E. T. W. de Sommerville. 1943. Observaciones realizados con cepas de *Trypanosoma cruzi* Chagas 1909 conservados sobre ratones blancos. Rev. Inst. Bact. Carlos Malbran, Buenos Aires, 12:37-59.

Dominguez, A., and J. A. Suarez. 1963. Untersuchungen über das intrakardiale vegetative Nervensystem bei Myocarditis chagasica. Z. Tropenmed. Parasit., 14:81-85.

Dussert, E., J. Faiguenbaum, and A. Neghme Rodriguez. 1939. La reacción de Machado en Chile; comunicación preliminar. Rev. Chile. Hig. Med. Prev., 2:197-203.

Fernandes, J. F., O. Castellani, and M. Okumura. 1966. Histopathology of the heart and muscles in mice immunized against *Trypanosoma cruzi*. Rev. Inst. Med. Trop. S. Paulo, 8:151-156.

Ferrero, C., C. Taborda, J. Schlliamser, L. G. Sacchetti, O. Astrada, O. Pessat, and W. Puszkin. 1957. Catastro serológico sobre enfermedad de Chagas-Mazza en el N. O. de Cordoba; valoración estadistica. Rev. Med. Cordoba, 45:477-486.

Fistein, B., and R. N. P. Sutton. 1963. Chagas' disease in the West Indies. Lancet, 1:330-331.

Freitas, G. de. 1955. Contribuição a imunoquímica dos tripanosomídeos. Thesis. Faculdade Fluminense de Medicina, Rio de Janeiro. 55pp.
———— 1957. Contribuição a imunoquímica dos tripanosomídeos. An. Fac. Fluminense Med., 5:113-141.
Friebel, H. A. 1952. Über den Einfluss von Cortison auf die Infektabwehr. (Versuche an trypanosomenkranken Mäusen). Arch. Exp. Path. Pharm., 216:515-535.
Fromentin, H., A. Dodin, and P. Destombes. 1967. Essai d'immunisation de la souris (hôte vertebre) contre *Trypanosoma cruzi*, par une suspension de triatome (hôte invertebre). Acta Tropica (Basel), 24:261-265.
Garavelli, H. J., and A. Pandiella. 1967. Estudio comparativo de la trypanolisis y la reacción de fijación del complemento en cobayos infectados con *Trypanosoma cruzi*. Medicina (Buenos Aires), 27:227-229.
Girola, R. A., G. W. de Martini, and A. Milic. 1968. La reacción de inmunofluorescencia en el diagnostico de la enfermedad de Chagas-Mazza. Bol. Ofic. Sanit. Panamer., 64:130-136.
Goble, F. C. 1965. Vaccine for Chagas' disease. J. A. M. A., 193:177.
———— E. A. Konopka, and J. L. Boyd. 1965. Sex of host as a factor in protozoal pathogenesis. *In* Progress in Protozoology, Abstracts. Second International Congress on Protozoology, London, 1965. Amsterdam, Excerpta Medica Foundation, International Congress Series No. 91, pp. 54-55.
Gonzaga, A. L., J. de A. Albernaz, and R. R. Alves. 1967. Rotina sorológica para a doença de Chagas em banco de sangue. Apreciação de resultados na Guanabara de 25,508 reações de fixação do complemento. Apêndice técnico. Arq. Brasil. Med., 54:289-301.
Gonzalez, S. M., A. S. Parodi, G. Schumuñis, A. Taratuto, O. Traversa, and J. F. Yanovsky. 1967. Histopatologia de los ratones vacunados para la enfermedad de Chagas experimental en el ratón. Primer Congreso Latinoamericano de Parasitologia, Santiago de Chile, Resumens, p. 36.
Gonzalez-Cappa, S. M., G. A. Schumuñis, O. C. Traversa, J. F. Yanovsky, and A. S. Parodi. 1968. Complement fixation tests, skin tests, and experimental immunization with antigens of *Trypanosoma cruzi* prepared under pressure. Amer J. Trop. Med. Hyg., 17:709-715.
———— G. A. Schumuñis, O. C. Traversa, J. F. Yanovsky, M. E. Etcheverry, and H. J. Garavelli. 1968. New technique for the preparation of *Trypanosoma cruzi* antigens. I. Effect of pressure on the antigen binding the complement. C. R. Soc. Biol. (Paris), 162:293.
Grassi, O. T., G. E. Guerrero, and M. R. Perez. 1967. Estudio comparativo de la distribución de las reacciones de Machado-Guerreiro y hemaglutinación positivas en diversas provincias argentinas. Prensa Med. Argent., 54:821-825.
Gutierrez-Hoyos, Y. 1962. Contribución al conocimiento de trypanosomiasis humano en Colombia. Estudio llevado a cabo en la region de Tibu (N. de Santander). Caldas. Med. Manizales, 3:39-56, 65-78.
Hauschka, T. S. 1949. Endotoxin aus *Trypanosoma cruzi* bei der Behandlung von Mäusetumoren. Krebsarzt, 4:152.
———— and M. B. Goodwin. 1949. Tratamento dos tumores malígnos do camondongo com endotoxina do *Trypanosoma cruzi*. Arq. Biol. (S. Paulo), 33:22.
Hoare, C. A., and F. G. Wallace. 1966. Developmental stages of trypanosomatic flagellates: A new terminology. Nature (London), 212:1385-1386.
Jedeloo, G. C., G. O. E. Lignac, A. J. Ligtenberg, and P. H. Van Hiel. 1951. The biotherapeutic action of *Trypanosoma cruzi* on tar carcinoma in mice. Acta Leidensia, 21:120:128.
Jörg, M. E. 1967. Posible intervencion de mecanismos inmunobiologicos en la patogenia de la miocarditis cronica aparasitica, atribuida a la tripanosomiasis cruzi. Primer Congreso Latinoamericano de Parasitologia, Santiago de Chile, Resumenes, P. 33.
Kagan, I. G. 1965. Evaluation of routine serologic testing for parasitic diseases. Amer. J. Public Health, 55:1820-1829.
———— L. Norman, and D. Allain. 1966. Studies on *Trypanosoma cruzi* isolated in the United States. A review. Rev. Biol. Trop. (Costa Rica), 14:55-73.
———— L. Norman, and E. C. Hall. 1966. The effect of infection with *Trypanosoma cruzi* on the development of spontaneous mammary cancer in mice. Medicina Tropical. Mexico, Talleres Graficos de Editorial Fournier, S.A., pp. 326-340.
Knierim, F., and J. Sandoval. 1967. Evaluación de la sensibilidad y especificidad de la

reacción de fijación del complemento (RFC) para enfermedad de Chagas. Primer Congreso Latinoamericano de Parasitologia, Santiago de Chile, Resumenes, p. 31.

——— and P. Saavedra. 1967. Comparición entre las reacciones de hemaglutinación y fijación del complemento para enfermedad de Chagas. Primer Congreso Latinoamericano de Parasitologia, Santiago de Chile, Resumenes, pp. 31-32.

Kolodny, M. H. 1939. The transmission of immunity in experimental trypanosomiasis (*Trypanosoma cruzi*) from mother rats to their off-spring. Amer. J. Hyg. 30(c):19-39.

Lacorte, J. G. 1938. A reação de Machado na moléstia de Chagas. Acta Med. (Rio de Janeiro), 1:264-274.

——— 1942. A reação de fixação do complemento aplicado à moléstia de Chagas (reação de Machado ou Machado Guerreiro). Acta Med. (Rio de Janeiro), 10:87-94.

Lange, D. E., and M. G. Lysenko. 1960. *In vitro* phagocytosis of *Trypanosoma lewisi* by rat exudative cells. Exp. Parasit., 10:39-42.

Laranja, F. S., E. Dias, E. Duarte, and J. Pellegrino. 1951. Observações clínicas e epidemiológicas sôbre a moléstia de Chagas no oeste de Minas Gerais. Hospital (Rio de Janeiro), 40:945-988.

Laszlo, H. P. 1950. Recherches préliminaires sur la composition chimique de la fraction spécifique soluble obtenue par la méthode de Fuller de *Schizotrypanum cruzi*. Hospital (Rio de Janeiro), 38:621-624.

——— 1952. Composição química da "substância solúvel e específica" do *Trypanosoma (Schizotrypanum) cruzi* e da *Leishmania brasiliensis*, extraída pelo metodo de Fuller. Nôvo meio de cultura para o crescimento dêsses flagelados. Brasil-Med., 66:101-106.

Lausi, L. 1958. Diagnóstico de la enfermedad de Chagas. Semana Med., 112:694-699.

Little, P. A., and Y. Subbarow. 1954. A practical liquid medium for cultivation of *Trypanosoma cruzi* in large volumes. J. Bact., 50:57-60.

Lomonaco, D. A., H. H. Oliveira, J. Kieffer, and R. R. Pieroni. 1966. Abnormal regulation of thyroid function in patients with chronic Chagas' disease. Acta Endocr., 53:162-176.

Lopes, E. R., A. Raphael, and V. Amato Neto. 1967. Reação de Guerreiro Machado em portadores de neoplasias malignas. Hospital (Rio de Janeiro), 71:221-224.

Loretti, G. A., and O. F. Franzani. 1954. Importancia de la reacción de fijación del complemento en el diagnostico de la enfermedad de Chagas. Nueva tecnica empleada en el Hospital Militar Central "Cirujano Mayor Dr. Cosme Argerich". Rev. Sanid. Milit. Argent., 53:218-225.

Machado, D. 1940. Diagnóstico laboratorial na doença de Chagas. Rev. Fluminense Med., 5:163-165.

Machado, O. L., S. Silva, and F. J. Rodrigues-Gomes. 1967. Dados serológicos das reações de grupo na toxoplasmose e na doença de Chagas. Primer Congreso Latinoamericano de Parasitologia, Santiago de Chile, Resumenes, p. 34.

Maekelt, G. A. 1957. Investigaciones de sangre de donantes mediante la reaccion de fijación de complemento para la enfermedad de Chagas. Acta Med. Venez., 5:104-107.

——— and V. A. Diaz. 1962. La especificidad del antigeno de *Schizotrypanum cruzi*, fijador de complemento, frente a la infección por *Trypanosoma rangeli*. Arch. Venez. Med. Trop. Parasit. Med., 4:183-193.

Manrique, I. J. 1950. Aspecto clinico local de la cardiopatia chagasica cronica. Rev. Ecuator. Hig. Med. Trop., 7:13-39.

Manso-Soto, A. E., G. A. Loretti, and C. Sosa Miatello. 1955. Antigeno chagasico liofilizado. Misión de Estudios de Patologia Regional Argentina, 26:15-20.

Marinkelle, C. J., and E. Rodriguez. 1968. The influence of environmental temperature on the pathogenicity of *Trypanosoma cruzi* in mice. Exp. Parasit., 23:260-263.

Mardsen, P. D., 1967. *Trypanosoma cruzi* infections in CFI mice. II. Infections induced by different routes. Ann. Trop. Med. Parasit., 61:62-67.

——— 1967. *Trypanosoma cruzi* infections in CF_1 mice. I. Mortality with different doses of trypanosomes. Ann. Trop. Med. Parasit., 61:57-61.

——— and J. W. C. Hagstrom. 1968. Experimental *Trypanosoma cruzi* infection in beagle puppies. The effect of variations in the dose and sources of infecting trypanosomes and the route of inoculation on the course of the infection. Trans. Roy. Soc. Trop. Med. Hyg., 62:816-824.

Martinez Colombres, V., C. Bocca Torres, R. Bilella, and P. Dobladez. 1952. Enfermedad de Chagas-Mazza en la infancia en la provincia de San Juan. Terceras Jornadas de la Sociedad Argentina de Pediatria, Tucuman, p. 395.

Martins, F. 1949. Modificações verificadas em sorodiagnósticos da doença de Chagas com o iodeto de sódio. Med. Cirurg. Farm., 163:656-659.

Mazza, S., and M. E. Jörg. 1940. Reproducción experimental de nodulos de histiocitosis del granuloma chagasico mediante el fenomeno de Schwartzman (Existencia de principio activo de activo de *Schizotrypanum cruzi* capaz de provocar hiperplasia y su confluencia plasmodial). Misión de Estudios de Patologia Regional Argentina, 47:3-18.

——— G. Basso, and R. Basso. 1942. Enfermedad de Chagas en primer periodo diagnostica da exclusivamente por biopsia de ganglio linfatico con hallazgo de parasitos leishmaniformes. Misión de Estudios de Patologia Regional Argentina, 63:3-48.

Mello, A., and N. R. Mello. 1965. A forma nervosa crônica de doença de Chagas. Rev. Inst. Adolfo Lutz, S. Paulo, 15:194-222.

Menezes, H. 1966. A importância do fator sexo na parasitemia e mortalidade de camundongos albinos com infecção experimental pelo *Trypanosoma cruzi*. Hospital (Rio de Janeiro), 70:991-994.

Miller, H., and W. H. Abelmann. 1967. Effects of dietary ethanol upon experimental trypanosomal (*T. cruzi*) myocarditis. Proc. Soc. Exp. Biol. Med., 126:193-198.

Moura Gonçalves, J. 1958. Complexo polissacaridopolipéptido de *Trypanosoma cruzi*. Proceedings of the Sixth International Congress on Tropical Medicine and Malaria (Lisbon), Vol. 3, pp. 246-247.

Muniz, J. 1962. Imunidade na doença de Chagas. Mem. Inst. Oswaldo Cruz, 60:103-147.

——— 1967. De l'emploi de la technique de double diffusion en tube (Oakley et Fulthorp) pour l'analyse des cultures de *Schizotrypanum cruzi* en développement. C.R. Soc. Biol. (Paris), 161:492-495.

——— 1967. Contribuição para um melhor conhecimento da ação patogênica do *S. cruzi* no organismo humano. Hospital (Rio de Janeiro), 72:675-700.

——— and G. de Freitas. 1945. Estudo sôbre o determinismo da transformação das formas sanguícolas do *Schizotrypanum cruzi* em critidias. I. Da existência de um fator responsável por essa metamorfose. Rev. Brasil. Med., 2:995-998.

——— and G. de Freitas. 1946. Realização "in vitro" do ciclo de *S. cruzi* no vertebrado, em meios de caldo-líquido peritonial. Rev. Brasil. Biol., 6:467-484.

——— and A. P. de Azevedo. 1950. Nôvo conceito da patogenia da doença de Chagas (Trypanosomiasis americana). Primera Reunión Panamericano Enfermedad de Chagas, Vol. 1, pp. 55-56.

——— and J. Gomes de Souza. 1959. Da ação anticomplementar dos antigenos constituídos por formas de cultivo do *S. cruzi*. Congreso Internacional sôbre Doença de Chagas, Rio de Janeiro. Resumo dos trabalhos, pp. 61-63.

——— R. R. L. Soares, S. Batista, and L. Quiroga. 1953. Evolução da imunidade humoral em cães infectados experimentalmente pelo *S. cruzi*. Rev. Brasil. Malar., 5:197-200.

Nattan-Larrier, L. 1921. Hérédité des infections expérimentales à *Schizotrypanum cruzi*. Bull. Soc. Path. Exot., 14:232-238.

Nussenzweig, V., V. Amato Neto, J. L. Pedreita de Freitas, and R. Sonntag. 1955. Moléstia de Chagas em bancos de sangue. Rev. Hosp. Clin. Fac. Med. Univ. S. Paulo, 10:265-283.

Packchanian, A. 1952. Purification of serologically active principles, particularly protein and polysaccharides, from *Trypanosoma cruzi*. Fed. Proc., 11:477-478.

Pan, C. T. 1968. Cultivation of the leishmaniform state of *Trypanosoma cruzi* in cell-free media at different temperatures. Amer. J. Trop. Med. Hyg., 14:823-832.

Passalacqua, C. de S. P., V. Amato Neto, I. Zata, and A. Damasco. 1953. Incidência da doença de Chagas entre candidatos a doadores de un banco de sangue de São Paulo. Inquérito sorológico. Hospital (Rio de Janeiro), 43:443-447.

Pedreira de Freitas, J. L. 1948. Dados atuais sôbre a distribuição de triatomídeos e moléstia de Chagas na Delegacia de Saúde de Sorocaba. Arq. Hig. Saúde Pública (S. Paulo), 13:93-96.

——— 1950. Reação de fixação do complemento para diagnóstico da moléstia de Chagas pela técnica quantitativa. Folia Clin. Biol. S. Paulo, 16:192-198.

——— 1951. Orientação para o diagnóstico das formas crônicas de moléstia de Chagas. Arch. Argent. Hig. Salúd Pública, 16:55.

——— 1952. Reação de fixação do complemento para diagnóstico da moléstia de Chagas pela técnica quantitativa; vantagens do método a sua aplicação em saúde publica. Hospital (Rio de Janeiro), 41:257-267.

——— 1960. Importancia de la enfermedad de Chagas para le salud publica. Bol. Ofic. Sanit. Panamer., 49:552-562.

——— 1961. Reação de fixação do complemento para diagnóstico da Moléstia de Chagas. An. Congr. Internac. Doença de Chagas, 2:557-569.

———— V. Amato Neto, A. Nesti, U. de Andrade e Silva, and F. X. Lima. 1950. Resultados de um inquérito sôbre moléstia de Chagas realizado no município de São Carlos (Estado de São Paulo, Brasil) e arredores. Folia Clin. Biol. S. Paulo, 16:150-157.

———— V. Amato Neto, and F. Fujioka. 1955. Reação de fixação do complemento com antigeno de Trypanosoma cruzi em transudatos. Hospital (Rio de Janeiro), 47:57-59.

Pellegrino, J. 1947. Influência de injeção intravenosa de antigeno de Schizotrypanum cruzi sôbre o electrocardiograma de cães na fase crônica da doença de Chagas experimental. Mem. Inst. Oswaldo Cruz, 45:521-535.

———— and S. S. Mesquita. 1947. A reação de fixação do complemento na doença de Chagas. I. Nota sôbre falsas reações positivas e duvidosas feitas com antigeno de cultura de "Schizotrypanum cruzi" em soros conservados em geladeira. Brasil-Med., 61:396-401.

———— and Z. Brener. 1951. A reação de precipitina com a fração polisacarídea isolada de formas de cultura de Leishmania brasiliensis e do Schizotrypanum cruzi na Leishmania tegumentar americana. Arq. Hig. Saúde Pública (S. Paulo), 2:56-62.

———— and Z. Brener. 1952. A reação de fixação do complemento na doença de Chagas. II. Observações sôbre o antigeno de Davis. Hospital (Rio de Janeiro), 42:423-434.

———— and Z. Brener. 1952. A reação de fixação do complemento na doença de Chagas. III. Observações sôbre as propriedades da fração polissacarídea isolada de formas de cultura do Schizotrypanum cruzi. Hospital (Rio de Janeiro), 42:553-559.

———— and Z. Brener. 1952. A reação de fixação do complemento na doença de Chagas. IV. Observações feitas em casos agudos de esquizotripanose. Hospital (Rio de Janeiro), 42:755-761.

———— and Z. Brener. 1952. A reação de fixação do complemento com antigeno de forma de cultura do Schizotrypanum cruzi na leishmaniose tegumentar americana. Hospital (Rio de Janeiro), 42:971-980.

———— and Z. Brener. 1953. A reação de precipitina com a fração polissacarídea isolada de formas de cultura do Schizotrypanum cruzi na infecção chagásica experimental no cão. Hospital (Rio de Janeiro), 43:113-117.

———— and Z. Brener. 1953. A reação de fixação do complemento com antigeno de formas de cultura do Schizotrypanum cruzi na doença de Chagas experimental no cão. Hospital (Rio de Janeiro), 43:481-483.

———— Z. Brener, and R. Jacomo. 1956. A reação de precipitina na fase aguda da doença de Chagas. Rev. Brasil. Malar., 8:246-252.

Peñalver, L. M., M. I. Rodriguez, M. Bloch, and G. Sancho. 1957. Tripanosomiasis en El Salvador. Trabajo presentado en el Séptimo Congreso Medico Centroamericano, Managua, Nicaragua.

Pera, J. S. 1951. O diagnóstico da cardiopatia crônica chagásica. Rev. Brasil. Med., 8:790-796.

Perez, L. 1962. La reacción de fijación del complemento. Su utilidad para el diagnostico en los crónicos de enfermedad de Chagas-Mazza. Rev. Fac. Med. Tucumán, 5:61-90.

Perez Reyes, R. 1950. Diferenciación serologica de algunas especies de la familia Trypanosomidae. Rev. Palud. Med. Trop. Mexico, 2:1-22.

Pifano, C. F. 1964. Aspectos de medicina tropical en Venezuela. Temas de catedra. Imprenta universitaria. Organizacion de Vienestar Estudiantil (OBE) Universidad Central, Caracas, Venezuela.

Pifano, F. 1954. El diagnostico parasitologico de la enfermedad de Chagas en fase cronica. Arch Venez. Patol. Trop. Parasit. Med., 2:121-156.

———— 1960. Algunos aspectos de la enfermedad de Chagas en Venezuela. Arch. Venez. Med. Trop. Parasit. Med., 3:73-99.

———— and G. Marcuzzi. 1950. Contribuición al estudio experimental de las miocardiopatias parasitarias de la region neotropico. Investigaciones histopatologicas sobre el miocardio de ratones blancos infectados experimentalmente con Schizotrypanosoma cruzi y Schistosoma mansoni, sometidos a dietas carentes en Vitamina B, y Factor P. P. Arch. Venez. Patol. Trop. Parasit. Med., 2:175-182.

Pittaluga, G. 1938. Les fonctions et les maladies du systeme reticulo-endothelial. Bruxelles-Med., 18:330-343.

Pizzi, P. T., and S. J. Chemke. 1955. Acción de la cortisona sobre la infección experimental de la rata por Trypanosoma cruzi. Biologica (Santiago), 21:31-58.

Pizzi, T. 1950. Trypanosoma cruzi y tumores: Revisión critica. Bol. Chile. Parasit., 5:10-12.

———— 1953. Sobre el problema de las formas delgadas de *Trypanosoma cruzi* (comunicación preliminar). Bol. Inform. Parasit. Chile., 8:26-30.

———— M. Rubio, and F. Knierim. 1954. Inmunologia de la enfermedad de Chagas. Bol. Chile. Parasit., 9:35-47.

Prager, R. 1953. Acción de la cortisona del acetato de cortisona y del cortone sobre el consumo de oxigeno de formas de cultivo de *Trypanosoma cruzi*. Bol. Chile. Parasit., 8:52-53.

Ramos, J., J. L. Pedreira de Freitas, and S. Borges. 1949. Moléstia de Chagas. Estudo clínico e epidemiológico. Arq. Brasil. Cardiol., 2:111-162.

Rezende, C. L., J. de Pellegrino, Z. Brener, and A. Canelas. 1954. Sôbre a transmissão transplacentária de infecção chagásica humana. Comportamento da reação de fixação do complemento com antigeno de *S. cruzi* em filhos de portadores de esquizotripanose na fase crônica. J. Pediat., 19:21-26.

Rodhain, J., and R. Resseler. 1947. Ensayo de diferenciación serológica entre tripanosomas y esquizotripanosomas. Med. Colon. (Madrid), 9:173-186.

Rodrigues da Silva, J., and Genaro de Queiroz. 1960. Investigações sôbre a doença de Chagas no Distrito Federal. Inquérito sorológicos entre acadêmicos de medicina. J. Brasil. Med., 2:483-488.

———— and Genaro de Queiroz. 1963. Investigações sôbre a doença de Chagas no Distrito Federal. Inquérito sorológico entre acadêmicos de medicina. An. Congresso Internac. Doença de Chagas, 4:1511-1516.

Romaña, C. 1960. Aplicacion de la techica de Kolmer-Boerner modificada a la reaccion de fijacion de complemento para el diagnostico de la enfermedad de Chagas. An. Inst. Med. Regional (Resistencia), 5:47-54.

———— 1963. Enfermedad de Chagas. Buenos Aires, Imprenta Lopez S. R. L.

———— and M. Conejos. 1946. Intradermo-reaccion con antigeno de *S. cruzi* en la leishmania tegumentaria americana. An. Inst. Med. Regional, 1:289-296.

———— and M. S. de Romaña. 1957. Valor comparativo de la reacción de fijación de complemento y del xenodiagnostico en un grupo de chagasicos crónicos. An. Inst. Med. Regional, 4:245-254.

Rosenbaum, M. B., A. J. Alverez, and J. A. Cerisola. 1957. El peligro de transmisión de la enfermedad de Chagas por transfusión sanguinea. Prensa Med. Argent., 44:3305-3308.

Roskin, G., and K. Romanova. 1936. Untersuchung über die Einwirkung der Protozoentoxine auf die Zellen maligner Geschwülste. Z. Krebsforschung, 44:375-383.

———— 1939. L'action des toxines sur le cancer expérimental. Acta Medica URSS, 2:138-144.

———— and K. Romanova. 1937. Traitement du cancer expérimental par les endotoxines des protozoaires. Bull. Biol. Med. Exp., 3:145-148.

———— and K. G. Romanova. 1938. Étude de l'action therapeutique des endotoxines des protozoaires sur le cancer experimental. Bull. Biol. Med. Exp., 6:118-120.

———— and K. Romanova. 1938-1939. Traitement du cancer expérimental par les endotoxines des protozoaires. Arch. Internat. Med. Exp., 13:379-384.

Rotberg, A. 1952. Contribuição para o estudo da alergia na leishmaniose tegumentar americana. Rev. Hosp. N.S. Aparecida, 5:1-88.

Rubio, U. M. 1954. Estudio de los factores que intervienen en la virulencia de una cepa de *Trypanosoma cruzi*. Acción de la cortisona en la capacidad de invasion y multiplicación del parasito. Biologica (Santiago), 20:89-125.

———— 1955. Influência de acetato de cortisona sobre la inoculencia y localización tisular de une nueva cepa de *Trypanosoma cruzi*. Estudio de la persistencia de los cambios observados. Biologica (Santiago), 21:75-89.

———— 1959. Natural and acquired immunity against *Trypanosoma cruzi* in the hamster (*Cricetus auratus*). Biol. Trab. Inst. Biol. Juan Noe Fac. Med. Univ. Chile, 27/28:95-116.

Salgado, F. 1947. Tratamento do câncer com a endotoxina do *Trypanosoma cruzi*. Rev. Brasil. Med., 4:385.

Sassen, F. A., and I. C. Arnt. 1959. A doença de Chagas no Rio Grande do Sul. Rev. Med. Rio Grande do Sul., 15:133-142.

Seneca, H. 1963. American trypanosomiasis or Chagas' disease. An. Congr. Internac. Doença de Chagas, 4:1485-1497.

Senekjie, H. A. 1943. Serological studies on American trypanosomiasis. Abstr. Theses Tulane Univ., 44:27.

———— 1943. Biochemical reactions. Cultural characteristics and growth requirements of *Trypanosoma cruzi*. Amer. J. Trop. Med., 23:523-531.

Serravalle, A. 1963. Contribuição ao estudo de serologia da doença de Chagas. An. Congr. Internac. Doença de Chagas, 4:1505-1509.

Shaw, J. J., and A. Voller. 1963. Preliminary fluorescent antibody studies on *Endotrypanum schaudinni*. Trans. Roy. Soc. Trop. Med. Hyg., 57:232-233.

———— and A. Voller. 1964. The detection of circulating antibody to Kala-azar by means of immunofluorescent techniques. Trans. Roy. Soc. Trop. Med. Hyg., 58:349-352.

Silva, I. I. 1954. Metodo de cultivo del *Trypanosoma (Schizotrypanum) cruzi* para la preparación de antigenos. An. Inst. Med. Regional (Tucuman), 4:71-75.

Silva, T. L. da, and O. Unti. 1952. Epidemiologia e profilazia da molestia de Chagas no Estado de Sao Paulo. Arq. Hig. Saúde Pública, (S. Paulo), 17:83-90.

Siqueira, A. F. de. 1964. Comparação de antigenos de *Trypanosoma cruzi* para reações quantitativas de fixação do complemento. Rev. Inst. Med. Trop. S. Paulo, 6:268-276.

———— J. Ferriolli, and J. Carvalheiro. 1966. Un antigeno soluvel presente no soro de ratos infetados com *Trypanosoma cruzi*. Nota Previa. Rev. Inst. Med. Trop. S. Paulo, 8:148.

Souza, S. L. de, and M. E. Camargo. 1966. The use of filter paper blood smears in a practical fluorescent test for American trypanosomiasis serodiagnosis. Rev. Inst. Med. Trop. S. Paulo, 8:255-258.

Strejan, G. 1965. Antibody heterogeneity to *Trypanosoma cruzi*. Experientia, 21:399.

Talice, R. V., F. Pick, and L. Perez Moreira. 1954. Tentativas de bioterapia por *T. cruzi* en casos humanos de tumores malignos; inoculación de *Trypanosoma cruzi* por via intraperitoneal en un caso de linfosarcoma de localizacion primaria mesenterica. An. Fac. Univ. Repub., Montevideo, 39:207-224.

———— S. Verissimos, J. J. Osimani, and M. E. Franca. 1952. Estudio epidemiologico sobre la enfermedad de Chagas de la zona endemica del Uruguay. Bol. Ofic. Sanit. Panamer., 33:595-620.

Taratuto, A. L., J. F. Yanovsky, G. A. Schumuñis, O. C. Traversa, S. M. Gonzalez-Cappa, and A. S. Parodi. 1968. Histopathology in Rockland mice immunized against American trypanosomiasis (Chagas' disease). Amer. J. Trop. Med. Hyg., 17:716-723.

Thiermann, E., G. Niedmann, and F. Naquira. 1958. *Toxoplasma* dye test and complement fixation test in 169 blood samples from individuals with Chagas infection. Biol. Trab. Inst. Biol. Juan Noe Fac. Med. Univ. Chile, 26:51-59.

Torrealba, J. F., and B. Italia Ramos. 1962. Otra nota sobre extracto de protozoarios y cancer. Gac. Med. Caracas, 70:213-242.

———— R. V. Pieretti, I. Ramos, A. Diaz Vazquez, and O. H. Pieretti. 1958. Encuesta sobre enfermedad de Chagas en la Penitenciaria General de Venezuela. Examin de 62 reclusos. Gac. Med. Caracas, 67:19-58.

———— C. de Roys, and B. Italia Ramos. 1962. Otra nota sobre extractos de protozoarios. Gac. Med. Caracas, 70:291-297.

Torres, C. M., and E. Duarte. 1948. Miocardite na forma aguda da doença de Chagas. Mem. Inst. Oswaldo Cruz, 46:749-793.

———— and B. M. Taveres. 1958. Miocardite no macaco *Cebus* após inoculações repetidas com *Schizotrypanum cruzi*. Mem. Inst. Oswaldo Cruz, 56:85-152.

Ucros Guzman, H., and C. Gerlein. 1953. Desviación del complemento en la trypanosomiasis americana. An. Soc. Biol. Bogota, 5:245-254.

———— and C. Gerlein. 1954. Desviación del complemento en la enfermedad de Chagas. An. Soc. Biol. Bogota, 6:85-89.

Unti, O., T. L. Da Silva, and A. A. deAguiar. 1952. Alguns dados sôbre a reação de Machado & Guerreiro na infância. Arq. Hig. Saúde Pública (S. Paulo), 17:529-534.

VanThiel, P. H. 1964. L'antagonisme entre *Trypanosoma cruzi* et *Spirillum minis*. Ann. Soc. Belg. Med. Trop., 44:347-351.

Voller, A. 1963. Immunofluorescent observations on *Trypanosoma cruzi,* Trans. Roy. Soc. Trop. Med. Hyg., 57:232.

Werner, H. 1954. Über die Frage der placentaren Trypanosomen-Infektionen und Übertragung von Trypanosomen und Antikörpern durch die Milch auf das Neugeborene. Z. Tropenmed. Parasit., 5:422-442.

Wood, F. D. 1934. Experimental studies on *Trypanosoma cruzi* in California. Proc. Soc. Exp. Biol. Med., 32:61-62.

Yanovsky, J. F., S. M. Gonzalez-Cappa, and H. J. Garavelli. 1967. Nouvelle réaction pour le diagnostic de la trypanosomiase americaine (maladie de Chagas). C. R. Soc. Biol. (Paris), 161:2066-2067.

Zeiss, H. 1920. Die Einwirkung menschlichen Serum auf menschenpathogene Trypanosomen. Arch. Schiffs. Tropen. Hyg., 24:73-92.

Zil'berblat, G. S., and A. S. Skorikova. 1963. A study on the activity of some lysate fractions of *Trypanosoma* cruzi in malignant cell suspensions (In Russian). Antibiotiki, 8:1040-1045.

Nonpathogenic Trypanosomes
of Rodents

PHILIP A. D'ALESANDRO

The Rockefeller University, New York, New York

INTRODUCTION

Trypanosomes of rodents comprise a large group of parasites with a cosmopolitan distribution. More than 80 species have been described (Davis, 1952; Galuzo and Novinskaya, 1961). With the exception of a few species, little is known about their life histories and host immunologic responses. The simi-

* Although not a rodent trypanosome, this species is included for comparative purposes.

larities of members of this group suggest, however, that they are very closely related. Comparisons of *Trypanosoma lewisi*, *T. duttoni*, *T. sigmodoni*, and *T. zapi*, the most studied species, have shown that although interesting differences in life histories occur, these are but variations on a basic theme. Therefore, it will probably be found that the considerable information now available on a few species is generally applicable to the whole group. It has been suggested, in fact, that all these parasites are really members of the same species and have adapted over many years to different rodent hosts (Roudsky, 1910b; Wenyon, 1926).

The most striking immunologic feature of rodent trypanosome infections is the host's control of parasitemia by inhibiting the reproduction of the parasites. This feature, perhaps more than any, distinguishes the group from all other trypanosomes and accounts for the usually benign or nonpathogenic nature of the infection. But it should be remembered that the term "nonpathogenic" does not pertain to all infections with rodent trypanosomes. In very young animals, for example, or under conditions of stress, infections may terminate fatally because of an inadequate immune response. On the other hand, the "pathogenic" African trypanosomes are frequently fatal in man and certain domestic animals, but they appear to show no pathogenicity in many wild game animals (Wenyon, 1926; Taliaferro, 1929; Ashcroft et al., 1959; Desowitz, 1960). Therefore, in both groups nonpathogenic infections occur, but it is not yet known whether these have a similar immunologic basis.

In the next section, *T. lewisi*, the most studied species of the group, will be discussed first in terms of the course of infection, acquired and innate immunity, other factors affecting the immune response, and host specificity. Other, less studied species will then be considered and compared with *T. lewisi*. In this way, using *T. lewisi* as a standard, the group as a whole can be more easily understood. Following this, the humoral factors of immunity, both trypanocidal and inhibitory, will be treated in detail, since these have been well-studied and appear to be of primary importance in the immune response. Cellular elements will also be mentioned where they are known to play a role. Finally, the reproduction-inhibiting antibody will be discussed at length because more than any other factor, it appears to be responsible for the uniqueness of rodent trypanosome infections. While much is known about the effects of this antibody, it continues to be the subject of controversy, due in part to our still incomplete knowledge of its mode of action.

LIFE CYCLES AND THE COURSE OF INFECTION IN THE VERTEBRATE HOST

Intermediate hosts are known for only several rodent trypanosomes (Wenyon, 1926; Davis, 1952). But in each case, the vector is a flea, and cyclical development is presumed to be similar to that of *T. lewisi* in the rat flea as described by Minchin and Thomson (1915). After ingestion in infected blood, the parasites undergo cyclical development in the stomach and rectum, and after several days infective (metacyclic) trypanosomes appear in the latter location. Infection of the vertebrate host occurs by ingestion of infected fleas or their feces. The trypanosomes then pass to the blood stream where they become established and develop extracellularly. Experimentally, infections can also be initiated by direct inoculation of infected blood.

Trypanosoma lewisi of the rat

This species was one of the first rodent trypanosomes to be discovered, being first noted over 100 years ago (*see* Laveran and Mesnil, 1912). Because of its wide distribution, accessibility, and ease of maintenance, it has been extensively studied and is considered the type species of the group.

Course of infection and acquired immunity. Differences in duration of the reproductive period, intensity and length of the parasitemia, and host response occur depending upon the strain of *T. lewisi* studied and other variables. Common features are evident, however, and Figure 1, from the work of

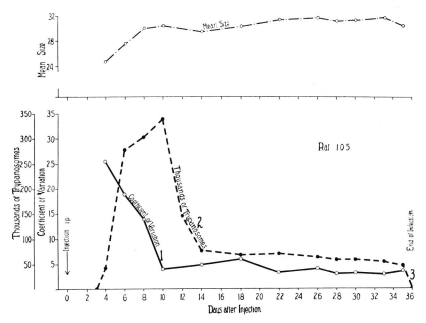

FIG. 1. A normal course of infection with *Trypanosoma lewisi* in the blood of the rat showing changes in parasite mean size, the coefficient of variation (CV), and numbers of parasites per cu mm of blood. The numerals indicate the three primary manifestations of acquired host immunity: (1) inhibition of reproduction by ablastin as reflected by the drop in the CV, (2) the first crisis in which the majority of the trypanosomes is destroyed by a trypanocidal antibody, and (3) the terminal crisis caused by a second trypanocidal antibody. (From Taliaferro. 1926. *J. Exp. Zool.*, 43:433.)

Taliaferro (1926), illustrates these. After an incubation period, the length of which depends upon the size of the inoculum (Augustine, 1941), parasites appear in the peripheral blood and show marked reproductive activity. After a sharp rise, the parasitemia reaches a peak between the seventh and tenth day. During this period, the intensity of reproduction is measured by determining the percentage of division forms* or by the more sensitive coefficient of variation (CV) method, which provides a statistical index of reproductive activity (Taliaferro and Taliaferro, 1922). The trypanosomes reproduce by multiple fission and show great variability in length during active multiplication. The CV is a measure of this variability. Thus, when it is high (about 25 percent) reproduction is intense; when it is low (about 3 to 5 percent) reproduction has ceased, and the parasites become extremely uniform in size, a so-called adult or inhibited population. As the parasitemia increases, the CV falls, indicating reduced reproductive activity caused by a reproduction-inhibiting antibody (Taliaferro, 1924). About the tenth day, when reproduction has virtually ceased (CV equaling 3 to 5 percent) due to the rising titer of the reproduction-inhibiting antibody (Coventry, 1925), a crisis occurs in which most of the parasites are killed by a trypanocidal antibody (Coventry, 1930). The surviving adult trypanosomes are resistant to this antibody, but because of the presence of the reproduction-inhibiting antibody they are unable to repopulate the blood. They continue to live in the blood for a period that may range from a few weeks to a few months until they are removed either gradually or suddenly by a second trypanocidal antibody that terminates the infection (Coventry, 1930). Following recovery, immunity is usually solid, sterile, and probably lifelong (Corradetti, 1963).

It has long been observed that reproduction occurs only during the first few days of the infection, after which only nonreproducing adults are found (Rabinowitz and Kempner, 1899; Laveran and Mesnil, 1901; McNeal, 1904; Brown, 1915; Steffan, 1921; Taliaferro, 1924). The marked morphologic changes that reflect this cessation of reproduction are illustrated in Figure 2 (Taliaferro, 1929). The parasites labeled "dividing trypanosomes" and "growth stages" are present during the early reproductive phase before the first crisis. They vary greatly in length (10 to 40μ) and have a high CV. The adult trypanosomes are found during the inhibited nonreproducing phase after the first crisis. Their CV is low and reflects an extreme uniformity in length (28 to 32μ).

That acquired humoral antibodies are responsible for cessation of reproduction and the trypanocidal responses has been well established by passive transfer experiments. Rabinowitz and Kempner (1899) first showed that the serum of recovered rats is protective for newly infected rats. This was later confirmed by Laveran and Mesnil (1900). However, it remained for Coventry (1930) to demonstrate the presence of two distinct trypanocidal antibodies. She found that serum taken after the first crisis is trypanocidal for divi-

---

*As used in this chapter, the term "division forms" refers to trypanosomes that are (1) in the actual process of fission, (2) small forms less than 20μ in length, and (3) broad, developmental forms; in short, those parasites in a reproducing population that are clearly not adults. (See Taliaferro et al., 1931.)

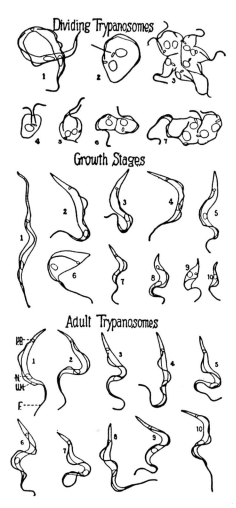

FIG. 2. Morphologic types of *Trypanosoma lewisi* occurring during the course of infection in the blood of the rat. Dividing trypanosomes (top) and growth stages (middle) appear during the early reproductive phase, and adult trypanosomes (bottom) appear later during the nonreproducing phase. Note the large variation in length of the dividing and growth stages and the extreme uniformity of the ablastin-inhibited adults. F—flagellum; N—nucleus; PB—parabasal body (or kinetoplast); UM—undulating membrane. ×1,000. (From Taliaferro. 1929. *The Immunology of Parasitic Infections*, p. 110. Courtesy of Appleton-Century-Crofts.)

sion forms but not for adults, and that serum taken after the terminal crisis is trypanocidal for all stages of the parasite. Taliaferro's (1924) classical experiments provided the first evidence that a true inhibition of reproduction occurs and that it results from an acquired humoral immunity distinct from the trypanocidal responses. He found that in normal rats inoculated with adult trypanosomes plus immune serum obtained from a donor after the first crisis, no reproduction of the parasites occurred; they remained unchanged in the blood at a constant level with a low CV until an actively acquired trypanocidal antibody terminated the infection. In control rats given normal serum, however, the adults began to reproduce, and normal infections resulted. Subsequently, Coventry (1925), using *in vivo* titration methods, demonstrated changes in titer of this reproduction-inhibiting factor during the course of infection. Thus, the titer showed a marked increase between the fifth and sixth day, reached a peak after the first crisis, and declined thereafter. Originally, Taliaferro (1924) called this humoral factor a "reaction product," but on the basis of later work (1932) that revealed its anti-body nature, he gave it the name "ablastin." Further studies by Taliaferro and others have confirmed and extended these observations (Taliaferro, 1938a,b; Culbertson, 1939b; D'Alesandro, 1959; Taliaferro and Pizzi, 1960).

There are, therefore, three distinct manifestations of acquired immunity in the rat (*see* Fig. 1), and all are due to humoral antibodies: (1) ablastin, which inhibits parasite reproduction, (2) a trypanocidal antibody responsible for the first crisis and specific for division forms, and (3) a second trypanoci-dal antibody that terminates the infection by killing adults. As far as can be tested, the titers of these antibodies vary independently (Coventry 1925, 1930; Taliaferro, 1932, 1941). They also have distinguishing physicochemi-cal and immunologic properties that will be discussed in a later section (*see* pp. 713-729).

Immunity to *T. lewisi* results not only from specific infection but also from inocluation with killed or attenuated blood and culture forms and deri-vatives of the parasites. Novy (1907) first reported successful immunization against trypanosomes and used culture forms killed by distilled water lysis in dialyzing sacs. It was later reported that Berkefeld filtrates of lysed cultures are not immunogenic, but that rats receiving one or more injections of living noninfective culture forms developed solid immunities within ten days (Novy et al., 1912). The majority of the animals showed parasites in their blood for 48 hours or less after vaccination, but no increase in numbers occurred. How-ever, when these trypanosomes were isolated, they were found to be nonin-fective for other rats and also failed to grow in culture. Successful immuniza-tion with attenuated culture forms has been reported more recently by Citri (1952) and Dusanic (1968).

Culbertson and Kessler (1939) vaccinated rats with formalin-killed blood-stream forms and obtained strong immunities with only a few injec-tions of antigen. Agglutinins were produced, and there was a rough correla-tion between the agglutinin titer and the degree of resistance to a challenge infection. The efficacy of formalin-killed antigen has been confirmed by Naiman (1944). Thillet and Chandler (1957) immunized rats with "meta-bolic products" produced by blood-stream forms incubated in a normal rat serum-saline mixture for 24 hours at room temperature. This antigen pro-duced better immunity than killed trypanosomes, for after challenge, animals vaccinated with the latter antigen developed light transient infections, whereas those vaccinated with the former were completely resistant. Recently, Sanders and Wallace (1966) used x-irradiated blood forms as vac-cine. The irradiated trypanosomes retained motility and multiplied in cul-ture but were noninfective. One injection with 10^7 parasites irradiated with 49,600 r produced complete immunity, and the authors point out the superi-ority of the irradiated vaccine to the killed vaccine used by Culbertson and Kessler (1939). Although meaningful comparisons of vaccines are not always possible because of inadequate quantitative data in earlier work (e.g., Novy et al., 1912) or unknown differences in strains of *T. lewisi* used, it is reason-able to assume that living attenuated blood or culture forms would produce better immunities than comparable killed materials. The relative effectiveness of metabolic antigens (Thillet and Chandler, 1957) and attenuated parasites has not yet been determined.

It is difficult to assess the roles of ablastin and the trypanocidal antibodies in the immunity produced by vaccines or indeed whether both types of antibody are formed. Frequently upon challenge, no parasites are ever found because they are destroyed so rapidly by hosts with strong immunities, and it is therefore impossible to determine whether ablastin is also present. On the other hand, when the immunity is not complete or when large overwhelming challenging doses are used, abortive or subnormal infections may result. In these cases, even when reduced reproductive activity may be evident and ablastin is therefore presumed to be present, because of the complementary actions of ablastin and the trypanocidal antibodies, it is difficult to determine their relative contributions to the immunity. To identify and quantitate the antibodies, *in vivo* titrations of the type used by Taliaferro (1924, 1932) and Coventry (1925, 1930) with immune serum from infected and recovered rats would have to be made with immune serum from vaccinated animals. This has not yet been done. The significance of experiments of this type, in terms of identification of ablastic and trypanocidal antigens, will be considered later (*see* pp. 724-725).

Under natural conditions, acquired immunity to *T. lewisi* results only from infection and from passive transfer of antibodies from immune mother rats to their nursing young. The latter type has been extensively studied by Culbertson (1938). Very little antibody is transferred *in utero* via the placenta, for the young of immune mothers nursed on normal mothers manifest little or no immunity. On the other hand, the young of normal mothers nursed on immune mothers promptly become resistant, indicating that most of the antibody is passed in the colostrum and milk. Young rats are able to absorb antibody from ingested milk for at least 15 days after birth (Culbertson, 1939a) and lose their acquired immunity within a few weeks after being weaned. It was later shown that mother rats immunized actively with formalin-killed parasites or passively by inoculation of immune serum can also confer resistance to their young (Culbertson, 1939b, 1941b).

Innate immunity as affected by age, sex, and diet. Although strains of *T. lewisi* have been described that produce fatalities in young and old rats alike (Brown, 1914), most strains are generally more pathogenic for young animals, as first reported by Jürgens (1902). Subsequent studies have confirmed this observation. Marmorston-Gottesman et al. (1930) noted that infections in young rats were more severe and at times terminated fatally with marked anemia. Latent *Bartonella* infections were also detected and complicated the results, but older animals showed a greater tolerance to the dual infections and never succumbed. Herrick and Cross (1936) studied *Bartonella*-free animals and recorded death rates of 80 to 90 percent in infected rats 30 days old or younger. Animals 40 days old always survived the infection and showed few if any ill effects. An unexplained observation was that suckling rats, regardless of age, usually survived infection even though the mothers were not immune. Duca (1939) found that over 70 percent of rats 25 days old or younger died from the infection, whereas less than 6 percent of those over 25 days of age died. Both old and young rats showed secondary anemias, but *Bartonella* was not found, leading Duca to postulate the existence of a hemolysin produced by the trypanosomes. Recently, Lincicome and Emejuaiwe (1963) reported higher parasitemias in young weanlings, but fatalities were not mentioned.

Although other factors may play a role in age resistance, the greater susceptibility of young rats to *T. lewisi* appears to result primarily from a poor antibody response. Culbertson and Kessler (1939) found that after immunization with formalin-killed blood forms, young rats less than 25 days old showed feeble agglutinin production and low resistance, sometimes succumbing to challenge infections as readily as nonvaccinated controls. Older rats, in contrast, promptly produced agglutinins and had good immunities. In a later study, Culbertson and Wotton (1939) measured ablastin production indirectly by determining the intensity of reproduction during the course of infection in rats of different ages. Rats 25 days of age or less usually succumbed to the infection and showed division forms with a high CV at the time of death, indicating poor ablastin formation. Older rats controlled parasite reproduction and survived. These results suggest that the greater capacity of older animals to produce antibodies, especially ablastin, is a major factor in age resistance.

Few studies have been made of sexual differences in resistance to *T. lewisi,* and some results are conflicting. Perla (1934) states briefly that female rats are definitely more resistant than males but gives few details. In a recent short note it is reported that parasitemias are greater in young adult males than in comparable female hosts, and that in gonadectomized young adults, sexual differences could not be demonstrated (Lincicome and Emejuaiwe, 1963). Herrick and Cross (1936) found that when young male rats 20 days old were given daily injections of estrogen for two weeks following infection, only 5 percent of the animals died; in contrast, over 80 percent of the controls succumbed. However, Lincicome and Emejuaiwe (1963) report that when normal and gonadectomized young adults were given supplements of homologous sex hormones, the trypanosomes grew better in females. Perla and Marmorston-Gottesman (1930) observed higher parasitemias in bilaterally gonadectomized adult male rats than in normal males, but the duration of the infections was unchanged. In similar experiments, Taliaferro et al. (1931) found castration had no demonstrable effect.

Diet can have a marked effect on resistance to *T. lewisi.* Adult rats fed an adequate diet supplemented with copper or iron or both show higher percentages of abortive and mild infections than controls (Perla, 1934). On the other hand, it was found that young rats fed a milk diet with copper have more severe infections and higher fatalities than animals fed milk alone. A complete explanation is not available, but Perla (1934) suggests that in the latter case, copper may act as a growth factor for the parasites, and in the former may aid hemoglobin synthesis thus countering secondary anemia.

Biotin-deficient rats have a lowered resistance to *T. lewisi*, and infections frequently terminate fatally when deficiencies are severe (Caldwell and György, 1943, 1947). Reproductive periods are prolonged, and there are delays in the crises, indicating lowered production of ablastin and the trypanocidal antibodies. These effects can be negated in moderately deficient hosts by the administration of biotin. Reduced ablastin formation has also been observed in pantothenate-deficient rats (Becker et al., 1943, 1947; Taylor and Becker, 1948). Recently, Lincicome and Shepperson (1965) reported enhanced parasitemias in thiamine-deficient hosts. Although all infections terminated fatally, it was observed that infected deficient animals survived about one week longer than uninfected deficient controls. The generally adverse effects of vitamin deficiencies on antibody formation in rats and other vertebrates is well known (*see* Axelrod and Pruzansky, 1955; Raffel, 1961).

Other factors affecting the immune response of the rat to *T. lewisi*— *Splenectomy and blockade of the reticuloendothelial system.* In the rat, the spleen forms a relatively large part of the reticuloendothelial system and plays an important role in antibody formation and phagocytosis. Consequently, splenectomy, blockade, or other stress factors that depress the reticuloendothelial system can interfere with the immune response and have an adverse effect on the course of infection. Regendanz and Kikuth (1927) first showed that ablastin formation is reduced by splenectomy. They found that parasite reproductive periods lasted several days longer than normally in splenectomized rats. In some cases reproduction never ceased, and infections terminated fatally. In a later study, Rengendanz (1932) confirmed these results and concluded that splenectomy alone can induce severe or fatal infections. Similar results were obtained by Perla and Marmorston-Gottesman (1930), but their studies, like those of Regendanz and Kikuth (1927), were complicated by the presence of latent concomitant *Bartonella* infections. Thus, they obtained 30 percent mortality in splenectomized adult rats with *Bartonella* alone, but mortalities increased to 100 percent when the *Bartonella*-infected rats were inoculated with *T. lewisi* seven days after splenectomy. Inoculation 48 days after splenectomy sharply reduced fatalities, but the intensity and duration of the parasitemias were greater than normal, indicating a reduced antibody response. Similarly enhanced parasitemias, but without fatalities, were reported recently by Haleem and Minton (1966). However, no mention was made of the time of splenectomy or whether the animals were *Bartonella*-free. Schwetz (1931) splenectomized rats during infection, and although division forms reappeared in some animals, he considered the effect doubtful.

Because latent *Bartonella* infections complicated the results of the early studies, the effects of splenectomy were re-examined by Taliaferro et al. (1931) in *Bartonella*-free and *Bartonella*-infected rats. Their thorough, carefully controlled, and definitive study showed that splenectomy alone does not have a marked effect on ablastin formation. They found that in young *Bartonella*-free rats, splenectomy may lengthen the reproductive phase of the parasites by a few days, but only if performed on the day of infection or within a few days after infection. Splenectomy at other times has little if any effect. In a few cases where ablastin formation was significantly reduced in splenectomized rats, additional stress factors such as paratyphoid infections and gestation were observed. In contrast, splenectomy of young *Bartonella*-infected rats can markedly lessen ablastin production if performed on the day of infection or within five to ten days after infection. The effect is slight if performed six days before infection or 21 days or later after infection. In some cases infections terminated fatally with the dual stress of *Bartonella* and splenectomy. A combination of India ink blockade and splenectomy was also found to interfere with ablastin formation.

Although splenectomy has little effect on ablastin production in *Bartonella*-free rats, it interferes more markedly with the formation of the terminal trypanocidal antibody as shown by Taliaferro et al. (1931), who observed infections of greater than normal duration in splenectomized animals. The delay in termination of infection was somewhat more pronounced in splenectomized *Bartonella*-infected rats.

The pathogenic infections with *T. lewisi* in splenectomized rats reported by Regendanz and Kikuth (1927), Linton (1929), Vassiliadis (1930), and Perla and Marmorston-Gottesman (1930) were undoubtedly due to the additional stress imposed by concurrent *Bartonella* infections. Taliaferro et al. (1931) found that all the splenectomized animals that died in their experiments either had *Bartonella* infections or, if *Bartonella*-free, had paratyphoid infections. Therefore, splenectomy alone does not induce fatal infections in healthy *T. lewisi*-infected rats or seriously impair the host immune response. However, when an additional stress factor such as *Bartonella* or paratyphoid infection, India ink blockade, or gestation is imposed on splenectomized animals, the host-parasite balance may be so disturbed that severe or fatal infections ensue.

X-irradiation.   The adverse effect of x-irradiation on acquired immunity is well known. Resistance is lowered because of injury to the phagocytic mechanism, depressed antibody synthesis, and destruction of lymphocytes that form a mesenchymal reserve from which macrophages and antibody-forming cells are derived (*see* Taliaferro and Taliaferro, 1951; Leone, 1962; Taliaferro et al., 1964). Naiman (1944) first demonstrated that total body irradiation alters the course of *T. lewisi* infections in rats. Her animals were given 300 to 500 r of x-rays on the day of infection and developed parasitemias two to eight times greater than normal. Ablastin production was markedly reduced, especially in young rats, which sometimes died of the infection, and formation of trypanocidal antibodies was affected as indicated by the prolonged duration of the elevated parasitemias. Irradiated animals also responded poorly to formalin-killed vaccine, but they were as well protected by passively transferred immune serum as normal controls. Elevated parasitemias in irradiated rats have been reported more recently by Jaroslow (1959), Herbert and Becker (1961), and Tempelis and Lysenko (1965). Infections frequently terminated fatally except in the experiments of the latter authors, who used lower doses of x-rays. Herbert and Becker (1961) attempted to reduce acquired immunity by irradiating recovered rats, but they found that animals so treated resisted reinfection. Similarly, Naiman (1944) could not induce relapses in recovered rats by irradiation, nor could Tempelis and Lysenko (1965) cause further interference with the production or action of ablastin and trypanocidal antibodies by subjecting their animals to a second dose of irradiation during the course of infection. Therefore, once a sufficient protective antibody level is attained, irradiation has little effect on the host-parasite balance, for it is known that the relatively low levels of x-rays that cause cell damage have no effect on formed antibody (*see* Luzzio, 1960; Taliaferro et al., 1964).

The elevated parasitemias observed in x-irradiated rats do not result from an increased reproductive rate. As first reported by Naiman (1944) and later confirmed by others (Jaroslow, 1959; Tempelis and Lysenko, 1965), the highest percentage of division forms attained in irradiated animals is similar to that observed in normal infections. The reproductive period may be extended because of delayed ablastin production, and this probably contributes to the elevated parasitemias, but more importantly, there is interference with the trypanocidal response. This probably results in part from damage to macrophages and, to a greater extent, from reduced production of trypanocidal antibodies, since Tempelis and Lysenko (1965) have shown that agglutinins are delayed in appearance and are of low titer in irradiated rats. Since the reproductive rate of *T. lewisi* is not enhanced in radiation-injured rats, this means that the trypanosomes reproduce at a maximal rate in normal hosts. Therefore, the rat appears to have no natural resistance to the reproduction of the parasites. This was first pointed out by Taliaferro and Pavlinova (1936), who used splenectomy and blockade to depress the reticuloendothelial system, and it is in contrast to mice infected with *T. duttoni*, which will be considered in a later section.

Intercurrent infections.   Dual infections with *T. lewisi* and another agent can have effects that range from beneficial to lethal. The most common partner is *Bartonella*, which is frequently latent in otherwise normal rats (Marmorston-Gottesman and Perla, 1930). In dual infections with this agent and *T. lewisi* as noted earlier, fatalities are common in young animals. Splenomegaly, anemia, and other pathologic symptoms frequently occur in young and adult rats alike. *T. lewisi* infection is thus similar in effect to splenectomy in that by imposing an additional stress on the host, latent *Bartonella* is activated (Marmorston-Gottesman et al., 1930).

Mixed infections with *T. lewisi* and pathogenic species of trypanosomes have been studied, but each species appears to have no effect on the development of the other, and the outcome is always fatal. Vassiliadis and Jadin (1930), for example, found that rats infected with *T. rhodesiense* alone died as quickly as rats infected with *T. lewisi* and *T. rhodesiense*. Together, the trypanosomes developed as they did in single infections. Similar results have been reported by Grillo and Schmitz (1935) in mixed infections with *T. lewisi* and *T. brucei*. In a more recent study, Tate (1951) infected rats with *T. equinum* at various intervals of up to six weeks after infection with *T.*

lewisi and found that animals with dual infections died as rapidly as those infected with *T. equinum* alone. Thus, antibody to *T. lewisi* present at the time of infection with *T. equinum* had no protective effect.

Infection with either *T. lewisi* or *Plasmodium berghei* is seldom fatal except in very young rats. In mixed infections, however, fatalities are frequent, even among older animals. Hughes and Tatum (1956b) reported 50 percent mortality in their experiments and found that both parasitemias, especially the malaria, were significantly increased in dual infections. In contrast, Jackson (1959) found that the two parasites did not significantly alter each other's course of infection, but did obtain a high mortality rate (68 percent), which he ascribed to very severe anemia. *P. berghei*, therefore, produces an effect similar to that of *Bartonella*.

Dual infections with *T. lewisi* and certain helminths are not fatal and appear to have no serious effects on the host. Ashley (1962) studied concurrent infections with *Nippostrongylus brasiliensis* and found that the trypanosome parasitemias followed a normal course and had no effect on the development of immunity to the worms. Rats with dual infections gained less weight and sometimes appeared to be in poorer condition than rats infected with worms alone, but host resistance was maintained. Rigby and Chobotar (1966) made a similar study of rats infected with *T. lewisi* and *Hymenolepis diminuta*. Host weight gains were not affected, and the trypanosomes showed a normal course of development. However, tapeworm growth was stunted. Since *H. diminuta* is a strictly intestinal parasite, the authors suggest that the trypanosomes have an indirect effect that may result from cross-reactions of worm antigens with antibodies to the trypanosomes, altered nutritive factors, or nonspecific stimulation of host defenses.

Spirillum minus infection in rats can have an antagonistic action toward *T. lewisi*. Tate (1951) found that when rats were infected with *T. lewisi* two to four weeks after inoculation with *S. minus*, the development of the trypanosomes was suppressed, and slight or subpatent infections resulted. Nevertheless, specific immunity to the trypanosomes developed, and the rats were resistant to reinfection. The nature of the antagonistic effect of the spirochetes is unknown. Tate (1951) suggests that trypanosomes are killed in some way by the spirochetes and then act antigenically to induce a specific immunity. Thus, the *S. minus* infections may act in a manner analogous to subcurative doses of trypanocidal drugs. Many pathogenic species of trypanosomes are also suppressed in mixed infections with spirochetes (*see* Goble and Singer, 1960).

Treatment with drugs, cortisone, and endotoxin.   Becker and Gallagher (1947) first demonstrated that sodium salicylate, administered by stomach tube, interferes with the ablastic response. In rats so treated, the parasite reproductive phase is prolonged, parasitemias are exalted, and infections may terminate fatally. Later studies have confirmed these findings (Becker and Lysenko, 1948; Saul and Becker, 1949; Lysenko, 1951; Zwisler and Lysenko, 1954; Meyers and Lysenko, 1956). Barnes (1951) has shown that in addition to sodium salicylate, salicylic acid and several of its derivatives can have an antiablastic effect. But in more recent studies, Becker (1961a,b) found that the *meta* and *para* isomers of salicylic acid, as well as certain dihydroxybenzoic acids, have no effect on the ablastic response. However, 2,4-dihydroxybenzoic acid antagonized the action of salicylic acid, for when these drugs were administered simultaneously, the activity of the salicylic acid was reversed, and reductions in parasitemias occurred. The antagonism is difficult to explain since the dihydroxy acid had no observable effect on parasitemias when administered alone. Treatment with sodium salicylate also delays the appearance of agglutinins to *T. lewisi* (Meyers and Lysenko, 1953).

Salicylates can diminish immune responses either by interfering with antibody production or antigen-antibody reactions (*see* Schwartz and Andre, 1962; Austen, 1963; Ambrose, 1966). Lysenko (1951) could find no evidence that salicylate combines with ablastin. Similarly, the addition of salicylate to immune sera from untreated animals has no effect on the titers of agglutinins to *T. lewisi* (Meyers and Lysenko, 1953), nor is the reinfection of immune salicylate-treated rats easily achieved (Becker and Lysenko, 1948; Herbert and Becker, 1961). These results indicate that salicylate does not react directly with formed antibody to the trypanosomes, but rather exerts its effects by interfering with antibody production.

Like salicylates, 6-mercaptopurine (6-MP) can suppress antibody synthesis (*see* Schwartz and Andre, 1962; Taliaferro et al., 1964). Atchley and Becker (1962) injected rats with 6-MP and expected the course of infection with *T. lewisi* to be similar to that observed in salicylate-treated animals. They found instead that both the density and the duration of the parasitemias were depressed. Furthermore, in contrast to recovered control animals which had solid immunities, reinfections were established in 30 percent of the drug-treated rats, indicating some interference with the immune response. However, since parasitemias were depressed in the initial infections, the 6-MP apparently also had a direct inhibitory effect on the trypanosomes. Nevertheless, Atchley and Becker (1962) report that the reproductive phase was as intense and almost as long in drug-treated rats as in controls. However, their method of measuring reproductive activity was a subjective "asterisk" rating system. Had a more sensitive method (e.g., CV) been used, a significant depression of activity might have been revealed, thus accounting for the lower parasitemias in the drug-treated animals. Another possibility is that 6-MP renders reproducing populations of trypanosomes more susceptible to removal from the circulation by nonspecific host defenses.

The suppression of antibody formation by cortisone is well known (*see* Taliaferro, 1957; McMaster and Franzl, 1961). The resistance of rats to pathogenic trypanosomes can be reduced by the hormone (Cantrell and Betts, 1956; Petana, 1964). Nevertheless, Herbert and Becker (1961) were unable to influence the immune response of the rat to *T. lewisi* by repeated cortisone administration. In similar experiments, however, Sherman and Ruble (1967) obtained prolonged parasite reproduction, elevated parasitemias, and frequent fatalities. Although the total amount of cortisone they administered to each rat was similar to that used by Herbert and Becker

(1961), unlike the latter, they began treatment two days prior to infection and gave larger though fewer doses. Therefore, the immune response was suppressed by allowing sufficient time for adequate amounts of cortisone to act before infection. But both Herbert and Becker (1961) and Sherman and Ruble (1967) found that repeated cortisone treatments to recovered immune rats did not permit reinfections to be established. The maintenance of immunity under these conditions is understandable since cortisone does not degrade formed antibody (see McMaster and Franzl, 1961). Suppression of antibody formation has also been reported by Patton and Clark (1968), who treated rats with dexamethasone, a synthetic corticosteroid. Treatments were started three days before infection, and the outcome was invariably fatal, but treated rats could be protected by passively transferred immune serum and peritoneal exudate cells (Patton, 1965).

Treatment with bacterial endotoxin can have effects that vary with the dosage schedule. Styles (1965) found that parasitemias were depressed when small serial doses of endotoxin were given before infection; in contrast, parasite levels were elevated when a single dose was given before or at the time of infection. The manner in which endotoxin can enhance either resistance or susceptibility to infection is unknown. According to Singer et al. (1964), antibodies developed to endotoxins are not known to cross-react with trypanosome antigens, but endotoxins do stimulate the reticuloendothelial system, and this enhanced activity may account for the increased resistance observed with adequate pretreatment. On the other hand, when there is insufficient time for the host to develop a tolerance to the endotoxin, the dual stress of the parasites and the toxin may depress resistance.

Adrenalectomy, hypophysectomy, thymectomy, and hypoxia. Bilateral adrenalectomy lowers resistance to *T. lewisi.* In the experiments of Marmorston-Gottesman et al. (1930), 70 percent of the operated infected rats died, whereas all control animals survived. However, at the time of death, parasitemias were not elevated, and in the 30 percent that survived, the parasite reproductive period, parasitemia peak, and duration of infection were not greater than in normal infections. Furthermore, the survivors resisted reinfection. Thus, adrenalectomy did not prevent antibody formation. The authors attribute the deaths to a lowered natural resistance of the host to toxic effects of the infection, for adrenalectomy has been observed to lower the resistance of the rat to toxins and chemical poisons (Perla and Marmorston, 1941). Similar results have been reported recently by Haleem and Minton (1966) who found, in addition, that all adrenalectomized infected rats survived when treated daily with moderate doses of cortisone, whereas almost 90 percent of the untreated control animals died. ACTH was ineffective, as expected, and the authors ascribe the protective action of cortisone to an antitoxic effect.

Hypophysectomy can have equally deleterious effects. Culbertson and Molomut (1938) found that the operation proved invariably fatal for infected rats, whereas only about 15 percent of uninfected controls died. Death of infected animals occurred at the height of the parasitemia, although the intensity of the infections at this time was not greater than in normal controls. Injection of anterior pituitary extract saved over 40 percent of the operated infected rats. In a later study, Molomut (1947) reported that the cause of death was not an impaired antibody response or an elevated parasitemia, but rather hypoglycemic shock. Blood sugar levels were found to be very low in operated infected rats due to the inability of the host to replace sugar stores depleted by the trypanosomes. In normal infections, blood sugar levels are not affected (Linton, 1929; Lysenko, 1951; Tempelis and Lysenko, 1965; Haleem and Minton, 1966).

In the experiments of Perla (1939), all hypophysectomized infected rats survived. However, the intensity and duration of the infections were greater than normal. Since the parasite reproductive period was not prolonged, the operation apparently impaired only the trypanocidal response. Infections followed a normal course in operated animals treated with pituitary extracts. Perla (1939) feels that the deaths reported by Culbertson and Molomut (1938) resulted from toxic effects due to their infecting their animals one week after operation when resistance is lowest, whereas he infected two to three weeks after. His data indicate that the effects of hypophysectomy result in part from atrophy of splenic and lymphoid tissue, as confirmed by recent studies (Keefe et al., 1967). Perla and Marmorston (1941) report that anterior pituitary extract contains a spleen-stimulating factor that causes splenomegaly and hyperplasia of other elements of the lymphoid-macrophage system. Thus, hypophysectomy can induce a condition similar to splenectomy. They also found that when such extracts were administered to normal rats, infections with *T. lewisi* were significantly shortened. Similarly, Herrick and Cross (1936) enhanced resistance to *T. lewisi* by implanting intramuscularly in young rats pituitary glands removed from nonimmune adults. Rats so treated survived the infection with no ill effects, whereas almost 90 percent of the normal control animals died. Young rats usually have a poor antibody response, and the primary effect of the implanted glands may have been to stimulate the lymphoid tissues. Therefore, the different explanations by Perla (1939) and Molomut (1947) for the lowered resistance of hypophysectomized rats may be equally valid. Because of the multiple functions of the hypophysis in controlling metabolism, infection at various times after hypophysectomy may exacerbate different metabolic defects that develop sequentially.

Thymectomy has been reported to enhance resistance to *T. lewisi*. Perla and Marmorston-Gottesman (1930) found that in thymectomized rats, the severity and duration of infection were diminished. The effect was somewhat more pronounced in young rats six weeks old than in adults. The results are difficult to explain. In rats of these ages, lymphoid tissues are sufficiently mature so that thymectomy should have no effect, or at most a slight depressive effect, on resistance (Miller, J. F., 1965), since thymectomy from the time of birth to three weeks of age has a progressively diminishing effect on suppression of the immune response (Jankovic et al., 1962).

The effects of hypoxia have been studied by Hughes and Tatum (1956a).

At simulated altitudes of 19,000 to 20,000 feet, parasitemias were elevated. At simulated altitudes of 22,000 feet, further enhancement occurred, and infections were invariably fatal, although death occurred when adults only were in the blood. In no case was there interference with the ablastic response, for the intensity and duration of the reproductive phase followed a normal course under all conditions. The elevated parasitemias and fatalities apparently resulted from an impaired trypanocidal response. Whether this was due to decreased formation of trypanocidal antibody or to reduced phagocytic activity is not known. However, the importance of humoral antibody is indicated by the observation that reinfections could not be established in recovered immune rats subjected to hypoxic conditions.

Trypanosoma lewisi **in heterologous hosts.** The nonpathogenic rodent trypanosomes display a high degree of host specificity that has been used almost exclusively for their speciation (Davis, 1952; Levine, 1965). Infections are difficult to establish in heterologous hosts, for as Davis (1952) has pointed out, "It has been demonstrated in countless experiments, involving almost every *lewisi*-like trypanosome that has ever been described, that these organisms, in general, are uninfective for animals other than the one in which they occur naturally and to which they have become apparently adapted." In instances where *T. lewisi* has been established in abnormal hosts, success has usually been achieved by modifying the host or the parasite in some way. Bruynoghe and Vassiliadis (1929), for example, found that field mice became susceptible after splenectomy, and some infections were fatal. Similarly, Schwetz (1933) was able to infect a splenectomized giant rat (*Cricetomys gambianus*).

Delanoë (1911a,b; 1912) infected mice with rat blood containing multiplying trypanosomes, but found that culture forms had greater infectivity. Although heavy infections resulted and some animals died, mouse-to-mouse passage was unsuccessful. Greater success was achieved by Roudsky (1910a,b; 1911a,c), who used a virulent strain of *T. lewisi* obtained by rapid passage from rat to rat. Infections were established in white mice, guinea pigs, field mice, voles, and rabbits. However, serial passage was possible only in white mice in which 75 subpassages were made. With successive passages, the percentages of positive infections and fatalities increased until at the 75th passage, these were 82 percent and almost 100 percent, respectively. Apparently, adaptation had occurred. Infections have also been established in guinea pigs with a normal strain of *T. lewisi* by Coventry (1929). Reproduction occurred and was eventually inhibited by ablastin, which was demonstrated by passive transfer to rats, but no significant increase in parasite numbers occurred, because of a continuous trypanocidal action. Attempts to enhance adaptation to the guinea pig by splenectomy, injections of normal rat serum, and passage from guinea pig to guinea pig were unsuccessful. Recently, pathogenic infections with *T. lewisi* in the gerbil have been reported (Juminer and Goudineau, 1960). Attempts have been made to establish *T. lewisi* in many additional species of vertebrates and in general have failed. A comprehensive review of the subject has been made by Lincicome (1958).

Heterologous hosts can sometimes be made susceptible to trypanosome infections by injecting them with serum proteins from the natural host. Desowitz and Watson (1952), for example, established *T. vivax* in rats in serial passage by giving supplementary inoculations of sheep serum. After 37 subpassages, the parasites lost their dependence upon the supplement and became adapted to the rat (Desowitz and Watson, 1953). Similar studies have been made of *T. lewisi* in the mouse by Lincicome (1963) and more recently by Mühlpfordt (1968). Daily supplements of rat serum are required and, unlike *T. vivax* in the rat, complete adaptation to the mouse has not occurred; after hundreds of subpassages, serum supplements are still necessary. Growth of *T. lewisi* can also be supported by sera from the hamster, guinea pig, and rabbit, but not as effectively as by rat serum. Sera from the horse, man, chicken, chinchilla, pig, dog, and cow have no effect (Lincicome and Francis, 1961). Low parasitemias occur in the mouse supplemented with rat serum, but if the mouse is also starved, parasite reproduction is enhanced, parasitemias are elevated, and fatalities may occur (Lincicome, 1958, 1959a,b). Thus, starvation increases susceptibility to infection. Recently, the factors in rat serum that allow growth of *T. lewisi* in the mouse have been identified by Greenblatt and Lincicome (1966) as the γ_2-globulins and the macroglobulins. Albumin has no effect. This is in contrast with *T. vivax* in the rat where both albumin and globulin have supplementary activity (Desowitz, 1954).

The nature of the insusceptibility of heterologous hosts to *T. lewisi* is not known. Roudsky (1911b) and Delanoë (1911c, 1912) believed that a natural immunity based on phagocytosis is responsible, since they observed the ingestion of trypanosomes by macrophages in the blood and the peritoneum of inoculated mice. Natural antibody has been found to be responsible for the resistance of the cotton rat to infection with *T. vivax* (Terry, 1957), but such antibody from abnormal hosts has not been demonstrated to *T. lewisi*. Culbertson (1934), for example, has shown that *T. lewisi* is not affected by human serum and yet is still uninfective for man. The manner in which serum supplements facilitate infection of abnormal hosts is not clear. The serum proteins may protect the trypanosomes against antibody of the heterologous host, blockade the reticuloendothelial system, and thereby suppress antibody formation, or supply essential nutrients the foreign host lacks. Serum from rats starved for two weeks shows a marked loss of supplementary activity in the mouse (Lincicome and Hinnant, 1962), suggesting a nutritional role. The fact that horse serum cannot substitute for rat serum indicates that rat serum does not act simply as a blockading agent of the reticuloendothelial system and also lends support to the nutritional hypothesis (Lincicome, 1958). However, serum proteins may coat the trypanosomes and have a protective function unrelated to nutrition, for it is known that well-washed *T. lewisi* retains rat serum proteins avidly (D'Alesandro, 1969) and that the parasites survive much longer *in vitro* in rat serum than in mouse serum (du Buy et al., 1966; Greenblatt and Shelton, 1968). Thus, the reduced activity of serum from starved rats may result from the lowered serum protein levels induced by starvation (Weimer et al., 1959a,b, 1963);

possibly, such sera also contain inhibitory substances. Similarly, sera from other animals such as the horse and hamster may either lack essential components or have them in reduced amounts. But it is more likely that the limited supplementary activity of other sera relative to rat serum (Lincicome and Francis, 1961) is really a reflection not of quantitative but rather qualitative differences that may affect the affinity of their proteins for the parasites. In a recent study it was found that the trypanosomes could be carried through several transfers in mice without rat serum supplements when grown in diffusion chambers to protect them from heterologous host cells (Greenblatt and Shelton, 1968). Growth under these conditions was greatly improved, however, when rat serum was provided, suggesting that in addition to supporting the parasites directly, homologous host serum proteins may depress the cellular defenses of the heterologous host. The problem has been thoroughly reviewed by Desowitz (1963) but is still unresolved.

Trypanosoma duttoni of the mouse

The course of infection with this trypanosome resembles that of *T. lewisi* in the rat but shows striking quantitative differences (Taliaferro and Pavlinova, 1936). The reproductive period is not as intense but is more prolonged with a much slower rise in parasitemia. The CV at the peak of reproduction is about 10 to 12 percent, half that of *T. lewisi*, and reproduction is inhibited very gradually and unevenly over a period of a week or more, rather than abruptly within a few days. The number of organisms at the peak of infection is ordinarily very much less than in *T. lewisi* infections, and there is a gradual decrease in numbers until all the parasites disappear, in contrast to the two sudden crises in the rat. The length of the infections with the two species is similar, as are the morphologic changes that accompany inhibition of reproduction.

Acquired humoral antibodies are produced during the course of infection. Taliaferro (1938a), using passive transfer techniques, demonstrated the presence of a specific ablastin and also showed in curative tests that serum from recovered mice has trypanocidal antibody. The latter is presumably responsible only for the termination of the infection, for no tests were made to determine whether trypanocidal antibody is present between the time the parasitemia starts its gradual decline and the end of the infection. Thus, in contrast with the two distinct trypanocidal antibodies produced by the rat to *T. lewisi* (Coventry, 1930), only one has been conclusively demonstrated to *T. duttoni*. Unquestionably, the decline in numbers before the infection ends indicates trypanocidal activity, but the nature of this activity and its relation to the trypanocidal antibody have yet to be determined.

Mice can be immunized specifically against *T. duttoni* by repeated injections of killed trypanosomes (Culbertson, 1941c), and can be protected against infection by injections of normal sheep serum (Taliaferro and Olsen,

1943). Normal rat serum is also trypanocidal to *T. duttoni* in the mouse (Taliaferro, 1938a), but the nature of the nonspecific protective factors is unknown. Baby mice passively acquire specific immunity via the colostrum and milk from immune mothers (Culbertson, 1940). Antibody is absorbed from the intestine for at least two weeks after birth, and mother mice passively immunized with immune serum can also transmit antibody to their young. Nonimmune young mice are reported to have heavier infections than older mice (Culbertson, 1941c), indicating the development of an age immunity similar to that of the rat to *T. lewisi*.

The immune response of the mouse to *T. duttoni* can be affected by factors that depress the reticuloendothelial system. Splenectomy, for example, when performed shortly before infection, delays the appearance of ablastin as indicated by a prolonged reproductive period (Galliard, 1933; Jaroslow, 1959). Splenectomy during the adult phase of the infection delays production of the terminal trypanocidal antibody, and infections last longer than usual (Galliard, 1933). Severe stress such as splenectomy plus India ink blockade (Taliaferro and Pavlinova, 1936), whole-body x- or neutron-irradiation, and India ink blockade plus x-irradiation (Jaroslow, 1955, 1959) can cause prolonged parasite reproduction, exalted parasitemias, and fatal infections. More importantly, however, the reproductive rate is enhanced, as indicated by a greatly elevated CV and a higher percentage of division forms. This contrasts with *T. lewisi*, which reproduces at the same rate in normal and stressed rats, and indicates that the mouse, unlike the rat, has a natural resistance to the reproduction of the trypanosomes. Taliaferro and Pavlinova (1936) first discovered this natural immunity when they observed that *T. duttoni* infections in splenectomized and blockaded mice are enhanced and become similar in rates of reproduction and intensity of parasitemias to *T. lewisi* infections in normal rats. The natural immunity of the mouse does not appear to be humoral but seems to be dependent upon a functional macrophage system, for Taliaferro (1938a) found that the intensity of parasite reproduction in splenectomized and blockaded mice is not reduced by the injection of normal mouse serum. However, the importance of humoral antibody to acquired immunity is illustrated by the observation that x-irradiation of mice 14 days after infection, when acquired ablastic immunity is well-developed, has no visible effect on the course of infection (Jaroslow, 1959).

Mixed infections with *T. duttoni* and pathogenic trypanosomes have been reported to make the nonpathogenic species virulent. Galliard (1934) used a strain of *T. gambiense* that did not cause death for at least 11 months, but he found that when mice were infected simultaneously with this relatively avirulent pathogen and *T. duttoni*, death occurred within seven days. *T. duttoni* was numerous with many division forms and resembled *T. lewisi* in the rat. At the time of death, *T. gambiense* was in low numbers, and death was therefore attributed to the large numbers of *T. duttoni*. These results contrast with those obtained from mixed infections with *T. lewisi* and pathogenic trypanosomes in the rat (*see* pp. 701-702). The enhanced virulence of *T. duttoni* in the mouse appears to result from a lowering of the natural immunity by the pathogenic species. A similar effect has been reported by Singer et al. (1964), who studied *T. duttoni* infections in mice treated with bacterial endotoxin. Mice made endotoxin-tolerant before infection had decreased parasitemias. However, endotoxin administration (one quarter of LD_{50} dose) seven days after infection, when acquired immunity is not yet well-developed, invariably resulted in death within 24 hours. Although it is not clear whether the parasites rendered the host more susceptible to the effects of the endotoxin or vice versa, death apparently resulted from a rapid depression of natural immunity.

Other types of stress can make *T. duttoni* infections fatal. Sheppe and Adams (1957) found that deaths occurred more frequently and significantly earlier among *T. duttoni*-infected mice than among controls when both groups were subjected to partial starvation and low temperatures or partial starvation alone. Although *T. duttoni* is considered a benign parasite, it was also observed that parasitized mice on full rations averaged only half as much weight gain as nonparasitized mice. Sheppe and Adams (1957) suggested, therefore, that even under favorable environmental conditions *T. duttoni* can have harmful effects on its host. This observation and conclusion differ from those of Lincicome and Shepperson (1963) who found that infected mice gained weight at a faster rate than uninfected mice. Similar accelerated weight gains have been reported to occur in rats infected with *T. lewisi* (Lincicome et al., 1963).

Like other rodent trypanosomes, *T. duttoni* shows marked host specificity. Roudsky (1912a) observed that rats inoculated with blood or culture forms of *T. duttoni* remained negative or had light transient infections. However, when he used a virulent strain obtained by rapid passage from mouse to mouse, infections with high parasitemias were readily established in rats. Thirteen subpassages were made, and fatalities were common. In spite of host specificity, *T. duttoni* and *T. lewisi* appear to have antigens in common since cross-immunity has been demonstrated. Roudsky (1912b) immunized a rat to a rat-adapted strain of *T. duttoni* by repeated injections of infected blood and found that it resisted infection with *T. lewisi*. Conversely, a rat immunized to *T. lewisi* resisted infection with rat-adapted *T. duttoni*. Similarly, mice can be immunized against *T. duttoni* by injections of *T. lewisi* vaccine (Culbertson, 1941c). The antibody basis of this cross-immunity has been demonstrated by Taliaferro (1938a) who found that the ablastic and trypanocidal antibodies of anti-*T. duttoni* mouse serum and anti-*T. lewisi* rat serum react with the heterologous species *in vivo*. A somewhat weaker cross-reaction of the trypanocidal antibodies also occurs *in vitro*.

Trypanosoma zapi of the Allen jumping mouse *(Zapus princeps alleni)*

This trypanosome has been studied in detail by Davis (1952), and the discussion that follows is based entirely on her work. The course of infection with *T. zapi* in general resembles that of *T. lewisi* more closely than that of *T. duttoni*. The reproductive period is as intense as that of *T. lewisi*, the parasitemia rises as rapidly, and the CV shows values and changes of the same magnitude. Inhibition of reproduction is not always as abrupt as in *T. lewisi* infections, but it occurs more quickly than in *T. duttoni* infections. The number of parasites at the peak of infection is very much less than in *T. lewisi* infections, and in this quantitative aspect, *T. zapi* resembles *T. duttoni*. Division forms are found during the early part of the infection, and adults are found later. However, unlike *T. lewisi* and *T. duttoni*, which show multiple- and binary-fission forms, *T. zapi* presents only binary-fission forms in the peripheral blood during the reproductive period. Multiple-fission forms occur at this time only in the capillaries of the lungs, heart, and spleen, and these apparently give rise to the stages found in the blood.

No attempt was made to demonstrate the presence of acquired humoral antibodies directly by passive transfer or other techniques, but the effects of splenectomy indicate that antibody plays an important role in controlling the infection. Thus, splenectomy shortly before infection prolongs the reproductive period and causes a slightly elevated parasitemia. Splenectomy during the adult phase of the infection results in a renewal of reproductive activity and a consequent increase in parasite numbers. In neither case, however, is the reproductive rate enhanced, and multiple-fission forms do not appear in the peripheral blood. Since a more severe stress such as splenectomy plus blockade was not imposed on the host, it is possible that the reproductive rate can be increased as it is in severely stressed mice infected with *T. duttoni*. Therefore, from these results, it is not clear whether or not the jumping mouse has a natural resistance to the reproduction of *T. zapi*. Nevertheless, the spleen plays a role in the development of acquired ablastic immunity, and in this respect the jumping mouse resembles the rat and the mouse.

The host specificity of *T. zapi* was demonstrated by its failure to infect laboratory rats and mice of various ages and two species of wild mice.

Trypanosoma nabiasi of the rabbit

Although not a rodent trypanosome, this species is included here because it has much in common with the rodent species and its host is closely related to rodents. As described by Ashworth et al. (1909), Channon and Wright (1927), Kroó (1936), and Grewal (1957), the course of infection is as follows. After an incubation period of five to twelve days, parasites appear in the blood and rapidly increase in number, reaching a peak within three to five days of their appearance. Thereafter, the parasitemia declines gradually until the infection terminates. The parasitemia is very much lower than in *T. lewisi* infections and is similar to those produced by *T. duttoni* and *T. zapi*. Division forms are never seen in the peripheral blood. Grewal (1957) has found that reproduction occurs only in capillaries of the spleen, is of short duration, and is most active during the rise in parasitemia. Division forms transform into adults before moving into the peripheral circulation, and for this reason only nonreproducing forms occur in the blood. However, during the reproductive period, the adults in the blood are somewhat atypical and show a greater variation in length than the adults found later (Grewal, 1957). Therefore, the CV undergoes changes similar to those reported for other members of this group even though division forms are not seen.

After recovery, rabbits are immune to reinfection (Channon and Wright, 1927; Kroó, 1936; Grewal, 1957), but humoral antibody has not been consistently demonstrated. Channon and Wright (1927), for example, could not protect normal rabbits against infection with passively transferred serum from recovered animals, nor could they detect any *in vitro* activity of immune blood against the parasites. Kroó (1936), however, demonstrated agglutinins in immune serum and also found that the new-born of immune mother rabbits have solid immunities that diminish gradually, presumably because of the loss of passively acquired antibody. Young nonimmune rabbits are reported to be more susceptible to infection than adults (Grewal, 1957). Ablastin has not yet been demonstrated, but an acquired immunity is assumed to be responsible for the cessation of reproduction.

Splenectomy shortly before infection or at the time of peak parasitemia does not appear to have any marked effect (Grewal, 1957). The parasite numbers may be slightly elevated, but the course of infection is essentially unchanged. Since Grewal (1957) could not find division forms in organs other than the spleen, it is not clear where the parasites reproduce in splenectomized hosts. Obviously, other sites are utilized, but no attempt was made to identify them. These results also indicate that the spleen is not as important to the rabbit for the development of acquired immunity as it is to the rat, mouse, and jumping mouse.

T. nabiasi shows marked host specificity. Attempts to infect mice, rats and guinea pigs have been unsuccessful (Ashworth et al., 1909; Channon and Wright, 1927). Splenectomized rats and guinea pigs also resist infection (Grewal, 1957). Limited studies of cross-immunity have shown than anti-*T. nabiasi* rabbit serum has no protective or curative effect on rats infected with *T. lewisi* (Grewal, 1957).

Trypanosoma sigmodoni of the cotton rat

Culbertson (1941a) has studied this species and found that infections last at least one month, with peak parasitemia occurring about one week after the six- to ten-day incubation period. Parasite numbers are much lower than in *T. lewisi* infections, and division forms are not seen in the peripheral blood. Reproduction may occur in the capillaries of organs and tissues, but as yet there is no evidence for this. However, the rise and fall of parasite numbers indicate that reproduction and subsequent host destruction of parasites do occur.

After recovery, cotton rats are immune to reinfection. Serum from immune cotton rats protects normal cotton rats from infection, but the types of antibodies in the immune serum have not been identified. Nine-day-old albino rats are susceptible to very mild infections with *T. sigmodoni* and after recovery resist infection with *T. lewisi*. Conversely, even though cotton rats inoculated with *T. lewisi* fail to develop patent infections, such animals acquire a partial immunity to *T. sigmodoni*. Thus, the two species are immunogenically related, although they are host-specific.

Other, less studied species

The course of infection with other rodent trypanosomes has been studied, but in many cases observations have been incomplete, and immunologic aspects, aside from host specificity, have been largely ignored. Reproductive stages followed by the appearance of adults have been described for *T. blanchardi* in the dormouse (Nájera Angulo, 1935) and *T. rabinowitschi* in the hamster (Regendanz, 1929; Zozaya, 1929). Ablastin has not been demonstrated in these infections, but it is very likely responsible for the observed cessation of reproduction. In cross-immunity studies, anti-*T. rabinowitschi* hamster serum failed to protect rats against *T. lewisi* (Rabinowitz and Kempner, 1899). Infections have also been studied, but reproductive stages have not been described, with *T. neotomae* of the wood rat (Wood, 1936) and an unnamed species from the collared lemming (Quay, 1955). Only adults have been found in the peripheral blood, and examinations of various tissues and organs have failed to reveal division forms. Reproduction may occur outside the circulation and last for only a few days as it does in *T. nabiasi* infections of rabbits, and the timing of tissue examinations could therefore be extremely important. Molyneux (1968), for example, recently demonstrated for the first time reproductive stages of *T. microti* in the appendix and of *T. evotomys* in the appendix and spleen by examining voles 24 hours after parasites first appeared in the blood. Like other members of this group, these species show marked host specificity. Wood (1936), for example, failed to infect six species of heterologous hosts with *T. neotomae*, and Zozaya (1929) and Regendanz (1929) could not infect rats and guinea pigs with *T. rabinowitschi*. But Nattan-Larrier and Noyer (1932) were able to infect new-born rats with metacyclic forms from old cultures of the latter species. However, infections were short lived, and only a few subpasses could be made. A thorough review of the biology of several rodent trypanosomes has been made by Davis (1952). Detailed studies of the vast majority of these parasites have not yet been made.

THE HUMORAL FACTORS OF IMMUNITY

This section is based, of necessity, almost entirely on studies of antibodies produced by the rat to *T. lewisi* because it is the only member of the group that has been thoroughly investigated. However, the results of more limited studies of antibodies to other species such as *T. duttoni* and *T. sigmodoni* are in general agreement, as far as they go, with the results obtained with *T.*

lewisi. As the immune responses to other members of the group are studied in detail, the results will very likely indicate that *T. lewisi* is a generally valid model for the whole group.

The evidence now available overwhelmingly indicates that ablastin and the trypanocidal antibodies are of primary importance in the immune response, with phagocytosis playing a subsidiary role (Taliaferro, 1929, 1932, 1938a). These humoral factors have distinguishing immunologic properties that were first clearly determined by Taliaferro (1932). Both types of antibody can be passively transferred to normal rats, and immune sera can be used protectively and curatively. In their mode of action, however, the antibodies differ fundamentally; the trypanocidal antibodies destroy the parasites, but ablastin only inhibits reproduction and has no apparent effect on the viability and motility of the flagellates. The trypanocidal antibodies have a marked affinity for the parasites and can be removed from immune serum by adsorption with living trypanosomes. But even after repeated adsorptions, immune serum retains its reproduction-inhibiting activity. Ablastin, therefore, appears to be *nonadsorbable.* The trypanosomes are sensitized upon exposure to trypanocidal serum for when subsequently washed and then injected into normal rats, they are quickly removed from the circulation and destroyed. In contrast, parasites incubated in ablastic serum reproduce normally when later injected into nonimmune rats, indicating that they have not been sensitized by their exposure to the reproduction-inhibiting antibody. It appears that for inhibition to occur, ablastin must be continuously present in the surrounding medium, but that such conditions do not permanently impair the ability to reproduce. These observations suggest that ablastin has a low avidity, a property that will be discussed later. Lastly, the trypanocidal antibodies show *in vitro* activity. In Taliaferro's (1932) original study, technical difficulties did not permit the demonstration of ablastic activity *in vitro*, but more recent attempts have been successful (D'Alesandro, 1962). Other studies support all these findings (Taliaferro, 1938a,b; Taliaferro and Pizzi, 1960; D'Alesandro, 1959, 1962, 1966).

The serum proteins of the rat show only quantitative changes after infection and subsequent immunization (Lysenko, 1951; Meyers and Lysenko, 1956; D'Alesandro, 1959; Lincicome and Watkins, 1965). Total protein increases from about 5 percent to 6 percent. Electrophoretic analysis of immune serum shows a relative decline of the albumin fraction, essentially unchanged α-globulins, and a marked rise in the β- and γ-globulin levels. Most of the latter increase is probably nonspecific, for when immune serum is adsorbed with trypanosomes and then analyzed electrophoretically, the globulin fraction shows only a slight decline (D'Alesandro, 1969).

The trypanocidal antibodies

After Coventry's (1930) demonstration of two distinct acquired trypanocidal antibodies, Taliaferro (1932) found that they are precipitated with the globulin fraction of immune rat serum. Later studies have shown, in addition, that both electrophoretically migrate between the β- and γ-globulins, but that the early trypanocidal antibody is a small 6S γG-globulin, and the terminal trypanocidal antibody is a 16S γM-macroglobulin (D'Alesandro, 1959). In the primary immune response of rats and other mammals, macroglobulins are usually produced first followed by γG-globulins (Harris, 1965; Tomasi, 1965; Santos and Owens, 1966; de Carvalho et al., 1967). Why the rat responds in the opposite manner to *T. lewisi* antigens is not known. Possibly, a small initial γM response occurs but was missed because the *in vivo* titration methods used to measure antibody activity lack sufficient sensitivity. However, the trypanocidal antibodies have different specificities, since the first kills division forms but has no effect on adults, which are killed by the second, and therefore represent two distinct immune responses. This means that the rat follows the classical pattern of an initial γM synthesis only in the second trypanocidal response and follows an atypical pattern during the first response. Mice and rats immunized with bovine serum albumin have also been reported to produce only γG antibody during the primary response (Cushing and Johnson, 1966; Banovitz and Ishizaka, 1967). Therefore, the sequence of antibody formation may vary with the antigen, the species, or both, and it is not rigidly fixed (*see* Dixon et al., 1966; Pike, 1967).

Division forms and adults differ antigenically, and the distinct physicochemical properties of their respective trypanocidal antibodies may also be a reflection of this difference. But more direct evidence of antigenic differences is provided by the old observation that adults surviving the first crisis are resistant to the early trypanocidal antibody (Taliaferro, 1924, 1932; Coventry, 1930) and therefore are really antigenic variants. In this respect, *T. lewisi* resembles the pathogenic species of trypanosomes that cause relapsing infections, but differs in that it appears to be limited to two antigenic types, while the relapsing species can give rise to many antigenic variants (Ritz, 1914; Taliaferro and Taliaferro, 1922; Taliaferro, 1929; Inoki, 1960; Watkins, 1964; Gray 1965a,b, 1966). Ablastin seems to be responsible for limiting the antigenic expression of the parasites by curtailing reproductive activity, and yet when new infections are initiated with antibody-resistant adults, reversion to the original antigenic form occurs when reproduction begins; a third antigenic type does not appear. This suggests that because of its long stabilizing association with ablastin, *T. lewisi* has evolved to a point where it is now capable of expressing only two antigenic types and has lost any ability it once may have had for greater antigenic variation. Nevertheless, neither stage of the parasite develops a resistance to ablastin, indicating that unlike the trypanocidal antigens, ablastinogen does not change throughout the infection.

The changes in trypanocidal antigens are associated with the morphologic changes that occur as division forms transform into adults. However, shortly before the first crisis (*see* Fig. 1), the CV is very low and practically all the trypanosomes appear to be adults, and yet most of them are destroyed when the crisis occurs. This means that in spite of their adult morphology, these parasites have division-form antigens, and only the survivors of the crisis have adult antigens. Therefore, before the first crisis, morphology alone is not an adequate basis for the identification of antigenic adults. The results of a recent study by Entner and Gonzalez (1966) support this conclusion. Using rabbit antisera to the two stages and immunodiffusion methods, they found that the morphologic change to adults precedes the antigenic change by a few days. That is, when adults first appear, they contain division-form antigens that are eventually replaced by adult antigens as the infection progresses. Although these studies were made with rabbit antisera, similar results would probably be obtained with rat immune sera. It appears, then, that when ablastin inhibits reproduction and transformation into morphologic adults occurs, the corresponding antigenic transformation has yet to begin, and only those parasites that complete the antigenic change before the first crisis escape destruction.

The mechanism of trypanocidal action has been the subject of controversy. On the basis of early studies it was believed that phagocytosis is of primary importance. Laveran and Mesnil (1901), for example, reached this conclusion after observing the phagocytosis of living *T. lewisi* in the peritoneal cavity of actively and passively immunized rats. Roudsky (1911b) and Delanoë (1911c, 1912) observed similar activity in mice inoculated with *T. lewisi* and came to the same conclusion. They were actually studying natural immunity since the mouse is normally refractory, but Delanoë (1912) obtained similar results when he used a susceptible strain of mice that developed an acquired immunity. Regendanz and Kikuth (1927) and Regendanz (1932) believed that ablastin is the only acquired humoral antibody produced by the rat and that after reproduction is inhibited, the parasites are removed from the blood by nonspecific phagocytosis. That specific trypanocidal factors are involved is no longer disputed, but the importance of phagocytosis to the initial destruction of parasites is difficult to determine.

W. H. Brown (1915) observed agglutination and phagocytosis of parasites during *T. lewisi* infections in rats and also noticed many disintegrating trypanosomes that were presumably destroyed by lytic antibody. Similar observations were made by Augustine (1943) in immune rats reinfected with large numbers of parasites. He concluded, however, that division forms are destroyed principally by phagocytosis and adults by agglutination and mechanical removal from the circulation. Others have stressed the importance of lysis in parasite destruction (McNeal, 1904; Manteufel, 1909; Taliaferro, 1932, 1938a). Depending upon the conditions used, the trypanocidal antibodies to *T. lewisi* show all the classical antibody reactions when studied *in vitro*. Agglutination was first demonstrated by Laveran and Mesnil (1900) and has been subsequently shown by many others (Culbertson and Kessler, 1939; Meyers and Lysenko, 1953; Thillet and Chandler, 1957; Tempelis and Lysenko, 1965; Lincicome and Watkins, 1965). Complement fixation (Marmorston-Gottesman et al., 1930), lysis (Taliaferro, 1932, 1938a), and opsonization (Lange and Lysenko, 1960) have also been demonstrated, as well as precipitation in double diffusion gels with hyperimmune rat serum and trypanosome extracts (D'Alesandro, 1969). Recently, it has been reported that the loss of intracellular material through leaching is accelerated by rat immune serum (du Buy et al., 1966). With anti-*T. duttoni* mouse serum, only agglutination and trypanolysis have been reported thus far (Taliaferro, 1938a).

In vivo, it is quite likely that several trypanocidal mechanisms are operative, especially agglutination, lysis, and phagocytosis, since these have been commonly observed. Taliaferro (1932) has suggested that the mode of action may depend upon the titer of trypanocidal antibodies. Thus, when it is high trypanolysis occurs, and when it is low phagocytosis predominates. There is some evidence to support this view, for Taliaferro (1932) could demonstrate lysis only occasionally with immune rat serum, but when hyperimmune sera were used, lysis occurred more consistently (Taliaferro, 1938a). There is little question, however, that humoral antibody is of primary importance to trypanocidal activity in that the parasites must first be sensitized before macrophage stimulation or other activities occur. In the *in vitro* studies of Lange and Lysenko (1960), for example, it was observed that immune serum adsorbed with trypanosomes no longer enhanced phagocytosis. But even when trypanolysis and agglutination occur, it is obvious that macrophage cells are eventually involved in the removal of parasite debris. Therefore, their role, though secondary, is an important one.

The relation of phagocytic cells to trypanocidal antibody in the removal of parasites from the peripheral circulation was studied by Taliaferro (1938b), who used splenectomized and blockaded rats that were passively immunized and then infected. Whereas the trypanosomes disappeared quickly from the blood of passively immunized normal rats, there was a slight but definite impairment of trypanocidal activity in the splenectomized and blockaded animals. This effect could be explained as resulting from a decrease in the complement level, thus preventing trypanolysis, or from a depression of phagocytic function that would impede removal of opsonized parasites. It was found, however, that trypanosomes sensitized with trypanocidal antibody before injection are as readily removed from the circulation in splenectomzied and blockaded rats as in normal animals. It is not known whether the ultimate disposal of the parasites is the same in both cases since they may be agglutinated and mechanically removed in the treated rats, but the results suggest that severe depression of the reticuloendothelial system interferes with the union of antigen and antibody *in vivo*. Similar results were obtained by Kuhn (1938) in a study of splenectomized and blockaded mice passively immunized against *T. equiperdum*. In a study by Koenig et al. (1965) of the dynamics of reticuloendothelial blockade, it was found that effective blockade is correlated with high circulating levels of the blockading agent. Possibly, such a condition interferes with the antigen-antibody reaction. More recent evidence implicates a loss of plasma opsonic activity (Pisano et al., 1968). A definite answer is not yet available, but the problem deserves further study.

The trypanocidal antibodies play an important role in protecting the host against reinfection. Taliaferro (1932) inoculated rats intravenously at various times after recovery from an initial infection and found in most cases that the parasites were destroyed before ablastin had a chance to act. In similar experiments, Augustine (1943) reinfected rats intraperitoneally and found that the trypanosomes appeared promptly in the blood. Although the parasites were destroyed and reinfections lasted for only a few minutes to a few days, he concluded that there is no effective mechanism to prevent passage of the trypanosomes from the peritoneum of the immune host to the blood. However, Augustine (1943) used massive inocula of about 400 to 800 million parasites and probably overwhelmed host defenses. In a similar study by Cox (1964), it was found that few if any trypanosomes passed to the blood when actively and passively immunized rats were challenged with substantially smaller inocula. Under natural conditions, it is unlikely that reinfections would be so massive as to overwhelm host immunity. But even in cases where trypanocidal antibody is weak and some parasites escape initial destruction, ablastin can effectively check the survivors until the host produces more trypanocidal antibody and terminates the infection. This complementary action is singularly effective in preventing relapses as well as reinfections.

Ablastin and inhibition of reproduction

It has been suggested by Taliaferro (1929) that the immunologic basis of nonpathogenic infections may be the formation by the host of ablastin plus trypanocidal antibody. In pathogenic infections, periodic crises may occur but are only temporarily successful because the few antibody-resistant survivors repopulate the blood and eventually kill the host. As described earlier, nonpathogenic infections can be made fatal by stress factors that interfere with ablastin formation, thus allowing uninhibited reproduction (see pp. 699-706). The most obvious difference, then, between the two types of infections is the apparent continuous reproductive activity of the pathogenic species, indicating the absence of an ablastic response (Taliaferro and Taliaferro, 1922). While it is certainly true that the pathogenic species also produce benign infections in many wild African game animals, the immunologic basis of this tolerance is unknown. Van Saceghem (1923) postulated the presence of a reproduction-inhibiting immune property in such infections, but as yet there is no evidence for this. Possibly, a balance is achieved between parasite reproduction and destruction such that a constant low parasitemia is maintained. Desowitz (1960), for example, was able to demonstrate trypanolytic antibody of low titer in a gazelle that had attained the reservoir state.

At present, ablastin has been demonstrated unequivocally by passive transfer only in *T. lewisi* and *T. duttoni* infections (Taliaferro, 1924, 1932, 1938a). Parasite populations made up of nonreproducing adults alone have been described in rodent hosts infected with other species mentioned earlier (see pp. 710-713), but it has only been inferred and not demonstrated that ablastin is responsible for cessation of reproduction in these infections. Similar observations have been made during infections in nonrodent hosts with other members of the *T. lewisi* group such as *T. primatum* of the macaque (Reichenow, 1917), *T. theileri* of cattle, and *T. melophagium* of sheep (Wenyon, 1926). It is very likely that ablastin is produced by all these hosts, and this suggests that the ablastic response is not peculiar to rodents but is a more widespread phenomenon. Nevertheless, ablastic immunity appears to be limited to nonpathogenic members of the *T. lewisi* group of trypanosomes, for although a few immune responses to other organisms show similarities, its combination of properties is unique (Taliaferro, 1948). Ascoli (1906, 1908), for example, studied anthrax in passively immunized guinea pigs and concluded that the serum exerts its protective action by inhibiting assimilative processes of the bacteria, thereby preventing germination and delaying capsule formation. He also observed that adsorption of antiserum with bacteria does not remove the protective property and that the bacteria are not sensitized by exposure to the serum. However, the inhibition of the anthrax bacteria was believed to cause the death of the organisms. In this latter aspect, the effect differs basically from the ablastic response in that after reproduction is inhibited, the trypanosomes can retain their motility and viability for long periods of time in the presence of ablastin, and they are destroyed only when a trypanocidal antibody intervenes. It is interesting that Ascoli called the anthrax immunity "antiblastic." Taliaferro (1932, 1948) was unaware of Ascoli's work when he proposed the term "ablastin."

Other antibodies have been described that resemble ablastin in that they also appear to be nonadsorbable. Campbell (1938a,b) has found that antisera from rats infected with *Cysticercus crassicollis* and from rabbits infected with *C. pisiformis* contain two protective properties: an early one that causes destruction of larvae before encystment, and a late one that destroys larvae after encystment. The former can be removed by adsorption with freshly ground larval worm material, but the latter cannot. Similarly, Oliver-Gonzalez (1941) observed that antibody against adult stages from rabbits infected with *Trichinella spiralis* is adsorbed slightly if at all with dried, powdered antigen from adult worms. In both cases, however, it is probable that adsorption was unsuccessful because the specific antigens are elaborated by living worms and are therefore absent or present only in low concentrations in dead worm material. The nonadsorbability of ablastin cannot be similarly explained. That is, if ablastin is not removed from immune serum because insufficient antigen is added, then the living trypanosomes used for the adsorption should be saturated with antibody. But the fact that these parasites reproduce when injected into normal hosts indicates that they have not been sensitized. This suggests that ablastin itself is different and that another phenomenon, avidity, is involved. Furthermore, the nonadsorbable antibodies in helminth infections have an effect fundamentally different from that of ablastin (Taliaferro, 1940a,b, 1948). Therefore, the ablastic response to nonpathogenic trypanosomes as presently known has no exact parallel in other systems.

The antibody nature of ablastin.   The unusual properties of ablastin may create doubts about calling it an antibody. Nevertheless, numerous studies have shown that except for its unique effects, ablastin has all the characteristics of conventional antibodies.

Physiochemical properties.   Taliaferro (1932) first demonstrated that ablastin is precipitated with the globulin fraction of immune rat serum. Subsequent electrophoretic studies have shown that on electrophoresis, it migrates between the beta- and gamma-globulins, and that it is a small 6S (γG) protein (D'Alesandro, 1959). Furthermore, a functional reticuloendothelial system is essential to the formation of ablastin. Factors that are known to suppress antibody formation, such as splenectomy, blockade, x-irradiation, and treatment with salicylates and cortisone, also impair the ablastic response (*see* pp. 699; 709). However, once ablastin is formed, it does not appear to be dependent upon cellular elements to exert its effects, for Taliaferro (1938b) found that splenectomized and blockaded rats are as effectively protected by passively transferred ablastin as normal animals.

Specificity.   Like other antibodies, ablastin shows marked specificity. Taliaferro (1932) observed that the pathogenic trypanosomes, *T. brucei*, *T. rhodesiense*, and *T. equiperdum*, reproduce freely in rats that have high titers of ablastin. Similarly, Tate (1951) found that rats immune to *T. lewisi* readily succumb to *T. equinum*. But with closely related species, there is some cross-immunity, for ablastic anti-*T. lewisi* rat serum and anti-*T. duttoni* mouse serum inhibit reproduction of the heterologous species *in vivo* (Taliaferro, 1938a).

In vitro and in vivo activity.   The early studies of ablastic activity were made *in vivo*. Although such techniques can be involved and lengthy, they provided the means to determine the functional role of ablastin in acquired immunity. Later attempts by Taliaferro (1932) to study the antibody *in vitro*, free of host complications, were unsuccessful because it was not possible to keep the trypanosomes alive and in good condition over sufficiently long periods of time to determine whether reproduction was affected. These technical difficulties have been overcome, and it is now possible to demonstrate that ablastin, like other antibodies, shows activity *in vitro* (D'Alesandro, 1962). *T. lewisi* can be grown as the blood-stream form in a tissue culture-type medium for approximately 24 hours at 37°C. If adult trypanosomes are inoculated into the medium when it contains normal rat serum, most of the parasites are in various stages of division after overnight incubation. But when ablastic serum is used, there is no reproduction, and the parasites remain in the viable adult stage. Similarly, when reproducing trypansomes are inoculated into the medium, they continue to reproduce in the presence of normal serum, but they are converted almost completely into nonreproducing adults when ablastin is present. Heat-inactivated ablastic serum does not lose its inhibitory activity *in vitro*, indicating that ablastin is not complement dependent. This could not be determined with *in vivo* methods. Lastly, ablastin has no effect on culture forms of *T. lewisi* growing at room temperature. Because of the specificity of ablastin and the similarity of the culture forms to the stages found in the insect vector, this means that basic antigenic changes occur during the life cycle of the trypanosome.

Combination with the parasites.   The one property of ablastin that has probably caused the greatest difficulty in accepting it as an antibody is its apparent lack of affinity for the trypanosomes. This property is useful in separating the trypanocidal antibodies from ablastin, which can then be studied alone (Taliaferro, 1932), but it is difficult to imagine how an antibody can have an effect without coming into contact with its antigen. Obviously, combination occurs, but, because of the low avidity of ablastin, it does so to such a small degree that it is not detectable by conventional methods.

However, with a new sensitive technique called immunoelectroadsorption (IEA), it has been possible to demonstrate what appears to be a reaction between ablastin and the trypanosomes (D'Alesandro, 1966). With IEA, developed by Mathot et al. (1964), antigen is deposited on a charged metallized glass slide, and the thickness of the layer in Angstroms is measured with an ellipsometer (Rothen, 1957). Then the charge on the slide is reversed, normal or immune serum proteins are deposited on the antigen, and the thickness of the serum protein layer is measured. The reaction is specific; homologous immune sera form significantly thicker layers than heterologous and normal sera. When rat immune sera are repeatedly adsorbed with living trypanosomes to remove all the trypanocidal antibodies and are then tested by IEA, the serum protein layers formed are thinner than those of the same sera before removal of the trypanocidal antibodies, but they are still significantly thicker than those of normal sera. This residual activity is believed to be due to ablastin, for these trypanocidal antibody-free sera still show undiminished ablastic activity *in vitro*. Further evidence is provided by the finding that when antiserum to *T. lewisi* from the rabbit, which produces trypanocidal antibody but no ablastin (Taliaferro, 1932; D'Alesandro, 1969), is similarly adsorbed to remove trypanocidal antibodies and then tested by IEA, values indistinguishable from those of normal rabbit serum are obtained.

Effects of ablastin on the trypanosomes—*Morphologic.*   In addition to inhibiting reproduction, ablastin induces other changes that are associated with the inhibited state of the parasites. The most obvious are morphologic. The change from division forms to adults early in the infection has been observed for many years and is one of the most striking features of the nonpathogenic rodent trypanosome infections. Noteworthy also is the extreme uniformity of the nonreproducing adults in size and appearance (*see* p. 694, Fig. 2). That ablastin is responsible for these marked morphologic changes is shown by experiments in which passively transferred immune serum, adsorbed to remove trypanocidal antibodies, causes reproducing *T. lewisi* to change into adults within one or two days, much sooner than in an uninfluenced infection (D'Alesandro, 1959; Taliaferro and Pizzi, 1960). A similar conversion can also be made to occur *in vitro* (D'Alesandro, 1962). Therefore, these changes are not an inherent part of the developmental pattern of the parasites but occur only when an extraneous agent, ablastin, appears.

Metabolic and biochemical.   The marked effects of ablastin on parasite metabolism began to be understood when Moulder (1948) demonstrated that *T. lewisi* adults utilize significantly less glucose than division forms but show greater oxygen uptake and have a larger RQ, indicating that the antibody changes the glucose metabolism from one of assimilation to one of maintenance. This has been confirmed by Pizzi and Taliaferro (1960), who found that division forms incorporate more C^{14} from labeled glucose than adults. Numerous additional studies have verified the increase in oxygen uptake that occurs with the appearance of ablastic immunity (Zwisler and Lysenko, 1954; Thurston, 1958; Lincicome and Hill, 1965; Lincicome and Smith, 1966; Lincicome and Warsi, 1966; Lincicome et al., 1968). Subsequently, it has been found that enzymes involved in carbohydrate metabolism are also affected by ablastin. Thus, lactic dehydrogenase levels are over three times higher in division forms than in adults, but the reduction is probably controlled indirectly, for ablastic serum has no apparent effect on the enzyme (D'Alesandro and Sherman, 1964). Enzymes of the hexose monophosphate shunt are also significantly higher in division forms, but enzymes of the Krebs cycle are at similar levels in both stages (D'Alesandro, 1966). These results suggest that ablastin induces reductions in levels of enzymes outside the Krebs cycle only, and that reproducing trypanosomes depend greatly on the glycolytic pathway and the hexose monophosphate shunt whereas adults have a greater reliance on the Krebs cycle. Supporting this conclusion are the observed rise in RQ from 0.7 to 0.9 when inhibition of reproduction occurs and the finding that sodium malonate, a Krebs cycle inhibitor, reduces the oxygen uptake of adults much more than that of division forms (Moulder, 1948).

The arrest of cell division and the changes in enzyme levels are also reflected by reductions in synthetic activity of ablastin-inhibited trypanosomes. Using labeled materials, Taliaferro and Pizzi (1960) found that in inhibited adults, nucleic acid synthesis is virtually stopped and protein synthesis is reduced to a low maintenance level. The latter finding aids in understanding how the parasites retain their viability and motility in the presence of ablastin. That these changes result from the action of the antibody was shown by passive transfer experiments in which ablastic serum simultaneously curtailed reproductive and synthetic activities. Therefore, cellular metabolism is profoundly altered by ablastin, and the effects of inhibition are evident at many levels.

Concepts of the nature and action of ablastin.   There has been some controversy about cessation of reproduction in rodent trypanosome infections. Taliaferro's (1924, 1932, 1948, 1963) belief that a true inhibition occurs and that ablastin is responsible has met with criticism. Alternative explanations have been proposed that assume the observed changes result from the action of conventional trypanocidal antibodies, and that ablastin plays only a minor part or does not exist. Among the first to question the role of ablastin was Augustine (1943) who studied the recovery of immune rats from reinfection with large numbers of *T. lewisi*. In some cases reinfections lasted a few days, and since parasite numbers showed no increase in spite of the presence of division forms, he concluded that control of the parasitemias resulted from a differential susceptibility of division forms to the trypanocidal antibodies. Thus, ablastin was presumed to be absent or inoperative because a selective removal of reproducing parasites could effectively limit the trypanosome population without restricting division. However, because of the large overwhelming numbers of trypanosomes inoculated into the immune rats, it is not surprising that reproduction sometimes occurred since there was probably a large excess of antigen relative to ablastin. Moreover, Augustine (1943) reinfected his animals at intervals ranging from two weeks to nine months after recovery from the first infection, and Coventry (1925) has shown that the titer of ablastin begins to decline before the initial infection is terminated.

The trypanocidal antibodies are unquestionably important in preventing reinfection, but the nature of the immunologic response will depend upon both the size of the inoculum and the relative titers of the trypanocidal antibodies and ablastin (see pp. 717-718). In some reinfections, in fact, Augustine (1943) could find no evidence of reproduction. In similar studies by Taliaferro (1932), when parasites were not immediately destroyed and remained visible in the blood for a few days, reproduction occurred in some rats but not in others. Furthermore, as Taliaferro (1948) has indicated, Augustine's results can be interpreted to show that ablastin does not exist because a static adult population could be maintained by selective removal of division forms. But he points out that such a view contains an inherent contradiction in that a population from which adults are removed as soon as they start to divide would not remain constant but would decrease.

A more recent criticism has been made by Ormerod (1963), who proposes a "two antigens hypothesis" to explain immunity to T. lewisi. It is similar to Augustine's interpretation in that it is based on selective destruction of division forms, which differ antigenically from adults. However, to explain the maintenance of a static population, it is suggested that whenever adults begin to divide and are removed, they are replenished by "low grade" reproduction occurring in blood vessels of the kidneys outside the peripheral circulation. Although division forms were found in these blood vessels during the reproductive phase of the infection, and even then with difficulty, it was not possible to demonstrate them during the adult phase. Therefore, there are no data to support the hypothesis. Furthermore, it is not explained how the cryptic division forms would escape destruction, since they would still be bathed by antibody-containing blood.

That division forms and adults are antigenically distinct is well established (see p. 715), but Ormerod's hypothesis that trypanocidal antibodies alone control the infection has other failings. While he does state that the idea of inhibition of growth "cannot be abandoned entirely, especially with reference to the adult form," he rejects the evidence that the falling CV during the first few days of the infection reflects a true inhibition of reproduction. He believes instead that as the titer of the trypanocidal antibodies increases and catches up with the rate of reproduction, the selective removal of division forms is accelerated until a population of uniform adults alone remains. At the observed peak of reproductive activity in *T. lewisi* infections, division forms make up 20 to 50 percent of the parasite population (Taliaferro, 1941; Jaroslow, 1959; Taliaferro and Pizzi, 1960; D'Alesandro, 1962; Tempelis and Lysenko, 1965; Sherman and Ruble, 1967). If the reproductive rate is undiminished as Ormerod assumes, and with a generation time of 9 to 14 hours for *T. lewisi* (Walker, 1964), "low grade" reproduction in the kidneys could not possibly maintain a replacement rate of this magnitude. Therefore, if inhibition of reproduction only appears to occur and selective killing is really responsible for the falling CV as Ormerod maintains, then either division forms should be found easily during the adult stage, or the infection should end shortly after the first crisis begins with such a high reproductive rate and its coupled selective destruction of division forms. But the postulated division forms could not be found, and infections usually continue considerably beyond the first crisis. Finally, in *in vitro* cultures, where cryptic reproduction cannot occur, ablastic serum inhibits reproduction without decreasing parasite numbers (D'Alesandro, 1962).

It has been suggested that ablastin is an enzyme and not an antibody. The observation that a pantothenic acid-deficient diet or the administration of salicylate interferes with the ablastic response to *T. lewisi* (Becker et al., 1943. 1947; Becker and Gallagher, 1947) led Becker and Gallagher (1947) to postulate that ablastin is an oxidative enzyme and pantothenic acid is its coenzyme. Thus, in the absence of the coenzyme during the deficiency, the enzyme cannot function, and administered salicylate displaces pantothenate and renders the enzyme inactive. But later studies have failed to provide any evidence that salicylate combines with ablastin (Lysenko, 1951). The effects of such treatment are more readily explained by the known depression of antibody synthesis by vitamin deficiencies and salicylates (*see* pp. 698-699; pp. 702-703).

Others have claimed that ablastin is an antibody to "metabolic products" of the trypanosomes. Thillet and Chandler (1957) incubated living *T. lewisi* in normal rat serum *in vitro* and collected a soluble, parasite-free antigen, which they believed to be ablastinogen. But when rats were immunized with this antigen and then challenged, the injected parasites were destroyed so quickly that it was not possible to demonstrate inhibition of reproduction. In other experiments, it was reported that when immune serum from recovered rats was adsorbed with the antigen and then passively transferred, it permitted "practically normal reproduction" to occur. It was therefore concluded that ablastin had been adsorbed. However, the adsorbed serum was administered in doses of 1 ml per 100 gm of body weight only, and it is known from other *in vivo* titration studies that larger doses are usually required before an effect is evident (Taliaferro, 1932; D'Alesandro, 1959). Therefore, although the formation of trypanocidal antibodies was unquestionably elicited by the antigen since sera from vaccinated rats also agglutinated parasites *in vitro*, there was no conclusive direct evidence that it stimulated ablastin formation or neutralized the antibody.

Attempts to substantiate these results with *in vitro* culture methods have been unsuccessful (D'Alesandro, 1962). Wilson (1962) has also repeated the experiments of Thillet and Chandler but found that immune serum is only "doubtfully adsorbable" with trypanosome metabolites. To resolve this problem satisfactorily, immune serum from vaccinated rats should first be thoroughly adsorbed with living parasites to remove trypanocidal antibodies and then tested *in vivo* and *in vitro* for ablastic activity. In this way, it can be determined whether ablastin has actually been produced. Although Taliaferro (1932) found that blood forms killed by freezing and thawing appear to stimulate only an ablastic immunity, the antigens in the vaccine were not identified, and no subsequent attempts to confirm these results have been reported (*see* pp. 696-697 for a discussion of vaccines).

On the basis of the Thillet and Chandler (1957) experiments, Chandler (1958) proposed that ablastin also shows trypanocidal activity. According to this view, there is no need to consider the presence of separate trypanocidal antibodies because ablastin first inhibits reproduction when its titer is low, and later, when the titer is sufficiently high, acts as an agglutinin to cause the first crisis. Incomplete destruction of the parasites at this time is attributed to the reduced population density that decreases the opportunities for contact in the blood and consequent agglutination and phagocytosis. But in view of the known antigenic differences between division forms and adults (*see* p. 715), a more reasonable explanation is that the survivors are spared because they are resistant to the trypanocidal antibody. There is ample evidence supporting the view that inhibition of reproduction and the first crisis are caused by two distinct antibodies, and not by ablastin alone as Chandler claimed. Saul and Becker (1949) observed in salicylate-treated rats that trypanocidal antibody was formed in amounts sufficient to cause a crisis despite the absence of ablastin, as indicated by a continuously high reproductive rate. Similar results have been reported with cortisone-treated rats (Sherman and Ruble, 1967). Therefore, since the antibody titer was high enough to cause a crisis, inhibition of reproduction should have occurred earlier when the titer was lower, as required by Chandler's hypothesis. Furthermore, all indications are that the titers of ablastic and trypanocidal activities vary independently, and this would not occur if only one antibody were involved* (Coventry, 1925, 1930; Taliaferro, 1932, 1941).

*Brown's (1915) observations and interpretations are relevant to these considerations and also have historical interest in that they predate Taliaferro's (1924) demonstration of ablastic immunity:

"There appears to be some distinction, however, between the mechanism limiting multiplication and that causing the destruction of trypanosomes in the rat's blood. In the usual infection of *Trypanosoma lewisi* we have evidence of what I regard as two distinct classes of immunological reactions, one of which is concerned with checking the multiplication of trypanosomes, as ordinarily understood, and the other in their destruction. That these phenomena are in reality separable is shown by the fact that in some infections multiplication in the peripheral blood may be completely checked early in the infection with no appreciable decrease in the numbers of trypanosomes or other evidence of their destruction for weeks or even months. On the other hand, in certain infections, . . . active multiplication may continue beyond its usual limits, while the number of trypanosomes in the peripheral blood continually diminishes with abundant evidence of vigorous destruction" (Brown, 1915).

Nevertheless, metabolic products may be important to the immune response. Soluble parasite antigens have been demonstrated in the serum of *T. lewisi*-infected rats (D'Alesandro, 1963). Weitz (1960) first described antigens of this type in experimental *T. brucei* infections and has called them "exoantigens." They have also been reported for other species of trypanosomes (Gray, 1961; Dodin and Fromentin, 1962; Seed, 1963; Gill, 1965; J. K. Miller, 1965). In most cases these antigens have immunogenic properties, but there is no evidence as yet that the *T. lewisi* exoantigens are involved in ablastin formation (D'Alesandro, 1966).

Despite the few criticisms of ablastic immunity, it is generally accepted that a true inhibition of reproduction occurs and that ablastin is responsible. But the nature of the antigen and the site of antibody activity have yet to be determined. It has been suggested that ablastinogen is a soluble enzyme released from the trypanosomes and provides hematin or protoporphyrin from host hemoglobin for use in the terminal respiration of the parasites (Chandler, 1958). Thus, by neutralizing the enzyme, ablastin restricts the availability of metabolites essential for growth and reproduction. This idea does not seem reasonable because adults consume more oxygen than division forms (*see* p. 722), and this would not occur if terminal respiration were depressed. Furthermore, there is no evidence that trypanosomes release extracellular enzymes for nutritional purposes. Others have compared the action of ablastin with that of dinitrophenols, which can inhibit cell division and stimulate oxygen uptake (Moulder, 1948; Lincicome and Hill, 1965). Presumably, such action would occur intracellularly.

As yet, it is not known whether ablastin acts within the cell by obstructing synthetic pathways, or whether it is active on the cell membrane where it impedes or regulates the passage of vital metabolites. There is no doubt that molecules as large as antibodies can enter trypanosomes. *T. lewisi* has been observed to ingest particulate lipid while circulating in the blood (Wotton and Becker, 1963), and *T. rhodesiense* ingests ferritin particles, which are localized in the area surrounding the invagination at the base of the flagellum (Brown, K. N., et al., 1965). The fact that lactic dehydrogenase from *T. lewisi* is not neutralized by ablastic serum does not preclude the possibility that the antibody functions intracellularly (D'Alesandro and Sherman, 1964); the reduced enzyme levels of adults could be a secondary effect resulting from a primary reaction between ablastin and other intracellular components.

Experiments to determine whether ablastin blocks vital metabolites at the cell surface have yielded inconclusive results (D'Alesandro, 1966). By dry emulsion autoradiography with adenine-H^3, the pool size of *T. lewisi* was studied. It was expected that if inhibition occurs on the cell membrane, adults would have no adenine pool and that division forms, which are actively synthesizing, would have one. However, no soluble adenine pool could be detected in either stage. Possibly, the method lacks adequate sensitivity, but in a comparative study by Williamson (1963) of the free amino acid levels of several species of trypanosomes, the level in adult *T. lewisi* was found to be "aberrantly low." Unfortunately, division forms were not included in his study. Nevertheless, the possibility that inhibition occurs at the cell surface cannot be dismissed, for the apparent absence of an adenine pool in division forms may result from a high synthetic rate that keeps the pool in a state of near depletion. Furthermore, if it is assumed that ablastin enters the parasites, it is difficult to conceive of the antibody being active intracellularly, for it would probably be isolated and eventually destroyed by enzymes. This is suggested by the studies of Brown, K. N., et al. (1965), who found that the ferritin ingested by *T. rhodesiense* was usually contained within membrane-limited organelles, which were interpreted as phagocytic vesicles and possibly part of a lysosomal system. Because of these considerations, it therefore seems more logical to assume that ablastin acts on the cell membrane. This view is also consistent with the evidence indicating that the antibody has a low avidity and that antibodies in general do not penetrate live cells in an active form (Coombs and Lachman, 1968).

How then can ablastic action be explained, especially the apparent lack of affinity of the antibody for the trypanosomes? It has been reported in several studies that there are no immediate changes in morphology or in metabolic activities when ablastin is allowed to act. For example, ablastic serum has no effect on the oxygen uptake of division forms in a Warburg respirometer (Moulder, as communicated to Taliaferro, 1948; Zwisler and Lysenko, 1954). Division forms also incorporate similar amounts of labeled adenine whether incubated in normal or ablastic serum *in vitro* for 30 minutes or less (D'Alesandro, 1966). That immediate effects could not be detected in these experiments is not surprising in view of the short exposures to ablastin and the extent of the changes that eventually occur. Thus, to transform division forms into adults *in vitro*, at least an overnight exposure to ablastin is required before the effect is marked (D'Alesandro, 1962). Long exposures are also required for *in vivo* transformation (*see* p. 721). Conversely, no immediate changes are evident when inhibited adults are transferred from ablastic to normal serum. *In vitro*, for example, adults incorporate similar amounts of labeled adenine whether incubated briefly in normal or ablastic serum (D'Alesandro, 1966), and reproduction does not begin for at least one day when infections are initiated with adults (Taliaferro, 1924; Augustine, 1941). But Taliaferro and Pizzi (1960) found that the highest rate of protein synthesis occurs in *T. lewisi* adults three hours after injection into normal rats while the parasites still have adult morphology and show no evidence of division. Taliaferro (1963) believes these results indicate ablastin is an extremely non-avid antibody, comparable to the normal Forssman hemolysin. He reasons that if this is so, high concentrations of ablastin would be required in the surrounding medium to maintain an adequate inhibitory amount combined with the parasites. Conversely, when low concentrations are present, as would occur when parasites are transferred from ablastic to normal serum, the combination dissociates, the trypanosomes are released from the inhibited state, and synthetic activity accelerates markedly. There-fore, it follows from these considerations that there would be no immediate changes when adults are removed from and division forms placed in ablastic serum, because with such a non-avid antibody, at least a few hours would be required to obtain a significant degree of dissociation or combination*.

The nonadsorbability of ablastin could also be accounted for by assuming that the antigen is masked or is not present in sufficient quantity. If the former condition prevails, it would be difficult to explain how the antibody can have an effect when the antigen is not accessible. In the latter instance, if it is also assumed that ablastin has a relatively high avidity, then com-bined antibody would be retained by parasites washed free of ablastic serum, even though small amounts of antigen were involved. Under these conditions, reproduction could not occur, even upon transfer to a normal host, because the trypanosomes would be permanently sensitized. Furthermore, Patton (1967) has shown that the inhibitory effect of ablastin on synthesis is revers-ible. Thus, incorporation of thymidine-H^3 *in vitro* by *T. lewisi* increases when ablastic serum is replaced by normal serum and ceases when normal serum is replaced by ablastic serum. This reversibility would not occur if an avid antibody were involved. Therefore, it is more reasonable to assume that ablastin has a low avidity for its antigen.

Left unanswered by these considerations, however, is the question of how ablastin inhibits reproduction. All indications are that the changes associated with ablastic inhibition, whether morphologic, in enzyme levels, rates of pro-tein and nucleic acid synthesis, glucose utilization, or respiration, are con-trolled by the antibody indirectly. Although it is possible that ablastin is a complex of antibodies, each directed toward a different metabolic process, it is more likely that only one vital process is affected directly and the others indirectly. Since it is reasonable to assume that ablastin acts on the cell sur-face, the affected process may well be the transport mechanism controlling the passage of vital metabolites across the cell membrane. Christensen (1962) believes that transport sites are exposed macromolecular structures embedded in the plasma membrane, and in recent studies transport proteins have been isolated and characterized (Pardee, 1968). These sites would therefore probably be antigenic. By combining with antigens at or near these sites, ablastin could impede or limit the passage of metabolites. Because of transport specificity, there are different types of sites, but probably only one type reacts with ablastin unless the different types have antigens in common. But in either case, the restrictions imposed by ablastin on the transport of vital metabolites would force the trypanosomes to assume a maintenance state. Therefore, although antigens associated with only one process would

---

*The allowance of a few hours for either dissociation or combination to occur is reasonable when it is remembered that non-avid antibodies dissociate rapidly and com-bine slowly. Thus, a dissociation time of a few hours for a non-avid antibody would be rapid when compared with that of an avid antibody, which might dissociate little if at all even after days. Similarly, the few hours required for a significant degree of com-bination to occur with a non-avid antibody would be slow when compared with the virtually instantaneous reaction of an avid antibody. For discussions of avidity, see Jerne (1951) and Talmage (1957).

be directly involved, many other changes would occur, but these would be secondarily acquired and characteristic of the inhibited trypanosomes. Moreover, because of the low avidity of ablastin, the effects of the antibody would not be immediately evident.

This concept of ablastin, though general and leaving many questions unanswered, is in reasonable agreement with present knowledge. Future studies of transport in trypanosomes and other cells may well provide additional insights. As yet, transport site structures have not been identified and isolated (Christensen, 1962), and this may explain the present difficulties in identifying ablastinogen. It is also possible that the apparent low avidity of ablastin is really a reflection of properties of the transport site antigens and not of the antibody *per se*. As more is learned about ablastin, its effects, and the nature and site of its antigen, a detailed explanation of ablastic action should be possible.

CONCLUSION

As a group, the nonpathogenic rodent trypanosomes are virtually unstudied. Of the more than 80 species described, only *T. lewisi* and a few other species have been examined in detail, usually from an immunologic point of view. But the marked similarities of members of this group suggest that the considerable information available on a few species is generally applicable to the whole group. The nonpathogenic nature of these parasites appears to have an immunologic basis, which is primarily humoral. Two types of host response occur: the first inhibits parasite reproduction, and the second is trypanocidal. The reproduction-inhibiting antibody, called ablastin, has a unique combination of properties found nowhere but in the *T. lewisi* group of trypanosomes; the trypanocidal antibodies are conventional. Although ablastin has been unequivocally demonstrated only with two species, it is probably produced against all members of the group and may very well be the distinguishing feature of nonpathogenic trypanosome infections. The apparent nonadsorbability of the antibody and the unsuccessful attempts to identify its antigen have caused controversy about its classification as an antibody, whether it indeed exists, and its mechanism of action, which is at present unknown. That ablastin is an antibody is difficult to deny in light of all the available evidence, but considerations of its mode of action must remain speculative, at least for the immediate future, in spite of the fact that much is known about its effects on the trypanosomes. It is quite possible, however, that the antibody reacts directly with the transport mechanism of the parasites thereby restricting the uptake of vital metabolites, and that all the changes associated with inhibition are secondarily acquired and result indirectly from this primary reaction. Future studies of transport and associated metabolic activities may well provide the key to understanding how this unique antibody works.

REFERENCES

Ambrose, C. T. 1966. Inhibition of the secondary antibody response *in vitro* by salicylate and gentisate. J. Exp. Med., 124: 461-482.

Ascoli, A. 1906. Zur Kenntnis der aktiven Substanz des Milzbrandserums. Z. Physiol. Chem., 48: 315-330.

——— 1908. Über den Wirkungsmechanismus des Milzbrandserums: Antiblastische Immunität. Zbl. Bakt. [Orig.], 46: 178-188.

Ashcroft, M. T., E. Burtt, and H. Fairbairn. 1959. The experimental infection of some African wild animals with *Trypanosoma rhodesiense, T. brucei* and *T. congolense*. Ann. Trop. Med. Parasit., 53: 147-161.

Ashley, W., Jr. 1962. The effect of a concurrent infection with *Trypanosoma lewisi* on the development and maintenance of acquired immunity to *Nippostrongylus brasiliensis* in rats. Proc. Helminth. Soc. (Washington), 29: 59-62.

Ashworth, J. H., J. P. MacGowan, and J. Ritchie. 1909. Note on the occurrence of a trypanosome (*Trypanosoma cuniculi*, Blanchard) in the rabbit. With a note on the experimental work. J. Path. Bact., 13: 437-442.

Atchley, F. O., and E. R. Becker. 1962. Depression of parasitemia in *Trypanosoma lewisi* infection of rats injected with 6-mercaptopurine. J. Parasit., 48: 578-583.

Augustine, D. L. 1941. The behavior of *Trypanosoma lewisi* during the early stage of the incubation period in the rat. J. Infect. Dis., 69: 208-214.

——— 1943. Some factors in the defense mechanism against reinfection with *Trypanosoma lewisi*. Proc. Amer. Acad. Arts Sci., 75: 85-93.

Austen, K. F. 1963. Immunological aspects of salicylate action–a review. *In* Salicylates. Dixon, A. St. J., Martin, B. K., Smith, M. J. H., and Wood, P. H. N., eds. Boston, Little, Brown and Co., pp. 161-169.

Axelrod, A. E., and J. Pruzansky. 1955. The role of the vitamins in antibody formation. Vitamins Hormones (N.Y.), 13: 1-27.

Banovitz, J., and K. Ishizaka. 1967. Detection of five components having antibody activity in rat antisera. Proc. Soc. Exp. Biol. Med., 125: 78-82.

Barnes, E. A. 1951. Effect of benzene and six selected salicylates on the development of immunity in *Trypanosoma lewisi* infection and on various aspects of the blood picture. Iowa State Coll. J. Sci., 26: 1-17.

Becker, E. R. 1961a. Effect of salicylates and related compounds on ablastic response in rats infected with *Trypanosoma lewisi*. I. Isomers of salicylic acid. J. Parasit., 47: 425-427.

——— 1961b. Effect of salicylates and related compounds on ablastic response in rats infected with *Trypanosoma lewisi*. II. Dihydroxybenzoic acids; antagonisms. J. Parasit., 47: 1007-1014.

——— and P. L. Gallagher. 1947. Prolongation of the reproductive phase of *Trypanosoma lewisi* by the administration of sodium salicylate. Iowa State Coll. J. Sci., 21: 351-362.

——— and M. G. Lysenko. 1948. Reinfection with *Trypanosoma lewisi* and recurrence of reproduction in recovered and near-recovered rats. Iowa State Coll. J. Sci., 22: 239-255.

——— M. Mauresa, and E. M. Johnson. 1943. Reduction in the efficiency of ablastic action in *Trypanosoma lewisi* infection by withholding pantothenic acid from the host's diet. Iowa State Coll. J. Sci., 17: 431-441.

——— J. Taylor, and C. Fuhrmeister. 1947. The effect of pantothenate deficiency on *Trypanosoma lewisi* infection in the rat. Iowa State Coll. J. Sci., 21: 237-243.

Brown, K. N., J. A. Armstrong, and R. C. Valentine. 1965. The ingestion of protein molecules by blood forms of *Trypanosoma rhodesiense*. Exp. Cell Res., 39: 129-135.

Brown, W. H. 1914. A note on the pathogenicity of *Trypanosoma lewisi*. J. Exp. Med., 19: 406-410.

——— 1915. Concerning changes in the biological properties of *Trypanosoma lewisi* produced by experimental means, with especial reference to virulence. J. Exp. Med., 21: 345-364.

Bruynoghe, R., and P. Vassiliadis. 1929. La splénectomie dans l'infection du *Tr. lewisi*. Ann. Soc. Belg. Med. Trop., 9: 191-195.

Caldwell, F. E., and P. György. 1943. Effect of biotin deficiency on duration of infection with *Trypanosoma lewisi* in the rat. Proc. Soc. Exp. Biol. Med., 53: 116-119.

———— and P. György. 1947. The influence of biotin deficiency on the course of infection with *Trypanosoma lewisi* in the albino rat. J. Infect. Dis., 81: 197-208.

Campbell, D. H. 1938a. The specific absorbability of protective antibodies against *Cysticercus crassicollis* in rats and *C. pisiformis* in rabbits from infected and artificially immunized animals. J. Immun., 35: 205-216.

———— 1938b. Further studies on the "nonabsorbable" protective property in serum from rats infected with *Cysticercus crassicollis*. J. Immun., 35: 465-476.

Cantrell, W., and G. D. Betts. 1956. Effect of cortisone on immunization against *Trypanosoma equiperdum* in the rat. J. Infect. Dis., 99: 282-296.

Chandler, A. C. 1958. Some considerations relative to the nature of immunity in *Trypanosoma lewisi* infections. J. Parasit., 44: 129-135.

Channon, H. A., and H. D. Wright, 1927. Observations on trypanosomiasis of rabbits, and its natural mode of transmission. J. Path. Bact., 30: 253-260.

Christensen, H. N. 1962. Biological Transport. New York, W. A. Benjamin, Inc.

Citri, N. 1952. Immunological observations on *Trypanosoma lewisi*. Bull. Res. Counc. Israel, 1: 99-100.

Coombs, R. R. A., and P. J. Lachman. 1968. Immunological reactions at the cell surface. Brit. Med. Bull., 24: 113-117.

Corradetti, A. 1963. Acquired sterile immunity in experimental protozoal infections. *In* Immunity to Protozoa. Garnham, P. C. C., Pierce, A. E., and Roitt, I., eds. Oxford, Blackwell Scientific Publications, pp. 69-77.

Coventry, F. A. 1925. The reaction product which inhibits reproduction of the trypanosomes in infections with *Trypanosoma lewisi*, with special reference to its changes in titer throughout the course of the infection. Amer. J. Hyg., 5: 127-144.

———— 1929. Experimental infections with *Trypanosoma lewisi* in the guinea-pig. Amer. J. Hyg., 9: 247-259.

———— 1930. The trypanocidal actions of specific antiserums on *Trypanosoma lewisi in vivo*. Amer. J. Hyg., 12: 366-380.

Cox, H. W. 1964. Immune response of rats and mice to trypanosome infections. J. Parasit., 50: 15-22.

Culbertson, J. T. 1934. The trypanocidal action of human serum: The relationship between the trypanocidal action of the serum and man's immunity to the trypanosomes pathogenic for animals. Ann. Trop. Med. Parasit., 28: 93-97.

———— 1938. Natural transmission of immunity against *Trypanosoma lewisi* from mother rats to their offspring. J. Parasit., 24: 65-82.

———— 1939a. The immunization of rats of different age groups against *Trypanosoma lewisi* by the administration of specific antiserum *per os*. J. Parasit., 25: 181-182.

———— 1939b. Transmission of resistance against *Trypanosoma lewisi* from a passively immunized mother rat to young nursing upon her. J. Parasit., 25: 182-183.

———— 1940. The natural transmission of immunity against *Trypanosoma duttoni* from mother mice to their young. J. Immun., 38: 51-66.

———— 1941a. Trypanosomiasis in the Florida cotton rat, *Sigmodon hispidus littoralis*. J. Parasit., 27: 45-52.

———— 1941b. Natural transmission of immunity against *Trypanosoma lewisi* from vaccinated mother rats to their young. J. Parasit., 27: 75-79.

———— 1941c. Immunity against Animal Parasites. New York, Columbia University Press.

———— and N. Molomut. 1938. Infection with *Trypanosoma lewisi* in the hypophysectomized rat. Proc. Soc. Exp. Biol. Med., 39: 28-30.

———— and W. R. Kessler. 1939. Studies on age resistance against trypanosome infections: III. Vaccination of rats against *Trypansoma lewisi* with special reference to the response of different age groups. Amer. J. Hyg. (Sec. C), 29: 33-43.

———— and R. M. Wotton. 1939. Studies on age resistance against trypanosome infections. VI. Production of ablastin in rats of different age groups after infection with *Trypanosoma lewisi*. Amer. J. Hyg. (Sec. C), 30: 101-113.

Cushing, R. T., and A. G. Johnson. 1966. γG antibodies appearing early in the primary response of the mouse. Proc. Soc. Exp. Biol. Med., 122: 523-525.

D'Alesandro, P. A. 1959. Electrophoretic and ultracentrifugal studies of antibodies to *Trypanosoma lewisi*. J. Infect. Dis., 105: 76-95.

———— 1962. *In vitro* studies of ablastin, the reproduction-inhibiting antibody to *Trypanosoma lewisi*. J. Protozool., 9: 351-358.

—— 1963. Soluble parasite antigens in the serum of rats infected with *Trypanosoma lewisi*. J. Protozool., 10 (Suppl.): 22.

—— 1966. Immunological and biochemical studies of ablastin, the reproduction-inhibiting antibody to *Trypanosoma lewisi*. Ann. N. Y. Acad. Sci., 129: 834-852.

—— 1969. Unpublished results.

—— and I. W. Sherman. 1964. Changes in lactic dehydrogenase levels of *Trypanosoma lewisi* associated with appearance of ablastic immunity. Exp. Parasit., 15: 430-438.

Davis, B. S. 1952. Studies on the trypanosomes of some California mammals. Univ. Calif. Publ. Zool., 57: 145-250.

de Carvalho, I. F., Y. Borel, and P. A. Miescher. 1967. Influence of splenectomy in rats on the formation of 19S and 7S antibodies. Immunology, 12: 505-516.

Delanoë, P. 1911a. Sur la réceptivité de la souris au *Trypanosoma lewisi*. C. R. Soc. Biol. (Paris), 70: 649-651.

—— 1911b. Sur l'existence des formes trypanosomes dan les cultures de *T. lewisi*. C. R. Soc. Biol. (Paris), 70: 704-706.

—— 1911c. Méchanisme de l'immunité naturelle de la souris a l'égard du *Trypanosoma lewisi*. C. R. Soc. Biol. (Paris), 70: 1041-1043.

—— 1912. L'importance de la phagocytose dans l'immunité de la souris a l'égard de quelques flagellés. Ann. Inst. Pasteur (Paris), 26: 172-203.

Desowitz, R. S. 1954. Studies on *Trypanosoma vivax*. X. The activity of some blood fractions in facilitating infection in the white rat. Ann. Trop. Med. Parasit., 48: 142-151.

—— 1960. Studies on immunity and host-parasite relationship. II. The immune response of antelope to trypanosomal challenge. Ann. Trop. Med. Parasit., 54: 281-292.

—— 1963. Adaptation of trypanosomes to abnormal hosts. Ann. N. Y. Acad. Sci., 113: 74-87.

—— and H. J. C. Watson. 1952. Studies on *Trypanosoma vivax*. III. Observations on the maintenance of a strain in white rats. Ann. Trop. Med. Parasit., 46: 92-100.

—— and H. J. C. Watson. 1953. Studies on *Trypanosoma vivax*. IV. The maintenance of a strain in white rats without sheep-serum supplement. Ann. Trop. Med. Parasit., 47: 62-67.

Dixon, F. J., J. Jacot-Guillarmod, and P. J. McConahey. 1966. The antibody response of rabbits and rats to hemocyanin. J. Immun., 97: 350-355.

Dodin, A., and H. Fromentin. 1962. Mise en évidence d'un antigène vaccinant dans le plasma de souris expérimentalement infectées par *Trypanosoma gambiense* et par *Trypanosoma congolense*. Bull. Soc. Path. Exot., 55: 128-138.

du Buy, H. G., C. L. Greenblatt, J. E. Hayes, Jr., and D. R. Lincicome. 1966. Regulation of cell membrane permeability in *Trypanosoma lewisi*. Exp. Parasit., 18: 231-243.

Duca, C. J. 1939. Studies on age resistance against trypanosome infections: II. The resistance of rats of different age groups to *Trypanosoma lewisi*, and the blood response of rats infected with this parasite. Amer. J. Hyg. (Sec. C), 29: 25-32.

Dusanic, D. G. 1968. Growth and immunologic studies on the culture form of *Trypanosoma lewisi*. J. Protozool., 15: 328-333.

Entner, N., and C. Gonzalez. 1966. Changes in antigenicity of *Trypanosoma lewisi* during the course of infection in rats. J. Protozool., 13: 642-645.

Galliard, H. 1933. Infections à *Trypanosoma duttoni* Thiroux chez les animaux splénectomisés. Bull. Soc. Path. Exot., 26: 609-613.

—— 1934. Les formes de multiplication de *Trypanosoma duttoni* Thiroux, au cours d'infections mortelles chez la souris. Ann. Parasit. Hum. Comp., 12: 273-277.

Galuzo, I. G., and V. F. Novinskaya. 1961. Tripanozomy zhivotnykh Kazakhstana. II. Tripanozomy gryzunov. *In* Prirodnaya Ochagovest' Boleznei i Voprosy Parazitologii. Galuzo, I. G., et al., eds. Alma-Ata, USSR, Izdat. Akademii Nauk, Kazakhstan SSR, pp. 151-172.

Gill, B. S. 1965. Properties of soluble antigen of *Trypanosoma evansi*. J. Gen. Microbiol., 38: 357-362.

Goble, F. C., and I. Singer. 1960. The reticuloendothelial system in experimental malaria and trypanosomiasis. Ann. N. Y. Acad. Sci., 88: 149-171.

Gray, A. R. 1961. Soluble antigens of *Trypanosoma vivax* and of other trypanosomes. Immunology, 4: 253-261.

———— 1965a. Antigenic variation in clones of *Trypanosoma brucei*. I: Immunological relationships of the clones. Ann. Trop. Med. Parasit., 59: 27-36.

———— 1965b. Antigenic variation in a strain of *Trypanosoma brucei* transmitted by *Glossina morsitans* and *G. palpalis*. J. Gen. Microbiol., 41: 195-214.

———— 1966. Antigenic variation in clones of *Trypanosoma brucei*. II: The drug-sensitivities of variants of a clone and the antigenic relationships of trypanosomes before and after drug treatment. Ann. Trop. Med. Parasit., 60: 265-275.

Greenblatt, C. L., and D. R. Lincicome. 1966. Identity of trypanosome growth factors in serum. II. Active globulin components. Exp. Parasit., 19: 139-150.

———— and E. Shelton. 1968. Mouse serum as an environment for the growth of *Trypanosoma lewisi*. Exp. Parasit., 22: 187-200.

Grewal, M. S. 1957. The life cycle of the British rabbit trypanosome, *Trypanosoma nabiasi* Railliet, 1895. Parasitology, 47: 100-118.

Grillo, J., and J. Schmitz. 1935. Chemotherapeutische Versuche bei Mischinfektionen mit zwei Trypanosomenarten. Z. Immunitätsforsch. 85: 203-217.

Haleem, M. A., and S. A. Minton. 1966. The effects of adrenalectomy and splenectomy on *Trypanosoma lewisi* infection in white rats. J. Trop. Med. Hyg., 69: 294-298.

Harris, T. N. 1965. Cellular sources of antibody: A review of recent developments. Med. Clin. N. Amer., 49: 1517-1531.

Herbert, I. V., and E. R. Becker. 1961. Effect of cortisone and X-irradiation on the course of *Trypanosoma lewisi* infection in the rat. J. Parasit., 47: 304-308.

Herrick, C. A., and S. X. Cross. 1936. The development of natural and artificial resistance of young rats to the pathogenic effects of the parasite *Trypanosoma lewisi*. J. Parasit., 22: 126-129.

Hughes, F. W., and A. L. Tatum. 1956a. Effects of hypoxia on rats infected with *Trypanosoma lewisi*. J. Infect. Dis., 98: 127-132.

———— and A. L. Tatum. 1956b. Effects of hypoxia and intercurrent infections on infections by *Plasmodium berghei* in rats. J. Infect. Dis., 99: 38-43.

Inoki, S. 1960. Studies on the antigenic variation in the Wellcome strain of *Trypanosoma gambiense*. I. Improvements in technique. II. On the first relapse appearing in mice treated with human plasma. Biken's J., 3: 215-228.

Jackson, G. J. 1959. Simultaneous infections with *Plasmodium berghei* and *Trypanosoma lewisi* in the rat. J. Parasit., 45: 94.

Janković, B. D., B. H. Waksman, and B. G. Arnason. 1962. Role of the thymus in immune reactions in rats. I. The immunologic response to bovine serum albumin (antibody formation, Arthus reactivity, and delayed hypersensitivity) in rats thymectomized or splenectomized at various times after birth. J. Exp. Med., 116: 159-176.

Jaroslow, B. N. 1955. The effect of X-irradiation on immunity of the mouse to *Trypanosoma duttoni*. J. Infect. Dis., 96: 242-249.

———— 1959. The effect of X or neutron irradiation, India ink blockade, or splenectomy on innate immunity against *Trypanosoma duttoni* in mice. J. Infect. Dis., 104: 119-129.

Jerne, N. K. 1951. A study of avidity based on rabbit skin responses to diphtheria toxin-antitoxin mixtures. Acta Path. Microbiol. Scand., 87 (Suppl.): 183.

Juminer, B., and J. A. Goudineau. 1960. Sensibilité de la gerbille (*G. hirtipes*) à *Trypanosoma lewisi*. Arch. Inst. Pasteur (Tunis), 37: 171-180.

Jürgens, R. J. 1902. Beitrag zur Biologie der Rattentrypanosomen. Arch. Hyg., 42: 265-288.

Keefe, F. B., S. I. Helman, and J. J. Smith. 1967. RES response to hypophysectomy in the rat. J. Reticuloendothel. Soc., 4: 177-189.

Koenig, M. G., R. M. Heyssel, M. A. Melly, and D. E. Rogers. 1965. The dynamics of reticuloendothelial blockade. J. Exp. Med., 122: 117-142.

Kroó, H. 1936. Die spontane, apathogene Trypanosomeninfektion der Kaninchen. Z. Immunitätsforsch., 88: 117-128.

Kuhn, L. R. 1938. The effect of splenectomy and blockade on the protective titer of antiserum against *Trypanosoma equiperdum*. J. Infect. Dis., 63: 217-224.

Lange, D. E., and M. G. Lysenko. 1960. *In vitro* phagocytosis of *Trypanosoma lewisi* by rat exudative cells. Exp. Parasit., 10: 39-42.

Laveran, A., and F. Mesnil. 1900. Sur l'agglutination des trypanosomes du rat par divers sérums. C. R. Soc. Biol. (Paris), 52: 939-942.

———— and F. Mesnil. 1901. Recherches morphologiques et expérimentales sur le trypanosome des rats (*Trypanosoma lewisi*, Kent). Ann. Inst. Pasteur (Paris), 15: 673-714.

———— and F. Mesnil. 1912. Trypanosomes et Trypanosomiases. Paris, Masson & Cie, 2nd ed.

Leone, C. A. 1962. Effects of Ionizing Radiations on Immune Processes. New York, Gordon and Breach Science Publishers.

Levine, N. D. 1965. Trypanosomes and *Haemobartonella* in wild rodents in Illinois. J. Protozool., 12: 225-228.

Lincicome, D. R. 1958. Growth of *Trypanosoma lewisi* in the heterologous mouse host. Exp. Parasit., 7: 1-13.

———— 1959a. Serial passage of *Trypanosoma lewisi* in the heterologous mouse host. I. Development in calorically-restricted hosts. J. Protozool., 6: 310-315.

———— 1959b. Observations on changes in *Trypanosoma lewisi* after growth in calorically-restricted and in normal mice. Ann. Trop. Med. Parasit., 53: 274-287.

———— 1963. Chemical basis of parasitism. Ann. N. Y. Acad. Sci., 113: 360-380.

———— and E. H. Francis. 1961. Quantitative studies on heterologous sera inducing development of *Trypanosoma lewisi* in mice. Exp. Parasit., 11: 68-76.

———— and J. A. Hinnant. 1962. Identity of trypanosome growth factors in serum. I. Alteration of factors in rat serum by host starvation. Exp. Parasit., 12: 128-133.

———— and S. O. Emejuaiwe. 1963. Influence of host sex and age on *Trypanosoma lewisi* populations. J. Parasit., 49 (5, Sec. 2): 23.

———— and J. Shepperson. 1963. Increased rate of growth of mice infected with *Trypanosoma duttoni*. J. Parasit., 49: 31-34.

———— and G. C. Hill. 1965. Oxygen uptake by *Trypanosoma lewisi* complex cells—I. L isolate. Comp. Biochem. Physiol., 14: 425-436.

———— and J. R. Shepperson. 1965. Experimental evidence for molecular exchanges between a dependent trypanosome cell and its host. Exp. Parasit., 17: 148-167.

———— and R. C. Watkins. 1965. Antigenic relationships among *Trypanosoma lewisi*-complex cells. I. Agglutinins in antisera. Parasitology, 55: 365-374.

———— and A. S. Smith. 1966. Oxygen uptake by *Trypanosoma lewisi*-complex cells—II. R and L isolates compared. Comp. Biochem. Physiol., 17: 59-68.

———— and A. A. Warsi. 1966. Oxygen uptake by *Trypansoma lewisi* complex cells—III. C isolate. Comp. Biochem. Physiol., 17: 871-881.

———— R. N. Rossan, and W. C. Jones. 1963. Growth of rats infected with *Trypanosoma lewisi*. Exp. Parasit., 14: 54-65.

———— A. A. Warsi, and C. M. Lee. 1968. Oxygen uptake of *Trypanosoma lewisi*-complex cells. IV. "E" and "Sp" isolates. Exp. Parasit., 23: 114-127.

Linton, R. W. 1929. Blood sugar in infections with *Trypanosoma lewisi*. Ann. Trop. Med. Parasit., 23: 307-313.

Luzzio, A. J. 1960. Effect of X rays on antibodies. J. Infect. Dis., 106: 87-90.

Lysenko, M. G. 1951. Concerning salicylate inhibition of ablastic activity in *Trypanosoma lewisi* infection. J. Parasit., 37: 535-544.

Manteufel, P. 1909. Studien über die Trypanosomiasis der Ratten mit Berücksichtigung der Übertragung unternatürlichen Verhältnissen und der Immunität. Arb. Gesundh. (Berlin), 33: 46-83.

Marmorston-Gottesman, J., and D. Perla. 1930. Studies of *Bartonella muris* anemia of albino rats. I. *Trypanosoma lewisi* infection in normal albino rats associated with *Bartonella muris* anemia. II. Latent infections in adult normal rats. J. Exp. Med., 52: 121-129,

———— D. Perla, and J. Vorzimer. 1930. Immunological studies in relation to the suprarenal gland. VIa. *Trypanosoma lewisi* infection in the normal rat. VIb. *Trypanosoma lewisi* infection in suprarenalectomized adult albino rats. J. Exp. Med., 52: 587-600.

Mathot, C., A. Rothen, and J. Casals. 1964. A new sensitive method for detecting immunological reactions. Nature (London), 202: 1181-1183.

McMaster, P. D., and R. E. Franzl. 1961. The effects of adrenocortical steroids upon antibody formation. Metabolism, 10: 990-1005.

McNeal, W. J. 1904. The life-history of *Trypanosoma lewisi* and *Trypanosoma brucei*. J. Infect. Dis., 1: 517-543.

Meyers, W. M., and M. G. Lysenko. 1953. Effect of sodium salicylate treatment on antibody titers in rats infected with *Trypanosoma lewisi*. Proc. Soc. Exp. Biol. Med., 84: 97-98.

────── and M. G. Lysenko. 1956. The effect of salicylate treatment on plasma proteins in rats infected with *Trypanosoma lewisi*. Exp. Parasit., 5: 1-21.

Miller, J. F. A. P. 1965. The role of the thymus in immune processes. Int. Arch. Allerg. Appl. Immun., 28: 61-70.

Miller, J. K. 1965. Variation of the soluble antigens of *Trypanosoma brucei*. Immunology, 9: 521-528.

Minchin, E. A., and J. D. Thomson. 1915. The rat trypanosome, *Trypanosoma lewisi*, in its relation to the rat flea, *Ceratophyllus fasciatus*. Quart. J. Micr. Sci., 60: 463-692.

Molomut, N. 1947. Mechanism responsible for lowered resistance of hypophysectomized rats to *T. lewisi*. J. Immun., 56: 139-141.

Molyneux, D. H. 1968. The reproductive stages of the trypanosomes of *Microtus agrestis* and *Clethrionomys glareolus*. Trans. Roy. Soc. Trop. Med. Hyg., 62: 464-465.

Moulder, J. W. 1948. Changes in the glucose metabolism of *Trypanosoma lewisi* during the course of infection in the rat. J. Infect. Dis., 83: 42-49.

Mühlpfordt, H. 1968. Untersuchungen über die experimentelle *Trypanosoma lewisi*-infektion der Maus. Z. Tropenmed. Parasit., 19: 73-82.

Naiman, D. N. 1944. Effect of X-irradiation of rats upon their resistance to *Trypanosoma lewisi*. J. Parasit., 30: 209-228.

Nájera Angulo, L. 1935. Sur le parasitisme de "*Trypanosoma Blanchardi*" et "*Hepatozoon lusitanicus*" n. sp. dans "*Eliomys lusitanicus*", en Espagne. Int. Congr. Zool., 3: 1921-1946.

Nattan-Larrier, L., and B. Noyer. 1932. Infection expérimentale du rat par le trypanosome du hamster. C. R. Soc. Biol. (Paris), 111: 887-889.

Novy, F. G. 1907. Immunity against trypanosomes. Proc. Soc. Exp. Biol. Med., 4: 42-44

────── W. A. Perkins, and R. Chambers. 1912. Immunization by means of cultures of *Trypanosoma lewisi*. J. Infect. Dis., 11: 411-426.

Oliver-Gonzalez, J. 1941. The dual antibody basis of acquired immunity in trichinosis. J. Infect. Dis., 69: 254-270.

Ormerod, W. E. 1963. The initial stages of infection with *Trypanosoma lewisi*; control of parasitaemia by the host. *In* Immunity to Protozoa. Garnham, P. C. C., Pierce, A. E., and Roitt, I., eds. Oxford, Blackwell Scientific Publications, pp. 213-227.

Pardee, A. B. 1968. Membrane transport proteins. Science, 162: 632-637.

Patton, C. L. 1965. Passive immunization against *Trypanosoma lewisi* using serum and peritoneal exudate cells in Dexamethasone-treated and untreated rats. J. Parasit., 51 (2, Sec. 2): 28.

────── 1967. Personal communication.

────── and D. T. Clark. 1968. *Trypanosoma lewisi* infections in normal rats and in rats treated with dexamethasone. J. Protozool., 15: 31-35.

Perla, D. 1934. The protective action of copper and iron against *Trypanosoma lewisi* infections in albino rats. Amer. J. Hyg., 19: 514-519.

────── 1939. Relation of hypophysis to spleen. III. Hypophysectomy and resistance to *Trypanosoma lewisi*. Proc. Soc. Exp. Biol. Med., 40: 91-94.

────── and J. Marmorston. 1941. Natural Resistance and Clinical Medicine. Boston, Little, Brown and Co., pp. 575-576, 585.

────── and J. Marmorston-Gottesman. 1930. Further studies on *T. lewisi* infection in albino rats. I. The effect of splenectomy on *T. lewisi* infection in albino rats and the protective action of splenic autotransplants. II. The effect of thymectomy and bilateral gonadectomy on *T. lewisi* infection in albino rats. J. Exp. Med., 52: 601-616.

Petana, W. B. 1964. Effects of cortisone upon the course of infection of *Trypanosoma gambiense, T. rhodesiense, T. brucei,* and *T. congolense* in albino rats. Ann. Trop. Med. Parasit., 58: 192-198.

Pike, R. M. 1967. Antibody heterogeneity and serological reactions. Bact. Rev., 31: 157-174.

Pisano, J. C., J. T. Patterson, and N. R. Di Luzio. 1968. Reticuloendothelial blockade: effects of Puromycin on opsonin-dependent recovery. Science, 162: 565-567.

Pizzi, T. and W. H. Taliaferro. 1960. A comparative study of protein and nucleic acid synthesis in different species of trypanosomes. J. Infect. Dis., 107: 100-107.

Quay, W. B. 1955. Trypanosomiasis in the collared lemming, *Dicrostonyx torquatus* (Rodentia). J. Parasit., 41: 562-565.

Rabinowitz, L. and W. Kempner. 1899. Beitrag zur Kenntnis der Blutparasiten, speciell der Rattentrypanosomen. Z. Hyg. Infektionskr., 30: 251-294.

Raffel, S. 1961. Immunity. New York, Appleton-Century-Crofts, 2nd ed.

Regendanz, P. 1929. Die multiple Teilung des *Trypanosoma criceti*, seine Entwicklung im Hundefloh and Übertragungsversuche auf den Hamster. Z. Parasitenk., 2: 44-54.
——— 1932. Über die Immunitätsvorgänge bei der Infektion der Ratten mit *Trypanosoma lewisi*. Z. Immunitätsforsch., 76: 437-445.
——— and W. Kikuth. 1927. Über die Bedeutung der Milz für die Bildung des vermehrungshindernden Reaktionsproduktes (Taliaferro) und dessen Wirkung auf den Infektionsverlauf der Ratten-Trypanosomiasis (*Tryp. lewisi*). Versuche der Übertragung des *Tryp. lewisi* auf die weisse Maus. Zbl. Bakt. [Orig.], 103: 271-279.
Reichenow, E. 1917. Parasitos de la sangre y del intestino de los monos antropomorfos africanos. Bol. Soc. Espan. Hist. Nat., 17: 312-332.
Rigby, D. W., and B. Chobotar. 1966. The effects of *Trypanosoma lewisi* on the development of *Hymenolepis diminuta* in concurrently infected white rats. J. Parasit., 52: 389-394.
Ritz, H. 1914. Über Rezidive bei experimenteller Trypanosomiasis. Deutsch. Med. Wschr., 40: 1355-1358.
Rothen, A. 1957. Improved method to measure the thickenss of thin films with a photoelectric ellipsometer. Rev. Sci. Instruments, 28: 283-285.
Roudsky, D. 1910a. Sur la réceptivité de la souris blanche à *Trypanosoma lewisi* Kent. C. R. Soc. Biol. (Paris), 68: 458-460.
——— 1910b. Sur le *Trypanosoma lewisi* Kent renforcé. C. R. Soc. Biol. (Paris), 69: 384-386.
——— 1911a. Sur la possibilité de rendre le *Trypanosoma lewisi* virulent pour d'autres rongeurs que le rat. C. R. Acad. Sci. (Paris), 152: 56-58.
——— 1911b. Mécanisme de l'immunité naturelle de la souris vis-à-vis du *Trypanosoma lewisi* Kent. C. R. Soc. Biol. (Paris), 70: 693-694.
——— 1911c. Action pathogène de *Trypanosoma lewisi* Kent, renforcé, sur la souris blanche. C. R. Soc. Biol. (Paris), 70: 741-742.
——— 1912a. Sur la réceptivité du *Trypanosoma duttoni* Thiroux. C. R. Soc. Biol. (Paris), 72: 221-223.
——— 1912b. Sur l'immunité croisée entre le *Trypanosoma lewisi* et le *Tr. duttoni* renforcé. C. R. Soc. Biol. (Paris), 72: 609-611.
Sanders, A., and F. G. Wallace. 1966. Immunization of rats with irradiated *Trypanosoma lewisi*. Exp. Parasit., 18: 301-304.
Santos, G. W., and A. H. Owens, Jr. 1966. 19S and 7S antibody production in the cyclophosphamide- or methotrexate-treated rat. Nature (London), 209: 622-624.
Saul, L. A., and E. R. Becker. 1949. Course of *Trypanosoma lewisi* infections in white rats treated with sodium salicylate. J. Parasit., 35: 54-60.
Schwartz, R., and J. Andre. 1962. The chemical suppression of immunity. In Mechanism of Cell and Tissue Damage Produced by Immune Reactions. Grabar, P., and Miescher, P., eds. New York, Grune and Stratton, Inc., pp. 385-409.
Schwetz, J. 1931. *Trypanosoma lewisi* et splénectomie. Ann. Parasit. Hum. Comp., 9: 10-14.
——— 1933. Trypanosomes rares de la région de Stanleyville (Congo Belge). Ann. Parasit. Hum. Comp., 11: 287-296.
Seed, J. R. 1963. The characterization of antigens isolated from *Trypanosoma rhodesiense*. J. Protozool., 10: 380-389.
Sheppe, W. A., and J. R. Adams. 1957. The pathogenic effects of *Trypanosoma duttoni* in hosts under stress conditions. J. Parasit., 43: 55-59.
Sherman, I. W., and J. A. Ruble. 1967. Virulent *Trypanosoma lewisi* infections in cortisone-treated rats. J. Parasit., 53: 258-262.
Singer, I., E. T. Kimble, III, and R. E. Ritts, Jr. 1964. Alterations in the host-parasite relationship by administration of endotoxin to mice infected with trypanosomes. J. Infect. Dis., 114: 243-248.
Steffan, P. 1921. Beobachtungen über der Verlauf den künstlichen Infektion der Ratte mit *Trypanosoma lewisi*. Arch. Schiffs. Tropenhyg., 25: 241-247.
Styles, T. J. 1965. Effect of bacterial endotoxin on *Trypanosoma lewisi* infections in rats. J. Parasit., 51: 650-653.
Taliaferro, W. H. 1924. A reaction product in infections with *Trypanosoma lewisi* which inhibits the reproduction of the trypanosomes. J. Exp. Med., 39: 171-190.
——— 1926. Variability and inheritance of size in *Trypanosoma lewisi*. J. Exp. Zool., 43: 429-473.
——— 1929. The Immunology of Parasitic Infections. New York, The Century Co.

———— 1932. Trypanocidal and reproduction-inhibiting antibodies to *Trypanosoma lewisi* in rats and rabbits. Amer. J. Hyg., 16: 32-84.

———— 1938a. Ablastic and trypanocidal antibodies against *Trypanosoma duttoni*. J. Immun., 35: 303-328.

———— 1938b. The effects of splenectomy and blockade on the passive transfer of antibodies against *Trypanosoma lewisi*. J. Infect. Dis., 62: 98-111.

———— 1940a. The mechanism of immunity to metazoan parasites. Amer. J. Trop. Med., 20: 169-182.

———— 1940b. The mechanism of acquired immunity in infections with parasitic worms. Physiol. Rev., 20: 469-492.

———— 1941. The immunology of the parasitic protozoa. *In* Protozoa in Biological Research. Calkins, G. N., and Summers, F. M., eds. New York, Hafner Publishing Co., Inc., pp. 830-889.

———— 1948. The inhibition of reproduction of parasites by immune factors. Bact. Rev., 12: 1-17.

———— 1957. Modification of the immune response by radiation and cortisone. Ann. N.Y. Acad. Sci., 69: 745-764.

———— 1963. Cellular and humoral factors in immunity to protozoa. *In* Immunity to Protozoa. Garnham, P. C. C., Pierce, A. E., and Roitt, I., eds. Oxford, Blackwell Scientific Publications, pp. 22-38.

———— and L. G. Taliaferro, 1922. The resistance of different hosts to experimental trypanosome infections with especial reference to a new method of measuring the resistance. Amer. J. Hyg., 2: 264-319.

———— and Y. Pavlinova. 1936. The course of infection of *Trypanosoma duttoni* in normal and in splenectomized and blockaded mice. J. Parasit., 22: 29-41.

———— and Y. P. Olsen. 1943. The protective action of normal sheep serum against infections of *Trypanosoma duttoni* in mice. J. Infect. Dis., 72: 213-221.

———— and L. G. Taliaferro. 1951. Effect of X-rays on immunity: A review. J. Immun., 66: 181-212.

———— and T. Pizzi. 1960. The inhibition of nucleic acid and protein synthesis in *Trypanosoma lewisi* by the antibody ablastin. Proc. Nat. Acad. Sci. U.S.A., 46: 733-745.

———— P. R. Cannon, and S. Goodloe. 1931 The resistance of rats to infection with *Trypanosoma lewisi* as affected by splenectomy. Amer. J. Hyg., 14: 1-37.

———— L. G. Taliaferro, and B. N. Jaroslow. 1964. Radiation and Immune Mechanisms. New York, Academic Press, Inc.

Talmage, D. W. 1957. The primary equilibrium between antigen and antibody. Ann. N.Y. Acad. Sci., 70: 82-93,

Tate, P. 1951. Antagonism of *Spirillum minus* infection in rats toward *Trypanosoma lewisi* and *T. equinum*. Parasitology, 41: 117-127.

Taylor, J., and E. R. Becker. 1948. Liver changes in pantothenate-deficient rats infected with *Trypanosoma lewisi*. J. Infect. Dis., 82: 42-44.

Tempelis, C. H., and M. G. Lysenko. 1965. Effect of X-irradiation on *Trypanosoma lewisi* infection in the rat. Exp. Parasit., 16: 174-181.

Terry, R. J. 1957. Antibody against *Trypanosoma vivax* present in normal cotton rat serum. Exp. Parasit., 6: 404-411.

Thillet, C. H., Jr., and A. C. Chandler. 1957. Immunization against *Trypanosoma lewisi* in rats by injections of metabolic products. Science, 125: 346-347.

Thurston, J. P. 1958. The oxygen uptake of *Trypanosoma lewisi* and *Trypanosoma equiperdum*, with especial reference to oxygen consumption in the presence of amino-acids. Parasitology, 48: 149-164.

Tomasi, T. B., Jr. 1965. Human gamma globulin. Blood, 25: 382-403.

van Saceghem, R. 1923. Le pouvoir empêchant dans les trypanosomiases. Bull. Soc. Path. Exot., 16: 733-735.

Vassiliadis, P. 1930. La fonction antiparasitaire de la rate décélée par la splenectomie. Arch. Intern. Med. Exp., 6: 89-118.

———— and J. Jadin. 1930. Influence du spirochetehispanicum sur l'infection à *Trypanosoma rhodesiense*. Ann. Soc. Belg. Med. Trop., 10: 133-136.

Walker, P. J. 1964. Reproduction and heredity in trypanosomes. A critical review dealing mainly with the African species in the mammalian host. Int. Rev. Cytol., 17: 51-98.

Watkins, J. F. 1964. Observations on antigenic variation in a strain of *Trypanosoma brucei* growing in mice. J. Hyg. (Camb.), 62: 69-80.

Weimer, H. E., R. T. Bell, and H. Nishihara. 1959a. Dietary protein and serum electrophoretic patterns in the adult rat. Proc. Soc. Exp. Biol. Med., 100: 853-855.
———— C. M. Carpenter, A. W. C. Naylor-Foote, R. W. McKee, and H. Nishihara.
1959b. Effects of inanition, protein depletion and repletion on serum lactic acid dehydrogenase levels in rats. Proc. Soc. Exp. Biol. Med., 101: 344-346.
———— J. F. Godfrey, R. L. Meyers, and J. N. Miller. 1963. Effects of food restriction
and realimentation on serum proteins: Complement levels and electrophoretic pat-
terns. J. Nutr., 81: 405-410.
Weitz, B. 1960. The properties of some antigens of *Trypanosoma brucei*. J. Gen. Micro-
biol., 23: 589-600.
Wenyon, C. M. 1926. Protozoology. New York, William Wood and Co., Vol. 1.
Williamson, J. 1963. The chemical composition of trypanosomes. Proc. 16th Int. Congr.
Zool., 4: 189-195.
Wilson, G. A. 1962. Metabolites of *Trypanosoma lewisi* as antigen of ablastin. M. S.
Thesis, Tempe, Arizona, Arizona State University.
Wood, F. D. 1936. *Trypanosoma neotomae*, sp. nov., in the dusky-footed wood rat and
the wood rat flea. Univ. Calif. Publ. Zool., 41: 133-144.
Wotton, R. M., and D. A. Becker. 1963. The ingestion of particulate lipid containing a
fluorochrome dye, Acridine Orange, by *Trypanosoma lewisi*. Parasitology, 53: 163-168.
Zozaya, C. 1929. Über das Trypanosoma des Hamsters (*Cricetus frumentarius*). Zbl.
Bakt. [Orig.], 110: 187-190.
Zwisler, J. B., and M. G. Lysenko. 1954. The oxidative metabolism of *Trypanosoma
lewisi* from salicylate treated infected white rats. J. Parasit., 40: 531-535.

Leishmanias

LESLIE A. STAUBER

Department of Zoology and Bureau of Biological Research, Rutgers University,
New Brunswick, New Jersey

INTRODUCTION

Leishmania is defined as the genus of the family Trypanosomatidae whose members exist in two morphologic types: (1) the amastigote (Hoare and Wallace, 1966), or Leishman-Donovan body, an intracellular parasite of the

This manuscript was largely prepared while on leave of absence from regular duties at Rutgers—The State University and during periods of residence at the Naval Medical Research Institute, Bethesda, Md. and the Gorgas Memorial Laboratory, Panama, Republica de Panama.

It is a pleasure to acknowledge indebtedness to the National Institute of Allergy and Infectious Diseases for Special Fellowship No. AI-37,396 and to the Rutgers Research Council for Faculty Fellowship No. 148 for the financial arrangements which made the leave of absence possible.

Dr. Clay G. Huff and the personnel at the Naval Medical Research Institute and Drs. Martin D. Young and Aristides Herrer of Gorgas Memorial Laboratory extended many courtesies during the writing. The U.S. Public Health Service under research grant AI-00092 and training grant AI-00187 (National Institute of Allergy and Infectious Diseases) generally supported the research conducted by my students and me that furnished most of the background experience for the writing. I am especially indebted to the students for their many contributions.

macrophages of vertebrates, and (2) the motile promastigote, or leptomonad, found in nature in the alimentary tracts of certain insects (phlebotomines). The promastigote form is the predominant form found in culture whether these cultures are seeded with amastigotes or promastigotes.

In the vertebrates, a large range of host responses has been observed from small accumulations of parasites in the skin of animals without visible lesions (Herrer et al., 1966) to fatal visceral involvement with large numbers of parasites in many organs of the body (Meleney, 1925). It is customary to separate cutaneous from visceral infections clinically, although it has long been recognized that even in the human, both early (leishmanioma: Kirk, 1938; Manson-Bahr, 1955) and late (post-kala-azar dermal leishmanoid: Brahmachari, 1922; Sen Gupta, 1962) cutaneous lesions may be associated with the typically visceral parasite. Likewise, many isolates of typically cutaneous parasites show some tendency to visceralize. In man, this is expressed as lymphangitis (Shanbron et al., 1956; Bureau et al., 1960) or appearance of metastatic lesions (Pacheco et al., 1961; Biagi, 1967), and in animals, as parasites cultured from blood (Hertig et al., 1956, 1957) or found in viscera (Garnham and Lewis, 1959; Disney, 1964). Kellina's recent work (1965) suggests that the capacity of cutaneous isolates to visceralize in animals may be generally associated with virulence. The visceral parasite from man is called *L. donovani*, though Adler (1964) still referred to the Mediterranean visceral parasite as *L. infantum*. Two cutaneous species are widely accepted: *L. tropica* in the Old World and *L. brasiliensis* in the New World. Variants of *L. tropica* are recognized as such (var. *major* and *minor*), but in the New World, chiefly because of the striking clinical differences observed from place to place, variants have often been called new species (e.g., *L. pifanoi*, *L. mexicana*). The criteria for taxonomic separation seem to be getting better and without doubt a general revision of the species will soon be validated in a way to satisfy scientists generally. Unlike malaria, the leishmaniases are much more nearly true zoonoses (Heisch, 1961; Garnham, 1965), and therefore the organisms studied in the laboratory in experimental animals are the species naturally infective to man. Other species exist, which are quite distinct from the above, and are found in lower animals, e.g., *L. enriettii* from the guinea pig, among several from mammals mostly still undescribed (Herrer, personal communication, 1968) and *L. tarentolae*, among several, from lizards (Brygoo, 1963).

In recent years useful reviews have been written on immunity in leishmaniasis (Manson-Bahr, 1961; Zuckerman, 1962; Adler, 1963a, 1964; Stauber, 1963a; Sen Gupta, 1965; Taliaferro and Stauber, 1968). There is much new work, and the following discussion will emphasize these newer findings.

INNATE IMMUNITY

Host Specificity

The peculiar distribution of *Leishmania donovani* in rodents, canids, and man suggests that many mammals are innately resistant to naturally acquired infection. On the other hand, the diversity of the canids and rodents infected in nature suggests a rather low level of specificity within the groups. Observations in the laboratory support these suggestions. For example, the common laboratory rabbit is refractory, but infections useful for experimental studies of *L. donovani* have been obtained in the mouse (*Mus musculus*), golden hamster (*Mesocricetus auratus*), Chinese hamster (*Cricetulus griseus*), cotton rat (*Sigmodon hispidus*), and chinchilla (*Chinchilla lanigera*) (Grun, 1958; Stauber, 1955, 1958, 1963a,b,c). None of these species of rodents (except the mouse) occurs naturally on the African continent, where the isolate of *L. donovani* (Khartoum strain) used in these studies was obtained. In the past couple of years, a few new kinds of mammals have been added to the list of those naturally infected with *L. donovani*: rats of genera *Rattus* and *Arvicanthis* (Hoogstraal et al., 1963), a mouse (*Acomys*), a genet (*Genetta g. senegalensis*), a serval (*Felis serval phillipsi*) (Hoogstraal and Dietlein, 1964), and a fox (*Vulpes v. alpherakyi*) (Maruashvili and Bardzhadze, 1966). Similar work has been reported recently with *L. tropica* in the U.S.S.R., where a hedgehog, *Hemiechinus auratus*, (Zvyagintseva, 1965) has been found naturally infected, and where a number of animals including the hedgehog have been tested for susceptibility (Ny, 1966).

In the Americas, the picture is more complicated. Here the rapidly increasing list of naturally infected mammals is even more varied, and in Panama alone it now includes seven animals all of different genera in four different orders of mammals. Added to the earlier rodent genera, *Proechimys* and *Hoplomys* (Hertig et al., 1956, 1957, 1958), are *Kannaboteomys*, *Dasyprocta*, *Agouti*, *Rattus*, *Heteromys*, *Zygodontomys*, *Ototylomys*, *Nyctomys*, and *Oryzomys* (Forattini, 1960; Alencar et al., 1960; Lainson and Strangways-Dixon, 1963, 1964; Kerdel-Vegas et al., 1966; Guimaraes and Costa, 1966). Natural infections have also been found in the kinkajou, *Potus flavus* (Thatcher et al., 1965a), the olingo, *Bassaricyon gabbii* (Gorgas Memorial Laboratory, 1968), the porcupine, *Coendou rothschildi* (Herrer et al., 1966), the sloths, *Choloepus hoffmanni* and *Bradypus griseus* (Herrer, personal communication, 1968), and the marmoset, *Sanguinus geoffroyi* (Gorgas Memorial Laboratory, 1967). The list is certain to be extended appreciably as methods of isolation get better and the search for infected animals is broadened. It is likely that many of the animals found infected in nature are sentinels of the presence of transmission of *Leishmania* (all species) rather than true zoonotic reservoir hosts.

Three other lists of mammals are part of the evaluation of susceptibility and immunity to the *Leishmania*. One is the list of host species shown susceptible to experimental infection. In an especially fruitful study with *L. brasiliensis*, Medina (1966) reported successful infections of the rodents, *Proechimys guyanensis*, *Dasyprocta rubrata*, the armadillo, *Dasypus novencinetus*, the paca, *Cuniculus paca*, and the monkey, *Cebus n. nigrivittatus*. He also reported that infections were produced in a bat, a land turtle, and a variety of lizards, although without the production of lesions. Parasites, still infective for hamsters, were recovered from the injected turtle and lizards at varying intervals of time. Similar recent work has been reported for *L. tro-*

pica (Lariviere, 1966) and for *L. donovani* (Heyneman and Mansour, 1963; Krampitz and Muhlpfordt, 1964; Popovic, 1965; Sati, 1962; Packchanian and Kelly, 1965).

The next list comprises those animals found not to have been infected in surveys of animals caught in the wild. In such surveys, the negative findings have much less value. The size and time of the sample and the sensitivity of the method of sampling are technical problems in such surveys, and the age and immune state are host factors which influence the results. Even for a species known to be capable of infection in nature, geographic location and time of sampling are important (e. g., *Proechimys* in Panama). Except for *Rhombomys* in endemic foci of *L. tropica major*, no infection rates in reservoir animals approach 100 per cent. Still, work of this nature is necessary, and for some more recent surveys, see Lainson and Strangways-Dixon, 1964, and Herrer et al., 1966. The same comments apply to studies in reservoir hosts of *L. donovani* (Torrealba and Torrealba, 1963) and of *L. tropica* in the Old World (Camerlynck et al., 1967).

The last list comprises those animals experimentally injected with isolates of *Leishmania*, which apparently did not become infected and are therefore presumed not to be susceptible. Again caution is needed in interpretation, especially with respect to the method of searching for parasites where no visible lesion exists, and with respect to the possible presence of an already immune state due to previous spontaneous recovery in the wild-caught animal. Stocks of animals from nonendemic foci or, better yet, laboratory-bred animals, are best used for such studies.

Factors altering innate immunity

Epidemiologic observations and laboratory experimentation indicate that a number of factors influence innate resistance to the *Leishmania*.

Age.   The age of the host, however, does not seem to be an important factor. In the human, where previous exposure can be certainly ruled out, infection with either cutaneous or visceral forms may occur at any age (Lainson and Strangways-Dixon, 1963). Thus, in the Mediterranean, where it was once called infantile anemia, and in Brazil and China, kala-azar is a disease of the young, but in India and the early Kenya outbreak (Fendall, 1953) and in the Sudan (van Peenen and Reid, 1963), adults are infected. The recent paper of Southgate and Oriedo (1962) gives a reasoned analysis of the age distribution for Kenya, where newly invaded communities show a different age-incidence than areas that have passed from epidemic to endemic status. The same is true for the cutaneous diseases (see especially the analysis by Herrer, 1962, of cutaneous leishmaniasis [uta] in Peru), where infection of young adults in military service (Walton et al., 1968) may be contrasted with infection of the young in the more classical description of Oriental sore. Risks of exposure to transmission or of previous infection, not age, seem to be the chief limiting factors. Experimentally, similar results have been obtained in our laboratory with *L. donovani*. Grun*, working with all ages of mice down to three days after birth, found almost no difference in resistance to *L. donovani*. Ott* came to the same conclusion, contrasting hamsters 1 to 2 and 6 to 7 months old infected by the standardized intracardial infection procedure (Stauber, 1955), and using an inoculum of 120,000 splenic amastigotes per gram of body weight. In Ott's trial, the group median counts were 15 versus 30 for one hour and 1,480 versus 4,687 for 12 days after inoculation, with median times to death of 50 versus 40 days for the young and old animals, respectively. Since two-fold differences in numbers are generally not statistically significant in this test, these data suggest, if anything, that older hamsters may be very slightly more susceptible. Mansour and McCoy* found similar results with puppies in contrast to adult dogs infected with one Mediterranean and two African isolates of *L. donovani*. Pedroso (1923), however, claimed that it was easier to produce lesions with *L. brasiliensis* in young dogs than in old dogs. Also, Adler (1962) claimed that *L. adleri* would infect baby mice and that he obtained infections of baby mice with avirulent cultures of *L. tropica*.

Sex. Risk of exposure rather than sexual difference has been used to explain the greater incidence of infection in males with some types of cutaneous leishmaniasis (Beltran, 1945, and Lainson and Strangways-Dixon, 1962, for chiclero ulcer; Barbosa et al., 1965, for mucocutaneous leishmaniasis; Herrer, 1951, for uta.) In many areas, kala-azar is more often a disease of children. Thus, emphasis has not been placed on sex differences in host resistance. Southgate and Oriedo (1962), in their careful epidemiologic analysis of kala-azar in Kenya, noted unexplained differences in the sex distribution of the cases studied. Also, the reports of Goble et al. (1965) and Goble (1966) showed that the female hamster is more resistant to visceral leishmaniasis than the male as measured by time to death or by development of edema. These observations suggest the need for a reexamination of this aspect of host resistance. It may be that the sex difference is related to resistance only in adult animals.

Race. The only report known to the present author that emphasizes racial differences in response to cutaneous infection is that of Walton (personal communication, 1967). He claims that in Bolivia, mucocutaneous involvements are almost exclusively found in Negroid people. Earlier, Pessoa (1941), although claiming there were no racial differences related to rates of infection (*see also* Lainson and Strangways-Dixon, 1962), noted racial differences in allergic responses to injections of dead leishmanial antigens. Negroes were found more reactive. How this relates to Walton's finding has yet to be put to experimental test in human leishmaniasis. The experiments of several workers in my laboratory (*see* Janovy, 1967) have shown that a leishmanioma can be induced by the injection of live *L. donovani* under the skin of mice previously sensitized to dead flagellates. Differences due to the race or strain of experimental animal have not been investigated to any ex-

* I wish to express my appreciation to Drs. John Grun, Karen J. Ott, Noshy S. Mansour, and John R. McCoy for use of unpublished data.

tent at present, though Grun (1958) and Franchino (1959) found slight observable differences in strains of mice infected intraperitoneally with splenic amastigotes of *L. donovani*.

Endocrinologic state of the host. Although some manipulation of host-parasite interaction in experimental visceral leishmaniasis has been attempted (Stauber et al., 1952; Franchino, 1959), the small changes produced were seen only after the injection of considerable amounts of active compounds. Adrenocorticosteroids were shown not to modify the edema that is part of the usual terminal syndrome in the infected hamster but, in proper concentrations, did decrease parasite numbers and splenic hyperplasia. It might be expected that a greater effect would be produced in the cutaneous infection in which the antiphlogistic action of the steroids could alter the inflammatory picture and might cause dissemination of the lesion. Ary et al. (1964) recently reported such an effect.

Nutritional state. Although kala-azar was associated early with poor nutritional states and Corkill (1949) stressed the probable role of protein deficiency, specific data were not available until the reports of Ritterson and Stauber (1949) and Actor (1958, 1960). Using standardized infection procedures in mice (and supplemented in part by trials in hamsters), Actor showed that specific deficiency states could produce significant effects on the course of infection in visceral leishmaniasis. Protein or pyridoxine deficiency decreased innate (early) and acquired resistance. Pantothenate deficiency at first increased host resistance, but, when the deficiency was continued, it later led to increased parasite burdens, probably by influencing the host's capacity to establish acquired resistance. Strangely, severe thiamine deficiency seemed not to affect the course of infection in the mouse. Protein deficiency studies showed an interesting contrast. In the hamster, the severely deficient state apparently increased host "resistance," but in the mouse it did the reverse. Actor reasoned that only where some degree of innate resistance already existed in the host (mouse) could it be decreased. In the extremely susceptible hamster, it was not possible to make its lack of resistance any less. The evidence even indicated that the severely protein-deficient hamster was a poorer host for *L. donovani*.

Environmental temperature. The two morphologic stages (promastigotes and amastigotes) of the leishmania are associated with different host environments (i.e., insect gut and vertebrate macrophages), which, among other conditions, differ in ambient temperature. In the mammal the temperature is high with a small diurnal range; whereas in the insect the temperature is usually lower and much more variable. Cultivation of leishmania *in vitro* is favored at lower temperatures (25 to 28°C), and the promastigote stage is seen. Growth at 37°C has not yet been achieved, but where approached (Trager, 1953; Lemma and Schiller, 1964), the parasite assumes the more nearly rounded aflagellate condition. This is also true in tissue culture (Frothingham and Lehtimoki, 1967), in which proper manipulation of temperature produces either promastigotes or amastigotes, and in which it even appears that 37° C is strongly inhibitory to the amastigote as well.

It is not surprising, then, that attempts have been made to alter the course of infection in hosts by manipulation of local body or environmental temperatures. Stauber (1953, 1963b) reported the effect of temperature on *L. donovani* in the hamster. He found that infected hamsters held at 36°C and 40 percent relative humidity were essentially cured of their infection, and that significant inhibition of parasite reproduction occurred even when animals were exposed to the 36°C environment every other day. He did not follow the details of concomitant changes in body temperatures. Attempted manipulations of body temperatures with pyrogens and dinitrophenol failed to inhibit infections. Baker and Gutierrez-Ballesteros (1957) showed similar environmental temperature effects with guinea pigs with lesions of *Leishmania enriettii*, Trejos et al. (1965) with mice infected with *Trypanosoma cruzi*, and Conti-Diaz and Mackinon (1961) with guinea pigs and *Blastomyces*. This same idea has been applied to human cutaneous infections (Gutierrez-Ballesteros, 1959) in which local heat treatment favored healing. More recently, Zeledon et al. (1965) showed that local skin temperature was related to success in inducing cutaneous infection of the hamster. They obtained lesions (ear, foot, nose, and tail) only where skin temperatures were below 30°C. They also "easily cured" foot lesions by subjecting the animals to daily exposures to ambient temperature environments of 37°C. Eliseev and Strelkova (1966) also studied the effects of ambient temperature on *Rhombomys opimus* and *Meriones libycus* and offer explanations for the effect on the course of infection and on transmission.

Intercurrent infections. It is well-known that infections of hosts in nature are often multiple, making diagnoses difficult. It used to be said that in some areas endemic for malaria and visceral leishmaniasis, if a patient with fever and splenomegaly did not respond to treatment with quinine, kala-azar should be strongly suspected. The concurrency of the infections was recognized without implying any affect of one upon the other. Experimental evidence for any influence of a second infection on the course of leishmaniasis is reported only by Konopka et al. (1961), who showed mycobacterial infections were inhibitory to the leishmania (and vice versa). Adler (1954) studied the opposite, i.e., the inhibitory effect of visceral leishmaniasis on *Plasmodium berghei* infection in the hamster. His evidence suggested no influence of *P. berghei* on visceral leishmaniasis in the hamster. The chronicity of the leishmanial infection makes an effect difficult to assess, but an approach like that of short-term chemotherapy (Stauber et al., 1958) or temperature (Stauber, 1963b) trials might be used to test for the influence of an intercurrent infection on the course of visceral leishmaniasis in experimental animals.

Little is also known of cutaneous infections, although it is generally assumed that gross contamination of the local lesions almost always occurs. The comment of Price and Fitzherbert (1965) that overlying infection of fungi were regularly present in nodular (lepromatous) leishmaniasis makes it desirable to learn what role, if any, such organisms play in the nature of the developing lesion or of host response to it.

So little is known about innate immunity to the leishmania and the factors which influence it that obviously much more work needs to be done. As for mechanisms, even less is understood.

ACQUIRED IMMUNITY

Cutaneous leishmaniasis

The clinical picture of the typical simple dermal lesion in leishmaniasis, progressing from macule to papule, to ulcer, to healing with scar formation, is descriptive of a self-limiting process. The histopathological picture, changing from early inflammatory exudate (chiefly mononuclear), to histiocytic development, to late invasion by lymphocytes and plasma cells, and finally to healing with or without fibrosis, supports the clinical observations and suggests that the host response is indeed one of acquired immunity. The species of parasite, species of host, strain of parasite (or virulence), and host condition all influence the outcome of the natural infection or of experiments conducted to test the effectiveness of the immunity to reinfection. This implies, as is well-known, that the lesion is progressive in some hosts with some strains (e.g., the *difusa* form of *L. brasiliensis*; Convit, 1958), but in other cases no appreciable lesion may be produced (Herrer, et al., 1966).

It is common knowledge that there is acquired immunity in cutaneous leishmaniasis, and in some parts of the world, successful "vaccination" procedures are based on the subcutaneous inoculation of living culture promastigotes for the induction of a lesion, which, upon spontaneous cure, leaves the host resistant to reinfection (Lawrow and Dubowsky, 1937; Senekji and Beattie, 1941; Berberian, 1944; Adler and Katzenellenbogen, 1952). The evidence states that promastigotes of *L. tropica* from culture injected into a nonimmune person will produce a suitable lesion (*nodosa*-type or "Oriental sore") that will take from 6 to 17 months to cure (Berberian, 1939; Senekji and Beattie, 1941; Sagher et al., 1955). If reinoculation is attempted before the initial lesion has healed, typical *nodosa* lesions are initiated. Reinoculation after cure produces a lesion which heals much sooner than the initial lesion, or often no lesion at all. Since parasites are not found two weeks after the reinoculation, the lesion is related to the hypersensitive state of the host and has been called a "Koch reaction," i.e., one which is "highly specific immunologically" although "a nonspecific inflammation" histologically.

In Kellina's (1966) study of 56 reinoculations, a wider range of response was noted depending on the virulence of the strain used in the reinoculation. Strains of low virulence produced only a delayed-type local skin reaction similar to that following the injection of killed promastigotes (as in the leishmanin test). With virulent strains, however, nodule formation occurred which was similar to the allergic tubercles seen by Kozhevnikov (1950) in natural infections. Parasites were scanty in these lesions, though there was evidence of their multiplication. Necrosis with ulcer formation occurred in some cases on reinoculation. Demina et al. (1965) found evidence of parasites persisting longer on reinoculation than did Adler and Zuckerman (1948), again probably reflecting the influence of parasite virulence.

In Belova's (1964) study of strain virulence, she confirmed Adler's earlier statements (see Adler, 1964) that new isolates had greater virulence and that virulence decreases with time of cultivation in the laboratory. In addition, she pointed out that old cultures in some cases produced atypical cutaneous leishmaniasis with a prolonged course and emphasized that freshly-isolated cultures should be preferred for "vaccines."

Several workers claim that protection may be conferred by using killed leptomonads, but they specify the need for several injections (Pessoa, 1941b; Pessoa and Pestana, 1941; de Sampaio, 1951). Coutinho (1954, 1955) obtained partial protection of guinea pigs to *L. enriettii* by immunization with several injections of killed promastigotes. Protection was measured by the reduction of mortality in the guinea pigs. Lainson and Bray (1964), however, failed to induce protection in hamsters or mice with *L. mexicana* killed in formol-saline.

Although several workers have clearly shown the existence of common antigens (see pp. 750; 756) among the leishmania, it is known that recovery from kala-azar does not protect against later inoculation with *L. tropica* (Manson-Bahr, 1961b). Thus, species specificity does exist. The Russian workers, Latyshev et al. (1951, 1953), also presented evidence for the existence of strain specificity. In central Asia, cutaneous leishmaniasis is represented by two main types—one producing "dry" lesions more like typical Oriental sore, and the other, "wet" lesions which appear sooner, ulcerate earlier, and go to recovery sooner (usually within six months). "Wet"-type lesions in the human confer protection against subsequent infection with "dry"-type parasites after recovery from a "wet"-type lesion. Some cross-protection is also induced by primary infection with "dry"-type lesions (Ansari and Mofidi, 1950). Kellina's work (1966) suggests an even broader spectrum of response correlated with virulence of the strain of parasite. Similar differences have been claimed among isolates of parasites from South American patients, although the tendency has been to call the different parasites from these isolates by specific names. Thus, Convit (1958) showed that recovery from infection with *L. brasiliensis* resulted in protection against challenge with the same organism but not to a heterologous strain of parasite designated on clinical grounds as a different species, *L. pifanoi*. He also claimed partial interspecific protection in the guinea pig using *L. brasilensis* in the initial infection and *L. enriettii* in the subsequent challenge. Lainson and Strangways-Dixon (1963) showed that for *L. mexicana*, recovery may even give protection against a second inoculation before the primary lesion heals. As has been already pointed out (Stauber, 1963a), it is much more difficult to deal quantitatively with the cutaneous infections since the variability of the measurement procedures is increased by the lack of a defined infective dose of parasites, the long incubation period (suggesting considerable but variable mortality of the parasites injected), the slow development of the lesion, and the uneven distribution of parasites in the lesion.

In spite of these difficulties, there has been steady progress in accumulating evidence to support the contentions that both group- and strain-specific responses occur. Lainson and Shaw (1966), using recent isolates of parasites, have shown *L. mexicana* and a Panamanian *Leishmania* to be antigenically distinct. The Panamanian parasite protects against the *L. mexicana*, but the *L. mexicana* does not seem to give even partial protection to the other.

Studies of this nature have also been performed with animals. Lainson and Bray (1966) recently used rhesus monkeys and found that they could obtain strong resistance to challenge with homologous parasites (in this case the inocula were amastigotes [LD bodies] from triturated nodules) and complete or partial cross-resistance to heterologous ones. They were comparing *L. mexicana* with typical and atypical *L. brasiliensis* (espundia and *difusa* strains). Medina (1966) has also studied the development of immunity to cutaneous leishmaniasis in several experimental animals, and Kretschmar (1965), immunity to *L. enriettii* in the guinea pig.

Not many attempts at cross-immunity have been made with strains of parasites from different continents, but Adler and Gunders (1964) report apparently complete cross-resistance to challenge with *L. mexicana* promastigotes in two volunteers infected naturally years before with *L. tropica*.

Relapsing or chronic cutaneous infections of the *recidivans* (Dostrovsky et al., 1952b), disseminated (*difusa*, Convit, 1958), or mucocutaneous types do not follow the general rules of immunity set forth above. They are often even very difficult to treat successfully. A wide variety of lesions is seen in such cases, ranging from relapsing types with satellite lesions around a primary sore to extensive tissue involvement (Galliard, 1962; Convit, 1958; Dostrovsky et al., 1952a). Their very relapsing or chronic nature indicates the host's incapacity to cure them by the acquisition of a satisfactory immune state. However, not all noncuring lesions are disseminating, and ear lesions persisting for many years have been reported numbers of times (Biagi et al., 1960; Lainson and Strangways-Dixon, 1963). Special conditions are invoked to explain such persistence among strains normally inducing solid immunity, such as sequestration of parasites in ear cartilage (Adler, 1965) and low skin temperature (Zeledon et al., 1965). It is not surprising to find that subsequent reinfection or inoculation of parasites during the active state leads to the production of another lesion. What is surprising is that the strain of parasite seems less important than the nature of the host's response, for Dostrovsky et al. (1952b) injected parasites of the *nodosa*-producing type into patients with *recidivans* lesions and obtained not *nodosa* but *recidivans* lesions. Later, Liban et al. (1955) injected *nodosa*-producing parasites into the skin of leprous patients who presumably had never had cutaneous leishmaniasis. The lesions clinically appeared to be the *nodosa*-type but histologically showed abundant parasites crowded into the foam cells, which are characteristic of lepromatous or prelepromatous lesions. Convit (1958) showed a lack of protection to inoculation with the *difusa*-type parasite after recovery from *brasiliensis*-type lesions. The reverse has apparently not been attempted, namely, the inoculation of *brasiliensis* parasites into a patient cured of *difusa* infection. It might be difficult to prove that the patient cured of *difusa* parasites is as free of parasites as is suspected in the case of the patient recovered from a *tropica* lesion.

Destombes (1960) and others (e.g., Convit et al., 1957) have pointed out the anergic or tolerant state of the host in these cases, even in the presence of large numbers of parasites. This is confirmed by the general failure of the host to show the typical positive response to the Montenegro, or leishmanin, test, although the skin becomes reactive early in the development of the more typical *tropica* cutaneous lesion and retains its positive reactivity for a long time. The leishmanin test even becomes positive in the *recidivans*-type infection (Dostrovsky and Sagher, 1946). Cahill (1965) claims that therapy resulted in a change to positive leishmanin tests in cases of Ethiopian disseminated cutaneous infection. In 1962, Sen Gupta reasoned that disseminated cutaneous infection of the African and American continents may in fact be the post-kala-azar dermal leishmanoid described years ago in India (Brahmachari, 1922). Much of the confusion noted above would be resolved if further study proves this to be the case.

The mechanisms of recovery in cutaneous leishmaniasis are not known. The shift of cell types in the lesions to include plasma cells (Adler, 1963a) suggests specific sensitization and antibody formation. Until recently, most workers have failed to demonstrate by laboratory procedures circulating antibodies in the sera of patients with cutaneous leishmaniasis (Chaffee, 1963). However, the reactivity of such sera with *T. cruzi* antigens (Sadun et al., 1963; Williams et al., 1963; Shaw and Voller, 1963) and the known group-specificity of the serologic tests were suggestive of low titer antibody. Recently, Convit and Kerdel-Vegas (1965), Shuikina (1965), and Walton et al., (1967) claimed that such antibodies (determined by the indirect fluorescent-antibody test) occur in the common forms of the disease but not in the disseminated variety of *L. brasiliensis*. Dostrovsky and Sagher (1946) successfully transmitted hypersensitivity to the skin by means of injection of patients' sera (*see also* Bray and Lainson, 1965a). This constitutes another kind of antibody demonstration, but none of these antibodies has yet been associated directly with protection of the host.

Several lines of evidence suggest that not all parasites in a local leishmanioma may be alive. Microscopically, parasites in some parts of the lesion appear to be degenerating. Recently, Strunk and Chaffee (1967) have shown that electron micrographs of cutaneous lesions in hamsters bear this out. They even see differences in the fate of *L. mexicana* and *L. brasilienesis* parasites in cutaneous lesions of the hamster. We also have shown (Hanson and Stauber, unpublished) that parasites from *L. mexicana* nodules from hamsters have remarkably low infectivity either intracardially or subcutaneously, and that promastigotes from culture produce cutaneous nodules sooner, even with many times fewer parasites. Three experiments have been run. In two, no parasites were found by microscopic examination at any time, although they were demonstrated in the spleen by culture techniques up to eight days after inoculation. The account of the other experiment is as follows: Intracardial injection of a dilution of ground nodules containing 121 million parasites per inoculum showed below threshold level of parasitization in the liver of two of seven animals (and no more than ten parasites per 1,000 liver cell nuclei in the heaviest one; the median value was four) one hour after inoculation. Such an inoculum of splenic parasites of *L. mexicana* (from a visceralizing infection) has been shown (unpublished) to result in ten times as many parasites in the liver. Since the time interval is so short (one to two hours) and the strain of *L. mexicana* visceralizes mildly, conditions should be satisfactory for finding more parasites if they were viable. Similarly, injection of nodule amastigotes often produces no nodules, whereas culture promastigotes of the same species of parasite nearly always do (*see also* Ercoli, 1961). The mechanism of this destruction is not known, though the work of Strunk and Chaffee is a beginning study.

The leishmanin test, produced by injection of from one to several million killed (phenolized or heat-inactivated) culture promastigotes of *Leishmania* spp., has now been conducted on hundreds of people since first described by Montenegro in 1926, and it has been used as a diagnostic aid, especially in mucocutaneous cases in South America. In surveys and other studies, there has been a high correlation of positive skin reactions with old healed scars (Sagher et al., 1955; Hertig et al., 1959; Navarrete and Biagi, 1960; Pifano, 1960, 1962; van Peenen and Dietlein, 1963; Cahill et al., 1965, and others). However, surveys usually show more positive reactions than can be documented from data on previous infections and even show positive reactions in some persons presumably never exposed to the risk of infection. The skin reaction plays a doubtful role in immunity. Its true nature has not yet been worked out and it may need better definition. It has been called both a delayed-type reaction and an Arthus reaction, although the two are different allergic states. Perhaps each state exists consecutively during infection. Boysia (1967) has made an attempt to clarify this situation by showing that leishmanial antigens (*L. mexicana* promastigotes and an alkaline extract of *L. donovani* promastigotes) are capable of inducing in the guinea pig proved delayed hypersensitivity in the strictest definition of the phrase. Boysia's criteria were: (1) no early skin response and peak response at 24 hours, (2) no passive transfer with serum from proved hypersensitive animals (PCA or reversed PCA), and (3) passive transfer using lymphoid cells from proved hypersensitive animals. Earlier, Adler and Nelken (1965) and Bray and Lainson (1965a) had attempted passive transfer of delayed-type skin reaction with leukocytes or whole blood. In Adler and Nelken's work, man-to-man passive transfer was attempted. Bray and Lainson showed that skin reactions could be obtained in rabbits and monkeys and made passive transfer attempts from man and monkeys. Their failures were probably due to transferring insufficient material (Boysia, 1967).

The antigens active in the leishmanin test are group-specific and may be elicited by lizard leishmania and *Strigomonas oncopelti* (Zeledon et al., 1960, 1961; Southgate and Manson-Bahr, 1967b), rodent strains of *L. donovani* (Manson-Bahr and Southgate, 1964), and even trypanosomal material (Pessoa and Cardoso, 1942). However, the differences found by Boysia (1967) in the delayed response to mexicana, donovani and tarentolae antigens is encouraging and should be pursued further.

In summary, acquired immunity to cutaneous leishmaniasis follows recovery from infection. When challenged again by live parasites, the dermal response in the immune host is considerably less than the original lesion. This is more true of homologous than heterologous strains of parasites, though virulence of strain and host responsiveness both play a role and may obscure the presence of a low degree of resistance. When challenged with dead parasites (or extracts of parasites), the host infected with cutaneous leishmaniasis, or recovered from it, responds with an allergic skin reaction (except in the case of disseminating-type lesions). Both immediate and delayed-type reactions may occur, since passive transfer of skin reactivity with either serum or lymphoid cells has been achieved. The reaction is at best only genus-specific. The role of the allergic reaction in the development of the lesion induced by challenge with live or dead parasites (*see* Lissia, 1965) is unknown, as is the responsiveness of the host to those allergens in the environment of the host which by contact (dermatitis-producing plants) or puncture (insect bites) commonly lead to allergic states.

Visceral leishmaniasis

Active immunity. Evidence for active immunity in man and lower animals has been slowly accumulating for a number of years. In man, the rarity of second cases, the occasional spontaneous recovery, the atypical and asymptomatic nonfatal infections, and the rare descriptions of nonvisceralization after a cutaneous infection with *L. donovani* parasites, all point to acquisition of immunity. In lower animals many reports of low grade and inapparent infections and of recovery after a period of parasitic patency also suggest acquired immunity. More carefully controlled experiments have been done recently.

Manson-Bahr's (1959, 1961) reports are still the only ones dealing with experimental proof of human resistance to reinfection with *L. donovani* parasites. Injection of human strain promastigotes induced formation of leishmaniomas in the human skin from which visceralization to typical kala-azar could occur. Similar cutaneous nodules were initiated upon introduction of promastigotes of animal strain origin (gerbil) but did not visceralize. If promastigotes of human or animal strain origin were injected into persons cured of kala-azar, only temporary nodules appeared from which live parasites could not be cultured. This is acquired immunity to challenge in the same sense as in cutaneous leishmaniasis. Complete cross-immunity to all rodent and human strains of *L. donovani* was obtained by Manson-Bahr, but all trials with several strains of *L. tropica* parasites gave more or less typical lesions with live parasites in them. Cross-immunity between *L. donovani* and *L. tropica* parasites, therefore, does not exist, although Senekji's early work suggested the opposite (Senekji, 1943).

Recovery from the primary leishmaniomas caused by rodent strains of *L. donovani* was shown to lead to protection against visceralization of human strains injected later. The same immune-type local lesion was produced during this challenge. Extended to field trial immunizations in Kenya, the results were disappointing. This does not seem to diminish the value of Manson-Bahr's original experiments. He and Southgate have more recently discussed the probable reasons for the apparent failure of the field trials (1964). Since then, new experimentation has disclosed interesting findings on cross-immunity to leishmanias in human subjects in Kenya. Southgate and Oriedo (1967) found areas where leishmaniasis had never occurred but where many people gave a positive leishmanin reaction. Some of these persons, injected with promastigotes of a dermotropic *L. donovani* strain from the ground squirrel (Southgate and Manson-Bahr, 1967b), gave the typical immune reactions described earlier from which live parasites could not be isolated. By contrast, volunteers with negative leishmanin reactions developed lesions typical of the nonimmune host which contained live parasites. Southgate and Manson-Bahr (1967a) have also shown that two persons previously inoculated with *L. adleri* from lizards developed positive skin reactions to other leishmanial antigens, including human strains of *L. donovani*. These same persons were shown to be immune to challenge injections of live promastigotes of *L. adleri* and *L. donovani*. Other persons with known experience with leishmania were immune to challenge with *L. adleri* promastigotes. Southgate and Oriedo (1967), in their epidemiologic study with the leishmanin test, showed that there seemed to be an inverse relationship between the presence of positive skin reactors and the occurrence of cases of clinical kala-azar. The sum of this evidence points to the likelihood that rodent and lizard leishmania can induce in man both cutaneous sensitivity to leishmanial antigens and immunity to kala-azar.

Stauber (1958) and his students (Franchino, 1959; Ott, 1964) used standardized infections in animals of varying susceptibility to test for immunity to superinfection. In the highly susceptible hamster, which eventually dies of the infection, no acquired resistance develops and superinfection appears not to influence the subsequent course of infection significantly. In the jird, mouse, and guinea pig, however, a condition of premunition develops when initial infections are reduced to near latency. Subsequent challenge with large numbers of parasites intravascularly shows that the immune host is able to control and dispose of the parasites more efficiently.

Taliaferro (1962) discussed defense reactions of the host during visceral leishmaniasis and noted that in general, the cellular reactions were not much different from those occurring in other similar visceral infections, even though some of the cells of the lymphoid-macrophage system were host cells for the parasite. He discussed the interplay between fixed mesenchymal reserves and various lymphoid cells, as well as the consequence of both the loss of lymphocytes by heteroplastic development and destruction and of the reparative lymphocytopoiesis set in motion to replace the lost cells. In this dual process, both macrophage and plasma cells dominate the picture at different times, the former as host cells and the latter involved in the globulin synthesis so characteristic of visceral leishmaniasis, even though the host may die of the infection (Stauber et al., 1954; Rossan, 1960).

Adler (1963a) and others describe similar cellular events for the local cutaneous lesion, which is, of course, less depleting of general mesenchymal reserves and usually goes on to recovery. Adler has also commented on the host response to the disseminated cutaneous infection (*see* Guimaraes, 1951). Here the heteroplastic development of macrophages seems to continue indefinitely and produces a "histiocytoma." The immune response does not set in, and, as Adler comments, "it may well be compared to complete immunological tolerance." On the other hand, where recovery from infection with the visceral parasite occurs, as in the jird (*Meriones unguiculatus*), the liver lesion appears more like the *L. tropica* dermal lesion (Stauber, 1958, and unpublished). It begins and remains sharply focal, and it goes through the changes in cell composition generally suggestive of the mild cutaneous lesion, with maximum reaction at 60 days and with considerable regression noticeable by the 120th day. In the spleen the follicles start to lose lymphocytes early in the infection. Germinal centers come to dominate the follicular appearance later, with many mitoses visible in the centers. This activity combined with the hyperplastic development of macrophages in the red pulp makes the low-magnification view of the spleen appear to be more homogeneous and devoid of any follicle-red pulp distinction. Plasma cells are found in both liver foci and splenic red pulp late in the infection when parasites are scarce.

Passive immunity. There are several ways in which passive transfer experimentation can contribute to understanding of immunity to the leishmania. Serum could be transferred and studied for its protective properties or for the demonstration in the recipient of antibodies and their significance for host resistance. In a similar fashion, lymphoid cells can also be passively transferred and tested. Most of these transfers have already been tried, and enough limited success has been achieved to encourage further work. For cutaneous leishmaniasis, the success of Dostrovsky and Sagher (1946) in passive transfer of hypersensitivity to the skin by serum should be noted, as well as the failures of Adler and Nelken (1965) and Bray and Lainson (1965a) to do so with leukocytes from persons recovered from the infection. In a more artificial but technically correct system, Boysia (1967) has more recently shown conclusively that delayed hypersensitivity can be induced in the guinea pig to leishmanial antigens (*L. mexicana* and *L. donovani*) and is passively transferred by cells from the lymph nodes and spleen of the sensitized guinea pigs.

Few attempts at passively transferring protection have been made for either cutaneous or visceral leishmaniasis (*see* Kretschmar, 1965, for a report of a recent failure), and the role of antibody in recovery from infection, if it has a role, is still unknown. The state of premunition in the visceral infection in some animals suggests either the presence of antibodies in low titer (as shown for malaria by the passive transfer experiments of Coggeshall and

Kumm [1937] and Cohen and McGregor [1963]) or some other, perhaps even physical, protective mechanism associated with antibody action (e.g., the presence of leishmania inside the host macrophage).

Stauber (1955), working with *L. donovani*, indicated that it might take as long as seven to eight days from the time of injection to time of release of parasites from host cells. He also found that cortisone seemed to increase the size of infected macrophages and the number of parasites within them, perhaps by preserving the integrity of the host cell membrane and thus preventing the release of parasites from it. Since contiguous macrophages occur in many sites and the transfer of material between them has now been demonstrated, it is easy to imagine perpetuation of infection in the presence of high-level host resistance. One can also imagine that the hamster or man, both very highly susceptible to the parasite, would not be the hosts of choice for passive transfer experiments and that large amounts of serum would need to be transferred in such a case.

Standardized infections are also needed to facilitate evaluation of transferred protection. Ott (1964) has made some progress along these lines by completing two successful experiments. In one, for example, sera from guinea pigs immune to *L. donovani* (at 60th day of infection) and parasites from hamster spleen were passed into test mice. Although both inocula had material heterologous to the mouse recipients, the passively immunized mice showed a lower peak infection and an earlier fall of parasite numbers in liver impression smears than did control mice receiving normal guinea pig serum or no serum. Earlier attempts at passive transfer of rabbit antibodies failed, but Adler's (1963b) report of the profound effects of rabbit antibodies, even in high dilution, on the growth, morphology, and differentiation of leishmania in culture suggests the need for new trials *in vivo*.

Miller and Twohy (1968) have recently reported passive transfer of protection to *L. donovani* using lymphoid cells from immunized animals and have shown counterpart effects in their cell culture system where macrophages from immune animals did not support parasite proliferation.

While an antibody basis for immunity is still unproved, the specific aspects of protection noted for cutaneous leishmaniasis and the passive transfers noted above suggest that these infections also follow the general rules of immunology, as Taliaferro (1962) indicated for tissue studies.

Serology—*Serum proteins.* It has long been known that infection with *L. donovani* leads to a derangement of the plasma (or serum) protein pattern (*see* reviews by Stauber, 1954; Rossan, 1960; also van Peenen and Miale, 1962; Lupasco et al., 1965; Rahmann, 1966; Chaves and Ferri, 1966; and Priolisi and Giuffre, 1967), and hyperglobulinemia was known to Lloyd and Paul as early as 1928. Some of the alterations are generally associated with severe infectious disease (e.g., a fall in albumin) or with tissue destruction (e.g., a rise in alpha-globulin), but the very large rise in gamma-globulin is as yet unaccounted for. The gamma-globulin may rise to a total of more than 50 g per liter in man and nearly this much in the chinchilla, and may represent more than 50 percent of the total serum protein. The material responsible for this increase is apparently not a distinctive protein, such as that found in myeloma, and at present is considered simply as excess gamma-globulin. The peak produced by electrophoretic separation appears broader than normal, which could be explained by the general increase of minor components or by the heterogeneities known to exist even for antibodies specific for a single antigen. The high gamma-globulin content (Gutman, 1948) along with the low albumin content (Most and Lavietes, 1947) are the probable bases for the formol-gel test (and similar tests) that are used widely in the clinic to assist in diagnosis of the visceral infection.

Man and the chinchilla usually die of visceral leishmaniasis. The golden hamster dies also, but its serum protein pattern is complicated by the loss of protein in urine during the developing amyloidosis in this animal (Ada and Fulton, 1948; Gellhorn et al., 1946). Both Howes (1966) and Schatz (personal communication, 1967) have shown that appreciable amounts of gamma-globulin, as well as albumin, are lost in the urine. Nevertheless, before death is imminent, significant increases in serum gamma-globulin have been found in infected hamsters (Rossan, 1960; Howes, 1966; Schatz, 1967). It would appear that the large amount of gamma-globulin produced by these hosts during infection is not protective antibody active against the leishmania. Taliaferro (1962) has emphasized Putnam's (1960) view that these abnormalities may be more quantitative than qualitative and that until we know much more about the many antigens inducing gamma-globulin synthesis during infection (parasite antigens, parasite product antigens, or altered host antigens), we have little basis for calling them abnormal globulins.

Serologic reactions. That the leishmania contain antigenic materials and that antibodies, as usually defined, are produced by hosts after injection or during infection are happily now well established. Much of the earlier work (*see* Taliaferro 1929) and some of the more recent studies (Adler, 1963b; Duxbury and Sadun, 1964; Bray and Lainson, 1965b, 1966; Schneider and Hertig, 1966) specialized in using rabbits for synthesizing the globulins for serologic tests. Adler's recent work on the influence of antibody (Adler, 1963b; Adler et al., 1966) on the form and development of leishmania in culture is unique and of great interest, not only for the basic understanding of reproduction and differentiation it provides, but also because he used it as a sensitive test for antigenic differences among the strains and species of *Leishmania* (*see also* Safyanova, 1966).

Of more direct interest to host resistance, there has been much recent progress in the study of antibodies in infected hosts. These include hemagglutinating systems in jirds (Rossan, 1959) and in humans (Bray and El-Nahal, 1966), other agglutinating systems (Pifano and Scorza, 1960; Sen and Mukerjee, 1961; Shuikina, 1965; Bray and Lainson, 1967), fluorescent-antibody studies (Herman, 1965; Oddo and Cascio, 1963; Sadun et al., 1963; Shaw and Voller, 1964; Duxbury and Sadun, 1964; Shuikina, 1965; Bray and Lainson, 1965b; Convit and Kerdel-Vegas, 1965; Demina et al., 1965; Walton et al., 1967) precipitation reactions by gel diffusion or immunoelectrophoresis (Chaffee, 1963; Garcia, 1965; Bray and Lainson, 1966; Chaves and Ferri, 1966; Schneider and Hertig, 1966), and complement-fixation reactions, mostly with mycobacterial antigens (Nussenzweig, 1957, 1958a,b,c; Nussenzweig et al., 1957a,b; Cunha et al., 1959, 1963; Alencar and Cunha, 1963; Alencar et al., 1966; Torrealba et al., 1963; Torrealba and Chaves-Torrealba, 1964; Khaleque, 1965) and some with flagellate antigens (Ranque and Duncan, 1964). The new immunoelectroabsorption technique has also been revealing since it shows specific antibody even in the infected hamster before proteinuria becomes too severe (Mathot et al., 1967).

Each of these tests has contributed to our knowledge and many are useful diagnostic tools. However, their specificity is generally low. Many of the reactions are group-reactive, especially within the family Trypanosomatidae. Homologous reactions are usually stronger than reactions with heterologous strains of parasites. Serologic groupings usually reveal either distinctions or similarities inconsistent with origin, pathogenicity, or histotropism. For example, in agglutination reactions, Bray and Lainson (1967) detected serologic differences between strains of *L. donovani* from India and Kenya, yet detected no differences between an *L. donovani* strain (dermal leishmanial) and an *L. tropica* (Israel). Schneider and Hertig (1966) did an extensive study of immunodiffusion reactions using Panamanian leishmania. They could arrange the strains into serotypes based on these reactions but, in like fashion, obtained inconsistencies. For example, some sandfly strains fell into groups but others showed more uncertain affinities. While "*L. mexicana* group" parasites and Peruvian uta parasites seemed distinguishable from the Panamanian human strains, two human strains from the same locale were also different. The very heterogeneity of the Panamanian strains as revealed by these studies emphasizes the work still necessary to clarify the antigenic structure of the *Leishmania*. Much less work has been done with the amastigotes than with the culture promastigotes. The amastigotes from tissue seem less antigenic and less cross-reactive than promastigotes. Some of these differences may be quantitative rather than qualitative. However, the immunodiffusion studies of Simpson (1967, 1968) support earlier agglutination findings of D'Alesandro (1954), Adler and Adler (1955), and the cultivation in antiserum studies by Adler et al. (1966). Simpson found at least three promastigote antigens in addition to the common antigens shared with the amastigotes. Not enough studies on specific adsorption have been performed (Menolasino and Hartman, 1954), although Bray and Lainson (1965b) state that specific adsorption completely eliminated positive fluorescent-antibody reactions. There is no evidence yet that "relapse" strains, or strain variation in the *T. brucei* sense, occurs in the *Leishmania*, although this is one possible interpretation of the differences noted by Sen and Mukerjee (1961) for visceral and post-kala-azar dermal parasites.

CONCLUSION

In many ways the *Leishmania* are typical as agents of disease and in the induction of immune responses. Their unique features probably stem more from their dimorphic structure, their peculiar host localizations, and their variation at strain-level than from species-level antigenic differences.

REFERENCES

Actor, P. 1958. Protein intake and visceral leishmaniasis in the golden hamster. M.A. Thesis, New Brunswick, N. J., Rutgers—The State University, 48 pp.
———— 1960. Protein and vitamin intake and visceral leishmaniasis in the mouse. Exp. Parasit., 10:1-20.
Ada, G., and J. D. Fulton. 1948. Electrophoretic studies in the serum of golden hamsters infected with Leishmania donovani. Brit. J. Exp. Path., 29:524-529.
Adler, S. 1954. The behavior of Plasmodium berghei in the golden hamster Mesocricetus auratus infected with visceral leishmaniasis. Trans. Roy. Soc. Trop. Med. Hyg., 48:431-440.
———— 1962. The behavior of a lizard Leishmania in hamsters and baby mice. Rev. Inst. Med. Trop. (São Paulo), 4:61-64.
———— 1963a. Immune phenomena in leishmaniasis. In Immunity to Protozoa. Garnham, P. C. C., Pierce, A. G., and Roitt, I., eds. Oxford, Blackwell Scientific Publications, pp. 235-245.
———— 1963b. Differentiation of Leishmania brasiliensis from L. mexicana and L. tropica. Rev. Inst. Salubr. Enferm. Trop., 23:139-152.
———— 1964. Leishmania. In Advances in Parasitology, Vol. 2. Dawes, B., ed. New York, Academic Press, Inc., pp. 35-96.
———— 1965. Immunology of leishmaniasis. Israel J. Med. Sci., 1:9-13.
———— and A. Zuckerman. 1948. Observations on a strain of Leishmania tropica after prolonged cultivation: notes on infectivity and immunity. Ann. Trop. Med. Parasit., 42:178-183.
———— and I. Katzenellenbogen. 1952. The problem of the association between particular strains of Leishmania tropica and the clinical manifestations produced by them. Ann. Trop. Med. Parasit., 46:25-32.
———— and J. Adler. 1955. The agglutinogenic properties of various stages of the Leishmanias. Bull. Res. Counc. Israel (correspondence), 4:396-397.
———— and A. E. Gunders. 1964. Immunity to Leishmania mexicana following spontaneous recovery from oriental sore. Trans. Roy. Soc. Trop. Med. Hyg., 58:274-277.
———— and D. Nelken. 1965. Attempts to transfer delayed hypersensitivity to Leishmania tropica by leucocytes and whole blood. Trans. Roy. Soc. Trop. Med. Hyg., 59:59-63.
———— A. Foner, and B. Montiglio. 1966. The relationship between human and animal strains of Leishmania from the Sudan. Trans. Roy. Soc. Trop. Med. Hyg., 60:380-386.
Alencar, J. E. de, and R. V. Cunha. 1963. Inquéritos sôbre calazar canino no Ceará—Novos resultados (Studies on canine Kala Azar in Ceara—New results). Rev. Brasil. Malar., 15:391-403.
———— E. P. Pessoa, and Z. F. Fontienele. 1960. Natural infection of Rattus rattus alexandrinus with Leishmania, probably L. brasiliensis, in an endemic area of cutaneous leishmaniasis, in Ceara, Brazil. Rev. Inst. Med. Trop. (São Paulo), 2:347-348.
———— A. Ilardi, and S. Pampiglione. 1966. La reazione di fissazione del complemento nella diagnosi della leishmaiosi viscerale: antigeni da batteri acido alcool resistenti. Parassitologia, 8:147-181.
Ansari, N., and C. Mofidi. 1950. A contribution to the study of "moist forms" of cutaneous leishmaniasis. Bull. Soc. Path. Exot., 43:601-607.
Ary, R. A., R. Zeledon, and W. Hidalgo. 1964. A case of verrucous leishmaniasis probably disseminated through the use of steroids and cured by glucantime. Acta Med. Costarricense, 7:105-111.
Baker, A. C., and E. Gutierrez-Ballesteros. 1957. Tratamiento experimental de las úlceras leishmaniasicas por el procedimiento del calor del vapor. Rev. Inst. Salubr. Enferm. Trop., 17:115-117.

Not all of these references were seen in the original, and not all are given titles in their original language.

Barbosa, W., M. dos R. e Silva, and P. C. Borges. 1965. Preliminary report on American mucocutaneous leishmaniasis in Goias state (Brazil). Rev. Goiana Med., 11:1-9.

Belova, E. M. 1964. Investigation of the virulence of different strains of the causative agent of zoonotic cutaneous leishmaniasis (in Russian). Med. Parazit. (Moskva), 33:666-670.

Beltran, E. 1945. Cutaneous leishmaniasis in Mexico, Lab. Digest, 9:1-5.

Berberian, D. A. 1939. Vaccination and immunity against oriental sore. Trans. Roy. Soc. Trop. Med. Hyg., 33:87-94.

―――― 1944. Cutaneous leishmaniasis (Oriental sore) I. Time required for development of immunity after vaccination. Arch. Derm. Syph., 49:433-435.

Biagi, F. F. 1967. Table on anatomo-clinical aspects of leishmaniasis (personal communication).

―――― F. J. Vargas, and J. Torres. 1960. Two new foci of cutaneous leishmaniasis in Mexico. Medicina, 10:410-413.

Boysia, F. 1967. Delayed hypersensitivity to leishmanial antigens in the guinea pig. Ph.D. Thesis, New Brunswick, N. J., Rutgers—The State University, 135 pp.

Brahmachari, U. N. 1922. A new form of cutaneous leishmaniasis dermal leishmanoid. Indian Med. Gazette, 57:125-127.

Bray, R. S., and H. M. S. El-Nahal. 1966. Antibody estimation by passive haemagglutination in malaria and leishmaniasis. Trans. Roy. Soc. Trop. Med. Hyg., 60:423-424.

Bray, R. S., and R. Lainson. 1965a. Failure to transfer hypersensitivity to Leishmania by injection of leucocytes. Trans. Roy. Soc. Trop. Med. Hyg., 59:221-222.

―――― and R. Lainson. 1965b. The immunology and serology of leishmaniasis. I. The fluorescent antibody staining technique. Trans. Roy. Soc. Trop. Med. Hyg., 59:535-544.

―――― and R. Lainson. 1966. The immunology and serology of leishmaniasis. IV. Results of Ouchterlony double diffusion tests. Trans. Roy. Soc. Trop. Med. Hyg., 60:605-609.

―――― and R. Lainson. 1967. Studies on the immunology and serology of leishmaniasis. V. The use of particles as vehicles in passive agglutination tests. Trans. Roy. Soc. Trop. Med. Hyg., 61:490-505.

Brygoo, E. R. 1963. Contributions à la connaisance de parasitologie des caméléons malgaches. Part 2. Ann. Parasit. Hum. Comp., 38:533-739.

Bureau, Y., Jarry, Barriere, and Litoux. 1960. Leishmaniose à localizations cutanées multiples et nodules lymphangitiques dissemenes. Bull. Soc. Franc. Derm. Syph., 67:67-68.

Cahill, K. M., G. R. Anderson, and N. Turegun. 1965. A leishmanin survey in southeast Turkey. Bull. W. H. O., No. 32, pp. 121-123.

―――― 1965. Leishmanin skin testing in Africa and the Middle East. E. Afri. Med. J., 42:213-220.

Camerlynck, P., P. Ranque, and M. Quilici. 1967. Intérêt des cultures systematiques et des subcultures dans la recherche des reservoirs de virus naturels de la leishmaniase cutanée. Med. Trop. (Marseille), 27:89-92.

Chaffee, E. F. 1963. Preliminary report on the Leishmania antigens. Proc. 7th Int. Congr. Trop. Med. Malaria, 2:309-310.

Chaves, J., and R. G. Ferri. 1966. Immunoglobulins in visceral leishmaniasis. Rev. Inst. Med. Trop. (São Paulo), 8:225-226.

Coggeshall, L. T. and H. W. Kumm. 1937. Demonstration of passive immunity in experimental monkey malaria. J. Exp. Med., 66:177-190.

Cohen, S., and I. A. McGregor. 1963. Gamma globulin and acquired immunity to malaria. In Immunity to Protozoa. Garnham, P. C. C., Pierce, A. E., and Roitt, I., eds. Oxford, Blackwell Scientific Publications, pp. 125-159.

Conti-Diaz, I. A., and J. E. Mackinon. 1961. Infección evolutiva e infección latente del cobaya por Blastomyces dematitidis condicionadas a la temperatura ambiente. An. Fac. Med. Montevideo, 46:280-282.

Convit, J. 1958. Leishmaniose tegumentaire difusa neuva entidad clinico y parasitaria. Rev. Sanid. Assis. Soc., 23:1-28.

―――― O. Reyes, and F. Kerdel-Vegas. 1957. Disseminated anergic American leishmaniasis. Report of three cases of a type clinically resembling lepromatous leprosy. Arch. Derm. (Chicago), 76:213-217.

―――― and F. Kerdel-Vegas. 1965. Disseminated cutaneous leishmaniasis. Inoculation to laboratory animals, electron microscopy, and fluorescent antibody studies. Arch. Derm. (Chicago), 91:439-447.

Corkhill, N. L. 1949. The activation of latent Kala-Azar in relation to protein metabolism. Ann. Trop. Med. Parasit., 43:261-267.

Coutinho, J. O. 1954. Preventive vaccination with dead leptomonads against leishmaniasis of guinea pigs due to Leishmania enriettii. Folia Clin. Biol. (São Paulo), 21:321-326.

——— 1955. Study of Leishmania enriettii-experimental infections. Folia Clin. Biol. (São Paulo), 23:91-102.

Cunha, R. V., A. F. S. Xavier, and J. E. de Alencar. 1959. Disproteinaemia in Kala Azar and its relations with complement fixation. Rev. Brasil. Malar., 11:45-54.

——— J. E. de Alencar, and F. B. Andrade. 1963. The use of a complement-fixation test for the diagnosis of canine Kala Azar in mass surveys. Rev. Brasil. Malar., 15:405-410.

D'Alesandro, P. A. 1954. A serological comparison of the leishmaniform and the leptomonad stages of Leishmania donovani. M. A. Thesis, New Brunswick, N. J., Rutgers— The State University, 42 pp.

Demina, N. A., O. I. Kellina, E. E. Shuikina, S. G. Vasina, and Z. I. Glazunova. 1965. Investigations on immunity in leishmaniasis. In Progress in Protozoology. Abstracts, 2nd Int. Conf. Protozool., London. International Congress Series No. 91. Amsterdam, Excerpta Medica Foundation, pp. 134-135.

De Sampaio, L. F. 1951. O aparecimento, a expansão, e o fim da leishmaniose no Estado de São Paulo. Rev. Brasil. Malar., 8:717-721.

Destombes, P. 1960. A "polar conception" of the lesions of cutaneous leishmaniasis. Bull. Soc. Path. Exot., 53:299-300.

Disney, R. H. L. 1964. Visceral involvement with dermal leishmaniasis in a wild-caught rodent in British Honduras. Trans. Roy. Soc. Trop. Med. Hyg. (Correspondence), 58:581.

Dostrovsky, A., and F. Sagher. 1946. The intracutaneous test in cutaneous leishmaniasis. Ann. Trop. Med. Parasit., 40:265-269.

———F. Sagher, and A. Zuckerman. 1952a. Isophasic reaction following experimental superinfection of Leishmania tropica. Arch. Derm. Syph., 66:665-675.

——— A. Zuckerman and F. Sagher. 1952b. Successful experimental superinfection of Leishmania tropica in patients with relapsing cutaneous leishmaniasis. Harefuah (J. Israel Med. Ass.), 43:29-30.

Duxbury, R. E., and E. H. Sadun. 1964. Fluorescent antibody test for the serodiagnosis of visceral leishmaniasis. Amer. J. Trop. Med. Hyg., 13:525-529.

Eliseev, L. N., and M. V. Strelkova. 1966. The effect of the environmental temperature upon the temperature of the skin and the course of cutaneous leishmaniasis in Rhombomys opimus Licht. and Meriones libycus Licht. Med. Parazit. (Moskva), 35:696-705.

Ercoli, N. 1961. Chemotherapeutic studies on cutaneous leishmaniasis. Proc. Soc. Exp. Biol. Med., 106:787-790.

Fendall, N. R. E. 1953. The history and character of the Kala-Azar outbreak in the Kitui District. E. Afr. Med. J., 30:269-285.

Forattini, O. P. 1960. On the natural reservoirs of American cutaneous leishmaniasis. Rev. Inst. Med. Trop. (São Paulo), 2:195-203.

Franchino, E. M. 1959. Factors influencing the course of infection of Leishmania donovani in the white mouse. Ph.D. Thesis, New Brunswick N. J., Rutgers—The State University, 74 pp.

Frothingham, T. E, and E. Lehtimoki. 1967. Leishmania in primary cultures of human amniotic cells. Amer. J. Trop. Med. Hyg., 16:658-664.

Galliard, H. 1962. Nodular and diffuse forms of cutaneous leishmaniasis. Scientific Reports of the Istituto Superiore di Sanita, 2:154-168.

Garcia, B. S. 1965. Antigenic components of Leishmania tropica. J. Philipp. Med. Ass., 41:647-652.

Garnham, P. C. C. 1965. The Leishmanias, with special reference to the role of animal reservoirs. Amer. Zool., 5:141-151.

——— and D. J. Lewis. 1959. Parasites of British Honduras with specific reference to leishmaniasis. Trans. Roy. Soc. Trop. Med. Hyg., 53:12-40.

Gellhorn, A., H. B. Van Dyke, W. J. Pyles, and N. A. Tupikova. 1946. Amyloidosis in hamsters with leishmaniasis. Proc. Soc. Exp. Biol. Med., 61:25-30.

Goble, F. C. 1966. Pathogenesis of blood protozoa. In Biology of Parasites. Soulsby, E. J. L., ed. New York, Academic Press, Inc., pp. 237-254.

———— E. A. Konopka, and J. L. Boyd. 1965. Sex of host as a factor in protozoal pathogenesis. In Progress in Protozoology. Abstracts, 2nd Int. Conf. Protozool., London. International Congress Series No. 91, Amsterdam, Excerpta Medica Foundation, p. 54.

Gorgas Memorial Laboratory. 1967. Leishmaniasis. In 38th Annual Report Gorgas Memorial Laboratory for 1966. pp. 7-11.

———— 1968. Leishmaniasis. In 39th Annual Report Gorgas Memorial Laboratory for 1967. pp. 10-11.

Grun, J. 1958. A study of experimental leishmaniasis in the mouse, Mongolian gerbil, hamster, white rat, cotton rat, and chinchilla. Ph.D. Thesis, New Brunswick, N. J., Rutgers—The State University. 82 pp.

Guimaraes, F. N. 1951. Experimental leishmaniasis. IV. Reproduction in hamsters C. auratus cutaneous nodulotumor of Amazon (Leishmania histiocytoma). Hospital (Rio de Janeiro), 40:665-676.

———— and O. R. Costa. 1966. Novas observacões sôbre a Leishmania isolada de "Oryzomys goeldi," na Amazonia (4.a nota). Hospital (Rio de Janeiro), 69:161-168.

Gutierrez-Ballesteros, E. 1959. Treatment of cutaneous leishmaniasis with vapour-heat. Study of 5 human cases. Rev. Inst. Salubr. Enferm. Trop. (Mexico), 19:317-328.

Gutman, A. B. 1948. The plasma proteins in disease. Advances Protein Chem., 4:156-250.

Heisch, R. B. 1961. Rodents as reservoirs of Arthropod-borne diseases in Kenya. E. Afr. Med. J., 38:257-261.

Herman, R. 1965. Fluorescent antibody studies on the intracellular form of Leishmania donovani grown in cell culture. Exp. Parasit., 17:218-228.

Herrer, A. 1951. Estudios sobre leishmaniasis tegumentaria en el Perú. IV. Observaciones epidemiológicas sobre la uta. Rev. Med. Exp., 8:45-86.

———— 1962. The incidence of uta (cutaneous leishmaniasis) among the child population of Perú. Scientific Reports of the Istituto Superiore di Sanita, 2:131-137.

———— 1968. Personal communication.

———— V. E. Thatcher, and C. M. Johnson. 1966. Natural infections of Leishmania and trypanosomes demonstrated by skin culture. J. Parasit., 52: 954-957.

Hertig, M., G. B. Fairchild, and C. M. Johnson. 1956. Leishmaniasis transmission—Reservoir project. In Annual Report Gorgas Memorial Laboratory for 1956, pp. 9-11.

———— G. B. Fairchild, and C. M. Johnson. 1957. Leishmaniasis transmission—Reservoir project. In Annual Report Gorgas Memorial Laboratory for 1957, pp. 7-11.

———— G. B. Fairchild, and C. M. Johnson. 1958. Leishmaniasis transmission—Reservoir project. In Annual Report Gorgas Memorial Laboratory for 1958, pp. 11-15.

———— G. B. Fairchild, C. M. Johnson, P. T. Johnson, E. McConnell, and W. J. Hanson. 1959. Leishmaniasis transmission—Reservoir studies. In Annual Report Gorgas Memorial Laboratory for 1959, pp. 5-11.

Heyneman, D., and N. S. Mansour. 1963. Leishmaniasis in the Sudan Republic. II. Laboratory infection of Egyptian and Sudanese rodents with strains of Leishmania donovani. J. Egypt. Public Health Ass., 38:37-46.

Hoogstraal, H., and D. R. Dietlein. 1964. Leishmaniasis in the Sudan Republic: Recent results. Bull. W. H. O. No. 31, pp. 137-143.

———— P. F. D. van Peenen, T. A. Reid, and D. R. Dietlein. 1963. Leishmaniasis in the Sudan Republic. 10. Natural infections in rodents. Amer. J. Trop. Med. Hyg., 12: 175-178.

Hoare, C. A., and F. G. Wallace. 1966. Developmental stages of trypanosomatid flagellates: A new terminology. Nature (London), 212:1385-1386.

Howes, H. L. 1966. Studies on the pathogenesis of Leishmania donovani in the golden hamster. Ph.D. Thesis, New Brunswick, N. J., Rutgers—The State University, 132 pp.

Janovy, J. J., Jr. 1967. Effects of cycloguanil pamoate against various Leishmania donovani infections. Proc. 42nd Ann. Meeting Amer. Soc. Parasit., p. 25.

Kellina, O. I. 1965. A comparative study of the virulence of Leishmania tropica major strains. Med. Parazit. (Moskva), 34:309-316.

———— 1966. Studies on immunity in cutaneous leishmaniasis. II. Local allergic reactions and survival of Leishmania in the skin after inoculation of Leishmania tropica major culture to immune persons. Med. Parazit. (Moskva), 35:679-686.

Kerdel-Vegas, F., F. Conde Jahn, E. Essenfeld-Yahr, J. J. Henríquez Andueza, C. E.

Machado-Allison, R. Darricarrere, and F. Castro Ramírez. 1966. Reservorio extrahumano de la leishmaniasis americana en Venezuela. Informe preliminar de la infección leishmanica de un ratón selvático del género Zygodontomys en la región de Ticoporo, Estado Barinas (with English summary). Gac. Med. Caracas, 74: 283-293.

Khaleque, K. A. 1965. Complement fixation test for Kala-Azar with an antigen prepared from acid fast bacillus. Pakistan J. Med. Res., 4: 234-240.

Kirk, R. 1938. Primary cutaneous sore in a case of Kala-Azar. Trans. Roy. Soc. Trop. Med. Hyg., 32: 271-272.

Konopka, E. A., F. C. Goble, and L. Lewis. 1961. Effect of prior infection with Leishmania donovani on the course of experimental tuberculosis in mice. Bact. Proc., p. 134.

Kozhenvikov. 1950. In Kellina, 1966.

Krampitz, H. E., and H. Muhlpfordt. 1964. Zur Empfanglichkeit einiger exothermophiler Nagetierenarten für die experimentelle Infection mit Leishmania donovani (Calcutta-Stamm) Z. Tropenmed. Parasit., 15: 267-278.

Kretschmar, W. 1965. Immunität bei der Leishmania enriettii—Infection des Meerschweinchens. Z. Tropenmed. Parasit., 16: 277-283.

Lainson, R., and J. Strangways-Dixon. 1962. Dermal leishmaniasis in British Honduras: Some host reservoirs of L. brasiliensis mexicana. Brit. Med. J., 1: 1596-1598.

———— and J. Strangways-Dixon. 1963. Leishmania mexicana: The epidemiology of dermal leishmaniasis in British Honduras. I. The human disease. Trans. Roy. Soc. Trop. Med. Hyg., 57: 242-265.

———— and J. Strangways-Dixon. 1964. The epidemiology of dermal leishmaniasis in British Honduras. II. Reservoir hosts of Leishmania mexicana among the forest rodents. Trans. Roy. Soc. Trop. Med. Hyg., 58: 136-153.

———— and R. S. Bray. 1964. Leishmania mexicana (Correspondence). Trans. Roy. Soc. Trop. Med. Hyg., 58: 94.

———— and R. S. Bray. 1966. Studies on the immunology and serology of leishmaniasis. II. Cross-immunity experiments among different forms of American cutaneous leishmaniasis in monkeys. Trans. Roy. Soc. Trop. Med. Hyg., 60: 526-532.

———— and J. J. Shaw. 1966. Studies on the immunology and serology of leishmaniasis. III. On the cross immunity between Panamanian cutaneous leishmaniasis and Leishmania mexicana infection in man. Trans. Roy. Soc. Trop. Med. Hyg., 60: 533-535.

Lariviere, M. 1966. Aspects cliniques et épidémiologiques de la leishmaniase cutanée au Senegal. Bull. Soc. Path. Exot., 59: 83-98.

Latyshev, N. I., and A. P. Kryukova. 1953. The genetic relationship between various species of Leishmania. Probl. Reg. Gen. Exp. Parasit. Med. Zool., 8: 211-215.

———— A. P. Kryukova, and T. P. Povalishina. 1951. Essays on the regional parasitology of Middle Asia. I. Leishmaniasis in Tadjikistan. Materials for the medical geography of Tadjik S.S.R. (Results of expeditions in 1945-1947). Probl. Reg. Gen. Exp. Parasit. Med. Zool., 7: 35-62.

Lawrow, A. P., and P. A. Dubowskoj. 1937. Über Schutzimpfungen gegen Hautleishmaniose. Arch. Schiffs. Tropenhyg., 41: 374.

Lemma, A., and E. L. Schiller. 1964. Extracellular cultivation of the leishmanial bodies of species belonging to the Protozoan genus Leishmania. Exp. Parasit., 15: 503-513.

Liban, E., A. Zuckerman, and F. Sagher. 1955. Specific tissue alteration in leprous skin. VII. Inoculation of Leishmania tropica into leprous patients. Arch. Derm. (Chicago), 71: 441-450.

Lissia, G. 1965. Osservazioni epidemiologiche, cliniche, terapeutiche e profilattiche sulla leishmaniosi cutanea in Sardegna. Minerva Derm., 40: 196-201.

Lloyd, R. B., and S. N. Paul. 1928. Protein graphs in K-A. Indian J. Med. Res., 16: 529-535.

Lupasco, G., A. Bossie-Agavriloaei, and L. Ianco. 1965. Study of electrophoretic changes in the serum proteins in experimental infection of the golden hamster (Cricetus auratus) with Leishmania donovani. Arch. Roumaines Path. Exp. Microbiol., 24: 527-536.

Manson-Bahr, P. E. C. 1955. A primary skin lesion in visceral leishmaniasis (Correspondence). Nature (London), 175: 433-434.

———— 1959. East African Kala-Azar with special reference to the pathology, prophylaxis and treatment. Trans. Roy. Soc. Trop. Med. Hyg., 53: 123-136.

———— 1961. Immunity in Kala-Azar. Trans. Roy. Soc. Trop. Med. Hyg., 55: 550-555.

———— and B. A. Southgate. 1964. Recent research on Kala-Azar in East Africa. J. Trop. Med. Hyg., 67: 79-84.

Maruashvili, G. M., and B. G. Bardzhadze. 1966. Natural foci of visceral leishmaniasis in Georgia. Med. Parazit. (Moskva), 35: 462-463.

Mathot, C., P. A. D'Alesandro, S. Scher, and A. Rothen. 1967. The immune response of golden hamsters to *Leishmania donovani* as tested by immunoelectroadsorption. Amer. J. Trop. Med. Hyg., 16:443-446.

Medina, R. 1966. Leishmaniasis experimental en animales silvestros. Derm. Venez., 5:91-119.

Meleney, H. E. 1925. The histopathology of Kala-Azar in the hamster, monkey and man. Amer. J. Path., 1:147-168.

Menolasino, N. J., and E. Hartman. 1954. Immunology and serology of some parasitic protozoan flagellates. II. The hemoflagellate protozoa, *Leishmania donovani* and *Trypanosoma cruzi*. J. Protozool., 1:111-113.

Miller, H. C., and D. W. Twohy. 1968. Cellular immunity to *Leishmania donovani*. Bact. Proc. p. 100.

Montenegro, J. 1926. Cutaneous reactions in leishmaniasis. Arch. Derm. Syph., 13:187.

Most, H., and P. H. Lavietes. 1947. Kala-Azar in American military personnel. Medicine, 26:221-284.

Navarrete, A. F., and F. F. Biagi. 1960. Leishmaniasis cutanea. Especificidad de la reacción intradérmica de Montenegro. Prensa Med. Mex., 25:2-4.

Nussenzweig, V. 1957. Reação de fixação do complemento para leishmaniose visceral com antigeno extraido do bacilo da tuberculose. Técnica, sensibilidade e especificação. Hospital (Rio de Janeiro), 51:217-226.

———— 1958a. Valôr da reação da fixação do complemento para leishmaniose visceral com antigeno extraido de bacilos de tuberculose. II. Relação entre a reatividade do sôro e os dados clínicos. Rev. Brasil. Malar., 10:251-258.

———— 1958b. Valôr de reação de fixação do complemento para leishmaniose visceral com antigeno extraido de bacilos de tuberculose. III. Variação da reatividade serica com o tratamento específico. Rev. Brasil. Malar., 10:259-266.

———— 1958c. Valôr da reação de fixação do complemento para leishmaniose visceral com antigeno extraido de bacilos de tuberculose. IV. Inibição da reação por excesso de sôro. Rev. Brasil. Malar., 10:267-274.

———— R. S. Nussenzweig, and J. E. de Alencar. 1957a. Leishmaniose visceral canina nos arredores de Fortaleza, Estado do Ceará: inquérito sorológico utilizado a reação de fixação do complemento com antigeno extraido do bacilo da tuberculose. Observações sôbre diagnóstico e epidemiologia da doença. Hospital (Rio de Janeiro), 52:111-129.

———— R. S. Nussenzweig, and J. E. de Alencar. 1957b. Leishmaniose visceral canina: reação de fixação do complemento com antigeno extraido do bacilo da tuberculose. Hospital (Rio de Janeiro), 51:325-332.

Ny, G. V. 1966. Susceptibility of some laboratory and wild mammals to infection with Uzbek strains of *Leishmania tropica major* isolated from gerbils (*Rhombomys opimus* Licht). Med. Parazit. (Moskva), 35:270-274.

Oddo, F. G., and G. Cascio. 1963. Il test di immuno-fluorescenza nella leishmaniosi viscerale e cutanea. Riv. Ist. Sieroterop. Ital., 38:139-145.

Ott, K. J. 1964. Aspects of immunity of laboratory rodents to *Leishmania donovani*. Ph.D. Thesis, New Brunswick, N. J., Rutgers—The State University, 130 pp.

Pacheco, M. M., F. R. Cespedes, and H. Calderon. 1961. Concomitant hepatic lesions in cutaneous leishmaniasis studied by liver biopsy. Acta Med. Costarricense 4:3-23.

Packchanian, A., and L. Kelly. 1965. Susceptibility of *Peromyscus californicus* to infection with *Leishmania donovani*. Texas Rep. Biol. Med., 23:767-775.

Pedroso, A. M. 1923. Infecção do cao pela Leishmania tropical. Rev. Med. São Paulo, 24:42-44.

Pessoa, S. B. 1941a. Dados sôbre a epidemiologia da leishmaniose tegumenta em São Paulo. Hospital (Rio de Janeiro), 19:389-409.

———— 1941b. Profilaxia de leishmaniose tegumenta no estado de São Paulo. Folia Med., 22:157-161.

———— and B. R. Pestana. 1941. Attempt to vaccinate against cutaneous leishmaniasis with killed organisms. Arq. Hig. (São Paulo), 6:141-147.

———— and F. A. Cardoso. 1942. Notas sôbre a imunidade cruzada na leishmaniose tegumentar e na moléstia de Chagas. Hospital (Rio de Janeiro), 21:187-193.

Pifano, C. F. 1960. Aspectos epidemiológicos de la leishmaniasis tegumentaria en la región neotrópica, con especial referencia a Venezuela. Arch. Venez. Med. Trop. Parasit. Med., 3:15-30.

———— 1962. La evaluación de la leishmaniasis tegumentaria americana en el Valle de Aroa, Estado Yaracuy, mediante el índice alérgico (intrademoreacción con ántigeno de *Leishmania brasiliensis*). Arch. Venez. Med. Trop. Parasit. Med., 4:25-35.

———— and J. V. Scorza. 1960. Aspecto inmunológico de las leishmanias que parasitan al hombre, con especial referencia a la *Leishmania brasiliensis pifanoi*, Medina and Romero, 1957. Arch. Venez. Med. Trop. Parasit. Med., 3:15-30.

Popovic, D. 1965. Befunde bei mit *Leishmania donovani* infizierten Zieseln (*Citellus citellus*). Angew. Parasit., 6:181-185.

Price, E. W., and M. Fitzherbert. 1965. Cutaneous leishmaniasis in Ethiopia. A clinical study and review of literature. Ethiopian Med. J., 3:57-83.

Priolisi, A., and L. Giuffre. 1967. Immunoelectrophoretic analysis of serum proteins of patients affected by kala-azar. Path. Microbiol. (Basel), 30:215-221.

Putnam, F. W. 1960. The Plasma Proteins. New York, Academic Press, Inc., Vol. 2, p. 345.

Rahman, M. A. 1966. Electrophoretic differential serum protein pattern in dermal leishmaniasis. Pakistan J. Med. Res., 5:73-81.

Ranque, J., and S. Dunan. 1964. Comportement antigenique de divers flagelles au cour des leishmanioses cliniques et expérimentales. Ann. Parasit. Hum. Comp., 39:117-130.

Ritterson, A. L., and L. A. Stauber. 1949. Protein intake and leishmaniasis in the hamster. Proc. Soc. Exp. Biol. Med., 70:47-50.

Rossan, R. N. 1959. The serum proteins of animals infected with *Leishmania donovani*, with special reference to electrophoretic patterns. Ph.D. Thesis, New Brunswick, N.J., Rutgers—The State University, 214 pp.

———— 1960. Serum proteins of animals infected with *Leishmania donovani*, with special reference to electrophoretic patterns. Exp. Parasit., 9:302-333.

Sadun, E. H., R. E. Duxbury, J. S. Williams, and R. I. Anderson. 1963. Fluorescent antibody test for the serodiagnosis of African and American trypanosomiasis in man. J. Parasit., 49:385-388.

Safyanova, V. M. 1966. Serological comparison of leptomonad strains isolated from sandflies with *Leishmania tropica* and leptomonads of reptiles. Med. Parazit. (Moskva), 35:686-695.

Sagher, F., S. Verbi, and A. Zuckerman. 1955. Immunity to reinfection following recovery from cutaneous leishmaniasis (Oriental sore). J. Invest. Derm., 24:417-421.

Sati, M. H. 1962. A new experimental host of *Leishmania donovani*. Exp. Parasit., 14:52-53.

Schatz, F. 1967. Personal communication.

Schneider, C. R., and M. Hertig. 1966. Immunodiffusion reactions of Panamanian *Leishmania*. Exp. Parasit., 18:25-34.

Sen, A. and S. Mukerjee. 1961. Observation on antigenic differentiation of leishmania parasites of kala-azar and post-kala-azar dermal leishmaniasis. Ann. Biochem. Exp. Med. (Calcutta), 21:105-108.

Senekji, H. A. 1943. Hematologic and immunologic studies on natural and induced leishmaniasis in paretics. Amer. J. Trop. Med., 23:53-58.

———— and C. P. Beattie. 1941. Artificial infection and immunization of man with cultures of *Leishmania tropica*. Trans. Roy. Soc. Trop. Med. Hyg., 34:415-419.

Sen Gupta, P. C. 1962. Pathogenicity of *Leishmania donovani* in man. Rev. Inst. Med. Trop. (São Paulo), 4:130-135.

———— 1965. Host-parasite relationship in *Leishmania donovani* infection in man. Parassitologia, 7:1-8.

Shanbron. E., R. Minton, C. Lester, and J. L. Correa. 1956. Visceral manifestations in American mucocutaneous leishmaniasis. Amer. J. Med., 20:145-152.

Shaw, J. J. and A. Voller. 1963. Preliminary fluorescent antibody studies on *Endotrypanum schaudinni*. Trans. Roy. Soc. Trop. Med. Hyg., 57:232-233.

———— and A. Voller. 1964. The detection of circulating antibody to Kala-Azar by means of immunofluorescent techniques. Trans. Roy. Soc. Trop. Med. Hyg., 58:349-352.

Shuikina, E. E. 1965. Use of indirect fluorescent-antibody technique in studies of cutaneous leishmaniasis. Med. Parazit. (Moskva), 34:576-582.

Simpson, L. 1967. Studies on the kinetoplast of the hemoflagellates. Ph.D. Thesis, New York, Rockefeller University, 201 pp.

———— 1968. The leishmania—leptomonad transformation of *Leishmania donovani*:

Nutritional requirements, respiration changes, and antigenic changes. J. Protozool., 15:201-207.

Southgate, B. A., and B. V. E. Oriedo. 1962. Studies in the epidemiology of East African leishmaniasis. 1. The circumstantial epidemiology of Kala-Azar in the Kitui district of Kenya. Trans. Roy. Soc. Trop. Med. Hyg., 56:30-47.

—— and B. V. E. Oriedo. 1967. Studies in the epidemiology of East African leishmaniasis. 3. Immunity as a determinant of geographical distribution. J. Trop. Med. Hyg., 70:1-4.

—— and P. E. C. Manson-Bahr. 1967a. Studies in the epidemiology of East African leishmaniasis. 4. The significance of the positive leishmanin test. J. Trop. Med. Hyg., 70:29-33.

—— and P. E. C. Manson-Bahr. 1967b. Studies in the epidemiology of East African leishmaniasis. 5. *Leishmania adleri* and natural immunity. J. Trop. Med. Hyg., 70:33-36.

Stauber, L. A. 1953. Some effects of host environment on the course of leishmaniasis in the hamster. Ann. N.Y. Acad. Sci., 56:1064-1069.

—— 1954. Application of electrophoretic techniques in the field of parasitic diseases. Exp. Parasitol., 3:544-568.

—— 1955. Leishmaniasis in the hamster. *In* Some Physiological Aspects and Consequences of Parasitism. Cole, W. H., ed. New Brunswick, N. J., Rutgers University Press, pp. 76-90.

—— 1958. Host resistance to the Khartoum strain of *Leishmania donovani*. Rice Institute Pamphlet No. 45, pp. 80-96.

—— 1963a. Immunity to leishmania. Ann. N.Y. Acad. Sci., 113:409-417.

—— 1963b. Leishmaniasis. Proc. XVI Int. Congr. Zool., 4:198-203.

—— 1963c. Some recent studies in experimental leishmaniasis. Sci. Rep. Ist. Super. Sanita, 2:68-75.

—— S. I. Mauer, and J. H. Leathem. 1952. Leishmaniasis in the hamster: Adrenal cortical hormones and the course of infection. J. Parasit., 38 (4, Sect. 2):11.

—— J. Q. Ochs, and N. H. Coy. 1954. Electrophoretic patterns of the serum proteins of chinchillas and hamsters infected with *Leishmania donovani*. Exp. Parasit., 3:325-335.

—— E. M. Franchino, and J. Grun. 1958. An eight-day method for screening compounds against *Leishmania donovani* in the golden hamster. J. Protozool., 5:269-273.

Strunk, S. W., and E. F. Chaffee. 1967. Differences in the in vivo intracellular destruction of two species of *Leishmania*. Electronmicrographs of leishmaniasis. Fed. Proc., 26:406.

Taliaferro, W. H., 1929. The Immunology of Parasitic Infections. New York, The Century Company.

—— 1962. Remarks on the immunology of leishmaniasis. Sci. Rep. Ist. Super. Sanita, 2:138-142.

—— and L. A. Stauber. 1968. Immunology of parasitic infections. *In* Research in Protozoology, Vol. 3. T. T. Chen, ed. New York, Pergamon Press, pp. 506-564.

Thatcher, V. E., C. Eisenmann, and M. Hertig. 1965a. A natural infection of *Leishmania* in the kinkajou, *Potos flavus*, in Panama. J. Parasit., 51:1022-1023.

—— C. Eisenmann, and M. Hertig. 1965b. Experimental inoculation of Panamanian mammals with *Leishmania brasiliensis*. J. Parasit., 51:842-844.

Torrealba, J. F., and J. W. Torrealba. 1963. Resultados de búsquedas de reservorios extrahumanos domésticos y silvestres de tripanosomiasis y leishmaniasis. Inoculación de animales con *L. donovani*. Recopilación, 7:305-315.

Torrealba, J. W. and J. Chaves-Torrealba. 1964. Empleo de antigeno de B.C.G. en la reacción de fijación del complemento para el diagnóstico de la leishmaniasis visceral. (Nota previa) Rev. Inst. Med. Trop. (São Paulo), 6:252-253.

—— J. F. Torrealba, R. T. Torrealba, M. Zerpa, J. Ramos, and C. E. Henriquez. 1963. Kala-azar canino en el Estado Guarico. Resultados de una encuesta en 1105 perros, empleando la técnica de reacción de fijación del complemento en sangre desecada, retirada con papel de filtro. Quince neuvos casos de kala-azar canino comprobados parasitológicamente. Folia Clin. Biol., 32:1-13.

Trager, W. 1953. The development of *Leishmania donovani in vitro* at 37° C. Effects of the kind of serum. J. Exp. Med., 97:177-188.

Trejos, A., M. A. De Urquilla, and A. R. Paredes. 1965. Influence of environmental temperature on the evolution of experimental Chagas' disease in mice. *In* Progress in Protozoology. Abstracts, 2nd Int. Conf. Protozool., London. International Congress Series No. 91. Amsterdam, Excerpta Medica Foundation, p. 144.

van Peenen, P. F. D., and I. L. Miale. 1962. Leishmaniasis in the Sudan Republic. 5. Serum proteins in Sudanese kala-azar. J. Trop. Med. Hyg., 65:191-195.

—— and D. R. Dietlein. 1963. Leishmaniasis in the Sudan Republic. 14. Leishmania skin testing in upper Nile Province. J. Trop. Med. Hyg., 66:171-174.

—— and T. P. Reid, Jr., 1963. Leishmaniasis in the Sudan Republic. 15. An outbreak of Kala-Azar in the Khor Falus area, Upper Nile Province. J. Trop. Med. Hyg., 66:252-254.

Walton, B. C. 1967. Personal communication.

—— D. A. Person, and R. Bernstein. 1968. Leishmaniasis in the U.S. military in the Canal Zone. Amer. J. Trop. Med. Hyg. 17:19-24.

—— W. H. Brooks, and I. de Arjono. 1970. Indirect fluorescent antibody test for the diagnosis of *Leishmania brasiliensis* infection. (In press).

Williams, J. S., R. E. Duxbury, R. I. Anderson, and E. H. Sadun. 1963. Fluorescent antibody reactions in *Trypanosoma rhodesiense* and *T. gambiense* in experimental animals. J. Parasit., 49:380-384.

Zeledon, R., W. Hidalgo, and H. X. De Hidalgo. 1960. Intradermoreacción de Montenegro con antígeno de *Strigomonas oncopelti*. Nota previa. Rev. Biol. Trop., 8:145-146.

—— W. Hidalgo, and H. X. De Hidalgo. 1961. Consideraciones cuantitatives sobre la intradermo-reacción de Montenegro con antígeno homólogo (*Leishmania*) y antígeno de *Strigomonas oncopelti*. Abstr. II. Congr. Latinoamer. Microbiol., p. 155.

—— E. De Monge, and E. Blanco. 1965. Temperature of the host skin and physiology of the parasite in the experimental infection by *Leishmania braziliensis* Vianna. *In* Progress in Protozoology. Abstracts, 2nd Int. Conf. Protozool., London. International Congress Series No. 91. Amsterdam, Excerpta Medica Foundation, pp. 133-134.

Zuckerman, A. 1962. Some observations on immunity to *Leishmania tropica*. Sci. Rep. Ist. Super. Sanita, 2:95-102.

Zvyagintseva, T. V. 1965. Finding of *Hemiechinus auritus* Gmel. infected with cutaneous leishmaniasis in Syrdarya Region of the Uzbek S.S.R. Med. Parazit. (Moskva), 34:347-349.

Primate Malaria

P. C. C. GARNHAM

Imperial College of Science and Technology, Ascot, England

INTRODUCTION

Malaria parasites are protozoa belonging to the subphylum Sporozoa and the class Coccidiomorpha. Their further classification is shown in Table 1. Details of their life cycle have been known since the end of the last century, and the systematic position of these organisms is now fully established. The use of the term "malaria parasites" has varied considerably, and, at one time, the term was applied to all pigmented or unpigmented species inhabiting for part of their life cycle the erythrocytes of the vertebrate host. Now, the expression is confined to pigmented parasites which undergo schizogony in the blood, while related organisms without this character have been removed to another family (Haemoproteidae). This is a reasonable step, because the

Table 1
Classification of the Haemosporidia

Class: Coccidiomorpha
Subclass: Coccidia
Order: Eucoccida
Family: Plasmodiidae
Genus: *Plasmodium*
Subgenera: *Plasmodium*
Laverania
Vinckeia
etc.

Family: Haemoproteidae
Genera: *Hepatocystis*
Nycteria
Polychromophilus
etc.

former group (i.e., those possessing schizonts in the blood) alone is responsible for "malaria," a disease entity accompanied by periodic fever. Parasites of the latter group produce no such symptoms because they do not multiply in the blood stream, and the primate species, at least, of this group are apparently nonpathogenic.

The true malaria parasites belong to the genus *Plasmodium*, i.e., sporozoan parasites which exhibit two types of schizogony in the vertebrate host—one (pigmented) in the erythrocytes and another in the tissues—and which undergo sporogony in the mosquito.

Until the discovery in 1947 and succeeding years of the tissue stages of the mammalian parasites, *Plasmodium kochi*, the common parasite of the lower primates, was included in the malaria parasites, but the demonstration of its peculiar exoerythrocytic cycle and the absence of erythrocytic schizogony led to its reclassification as a member of the Haemoproteidae under the name of *Hepatocystis kochi*. Six or more species of this genus occur in the Old World, but so far none have been found in the Americas. The immune response to these infections has been little studied, but it is apparently very different from that of the true malaria parasite and the problem is omitted from consideration here.

The supralemuroid primate malaria parasites belong to two subgenera of the genus *Plasmodium*—*Plasmodium (Plasmodium)* and *Plasmodium (Laverania)*. The third subgenus, *Plasmodium (Vinckeia)*, is found in lemurs and nonprimate mammals (Garnham, 1964). Only two species of Plasmodium (*P. girardi* and *P. lemuris*) are known to occur in lemurs, and observations of these have been too few to have any bearing on the subject of immunity, except for the finding, constant in all forms of mammalian malaria, that splenectomy produces an immediate fall in immunity, with the production of a relapse (Bück et al., 1952).

This chapter is thus devoted to primate parasites belonging to the subgenera *Plasmodium* and *Laverania*. The former contains parasites which undergo schizogony of two types, one in red blood cells and the other in parenchymatous cells of the liver with the production of more than a thousand merozoites in *successive* generations of exoerythrocytic schizonts, and which undergo gametogony with *round* gametocytes. The subgenus *Laverania* is defined as containing parasites which undergo schizogony of two types, one in red blood cells and the other in parenchymatous cells of the liver, with the production of many more than a thousand merozoites in a *single* generation of exoerythrocytic schizonts, and which undergo gametogony with *crescentic* gametocytes.

Excluding the lemurs, the primates consist of the Old World and New World monkeys, the lower and higher apes, and man. With the exception of the human malaria parasites, the primate parasites have a restricted geographic distribution, which is often much less than the range of the host itself. Thus, *Plasmodium simium* of lower monkeys is limited to a small area in southern Brazil, *P. gonderi* of mangabeys and drills only occurs in a few places in West Africa, and the parasites of chimpanzees are largely confined to the West African coastal forests. The hosts themselves, on the other hand, are present throughout almost all of the respective continents. Sometimes, however, the parasite accompanies the host nearly everywhere, such as *P. inui* in *Macaca irus* in the Orient.

Such geographic considerations have an important bearing on the specific status of a parasite in a particular host. There has been a general tendency to regard many parasites as strictly host-specific in nature; in other words, the abnormal host possesses a greater or lesser degree of natural immunity to a parasite not its own. In particular, it was thought that malaria parasites were unlikely to jump from one category of primates to another. The species infecting Old World monkeys were thought to infect with difficulty those of the New World. Neither of them infect the apes, and the ape parasites were considered to be largely nontransmissible to man. It appeared that natural immunity barred their passage, though sometimes this resistance could be overcome by removal of the spleen. Today, though, experimental work on a large scale has shown that there are many exceptions to the above concepts. Man is easily infected with many simian species and marmosets with human species, and the exoerythrocytic stages of the parasites often possess a host range much wider than the original, though the erythrocytic stages may remain strictly host specific.

The cradle of primate malaria appears to be the East Indies, and in this region, the largest number of species and the greatest range of hosts are to be found. In the jungle, teeming with potential mosquito vectors, the environment is entirely favorable to multiplication of the organisms and to their speciation. Thus, many kinds of monkeys act as hosts of *P. cynomolgi* or *P. inui*, and, because of the varying response of these different hosts to the parasite, the latter reacts in time by minor changes, at first below a taxonomic level, but later reaching subspecific and eventually specific order. And in these combinations, varying degrees of natural immunity will be met. An analo-

Table 2
Plasmodium spp. of Monkeys

Species	Natural Host	Distribution
P. knowlesi	Macaca irus, M. nemestrina, Presbytis melalophos, (Man)	Malaya, East Indies, Taiwan and Philippines
P. coatneyi	M. irus	Malaya
P. fragile	M. sinica, M. radiata	Ceylon, India
P. cynomolgi cynomolgi	M. irus, M. nemestrina, Presbytis spp.	Philippines, East Indies, Pakistan
P. c. bastianellii	M. irus	Malaya
P. c. cyclopis	M. cyclopis	Taiwan
P. c. ceylonensis	M. sinica	Ceylon and India
P. simium	Alouatta fusca, (Man)	S. Brazil
P. fieldi	M. nemestrina, M. irus	Malaya
P. simiovale	M. sinica	Ceylon
P. gonderi	Cercocebus spp., Mandrillus leucophaeus	West Africa
P. inui	M. irus, M. nemestrina, M. assamensis, M. cyclopis, Presbytis spp., Cynopithecus niger	East Indies, Taiwan, Indochina, and Philippines
P. shortti	M. radiata, M. sinica	India, Ceylon
P. brasilianum	Cacajao, Alouatta spp., Ateles spp., Cebus spp., Saimiri spp., Lagothrix spp.	South and Central America

gous picture undoubtedly exists among the anopheline hosts, which exhibit various degrees of natural resistance and susceptibility. A proper understanding of natural immunity in primate malaria necessitates a full analysis of the whole biocenose.

Tables 2 and 3 give lists of the malaria parasites of monkeys and of the hominoids, respectively, together with their natural host range and geographic distribution.

During the course of evolution of the three components—primate, *Anopheles*, and *Plasmodium*—presence or absence of immunity must have played a large part in hindering or facilitating the establishment of new combinations. The writer (Garnham, 1963) attempted to illustrate some of them in evolutionary trees and diagrams; it might be thought that the feeble susceptibility of man (at the top of the tree) to many parasites of monkeys (at the bottom) indicated a gradual acquisition of immunity, but, unfortunately, the intervening primates appear to be less, and not more, susceptible than man. However, in studying the ontogeny of the parasite, the principle seems to emerge that in general, the more primitive stages of its life cycle are able to persist in hosts up (or down) the scale. Thus, the human *P. vivax* grows perfectly as an exoerythrocytic schizont in the liver of a chimpanzee, though the latter animal is largely immune to the blood stages (Rodhain, 1956; Bray, 1957b) *P. cynomolgi* of the Old World macaques is unable to infect the

Table 3
Plasmodium spp. in Hominoids

Species	Natural Host	Distribution
P. vivax	Man	Cosmopolitan
P. schwetzi	Chimpanzee, Gorilla	West and Central Africa
P. ovale	Man	Cosmopolitan
P. pitheci	Orangutan	East Indies
P. youngi	Hylobates lar	Malaya
P. eylesi	Hylobates lar	Malaya
P. jefferyi	Hylobates lar	Malaya
P. hylobati	Hylobates moloch, H. concolor	East Indies, Indochina
P. falciparum	Man	Cosmopolitan
P. reichenowi	Chimpanzee, Gorilla	West and Central Africa
P. malariae	Man, Chimpanzee	Cosmopolitan

erythrocytes of *Cebus* monkeys, but readily invades the parenchyme of their livers (Garnham and Bray, 1956). The sporozoites of several species of *Plasmodium* of Oriental macaques have been shown by Beye et al. (1961) to infect man easily, though man exhibits a considerable degree of immunity to the later blood stages, of which he quickly and spontaneously becomes cured. Curiously enough, this immunity does not extend to the toxic effects of the parasite because the signs and symptoms of the disease may be severe in the zoonotic infection.

It would be unwise to generalize too much from the above experiments since the reverse process does not necessarily occur: rhesus monkeys appear to be totally immune to all stages of *P. vivax* (Garnham and Bray, 1956). Perhaps the more highly evolved host (man) still retains a phylogenetic susceptibility to the ancestral species (from monkeys), but Old World monkeys, never having experienced human infections in their phylogeny, are totally immune to the more highly evolved parasites.

Natural immunity against and susceptibility of different species of *Anopheles* to the various malaria parasites appear to follow different laws. Parasites with a cosmopolitan distribution, such as those species infecting man, have been brought into contact in the course of time with different species of *Anopheles* and have overcome immune barriers in many of them. Malaria parasites of a limited range, like *P. reichenowi* and *P. schwetzi* of chimpanzees, *P. simium* of howler monkeys, or *P. fieldi, P. coatneyi*, and other species occurring in Malayan macaques and gibbons, infect with difficulty, or not at all, the usual laboratory-bred species of *Anopheles*; they are restricted to their own special sylvatic partners.

The immune mechanism is entirely different in the invertebrate host. Acquired immunity to malaria parasites has been shown to be absent in the mosquito (Garnham, 1955). Innate immunity, on the other hand, affects the sporogonic process in various ways. The mosquito may be nearly completely immune, only allowing fertilization of the macrogamete and formation of the ookinete to take place in the lumen of the midgut; development then ceases and the ookinetes are excreted, or the ookinete may manage to penetrate the epithelium and start to grow as an oocyst, only to become arrested a few days later and converted into Ross's black spores. Lastly, the immune mechanism may not become manifest until the mature oocyst ruptures and the sporozoites come into contact with the lethal hemocoelomic fluid, in which either they are immediately destroyed or a few manage to reach the salivary glands, where they remain, for a day or less, probably in nonviable form.

The subject of immunity to protozoa in invertebrates has been greatly neglected, yet it is of fundamental importance and presents a challenge to the parasitologists and immunologists, who might read with advantage the monographs of Steinhaus (1963) and of Weiser (1966) as a relaxation from their studies of the globulins of the vertebrate host.

NATURAL IMMUNITY

Natural immunity in primate malaria is influenced by many circumstances, which vary from genetic factors to extraneous conditions of all sorts, but probably the most important single factor affecting the vertebrate host is the spleen. The roles of this organ and of some other major factors are considered below.

The influence of the spleen

Natural immunity against closely related species of primate malaria, which are not normal parasites of the host, depends on an intact and well-functioning lymphoid-macrophage system, and particularly, on the spleen. If splenectomy is performed, either for the treatment of some disorder in man or experimentally in other primates, the animal loses its immunity and develops a severe infection on inoculation with the abnormal malaria parasite. Chimpanzees react in this way to *P. vivax*, *P. falciparum*, or *P. ovale* (Hoare 1965), human species to which the ape is otherwise largely insusceptible. Splenectomized marmosets (*Saguinus geoffroyi*) are fully susceptible to *P. vivax*, developing high parasitemias, accompanied by gametocytes which were shown by Porter and Young (1966) to be capable of infecting mosquitoes.

Immunity probably has been completely abolished in the foregoing instances, since one of the most sensitive indexes of the presence of immunity in the host is the viability of gametocytes, i.e., their infectivity to mosquitoes. In normal infections in a susceptible primate, the gametocytes are viable up to the time of the immune crisis, when, although remaining in large numbers in the circulation, they rapidly lose their power to infect *Anopheles*. Later in the disease, when immunity is not so high, the gametocytes may regain their infectivity. Hawking et al. (1966) noted that the infectivity to mosquitoes of a langur strain of *P. cynomolgi* rose from the sixth day to a maximum on the ninth day; then on the tenth day when the crisis occurred, infectivity sank to zero, only to rise to a smaller peak later in the infection, perhaps because of some antigenic variation in the parasite to which immunity had not yet been acquired.

Removal of the spleen invariably activates latent infection of primate malaria, but extirpation of this organ does not necessarily render one species of animal susceptible to the parasites of another. It might be thought that a close phylogenetic connection between the animals would facilitate the widening of susceptibility after splenectomy, but this can scarcely be the case when one considers the ability of the human plasmodium, *P. vivax*, to infect the quasi-lemuroid marmoset and its inability to infect even the liver of the splenectomized rhesus monkey. No reasonable explanation for these anomalies is forthcoming, and much further experimental work is needed to indicate the exact and special role of the spleen in maintaining natural immunity. This was the problem to which Laveran (1893) drew attention seventy years ago, and Fabiani (1966) has indicated the complexity of the problem today, mentioning that the liver is even more active than the spleen in defense, but that the latter organ is better placed anatomically in the circulatory system to effect phagocytosis.

Genetic factors

In the continual battle between a pathogenic parasite and its host, both elements attempt to react in a manner favorable to themselves. The parasite may try to mutate into strains against which the immunity mechanism of the host is unadapted, and the host attempts by natural selection to preserve members which are less susceptible to the infection.

Speciation of the parasite may be a response to an unfavorable environment in the host and has been discussed above in relation to phylogeny. In individual infections, the parasite may try to evade destruction by "antigenic variation." This process has been investigated by Brown and Brown (1966) in *P. knowlesi* infections in rhesus monkeys. Since the phenomenon throws light on the possible genetics of malaria infections, it is discussed here rather than under acquired immunity. Monkeys suffering from *P. knowlesi* malaria and treated with small doses of mepacrine quickly acquire an immunity to the initial parasitaemia; then either a parasite mutation occurs or resistant parasites survive to which the monkeys are not immune and a relapse ensues. Such antigenic variants continue to be produced, against which relapse-specific agglutinins are formed.

The apparent natural selection of resistant or less susceptible members of the primate host has only been studied in human malaria, and here only in observations on the contrast between the reaction of the Caucasian and African populations to malignant tertian malaria. During the last century and until recent years, the difference in the response of these two races to *P. falciparum* was marked. It was well recognized that the West Africans, for instance, showed few or no signs of disease, while the Europeans, in the same locality, were decimated by malaria. Weatherall (1965) gives a vivid account of what happened to the Europeans who were involved in opening up Central Africa during the nineteenth century. Of the Mungo Park expedition in 1803, 35 out of 44 Europeans died of malaria; the naval exploration of the Congo in 1816 lost 18 out of 44 Europeans through the disease; and another expedition to the Niger in 1841 suffered 42 fatal casualties out of a force of 145. The Africans, on the other hand, were largely unaffected, presumably because of natural selection after countless centuries of exposure to the infection. The contrast in the susceptibility of the two races is less obvious today than in the past because, first, the European now lives under the umbrella of antimalarial protection in one form or another and need never contract the disease, and, second, the African is also influenced by the new weapons in use against the infection so that he is both losing his immunity by less frequent exposure and enhancing it by carefully adjusted drug administration, while preserving at the same time his partial racial tolerance. Probably, the Caucasian now suffers less from the disease, and the African more.

Variations of a genetic origin in natural immunity are also seen in the invertebrate host of primate malaria. The phenomenon was first investigated by Clay Huff (1922) in his classic experiments on *Culex pipiens* and *P. cathemerium*, in which he was able to breed by selection, naturally resistant and naturally susceptible populations of the mosquito. The character was found to be recessive and was accompanied by such a loss of vigor that the special colonies finally died out. A similar picture has often been observed in primate malaria parasites in which the less suitable anopheline hosts may show, under experimental conditions, infection rates of 30 percent or less, 70 percent or more of the group proving resistant to the parasite.

The writer has recently been faced with the problem of natural immunity to *P. cynomolgi*, which suddenly arose in a long-established colony of *A. labranchiae atroparvus* of English origin (from the Essex marshes). The results were so striking that a new colony of the same species of mosquito was set up from eggs of a Rumanian origin (from the outskirts of Bucharest), and the infection rates in the two colonies were compared after simultaneous feeds on the donor monkey. Table 4 gives the results of several such experiments. There was never a complete natural immunity in the English colony and when attempts were made to breed mosquitoes from eggs selected from mosquitoes which had failed to become infected, no increase in the proportion of resistant specimens was obtained. Such experiments are tedious and long, and it is too soon to come to any final conclusion. Moreover, it is important to bear in mind that other factors in addition to a sudden mutation may lead to an apparent development of natural immunity. The writer (1956), for instance, noted that the presence of an infection of the microsporidian *Plistophora culicis* in his colonies of *A. labranchiae atroparvus* seriously impeded the progress of sporogony of the malaria parasite, and such

Table 4

Susceptibility of Strains of *A. labranchiae atroparvus* to *P. cynomolgi*

Monkey No.	Percent Infected		Number of Oocysts (in infected guts)		Infectivity of Sporozoites	
	Normal†	Abnormal†	Normal†	Abnormal†	Normal†	Abnormal†
276*	100	66	110	60	+	+
314	79	16	not counted		not tested	
318*	100	0	not counted		not tested	
374	73	64	51	14	+	−
375	45	23	5	2	+	−
385	40	45	8	5	+	+
387	74	66	not counted		+	+
405	44	30	15	5	not tested	
455	96	83	100	33	not tested	

* *P. cynomolgi ceylonensis*; others *P. c. bastianellii*.
† The "normal strain" was either the Horton or the Bucharest strain; the "abnormal strain" was the strain which is probably losing its susceptibility at the London School of Hygiene and Tropical Medicine.

resistance to infection due to the presence of a microsporidian has been noted by various workers since that time. Viruses, rickettsiae, and other agents may also exert a similar effect. Bertram et al. (1964) reported a detrimental action of Semliki Forest virus on *P. gallinaceum* in *Aedes aegypti*.

A genetic factor of considerable interest is the insusceptibility of the West African Negro to both *P. vivax* and *P. cynomolgi*. The Bantu has no natural immunity, but the pure Negro inhabitants of the country between Senegal and the Cameroons are almost totally insusceptible to these parasites. Even after centuries of residence in the U.S.A., natural immunity in the Negro persists, as was demonstrated by Young et al. (1955), but admixture of Caucasian blood results in less complete resistance and 23 percent of so-called Negroes can now become infected. The phenomenon is so well-known that *P. vivax* is never used for malaria therapy in Negroes suffering from cerebral syphilis, and this species is replaced by *P. falciparum* or *P. ovale*. It is significant that the Negro has also been shown by Beye et al. (1961) to be naturally immune to *P. cynomolgi bastianellii*, although the Negro is as susceptible as any other race to other species of simian malaria parasites. This result provides further confirmation of the close relationship between *P. vivax* and *P. cynomolgi*. Neither special types of hemoglobin nor other blood abnormalities appear to play any part in the natural immunity of West African Negroes to *P. vivax*, and the phenomenon remains just as much of a mystery today as in 1949 when Brumpt first drew attention to it.

In recent years, various genetic traits have been shown to confer a degree of natural immunity to *P. falciparum* in the otherwise unfortunate possessors of the abnormalities. The best known example is the replacement of normal hemoglobin by sickle-cell hemoglobin, and this appears to inhibit the multiplication of *P. falciparum*. The homozygote is severely affected by the condition and dies young, but the heterozygote suffers less and is more resistant to the parasite than the normal individual and survives better in a population exposed to hyperendemic malaria. Such populations thus contain a high proportion of people with the sickle-cell trait, and Allison (1963) has pointed out the coincidence of the two conditions in the tropical and subtropical parts of the world. Other genetic abnormalities, including glucose-6-phosphate enzymopenia, hemoglobin C, and thalassemia, are also thought to confer a degree of natural immunity against infections of *P. falciparum*, though the evidence is less convincing than in the case of sickle-cell anemia.

Other factors concerned in natural immunity

In any study of immunity, the role of the age of the host must be taken into consideration, and although this factor is probably less significant in primate than in rodent or avian malaria, it has still to be reckoned with in experimental work. As a rule, the younger the animal, the less is the degree of natural immunity, but, strangely enough, some infections, such as those due to *P. falciparum* or *P. knowlesi*, prove to be as fatal to the adult as to the infant. However, in other primate malaria species, the parasitemia reaches a higher level in younger than in older animals. In regard to the invertebrate host, it appears that the young mosquito is rather more susceptible than the aged, in which infection rates tend to be lower.

Maegraith et al. (1952) disclosed an unusual and almost absolute degree of natural immunity to malaria if animals were placed on a strict milk diet, and rodents were thereby shown to be practically immune to *P. berghei*. Bray and Garnham (1953) extended the experiments to monkeys and demonstrated that the rhesus on a milk diet is immune to the blood stages of *P. cynomolgi*, though susceptible to the exoerythrocytic stages. Later Colbourne (1956) investigated the effect of a milk diet on human malaria and obtained conflicting results; the observations were made in West Africa, where it was impossible to ensure that the children did not receive any food other than milk. Kretschmar (1966), however, showed that the parasitemia of Nigerian infants remained unusually low as long as they were kept on a pure milk diet. The malaria parasite is essentially dependent upon *p*-aminobenzoic acid. This substance is absent in milk, and Hawking (1953) showed that if it was added to the diet, the animal immediately lost its immunity and a normal infection arose. The effect of the deprivation of metabolites on human malaria is also seen in famine-stricken populations. The parasite, as well as the host, becomes undernourished; there is interference with growth of the organism, and the people suffer much less than usual from the disease. Competition for metabolites by other infective agents may also render an animal largely immune to the malaria parasite, the latter usually coming off worse.

Totally extraneous factors may be responsible for the apparent immunity of certain groups of the population. Muirhead-Thomson (1951, 1954) suggested that one cause of the immunity of African infants in a hyperendemic locality is their much-diminished exposure to mosquito bites; not only is there a much smaller area of skin for the mosquito to feed upon, but the infant is swaddled with clothes and may even smell less attractively to the mosquito than older individuals. MacDonald (1957) points out that the parasite rate in infants in tropical Africa is unexpectedly low in comparison with the estimated number of infective bites. This immunity is due to many causes, including the above, and probably also to natural racial immunity, the presence of protective traits like hemoglobin S, a milk diet, and passive immunity inherited from the immune mother.

ACQUIRED IMMUNITY

Some of the earliest conceptions of immunity to infections in general were derived from studies on primate malaria. The "salting" of old residents in the tropics was well-recognized, and Metchnikov, Koch, and others were aware of the great significance of this disease in their studies on immunity. The phenomena were quickly classified into two principal categories, active and passive immunity, and the former was shown to be based on the cellular reaction of the vertebrate host and the production of antibodies.

Passive immunity is of minor importance in malaria, though it may play a part in protecting children from the more severe effects of the disease. Antibodies pass across the placenta to the fetal circulation, while small amounts may be secreted in the milk, but the latter route is less important in primate than in rodent malaria (Bruce-Chwatt, 1963). Experimentally, it has been shown that the administration in sufficient quantity of immune gamma-globulin has a marked antiparasitic effect, and this action is discussed below under humoral immunity.

The lymphoid-macrophage system occupies a central place in acquired immunity. The various mobile cells responsible for phagocytosis are developed from it, while another line (probably chiefly via plasma cells or plasmatoid lymphocytes) is concerned with the production of the antibodies. The other important source of phagocytic activity arises from the specialized endothelial cells lining the sinusoids of the liver, the sinuses of the spleen, the alveoli of the lungs, and the blood spaces in the bone marrow.

The acquisition of immunity to primate malaria takes about a week to ten days and varies according to the species of parasite. Sergent's (1963) complicated hypothesis of the immune reaction in this disease is largely based on observations on avian and later on rodent malaria, but it is also applicable to infections in primates. Primate reactions fall into three principal categories, as follows:

1. *Little immunity and a rapidly fatal outcome.* This is the picture seen *par excellence* in infections of *P. knowlesi* in rhesus monkeys, and to a lesser extent in malaria due to *P. coatneyi* and *P. fragile. P. knowlesi* has a quotidian cycle of erythrocytic schizogony, and within a few days after infection,

the parasitemia has reached such a height and toxic manifestations have become so severe that the animal dies before the protective mechanism can take effect in this abnormal host. In the natural host, *M. irus*, the reaction is less severe, presumably because of the existence of some racial tolerance, and premunition (*see* below) is acquired. *P. coatneyi* and *P. fragile* are related to *P. knowlesi* but have a tertian periodicity. Their multiplication rate in the blood stream is therefore less rapid, and a few rhesus monkeys manage to acquire enough immunity to survive.

2. *True immunity and complete cure.* The clearest picture of this condition is seen under experimental conditions when an animal is infected with an abnormal parasite. Thus, if man is inoculated with *P. cynomolgi bastianellii* or another similar parasite, he suffers from a short infection which disappears spontaneously, and this is followed by a sterile residual immunity. Deschiens and Benex (1965) discuss such parasitic engagements, or "*impasses,*" and point out the benign or abortive nature of the process. The same response occurs both after blood- and sporozoite-induced infections. Under natural conditions in a fully susceptible host, the course of the infection is largely determined by the persistence or disappearance of secondary exoerythrocytic schizonts in the liver, together with the actual duration of the residual immunity, which is rarely permanent. This problem is related to the theory of relapses and is discussed separately below.

P. vivax and *P. ovale* in man react in much the same way immunologically, though there are many strains of the former and only a few of the latter. The primary attack of each is followed by a "sterile" immunity of short duration at the end of which a relapse occurs. This succession of events continues for several years until the liver cycle dies out, and the infection disappears.

3. *Premunition and chronicity of infections.* This response is frequently seen in primate malaria, and it has been analyzed in great detail by Sergent (1963) in avian malaria. *P. inui* infections in Oriental macaques offer excellent material for studying the phenomenon. The primary infection is relatively mild. Parasitemia reaches a low peak when premunition ensues. The lymphoid-macrophage system becomes sensitized and hyperplastic. It remains permanently in this condition so that the majority of, but not all, the parasites are destroyed. According to Sergent, all newcomers of the same strain will be immediately killed. If the infection is sterilized by administering a suitable drug, the animal at once loses its premunition and becomes susceptible. Premunition of this type is seen both in experimental infections of rhesus monkeys and in the natural host. *P. shortti*, *P. knowlesi*, *P. fragile*, and *P. simiovale* provoke premunition in Asian macaques, and *P. schwetzi* and *P. reichenowi*, in chimpanzees. Premunition may be so effective that parasites become almost undetectable in blood films, but splenectomy will cause a temporary breakdown in immunity, and a succession of unsuspected parasites of various species may, after such an operation, be revealed. Dissanaike (1965) detected latent infections of *P. cynomolgi ceylonensis*, *P. fragile*, *P. simiovale*, and *P. shorttii* in single specimens of *M. sinica* after removal of the spleen.

All the above species continue to flourish in the host for years, with minor exacerbations from time to time. The human parasite, *P. falciparum*, behaves rather differently; true relapses do not arise in infections with this species due to the apparent absence of secondary exoerythrocytic schizogony. Recrudescences of the blood infection occur for one or two years (or possibly more), during which time the person is in a state of premunition that terminates when the last parasite disappears.

The relapse phenomenon in primate malaria is closely concerned with immunity, and at least four theories have been advanced (Garnham, 1966b) to account for this highly characteristic feature of the disease. Two of the theories depend upon the assumption that relapses originate from erythrocytic forms of the parasite, and the other two are based on their supposed origin from an exoerythrocytic source. It is necessary to discuss these briefly in particular reference to immunity:

1. *Blood origin of relapses*. This was the old theory of Marchiafava and Bignami (1894) and has been revived today by Corradetti (1965). It simply assumes that parasites persist in small numbers in the circulation or in the deep vascular spaces in the intervals between attacks and that when immunity declines (as demonstrable today by various serologic reactions), the parasites multiply and a relapse occurs (upper half of Fig. 1). Brown and Brown (1966) suggested an interesting modification of this theory by assuming that among the few parasites persisting after the primary attack, mutants or variants developed which gave rise to the subsequent relapses (*see* p. 773 and lower half of Fig. 1).

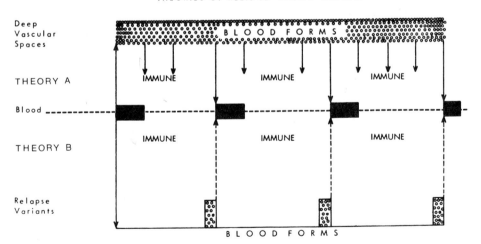

FIG. 1. Solid black represents multiplying parasites in peripheral blood (primary attack and three relapses), which meet the immune barrier at intervals (shown by arrows). In Theory A, parasites continue to multiply in deep vascular spaces and relapse in peripheral blood on decline of immunity. In Theory B, parasites respond by survival of variants (three are shown) which, on multiplication, provoke the relapses in peripheral blood when immunity declines.

2. *Exoerythrocytic origin of relapses.* Shortt and Garnham (1948a) described exoerythrocytic schizonts of *P. cynomolgi* in the liver of monkeys at the time of relapse (between 102 and 105 days after sporozoite-induced infections), and suggested that during the interval, a tissue cycle progressed in the liver, which was entirely unaffected by the immunity that developed against the blood stages of the parasite. Showers of merozoites were thought to be thrown into the circulation every eight days (on the rupture of the exoerythrocytic schizonts), only to meet with immediate destruction by means of the immune mechanism. Then, when the latter effect declined, the merozoites were able to multiply unhindered in the blood and a relapse occurred (upper half of Fig. 2). Unfortunately, further consideration shows that there are certain difficulties in accepting this explanation *in toto.* For example, the existence of strains of *P. vivax* with incubation periods delayed for 8 months or more, with no parasitemia (and no positive serologic reactions) in the interim, is almost impossible to explain by this theory, particularly since the patient is well known to be fully susceptible to *blood* forms of the homologous species if these are inoculated at any time throughout the delayed incubation period. In other words, immunity cannot be the explanation of the phenomenon, but instead it is thought to be due to the survival of dormant sporozoites or their immediate successors in the liver. Then, at an unknown biologic signal, the delayed primary attack occurs. This theory also offers a plausible explanation of successive relapses, as shown in the lower half of Figure 2.

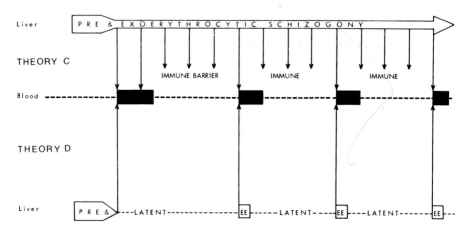

FIG. 2. Solid black represents multiplying parasites in peripheral blood (primary attack and three relapses), which meet the immune barrier at intervals as shown by arrows. In Theory C, parasites continue to multiply by exoerythrocytic schizogony in the liver and provoke relapses (three are shown) in peripheral blood on decline of immunity. In Theory D, exoerythrocytic parasites remain latent in the liver until an unknown stimulus reactivates them and causes a relapse (three are shown).

Physical basis of acquired immunity

The importance of cellular immunity or phagocytosis in primate malaria cannot be overemphasized. It constitutes a problem in histology, of which only the superficial aspects have really been studied. Yet nobody who has observed the tremendous activity of the lymphoid-macrophage system, as seen in the spleen and other organs of monkeys infected with *P. brasilianum*, *P. cynomolgi*, or *P. knowlesi* (Taliaferro and Mulligan, 1937), in the liver of young children dying of *P. falciparum* malaria, or in the placentas of infected African women (Fig. 3), could fail to appreciate the essential role of phagocytosis in this disease. Modern malaria research has practically neglected this subject with respect to the primate malaria species, although techniques are now available for the study of the sensitization and hyperplasia of lymphoid-macrophage cells under the influence of *Plasmodium* spp. *in vitro* and of the functional activity of the cells *in vivo*. On the other hand, humoral immunity in primate malaria has received much attention in recent years with regard to the isolation and immunologic properties of the antibodies, the nature of the antigens responsible for their production, and new serologic reactions. This work has been done largely for the practical objective of finding a protective vaccine for use in human malaria in holoendemic localities.

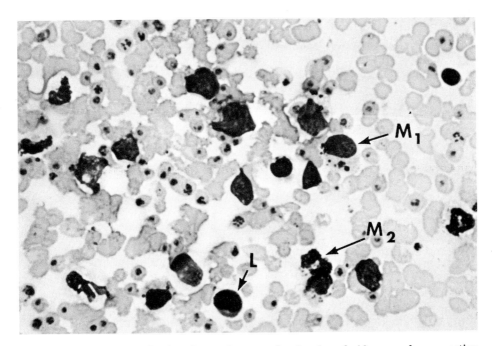

FIG. 3. Photomicrograph of a placental smear showing lymphoid-macrophage reaction to infection of *P. falciparum*. Many erythrocytes contain developing parasites. M₁—Macrophage with pigment; M₂—Macrophage with parasites; L—Lymphocyte.

Modern work on humoral immunity in primate malaria chiefly stems from the experiments of Cohen and McGregor (1963) in The Gambia. They isolated immunoglobulin (IgG) from the sera of the adult inhabitants who were highly immune to the local strains of *P. falciparum, P. malariae*, and *P. ovale*. The substance was then administered in large doses (1.2 to 2.5 g of gamma-globulin) to local infants suffering from acute and heavy infections of *P. falciparum* malaria, and within 9 days the parasitemia had disappeared, though parasites usually returned in 12 weeks. These experiments pinpointed the precise nature of the antiparasitic substance. Much earlier, Coggeshall and Kumm (1937) had shown that the crude serum from monkeys recovered from infections of *P. knowlesi* had both protective and curative properties.

The Gambian investigations were extended and confirmed. Moreover, McGregor and Carrington (1963) demonstrated that the West African immunoglobulin was nearly as effective in abolishing parasitemia in East African children as it was in the local population from which the serum had been derived. This unexpected result indicated either that there is not such a great heterogeneity of strains of *P. falciparum* as is generally thought, or that the large doses contained sufficient general antiparasitic substance to effect a cure.

In a continuation of this work, McGregor et al. (1966) showed that schizonts of *P. falciparum*, derived from highly infected placentas, contained an antigen which reacted strongly in gel-diffusion tests with the homologous IgG. The subject of antigenic analysis is discussed further on pp. 786-788.

The application of immunoelectrophoretic techniques to immune serum in primate malaria has revealed the existence of several immunoglobulins in addition to IgG. Little is known about the functional activity of the different elements, and the subject as a whole is in a state of flux. Neither the precise chemical composition nor the origin of the actively antiparasitic immunoglobulin is known, and probably the large-scale manufacture of an antimalarial vaccine must await the solution of these problems.

Stages of the parasite affected by acquired immunity

Acquired immunity in primate malaria is largely directed against the asexual parasites in the blood. The actual stage of schizogony most susceptible to the influence of immunity is probably the naked merozoite (the product of the ruptured schizont) before a new erythrocyte is invaded. At least, this is the stage which is in closest contact with humoral antibodies. On the other hand, the infected corpuscle acts as a target for phagocytic activity, and phagocytes, containing all stages of the parasite from rings to schizonts, are often seen.

Gametocytes in human malaria, and particularly the crescents of *P. falciparum*, circulate apparently unharmed and are affected only indirectly by immunity, i.e., by the destruction of their precursors in the blood. In some simian infections, as mentioned above (p. 772), the onset of immunity produces a rapid loss of viability of the gametocytes, although the numbers are unaffected.

Immunity is well-known to be without influence on the exoerythrocytic stages of the malaria parasites of man, chimpanzee, and monkeys. Shortt and Garnham (1948b) showed that a man who was immune to the blood stages of the Madagascar strain of *P. vivax* developed plentiful exoerythrocytic schizonts in his liver. Garnham and Bray (1956) carried out a quantitative experiment on two groups of rhesus monkeys, one immune and the other susceptible to *P. cynomolgi*, and found that approximately the same number of exoerythrocytic schizonts developed in each category after the inoculation of equal numbers of sporozoites; if anything, the immune monkeys had a larger number of the tissue forms. Lupascu et al. (1967) demonstrated that a chimpanzee in a state of premunition to a Rumanian strain of *P. malariae* developed a heavy infection in the liver of exoerythrocytic schizonts after the intravenous injection of large numbers of sporozoites of the homologous strain.

When the exoerythrocytic schizont ruptures, the area is at once invaded by large numbers of phagocytes: first, polymorphonuclear leukocytes, then lymphoid-macrophage cells, and finally fibroblasts appear, and the focus, which may be 250µ or more in extent (Fig. 4), disappears within a few days. Until the rupture takes place, the exoerythrocytic schizont is unaffected by immunity, however active it may be. Very rarely the relapse bodies

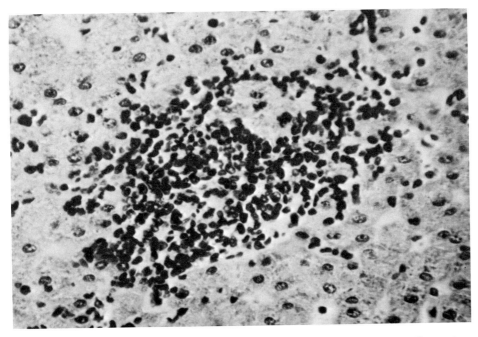

FIG. 4. Photomicrograph of a section of liver showing cellular response to the rupture of a *P. malariae* exoerythrocytic schizont.

(secondary exoerythrocytic schizonts) of *P. cynomolgi* may be seen surrounded by a zone of reaction up to 50μ in width and consisting largely of lymphocytes and plasma cells. One such schizont (45 by 30μ) appeared to be practically unaffected by the cellular activity around it: it possessed the usual convoluted outer membrane characteristic of the relapse form and caused by fissures in the cytoplasm (Fig. 5), and it showed, in addition, a curious retreat of the nuclei from the surface of the schizont, leaving a bare area of cytoplasm on the outside. Another schizont in the same material exhibited extremely elongated and attenuated nuclei; these were 4μ in length and resembled tubercle bacilli (Fig. 6). Such an appearance in exoerythrocytic schizonts has never been seen before, and possibly represents a phenomenon associated more with latency than with acquired immunity.

The sporogonic stages do not give rise to acquired immunity in the anopheline host, though the mosquitoes are affected in various ways by natural immunity.

In summary, it may be stated that acquired immunity acts on the asexual stages in the blood, but has no influence on the exoerythrocytic cycle in the liver of the primate or on the sporogonic stage in the mosquito, whereas natural immunity may affect all stages except the zygote and the exoerythrocytic. Immunity is most effective when the parasite is in contact with the body fluids, e.g., at the time when the sporozoites invade the hemocoelomic cavity of the mosquito or the merozoites escape into the plasma of the primate (Garnham, 1966).

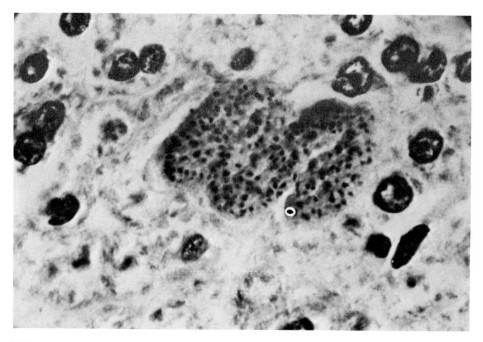

FIG. 5. Photomicrograph of section of liver showing a "relapse schizont" of *P. cynomolgi.*

TESTS FOR THE PRESENCE OF IMMUNITY

The presence or absence of immunity may most simply be observed by challenging the animal with parasites of the homologous strain. If the recipient develops an infection, then immunity is lacking; if there is no infection, the animal is clearly immune. The writer (Garnham, 1963) has pointed out that in nature, the results of such challenges may be measured in human populations by estimating the parasite rates at different ages when typical curves of incidence are obtained. Deliberate inoculation of parasites into the immune animal can be carried out, and cross-immunity of different strains or species thus ascertained.

The primate parasites tend to fall into two principal groups according to their response to challenge. The first group, of which *P. vivax* and *P. cynomolgi* may be taken as examples, exhibit a strictly homologous immunity. A man who has recovered from the Madagascar strain of *P. vivax* is immune to the homologous strain on reinoculation (Shortt and Garnham, 1948b), and a similar reaction is seen with various American strains of this species (Taliaferro, 1949). But if the challenge is made with a heterologous strain, no cross-immunity occurs and a man immune to the Chesson strain of *P. vivax* is found to be susceptible to the St. Elizabeth; there is also no cross-

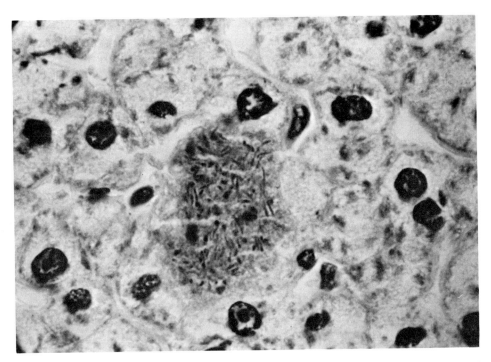

FIG. 6.   Photomicrograph of section of liver showing a relapse schizont of *P. cynomolgi* with bacilliform nuclei.

immunity between the Madagascar and Cameroons strains (Shute, 1946). Similarly, different strains or subspecies of *P. cynomolgi* confer no protection on monkeys infected with the heterologous parasite, as was clearly demonstrated in the writer's laboratory, with *P. cynomolgi, P. cynomolgi bastianellii, P. cynomolgi ceylonensis*, and a new langur strain (Voller et al., 1966).

The second group of species appears to possess some common antigens in that immunity is much less specific and the immunity derived from one parasite may be partially effective against challenge with another. This phenomenon was well demonstrated by Ciuca et al. (1947) in Rumania, where they reported that patients undergoing malaria therapy who had come from malarious zones of the country were immune to *P. knowlesi*, though others who had not previously been exposed to malaria were fully susceptible. Such partial cross-immunity is shared by the simian malaria parasites, *P. knowlesi, P. coatneyi, P. fragile*, and probably by *P. malariae*, and a degree of affinity also exists between *P. inui* and *P. shortti*. The protection is usually by no means complete, and the cross-immunity may easily be masked if too large a challenging dose is given.

Serologic reactions in malaria

Many attempts have been made to adapt the classical serologic methods to the diagnosis of malaria, and Fulton (1968) and Saliou (1964) have summarized the tests which at one time or another have been used in human and simian infections. The complement-fixation test was employed by Coggeshall and Eaton (1938), using an antigen prepared from *P. knowlesi*, and it gave positive results with a variety of species of malaria. This group reaction has since been repeatedly confirmed, and although Pautrizel and Nien (1958) showed that the test was capable of providing a clear picture of the rise and fall of immunity in rodent malaria, the method has largely fallen into disuse. The same fate has overtaken agglutination and precipitin tests, although the much less specific Henry's reaction of melanoflocculation still continues to be used in North Africa and at a few centers in France.

In recent years, three further methods have been introduced for the study of humoral immunity: the indirect fluorescent-antibody tests (FA), the hemagglutination reaction, and diffusion in gel against special antigenic fractions. Only the first of these is to any extent standardized, and the FA has been shown to be a most valuable tool in malaria research and of great potential value in the diagnosis of human infections (Tobie and Coatney, 1961).

The fluorescent-antibody test is capable of detecting antibodies in up to high dilutions of the immune serum, but it is not very specific and heterologous sera may only differ in two-fold dilutions. *P. cynomolgi bastianellii*, for instance, acts as an excellent antigen for all the human and simian species of malaria parasites (Tobie et al., 1962, 1963; Voller, 1962). This fact alone indicates that the FA does not measure "protective" antibodies since fluorescent antibodies of *P. falciparum* react strongly with *P. c. bastianellii* although no cross-immunity exists between these two parasites. Also, Rey (1966) found high titers in *fatal* cases of *P. falciparum* malaria in which immunity must have been absent. Nevertheless, the reaction follows closely both the curves of the complement-fixation reaction and the progress of immunity in a population exposed to holoendemic malaria. Furthermore, Voller (1964) showed that the curative IgG itself produced a strong fluorescence.

Voller and Bray (1962) noted that the immune reaction was marked in the umbilical cord blood (as the result of the passage of antibodies from the immune mother), was still present in the new-born child for the first weeks, and then faded, only to return later in infancy and reach its height in adults. Such a curve follows the classical concept of immunity in Africans, but it is quite unlike the results of FA in experimental malaria. In volunteers infected with *P. vivax*, *P. c. bastianellii*, and other species, the recipients respond with a rapidly rising titer which reaches a maximum height after about 10 days' patency. The titer then slowly declines and becomes negligible after about a year. But if the patient is challenged in the interim, the titer quickly regains its former height and stays for some considerable time at a high level (Kuvin et al., 1962). Yet the native African takes years, instead of days, of constant infection to reach the same point.

The fluorescent-antibody test is usually employed to measure the amount of antibody present in the serum. The antigen is contained in the erythrocytic stage of the organism and fluorescence is exhibited principally by the outer membrane and the cytoplasm of the parasite but not by the nucleus or the pigment. A vivid reaction is also given by the infected erythrocyte itself, particularly by the lesions (clefts or dots) of its membrane, in which, according to Voller and Bray (1962), antigen from the parasite is deposited.

Other stages of the malaria parasite also react in the fluorescent-antibody test. Corradetti et al. (1964) showed that sporozoites are an effective antigen and suggested that the test might be used for identifying the species of sporozoites obtained from mosquitoes captured in nature. Ingram and Carver (1963) were able to obtain fluorescence of the exoerythrocytic stages of *P. cynomolgi bastianellii* after application of the test. Voller and Taffs (1963) succeeded with tissue forms of *P. gallinaceum*, but not with those of the primate species. The material for such tests must not be exposed to ordinary histologic reagents but should be prepared by the freeze-substitution technique. El-Nahal (1967) tested the exoerythrocytic schizonts of *P. berghei yoelii* against sera immune to the blood stages of the homologous parasite and other rodent parasites and against those of *P. cynomolgi bastianellii*; the former gave a strong reaction, the latter a negative. Serum immune to sporozoites of *P. berghei yoelii*, strangely enough, failed to produce fluorescence in the tissue forms of the same species.

The hemagglutination test of Stein and Desowitz (1964) appeared to offer a more specific serologic reaction than the FA. Immune sera were found to react in the highest dilutions to the homologous antigen attached to the tanned sheep's corpuscles. Unfortunately, the reaction is often positive in nonimmune serum up to titers of 1:500. Further improvements in the technique of the test will be necessary before it can be accepted for general use.

The gel-diffusion technique was employed by McGregor et al. (1966) with immune serum and various antigen samples. Schizonts of *P. falciparum* from infected placentas were purified and, after lyophilization, were disintegrated in a Hughes press. Another antigen was prepared from blood containing the trophozoite (ring) stages of the parasite. Lines of precipitation were obtained most strongly with the former, possibly because the schizont contains so much more material than the tiny ring, or because the antigen does not appear until late in schizogony. There was no correlation between the results of this test and the FA, probably because a different antibody is concerned. The gel-diffusion test may well be extended to other host-parasite combinations, with immune serum of known antecedents and with cultured parasites, and a fruitful line of research may be anticipated.

The humoral basis of acquired immunity lies in the plasma proteins, of which IgG appears to be the most important. In an experimental study of *P. falciparum* malaria in volunteers and in splenectomized chimpanzees, Sadun et al. (1966) noted that the changes in the globulins differed in the two groups: the rise in IgG was similar, but there was a decrease of α_2-globulin and an increase of β-globulin in the man, and an increase of α_2-globulin and a decrease of β-globulin in the ape. This discrepancy may throw light on the role of the spleen in the origin of these different globulins. The amount of γ-globulin coincides with the titer of the FA; both rise and fall simultaneously in the course of the infection. There is also evidence that the complement-fixation reaction and the hemagglutination test measure the same process, but none of these serologic procedures appears to denote protective antibodies, which at present can only be detected by clumsy cross-immunity reactions or by the administration of purified antisera *in vivo*.

REFERENCES

Allison, A. C. 1963. Inherited factors conferring resistance to protozoa. *In* Immunity to Protozoa. Garnham, P. C. C., Pierce, A. E., and Roitt, I., eds. Oxford, Blackwell Scientific Publications, pp. 109-122.

Bertram, B., M. G. R. Varma, and J. R. Baker. 1964. Partial suppression of malaria parasites and the transmission of malaria in *Aedes aegypti gallinaceum* Brumpt. Bull. W. H. O., No. 31, pp. 679-697.

Beye, I. K., M. E. Getz, G. R. Coatney, H. A. Elder, and D. E. Eyles. 1961. Simian malaria in man. Amer. J. Trop. Med., 10:311-316.

Bray, R. S. 1957a. Studies on the exoerythrocytic cycle in the genus *Plasmodium*. Memoir 12. London, H. K. Lewis.

———— 1957b. Studies on malaria in chimpanzees. II. *Plasmodium vivax*. Amer. J. Trop. Med., 6:514-520.

———— and P. C. C. Garnham. 1953. Effect of milk diet on *P. cynomolgi* infections in monkeys. Brit. Med. J., 1:1200-1201.

Brown, K. N., and I. N. Brown. 1966. Antigen variation in simian malaria. Trans. Roy. Soc. Trop. Med. Hyg., 60:358-363.

Bruce-Chwatt, L. J. 1963. Congenital transmission of immunity in malaria. *In* Immunity to Protozoa. Garnham, P. C. C., Pierce, A. E., and Roitt, I., eds. Oxford, Blackwell Scientific Publications, pp. 89-108.

Brumpt, E. 1949. The human parasites of the genus *Plasmodium. In* Malariology. Boyd, M. F., ed. Philadelphia, W. B. Saunders and Co., Vol. 1, pp. 65-121.

Bück, G., J. Coudurier, and J. J. Quesnel. 1952. Sur deux nouveaux *Plasmodium* obsérvés chez un lemurien de Madagascar splénectomisé. Arch. Inst. Pasteur d'Algérie, 30: 240-246.

Ciuča, M., M. Chelarescu, A. Sofleta, P. Constantinescu, E. Teriteanu, P. Cortez, G. Balanovschi, and M. Ilies. 1947. Studies on Immunity in Malaria. Bucharest.

Coggeshall, L. T., and H. W. Kumm. 1937. Demonstration of passive immunity in experimental monkey malaria. J. Exp. Med., 66: 177-189.

——— and M. D. Eaton. 1938. The complement fixation reaction in monkey malaria. J. Exp. Med., 67: 871-882.

Cohen, S., and I. A. McGregor. 1963. Gamma-globulin and acquired immunity in malaria. *In* Symposium on Immunity to Protozoal Diseases. Garnham, P. C. C., Pierce, A. E., and Roitt, I., eds. Oxford, Blackwell Scientific Publications, pp. 123-159.

Colbourne, M. 1956. Does milk protect infants against malaria? Trans. Roy. Soc. Trop. Med. Hyg., 50: 82-90.

Corradetti, A. 1965. The origin of relapses in human and simian infections. Med. Parazit. (Moskva), 34: 673-677.

——— F. Verolini, A. Sebastiani, A. M. Proietti, and L. Amatis. 1964. Fluorescent antibody testing with sporozoites of plasmodia. Bull. W.H.O., No. 30, pp. 747-750.

Deschiens, R., and J. Benex. 1965. Les interactions hôtes-parasites et les engagements parasitaires abortifs. II. Les engagements parasitaires abortifs ou "impasses parasitaires." Bull. Soc. Path. Exot., 58: 590-630.

Dissanaike, A. S. 1965. Simian malaria parasites of Ceylon. Bull. W.H.O., No. 32, pp. 593-597.

El-Nahal, H. M. S. 1967. Fluorescent antibody studies on the pre-exoerythrocytic schizonts of *Plasmodium berghei yoelii* and *P. cynomolgi* langur strain. Trans. Roy. Soc. Trop. Med. Hyg., 61: 8-9.

Fabiani, M. G. 1966. Rôle de la rate dans l'immunité antipaludéenne. Bull. Soc. Path. Exot., 59: 605-648.

Fulton, J. D. 1968. Diagnosis of protozoal infections. *In* Clinical Aspects of Immunology. Gell, P. G. H., and Coombs, R. R. A., eds. Oxford, Blackwell Scientific Publications, 2nd Ed., pp. 133-160.

Garnham, P. C. C. 1955. The comparative pathogenicity of protozoa in their vertebrate and invertebrate hosts. *In* Fifth Symposium Society of General Microbiology. Cambridge, Cambridge University Press, pp. 191-206.

——— 1956. Microsporidia in laboratory colonies of *Anopheles.* Bull. W.H.O., 15: 845-847.

——— 1963. Distribution of simian malaria parasites in various hosts. J. Parasit., 49: 905-911.

——— 1964. The subgenera of *Plasmodium* in mammals. Ann. Soc. Belg. Med. Trop., 44: 267-272.

——— 1966a. Pathological features of the Haemosporidia. Med. Parazit. (Moskva), 43: 688-694.

——— 1966b. Immunity against the different stages of malaria parasites. Bull. Soc. Path. Exot., 59: 549-557.

——— and R. S. Bray. 1956. Influence of immunity upon the stages (including the exoerythrocytic schizonts) of mammalian malaria parasites. Rev. Brasil. Malar., 8: 151-160.

Hawking, F. 1953. Milk diet, para-aminobenzoic acid and malaria (*P. berghei*). Brit. Med. J., 1: 1201-1202.

——— M. J. Worms, K. Gammage, and P. A. Goddard. 1966. The biological purpose of the blood-cycle of the malaria parasite, *Plasmodium cynomolgi.* Lancet, 2: 422-444.

Hoare, C. A. 1965. The relationship between simian and human malarial infections. Med. Parazit. (Moskva), 34: 678-682.

Huff, C. G. 1922. The effects of selection upon susceptibility to bird malaria in *Culex pipiens.* Ann. Trop. Med. Parasit., 23: 427-439.

Ingram, R. L., and R. K. Carver. 1963. Malaria parasites: Fluorescent antibody technique for tissue stage study. Science, 139:405-406.

Kretschmar, W. 1966. Die Bedeutung der *p*-Aminobenzoesäure für den Krankheitsverlauf und die Immunität bei der Malaria im Tier (*Plasmodium berghei*) und im Menschen (*Pl. falciparum*). II. Untersuchungen an naturlich ernahrten Kleinkindern in Nigeria. Z. Tropenmed. Parasit., 17: 375-390.

Kuvin, S. F., J. E. Tobie, C. B. Evans, G. R. Coatney, and P. G. Contacos. 1962. Antibody production in human malaria as determined by the fluorescent antibody techniques. Science, 135:1130-1131.

Laveran, A. 1893. Paludism. London, The New Sydenham Society.

Lupascu, G., P. Constantinescu, E. Negulici, P. C. C. Garnham, R. S. Bray, R. Killick-Kendrick, P. G. Shute, and M. Maryon. 1967. The late primary exoerythrocytic stages of *Plasmodium malariae*. Trans. Roy. Soc. Trop. Med. Hyg, 61:482-489.

MacDonald, G. 1957. The Epidemiology and Control of Malaria. London, Oxford University Press.

Maegraith, B. G., J. Deegan, and E. S. Jones. 1952. Suppression of malaria (*P. berghei*) by milk. Brit. Med. J., 2:1382-1384.

Marchiafava, E., and A. Bignami. 1894. On Summer-Autumn Malarial Fevers. London, The New Sydenham Society.

McGregor, I. A., and S. D. Carrington. 1963. Treatment of East African *P. falciparum* malaria with West African human γ-globulin. Trans. Roy. Soc. Trop. Med. Hyg., 57:170-175.

———— P. J. Hall, K. Williams, C. L. S. Hardy, and M. W. Turner. 1966. Demonstration of circulating antibodies to *Plasmodium falciparum* by gel-diffusion techniques. Nature (London), 201:1384-1386.

Muirhead-Thomson, R. C. 1951. The distribution of anopheline mosquito bites among different age groups, a new factor in malaria epidemiology. Brit. Med. J., 1:1114.

———— 1954. Differential biting habits of the vectors as a factor in the age distribution of mosquito-borne filariasis. J. Trop. Med. Hyg., 57:107-112.

Pautrizel, R., and N. V. Nien. 1958. Mise en évidence d'anticorps chez le rat parasitisé par *P. berghei* à l'aide d'un antigène préparé avec du sang de rat impaludé. Bull. Soc. Path. Exot., 46:671-673.

Porter, J. A., and M. D. Young. 1966. Susceptibility of Panamanian primates to *Plasmodium vivax*. Milit. Med., 131(Suppl.):952-958.

Rey, M. M. 1966. Des expressions cliniques du paludisme à *P. falciparum* chez l'enfant noir africain. Bull. Soc. Path. Exot., 59:651-657.

Rodhain, J. 1956. Paradoxical behaviour of *Plasmodium vivax* in the chimpanzee. Trans. Roy. Soc. Trop. Med. Hyg., 50:287-291.

Sadun, E. H., J. G. Williams, and L. K. Martin. 1966. Serum biochemical changes in malarial infections in men, chimpanzees and mice. Milit. Med., 181 (Suppl.):1094-1106.

Saliou, P. 1964. Diagnostic sérologique du paludisme humain par l'immuno-fluorescence. Lyon, Bosc.

Sergent, E. 1963. Latent infection and premunition. *In* Symposium on Immunity to Protozoal Diseases. Garnham, P. C. C., Pierce, A. E., and Roitt, I., eds. Oxford, Blackwell Scientific Publications.

Shortt, H. E., and P. C. C. Garnham. 1948a. Demonstration of a persisting exoerythrocytic cycle in *Plasmodium cynomolgi* and its bearing on relapses. Brit. Med. J., 1:1225-1228.

———— and P. C. C. Garnham. 1948b. The pre-exoerythrocytic development of *Plasmodium cynomolgi* and *Plasmodium vivax*. Trans. Roy. Soc. Trop. Med. Hyg., 41:785-795.

Shute, P. G. 1946. Latency and long term relapses in benign tertian malaria. Trans. Roy. Soc. Trop. Med. Hyg., 40:189-200.

Stein, B., and R. S. Desowitz. 1964. The measurement of antibody in human malaria by a formalinized tanned sheep cell hemagglutination test. Bull. W.H.O., 30:45-49.

Steinhaus, E. A., ed. 1963. Insect Pathology. New York, Academic Press, Inc., Vols. 1 and 2.

Taliaferro, W. H. 1949. *In* Malariology, Vol. 2. Boyd, M. F., ed. Philadelphia, W. B. Saunders and Co., pp. 935-965.

———— and H. W. Mulligan. 1937. The histopathology of malaria with special reference to the functions and origins of the macrophages in defence. Indian Medical Research Memoir No. 29, pp. 1-138.

Tobie, J. E., and G. R. Coatney. 1961. Fluorescent antibody staining of human malaria parasites. Exp. Parasit., 11: 128-132.

———— S. F. Kuvin, P. G. Contacos, G. R. Coatney, and C. B. Evans. 1962. Fluorescent antibody studies on cross reactions between human and simian malaria in normal volunteers. Amer. J. Trop. Med. Hyg., 11: 589-596.

———— S. F. Kuvin, P. G. Contacos, G. R. Coatney, and C. B. Evans. 1963. Cross reactions in human and simian malaria. In Symposium on malaria, Part II. J.A.M. A., 184: 945-947.

Voller, A. 1962. Fluorescent antibody studies on malaria parasites. Bull. W.H.O., No. 27, pp. 283-287.

———— 1964. Comments on the detection of malaria antibodies. Amer. J. Trop. Med. Hyg., 13 (Suppl.) : 204-208.

———— and R. S. Bray. 1962. Fluorescent antibody staining as a measure of malaria antibody. Proc. Soc. Exp. Biol. Med., 110: 907-911.

———— and L. F. Taffs. 1963. Fluorescent antibody staining of exoerythrocytic stages of Plasmodium gallinaceum. Trans. Roy. Soc. Trop. Med. Hyg., 57: 32-33.

———— P. C. C. Garnham, and G. A. T. Targett. 1966. Cross immunity in monkey malaria. J. Trop. Med. Hyg., 69: 121-127.

Weatherall, R. 1965. Malaria and the opening-up of Central Africa. Nature (London), 5015: 1267-1269.

Weiser, J. 1966. Nemoci Hmyzu. Prague, Czechoslovak Academy of Sciences Publ. House.

Young, M. D., D. E. Eyles, R. W. Burgess, and G. M. Jeffery. 1955. Experimental testing of the immunity of Negroes to Plasmodium vivax. J. Parasit., 41: 315-318.

Malaria of Lower Mammals

AVIVAH ZUCKERMAN

Department of Parasitology, Hebrew University, Jerusalem, Israel

This study was supported in part by the U.S. Public Health Service through grant
AI-02859 from the National Institute of Allergy and Infectious Diseases.

INTRODUCTION: THE RODENT MALARIAS AS IMMUNOLOGIC TOOLS

In 1948, with the description of the first species of rodent malaria isolated by Vincke and Lips from the African jungle tree rat, *Thamnomys surdaster*, a new chapter was opened in malariologic research. Until that time, the only plasmodia available for extensive experimentation were parasites of birds, e.g., of the chicken, the duck and the canary. Extensive studies on the simian malarias were limited by the expense involved. While a very impressive body of information had been amassed on the immune reactions of avian hosts to their plasmodia, the projection of these results by analogy onto a mammalian host, man, was always accompanied by legitimate misgivings. It is, incidentally, worthy of note that despite these misgivings immune processes in avian and mammalian hosts have proved to resemble one another closely at many points.

The first rodent plasmodium, *Plasmodium berghei*, was soon transmitted to laboratory rats and mice, in which it provided convenient models of both fulminating and chronic infections. Unlimited experiments on the immune reactions of a plasmodium in a mammalian host could now be undertaken.

Several years later, a second rodent plasmodium, *Plasmodium vinckei*, was isolated (Rodhain, 1952), and studies on it quickly accumulated. In contrast, *Plasmodium inopinatum* (Resseler, 1956) has not become established as a laboratory tool. The newly isolated *Plasmodium metastaticum* (Raffaele, 1965) and *Plasmodium chabaudi* (Landau, 1965) are now also available for study.

A series of reviews on the rodent plasmodia has appeared (Draper, 1953; Thurston, 1953; Vincke et al., 1953b; Fabiani, 1959; Sergent, 1959; Ciuca et al., 1964), and symposia were published by the Indian Journal of Malariology in 1954 (Singh, 1954), and by the Annales de la Société Belge de Médecine Tropicale in 1965 (Jadin, 1965). Recent studies are further reviewed by Zuckerman (1969a).

The rodent plasmodia, and particularly *P. berghei* and *P. vinckei*, have already amply fulfilled their promise as models for the exploration of numerous problems in the immunology of mammalian malaria. Their value as models emerges clearly when it is noted that analogies with human and simian malarias can be drawn at almost every point.

Most of the studies on immune reactions to the rodent plasmodia have been carried out with *P. berghei*, and some with *P. vinckei*. This discussion will therefore deal almost exclusively with these two parasites.

INNATE IMMUNITY: THE RODENT MALARIAS IN VARIOUS HOSTS

When a series of hosts are exposed to a given plasmodium, their initial reactions to contact with the same parasite may range from negligible to fatal (i.e., their innate immunity ranges from very effective to negligible, respectively). As in most other infections, the reasons for the differences in innate immunity to the rodent plamodia have rarely been analyzed, and the unadorned record of varying susceptibilities is usually all that is available. All of the common laboratory rodents and a series of exotic species of rodents, as well as other mammals and even birds, have been exposed to *P. berghei.*

Among the adult, intact rodents generally developing fatal infections of *P. berghei* are the mouse (Vincke and Lips, 1948; Sergent and Poncet, 1950, 1955a,c; Mercado and Coatney, 1951; Vincke et al., 1953a; Durand and Mathis, 1955; Radacovici et al., 1958; Sergent, 1959; Weiss, 1965), the hamster (Adler et al., 1950; Durand and Mathis, 1951; Vincke et al., 1953a; Thurston, 1953), the multimammate rat (Cowper and Woodward, 1958), and the laboratory-bred *Thamnomys* (Yoeli and Most, 1964). Of particular interest is the fulminating infection of *P. berghei* in the muskrat (Wellde et al., 1966) in view of the relatively large size of the host and the large yield of infected blood which can therefore be obtained from it.

Among the adult, intact rodents developing chronic infections with relatively lower mortality rates are the rat (Vincke and Lips, 1948; Galliard and Lapierre, 1950; Sergent and Poncet, 1950, 1955a,c; Vincke et al., 1953a; de Smet and Frankie, 1954a; Radacovici et al., 1958; Sergent, 1959), the cotton rat (Rodhain, 1949; Vincke et al., 1953a; Thurston, 1953), and the field vole (Adler et al., 1950; Zuckerman and Yoeli, 1951; Mercado and Coatney, 1953; Thurston, 1953).

Among the adult, intact rodents with either transient negligible parasitemias or in which *P. berghei* gains no demonstrable foothold at all are the guinea pig (Vincke and Lips, 1948; Raffaele and Baldi, 1950; Sergent and Poncet, 1951b, 1955c; Satya Prakash et al., 1952; Thurston, 1953; Sergent, 1959), the jird (Sergent and Poncet, 1950, 1951a, 1955c; Thurston, 1953; Durand and Mathis, 1955; Sergent, 1959), the squirrel (Ramakrishnan and Satya Prakash, 1951; Thurston, 1953), the gerbil, *Dipodillus* (Durand and Mathis, 1955; Sergent and Poncet, 1956b; Sergent, 1959), and the spiny mouse, *Acomys* (Beer, 1961). The rabbit, though not a rodent, is also affected only slightly or not at all (Vincke and Lips, 1948; Raffaele and Baldi, 1950; Deschiens and Lamy, 1951; Satya Prakash et al., 1952; Thurston, 1953; Fabiani and Orfila, 1958). It has been pointed out (Wellde et al., 1966) that none of the Hystricomorpha exposed to *P. berghei* (including the capybara, the agouti, the nutria, the chinchilla, the paca, and the guinea pig) nor any of the Sciuromorpha (including the prairie dog, the ground hog, and the squirrel) is susceptible.

Numerous other wild rodents, for which only scattered observations are available, are so far regarded as only moderately susceptible to *P. berghei* (Vincke et al., 1953a; de Smet and Frankie, 1954a).

The hedgehog, *Erinaceus* (Sergent and Poncet, 1957b; Sergent, 1959) and several species of bats (van Riel, 1950; Rodhain, 1953b; Corradetti et al., 1959) are relatively refractory to *P. berghei*, though several other species of bat are very susceptible (Rodhain, 1953b).

Ungulates, such as lambs, pigs, and calves (Durbin, 1951); carnivores, such as puppies, kittens (Durbin, 1951) and a mongoose (Satya Prakash et al., 1952); and marsupials, such as the bandicoot (Satya Prakash et al., 1952) and the opossum (Wellde et al., 1966), are uniformly refractory. In contrast, three species of primate, including the rhesus monkey, are susceptible to *P. berghei* (Wellde et al., 1966).

Chicks resist infection with *P. berghei* (Durbin, 1951). *P. berghei* inoculated into chick, duck, and goose embryos fails to invade the erythrocytes of the chick but succeeds in invading those of the other two embryonic avian hosts (McGhee, 1954).

Clear differences in innate immunity to the rodent malarias thus obviously exist among host species. In addition, differences among individuals of the same species can also be demonstrated. A series of extrinsic and intrinsic factors (reviewed in Zuckerman, 1968) may affect innate immunity.

AGE IMMUNITY

An important factor in the innate immunity of a rodent to a plasmodium is the host's age. In general, since the mechanism for the development of acquired immunity is less effective in the immature animal than in the adult, the period during which only nonspecific innate immune factors come into play is longer in the young than in the adult animal. Therefore, the younger the animal, the higher is its susceptibility. This has been shown to be the case in *P. berghei* infections in rats (Raffaele and Baldi, 1950; Hsu and Geiman, 1952; Galliard and Lapierre, 1954; Zuckerman and Yoeli, 1954; Singer et al., 1955; Zuckerman, 1957), in hamsters (Hsu and Geiman, 1952), and in jirds (Durand and Mathis, 1955); as well as in *P. vinckei* infections in rats (Zuckerman, 1958).

A measure of age immunity to *P. berghei* has been reported in mice by Hsu and Geiman (1952), by Greenberg et al. (1953), and by Wellde et al. (1966), but Galliard and Lapierre (1954) and F. E. G. Cox (1965) claimed that the young and the adult mouse were equally susceptible to infection. An important cause of age immunity in *P. berghei* infections is the fact that circulating polychromasia, a feature of the blood picture of the young rodent, wanes with advancing age. Polychromasia predisposes the animal to infection, since *P. berghei* merozoites invade reticulocytes in preference to other erythrocytes.

ACQUIRED IMMUNITY

Chronic infection and latency

Plasmodial infections in which parasitemia advances unchecked until the host succumbs are termed "fulminating infections." In them the parasite counts rise steadily, innate immunity is ineffective in holding the parasitemia in check, and signs of the development of specific acquired immunity, such as crisis or the appearance of demonstrable circulating antibodies, are lacking (Fabiani, 1954a). The mouse, the hamster, and a number of rodents not commonly in use in the laboratory usually develop fulminating infections when exposed to *P. berghei*.

In contrast to these are infections exemplified by those of the rat and several other hosts, in which the infected animal tends to recover following a crisis or a turning point in the parasite count. At the time of the crisis, and often preceding it by several days, antiplasmodial antibodies appear in the circulating blood (*see* pp. 804-805). Parasitemia curves descend from the critical peak parasitemia at a more or less rapid rate, depending on the degree of acquired immunity. A protracted period of relatively stable equilibrium between parasitic multiplication and host defenses, known as the chronic state, may now ensue. Eventually the parasites may be so effectively suppressed by acquired immune mechanisms as to disappear from view when sought by ordinary microscopic means. The infection is now said to be latent, but the presence of subpatent numbers may still be demonstrated by subinoculation or splenectomy. The host's immune state, constantly primed by the unabated multiplication of residual parasites, is defined as premunition (Sergent, 1950). Premunition may develop in rats with *P. berghei* even if the initial infection was so mild as to be inapparent microscopically throughout (Sergent, 1954a). Most intact adult rats infected with *P. berghei* achieve latency following an initial infection such as that outlined above (Fabiani et al., 1952b; Fabiani, 1954a; Sergent, 1954b; Cox, 1964b).

In contrast, splenectomized rats are usually unable to suppress their infections to the latent state, and a low-grade, chronic, patent infection persists in them indefinitely (Corradetti, 1950; Zuckerman and Yoeli, 1954; Corradetti and Verolini, 1960).

Hosts normally succumbing to fulminating infection are not necessarily devoid of the ability to produce an immune response. The untreated infection overwhelms and kills such a host before it can call its potentially effective immune mechanism into action. Thus, certain drugs are capable of suppressing overt parasitemia without necessarily eradicating infection. They thereby give the treated host the time to build up an immune reaction and to establish either the chronic or even the latent state. Among such drugs are atabrine (Cox, 1957, 1958, 1959, 1964b), chloroquine (Carrescia and Arcoleo, 1957), or primaquine (Briggs et al., 1960). Intervention by sulfadiazine in rats (Satya Prakash, 1959, 1960b) or mice (Satya Prakash, 1960a) too early in the course of their infections with *P. berghei* interfered with the acquisition of immunity. The chronic or latent states may similarly be induced in otherwise highly susceptible hosts by feeding them a diet deficient in certain nutrients required by the plasmodium, thus partially inhibiting parasitemia and thereby giving the acquired immune mechanism time to attain an effective level (Schindler and Mehlitz, 1965).

Immunity to superinfection

Rodent hosts with chronic or latent infections are immune to reinoculation with the same strain of plasmodium. This is one of the characteristics of premunition as defined by Sergent (1950, 1963). The fact has been repeatedly confirmed for rats with *P. berghei* (for example, by Vargues and Fabiani, 1951; Ramakrishnan et al., 1951; Fabiani et al., 1952a,b; de Smet and Frankie, 1954a; Sergent and Poncet, 1955a, 1961; Cowper and Woodward, 1959; Sergent, 1959). It has also been recorded for the field vole, *Microtus* (Zuckerman, 1953), for the pouched rat, *Cricetomys*, and for the African tree rat, *Thamnomys* (de Smet and Frankie, 1954a).

Immunity to reinoculation with *P. berghei* has also been demonstrated in mice which, by one means or another, have been made to survive initial infection. Lapierre (1954) reported that five mice surviving after treatment with nivaquine were immune to reinoculation. Similar results were observed for mice treated with atabrine (mepacrine) (H. W. Cox, 1957, 1958; F. E. G. Cox, 1965), with 8-aminoquinolines (Box and Gingrich, 1958), with primaquine (Briggs et al., 1960), with sulfadiazine (Satya Prakash, 1960a) and with chloroquine (F. E. G. Cox, 1965). At least in the cases reported by Briggs et al. (1960) and by Satya Prakash (1960a), it is clear that some mice were not radically cured by the drugs but instead harbored latent infections at the time of reinoculation. Untreated mice of a relatively nonsusceptible strain, the NMRI strain, resist superinfection with *P. berghei* (Kretschmar, 1962; Gail and Kretschmar, 1965). Similarly, mice which survived initial infection due to having been fed a diet which partially suppresses *P. berghei* are immune to superinfection (Schindler and Mehlitz, 1965).

All the parasites introduced at reinoculation are not immediately removed from the circulation, and some still circulate for a few days after challenge (Vargues and Fabiani, 1951; Krishnaswami et al., 1953; Corradetti et al., 1961b).

Repeated reinoculation has generally been reported to reinforce the extent of premunition, as evidenced by the level and duration of parasitemia following challenge in rats with *P. berghei* (Krishnaswami et al., 1953; Fabiani, 1954a,b; Corradetti et al., 1961b; Kretschmar, 1962). Such reinforcing of immunity to superinfection has also been reported in mice (Satya Prakash, 1960a). However, Sergent and Poncet (1955c) found that a series of rats receiving six reinoculations eventually developed positive parasitemias. They concluded that these rats had become sensitized rather than progressively more immune to superinfection.

Relapses

Blood films from intact rodents which have achieved latency may remain microscopically negative for weeks or months. Occasionally, however, the vigilance of the premunizing mechanism is breached and a shower of microscopically demonstrable parasites appears in the circulation. This is known as a relapse. The immune process, alerted and reinforced by this now patent infection, again suppresses parasitemia, the relapse is terminated, and latency is resumed. Spontaneous recrudescences of this sort lasting for several days were reported in rats with *P. berghei* as occurring one to three weeks after the onset of latency following initial infection (Black, 1951). They are a regular feature of *P. berghei* infections in rats.

As long as spontaneous relapses occur, they bear witness to the fact that the host's body has not yet eradicated infection. Corradetti (1959) pointed out that once radical cure of *P. berghei* has been achieved in rats, about 50 days following initial exposure and thereafter, relapses can obviously no longer occur.

Mice surviving *P. berghei* infection with the aid of primaquine generally relapsed from the latent state to a protracted chronic state (Briggs et al., 1960). Though they were more immune than they had been before inoculation and remained alive despite a patent infection of long duration, their premunition was too weak to be suppressive. The precarious immune situation of these drug-treated mice is emphasized by comparing them with the stable condition of several hundred NMRI mice surviving infection with *P. berghei* (Kretschmar, 1963a). The latter group, a relatively nonsusceptible strain of mouse, was never observed to suffer spontaneous relapses.

The interesting suggestion has been made (Cox, 1959, 1962) that relapse strains of *P. berghei* in atabrine-treated intact mice differ in some fundamental way from the parent strains, since relapse variants can reproduce in hosts which are immune to the parent strain.

Duration of acquired immunity

As long as parasites persist, premunition is maintained. Few have studied the duration of latency systematically, but available observations show that it may be very long-lived in certain host strains and relatively short in others. As an extreme example of protracted latency, parasites were demonstrated in the bone marrow and kidney of a rat with latent *P berghei*, which died of old age at 19 months (Sergent and Poncet, 1955b). Similarly, mice having a latent infection with an avirulent strain of *P. berghei* were still highly immune when challenged with a virulent strain 19 months later (Weiss, 1965).

Radical cure and residual immunity

All are agreed that as long as parasites persist, premunition is maintained. But there is some disagreement as to whether any sterile residual immunity remains after all the parasites have been eradicated from a host with rodent malaria. In fact, an important point in the debate has been whether even the most stringent criteria devised to date for radical cure are reliable (Sergent and Poncet, 1955b, 1956a; Sergent, 1963).

In addition to the microscopic absence of parasites from the peripheral blood of infected rodents, criteria for radical cure of malaria have included the absence of relapse following splenectomy (Black, 1951; Zuckerman and Yoeli, 1951; Corradetti, 1952, 1959, 1963; Zuckerman, 1953; Beer, 1961; Garza and Box, 1961; Kretschmar, 1963a; Weiss and DeGiusti, 1966), the absence of infection in mice or rats after the inoculation of suspected blood or ground splenic tissue (Zuckerman and Yoeli, 1951; Corradetti, 1952, 1959, 1963; Zuckerman, 1953; Corradetti and Verolini, 1957; Beer, 1961; Garza and Box, 1961; Weiss and DeGiusti, 1966), and the development of normal infections following challenge in mice previously exposed to blood or splenic tissue from an animal suspected of having achieved cure (Zuckerman and Yoeli, 1951; Zuckerman, 1953).

Employing the above criteria in various combinations, numerous workers have reported radical cure in the rodent malarias. Corradetti (1950, 1952, 1955) and Corradetti et al. (1954b, 1961a) found that rats infected with *P. berghei* eradicated the infection within 50 to 60 days after the end of the primary attack. Cure of rats in 50 days was confirmed by Black (1951). Fabiani (1954a) recorded radical cure in rats in about 2 to 3 months, and Draper (1954) at about 4 months after inoculation. Zuckerman and Yoeli (1951) reported spontaneous radical cure of *P. berghei* in field voles (*Microtus guentheri*) about 30 days after inoculation. Radical cures of *P. berghei* in the pouched rat, *Cricetomys ansorgei* (de Smet and Frankie, 1954b), in the spiny mouse, *Acomys cahirinus* (Beer, 1961), in NMRI mice (Kretschmar, 1962), and in mice recovering from an avirulent strain of *P. berghei* (Weiss and DeGiusti, 1964b) have all been recorded.

Residual sterile immunity persists in rodent hosts for a time following radical cure as established by the above criteria. For example, rats remained resistant to superinfection for more than 150 days after achieving cure (Corradetti, 1952). Furthermore, rodents splenectomized to prove the occurrence of cures may develop either chronic, negligible, or no perceptible infection on challenge. This is true of both rats (Corradetti, 1950, 1955) and voles (Zuckerman, 1953), and it represents a very significant measure of resistance since infections were regularly more severe in rats and were fatal in voles splenectomized before initial exposure to the parasites. Some cured, splenectomized voles were even capable of re-eradicating their challenge infections after many months in the chronic state.

Corradetti and Verolini (1957) and Corradetti (1959, 1963) believe that residual immunity following cure of *P. berghei* in rats probably lasts for the life of the cured animal, although Draper (1954) observed that it wanes after 15 to 18 months. In mice recovering from an avirulent strain of *P. berghei*, sterile residual immunity lasted for at least 8 months (Weiss and DeGiusti, 1964b, 1966). In some voles, residual immunity waned gradually over a period of months (Zuckerman, 1953).

Sergent himself has interpreted the noninfectivity to mice of blood or ground tissue as an indication of cure in a jird, *Meriones shawi* (Sergent and Poncet, 1951a), in three gerbils, *Dipodillus campestris* (Sergent and Poncet, 1956b), and in 13 rats (Sergent, 1959). He also used the same criterion to demonstrate resistance to initial infection in a guinea pig (Sergent and Poncet, 1951b). However, Sergent and Poncet (1955b) warned that a negative result of the subinoculation test is inconclusive in proving cure, since initially negative results have occasionally been followed by positive ones when the same test was repeated in the same animal (Sergent, 1959). Sergent further maintains that even splenectomy and the subinoculation of extirpated tissues are inconclusive tests, and he does not consider that radical cure has been unequivocally demonstrated (Sergent, 1963). Deschiens and Lamy (1965) share Sergent's view, and some misgivings as to the demonstration of cure in rodent malaria are also expressed by Satya Prakash (1960b).

Since the criteria of cure employed by himself and others are not regarded by Sergent and his coworkers as reliable, and since no alternative criteria exist, the debate about the existence of cures is now at a stalemate. The debate has been presented in detail and the problem is crucial. Those who consider that sterile immunity exists in rodent malaria see the mechanism of rodent malarial immunity as basically similar to that in most other microbial diseases. Those who deny the existence of sterile immunity see it as basically dissimilar. We face the perennial difficulty of proving a negative point, in this case, that parasites are *not* present at a certain stage following inoculation. In this situation the best that we can do is to arrive at a tentative conclusion based on the evidence obtained using the criteria at hand.

VARIATIONS IN THE VIRULENCE OF RODENT PLASMODIAL STRAINS AFTER PASSAGE THROUGH TISSUE CULTURE

Weiss and DeGiusti (1964a,b, 1966) and Weiss (1965) have succeeded in modifying the virulence of a strain of *P. berghei* by passaging infected rat tissue through tissue culture containing heterologous serum. Infected rat bone marrow or liver were explanted into a medium containing lamb, calf, or hamster serum for 48 hours. The explants induced normal infections when implanted into rats. However, while they were still infective to mice, the strain was now distinctly less virulent in mice than was the parent strain or than was a control strain maintained in tissue culture in the presence of homologous rat serum. Survival times of mice receiving the modified strain were longer than in controls receiving the parent strain. After several serial passages from rat to culture to rat, 80 percent of the recipient mice recovered and were resistant to reinoculation. Furthermore, they also resisted exposure to the virulent parent strain.

Following a long series of passages through rats, the virulence of the modified strain reverted to that of the parent strain.

Exposure to heterologous serum in tissue culture may have suppressed certain antigenic variants within the original antigenically heterogeneous population of plasmodia. Antigens responsible for virulence may have characterized the variants which were suppressed. Alternatively, the modified strain may have consisted of a variant containing more protection-inducing antigenic groupings than the parent strain. The antigenic comparison of the parent and variant strains may help to resolve this question.

CROSS-IMMUNE REACTIONS AMONG STRAINS AND SPECIES

Complete cross-immunity has been recorded between strains of *P. berghei*, even though certain biologic differences (for example, the production of gametocytes) have been noted between them (Fabiani and Fulchiron, 1952; Krishnaswami et al., 1953).

In contrast, cross-immunity between species of rodent plasmodia has not been reported, except in the problematical case of *P. chabaudi* and *P. vinckei*, discussed below. Thus, *P. vinckei* and *P. berghei* do not cross-protect, and mice recovered from the former are completely susceptible to the latter (Rodhain, 1953a, 1954b; Fabiani and Orfila, 1959, 1961). Similar results were obtained in a hamster and a fruit bat (Rodhain, 1953a). Rats of varying age which had recovered from *P. berghei* were completely susceptible to *P. vinckei* (Rodhain, 1954a, b). Fabiani and Orfila (1961) recorded feeble protection against *P. berghei* in 7 out of 21 rats recovered from *P. vinckei*, but Garnham (1962), commenting on this result, was of the opinion that it "did not invalidate Rodhain's opinion that immunologically *P. berghei* and *P. vinckei* behave as different species." Thus, the biologic characteristic of lack of cross-protection has been used as a criterion in establishing the specific status of the two organisms.

The fact that mice with chronic *P. chabaudi* (which are completely susceptible to *P. berghei*) are highly resistant to *P. vinckei* (Nussenzweig et al., 1966) does not fit the above pattern. The following facts may shed light on this problem. A feature which was originally thought to distinguish *P. chabaudi* from *P. vinckei* is the relatively low mortality rate of the former in mice. In a recent study by Ott and Stauber (1966), mice infected with *P. chabaudi* from two different sources were found to harbor a concomitant infection with *Eperythrozoon coccoides*. In this situation, *P. chabaudi* infections were mild and mortality low. However, when *E. coccoides* was eliminated by chemotherapy, leaving the plasmodial strain uncontaminated, *P. chabaudi* was now found to produce fulminating fatal infections in mice, indistinguishable from those of *P. vinckei*. It is possible that the strains of *P. chabaudi* isolated in Africa were uniformly associated with *E. coccoides*. Landau, who described *P. chabaudi* in 1965, now considers it possible that this parasite may prove to be a subspecies of *P. vinckei* (Landau and Killick-Kendrick, 1966). Were this so, the positive cross-protection between the two (being intraspecific) would not contrast with the lack of cross-protection between *P. berghei* and *P. vinckei* (which is interspecific). It may be relevant that the disc electrophoretic pattern of *P. vinckei* is similar but not identical to that of a sample of *P. chabaudi* (Spira and Zuckerman, 1966).

Newer methods of antigenic analysis of the rodent plasmodia have included fluorescent-antibody, hemagglutination, and immunoelectrophoresis techniques. Cross-reactions between *P. berghei* and *P. vinckei* have been demonstrated using the fluorescent-antibody technique (Voller, 1964a) and the hemagglutination technique (Bray, 1965). While these tests indicate the fact that certain antigens are shared by the two species, it has repeatedly been emphasized that the antibody being demonstrated by them in such comparisons may be associated with other plasmodial antigens and not necessarily with the antigen which induces protection (Voller, 1964a,b; Bray, 1965; Desowitz et al., 1966).

Comparison of *P. berghei* with *P. vinckei* by immunoelectrophoresis (Zuckerman, 1964a; Zuckerman and Spira, 1965) also demonstrated the fact that most of their antigens are shared. However, each of the two plasmodia has at least one precipitinogen not shared by the other. Hosts can recover from infection with each of the two plasmodial species, and protective antibody against the homologous parasite must therefore be produced. If the antigen inducing the production of protective antibody were *shared*, the two species would be expected to cross-protect. Since they do not cross-protect, the *unshared* antigens demonstrated by immunoelectrophoresis are in each case suspected of being those which induce the formation of species-specific protective antibody.

A soluble antigen of *P. knowlesi* in the plasma of infected monkeys protected rats against *P. berghei* (Cox, 1966).

HUMORAL ASPECTS OF IMMUNITY TO THE RODENT MALARIAS

Serum proteins during infection

The recovery of rats from *P. berghei* is associated with a rise in serum euglobulins (Fabiani et al., 1952b; de Smet, 1955). Corradetti et al. (1954a, 1955) reported that it is the gamma-globulin level which rises, while the total serum nitrogen remains relatively constant. The rise in gamma-globulin during the infection of rats with *P. berghei* was confirmed by Ciuca et al. (1964) and by Isfan and Ianco (1964). The rise in serum globulins was even more striking in infected *Cricetomys* than in rats (de Smet, 1955).

Woodruff (1957) noted that the gamma-globulin titer in the sera of rats with *P. berghei* was further augmented by reinoculation. He took this fact to mean that the rise in gamma-globulin is at least in part due to the formation of antiplasmodial antibody. Causse-Vaills et al. (1961) considered the pro-

804   IMMUNITY IN MAMMALIAN HOSTS

tective antibody to be associated with the beta- and gamma-globulin fractions of the serum.

Sadun et al. (1965) state that there is little change in the serum protein pattern of untreated mice succumbing to *P. berghei*. On the other hand, the amount of gamma-globulins increased in the serum of *P. berghei*-infected mice which had been cured with the aid of 8-aminoquinolines; and, as in rats, the gamma-globulin titer was augmented by reinoculation (Box and Gingrich, 1958). Similarly, challenge was accompanied by a marked gamma-globulin response in mice in which *P. berghei* was reduced to a chronic state with the aid of primaquine (Briggs et al., 1960). Finally, both beta- and gamma-globulin titers rose in NMRI mice surviving infection with *P. berghei* (Gail and Kretschmar, 1965).

While there is general agreement that gamma-globulins rise in the course of recovery of rodents from infection with *P. berghei*, we do not yet know what proportion of this augmented gamma-globulin represents antiplasmodial antibody, nor do we know what proportion of the plasmodial antibody is protective. The urgent need for defining these proportions and for specifically distinguishing protective antibody from among the total array of antiplasmodial antibodies has been pointed out and reiterated by many (Jeffery et al., 1964; Schindler, 1965; Voller, 1964a,b; Gail and Kretschmar, 1965; Schindler and Mehlitz, 1965; Sodeman and Jeffery, 1965; Desowitz et al., 1966).

Demonstration of antiplasmodial antibody

Methods for demonstrating antiplasmodial antibody have recently been reviewed (Tobie, 1964; Zuckerman and Ristic, 1966). Those dealing with the rodent malarias include both the older immunologic techniques and the more recent ones, some of which, such as the fluorescent-antibody technique, hemagglutination and immunoelectrophoresis, are discussed below. There they are viewed as tools in exploring the antigenic structure of the rodent plasmodia. Shifting our point of view, we may here consider the same studies as demonstrations of the presence of antiplasmodial antibody with the aid of plasmodial antigen. Where a specific relationship exists between two molecules, as between antigen and antibody, the study of one is linked at every point with the study of the other.

Complement-fixing antibody was found in the sera of rats with *P. berghei* at and after crisis and well into latency (Vargues et al., 1951). In this study an extract of ground infected rat liver served as antigen (Vargues, 1951). Similar results were recorded using as antigen a frozen and thawed preparation of parasites from infected rat blood freed from their erythrocyte hosts by lysis and tryptic digestion (Pautrizel and Nguyen Vinh Nien, 1953). Reactions to a high titer were obtained with the sera of hyperimmune rats. But Schindler (1965) and Schindler and Mehlitz (1965) have pointed out the fact that complement-fixing antibody against *P. berghei* in NMRI mice, detectable throughout infection, is not protective antibody. In the older literature on malarial immunology (*see* Taliaferro, 1949, for a review), the complement-fixing reaction was already recognized as a group- rather than a species-specific reaction, while protective antibody is species-specific.

A nonprotective anti-*P. berghei* antibody present in the sera of normal mice but not of normal rats was demonstrated by the fluorescent-antibody technique (Sodeman and Jeffery, 1965). The same technique served to detect an antigen-antibody complex occurring *in vivo* in rats with *P. berghei* (Kreier and Ristic, 1964).

Antiplasmodial antibody has also been demonstrated in rodent malaria by double diffusion in gel (Zuckerman et al., 1965b). Precipitins were found in the sera of rats with *P. berghei* throughout initial infection and latency, beginning several days before crisis. Titers rose following superinfection, and particularly following the immunization of rats with a cell-free extract of *P. berghei* before challenge with viable parasites. The precipitins were specifically anti-*P. berghei*, and did not react with extracts of *P. vinckei* (Goberman and Zuckerman, 1966). Cox (1966) has also employed double diffusion in gel to demonstrate anti-rodent-plasmodial antibody.

Passive transfer of immunity

The host-parasite combination of choice in the study of protective antibody must obviously be comprised of a parasite yielding a perceptible parasitemia in a host which recovers from infection. Fulminating infections are barred, since the given host is unable to protect itself against the given plasmodium, and is therefore unlikely to be a good producer of protective antibody against it. At the other extreme, infections which can scarcely establish themselves in the face of highly efficient innate immune mechanisms are unlikely to induce a marked specific acquired immune response before they are eradicated.

The laboratory model most extensively used in studying protective antibody in the rodent malarias has therefore been *P. berghei* in the rat. The sera of rats with *P. berghei* collected after parasitic crisis were only slightly protective in uninfected rats; while sera from hyperimmune rats after numerous superinfections had a marked suppressive effect. A daily series of doses of hyperimmune serum retarded the onset of patency by several days, but it did not prevent parasitemia from eventually developing (Fabiani and Fulchiron, 1953a; Fabiani and Orfila, 1956).

Similar protection against *P. berghei* was afforded to infected mice by hyperimmune rat serum (Martin et al., 1966). However, despite a significant delay in the onset of patency, treated mice eventually succumbed to high parasitemia (Briggs et al., 1966). The protective effect of the immune rat serum in mice was a function of the number of superinfections to which the serum donor had been exposed (Briggs et al., 1966). In contrast to the sera of infected rats, those of infected mice were nonprotective (Fabiani, 1954a).

Causse-Vaills et al. (1961) reported that protection was associated with the beta- and gamma-globulin fractions of immune rat serum, and not with the alpha-globulin fraction or the albumin fraction.

Another instance of the passive transfer of protection against a rodent plasmodium concerns an entirely different type of mechanism. Sera from uninfected adult rabbits inoculated into rats or mice delayed the onset of *P. berghei* parasitemia (Fabiani and Orfila, 1958). Such sera also killed *P. berghei in vitro*. This antiplasmodial effect is obviously due to an innate factor in rabbit serum and is not associated with acquired immunity, which presupposes previous contact with the parasite. In an ingenious experiment in which a certain number of rabbit erythrocytes introduced into the peritoneum of an infected mouse became infected with *P. berghei*, the authors demonstrated that the resistance of the rabbit to this parasite is due to the destructive serum factor rather than to the inability of the rabbit erythrocyte to support the growth of *P. berghei*.

Congenital passage of protective antibody

A special case of the passive transfer of antiplasmodial antibody in the rodent malarias is the passage of antibody from mother to offspring, either transplacentally or via the milk. Female rats hyperimmune to *P. berghei* during gestation gave birth to litters relatively resistant to infection (Bruce-Chwatt, 1954; Bruce-Chwatt and Gibson, 1956). The protective factor was transferred chiefly, but not exclusively, through the milk, which was proved by interchanging litters between immune and normal female rats. The measure of protection transmitted in this way was very considerable. Bruce-Chwatt (1963), reviewing the rodent malarias as part of the general field of congenital passive transfer of immunity in malaria, emphasized the point that the more immune the rat mother, the more effective the passive transfer of protective antibody to the offspring.

These results were essentially confirmed by Serguiev and Demina (1957), by Demina (1958), by Radicovici et al. (1958), and by Isfan and Ianco (1964). Terry (1956) also confirmed the protection conferred on the offspring of immune mother rats, but he pointed out that this protection gradually disappeared a few weeks after the litters were weaned. He also observed that feeding immune rat serum to newborn rats had a protective effect against *P. berghei* until the litters were weaned but not thereafter, when weanling rats cease to be capable of absorbing antibody through the gut wall.

Kretschmar (1962) and Gail and Kretschmar (1965) noted that sterile residual immunity retained by NMRI mice following the eradication of *P. berghei* was not transmitted to their offspring either via the placenta or via the milk. Similarly, mice radically cured of *P. vinckei* with the aid of chloroquine or mepacrine, while themselves resistant to reinoculation, were unable to transmit this sterile immunity to their offspring (F. E. G. Cox, 1965). On the other hand, Adler and Foner (1965) immunized mice against an avirulent strain of *P. vinckei*, then exposed them to a virulent strain. Their direct offspring, as well as foster offspring fed by immune mothers, were relatively resistant, and 34 percent of them survived challenge infection.

Neutralization test

In view of the growing concern with defining and characterizing protective antibody, the advantages which a neutralization test could confer on malarial research are self-evident. Considering the ease with which the rodent malarias are manipulated in the laboratory, it is natural that such a test should have been sought for them. However, an effective neutralization test for a rodent plasmodium is not yet available.

Schindler (1965) exposed *P. berghei* isolated from mouse red cells to NMRI mouse serum with a high complement-fixing titer. The parasites' viability was not affected by contact with the antiserum.

It is necessary to be on guard against antierythrocyte antibody in designing a possible neutralization test. Cox (1964a), for instance, found that incubating rat or mouse blood infected with *P. berghei* with homologous antiserum against normal rat or mouse erythrocytes, respectively, destroyed the viability of the parasites. Similarly, Zuckerman et al. (1966) first worked with anti-*P. berghei* rat serum obtained following the inoculation of infected mouse blood. Mouse erythrocytes infected with *P. berghei* incubated with such immune anti-*P. berghei* rat serum were no longer infective when inoculated intraperitoneally into mice, but were infective if inoculated intravenously. Exposure of infected mouse erythrocytes to anti-mouse erythrocyte rat serum had the same effect. In contrast, exposure *in vitro* of infected rat erythrocytes to homologous rat antiserum was ineffective, and such parasites were viable even if inoculated intraperitoneally in mice. The rat antiserum obtained using an inoculum of mouse blood apparently contained anti-mouse-erythrocyte opsonin, but was not directly parasiticidal. Phagocytosis of the infected mouse erythrocytes was therefore induced in the peritoneum, but parasites directly introduced into the blood stream by-passed the phagocytic peritoneal barrier, and they were capable of invading clean, unopsonized red cells in the circulation. In fact, despite the negative results of the intraperitoneal inoculation of infected mouse blood after exposure to immune rat serum, the rat serum had not been parasiticidal *in vitro*.

CELLULAR ASPECTS OF IMMUNITY TO THE RODENT MALARIAS

Importance of the lymphoid-macrophage system

From the very beginning of research on the defense mechanisms in rodent malarias, the crucial importance of the lymphoid-macrophage system, and particularly of the spleen, has been recognized (Corradetti, 1950). This is

directly in line with defense reactions in other malarias (Taliaferro, 1949.)
Cellular and humoral defenses are interrelated. Thus, not only is phagocytosis, the chief mechanism of defense, carried out by cellular elements of the
blood-filtering organs, the macrophages, and their precursors, but also the
specific humoral factors in defense, the antibodies, are products of the same
cell lines. Elements of the lymphoid-macrophage system are therefore essential in establishing and maintaining acquired immunity to the rodent malarias (Zuckerman and Yoeli, 1951). In the *establishment* of acquired immunity, the spleen has generally been considered indispensable; but in its
maintenance the spleen can sometimes be dispensed with, and other lymphoid-macrophage elements may take over its functions (Zuckerman, 1953;
Fabiani and Fulchiron, 1954b; Fabiani, 1954a).

Splenomegaly was soon recognized as a characteristic of the immune
process in rodent malaria, as in other malarias (Vincke and Lips, 1948).
Ramakrishnan (1952) observed progressive enlargement of the rat spleen in
P. berghei infections. At and after crisis, the enlarged spleen was about 10
times normal size. It regressed during latency, though it remained somewhat
enlarged for months. Splenomegaly occurred in infected mice as well, but was
less marked in them. Similar results in rats and mice infected with *P. berghei*
were observed by Sergent and Poncet (1955a), and in rats with *P. berghei*
by Cox et al. (1966) and George et al. (1966). Infected rat spleens which
reached 20 times the normal size at the height of splenomegaly have been
observed (Zuckerman et al., 1964; Zuckerman, 1966). In mice, a large proportion of the observed splenomegaly is due to the proliferation of hematopoietic tissue (Singer, 1954c; Kretschmar and Jerusalem, 1963). Some, but
very much less, hematopoiesis is also observed in the infected rat spleen
(Zuckerman, 1966), in which hypertrophy of lymphoid-macrophage elements is marked.

Phagocytosis is the means by which infected red cells are removed from
the circulation by macrophages in the primary blood filters, particularly the
spleen and liver (Singer, 1954c; Jerusalem, 1964; Kretschmar, 1964;
Schroeder et al., 1965; Cox et al., 1966; Zuckerman, 1966). Such phagocytosis is particularly marked at and after crisis (Corradetti and Rigoli, 1963;
Zuckerman, 1966). Parasites exposed to other phagocytes in the presence of
antibody are also promptly engulfed. Thus, *P. berghei*, inoculated intraperitoneally into hyperimmune rats, underwent intense phagocytosis by peritoneal macrophages (Fabiani and Fulchiron, 1953b).

Depressing the function of the lymphoid-macrophage system in rats with
P. berghei, e.g., by hypoxia (Hughes and Tatum, 1956), led to intensification
of infection.

Effect of splenectomy on rodent malaria

When the spleen of an animal is extirpated, a large population of
lymphoid-macrophage cells is removed from the body, and the animal, if
healthy, is capable of surviving the operation indefinitely. This operation

therefore enables the investigator to reduce the extent of the lymphoid-macrophage system significantly though not eliminating it. As a result, it is possible to study the importance of this system in various disease states.

For example, the effect of splenectomy on the immunity of a variety of hosts to the rodent malarias has been extensively studied. The early literature was reviewed by Thurston (1953).

The timing of splenectomy with respect to that of initial exposure to the parasite affects the outcome of the infection. For instance, *P. berghei* causes a mild infection in the intact cotton rat; but if the cotton rat is splenectomized before inoculation, the infection subsequently induced is severe and often fatal (Rodhain, 1949, 1951). The same is true of the adult rat with *P. berghei* (Galliard and Lapierre, 1950; Fabiani and Fulchiron, 1954a; Zuckerman and Yoeli, 1954; Spira and Zuckerman, 1965); of the vole, *Microtus guentheri*, with *P. berghei* (Zuckerman, 1953); of the spiny mouse, *Acomys cahirinus*, with *P. berghei* (Beer, 1961); and of the rat with *P. vinckei* (Fabiani et al., 1958). However, in contrast to the consensus, Satya Prakash (1961) found that splenectomized rats were no more susceptible to *P. berghei* than were intact rats.

Splenectomy performed later, during latency, induces relapses of *P. berghei* of varying severity. Death may ensue, or a protracted chronic state may be established, depending on the degree of immunity which the individual host has acquired by the time the spleen is removed. In general, the longer the latent period before splenectomy, the better the chances of survival after the operation, as measured either by the severity of the relapses induced by splenectomy or as measured by resistance to reinoculation (Rodhain, 1949, 1951, for the cotton rat; Galliard and Lapierre, 1950; Fabiani et al., 1951, 1952a, b; Fabiani and Fulchiron, 1954b; Fabiani, 1954b; Corradetti and Verolini, 1960, for the rat; Zuckerman and Yoeli, 1951, and Zuckerman, 1953, for the vole). NMRI mice with latent *P. berghei* suffered severe relapses and numerous deaths after splenectomy (Kretschmar, 1963a). Mice surviving *P. berghei* infection with the aid of drugs and then splenectomized during latency succumbed following challenge (Box and Gingrich, 1958). Mice (Fabiani and Orfila, 1959) and rats (Fabiani et al., 1957) splenectomized after recovering from *P. vinckei* also succumbed to fatal relapse.

Whereas the intact rat with a chronic *P. berghei* infection is capable ultimately of achieving latency, the chronically infected splenectomized rat is unable to do so (Carrescia and Negroni, 1954; Zuckerman and Yoeli, 1954; Satya Prakash, 1961; Spira and Zuckerman, 1961; Cantrell and Moss, 1963; Martin et al., 1966). The splenectomized NMRI mouse with *P. berghei* is also unable to suppress chronic infection to latency (Kretschmar and Jerusalem, 1963). The same is true of the splenectomized mouse with *P. vinckei* (F. E. G. Cox, 1965). While this is generally true of voles as well, a few cases are on record in which voles achieved radical cure after many months of chronic infection (Zuckerman, 1953).

Removal of the spleen therefore interferes greatly with the acquisition of immunity in the rodent malarias, as well as with the maintenance of the infection at the suppressed latent level.

When no relapse follows splenectomy, the host is considered by most authors to have totally eradicated the infection at the time of the operation. This situation arises in rats with *P. berghei* about 50 days after the termination of the primary attack (Corradetti, 1950, 1952, 1955; Corradetti and Verolini, 1957), in voles (*Microtus guentheri*) after about 30 days (Zuckerman and Yoeli, 1951), and in NMRI mice late in latency (Kretschmar, 1963a). The fact that such nonrelapsing hosts develop low-grade chronic infections on reinoculation, despite the absence of their spleens, has been interpreted as indicating that they possess a measure of sterile immunity following cure (Corradetti, 1950, 1955; Zuckerman, 1953; Corradetti and Verolini, 1957; Kretschmar, 1963a). Since the spleen is absent, other elements of the lymphoid-macrophage system must be responsible for this partially immune state.

The adult rabbit, even if splenectomized, is quite insusceptible to *P. berghei* (Fabiani and Orfila, 1958). Similarly, the splenectomized spiny mouse, *Acomys cahirinus*, is refractory to *P. vinckei* (Beer, 1961).

Paradoxically, infection rates in some splenectomized rodents tend to be lower than those in their intact counterparts (mice: Singer, 1954a; Fabiani and Orfila, 1955a; Lapierre et al., 1958; and young rats: Zuckerman and Yoeli, 1954; Cantrell and Moss, 1963; Spira and Zuckerman, 1965). However, despite lower parasitemias, mortality rates were not reduced in such splenectomized animals. Singer (1954a) has suggested that in the mouse the suppression of parasitemia following splenectomy may be due to the fact that the infected mouse spleen is a locus of intense erythropoiesis. Removal of the spleen therefore eliminates an important source of reticulocytes, which are the host cells preferentially invaded by *P. berghei* merozoites. Fabiani and Orfila (1955a) found that the reticulocytic response to the anemia of infection was indeed suppressed in splenectomized mice.

Abnormal parasites with a reduced number of nuclear divisions, with augmented accumulation of malarial pigment, and with poorly staining cytoplasm ("crisis forms") have been described in unusually high numbers in splenectomized rodents with *P. berghei* (rats: Satya Prakash, 1961; Spira and Zuckerman, 1961, 1965; and spiny mice: Beer, 1961). Crisis forms were interpreted as parasites which had been injured but not destroyed as merozoites in transit through the plasma from one erythrocyte to another. Such injured forms, relatively promptly filtered out of the blood stream in the intact animal, tend to circulate for longer periods after the spleen, a primary blood filter, has been removed (Spira and Zuckerman, 1965).

In contrast to splenectomy, adrenalectomy cannot be tolerated by the rat infected with *P. berghei*, and adrenalectomized infected rats die within a matter of days (Fabiani and Izzo, 1952). The same is true of malarious mice (Fabiani and Orfila, 1955b).

Anemia and hematopoiesis during rodent plasmodial infection

Since plasmodia attack and destroy erythrocytes, anemia is obviously a factor in the pathology of malaria. In addition, numerous erythrocytes, in excess of those invaded by plasmodia, are destroyed in the course of many malarial infections (reviewed by Zuckerman, 1963, 1964b, 1966). In response to the anemia of malaria, erythropoiesis is stimulated both in the bone marrow and ectopically at other sites. Reticulocytosis in the circulating blood ensues. Certain plasmodia exhibit a marked preference for invading erythrocytes of a strictly delimited age (Zuckerman, 1957). The temporal interplay of the three variables, anemia, compensatory reticulocytosis, and the age of invaded erythrocytes, has a definite and sometimes a decisive bearing on the susceptibility of a given host to a given plasmodium. This complex of problems has been extensively investigated in the rodent malarias.

The anemia induced by an attack of rodent malaria is conspicuously in excess of that attributable to parasitic sporulation. This has been shown for *P. berghei* in mice (Greenberg and Coatney, 1954; Jerusalem, 1964; Kretschmar, 1964), *P. berghei* in rats (Zuckerman, 1957; Cox et al., 1965; George et al., 1966), and *P. vinckei* in rats (Zuckerman, 1958). Anemia, with its attendant anoxia, rather than overwhelming parasitemia, is often the direct cause of death in the rodent malarias.

The excessive anemia observed in the rodent malarias is correlated with the removal of great numbers of unparasitized as well as parasitized erythrocytes from the circulation by erythrophagocytosis. This occurs in the blood-filtering organs of the lymphoid-macrophage system, primarily but not exclusively in the spleen (Kretschmar and Jerusalem, 1963; Jerusalem, 1964, 1965; Kretschmar, 1964; Zuckerman et al., 1964; Cox et al., 1965, 1966; Zuckerman, 1966). The immediate cause of this extensive erythrophagocytosis is discussed below on pp. 812-815.

As in other malarias, the bone marrow is stimulated by anemia to compensatory erythropoiesis (Corradetti and Rigoli, 1961). In addition, ectopic erythropoiesis is very conspicuous in the infected mouse spleen (Singer, 1954c; Kretschmar and Jerusalem, 1963), and it has also been observed in the infected rat spleen, but to a much more limited extent than in mice (Zuckerman, 1966). In rats the liver is an important locus of extramedullary erythropoiesis (Corradetti and Rigoli, 1961). Compensatory circulating reticulocytosis is the product of such stimulated erythropoiesis.

Splenectomy of the malarious mouse removes an important potential site of ectopic erythropoiesis. Circulating reticulocytosis is thereby suppressed (Fabiani and Orfila, 1955a; Kretschmar and Jerusalem, 1963). This has been interpreted as the reason for the lower parasitemias observed in splenectomized mice with *P. berghei* as compared with intact ones (Singer, 1954a; Kretschmar and Jerusalem, 1963). The fact that mortality rates were not lowered despite the suppression of parasitemia again demonstrates that the direct cause of death in the rodent malarias is not necessarily overwhelming parasitemia.

P. berghei has a very marked preference for invading reticulocytes (Zuckerman, 1957; Kretschmar, 1964). Consequently, circulating reticulocytosis in rodents with *P. berghei* enhances the intensity of early parasitemia during the period when only innate immune mechanisms are available to control the infection (Zuckerman, 1957; Corradetti and Rigoli, 1961). However, when acquired immune mechanisms supervene, most sporulating merozoites are filtered out of the blood before they can invade new host cells. It follows that reticulocytosis after crisis no longer endangers the host.

The timing of the reticulocytic response *vis-à-vis* that of the acquisition of immunity plays an important role. Compensatory reticulocytosis begins in rats of all ages about a week after inoculation with *P. berghei*. Acquired immunity (parasitic crisis) develops after about a week in adult rats, but it is delayed until at least the end of the second week in immature rats. In young rats, augmented numbers of reticulocytes are therefore exposed to and freely invaded by plasmodia for about a week before effective acquired immunity suppresses the invasion of clean host cells. This delay in the development of acquired immunity in the young as compared to the mature rat therefore constitutes a factor in the age immunity of the rat to *P. berghei* (Zuckerman, 1957). That it is not the only factor governing age immunity in rodent malaria is attested by the observation that rats also have a clear age immunity to *P. vinckei*, which invades all available erythrocytes at random, and is therefore not likely to be exclusively governed by compensatory reticulocytosis (Zuckerman, 1958).

Manipulating reticulocytosis by extraneous means directly affects parasitemia. Thus, enhancing initial reticulocytosis by treatment with phenylhydrazine (Singer, 1954a) or with anti-mouse-erythrocyte rabbit serum (Schwink, 1960) intensifies parasitemia in the mouse with *P. berghei* without reducing survival time. Activating latent bartonellosis in rats by splenectomy induces reticulocytosis which, in turn, intensifies *P. berghei* parasitemia (Fabiani et al., 1952a; Hsu and Geiman, 1952). In contrast, treatment of the *P. berghei* infected mouse (Singer, 1954b) or the *P. berghei* infected rat (Jackson, 1955) with cortisone suppresses both reticulocytosis and parasitemia, and prolongs the survival time. Again, lower parasitemia is not associated with a lower mortality rate in the cortisone-treated rat (*see also* pp. 818-819).

THE CASE FOR AUTOIMMUNIZATION IN RODENT MALARIA

The excessive anemia associated with plasmodial infections is apparently a fundamental feature of malarial pathology, since it has been observed in avian, simian, and human malarias, as well as in the rodent malarias (reviewed in Zuckerman, 1964b, 1966). Several possible mechanisms were suggested in the above reviews to account for this excessive destruction of erythrocytes, none of which necessarily excludes the others. These hypotheses are: (1) the coating of normal circulating erythrocytes with soluble parasitic antigen, (2) the sharing of antigen by erythrocytes and plasmodia, (3) the production of tissue lysins, (4) the effect of hypersplenism, and (5) an autoimmunization of the host against its own erythrocytes, possibly antigenically altered after having harbored plasmodia. A body of evidence relating to this problem has been accumulated using the rodent malarias as test cases.

It is noteworthy that several features of the excessive anemia in rodent malaria suggest that it is governed by an immune mechanism, and any postulated explanation should take account of this point (Zuckerman, 1966). For example, Singer (1954b) and Kretschmar (1965b) showed that treatment of P. berghei infected mice with cortisone, which is known to depress immune functions in general, leads to partial suppression of anemia. Moreover, splenectomy of the rat with P. berghei delays but does not cancel excessive blood loss (Spira and Zuckerman, 1961, 1965). Excessive anemia might thus be one of the immune functions of the spleen eliminated by splenectomy but later taken over by other elements of the lymphoid-macrophage system. A third line of evidence concerns the fact that the stimulated erythrophagocytosis in the lymphoid-macrophage system is apparently the direct cause of the excessive anemia in rats with P. berghei (Zuckerman et al., 1964; Cox et al., 1965, 1966; Zuckerman, 1966). All types of circulating erythrocytes, parasitized and unparasitized, are engulfed. In fact, the latter greatly outnumber the former. The entire erythron of the infected rat thus behaves as if it were sensitized. Kretschmar (1964, 1965b) and Jerusalem (1964, 1965) considered the excessive anemia of NMRI mice with P. berghei to be an immune phenomenon associated with stimulated erythrocytosis in the spleen and other blood-filtering organs. In this case infected polychromatophile erythrocytes were preferred, but mature and uninfected erythrocytes were also engulfed. They referred to the mechanism as one of "autoaggression."

The hypothesis of autoimmunization, around which most of the discussion has centered, has been challenged as unnecessarily complicated and speculative. Since spleen size increases during infection (see p. 808), the possibility was suggested that nonspecific hypersplenism may contribute to the anemia of malaria (Kretschmar and Jerusalem, 1963; Zuckerman, 1964b, 1966). In view of the fact that autoimmune antibody had not been unequivocally demonstrated, George et al. (1966) took the stand that the hemolytic anemia of rats with P. berghei could be explained exclusively on the basis of hypersplenism "without an autoimmune component."

However, the experimental demonstration of autoimmune antibodies now invalidates the charge that an autoimmune component in the excessive anemia of rodent malaria is merely speculative. This demonstration has had a checkered career. The erythrocytes of rats with P. berghei were first shown at the peak of the excessive anemia to be Coombs-positive (Zuckerman, 1960), and this was thought to be compatible with an autoimmune hypothesis. This observation was confirmed for rats with P. vinckei (Zuckerman and Spira, 1961). However, in the same study, the reticulocyte per se in uninfected rats also proved to be Coombs-positive. Since peak anemia in the rodent malarias was always accompanied by reticulocytosis, the positive Coombs test in this situation was equivocal: it could be demonstrating autoantibody, reticulocytes, or both.

Although the Coombs test as an indicator only of autoantibody could not serve during reticulocytosis, the autoantibody hypothesis was not ruled out. Even assuming their sequestration for a time, reticulocytes are not all doomed to destruction in the blood-filtering organs, since if they were, there could be no recovery from reticulocytic states. Inasmuch as the excessive anemia of rodent malaria reflects the destruction of vast numbers of erythrocytes, some sensitizing mechanism which prepares them for destruction is logically indicated. This mechanism could be coating with autoantibody (Zuckerman, 1963).

Cox et al. (1965, 1966) have demonstrated the agglutination of trypsin-treated normal rat erythrocytes by the serum of some but not all rats with *P. berghei.* They found a correlation in time among the presence of autohemagglutinin, erythrophagocytosis, and anemia, and they suggested that a causal relationship might exist among these factors. Kreier et al. (1966), also working with trypsinized autologous and homologous rat erythrocytes, have demonstrated an autohemagglutinin produced in rats during infections with *P. berghei.* The antibody, a cold agglutinin, can be eluted from the erythrocytes of infected rats at 37°C. It occurs in all rats studied at the time of anemia, after crisis, during the chronic state, and early in latency. The following features are identical for the appearance of autohemagglutinin (Kreier et al., 1966) and for stimulated erythrophagocytosis in rats with *P. berghei* (Zuckerman, 1966):

1. They became positive early in patency and remain positive throughout patency.
2. They reach their peaks at peak anemia, which is near or after peak parasitemia.
3. They return to normal levels rather rapidly with the onset of latency.

Any explanation of excessive anemia in the rodent malarias must take into account the fact that it frequently is most marked when parasitemias are declining or even negligible (Zuckerman, 1957, 1958, 1966; Cox et al., 1966). The fact that excessive anemia and erythrophagocytosis wane as latency progresses has been interpreted in the framework of the autoimmune hypothesis as due to the gradual disappearance of autoantigen and, consequently, of autoantibody. Thus, as plasmodia are suppressed by acquired antiplasmodial immunity, they would cease to induce the changes in the constituents of their host erythrocytes which are recognized by the antibody-forming cells as "non-self" antigens (Cox et al., 1966; Zuckerman, 1966).

With the demonstration of autoimmune antibody, the chief obstacle to accepting autoimmunity as a factor contributing to rodent malarial anemia is removed. As pointed out above, another such factor may be hypersplenism. It is impossible at the present state of our knowledge to quantitate the contributions of either. Motulsky et al. (1958) have pointed out that the damage caused by erythrocytic stasis in a hypersplenic spleen may be aggravated by sensitization of the erythrocytes.

Soluble parasitic antigen has been demonstrated in the sera of malarious rodents (Cox, 1966). Cox believes that this type of soluble antigen may be "toxic" to erythrocytes and may contribute to the anemia of malaria.

In the light of all the above, several factors may contribute to rodent malarial anemia:

1. parasitic sporulation;
2. a specific autoimmune component, an autohemagglutinin;
3. a possible nonspecific, hypersplenic component;
4. a possible component due to soluble antigen "toxic" to erythrocytes, whose mode of action is still conjectural.

In the case of factor 1, the erythrocytes are presumably destroyed intravascularly, and the debris filtered out in the lymphoid-macrophage system. In the cases of factors 2 and 3, the mechanism of destruction appears to be erythrophagocytosis in the lymphoid-macrophage system.

There is no evidence that tissue lysins or the sharing of antigen by erythrocytes and plasmodia contribute to the anemia of rodent malaria.

ANTIGENIC ANALYSIS OF THE RODENT PLASMODIA

Several analytic techniques have been applied to the study of the antigenic constitution of plasmodia in recent years. Among a series of avian and mammalian parasites, the rodent plasmodia have also been tested either in exploring individual antigenic compositions or in studying cross-reactions among species or strains (see pp. 802-803, and a review by Zuckerman and Ristic, 1968).

The first of the newer analytic techniques applied to the rodent malarias was the fluorescent-antibody test (FA) (Brooke et al., 1959). Films of rat blood infected with P. berghei were flooded with hyperimmune rat serum conjugated with fluorescein isocyanate. The parasites' cytoplasm fluoresced brilliantly against a vaguely visible background of erythrocytes. Voller (1962) confirmed this observation for a series of avian and mammalian plasmodia, including P. berghei. He also noted fluorescent stippling in the erythrocytes infected with P. berghei, and he considered these points to be foci of antigen in the host cell (see also Voller, 1964a). He found that P. berghei yielded weak cross-reactions with human and simian plasmodia. Voller (1964b) reviewed the contribution of the FA test to malarial research, with particular emphasis on cross-reactions among species. Such cross-reactions frequently occur, but are not proof of functional cross-immunity. This point was also emphasized by Jeffery et al. (1964).

Before any other analytic techniques could be applied, it was necessary to devise methods for obtaining antigenic material relatively uncontaminated with host-cell antigens in a standard and replicable manner. This problem has been approached in several ways (reviewed in Zuckerman and Ristic, 1968), and is still under active consideration. Chemical (saponin, DNase), immunochemical (hemolysin), and physical (osmotic lysis, French press) techniques have been employed in attempting to divest the plasmodium of its enveloping erythrocyte. The completely pure plasmodial product has yet to be prepared, but much information has been accumulated using the relatively crude products already available.

The hemagglutination technique was introduced into malariology by Desowitz and Stein (1962), using *P. berghei* and homologous rodent antiserum as test objects. This method was quickly applied to other mammalian malarias, including those of man (Stein and Desowitz, 1964; Bray, 1965; Desowitz, 1965; reviewed by Desowitz et al., 1966). One advantage of the method is the fact that very minute quantities of antigen suffice in carrying out the test. *P. berghei* antigen yielded low titer cross-reactions with antisera from malarious human beings, whereas tests employing homologous human plasmodial antigen and antibody yielded much higher titers. However, since *P. berghei* is obtainable with relative ease, Stein and Desowitz (1964) envisaged its use in routine testing for human malaria. They considered a low 1:400 titer of tanned erythrocytes coated with *P. berghei* antigen in human serum as indicative of malarial infection in the human serum donor. However, as pointed out above, a positive hemagglutination test does not necessarily indicate that the host has developed protective immunity.

In contrast, the relatively less sensitive gel-diffusion technique may be pointing towards this objective. When rat immune serum containing precipitins to *P. berghei* demonstrable by double diffusion in gel is adsorbed with cell-free extracts of *P. berghei* and *P. vinckei*, respectively, the precipitins are removed by the former but not by the latter, i.e., they arise in response to an unshared antigen (Goberman and Zuckerman, 1966). It was noted above that the unshared antigens of *P. berghei* and *P. vinckei* are suspected of being those inducing protection.

Electrophoretic separation of the components of plasmodial extracts is a further step in the direction of the analysis of each antigen as a separate entity. With some confidence we may hope ultimately to associate the protection-inducing property of each plasmodium with a given specific antigenic factor or factors. The more discriminating the separatory technique, the more precise will be this pinpointing.

Immunoelectrophoresis of a rodent plasmodium, *P. vinckei*, revealed the presence of 6 to 8 precipitinogens (Spira and Zuckerman, 1962). *P. berghei* proved to have a similar number (Banki and Bucci, 1964a, b), most of which were shared by the two rodent plasmodia (Zuckerman, 1964a; Zuckerman and Spira, 1965). The fact that each also contained species-specific precipitinogens was discussed above.

Disc electrophoresis can discriminate between protein components in a complex mixture with even greater precision than immunoelectrophoresis. Thus, cell-free preparations of *P. berghei* contain as many as 10 (Chavin, 1966) or even 14 or 15 distinct protein bands when contaminant host components are subtracted from the total array of proteins (Sodeman and Meuwissen, 1966; Spira and Zuckerman, 1966). The protein patterns obtained by these different groups of workers using this technique have been similar and replicable. *P. vinckei* contains a similar number of protein components (Spira and Zuckerman, 1966).

The antigenic analysis of strains of plasmodia, especially by disc electrophoresis, should be capable of shedding light on several current problems in the immunology of the rodent malarias:

1. Are relapse strains of rodent malaria antigenically distinct from the parent stock? (Cox, 1959, 1962).
2. Are strains of rodent malaria whose virulence has been modified by passage through tissue culture antigenically distinct from the parent stock? (Weiss and DeGiusti, 1964a,b).
3. Are strains of rodent malaria whose virulence has been modified by passage through an unusual vector antigenically distinct from the parent stock? (Raffaele, 1965).
4. What is the antigenic relationship between two rodent plasmodia with similar biologic characteristics? (Landau and Killick-Kendrick, 1966).

INFLUENCE OF INTRINSIC HOST FACTORS ON RESISTANCE TO THE RODENT PLASMODIA

The ability of a parasite to establish and maintain itself within a host species (i.e., the virulence of the parasite) does not depend exclusively on any single characteristic of either the parasite or the host, but is rather the resultant of a series of characteristics of both partners. The balance among these interacting factors is different and specific for each host-parasite combination. Varying any one of them (e.g., the age or the genetic constitution of the host, or the antigenic composition of the parasite) may affect the final balance struck between the two organisms.

The genetic constitution of the host is one of the factors affecting the virulence of a given strain of rodent plasmodium (reviewed by Bruce-Chwatt, 1965). For instance, infections with the same strain of *P. berghei* in a series of homozygous inbred lines of mouse varied in a constant manner with the mouse line employed (Greenberg et al., 1953; Greenberg and Coatney, 1954). Parasitemia levels, mortality rates, and survival times were the parameters measured. Hybridization experiments confirmed the view that the differences in susceptibility among inbred mouse lines are functions of their genetic constitutions (Greenberg and Kendrick, 1958).

Bruce-Chwatt (1965), reviewing information on the resistance of inbred mouse strains to *P. berghei*, pointed out that pure lines fall into several distinct and stable categories with regard to susceptibility, and that a number of genes probably act independently to determine susceptibility in each inbred line. An inbred mouse line with particularly low susceptibility to *P. berghei* is the NMRI line, more than 10 percent of which actually recover spontaneously (Kretschmar, 1962). The conclusions based on blood-induced infections were confirmed for sporozoite-induced infections of *P. berghei* in inbred mice (Most et al., 1966).

Though homozygous inbred strains of rat were not available for study, the selection of diverging lines with high and low susceptibilities to *P. vinckei* in the course of 16 generations of brother-and-sister matings strongly suggests that a genetic factor or factors is involved in the susceptibility of this host to this parasite (Zuckerman, 1968).

Host diet may have a decisive effect on resistance to the rodent plasmodia (reviewed by Zuckerman, 1968). Numerous corroborations have followed the demonstration that a milk diet attenuates *P. berghei* malaria (Maegraith et al., 1952), and that the suppressive factor is the absence of *p*-aminobenzoic acid (PABA) from milk (Hawking, 1953). Similar results were obtained with meat diets (Adler and Gunders, 1965). Mice normally succumbing to malaria can survive with low infections on a diet deficient in PABA, and at the same time they are capable of developing a measure of acquired immunity to reinfection (Schindler, 1965; Adler and Gunders, 1965; Kretschmar, 1965a; Schindler and Mehlitz, 1965).

INFLUENCE OF EXTRANEOUS FACTORS ON RESISTANCE TO THE RODENT PLASMODIA

In addition to intrinsic characteristics of the parasite and of the host, certain extraneous factors may affect the interplay between host and parasite (i.e., the resistance of the former to the latter). Such extraneous influences may be physical (irradiation), chemical (drug treatment), or biologic (intercurrent infection).

X-irradiation damages the erythropoietic system of the mouse (Singer, 1953) and of the rat (Verain and Verain, 1957) infected with *P. berghei*. The x-irradiated host therefore fails to produce the usual number of circulating reticulocytes to replace the erythrocytes destroyed during infection. If irradiation is done early in the infection, resultant parasitemias are low. The host is affected by the radiation and not the parasite, since parasites irradiated *in vitro* remain unaffected and viable (Verain and Verain, 1957).

Cortisone is known to inhibit the immune responses of numerous hosts to infectious agents, but its effect in rodent malaria is debatable. In confirmation of its ability to inhibit immunity, Findlay and Howard (1952) and Fabiani and Orfila (1955b) found that cortisone exacerbated *P. berghei* infections in mice. Parasitemias were higher and more rapidly fatal in their treated mice, and spleens were smaller than in untreated controls, suggesting inhibition of the usual cellular response.

It is, however, noteworthy that certain other experiments do not verify the depressing effect of cortisone on the host's immunity to rodent malaria. Fulton (1954) gave cortisone to both rats and mice infected with *P. berghei* and in nearly all cases observed no intensification of infection, although he found the drug to be very toxic. Roberts (1954a) obtained similar results with mice and hamsters infected with *P. berghei*. Singer (1954b) and Jackson (1955) found that cortisone inhibited parasitemia in mice and rats, respectively; and they inferred that the drug affects parasitemia indirectly by reducing the production of reticulocytes. Jackson differentiated between the above inhibition of parasitemia and the fact that mortality rates in cortisone-treated rats are high. The former effect was thought to be due to

inhibition of erythropoiesis; the latter, to inhibition of lymphoid proliferation. Roberts (1954b) found that cortisone actually enhances protection
against *P. berghei* in mice. Thus, normal mouse serum, *P. berghei* infected
mouse serum, or serum from mice treated with cortisone alone have practically no effect on *P. berghei* in mice; whereas serum from *P. berghei*
infected mice receiving cortisone produces a marked reduction in parasitemia, lasting for several days. Cantrell and Kendrick (1963) observed that
treatment with cortisone or hydrocortisone reduces *P. berghei* parasitemia by
25 percent. The suppressive effect of cortisone on rodent malarial anemia was
discussed above.

The effect of intercurrent infection on rodent resistance to malaria
depends largely on the reaction of host tissues to the initial infection. Various intercurrent infections may aggravate, ameliorate, or have no perceptible effect on rodent malaria. Thus, bartonellosis in rats induces anemia,
which is followed by compensatory reticulocytosis. The latter favors the
exacerbation of rodent plasmodial infection (Fabiani et al., 1952a; Hsu and
Geiman, 1952). Prior infection of the vole, *Microtus guentheri*, with *Schistosoma mansoni* intensifies and prolongs later *P. berghei* parasitemia (Yoeli,
1956). Concurrent infections of *P. berghei* and *Trypanosoma lewisi* tend to
exacerbate each other (Hughes and Tatum, 1956). This was attributed to
depression of the function of the lymphoid-macrophage system. However,
Jackson (1959), working with the same two parasites, *P. berghei* and *T.
lewisi*, reported that in the rat, the two infections develop normally and independently of one another.

Some intercurrent infections have little perceptible effect on rodent
malaria. As an example, mice which had recovered from infection with rodent
spirochetes were fully susceptible to *P. berghei*, and vice versa (Colas-Belcour
and Vervent, 1954). Similarly, most rats with *P. berghei* and *Spirochaeta
hispanica* developed normal infections of both organisms, although in a few
the double infections were more severe than in the singly infected controls
(Sergent, 1957; Sergent and Poncet, 1957a). Mortality due to leukemia (L-
1210) in mice was not affected by prior exposure to *P. berghei* (Nadel et al.,
1954). In the reciprocal experiment (i.e., exposure first to leukemia and later
to *P. berghei*), the malaria had a slightly inhibitory effect on the leukemia
in that death was delayed from day 10 to day 12. Infection of mice with
influenza-A virus had no effect in mice on later parasitemia due to *P. berghei*
(Yoeli et al., 1955). Infection with *Eperythrozoon coccoides* had either no
observable effect on the development of immunity to *P. berghei* in NMRI
mice (Kretschmar, 1963b), or only a slight suppressive effect on its development in conventional mice (Peters, 1965).

Finally, some intercurrent infections may actually ameliorate the course
of rodent malaria. For example, visceral leishmaniasis, which induces lymphoid-macrophage hyperplasia, tends to protect against later exposure to
rodent plasmodia. Thus, hamsters with *Leishmania infantum* were markedly
protected against *P. berghei*, which generally induces fulminating, fatal
infections in this host (Adler, 1954). In more than half of the doubly

infected hamsters, survival times were significantly prolonged, and in about half, plasmodial infections were actually nonfatal or even negligible. Similarly, infection of mice with West Nile virus or with ornithosis virus partially suppressed *P. berghei* (Yoeli et al., 1955). The suppressive effect of *Eperythrozoon coccoides* on *Plasmodium chabaudi* (Ott and Stauber, 1966) has already been discussed above.

VACCINATION AGAINST RODENT PLASMODIA

Although killed avian malarial parasites have been reported to have an immunizing effect (Thomson et al., 1947), Sergent (1959) believed that killed parasites do not vaccinate against malaria.

Among rodents, the mouse has been observed to be incapable of producing a protective response against extracts of *P. berghei* (Schindler, 1965; Cox, 1965), although complement-fixing antibody was produced (Schindler, 1965). In contrast, a significant measure of protection develops in young rats treated with a cell-free extract of *P. berghei* before challenge with viable parasites (Hamburger, 1965; Zuckerman et al., 1965a). Up to three immunizing doses gave progressively better results, but more than three were no more effective than three doses of vaccine. The onset of patency was delayed, and the duration of patency, peak parasitemias, and mortality rates were all reduced. An immunogenic effect against *P. berghei* was obtained in rats by the injection of a soluble *P. knowlesi* antigen found in the plasma of monkeys during acute infection (Cox, 1966). Other similar results have recently been reviewed (Zuckerman, 1969b).

Attempts at identifying the immunizing antigen in a cell-free extract of plasmodium gain impetus from the fact that such an extract can invoke a protective response in vaccinated rodents.

REFERENCES

Adler, S. 1954. The behaviour of *Plasmodium berghei* in the golden hamster *Mesocricetus auratus* infected with visceral leishmaniasis. Trans. Roy. Soc. Trop. Med. Hyg., 48:431-440.
——— and A. Foner. 1965. Transfer of antibodies to *Plasmodium vinckei* through milk of immune mice. Israel J. Med. Sci., 1:988-993.
——— and A. E. Gunders. 1965. Immunization of mice against a virulent strain of *Plasmodium vinckei* by artificial mild infections on a diet deficient in para amino benzoic acid. Israel J. Med. Sci., 1:441.
——— M. Yoeli, and A. Zuckerman. 1950. Behaviour of *Plasmodium berghei* in some rodents. Nature (London), 166:571.
Banki, G., and A. Bucci. 1964a. Researches on the antigenic structure of *Plasmodium berghei*. Parassitologia, 6:251-257.
——— and A. Bucci. 1964b. Antigenic structure of *Plasmodium cynomolgi* and its relationship with the antigenic structure of *Plasmodium berghei*. Parassitologia, 6:269-274.
Beer, G. 1961. The behaviour of *Plasmodium berghei* and *Plasmodium vinckei* in the spiny mouse *Acomys cahirinus*. Bull. Res. Counc. Israel, 9E:37-38.

Black, R. H. 1951. Parasitic recrudescences in trophozoite-induced *Plasmodium berghei* infections in the albino rat. Ann. Trop. Med. Parasit., 45:199-206.

Box, E. D., and W. D. Gingrich. 1958. Acquired immunity to *Plasmodium berghei* in the white mouse. J. Infect. Dis., 103:291-300.

Bray, R. S. 1965. The Stein and Desowitz haemagglutination test for the detection of antibodies to *Plasmodium berghei* and *Plasmodium vinckei*. Ann. Soc. Belg. Méd. Trop., 45:397-404.

Briggs, N. T., B. L. Garza, and E. D. Box. 1960. Alterations of serum proteins in mice acutely and chronically infected with *Plasmodium berghei*. Exp. Parasit., 10:21-27.

——— B. T. Wellde, and E. H. Sadun. 1966. Effects of rat antiserum on the course of *Plasmodium berghei* infection in mice. Milit. Med., 131 (Suppl.):1243-1249.

Brooke, M. M., G. R. Healey, and D. M. Melvin. 1959. Staining *Plasmodium berghei* with fluorescein tagged antibodies. Proc. 6th Int. Congr. Trop. Med. Malar., 7:59-60.

Bruce-Chwatt, L. J. 1954. *Plasmodium berghei* in the placenta of mice and rats. Transmission of specific immunity from mother rats to litters. Nature (London), 173:353-354.

——— 1963. Congenital transmission of immunity in malaria. *In* Immunity to Protozoa. Garnham, P. C. C., Pierce, A. E., and Roitt, I., eds. Oxford, Blackwell Scientific Publications, pp. 89-108.

——— 1965. Les souches de souris resistantes au *Plasmodium berghei*. Ann. Soc. Belg. Méd. Trop., 45:299-312.

——— and F. D. Gibson. 1956. Transplacental passage of *Plasmodium berghei* and passive transfer of immunity in rats and mice. Trans. Roy. Soc. Trop. Med. Hyg., 50:47-53.

Cantrell, W., and L. P. Kendrick. 1963. Cortisone and antimalarial drug activity against *Plasmodium berghei*. J. Infect. Dis., 113:144-150.

——— and W. G. Moss. 1963. Partial hepatectomy and *Plasmodium berghei* in rats. J. Infect. Dis., 113:67-71.

Carrescia, P. M., and G. Arcoleo. 1957. Immunity to *Plasmodium berghei* in infections running a chronic course induced by chloroquine. Riv. Malariol., 36:51-63.

——— and G. Negroni. 1954. Infezioni da *Plasmodium berghei* in ratti splenectomizzatti e mantenutti à dieta lattea. Riv. Malar., 33:261-272.

Causse-Vaills, C., J. Orfila, and M. G. Fabiani. 1961. Fractionnement électrophorétique des protéines et pouvoir protecteur du sérum du rat blanc immunisé contre *Plasmodium berghei* è una immunità assoluta. Riv. Parassit., 18:65-68.

Chavin, S. I. 1966. Studies on the antigenic constituents of *Plasmodium berghei*. I. Immunologic analysis of the parasite constituents. Milit. Med., 131 (Suppl.):1124-1136.

Ciuca, M., E. Radovici, A. Cipiea, T. Isfan, and L. Ianco. 1964. Aspects cellulaires et sérobiochimiques de l'immunité du rat blanc (*Rattus norvegicus*) infecté au *Plasmodium berghei*. Arch. Roumaines Path. Exp. Microbiol., 23:5-22 (*In* Trop. Dis. Bull., 1965, 62:13-14).

Colas-Belcour, J., and G. Vervent. 1954. Sur des infections mixtes de la souris à spirochètes récurrents et *Plasmodium berghei*. Bull. Soc. Path. Exot., 47:493-497.

Corradetti, A. 1950. Particolari fenomeni immunitari nell' infezione da *Plasmodium berghei*. Riv. Parassit., 11:201-209.

——— 1952. Études de pathologie et d'immunologie comparées dans le paludisme de l'homme et des animaux. Riv. Malar., 31:129-134.

——— 1955. Studies on comparative pathology and immunology in Plasmodium infections of mammals and birds. Trans. Roy. Soc. Trop. Med. Hyg., 49:311-333.

——— 1959. Relapses and immunological course in Plasmodium infections. Parassitologia, 1:91-96.

——— 1963. Acquired sterile immunity in experimental protozoal infections. *In* Immunity to Protozoa. Garnham, P. C. C., Pierce, A. E., and Roitt, I., eds. Oxford, Blackwell Scientific Publications, pp. 69-77.

——— and E. Rigoli. 1961. Behaviour of the hematopoietic and R. E. systems in the albino rat during the 4th and 7th days of a fatal infection by *Plasmodium berghei*. Parassitologia, 3:87-95.

——— and E. Rigoli. 1963. Comportamento dei sistemi ematopoietico e reticoloendoteliale in ratti albini infetti di *Plasmodium berghei* nella seconda settimana e dopo un mese dalla crisi parassitolitica. Parassitologia, 5:53-59.

——— and F. Verolini. 1957. Dimostrazione che l'immunità acquisita del ratto albino al *Plasmodium berghei* è una immunità assoluta. Riv. Parassit., 18:65-68.

——— and F. Verolini. 1960. Decorso della reinfezione da *Plasmodium berghei* in ratti albini precedentemente infettati guariti e splenctomizzati. Parassitologia, 2:99-103.

——— G. Toschi, and F. Verolini. 1954a. Comportamento dei componenti proteici del siero durante l'attacco primario nei ratti infetti da *Plasmodium berghei*. Riv. Parassit., 15:141-150.

——— F. Verolini and G. Toschi. 1954b. Pathological and immunological host-parasite relationships between the albino rat and *Plasmodium berghei*. Indian J. Malar., 8:391-394.

——— G. Toschi and F. Verolini. 1955. Comportamento dei componenti proteici del siero durante l'attacco primario nei ratti infetti da *Plasmodium berghei*. Rendiconti, Istituto Superiore di Sanità, 18:246-255.

——— F. Verolini, and M. Rostirolla. 1959. Durata della sopravvivenza di *Plasmodium berghei* nel pipistrello insettivoro italiano *Miniopterus schreibersii*. Riv. Parassit., 20:255-257.

——— F. Verolini, I. Neri, C. Palmieri, A. M. Proietti, and L. Amati. 1961a. Determinazione del tempo di persistenza di *Plasmodium berghei* nell' ratto albino dopo la fine dell' attacco primario. Parassitologia, 3:77-79.

——— F. Verolini, C. Palmieri, I. Neri, C. Cavallini, and L. Amati. 1961b. Durata della sopravvivenza di *Plasmodium berghei* reinoculato in ratti albini resi immuni dalla guarigione dell' attacco primario. Parassitologia, 3:81-86.

Cowper, S. G., and S. F. Woodward. 1958. A note on infection of the multimammate rat *Rattus (Mastomys) natalensis erythroleucus* with *Plasmodium berghei*. W. Afr. Med. J., 7:151-153.

——— and S. F. Woodward. 1959. Observations on *Plasmodium berghei* infection in white rats: blood changes and acquired resistance. Ann. Trop. Med. Parasit., 53:103-112.

Cox, F. E. G. 1965. Acquired immunity to *Plasmodium vinckei*. *In* Progress in Protozoology. II. International Conference on Protozoology, London. International Congress Series No. 91, Amsterdam, Excerpta Medica Foundation, p. 167.

Cox, H. W. 1957. Observations on induced chronic *Plasmodium berghei* infections in white mice. J. Immunol., 79:450-454.

——— 1958. The roles of time and atabrine in inducing chronic *Plasmodium berghei* infections of white mice. J. Immun., 81:72-75.

——— 1959. A study of relapse *Plasmodium berghei* infections isolated from white mice. J. Immun., 82:209-214.

——— 1962. The behavior of *Plasmodium berghei* strains isolated from relapsed infections of white mice. J. Protozool., 9:114-118.

——— 1964a. Comments on autoimmunity in malaria. Amer. J. Trop. Med. Hyg., 13(Suppl.):225-227.

——— 1964b. Measurement of the acquired resistance of rats and mice to *Plasmodium berghei* infections. J. Parasit., 50:23-29.

——— 1966. A factor associated with anemia and immunity in *Plasmodium knowlesi* infections. Milit. Med., 131 (Suppl.):1195-1200.

——— W. F. Schroeder, and M. Ristic. 1965. Erythrophagocytosis associated with anemia in rats infected with *Plasmodium berghei*. J. Parasit., 51(sec. 2):35-36.

——— W. F. Schroeder, and M. Ristic. 1966. Hemagglutination and erythrophagocytosis associated with the anemia of *Plasmodium berghei* infections of rats. J. Protozool., 13:327-332.

Demina, N. A. 1958. The study of immunity to *Plasmodium berghei*. II. The mechanism of transmission of immunity to *Plasmodium berghei* from immune rats to their offspring. Med. Parazit. (Moskva), 27:319-329.

Deschiens, R., and L. Lamy. 1951. Infection expérimentale du lapin par *Plasmodium berghei*. Bull. Soc. Path. Exot., 44:405-409.

——— and L. Lamy. 1965. Aspects de l'immunité dans les infestations à *Plasmodium berghei*. Ann. Soc. Belg. Méd. Trop., 45:427-434.

Desowitz, R. S. 1965. Recent investigations on the use of the hemagglutination test in malaria. *In* Progress in Protozoology. II. International Conference on Protozoology, London. International Congress Series No. 91. Amsterdam, Excerpta Medica Foundation, p. 169.

——— and B. Stein. 1962. A tanned red cell hemagglutination test, using *Plasmodium berghei* antigen and homologous antisera. Trans. Roy. Soc. Trop. Med. Hyg., 56:257.

———— J. J. Saave, and B. Stein. 1966. The application of the indirect haemagglutination test in recent studies on the immuno-epidemiology of human malaria and the immune response in experimental malaria. Milit. Med., 131 (Suppl.):1157-1166.

Draper, C. C. 1953. *Plasmodium berghei*: A bibliography of published papers up to April 1953. London, Ross Institute, pp. 1-10.

———— 1954. The duration of residual immunity following spontaneous cure of *Plasmodium berghei* in rats. Parasitology, 44:338-341.

Durand, P., and M. Mathis. 1951. Sensibilité du hamster doré au *Plasmodium berghei*. C. R. Soc. Biol. (Paris), 145:29-31.

———— and M. Mathis. 1955. Sensibilité de trois rongeurs sauvages tunisiens, *Mus musculus spretus, Dipodillus campestris* et *Meriones shawi,* au *Plasmodium berghei*. Arch. Inst. Pasteur (Tunis), 32:17-24.

Durbin, C. G. 1951. Attempts to transfer *Plasmodium berghei* to domesticated animals. Proc. Helminth. Soc. (Washington), 18:108-110.

Fabiani, G. 1954a. Le paludisme expérimental des rongeurs. Son intérêt en immunologie et en pathologie générale. Bulletin de l'Association des Diplomés de Microbiologie de la Faculté de Pharmacie de Nancy, 56:1-16.

———— 1954b. Immunology of *Plasmodium berghei*. Indian J. Malar., 8:347-362.

———— 1959. Le paludisme expérimental (à *Plasmodium berghei* et à *Plasmodium vinckei*). Son intérêt en immunologie générale. Algérie Med., 63:793-799.

———— and G. Fulchiron. 1952. Démonstration et analyse de l'immunité croisé entre deux souches de *Plasmodium berghei*. C. R. Soc. Biol. (Paris), 146:435-437.

———— and G. Fulchiron. 1953a. Démonstration in vivo de l'existence d'un pouvoir protecteur dans le sérum de rats guéris de paludisme expérimentale. C. R. Soc. Biol. (Paris), 147:99-103.

———— and G. Fulchiron. 1953b. Comportement des hématozoaires de réinoculation dans la cavité péritonéale de rats guéris d'infection à *Plasmodium berghei*. Mise en évidence de la phagocytose des parasites. C. R. Soc. Biol. (Paris), 147:103-106.

———— and G. Fulchiron. 1954a. Influence de la splénectomie sur la résistance naturelle et l'apparition de l'immunité au cours du paludisme expérimental du rat blanc. C. R. Soc. Biol. (Paris), 148:530-533.

———— and G. Fulchiron. 1954b. Influence de la splénectomie sur le maintien de l'immunité spécifique au cours du paludisme expérimental du rat blanc. C. R. Soc. Biol. (Paris), 148:673-675.

———— and Izzo, M. A. 1952. Influence de la surrénalectomie sur le paludisme du rat blanc infecté expérimentalement par *Plasmodium berghei*. C. R. Soc. Biol. (Paris), 146:1155-1157.

———— and J. Orfila. 1955a. Influence de la splénectomie sur le paludisme expérimental à *Plasmodium berghei* de la souris blanche. C. R. Soc. Biol. (Paris), 149:87-90.

———— and J. Orfila. 1955b. Étude physiologique des surrénales dans le paludisme expérimental de la souris blanche. C. R. Soc. Biol. (Paris), 149:674-677.

———— and J. Orfila. 1956. Recherche du pouvoir séroprotecteur chez le rat infecté expérimentalement par *Plasmodium berghei*. C. R. Soc. Biol. (Paris), 150:1182-1184.

———— and J. Orfila. 1958. Résistance naturele du lapin à l'infection expérimentale par *Plasmodium berghei*. Analyse des facteurs immunologiques. Ann. Inst. Pasteur (Paris), 94:428-434.

———— and J. Orfila. 1959. Infection expérimentale de la souris blanche par *Plasmodium vinckei*. Bull. Soc. Path. Exot., 52:618-630.

———— and J. Orfila. 1961. Démonstration d'une immunité croisée dans les infections à *Plasmodium berghei* et à *Plasmodium vinckei*. C. R. Soc. Biol. (Paris), 155:483-485.

———— R. Vargues, P. Grellet, and J. Clausse. 1951. Influence de la splénectomie sur des rats blancs spontanément guéris d'une infection expérimentale à *Plasmodium berghei*. C. R. Soc. Biol. (Paris), 145:1131-1134.

———— J. Clausse, and G. Fulchiron. 1952a. Influence de la réticulocytose sanguine sur l'évolution du paludisme chez les rats immunisés at splénectomisés. C. R. Soc. Biol. (Paris), 146:1587-1589.

———— R. Vargues, P. Grellet, G. Fulchiron, and A. Verain. 1952b. Le paludisme expérimental du rat blanc à *Plasmodium berghei*. Bull. Soc. Path. Exot., 45:524-539.

———— J. Orfila, and G. Bonhoure. 1957. Effet de la splénectomie sur le paludisme de rats blancs précédemment infectés par *Plasmodium vinckei*. C. R. Soc. Biol. (Paris), 151:2135-2137.

———— J. Orfila and G. Bonhoure. 1958. Influence de la splénectomie sur la résistance naturelle du rat blanc à *Plasmodium vinckei*. C. R. Soc. Biol. (Paris), 152:337-339.

Findlay, G. M., and E. M. Howard. 1952. Cortisone and *Plasmodium berghei* infection in mice. Nature (London), 169:547.

Fulton, J. D. 1954. Cortisone and *Plasmodium berghei* infection in rodents. Ann. Trop. Med. Parasit., 48:314-317.

Gail, K., and W. Kretschmar. 1965. Serumeiweissveränderungen und Immunität bei der Malaria *(Plasmodium berghei)* in der Maus. Naturwissenschaften, 16:480.

Galliard, H., and J. Lapierre. 1950. Effets de la splénectomie sur l'évolution et les rechutes de l'infection à *Plasmodium berghei* chez le rat blanc. C. R. Soc. Biol. (Paris), 144:402-403.

———— and J. Lapierre. 1954. Investigations on immunity to *Plasmodium berghei* infection in mice. Indian J. Malar., 8:363-368.

Garnham, P. C. C. 1962. Comment on Fabiani, G., and Orfila, J., 1961. Trop. Dis. Bull., 59:527-528.

Garza, B. L., and E. D. Box. 1961. Evolution of test of cure procedures in mice treated for *Plasmodium berghei* infections. Amer. J. Trop. Med. Hyg., 10:804-811.

George, J. N., E. F. Stokes, D. J. Wicker, and M. E. Conrad. 1966. Studies of the mechanism of hemolysis in experimental malaria. Milit. Med., 131 (Suppl.):1217-1224.

Goberman, V., and A. Zuckerman. 1966. Dynamics of the formation of antiplasmodial precipitins in rats infected with *Plasmodium berghei*. J. Protozool., 13 (Suppl.):34.

Greenberg, J., and G. R. Coatney. 1954. Some host-parasite relationships in *Plasmodium berghei* infections. Indian J. Malar., 8:313-325.

———— and L. P. Kendrick. 1958. Parasitemia and survival in mice infected with *Plasmodium berghei*. Hybrids between Swiss (high parasitemia) and STR (low parasitemia) mice. J. Parasit., 44:592-598.

———— E. M. Nadel, and G. R. Coatney. 1953. The influence of strain, sex and age of mice on infection with *Plasmodium berghei*. J. Infect. Dis., 93:96-100.

Hamburger, J. 1965. Active immunization of rats against *Plasmodium berghei* malaria. M.S. Thesis, Hebrew University, Jerusalem, Israel.

Hawking, F. 1953. Milk diet, para amino benzoic acid and malaria *(Plasmodium berghei)*. Preliminary communication. Brit. Med. J., 1·1201-1202.

Hsu, D. Y. M., and Q. M. Geiman. 1952. Synergistic effect of *Haemobartonella muris* on *Plasmodium berghei* in white rats. Amer. J. Trop. Med. Hyg., 1:747-760.

Hughes, F. W., and A. L. Tatum. 1956. Effects of hypoxia and intercurrent infections on infections by *Plasmodium berghei* in rats. J. Infect. Dis., 99:38-43.

Isfan, T., and L. Ianco. 1964. Contribution à l'étude de la transmission de l'immunité de la rate à ses petits infectés avec *Plasmodium berghei*. Arch. Roumaines Path. Exp. Microbiol., 23:783-796 (*In* Trop. Dis. Bull., 1966, 63:261).

Jackson, G. J. 1955. The effect of cortisone on *Plasmodium berghei* infections in the white rat. J. Infect. Dis., 97:152-159.

———— 1959. Simultaneous infections with *Plasmodium berghei* and *Trypanosoma lewisi* in the rat. J. Parasit., 45:94.

Jadin, J., ed. 1965. Colloque international sur le *Plasmodium berghei*. Ann. Soc. Belg. Méd. Trop., 45:251-496.

Jeffery, G. M., W. A. Sodeman, and W. E. Collins. 1964. Fluorescent antibody studies in experimental malarias. III. Limitations of the fluorescent antibody technique. Proc. 1st Int. Congr. Parasit., Rome, 1:229-230.

Jerusalem, C. 1964. Über die Anämiegenese bei der Malariainfektion *(Plasmodium berghei)* von NMRI Mäusen. Z. Tropenmed. Parasit., 15:371-385.

———— 1965. Histo- und biometrische Untersuchungen zur Frage der Autohaemaggression bei Infektion mit *Plasmodium berghei*. Ann. Soc. Belg. Méd. Trop., 45:405-418.

Kreier, J. P., and M. Ristic. 1964. Detection of a *Plasmodium berghei* antibody complex formed *in vivo*. Amer. J. Trop. Med. Hyg., 13:6-10.

———— H. Shapiro, D. Dilley, I. P. Szilvassy, and M. Ristic. 1966. Autoimmune reactions in rats with *Plasmodium berghei* infection. Exp. Parasit., 19:155-162.

Kretschmar, W. 1962. Resistenz und Immunität bei mit *Plasmodium berghei* infizierten Mäusen. Z. Tropenmed. Parasit., 13:159-175.

———— 1963a. Weitere Untersuchungen über die Immunität bei der Nagetiermalaria. Z. Tropenmed. Parasit., 14:41-48.

———— 1963b. Die Abhängigkeit des Verlaufs der Nagetiermalaria (*Plasmodium berghei*) in der Maus von exogenen Faktoren. I. Interferierende Bartonellosen. Z. Versuchstierkrank., 3:151-166.

———— 1964. Parasitendichte und Erythrozytenverlust bei der Malaria (*Plasmodium berghei*) in der Maus. Z. Tropenmed. Parasit., 15:386-399.

———— 1965a. The effects of stress and diet on resistance to *Plasmodium berghei* and malaria immunity in the mouse. Ann. Soc. Belg. Méd. Trop., 45:325-343.

———— 1965b. Der Verlauf der Malaria (*Plasmodium berghei*) in hochresistenten Mäusestämmen. Z. Versuchstierkrank., 6:108-119.

———— and C. Jerusalem. 1963. Milz und Malaria. Der Infektionsverlauf (*Plasmodium berghei*) in splenektomierten NMRI Mäusen und seine Deutung anhand der histopathologischen Veränderungen der Milz nichtsplenektomierten Mäuse. Z. Tropenmed. Parasit., 14:279-310.

Krishnaswami, A. K., Satya Prakash, and S. P. Ramakrishnan. 1953. Studies on *Plasmodium berghei*. XII. Attempts to estimate in vivo the acquired immunity in albino rats. Indian J. Malar., 7:103-106.

Landau, I. 1965. Description de *Plasmodium chabaudi* n. sp., parasite de rongeurs africains. C. R. Acad. Sci. (Paris), 260:3758-3761.

———— and R. Killick-Kendrick. 1966. Note préliminaire sur le cycle évolutif des deux Plasmodium du rongeur *Thamnomys rutilans* de la République Centrafricaine. C. R. Acad. Sci. (Paris), 262:1113-1116.

Lapierre, J. 1954. *Plasmodium berghei* chez la souris. Apparition d'un état d'immunité à la suite de traitements répétés par la nivaquine au cours des rechutes. Bull. Soc. Path. Exot., 47:380-387.

———— M. Sretenovic, and J. J. Rousset, 1958. Influence de la splénectomie sur la réticulocytose au cours de l'infection à *Plasmodium berghei* chez la souris blanche. Bull. Soc. Path. Exot., 51:897-901.

McGhee, R. B. 1954. The infection of duck and goose erythrocytes by the mammalian malaria parasite *Plasmodium berghei*. J. Protozool., 1:145-148.

Maegraith, B. G., T. Deegan, and E. S. Jones. 1952. Suppression of malaria (*Plasmodium berghei*) by milk. Brit. Med. J., 2:1382-1384.

Martin, L. K., A. Einheber, R. F. Porro, E. H. Sadun, and H. Bauer. 1966. *Plasmodium berghei* infections in gnotobiotic mice and rats: parasitologic, immunologic, and histopathologic observations. Milit. Med., 131(Suppl.):870-890.

Mercado, T. I., and G. R. Coatney. 1951. The course of the blood-induced *Plasmodium berghei* infection in white mice. J. Parasit., 37:479-482.

———— and G. R. Coatney. 1953. The course of the blood-induced *Plasmodium berghei* infection in the meadow mouse *Microtus pennsylvanicus pennsylvanicus* and certain small rodents. Amer. J. Trop. Med. Hyg., 2:39-46.

Most, H., R. S. Nussenzweig, J. Vanderberg, R. Herman, and M. Yoeli. 1966. Susceptibility of genetically standardized (JAX) mouse strains to sporozoite and blood-induced *Plasmodium berghei* infections. Milit. Med., 131 (Suppl.):915-918.

Motulsky, A. G., F. Casserd, E. R. Giblett, G. O. Broun, and C. A. Finch. 1958. Anemia and the spleen. New Eng. J. Med., 259:1164-1169, 1215-1218.

Nadel, E. M., J. Greenberg, and G. R. Coatney. 1954. The effect of malaria (*Plasmodium berghei*) on leukemia L-1210 in mice. J. Infect. Dis., 95:109-113.

Nussenzweig, R. S., M. Yoeli, and H. Most. 1966. Studies on the protective effect of *Plasmodium chabaudi* infection in mice upon a subsequent infection with another rodent malaria species, *Plasmodium vinckei*. Milit. Med., 131(Suppl.):1237-1242.

Ott, K. J., and L. A. Stauber. 1966. Influence of *Eperythrozoon coccoides* on the course of infection of *Plasmodium chabaudi* in the mouse. Personal communication.

Pautrizel, R., and Nguyen Vinh Nien. 1953. Mise en evidence d'anticorps chez le rat parasité par *Plasmodium berghei* à l'aide d'un antigène préparé avec du sang de rat impaludé. Bull. Soc. Path. Exot., 46:671-673.

Peters, W. 1965. Competitive relationship between *Eperythrozoon coccoides* and *Plasmodium berghei* in the mouse. Exp. Parasit., 16:158-166.

Radacovici, E., T. Isfan, L. Iancu, and M. Dinculescu. 1958. Cercetari privind *Plasmodium berghei*. Studii si Cercetari Inframicrobiol., Microbiol. si Parasitol., 9:139-148.

Raffaele, G. 1965. Addatamento allo suiluppo nel pollo di *Plasmodium berghei*. Riv. Malar., 44: 1-8.

—— and A. Baldi. 1950. Sulla morfologia e sulla trasmissione di *Plasmodium berghei*. Riv. Malar., 29: 341-347.

Ramakrishnan, S. P. 1952. Studies on *Plasmodium berghei*. VII. Spleen size in albino mice and rats with blood-induced infections. Indian J. Malar., 6: 189-198.

—— and Satya Prakash. 1951. Susceptibility of the Indian garden squirrel (*Sciurus palmarum*) to *Plasmodium berghei* and its asexual periodicity. Nature (London), 31: 533.

—— Satya Prakash, and A. K. Krishnaswami. 1951. Studies on *Plasmodium berghei*. III. Latency, relapse and immunity in albino rats with blood-induced infections. Indian J. Malar., 5: 447-454.

Resseler, R. 1956. Un nouveau plasmodium de rat en Belgique: *Plasmodium inopinatum*. Ann. Soc. Belg. Méd. Trop., 36: 259-263.

Roberts, O. J. 1954a. The effect of cortisone on *Plasmodium berghei* infections. Parasitology, 44: 58-64.

—— 1954b. The effect of cortisone on *Plasmodium berghei* infections. Parasitology, 44: 438-445.

Rodhain, J. 1949. Le comportement du cotton rat vis-à-vis du *Plasmodium berghei*. Ann. Soc. Belg. Méd. Trop., 29: 483-489.

—— 1951. Le comportement du "cotton rat" vis-à-vis du *Plasmodium berghei*. Note complémentaire. Ann. Soc. Belg. Méd. Trop., 31: 289-296.

—— 1952. *Plasmodium vinckei* n. sp., un deuxième plasmodium parasite de rongeurs sauvages au Katanga. Ann. Soc. Belg. Méd. Trop., 32: 275-279.

——1953a. La spécificité biologique du *Plasmodium vinckei*. Ann. Inst. Pasteur (Paris), 84: 672-683.

—— 1953b. La réceptivité de quelques roussettes africaines à *Plasmodium berghei*. Bull. Soc. Path. Exot., 46: 315-318.

—— 1954a. Absence d'immunité croisée entre *Plasmodium berghei* et *Plasmodium vinckei* dans les infections chez les jeunes rats. C. R. Soc. Biol. (Paris), 148: 1519-1520.

—— 1954b. The absence of cross immunity between *Plasmodium berghei* and *Plasmodium vinckei*. Indian J. Malar., 8: 369-373.

Sadun, E. H., J. S. Williams, F. C. Meroney, and G. Hutt. 1965. Pathophysiology of *Plasmodium berghei* infection in mice. Exp. Parasit., 17: 277-286.

Satya Prakash. 1959. Studies on *Plasmodium berghei*. XXVI. The minimum duration of patent primary parasitemia in albino rats for the development of immunity to resist reinfection. Indian J. Malar., 13: 137-144.

—— 1960a. Studies on *Plasmodium berghei*. XXVII. Duration of patent primary parasitemia necessary for the development of measurable acquired immunity, if any, in the albino mice. Indian J. Malar., 14: 165-170.

—— 1960b. Studies on *Plasmodium berghei*. XXVIII. The duration of immunity due to a single untreated *Plasmodium berghei* infection in albino rats. Indian J. Malar., 14: 283-290.

—— 1961. Studies on *Plasmodium berghei*. XXX. Effects of splenectomy on the course of blood-induced infection in rats. Indian J. Malar., 15: 107-114.

—— A. K. Krishnaswami, and S. P. Ramakrishnan. 1952. Studies on *Plasmodium berghei*. V. On the host range in blood-induced infections. Indian J. Malar., 6: 175-182.

Schindler, R. 1965. Resistenz und Immunität bei der *Plasmodium berghei* Infektion der Maus. Ann. Soc. Belg. Méd. Trop., 45: 289-298.

—— and D. Mehlitz. 1965. Untersuchungen über die Bedeutung Komplementbildender Antikörper für die *Plasmodium berghei* Infektion der Maus. Z. Tropenmed. Parasit., 16: 30-49.

Schroeder, W. F., H. W. Cox, and M. Ristic. 1965. Mechanism of anemia resulting from *Babesia rodhaini* and *Plasmodium berghei* infections in rats. Progress in Protozoology. II. International Conference on Protozoology, London. International Congress Series No. 91. Amsterdam, Excerpta Medica Foundation, p. 182.

Schwink, T. N. 1960. The effect of antierythrocytic antibodies upon *Plasmodium berghei* infection in white mice. Amer. J. Trop. Med. Hyg., 9: 293-296.

Sergent, E. 1950. Definition de l'immunité et de la prémunition. Ann. Inst. Pasteur (Paris), 79: 786-797.

—— 1954a. Observations d'infection latente d'emblée avec prémunition corrélative dans le paludisme expérimentale à *Plasmodium berghei* du rat blanc. C. R. Acad. Sci. (Paris), 239: 524-525.

—— 1954b. Experimental study on the immunology of malaria due to *Plasmodium berghei*. Indian J. Malar., 8: 333-346.

—— 1957. De la coexistence, chez le même malade, de la fièvre récurrente et du paludisme. Z. Tropenmed. Parasit., 8: 242-245.

—— 1959. Réflexions sur l'épidémiologie et l'immunologie du paludisme. Arch. Inst. Pasteur (Algérie), 37: 1-52.

—— 1963. Latent infection and premunition. Some definitions of microbiology and immunology. *In* Immunity to Protozoa. Garnham, P. C. C., Pierce, A. E. and Roitt, I., eds. Oxford, Blackwell Scientific Publications, pp. 39-47.

—— and A. Poncet. 1950. De la virulence pour le mérion, rongeur nord-africain, de *Plasmodium berghei*. Arch. Inst. Pasteur (Algérie) 28: 323-334.

—— and A. Poncet. 1951a. De la longue durée de l'infection latente métacritique dans le paludisme expérimental à *Plasmodium berghei* du mérion nord-africain. Arch. Inst. Pasteur (Algérie), 29: 269-272.

—— and A. Poncet. 1951b. De la "resistance innée" du cobaye au paludisme des rongeurs à *Plasmodium berghei*. Arch. Inst. Pasteur (Algérie), 29: 273-276.

—— and A. Poncet. 1955a. Étude expérimentale du paludisme des rongeurs à *Plasmodium berghei*. I. Incubation. Accès aigu. Arch. Inst. Pasteur (Algérie), 33: 71-77.

—— and A. Poncet. 1955b. Étude expérimentale du paludisme des rongeurs à *Plasmodium berghei*. II. Stade d'infection latente métacritique. Arch. Inst. Pasteur (Algérie), 33: 195-222.

—— and A. Poncet. 1955c. Étude expérimentale du paludisme des rongeurs à *Plasmodium berghei*. III. Résistance innée. Arch. Inst. Pasteur (Algérie), 33: 287-306.

—— and A. Poncet. 1956a. Étude expérimentale du paludisme des rongeurs à *Plasmodium berghei*. IV. Résistance acquise. Arch. Inst. Pasteur (Algérie), 34: 1-51.

—— and A. Poncet. 1956b. Note sur la résistance innée à *Plasmodium berghei* de gerbilles de l'Afrique du Nord. Arch. Inst. Pasteur (Algérie), 34: 494-495.

—— and A. Poncet. 1957a. Étude expérimentale de l'association chez le rat blanc de la spirochètose hispano-nord-africaine et du paludisme des rongeurs à *Plasmodium berghei*. Arch. Inst. Pasteur (Algérie), 35: 1-23.

—— and A. Poncet. 1957b. Résistance innée du hérisson au paludisme des rongeurs à *Plasmodium berghei*. Arch. Inst. Pasteur (Algérie), 35: 203.

—— and A. Poncet. 1961. De la résistance acquise contre le paludisme des rongeurs à *Plasmodium berghei* par des rats blancs qui ont survécu à une première atteinte. Arch. Inst. Pasteur (Algérie), 39: 116-118.

Serguiev, P. G., and N. A. Demina. 1957. Studies of immunity to *Plasmodium berghei* infection. I. The transmission of acquired immunity against *Plasmodium berghei* from female rats to their offspring. Indian J. Malar., 11: 129-138.

Singer, I. 1953. Effect of x-irradiation on infections with *Plasmodium berghei* in the white mouse. J. Infect. Dis., 92: 97-104.

—— 1954a. Effect of splenectomy or phenyl hydrazine on infections with *Plasmodium berghei* in the white mouse. J. Infect. Dis., 94: 159-163.

—— 1954b. The effect of cortisone on infections with *Plasmodium berghei* in the white mouse. J. Infect. Dis., 94: 164-172.

—— 1954c. The cellular reactions to infections with *Plasmodium berghei* in the white mouse. J. Infect. Dis., 94: 241-261.

—— R. Hadfield, and M. Lakonen. 1955. The influence of age on the intensity of infection with *Plasmodium berghei* in the rat. J. Infect. Dis., 97: 15-21.

Singh, J., Editor. 1954. Symposium on *Plasmodium berghei*. Indian J. Malar., 8: 237-394.

Smet, R. M. de. 1955. Variations du rapport protéines totales: globulines du sérum lors de l'infection par *Plasmodium berghei*. Bull. Soc. Path. Exot., 48: 385-389.

—— and G. Frankie. 1954a. Quelques observations sur l'immunité vis-à-vis du *Plasmodium berghei*. Ann. Soc. Belg. Méd. Trop., 34: 881-891.

—— and G. Frankie. 1954b. Some observations about immunity to *Plasmodium berghei*. Indian J. Malar., 8: 375-390.

Sodeman, W. A., and G. M. Jeffery. 1965. Immunofluorescent studies of *Plasmodium berghei*: A "natural" antibody in white mice. Amer. J. Trop. Med. Hyg., 14: 187-190.

—— and J. H. E. T. Meuwissen. 1966. Disc electrophoresis of *Plasmodium berghei*. J. Parasit., 52: 23-25.

Spira, D., and A. Zuckerman. 1961. Blood loss and replacement in splenectomized rats infected with *Plasmodium berghei*. Bull. Res. Counc. Israel, 9E: 71.

—— and A. Zuckerman. 1962. Antigenic structure of *Plasmodium vinckei*. Science, 137: 536-537.

—— and A. Zuckerman. 1965. Blood loss and replacement in plasmodial infections. VI. *Plasmodium berghei* in splenectomized rats. J. Infect. Dis., 115: 337-344.

—— and A. Zuckerman. 1966. Recent advances in the antigenic analysis of plasmodia. Milit. Med., 131 (Suppl.) : 1117-1123.

Stein, B., and R. S. Desowitz. 1964. The measurement of antibody in human malaria by a formolized tanned sheep cell haemagglutination test. Bull. W. H. O., No. 30, pp. 45-49.

Taliaferro, W. H. 1949. Immunity to the malaria infections. *In* Malariology. Boyd, M. F., ed. Philadelphia, W. B. Saunders Co., Vol. 2, pp. 935-965.

Terry, R. J. 1956. Transmission of antimalarial immunity (*Plasmodium berghei*) from mother rats to their young during lactation. Trans. Roy. Soc. Trop. Med. Hyg., 50: 41-47.

Thomson, K. J., J. Freund, H. E. Sommer, and A. W. Walter. 1947. Immunization of ducks against malaria by means of killed parasites with or without adjuvants. Amer. J. Trop. Med., 27: 79-105.

Thurston, J. P. 1953. *Plasmodium berghei*. Exp. Parasit., 2: 311-332.

Tobie, J. E. 1964. Detection of malaria antibodies—immunodiagnosis. Amer. J. Trop. Med., 13 (Suppl.) : 195-203.

Van Riel, J. 1950. Le comportement de *Roussettus leachi* vis-à-vis du *Plasmodium berghei*. Ann. Inst. Pasteur (Paris), 79: 772.

Vargues, R. 1951. Étude sérologique de l'infection expérimentale du rat blanc par *Plasmodium berghei*: disparition d'alexine. Présence d'anticorps fixant le complément. C. R. Soc. Biol. (Paris), 145: 1134-1136.

—— and G. Fabiani. 1951. La réinoculation intracardiaque de *Plasmodium berghei* chez les rats guéris d'une infection première. C. R. Soc. Biol. (Paris), 145: 1521-1523.

—— G. Fabiani, and G. Fulchiron. 1951. Étude sérologique de l'infection expérimentale du rat blanc par *Plasmodium berghei*. Variations quantitatives de la sensibilisatrice et d'alexine au cours de la maladie. C. R. Soc. Biol. (Paris), 145: 1298-1300.

Verain, A., and A. Verain. 1957. *Plasmodium berghei* et rayons X. C. R. Soc. Biol. (Paris), 151: 1164-1166.

Vincke, I. H., and M. Lips. 1948. Un nouveau plasmodium d'un rongeur sauvage du Congo, *Plasmodium berghei*. Ann. Soc. Belg. Méd. Trop., 28: 97-105.

—— E. M. E. Peeters, and G. Frankie. 1953a. Evolution du *Plasmodium berghei* et *vinckei* chez differents mammifères. Ann. Soc. Belg. Méd. Trop., 33: 269-282.

—— E. M. E. Peeters, and G. Frankie. 1953b. Essai d'étude d'ensemble sur le *Plasmodium berghei*. Institut Royale Colonial Belge Bulletin des Séances, 24: 1364-1406.

Voller, A. 1962. Fluorescent antibody studies on malaria parasites. Bull. W. H. O., No. 27, pp. 283-287.

—— 1964a. Comments on the detection of malaria antibodies. Amer. J. Trop. Med. Hyg., 13 (Suppl.) : 204-208.

—— 1964b. Fluorescent antibody methods and their use in malaria research. Bull. W. H. O., No. 30, pp. 343-354.

Weiss, M. L. 1965. Development and duration of immunity to malaria (*Plasmodium berghei*) in mice. Progress in Protozoology. II. International Conference on Protozoology, London. International Congress Series No. 91. Amsterdam, Excerpta Medica Foundation, p. 168.

—— and D. L. DeGiusti. 1964a. The effect of different sera in the culture medium on the behaviour of *Plasmodium berghei* following serial passage through tissue culture. J. Protozool., 11: 224-228.

—— and D. L. DeGiusti. 1964b. Modification of a malaria parasite (*Plasmodium berghei*) following passage through tissue culture. Nature (London), 201: 731-732.

—— and D. L. DeGiusti. 1966. Active immunization against *Plasmodium berghei* malaria in mice. Amer. J. Trop. Med. Hyg., 15: 472-482.

Wellde, B. T., N. T. Briggs, and E. H. Sadun. 1966. Susceptibility to *Plasmodium berghei*: parasitological, biochemical and hematological studies in laboratory and wild animals. Milit. Med., 131 (Suppl.) : 859-869.

Woodruff, A. W. 1957. Serum protein changes induced by *Plasmodium berghei* infection in rats and *Plasmodium knowlesi* infection in monkeys. Trans. Roy. Soc. Trop. Med. Hyg., 51:419-424.

Yoeli, M. 1956. Some aspects of concomitant infections of plasmodia and schistosomes. I. The effect of *Schistosoma mansoni* on the course of infection of *Plasmodium berghei* in the field vole. Amer. J. Trop. Med. Hyg., 5:988-999.

———— and H. Most. 1964. A study of *Plasmodium berghei* in *Thamnomys surdaster*, and in other experimental hosts. Amer. J. Trop. Med. Hyg., 13:659-663.

———— Y. Becker, and H. Bernkopf. 1955. The effect of West Nile virus on experimental malaria infection (*Plasmodium berghei*) in mice. Harefuah (J. Israel Med. Ass.), 49:116-119.

Zuckerman, A. 1953. Residual immunity following radical cure of *Plasmodium berghei* in intact and splenectomized voles (*Microtus guentheri*). J. Infect. Dis., 92:205-223.

———— 1957. Blood loss and replacement in plasmodial infections. I. *Plasmodium berghei* in untreated rats of varying age and in adult rats with erythropoietic mechanisms manipulated before inoculation. J. Infect. Dis., 100: 172-206.

———— 1958. Blood loss and replacement in plasmodial infections. II. *Plasmodium vinckei* in untreated weanling and mature rats. J. Infect. Dis., 103:205-224.

———— 1960. Autoantibody in rats with *Plasmodium berghei*. Nature (London), 185:189-190.

———— 1963. Immunity to malaria with special reference to red-cell destruction. *In* Immunity to Protozoa. Garnham, P. C. C., Pierce, A. E., and Roitt, I., eds. Oxford, Blackwell Scientific Publications, pp. 78-88.

———— 1964a. The antigenic analysis of plasmodia. Amer. J. Trop. Med. Hyg., 13(Suppl.):209-213.

———— 1964b. Autoimmunization and other types of indirect damage to host cells as factors in certain protozoan diseases. Exp. Parasit., 15:138-183.

———— 1966. Recent studies on factors involved in malaria anemia. Milit. Med., 131(Suppl.):1201-1216.

———— 1968. Basis of host-cell-parasite specificity. *In* Infectious Blood Diseases of Man and Animals. Weinman, D., and Ristic, M., eds. New York, Academic Press Inc., pp. 23-36.

———— 1969a. Current status of the immunology of malaria and of the antigenic analysis of plasmodia. Bull. W.H.O., 40:55-66.

———— 1969b. Vaccination against plasmodia. Israel J. Med. Sci., 5:429-434.

———— and M. Ristic. 1968. Blood parasite antigens and antibodies. *In* Infectious Blood Diseases of Man and Animals. Weinman, D., and Ristic, M., eds. New York, Academic Press Inc., pp. 79-122.

———— and D. Spira. 1961. Blood loss and replacement in malarial infections. V. Positive antiglobulin tests in rat anemias due to the rodent malarias (*Plasmodium berghei* and *Plasmodium vinckei*), to cardiac bleeding, and to treatment with phenylhydrazine hydrochloride. J. Infect. Dis., 108:339-348.

———— and D. Spira. 1965. Immunoelectrophoretic comparison of plasmodial antigens. World Health Organization/Mal/407.65,1-10.

———— and M. Yoeli. 1951. The effect of splenectomy on the course of *Plasmodium berghei* infections in *Microtus guentheri*. J. Infect. Dis., 89:130-142.

———— and M. Yoeli. 1954. Age and sex as factors influencing *Plasmodium berghei* infections in intact and splenectomized rats. J. Infect. Dis., 94:225-236.

———— D. Spira, and N. Schulman. 1964. The phagocytic load of splenic macrophages and their precursor cells in rats infected with *Plasmodium berghei*. Proc. 1st Int. Congr. Parasit., Rome, p. 245.

———— J. Hamburger, and D. Spira. 1965a. Active immunization of rats against rodent malaria with a non-living plasmodial product. *In* Progress in Protozoology. II. International Conference on Protozoology, London. International Congress Series No. 91. Amsterdam, Excerpta Medica Foundation, pp. 50-51.

———— N. Ron, and D. Spira. 1965b. The demonstration of antiplasmodial antibody in rats by means of gel diffusion. *In* Progress in Protozoology. II. International Conference on Protozoology, London. International Congress Series No. 91. Amsterdam, Excerpta Medica Foundation, pp. 167-168.

———— D. Spira, and A. Shor. 1966. Unpublished data.

Babesiosis and Theileriosis

MIODRAG RISTIC

Department of Veterinary Pathology and Hygiene, College of Veterinary Medicine,
University of Illinois, Urbana-Champaign, Illinois

Portions of this study were supported by grants AI-03315 and HE-10609 from the U.S. Public Health Service, and by contract DADA17-70-C-0044 from the U.S. Army Research and Development Command.

INTRODUCTION

General considerations

Babesia and *Theileria* species are protozoan blood parasites that invade a variety of mammalian hosts. These parasites seem to be highly host specific and are primarily transmitted in nature by ticks. In tropical and subtropical areas of the world, certain *Babesia* and *Theileria* species cause economically important diseases in cattle. *Babesia bigemina*, the causative agent of "Texas fever", was the first protozoan parasite shown to be transmitted by an arthropod vector (Smith and Kilborne, 1893). In the United States, systematic control of the tick *Boophilus annulatus* resulted in the elimination of clinical forms of bovine babesiosis, although the disease still remains a major threat to cattle industries in many other countries of the five continents. Sporadically occurring *Babesia canis* infections of dogs have been found in the United States during the last two decades and, recently, babesiosis of horses, caused by *Babesia caballi*, was described in Florida (Sippel et al., 1962). Infections of cattle with *Theileria annulata* are known to occur throughout North Africa, the Middle and Far East, and the U.S.S.R. Conversely, infections with *Theileria parva*, or African East Coast fever, are limited to the African continent south of 10 degrees north of the equator in East, Central, and South Africa. The only two known cases of theileriosis in the United States are the case, as described by Splitter (1950), of *Theileria mutans* in an ox, and the case identified by Kreier et al. (1962) as *Theileria cervi* in erythrocytes of a splenectomized deer.

Recent developments

The last decade has witnessed great progress toward a better understanding of the biologic properties of *Babesia* and *Theileria* parasites by applying up-to-date methods in immunology, serology, and immunochemistry to their study. Only recently have we begun to acquire more specific knowledge about immunopathogenesis of babesial and theilerial infections. Several serodiagnostic procedures have been developed for detecting subclinical forms of babesiosis, and certain antigens from the blood of animals with acute babesial infections have been isolated that proved to be useful in producing sterile immunity. It is now evident that an immune antibody similar to that observed in bacterial and viral infections also seems to operate in babesial infections. This antibody, apparently developed against an antigen associated with a specific stage of parasitic development, appears to be more important in maintaining an immune state than are the antibodies against the parasite *per se*.

For many years it was suspected that an autoimmune process might operate in hemotropic infections. This process would be responsible for the occurrence of the anemia frequently observed in the absence of a high parasitemia. "Black water fever" is an example of a syndrome in which an autoimmune process was suspected to operate. The mechanism underlying the process depends on the host erythrocytes and other tissue cells being altered during infection to the extent that they acquire additional and different antigenic specificities which, in turn, stimulate the formation of antibodies that react with both altered and normal host tissues. The existence of autohemagglutinins was demonstrated in anaplasmosis, babesiosis, and malaria (Ristic, 1961; Mann and Ristic, 1963a,b; Cox et al., 1966; Schroeder et al., 1966). Recently, it has become apparent that serum components other than autohemagglutins may act as opsonins bringing about erythrophagocytosis (Schroeder, 1966; Schroeder and Ristic, 1968a). These findings introduced new insight into the mode by which an infectious agent can bring about damage to the host. In fact, these findings indicate that the pathology of immunologic and autoimmunologic processes in blood diseases was initiated by the infection *per se* and then followed an independent course, as typified by their persistence in the absence of an appreciable parasitemia (Schroeder and Ristic, 1968b).

In recent years, four human cases of babesial infection have been described (Skrabalo and Deanovic, 1957; Scholtens et al., 1968; Fitzpatrick et al., 1968; Western et al., 1969). The most significant history of three of these patients, two of whom died, was the splenectomy performed on them prior to the onset of the disease. Thus, it appears that the absence of the spleen may facilitate development of fulminating babesial infections in man. The history of the most recent case (Western et al., 1969), however, indicates that the disease may also develop in intact, nonsplenectomized humans. These findings point to the zoonotic potential of certain species of *Babesia* and suggest that babesiosis should be added to the list of zoonotic diseases.

Considerable progress has been made in devising tissue culture systems for *in vitro* propagation of *Theileria* species. Scientists are now in a position to conduct more critical studies into the growth properties and host-cell relationships of obligate intracellular blood protozoan parasites. Tissue culture studies of *Theileria* indicate that the parasite apparently stimulates the host cell to divide at an increasing rate. It is now apparent that lymphoid hyperplasia in cattle infected with *T. parva* largely arises from mitotic division of lymphoid cells, most of which are readily invaded by the parasite (Hulliger, 1965).

These and other newer developments symbolize the beginning of a new era of investigation into these long-known problems. It is hoped that the results of these and future studies will lead to better understanding of the principles governing the development, maintenance, and survival of these parasites.

RESISTANCE AND IMMUNITY IN *Babesia* AND *Theileria* INFECTIONS

Resistance to infection

Innate resistance. There are basically three types of resistance associated with *Babesia* and *Theileria* infections. First to be considered is that type of resistance which is innate to a given species. For example, the rabbit is completely resistant to babesial infections by either artificial or natural exposure to the agent.

Natural resistance. The second type, natural resistance, could be defined as that resistance which develops in susceptible, intact hosts and it implies that a specific organ plays a vital role in protecting the whole organism against fatal infection with *Babesia* or *Theileria*. An excellent example of this type of resistance is the case in Yugoslavia in which a human being was found to be infected with *Babesia bovis* (Skrabalo and Deanovic, 1957). This individual developed clinical symptoms of babesiosis 14 days after a *B. bovis* outbreak occurred among cattle in the same district in which the patient's farm was located. The entire area was heavily infested with *Dermacentor silvarum* and *Ixodes ricinus* ticks. Since none of the other cattlemen in this area developed the disease, the patient's susceptibility to a fulminating infection with fatal outcome was ascribed to the splenectomy performed on him several years earlier. Recently, Garnham and Bray (1959) drew attention to the fact that splenectomy could also make primates become susceptible to *Babesia* infection. Thus, it appears that both human beings and primates possess a degree of resistance to infections with *Babesia*. However, splenectomy can apparently reduce this resistance by increasing the host's susceptibility to infection. For some time it has been known that latent *B. bigemina*, and *T. annulata* infections of cattle could be easily activated into acute infections by splenectomy. It is, therefore, evident that the spleen is a vital natural body defense against babesial and theilerial infections and apparently essential for the development of natural resistance.

Age resistance. The third type of resistance to babesial and theilerial infections is associated with the age of the host. Although cattle up to 6 months of age are susceptible to infections with various species of *Babesia* and *Theileria*, they possess considerable parasitic tolerance as indicated by the moderate parasitemia which usually is not accompanied by severe clinical signs of the disease. Occasionally, this natural age resistance is further fortified by immunity passed from immune mother to offspring via ingested colostrum. Riek (1963) demonstrated a direct correlation between the presence and concentration of complement-fixing antibodies to *B. bigemina* and *B. argentina* in the colostrum and in the sera of calves after sucking on immune mothers. Hall (1960) artificially infected a group of pregnant cattle with *B. argentina* and found that all calves from noninfected mothers were more severely affected when challenged 2 to 52 days after birth than any of the calves in the infected group. The possibility that immunity was conferred by prenatal infection was ruled out by obtaining blood, at birth, from calves of infected mothers and inoculating it into susceptible splenectomized calves. The procedure did not produce infection in the recipients, indicating that a passive immunity had protected the calves from clinical symptoms.

The race of cattle has been considered as a factor influencing their resistance to *Babesia* or *Theileria* infection, but it has no experimental evidence in its favor. Daly and Hall (1955) suggested that very mild infections with *B. argentina* were observed in purebred Afrikander and Zebu cattle, as compared to more severe disease signs observed in Santa Gertrudis cattle, following inoculation of these animals with equal doses of infective blood. Conversely, Arnold (1948) observed that Brahman or European breeds of cattle imported from tick-free areas of the United States into Jamaica soon developed equally severe signs of babesiosis. According to Barnett (1963), the wide variation in resistance to *Theileria* infection observed among these races of cattle is due to local selection rather than to any breed or race resistance. He considers the age at which infection is experienced also to be a significant factor in resistance to later infections. For example, Zebu cattle in the enzootic East Coast fever areas of East Africa show a high natural resistance to *T. parva* because they experienced the infection during calfhood when mortality is low.

Infection immunity and sterile immunity

In general, immunity to babesial species is based on the principle of infection immunity in which, following the host's recovery from the initial infection, the parasite persists in the host's peripheral blood as a latent infection. In cattle, these latent infections may last for at least one (Seddon, 1952) to 12 years (Neitz, 1956). It is not clear whether the initial infection alone contributes to the long-term persistence of latent infection or whether the reinfections of cattle in enzootic areas are responsible for it. In certain babesiosis enzootic areas, infection of young calves is used as a means of protecting them against the occurrence of a fulminating and frequently fatal disease when they are older.

Apart from infection immunity, sterile immunity with or without previous infection apparently also operates in babesiosis. There have been several reports describing resistance to clinical reinfection in cattle that no longer carry latent infections (Arnold, 1948; Davies et al., 1958; Riek, 1963; 1968). Also, sufficiently effective sterile immunity was conferred by immune mothers to their nursing calves to protect the calves from showing clinical symptoms of babesiosis when challenged (Hall, 1960). More recently, a purified antigen isolated from the serum of dogs acutely infected with *B. canis* was found to be immunogenic in susceptible dogs (K. H. Sibinovic et al., 1967b). An inverse relation was shown between the concentration of antibody produced in response to the antigen and the degree of parasitemia caused by challenge infection. The antigen was considered to be a metabolite rather than an integral component of the parasite, and it appeared in the plasma of infected animals during the acute stage of infection when vigorous reproduction of babesial parasites is underway (K. H. Sibinovic, 1966).

Evidence that sterile immunity to clinical infection with *B. canis* can be produced in susceptible dogs raises a question regarding the circumstances under which sterile immunity to bovine babesiosis develops in the field. Also, an explanation is needed for the fact that not all animals that recover from latent infection develop a sterile immunity sufficiently protective to enable them to withstand clinical reinfection.

In contrast to the apparently short-lasting sterile immunity to babesial species, the immunity to *T. parva* is long-lasting and apparently a sterile one. This, however, is not true of the immunity to *T. annulata* and *T. mutans*. These parasites persist in clinically recovered animals, and for many years such animals remain a source of reinfection for ticks.

The exact mechanism by which sterile immunity to *T. parva* develops is not clearly understood. The apparent effectiveness of serum therapy reported by some workers (Agaev, 1958; Robson, 1961) led them to believe that a protective antibody developed in the serum of animals surviving *T. parva* infection. However, according to Barnett (1963), the experimental evidence for the existence of such an antibody in animals recovered from *T. annulata* or *T. parva* infections has not been conclusively demonstrated and no experimental work on the subject has been carried out with *T. mutans*. The concept of true sterile immunity following an infection with *T. parva* has recently been questioned (Barnett, 1955; Barnett and Brocklesby, 1966).

Histopathologic studies of the lymph nodes of cattle that recovered from acute *T. parva* infection usually show hypertrophy of lymphocytes having very dense cytoplasm with accumulations in it of azurophilic granules which are probably degenerated schizonts. No evidence for macrophage production and phagocytosis of schizonts was observed, indicating that the phagocytic cell elements are probably not directly involved in residual immunity to *T. parva*. According to Barnett (1965), immunity to *T. parva* appears to be a tissue immunity with the lymphocytic cells involved in limiting and eliminating the parasites. This opinion is supported by the tissue culture studies of immunity to *T. parva* (Hulliger, 1965; Hulliger et al., 1966).

Immunologic principles operating in *Babesia* or *Theileria* infections can be summarized as follows: 1. Except for the apparently sterile immunity to *T. parva*, immunity to other *Theileria* species and also to *Babesia* appears to be based on infection immunity characterized by a latency of variable duration. 2. Animals in which latency has been destroyed or eliminated possess little to no residual sterile immunity, but if some sterile immunity persists, then the animal can resist clinical reinfection. 3. There is indication that sterile immunity from *Babesia* infection depends, at least in part, on the presence of protective serum antibody.

It would be logical to assume from studies of the pathogenesis of babesiosis that the parasite and its various developing forms maximally stimulate the host's defense mechanisms during acute infection when massive numbers of parasites invade the host's entire blood vascular system. This antigenic stimulation usually continues, although probably at lower levels, throughout subclinical relapses of the infection. In these periods, the gradual increase of circulating antibody and intense proliferation of macrophages render it increasingly difficult for the parasite to infect normal erythrocytes. When infection does occur, it is confined to a small percentage of erythrocytes. At this stage, however, a certain number of organisms would escape the host's defenses and continue to perpetuate the infection, thus providing for continued antigenic stimulation. The low level of parasite development that occurs in an immunologically competent host, without causing the appearance of detectable clinical manifestations, is referred to as a "carrier stage." The duration of the carrier state depends on the chance infection of new erythrocytes. If the residual infection in the host's circulating erythrocytes is destroyed, it is not possible to transmit the infection further by blood subinoculation into a susceptible animal, and such a host is referred to as being free of babesiosis.

Some of these *Babesia*-free animals, however, possess a considerable degree of acquired resistance to reinfection. This observation can be explained in the following ways: 1. Some individual animals undergo greater antigenic stimulation than others as a result of the intensity of parasitemia present during the acute infection and of the virulence and antigenicity of the invading parasite. 2. In certain animals, although the presence of the parasite cannot be demonstrated by blood transmission experiments, the parasite may continue to exist in tissue cells of organs such as liver, spleen, bone marrow, and brain. In birds the latter organ has been shown to harbor *Plasmodium gallinaceum* after the parasite was eliminated from the blood vascular system (Huff, 1957).

Role of the spleen

One basic immunogenic difference between *Babesia* and *T. parva* is illustrated by the role that the spleen plays in the development of acquired immunity to infection with these organisms. The state of nonsterile immunity in animals infected with *Babesia* species can easily be broken by splenectomy (Miessner, 1931). Contrary to this is the observation that a loss of immunity to infection with *T. parva* cannot be induced by splenectomy (Du Toit, 1928). Therefore, in babesial infections it is evident that the spleen plays a vital dual role in the defense of the body. First, it is the principal organ involved in limiting the uncontrolled spread of the infecting agent during the acute phase of the infection. This role is best illustrated by the fact that if splenectomized and nonsplenectomized calves are each injected with comparable numbers of parasites, the splenectomized animals undergo a more severe attack which is frequently fatal, while the nonsplenectomized calves show less severe signs of the disease and usually survive. The second role of the spleen is to maintain continuous control of parasitic crises during the convalescent and carrier phases of babesial infections. This function possibly contributes to the production and maintenance of the extrasplenic cellular and humoral elements necessary to control the infection efficiently at the latent level.

This paramount role of the spleen in the mechanism of babesial immunity is partly responsible for the difficulty one encounters in clearly defining the susceptibility of certain animal species to infection with *Babesia* species. The best example of this is the recent observation that both splenectomized man and chimpanzees were subject to a fulminating and fatal infection with *Babesia* species (Skrabalo and Deanovic, 1957; Garnham and Bray, 1959). These investigators studied the role of the spleen in human and primate resistance extensively and proposed that people and primates living in babesiosis enzootic, tick-infested areas may harbor latent *Babesia* infections. These infections may be responsible for some unknown pathogenic effect that frequently affects farm workers, such as multiple sclerosis (Garnham and Bray, 1959). Under these circumstances, it is evident that there is a need for the development of a serodiagnostic procedure to detect an antibody to *Babesia*, rather than to detect the parasite itself. Fortunately, several such diagnostic procedures have recently been developed. The implementation of these tests with other sensitive tools for detecting *Babesia* species promises to play an important role in studying the epidemiology of babesiosis. The results of the capillary-tube latex-agglutination (CTLA) test, to be described later, served as supporting evidence for the identification of a second human case of babesiosis, also to be described later.

In cattle that survive infections with *T. parva*, the sterile immunity apparently is not affected by splenectomy. However, such immunity does not seem to exist in infections with other species of *Theileria*, such as *T. annulata* and *T. mutans*. The immunity involved in infection with the latter two parasites seems to follow the pattern of infection immunity typical of *Babesia*, i.e., a relapse of the infection can be caused by splenectomy. These immunogenic differences between *T. parva* and other *Theileria* species indicate some of the basic differences that probably exist between these parasites with reference to the pathogenesis of the disease they cause, the tissues they selectively invade, and the defense forces they stimulate. In the case of *T. parva*, the cellular tissue immunity seems to be the vital defense force preventing reinfection.

Babesia

General features

Babes (1888) first observed *Babesia* parasites in the blood of African cattle showing signs of hemoglobinuria. This author named the parasites *Haema-*

tococcus bovis in the belief that he had succeeded in propagating them *in vitro*. The parasite was renamed *Babesia bovis* by Starcovici (1893). In 1893, Smith and Kilborne studied Texas Fever of cattle in the United States and recognized the role of ticks as biologic vectors of the causative agent. These authors clearly recognized the protozoan nature of the agent and proposed the name *Pyrosoma bigeminum*. This was later changed to *Babesia bigemina* by Starcovici (1893).

Transmission of babesiosis in nature is accomplished through arthropods such as hard ticks of the genera *Rhipicephalus, Ixodes, Boophilus, Haemaphysalis, Hyalomma*, and *Dermacentor*. Blood-sucking flies, such as *Stomoxys* and *Tabanus* species, have been implicated as mechanical vectors (Abramov, 1952; Neitz, 1956). A developmental cycle in arthropods has not been satisfactorily determined. Smith and Kilborne (1893) demonstrated transovarial transmission of *B. bigemina* in *Boophilus annulatus*. Dennis (1932) reported that *B. bigemina* underwent morphologic changes in *B. annulatus*. The results of recent studies by Riek (1968) and by Friedhoff and Scholtyseck (1968) indicate that *Babesia* parasites develop similarly to those belonging to the class of Sporozoa.

Infections of dogs with *B. canis* have been reported to occur in a number of localities in the United States, e.g., Florida (Sanders, 1937), Texas (Merenda, 1939), Virginia (Grogan, 1953), California (Alperin and Bevins, 1963), and Illinois (Ristic, 1965, unpublished data).

Equine babesiosis, thought to be caused by *B. caballi*, was first described in the United States by Sippel et al. (1962). The disease was diagnosed in 97 horses from Florida based on examination of Giemsa-stained blood films. Maurer (1962) described equine babesiosis as a "newly emerging disease in the United States."

Studies of the parasites present in *Babesia*-infected horse blood from Florida were conducted using a fluorescent-antibody technique. Parasites resembling *B. caballi* constituted a majority of the parasite population. Forms typical of *Babesia equi* were also observed. Thus, it was concluded that infected equine blood from Florida contained both species of parasites (Ristic et al., 1964). Diagnosis of the acute phase of infection is made by examining stained blood films. During this brief period, the percentage of erythrocytes containing the parasite is low, seldom exceeding 4 to 6 percent. Horses which recover from the acute infection enter latency and become healthy carriers. In these animals, parasites cannot readily be found in blood films with any of the staining techniques.

Serologic diagnosis

Complement-fixation (CF) tests. A complement-fixation (CF) test for the diagnosis of equine babesiosis was described by Hirato et al. (1945). The antigen, consisting of stromata of erythrocytes from an acutely infected horse, was used to detect serum antibody. In one case, complement-fixing antibody persisted for at least 100 days following infection of the animal. Recently, Holbrook (1965) used the CF test to diagnose equine babesiosis in the United States.

Mahoney (1962) prepared an antigen from water-lysed erythrocytes of cattle acutely infected with *B. argentina* and *B. bigemina*. The antigen was shell-frozen in 1.0 ml quantities at −79°C and then preserved at −20°C. Homologous antibodies became detectable in the CF test within 12 to 34 days following infection. No serologic cross-reaction was observed between *Babesia rodhaini* and *B. canis* using the antigen of the latter parasite. Lyophilization was found to be an efficient method for long-term preservation of the antigen.

By means of immunohemolysis and, more recently, by exposure to 0.3 per cent saponin, Schindler and Dennig (1962 a,b) prepared a complement-fixing antigen from erythrocytes of dogs acutely infected with *Babesia canis*. The antibody became detectable in the CF test within 12 to 34 days following infection. As in the case of *B. argentina* and *B. bigemina*, no serologic cross-reaction was observed between *B. rodhaini* and *B. canis* using the antigen of the latter parasite. Lyophilization was again found to be an efficient method for long-term preservation of the antigen.

Capillary-tube agglutination (CA) test. Using a technique similar to that employed for preparation of *Anaplasma* capillary-tube agglutination (CA) antigen (Ristic, 1962), a CA antigen was prepared from *Babesia*-infected erythrocytes and used for the demonstration of agglutinating antibodies in sera of infected horses (Ristic, 1964, unpublished data). Agglutinating antibodies were detected in 19 of 20 known infected horses from Florida and Georgia. However, the *Babesia* CA antigen was highly perishable and, therefore, was of little practical value.

A modification of the above method was recently used to prepare a more stable CA antigen from erythrocytes of dogs infected with *Babesia canis* (Ristic et al., 1969a). The antigen was preserved in lyophilized form and was reconstituted for use when needed. Reconstituted antigen remained stable for at least one month when kept at 4°C. Employed in a capillary-tube agglutination (CA) test, the antigen was found useful for detection of subclinical forms of canine babesiosis. More recently, the test was applied to diagnose a fourth human case of babesiosis (Western et al., 1969; Healy et al., 1969; Ristic et al., 1969b). The advantages of the CA test are simplicity, economy, and speed of performance. The test may be useful to practicing veterinarians in the prevention and control of canine babesiosis.

Fluorescent-antibody (FA) techniques. The use of fluorescein-labeled anti-*Babesia* (Florida isolate) globulin for detecting *Babesia* parasites in the blood of infected horses was described by Ristic et al. (1964). The specific serologic staining of different structural and developmental features revealed that the Florida isolate of *Babesia* probably contained both *B. caballi* and *B. equi* (Ristic et al., 1964). It was anticipated that all growth stages of *Babesia* that were capable of stimulating antibody production in infected horses should have been revealed by the FA technique (Figs. 1-4).

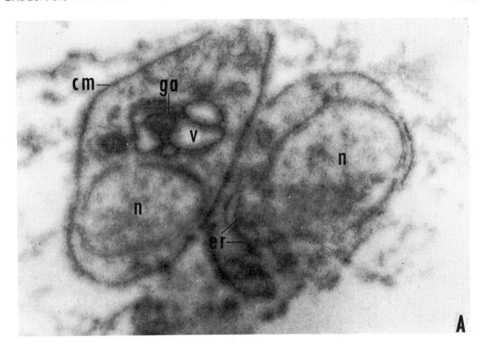

FIG. 1.   *A.* Electron micrograph of a section through two *Babesia* parasites in a lysed equine erythrocyte. The parasites are bounded by a single cytoplasmic membrane (cm). In the cytoplasm of the parasites are seen endoplasmic reticulum (er), vacuoles (v), and Golgi apparatus (ga). The nuclei (n) have double membranes and are situated eccentrically, indicating that the poles of the parasites are reversed. Reduced 10 percent from $\times$ 30,000. *B.* Two parasites in a situation comparable to those in (*A*). Fluorescent-antibody stain; Reduced 10 percent from $\times$ 920.

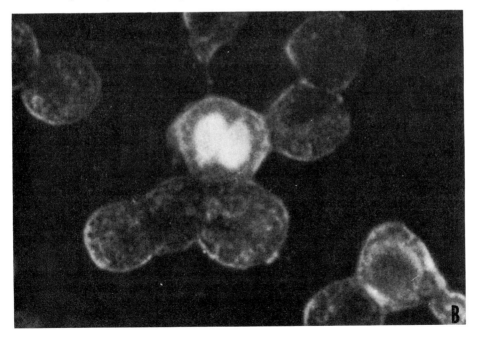

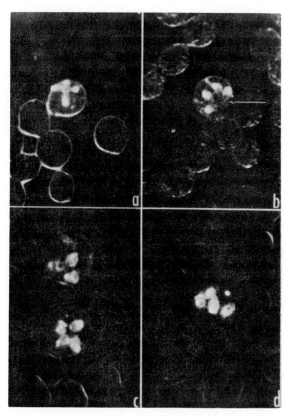

FIG. 2. *Babesia equi* in various stages of multiplication and stained with fluorescein-labeled antibody. *A*. An early stage of multiplication by budding into four units, known as the "Maltese cross" form; *B*. Newly formed parasites separated in four directions with the rounded ends oriented toward the erythrocyte's periphery; *C*. and *D*. Four newly formed, irregularly arranged parasites. Fluorescent-antibody stain; × 650.

Ristic and Sibinovic (1964) described a one-step fluorescence inhibition test for diagnosing equine babesiosis. The procedure of Cherry et al. (1960) for the one-step fluorescence inhibition test was modified by using plastic cups for deposition of reactants employed in the test. The modification gave the advantage of permitting maximal contact between antigen and antibody. Sera from 14 known *Babesia* carriers and from 10 apparently normal horses were studied in the test. All positive sera caused a degree of inhibition of fluorescence that ranged from complete inhibition with parasites not visible, to partial inhibition with only contours of the parasites visible. With eight of the negative sera, inhibition of the fluorescence was not observed. Two of the sera from normal horses, however, caused inhibition of fluorescence equal to that observed with the sera from some positive horses. Heat inactivation (56°C for 30 minutes) of sera from positive horses did not alter the inhibition of specific fluorescence. Addition of 1:200 phenol or 1:10,000 thimerosal to heat-inactivated positive sera resulted in an increase of nonspecific fluorescence.

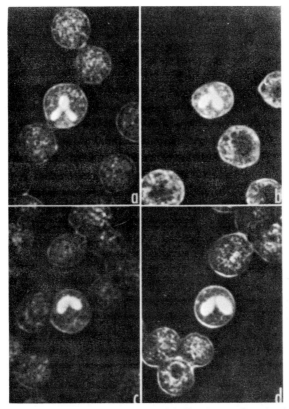

FIG. 3. *Babesia caballi* in various stages of multiplication and stained with fluorescein-labeled antibody. *A.* In an early stage of multiplication by binary fission, two daughter cells formed; *B.* and *C.* There was progressive separation and maturation of the daughter cells; and *D.* Two completely separated parasites formed. Fluorescent-antibody stain; × 700.

Recently, Madden and Holbrook (1968) used the indirect fluorescent-antibody technique to detect carrier horses experimentally infected with *B. caballi* and to study the serologic relationship between *B. caballi* and *B. equi.* There was no cross-reaction between these parasites when strain-specific sera from carrier horses were used.

Gel-precipitation (GP) test. By means of precipitation with protamine sulfate, a soluble antigen, termed the PS antigen, was obtained from erythrocytes of horses acutely infected with *B. caballi* and *B. equi*, a mixed strain known as the Florida isolate (Ristic and Sibinovic, 1964). The interaction of the PS antigen in gel with sera of affected horses demonstrated the presence of a precipitating antibody in horses with babesiosis. Acute or subclinical latent phase sera gave equal precipitation reactions. The specificity of the GP test was shown by the absence of reactions with sera from horses experiencing other infections, including viral infectious anemia.

Antibodies to the PS antigen were first demonstrable at 17 days postinfection. The antibody persisted for at least 15 months after infection.

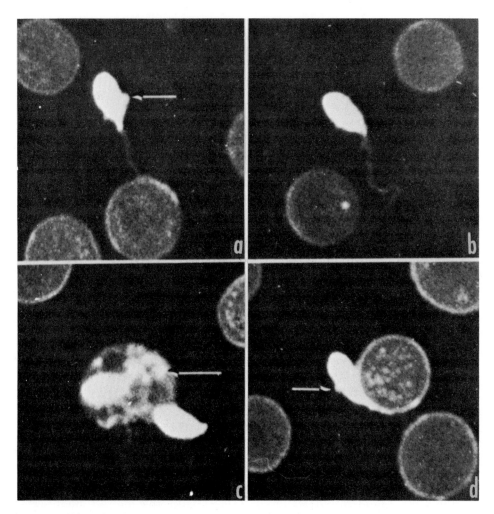

FIG. 4.   Tailed forms of *Babesia* strained with fluorescent antibody. *A*. One free parasite has a protuberance on its body (arrow). *B*. Notice the length of the tail on another free parasite. *C*. An erythrocyte containing two parasites is shown, one of which is partially outside the erythrocyte; the intraerythrocytic parasite has its tail twisted to form a loop (arrow). *D*. A parasite is attached to the erythrocytic membrane. Its tail encircles one-third of the circumference of the erythrocyte. The body of the parasite shows a protuberance (arrow). Fluorescent-antibody stain; × 1200.

Preparation of protamine sulfate (PS) antigen.   The technique for preparing PS antigen is a modification of a method used for preparing a similar antigen from *Anaplasma marginale* (Ristic et al., 1963; Ristic and Mann, 1963).

An acutely infected splenectomized horse, with one or more *Babesia* parasites in approximately 14 percent of its erythrocytes, was exsanguinated under deep anesthesia. The blood was collected in an equal volume of sterile Alsever's solution. Three washings of the erythrocytes were accomplished by centrifugation at 1,500 g after successive suspensions in physiologic salt solution. Subsequently, three volumes of physiologic salt solution were added to each volume of packed erythrocytes, and the suspension was sonically oscillated twice in a continuous-flow ultrasonicator with a current output of 4.5 amperes and a lysate flow of 50 ml per minute. The oscillated material was sedimented at 3,300 g for 30 minutes in a refrigerated centrifuge. To each 100 ml of the supernatant lysate, 0.5 g of protamine sulfate dissolved in 10 ml of distilled water was added. The mixture was left at 4°C for 2 hours, then centrifuged at 3,300 g for 30 minutes, and the sedimented precipitate was collected. Two volumes of phosphate-buffered physiologic salt solution (pH 9.0) were added to each volume of the precipitate. The precipitate was homogenized with a TenBroeck glass grinder and centrifuged at 12,100 g for 30 minutes. The supernatant fluid was the precipitinogen used in the GP test. The precipitinogen was routinely stored in 1 to 2 ml quantities at −65°C. During use, the precipitinogen was maintained at 4°C. *Properties of protamine sulfate (PS) antigen.* Paper electrophoretic studies of the PS antigen revealed four separate bands, I, II, III, and IV. Band II varied in intensity depending upon the pH of the buffer used in the electrophoretic system. The antigenic activity was destroyed by trypsin and taka-diastase. Analytic ultracentrifugation of the PS antigen revealed a sedimentation rate of 12 svedberg units.

The antigen was thermostable, withstanding boiling for 30 minutes. Serologic reactivity was retained for at least two weeks when the antigen was treated with either 1:500 phenol or 1:20,000 thimerosal. Antigen stored at −65°C was still serologically reactive 15 months later. On the basis of these findings, the soluble PS antigen is thought to be a mucoprotein (S. Sibinovic, et al., 1966).

Passive hemagglutination (HA) test. Heated PS antigen was adsorbed onto intact sheep erythrocytes and these cells were then used in a passive hemagglutination (HA) test for detection and titration of antibodies in serum of horses infected with *B. caballi* (S. Sibinovic et al., 1969). Reactions were observed with convalescent sera from horses infected with *B. caballi* but not with convalescent sera from *B. canis* or *B. rodhaini* infections.

Soluble serum antigens in animals with babesial infections

The observations made by independent workers studying infections with different blood parasites indicate that in certain hemoparasitic diseases, an antigen-antibody system exists which resembles that of the neutralizing and protective phenomena frequently observed in bacterial and viral diseases. D'Alesandro (1963) reported a soluble antigen present in rats infected with *Trypanosoma lewisi*, and Seed and Weinman (1963) found a similar antigen in sera of mice infected with *Trypanosoma rhodesiense*. There was evidence that these antigens may have elicited production of protective antibodies.

K. H. Sibinovic et al. (1965) found a soluble antigen in sera of horses acutely infected with *B. caballi*. Antibodies against this antigen were demonstrated by the slide gel-diffusion technique. Serum from an acutely infected horse was used as the antigen, and sera from convalescing horses were used as antibody. Of 32 fractions obtained by continuous-flow electrophoresis of post-infection serum, 7 contained an antigen not found in pre-infection serum. Two of the fractions reacted with the serum from a carrier horse when tested by the slide gel-diffusion technique. In the immunoelectrophoretic system, the antigens disappeared from the sera of infected horses approximately one month after experimental infection. Antibodies to the soluble *Babesia* antigens became demonstrable at 3 months after infection and persisted for at least an additional 7 months. The time of appearance of antibodies to serum antigens coincided with the beginning of the carrier stage of infection when immunity against reinfection is usually demonstrable. Thus, one may speculate that a similarity exists between the soluble antigen-antibody complex occurring in infections with *Babesia* and a similar complex recently demonstrated in *T. lewisi* infections (D'Alesandro, 1963). It is possible that the antigen described in the present study may be similar to the *T. lewisi* soluble antigen, and that it also stimulates production of immune antibody in infected horses.

Isolation and purification of serum antigens. The antigens found in the sera of horses, dogs, and rats with acute babesiosis were isolated and purified by means of ultracentrifugation and column fractionation, (K. H. Sibinovic et al., 1967a). In the process, the antigens were separated from lipids, lipoproteins, albumin, blood pigment, alpha-globulins and a majority of the beta- and gamma-globulins.

The babesial serum antigens from the horse, dog, and rat were further separated into two fractions by zonal density-gradient centrifugation. Fraction A, found in the 25 percent sucrose concentration, was slow moving and appeared to migrate as a gamma-globulin when tested by means of paper electrophoresis. Fraction B, found in the 40 percent sucrose concentration, moved more rapidly and in a manner similar to the beta-globulins.

Analytic ultracentrifugation studies of the babesial serum antigens also revealed that they consisted of two fractions with significantly different sedimentation coefficients (Fig. 5). Further study showed that fraction A, obtained by zonal density-gradient centrifugation, was identical to the component with the lower sedimentation coefficient and that fraction B was identical to the component with the higher sedimentation coefficient.

Biophysical and biochemical characteristics of serum antigens. A study of the biophysical and biochemical characteristics of the babesial serum antigens indicated that fraction A was a lipoprotein and fraction B was a muco-lipoprotein (K. H. Sibinovic et al., 1967a). The serologic activity of both fractions was destroyed by dialysis against distilled water, by sodium chloride concentrations of over 5 percent, and by a pH above 9.0. Fraction A precipitated in acetate buffers at pH 4.4 to 6.0, and it remained serologically reactive when redissolved by dialysis against 0.1 molar sodium chloride.

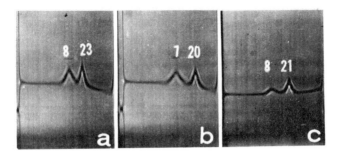

FIG. 5. Sedimentation patterns of babesial serum antigens diluted to give an optical density of 0.5 at 280 mμ and centrifuged at 56,000 rpm in the Beckman Analytical Ultracentrifuge equipped with a Schlerin optical system: A. Horse-origin babesial serum antigen, at 16 minutes; B. Dog-origin babesial serum antigen, at 24 minutes; C. Rat-origin babesial serum antigen, at 16 minutes. (Courtesy of Dr. K. H. Sibinovic.)

Aminoacid analysis by paper chromatography showed that this fraction contained all the aminoacids except proline and methionine. Serologic reactivity was destroyed by treatment with papain, trypsin, lipase, and lecithinase C. Fraction B was not precipitated in acetate buffers, and on aminoacid analysis, it was shown to lack proline and histidine. Serologic reactivity was destroyed by taka-diastase, as well as by those enzymes which destroyed fraction A, suggesting that the "muco" component present in fraction B was absent in fraction A.

Immunoelectrophoretic studies of the babesial serum antigens also revealed the presence of two fractions. The degree of parasitemia, however, appeared to influence the number of fractions obtained since antigens from dogs or rats with more than 50 percent and horses with more than 10 percent parasitized erythrocytes gave up to 9 lines of precipitation when reacted with specific antisera by means of immunoelectrophoresis.

Serologic specificity of serum antigens. Serologic specificity of the babesial serum antigens was tested by gel precipitation against convalescent sera from horses infected with *B. equi* and *B. caballi*, from dogs infected with *B. canis*, and from rats infected with *B. rodhaini* parasites. The antigens reacted with homologous and heterologous convalescent sera but not with sera of noninfected animals. Lines of identity were evident within the A fractions of horse, dog, and rat antigens, as well as within the B fractions. Lines of identity were absent between the A and B fractions (K. H. Sibinovic et al., 1967b).

Effect of antibodies to serum antigens on the infectivity of *Babesia*. When infected erythocytes were mixed with antiserum produced against babesial serum antigens and immediately injected into dogs (*B. canis*-infected erythrocytes) or rats (*B. rodhaini*-infected erythrocytes), the animals developed typical babesiosis. When injected with erythrocyte suspensions incubated with this antiserum at 37°C for 30 minutes, the animals developed mild babesiosis with low degrees of parasitemia, moderate anemia, and only slightly elevated temperatures. Animals that received erythrocyte suspensions incubated with the antiserum for 60 minutes at 37°C did not develop clinical signs of babesiosis and parasites were not found in the peripheral blood.

Studies of the *in vitro* effects on *Babesia* of immunoglobulins to serum antigens showed that the primary effect was agglutination of the infected erythrocytes or of the parasites freed by ultrasonic oscillation. Inoculation of these agglutinated parasites into susceptible animals did not result in an infection in the animals. Normal sera and normal globulins did not agglutinate infected erythrocytes or parasites from the erythrocytes, nor were normal erythrocytes agglutinated by the immunoglobulins (K. H. Sibinovic, 1966).

Application of the fluorescent-antibody (FA) technique to the study of serum antigens. Several experiments have been conducted using the FA technique in an effort to ascertain the origin of the serum antigens. The results of these studies indicated that the antigen is present in the cytoplasm of the infected erythrocyte. Since the maximal concentration of these antigens was observed at the peak of parasitemia when the erythrocytes become increasingly fragile and hemolysis usually takes place, one may conclude that the origin of the serum antigen is the infected erythrocyte.

Following intravenous injection of babesial serum antigen from dogs or rats into normal rats, rat erythrocytes fluoresced within 15 minutes. A "doughnut-like" halo effect was first seen within 10 minutes after injection. Subsequently collected samples revealed intense fluorescence of the entire erythrocytic surface. There was no fluorescence of erythrocytes collected 8 to 10 hours after injection (K. H. Sibinovic, 1966).

Role of antibody to serum antigens on the course of parasitemia. Titration of the serum antigen and its antibody in the course of babesial infection revealed that the antibody titer is inversely related to the severity of parasitemia and the concentration of serum antigen. Titrations of the antigen and antibody were accomplished by means of a bentonite agglutination (BA) test (K. H. Sibinovic et al., 1966) using bentonite particles sensitized with antibody or antigen, respectively. From these studies it was ascertained that in infected animals the disappearance of the antibody to serum antigen was followed by the appearance of parasitemia and serum antigen, which then resulted in the reappearance of antibody and disappearance of both parasitemia and the serum antigen (K. H. Sibinovic et al., 1967b). It is now evident that the antibody to serum antigen developed in the course of infection has a suppressive and controlling effect on the extent of parasitemia.

The exact mechanism by which the protective antibody operates is not clearly understood. It appears, however, that the serum antigen against which the antibody is directed represents a substance intimately associated with the development of the parasite, and that its reaction with specific antibody may have interfered with the completion of the parasite's cycle of development.

A capillary-tube latex-agglutination (CTLA) test for babesiosis. The serum antigens isolated from dogs with acute babesiosis were adsorbed to latex particles having an average diameter of 0.81 μ, in accordance with the method described by Todorovic et al. (1967) for adsorption of plasmodial antigens. The sensitized latex particles were used as agglutinogens in a capillary-tube latex-agglutination (CTLA) test for titration of antibodies in sera from dogs infected with *B. canis*. Due to the fact that the soluble babesial antigens serologically cross-react with other members of the genus, the CTLA test was used for detection and titration of antibodies to several babesial species.

The earliest detection of antibodies in infected dog serum occurred at approximately 15 days following infection, they reached a maximal titer of 1:640 about two months later, and persisted at titers of 1:40 to 1:80 during the next four months. The persistence of serum agglutinins was generally correlated with the persistence of an active carrier stage which, in some cases, terminated between 8 and 18 months post-infection and, in other cases, persisted as long as three years post-infection.

The CTLA test has also been successfully used for investigating the incidence of subclinical canine babesiosis in dogs. Serum samples from 65 dogs, purchased for experimental use from various localities in Illinois, were examined by the CTLA test. Samples from two of the dogs were positive. Splenectomy was performed on one dog and it relapsed with babesiosis two and a half weeks later. Eighteen days later, a maximum parasitemia of 11 percent was observed in the peripheral blood of this dog.

From these preliminary observations, it was concluded that the CTLA test for canine babesiosis is a useful tool for diagnosing clinical and subclinical forms of the disease. Furthermore, it appears that the subclinical form of babesiosis occurs rather frequently in dogs and can be accurately identified by this test.

Serologic diagnosis of human babesiosis. The CTLA and CA tests were applied to the diagnosis of babesiosis in man. For example, besides the first authentic human case of babesiosis described by Skrabalo and Deanovic (1957), another such case was recently brought to our attention* wherein a 46-year-old Caucasian male San Francisco resident was admitted to the hospital in June, 1966. This patient's serum was examined, using the FA technique, for malarial antibodies, and it was found negative to ten malarial antigens, including those of the four human species of malaria. Additional examination of blood from this patient by the *Babesia* research team at the United States Department of Agriculture revealed that the forms of the parasites in question resembled *B. caballi* and *B. equi*. His serum, examined by the CTLA test, showed a titer of 1:80, positive dog serum reacted at 1:160, and five control human sera showed no reaction at a 1:2 dilution.

The most significant part of this patient's medical history was that a

* The history of the patient and his serum sample were provided by Dr. E. H. Braff, San Francisco Department of Public Health, San Francisco, California, and by Dr. R. G. Scholtens, Parasitic Diseases Section, Epidemiology Branch, Communicable Disease Center, United States Public Health Service, Chamblee, Georgia. The report on this case is found in the Morbidity and Mortality Weekly Report, January 7, 1967, p. 8, of the C.D.C., U.S.P.H.S., Atlanta, Georgia.

splenectomy was performed in 1964 to relieve a hereditary spherocytosis. This history is nearly identical to that of the previous case of human babesiosis described by Skrabalo and Deanovic (1957).

The third human case of babesiosis was described by Fitzpatrick et al. (1968) and again concerned a splenectomized person.

Recently, the fourth human case of babesiosis was brought to our attention* and involved a person who had not had a splenectomy. A 59-year-old widow from New Jersey was admitted to a hospital in July, 1969, with a two-week history of fever, headache, malaise, and weakness (Western et al., 1969). Intraerythrocytic *Babesia* parasites were observed in stained blood films of the patient. Epidemiologic investigation revealed that during the summer on Nantucket Island, Massachusetts, the patient's dog was frequently invaded by ticks, and the patient herself once removed a deeply embedded tick from her chest. Healy et al. (1969) inoculated various laboratory animals with the patient's blood and established babesial infection in a hamster.

In our laboratory, *Babesia* was isolated in a splenectomized rhesus monkey inoculated with the patient's blood. Four additional passages of the parasite were made in splenectomized rhesus monkeys. Acute babesiosis, characterized by severe anemia and parasitemia, was observed in these animals.

Paired serum samples were obtained from the patient during the disease and approximately three weeks later. The first sample was negative, but the second was positive by the CA test using *B. canis* antigen. Also, the serum from the patient's dog was positive by the test. Sera from a donkey and a horse were negative.

From these studies, it could be concluded that latent infections with certain *Babesia* species probably do exist in human beings, and that clinically demonstrable fulminating infections are often observed when the spleen, which appears to play a vital role in the defense against babesial infections, is removed.

Immunogenic properties of serum antigens. The immunogenic activity of the antigens was extensively tested in rats and dogs (K. H. Sibinovic, 1966). When dogs were immunized with babesial serum antigens of dog or rat origin, they were protected against challenge with *B. canis* for at least 9 months. The animals apparently became susceptible to challenge infection at the time when the hemagglutination titer fell below 40. When rats were immunized with babesial serum antigen of rat origin or with fraction B of horse origin, the animals showed partial resistance against challenge with *B. rodhaini*. In these animals, the degree of parasitemia was the criterion for

* The history of the patient and her blood samples were provided through the courtesy of Dr. G. R. Healy, Chief, Helminthology and Protozoology Unit, Parasitology Section of the National Communicable Disease Center, United States Public Health Service, Atlanta, Georgia. These samples were obtained from the patient by Dr. Gordon D. Benson, Department of Medicine, Rutgers Medical School. The report on this case is found in CDC Veterinary Public Health Notes, September, 1969, p. 3. A paper on the subject by Western et al. (1969) is in press for the New England Journal of Medicine.

evaluation of protection; however, when anemia was considered the criterion, the protection was not significant. The antisera prepared in homologous species against babesial serum antigens of dog or rat origin produced complete protection for periods up to 45 days when administered in a 20 ml dose to dogs and in a 3 ml dose to rats. Also, the antisera prepared against horse antigen produced significant protection in these animals. Pyrexia and mild leukocytosis were the only adverse reactions seen in these trials.

Autoimmunization and anemia

Autohemagglutinins. An outstanding feature of erythrocytic infections, including babesiosis, is the occurrence of anemia that is often not proportional to the prevailing parasitemia. This observation led many workers to suspect that the anemia may be, in part, of immunologic origin. A study of the macrocytic anemia occurring in calves infected with *A. marginale* revealed the presence of erythrocyte-bound and free-serum autohemagglutinins during the acute and convalescent phases of infection (Ristic, 1961; Mann and Ristic, 1963 a,b). The hemagglutinins occurred during the anemic crisis and reacted with autologous and homologous trypsin-treated erythrocytes (Schroeder and Ristic, 1965). The onset of erythrophagocytosis in the spleen and bone marrow of *Anaplasma*-infected calves seemed to be associated with the initial appearance of free-serum hemagglutinins (Kreier et al., 1964).

In earlier studies, Morton and Pickles (1947, 1951) and Wiener and Klatz (1951) found that treating animal erythrocytes with proteolytic enzymes, such as trypsin, papain, and ficin, results in an antigenic alteration of these cells similar to that caused by bacterial enzymes. They then used proteolytic enzyme-altered erythrocytes in a hemagglutination test to detect incomplete Rh antibodies. Antisera from patients with acquired hemolytic anemia were shown to react with enzyme-treated erythrocytes (Henningsen, 1949; Mabry et al., 1956 a,b). Following the injection of autologous trypsin-treated erythrocytes in rabbits, hemagglutinins developed that reacted *in vitro* with the treated erythrocytes (Dodd et al., 1953; Smith et al., 1954; Wallace et al., 1955). Treatment of bovine erythrocytes with trypsin uncovered antigenic sites that then reacted with certain of the isoantibodies of cattle, with the antibody from patients with infectious mononucleosis, or with free-serum hemagglutinins from the sera of calves infected with *Anaplasma* (Burnet and Anderson, 1946; Stone and Miller, 1955; Tomsick and Baumann-Grace, 1960; Mann and Ristic, 1963 a,b).

Serum hemagglutinins that reacted with trypsin-treated erythrocytes were detected in the sera of rats infected with *B. rodhaini* (Schroeder et al., 1966) by utilizing a technique developed by Morton and Pickles (1947) and modified by Mann and Ristic (1963b). Four and one-half ml of a 0.25 percent trypsin solution were added to 0.5 ml of washed, packed erythrocytes. Rat erythrocytes were incubated for 10 minutes at 25°C and bovine erythrocytes were incubated for 20 minutes at 37°C. Treated cells were then washed 3 times, and a 2 percent saline suspension of the cells was prepared. In conducting the test, 0.2 ml of 2 percent trypsin-treated erythrocytes was added to an equal volume of two-fold serially diluted inactivated serum and the mixture was incubated at 25°C for 4 hours. The formation of a single clump that did not readily break up upon mild agitation of the tube was taken to represent a positive agglutination reaction. A negative test was characterized by the uniform resuspension of erythrocytes in serum following mild agitation of the tube.

Erythrophagocytosis and anemia. Erythrophagocytosis is considered a normal physiologic function of cells of the reticuloendothelial system (RES) and is believed to assist in the removal of aged erythrocytes (Bessis, 1962). An increase in erythrophagocytosis is frequently observed in immunopathologic conditions such as acquired hemolytic anemia and paroxysmal nocturnal hemoglobinuria (Dacie, 1962). It has been understood that the immunologic mechanism responsible for the increased removal of erythrocytes was an antigen-antibody reaction between altered erythrocytes and corresponding antibodies, respectively.

The possibility that serum factors and cellular response are an expression of autoimmune reactions to erythrocytic infections was proposed by Oliver-Gonzales (1944). He demonstrated autoantibodies in the sera of patients with "black water fever" and stated that infected erythrocytes might have been sufficiently altered to act as autoantigens which stimulate the formation of antibodies against noninfected erythrocytes. Zuckerman (1958, 1960, 1964) concluded that the development of anemia and of a positive Coombs' test, and the demonstration of erythrophagocytosis during the course of rodent malaria, were compatible with the idea that such rats had become immune to their own erythrocytes. Ristic (1960) demonstrated an erythrocyte-bound autohemagglutinin associated with macrocytic anemia in anaplasmosis and postulated that the autohemagglutinin may play a role in the development of the anemia.

Recent studies with trypsin-treated erythrocytes revealed that they are more readily phagocytized by cells of the RES than are intact erythrocytes (Vaughan and Boyden, 1964). Rao and Ristic (1963) studied the sialic acid content of the serum of cattle infected with the erythrocytic parasite *A. marginale*. They concluded that the ability of *Anaplasma* to desialize erythrocytic mucoproteins may help to explain one of the autoimmune processes in anaplasmosis (Ristic, 1961). It has been established that desialization of mucoproteins greatly enhanced the antigenicity of these otherwise antigenically poor complexes (Athineos et al., 1962).

The appearance of serum autohemagglutinins in anaplasmosis was associated with a sharp decrease of hematocrit values (Schroeder and Ristic, 1965). Kreier et al. (1964) observed that the appearance of hemagglutinins was followed by the phagocytosis of predominantly infected erythrocytes in the spleen and bone marrow. Based on these observations, Schroeder et al. (1966) investigated the role of autohemagglutinins in the pathogenesis of anemia resulting from *B. rodhaini* infections in rats. Their experiments revealed that the severity of anemia associated with *B. rodhaini* infections was not directly correlated with the extent of the parasitemia. Anemia was invariably maximal on the 11th or 12th day after inoculation, irrespective of the degree of parasitemia.

Hemagglutinins were found in the sera of a number of *Babesia*-infected rats 9 and 11 days after infection. When present, they were associated with both the anemia and the onset of erythrophagocytosis in the spleen and bone marrow. The hemagglutinins reacted *in vitro* with both autologous and homologous trypsinized erythrocytes at a titer of 1:32. In general, the anemia associated with *B. rodhaini* infections of rats was more closely related to splenomegaly, to erythrophagocytosis, and to autohemagglutinins than it was to parasitemia. On the basis of these results, Schroeder et al. (1966) concluded that the observed anemia may be partially a result of autoimmunization, with serum autohemagglutinins acting as opsonins in erythrophagocytosis.

These findings generally agree with those of Maegraith et al. (1957), who observed that in *B. canis*-infected puppies, the severity of anemia was not always commensurate with the degree of parasitemia. Maegraith and co-workers suggested that the anemia in these animals was due to two factors: (1) the tissue destruction by the parasite *per se*, and (2) the removal or destruction of erythrocytes by immune factors. The latter effects become evident only in animals with a slight parasitemia.

Opsonins and *in vitro* erythrophagocytosis. On the assumption that autohemagglutinins in the sera of rats infected with *B. rodhaini* might opsonize erythrocytes and that subsequent phagocytosis contributed to the development of anemia, Schroeder (1966) conducted a series of experiments designed to elucidate this hypothesis.

The opsonic activity of serum for normal homologous erythrocytes was detected by an *in vitro* test which was a modification of a technique developed by Perkins and Leonard (1963). Peritoneal exudate was obtained from 20 white Swiss mice of both sexes following stimulation of exudate by injecting each mouse intraperitoneally with 1 ml of a 2 percent aqueous suspension of corn starch on two consecutive days (Bennett et al., 1963). On the fourth day, 4 ml of heparinized saline solution were injected intraperitoneally into each mouse. The mice were anesthetized, their abdomens were opened, and the exudate was collected with a capillary pipette. The peritoneal exudates contained less than 10 mouse erythrocytes per 100 macrophages. Two-tenths milliliter of a 1 percent suspension of normal washed erythrocytes was added to 0.5 ml of the exudate suspension, and the mixture was centrifuged for 5 minutes at 1,000 rpm in a size 2 Model V International Centrifuge. The supernate was discarded and 0.2 ml of test serum was added. The mixture was resuspended and incubated for 30 minutes in a 37°C waterbath. A drop of the incubated cell suspension was placed on a glass slide, a coverslip applied, and the wet preparation was examined microscopically under oil immersion for evidence of erythrophagocytosis (Fig. 6).

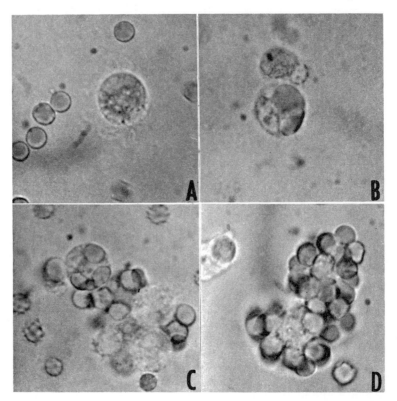

FIG. 6. Unstained suspensions of mouse peritoneal exudate cells and rat erythrocytes in various homologous serum samples: *A*. No erythrophagocytosis in preinfection serum; *B*. Phagocytosis of normal rat erythrocytes in serum from a *Babesia*-infected rat and *C*. From a Plasmodium-infected rat. *D*. Immune adherence of *Plasmodium*-infected rat serum. × 800. (Courtesy of Dr. W. F. Schroeder.)

The degree of opsonic activity of serum samples was measured by determining: (1) the percentage of phagocytes that contained one or more erythrocytes at any dilution, and (2) the highest dilution of serum in which at least 3 percent of the phagocytes contained erythrocytes. This dilution was expressed as the opsonic titer of the serum.

The titers of opsonins and hemagglutinins for trypsin-treated erythrocytes were compared with the onset and duration of anemia in two groups of rats, one infected with *B. rodhaini* and the other with *P. berghei*. The opsonins, however, could only be demonstrated *in vitro* in sera absorbed with normal intact or trypsin-treated erythrocytes. Thus, it appeared that sera which contained opsonins also contained a factor that interfered with the *in vitro* demonstration of erythrophagocytosis.

Interfering factors, hemagglutinins, and opsonins were selectively removed from the serum by absorbing it at 25° and 37°C, respectively, with homologous intact and trypsin-treated erythrocytes. It is apparent from the study that these substances occur free in the serum and may be isolated in a form suitable for their physiochemical characterization. Schroeder (1966) indicated, however, that the mechanism by which interfering factors act to prevent erythrophagocytosis *in vitro* requires further studies. According to the author, hemagglutinins did not appear to sensitize erythrocytes to phagocytosis or to interfere with the phagocytic process; thus their role in the pathogenesis of anemia remains unexplained.

Theileria

Immunity in East Coast fever

East Coast fever is a tick-borne, usually fatal disease of cattle caused by *T. parva* (Theiler, 1904). The disease is characterized by acute changes in temperature and a lymphoid hyperplasia, followed by exhaustion of the lymphoid tissues and leukopenia. There is an approximately 10-day period during which a *T. parva*-infected animal can serve as a further source of infection. During this period, the animal is generally feverish. However, after the infected animals recover, they appear to be refractory to reinfection by ticks. Recovery from the infection during calfhood usually results in a solid immunity which lasts for at least two years. Thereafter, reactions to reinfection tend to be more severe. The duration and the degree of immunity apparently cannot be correlated with the severity of the initial infection (Barnett, 1968; Wilde, 1967).

Studies by Neitz (1953) and Barnett and Brocklesby (1958) demonstrated that when an aureomycin by-product, called aurofac, is administered orally at the time of infection and throughout the course of disease until recovery, a durable, sterile immunity is produced. Apparently, the drug is protozoostatic rather than protozooicidal, and continuous therapy must be maintained from the time of infection until recovery. Even briefly discontinued administration of the drug during infection results in increased virulence of the organism, and subsequent use of the drug will not control the course of the disease. Immunity resulting from drug-assisted recoveries appears to be as strong as that following natural recovery. This immunization method is rather expensive and cumbersome, and it is therefore only applied to certain types of particularly valuable animals.

Based upon results of earlier work by Neitz (1957, 1964) and others, Jarrett et al. (1964) attempted to perpetuate infectious *T. parva* continuously by implanting suspensions of diseased lymph nodes or splenic tissue suspensions intraperitoneally into susceptible cattle, using similar techniques. From their preliminary studies, the authors concluded that it was practical to infect cattle with *T. parva* without using ticks, but they also mentioned that much work remained to be done in identifying, quantitating, and purifying the infective and/or immunogenic stage of *T. parva*. More recently, Brocklesby et al. (1965) used splenic tissues from cattle with tick-induced *T. parva* (Muguga) infection to immunize susceptible cattle against East

Coast fever. Apparently, a significant degree of immunity was provided by the method. These authors concluded that further experiments may result in isolation of the immunogenic phase of the life cycle of the parasite.

Immunologic basis of hematologic changes. According to Brown et al. (1965), the most frequent hematologic abnormalities in cattle infected with *T. parva* are panleukopenia, thrombocytopenia, and a relative decrease in erythropoietic elements. During the course of theileriosis, retardation of the rate of granulocyte maturation and an apparent lymphocytosis in the bone marrow are observed. It was the opinion of the above authors that intralymphocytic parasites are not primarily responsible for the hematologic abnormalities described. Studies of the bone marrow (Brown et al., 1966) of cattle infected with *T. parva* indicate that halting the maturation of cellular precursors may be of major importance as a factor contributing to leukopenia, thrombocytopenia, and anemia (Wilde, 1966, 1967). This author considered the possibility of cytotoxic agents affecting both leukocyte and erythrocyte precursors. However, a series of experiments using large volumes of serum and/or whole blood or homogenates of infected tissue cells failed to induce leukopenia in susceptible cattle inoculated with these preparations. These findings stimulated Brown et al. (1966) to suggest that an autoimmune mechanism operating against lymphoid cells may be responsible for the cellular destruction observed. This mechanism could be visualized as a classical model of autoimmunization whereby the parasitized cells are so modified by the schizont that they become unrecognizable as "self" components. Under these circumstances, autoantibodies formed against these altered cells may fail to distinguish between parasitized and nonparasitized cells. "The morphologic similarity between lymphoblasts, plasmablasts and haemocytoblasts would appear to permit this unwitting resistance within the infected animal if it is indeed a mistake to be taken to its ultimate end" (Brown et al., 1966).

In view of the information available concerning the role of an autoimmune process in erythrocytic infections, i.e., anaplasmosis (Ristic, 1961; Mann and Ristic, 1963 a,b) and babesiosis (Schroeder et al., 1966), it is also possible that in theileriosis certain disease syndromes are not solely brought about through direct action of the parasite. Under such circumstances, infection with *T. parva* may serve as a trigger mechanism initiating a series of autoimmune sequences which, in turn, are responsible for hematologic abnormalities similar to those observed in anaplasmosis and babesiosis. In contrast to *Anaplasma* infections in which only mature erythrocytes seem to be invaded by the organism, in theileriosis both lymphatic and erythroid elements are affected. Consequently, with theileriosis, one may expect that damage resulting from an autoimmune process would appear as abnormalities in myeloid and erythropoietic tissues.

Consideration of the immune mechanism*—*Investigations in vivo.* According to Wilde et al. (1966), the results of experiments aimed at immu-

---

*This author wishes to acknowledge unpublished material graciously made available by Drs. J. K. H. Wilde and C. G. D. Brown (of the Wellcome Research Laboratory, Kabete, Kenya) which has been of great assistance in preparing this section.

nizing cattle by mechanical transmission of infected tissues are unpredictable enough to render the method of limited practical value. The unpre-
dictability of the results seems to arise, partially, from the lack of exact
knowledge about the identity of the immunogenically active stage of the
parasites. Dead schizonts injected into susceptible animals do not stimulate
development of immunity. Evidence further indicates that schizonts removed from the host cell cannot initiate infection. Apparently, some degree
of actual parasite development must be established in the host before an
immune response is stimulated. The sporozoite seems to be the stage of the
parasite cycle most capable of becoming readily established in the susceptible bovine host. Injection of sporozoites into the bovine host in the form of
emulsified salivary glands from partially-fed infected ticks may result in
infection with a sterile, residual immunity later developing in animals which
recover. Occasionally, an immune response can be experimentally induced
following an infection caused by inoculation of infected hyperplastic lymphatic material into susceptible cattle. In this case, however, the true nature
of the infectious particles is not clearly defined.

In addition to the infection and the immunity associated with parasitic
stages of the lymphoid tissue, there is an infection and apparently resultant
immunity associated with the erythrocytic forms of the parasite. Neitz
(1959, 1964) has succeeded in establishing the erythrocytic infection by injecting infected blood into a susceptible bovine host. This infection, however,
did not result in a resistance against tick-induced disease.

These and other observations concerning the pathogenesis of East Coast
fever have led Barnett (1963) to consider the disease as having two clinical
phases. The first phase is characterized by schizogony in the lymphatic tissue, during which time the animal shows elevated body temperature and
general clinical depression. In the second phase, clinical recovery takes
place, schizonts disappear rapidly, and body temperature returns to normal;
however, the erythrocytic parasites persist and even increase in number.
This observation, and others, prompted Barnett (1963) to postulate that different immune mechanisms are involved in each phase, and if antibody production occurs, then the antibodies produced by the two phases are serologically different (Fig. 7). Schindler and Wokatsch (1965) showed by
means of the indirect fluorescent-antibody method that fluorescence was not
confined to the intraerythrocytic parasites but that lymphocytic stages
(Koch's bodies) gave even more intense fluorescence. The latter finding
is consistent with Barnett's hypothesis of the existence of "two antigen-
antibody systems," since it is possible that sera used by Schindler and
Wokatsch (1965) contained both types of antibody. In addition, by introducing this hypothesis, Barnett questioned the existence of protective serum
antibody in animals with *Theileria* infections. The administration of immune
sera or immune gamma-globulins to clinical cases of *T. parva* did not produce
convincing evidence of protection (Barnett, 1968).

Investigations with the parasite propagated in vitro. Considerable progress has been made in devising tissue culture systems for *in vitro* propagation of *Theileria*. Some of the most successful efforts along these lines have

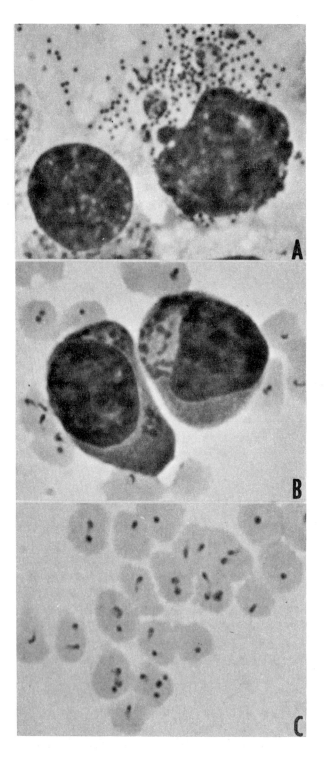

FIG. 7. Lymphatic and erythrocytic phases of *Theileria parva* in impression smears stained by the Giemsa method. *A.* Cells of parotid lymph node infected by macro- and microschizonts with the latter forms being released to invade erythrocytes. *B.* Two splenic lymphocytes with developing macroschizonts. *C.* Various erythrocytic forms. Giemsa stain; × 3,000. (Courtesy of Dr. C. G. D. Brown.)

been with *T. annulata*. Working independently, Tsur and Adler (1965) and Hulliger (1965) propagated *T. annulata* and *T. parva* through serial passages in monocytic tissue cells. The most intriguing observation was that only those bovine monocytes which were infected *in vivo* continued to multiply and support *in vitro* propagation of the parasites. In contrast, noninfected monocytes, although they originated from infected animals, had less or no tendency for *in vitro* growth. Hulliger (1965) propagated *Theileria* in tissue cultures consisting of splenic cells derived from infected animals and monolayers of baby hamster kidney cells. Multiplication of *Theileria* took place in the bovine cells only.

On the basis of early studies by Gonder (1910) and many subsequent investigators, the controversial proposal was made that parasite multiplication takes place by schizogony and that the the schizont breaks into single merozoites which infect new lymphatic cells. Studies on the multiplication of *Theileria* species in tissue cultures (Hulliger, 1965) suggested that division of single theilerial particles takes place by binary, not multiple, fission. The 30 to 40 hours needed for division of a single parasite particle seem to be equal to the time needed for division of the host cell. The *Theileria* particles did not seem to divide synchronously, and there was no indication that division of these particles occurs simultaneously with the division of the host cell. When tissue cultures were grown at higher temperatures, the multiplication of the host cells was slowed down, very large parasites ensued, and microschizonts developed. At this stage, Hulliger et al. (1966a) noted disintegration of the host cells, with the separation of single parasites consisting of one nucleus with an enveloping cytoplasmic body.

According to Wilde et al. (1966), subcutaneous administration of *T. parva*-infected tissue cultures into susceptible bovine animals readily produced infections characterized by the appearance of macroschizonts in the lymphoid tissues. The parasite, however, does not complete the cycle to the extent of producing erythrocytic forms. Animals recovered from tissue-culture infections were found fully susceptible to tick-transmitted East Coast fever. On the other hand, these animals were immune to further infection with the tissue culture form of the parasite. Consequently, Wilde and co-workers (1966) postulated that in the process of its adaptation to the tissue culture environment, immunogenically important antigens of the parasite were dissociated.

The possibility that the tissue-culture-propagated organisms were simply transferred into new hosts without actually developing in them was studied by Wilde et al. (1966). In their experiments, parasites which were propagated in male or female tissue culture cells were injected into susceptible female and male cattle, respectively. In both cases, infected lymphatic cells of the sex opposite to that contained in the inoculum were recovered from host animals.

The effects of "immune" sera and of "immune" cells on multiplication of *Theileria* propagated in tissue cultures and on their infectivity for cattle were investigated by Hulliger et al. (1965). Cells infected with *T. parva* were grown with and without "immune" sera secured from convalescent animals. Three animals which were inoculated with cells cultivated in "immune" sera developed even more severe theileriosis than did the two animals which were inoculated with tissue grown in a control serum obtained from susceptible animals. Also, multiplication of *Theileria*-infected cells in the presence of "immune" sera was compared with multiplication in control serum. No significant differences in multiplication rate of the cells were noted, and no indication of an effect due to "immune" sera on the intracellular form of the parasite was found.

In an attempt to explore the immune mechanism in *T. parva* infections, Hulliger et al. (1965) offered several possible working hypotheses. They also compared the immune tissue mechanism known to exist in other obligate intracellular parasites, e.g., viruses and *Mycobacterium tuberculosis*, with that of *T. parva*. No reasonable comparison was possible simply on the ground that *Mycobacteria* and viruses can be subject to destruction by an immune factor in the process of entering new cells. No extracellular invading forms of *Theileria* were noted in tissue cultures, and there was no evidence that the parasite affects its host cell in any adverse way. In fact, the parasite seems to stimulate division of its host cell. However, in animals undergoing an immune reaction following recovery from *T. parva* infection, degenerating parasites can very often be seen within healthy-looking cells. This and other experimental evidence obtained by Hulliger et al. (1965) strongly suggest that the immune factor in *T. parva* is formed within the parasitized cell and can act directly on the parasite. The authors, however, feel that additional evidence will be needed to support this concept. It was concluded that with *Theileria*, immunity is cell-bound rather than humoral (Wilde, 1967).

Theileria annulata infections

In contrast to *T. parva*, with which artificial infections are relatively difficult to produce, deliberate infection with *T. annulata* using blood from carrier animals is easily accomplished. The mortality resulting from such infections is lower than that resulting from natural exposure. Animals which recover from acute infections usually become carriers of the infection.

On the basis of differences in virulence, several strains of *T. annulata* have been identified. When less virulent strains were used to vaccinate cattle against challenge with more virulent strains, partial protection was demonstrated. This finding led the investigators to believe that in addition to their differences in virulence, these strains also differ antigenically.

A comparative evaluation of the immune principle and pathogenesis of the disease observed in infections with *T. parva*, *T. annulata*, and *T. mutans* is summarized in Table 1. In view of the fact that infection immunity is the immune mechanism operational in infections with *T. annulata*, vaccinations with this organism by means of deliberately infecting young calves have been practiced (Barnett, 1968). Animals with immunity to *T. annulata*

Table 1

Immunologic and Clinical Features of Theilerial Infections

Features	T. parva	T. annulata	T. mutans
Type of immunity	sterile	infection	infection
Cross-immunity with other strains	none	none	none
Mortality	90 to 100%	10 to 80%	less than 1%
Anemia	oligocythemia	present	very mild
Average duration of disease	15 days	10 days	5 days

achieved by natural or artificial means can best be identified by sub-inoculating blood from these suspected cases into susceptible cattle. Splenectomy of suspected *T. annulata*-infected animals can also be used as a means of diagnosing this infection. In infected animals, relapse of the infection usually follows within three to four weeks after splenectomy (Neitz and Jansen, 1956).

Theileria mutans infections

Theileria mutans infections of cattle are generally benign and nonfatal. The disease is manifested by transitory anemia and occasional swelling of the superficial lymphatic glands. All recovered animals develop long-lasting premunition. Within the same strain, however, there seems to be a difference between immunity to erythrocytic infection and immunity to the schizogonous phase. Neitz (1957) demonstrated that cattle infected with the blood phase of the parasite were susceptible to the schizogonous stage of the parasite when exposed to ticks naturally infected with *T. mutans*. In the field, however, most of the cattle infected with *T. mutans* seem to be immune to the both phases of the parasite. As in infections with *T. annulata*, immunity in *T. mutans* infections can be interrupted by splenectomy and will result in the reappearance of *T. mutans* in the peripheral blood and of Koch's bodies in the lymphatic glands. Neitz (1957) reported that immunity to *T. mutans* can also be interrupted by babesiosis, rinderpest, and other infectious diseases. Also, animals that have recovered from a natural *T. mutans* infection are fully susceptible to *T. parva* and *T. annulata* (Neitz, 1957).

Theileria species in the United States

There are only two reports describing infections with *Theileria* in the United States; one is of *T. mutans* in an ox (Splitter, 1950) and the other of *Theileria* species in a deer (Kreier et al., 1962).

The occurrence of *T. mutans* in native cattle in the United States indicates that one or more species of ticks are present which are capable of transmitting the organism. It can be expected that these vectors may also transmit the other more pathogenic species of *Theileria* should they be introduced to this country.

Theileria species in deer.   There have been only seven known descriptions of infections with *Theileria* species in deer. All the deer were native to India, Portugal, Indochina, Russia, or Japan (Neitz, 1957).

Pathogenesis of the disease.   During the course of a routine hematologic examination of a splenectomized deer (No. 321) for anaplasmosis, we observed large numbers of intraerythrocytic parasites identified as *Theileria* sp. (Kreier et al., 1962). The identification was based on morphologic features of the organism in Giemsa-stained blood films. The time from splenectomy until the first parasites appeared in the erythrocytes was four weeks. The animal's previous clinical history was not available, but it appears that the animal must have been in a true carrier stage, since the infection appeared after splenectomy and while the animal was in isolation. Theileriosis was produced in a second splenectomized deer by intravenous injection of 1 ml of infected blood from deer 321. A sheep and a splenectomized calf which were injected intravenously with 40 ml of *Theileria* sp.-infected blood from deer 321 did not develop theileriosis. Parasites were not observed in the erythrocytes, and clinical signs were absent.

In deer 321, in which the parasite was discovered, severe anemia developed, and a maximum of 50 per cent of the erythrocytes contained one or more parasites. The anemia was microcytic and hypochromic. The mean corpuscular volume (MCV) before clinical infection was 36.0 cu μ, and the mean corpuscular hemoglobin (MCH) was 12.6 $\mu\mu$g; at the point of maximal infection a MCH content of 9.3 $\mu\mu$g was observed. During the subsequent four weeks, the MCV continued to decrease, reaching a low value of 18.0 cu μ shortly before the animal died.

In the deer infected with the blood from deer 321, parasites were first detected in the erythrocytes after an incubation period of four weeks. The percent of infected cells increased rapidly for about 12 days, until a maximum of 50 percent of the erythrocytes contained parasites. Thereafter, there was a slight decrease in the percent of infected erythrocytes, but more than 25 percent of the erythrocytes still contained parasites when the animal died six weeks later. The erythrocyte count, hemoglobin content, and packed cell volume decreased rapidly as the parasite count increased. The total white blood cell count increased slightly during the course of the infection; this may have been due to a pyogenic infection which developed in one hock after an injury was sustained by the deer while it was being restrained.

Morphologic and taxonomic features of the parasite.   In Giemsa-stained preparations, the parasite appeared to be somewhat pleomorphic. In most of the parasites, both nuclear and cytoplasmic components could be seen. The cytoplasm stained light blue, and the nuclear region stained a deep purple-red. Parasites were comma-shaped, bipolar, tailed, *Anaplasma*-like, or resembled safety pins and dumbbells.

Ultra-thin sections of infected erythrocytes examined by electron microscopy revealed that the parasite had a complex structural organization. It had a distinct double plasma membrane and a large nucleus occupying one end of the body. The nucleus was also delineated by a double membrane. A number of membranous profiles were present in the cytoplasm, some of which morphologically resembled the elements of an endoplasmic reticulum. Also observed were an electron-lucid polar body located at the end opposite the nucleus and a mitochondrion-like body with incomplete, centrally placed double membranes. The nucleus, cytoplasm, and polar body seen in ultra-thin sections could be identified in many of the parasites stained by the Giemsa method (Fig. 8).

The *Theileria* sp. described in this report has not yet been assigned to any particular species. It can be said, however, that it is not *T. mutans* because it occurred in deer and could not be transmitted to the ox or sheep, whereas the *T. mutans* found by Splitter (1950) in an ox could be maintained only in cattle. Pathogenicity presents another difference between this parasite and that found by Splitter. Our recent studies indicate that deer inoculated with infected blood or lymph node preparations frequently develop a rapidly progressing and fatal disease. Signs of severe intoxication were associated with this infection. The presence of a toxin acting on the bone marrow would explain the microcytic, hypochromic anemia. An alternative explanation for the character of the anemia could be that the *Theileria* infection caused erythrocyte destruction, but that the erythropoietic response to the anemia was modified by an iron deficiency. The infected animals developed a clinical syndrome similar to that described for East Coast fever.

Histochemical and serologic staining of the parasite.   The chromatin bodies of *Theileria* gave a pink reaction in the Feulgen test for DNA, a dark blue one with toluidine blue, and a yellow one with acridine orange. A reaction was also obtained with acridine orange and toluidine blue stains for RNA. The parasites were stained blue in the mercuric-bromphenol blue test for basic protein, but tests for arginine and tyrosine were negative. No polysaccharides could be demonstrated in the parasites by the periodic-acid Schiff technique. The Prussian-blue test revealed iron in the form of minute dark blue granules in the cytoplasm, and lipids were detected in both the nucleus and cytoplasm of the organism by sudan black B stain in 70 percent alcohol. The test for calcium was negative (Schaeffler, 1962).

Staining of the *Theileria* by the FA method gave no serologic cross-reaction with *A. marginale* or *Eperythrozoon ovis* (Kreier et al., 1962). Schaeffler (1963), following the method of Ristic (1962), prepared agglutinating antigen from *Theileria cervi* and used it in the capillary-tube agglutination (CA) test to detect serum agglutinins.

CONCLUSION

The last decade has witnessed great strides in the application of immunologic principles and techniques to the study of these erythrocytic protozoa.

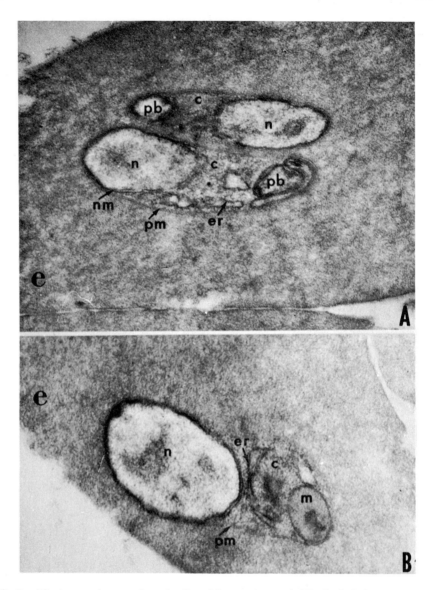

FIG. 8. Electron micrographs of ultra-thin sections of *Theileria*-infected deer ery-throcytes: erythrocyte (e); cytoplasm of the parasite (c); organelle of unknown type, possibly a mitochondrion (m); nucleus (n); endoplasmic reticulum (er); nuclear mem-brane (nm); polar body (pb); and plasma membrane (pm). × 60,000.

It became evident from the results of preliminary studies that immunologic mechanisms governing host-parasite relationships in these protozoa are in many respects similar to those operating in infections with other intracellular obligate parasites, such as viruses and rickettsiae.

An apparently immune antibody has been demonstrated in babesial infec-tions. Although the exact mechanism by which this antibody acts is not clearly understood, all indications are that it acts by interrupting a specific sequence in the cycle of parasitic development, thus interfering in a yet unknown way with the invasive properties of the parasite.

The application of immunologic principles to the study and understanding of pathologic changes is now recognized in medical sciences as the field of immunopathology. This discipline seems to be most applicable to the study of infections with erythrocytic parasites. We are now beginning to understand that factors other than the parasite *per se* may be responsible for the destruction and removal of erythrocytes. These complicated immunologic processes, which are obviously initiated by the infection, may bring about pathologic manifestations, the intensity of which does not necessarily depend on the mass of parasitic population.

Finally, the successful propagation of *Theileria* species in tissue cultures provides a useful system for studying the growth requirements and immunologic principles pertaining to the relationship of the host cell and the intracellular parasite. A phenomenon observed in these preliminary studies was that only those bovine monocytes infected *in vivo* continued to multiply and support the *in vitro* reproduction of *Theileria*. This observation poses many intriguing questions. Numerous studies with bacterial and animal viruses have clearly shown that replicating viral particles affect protein synthesis and other metabolic processes of the living host cell. This is the first time that an obligate intracellular protozoan parasite has been observed to affect the host cell in a similar manner.

Preliminary observations concerning the immune mechanism in *T. parva* infections indicate that circulating antibody has little effect on parasitic development. This may be due to the fact that the invasive phase of development is not associated with the extracellular phase of the parasite, i.e., the dividing *Theileria* units are reapportioned among newly formed daughter cells. Therefore, it appears reasonable to speculate that an intracellular factor of unknown nature may be involved in governing the development of local tissue and of general host immunity. The existence and the nature of this immune factor pose intriguing questions for future investigation.

There is a continuously growing interest in applying immunology and related disciplines to the study of erythrocytic parasites. These efforts should provide some of the fundamental information for a better understanding of the parasitic nature of these species.

REFERENCES

Abramov, I. V. 1952. Summary of the 36th plenary session of the USSR Lenin Agricultural Academy, Veterinary section on protozoan diseases. Veterinariya (Moscow), 29:55-57 (Abstr.: Vet. Bull., 1953, 23:140).

Agaev, A. A. 1958. Blood transfusion in the treatment of bovine theileriasis (In Russian). Veterinariya (Moscow), 35:42-44.

Alperin, A. L., and Bevins, N. F. 1963. Babesiosis in a California dog. J. Amer. Vet. Med. Ass., 143:1328-1330.

866   IMMUNITY IN MAMMALIAN HOSTS

Arnold, R. M. 1948. Resistance to tick-borne disease (Correspondence). Vet. Rec., 60:426.

Athineos, E., M. Thornton, and R. J. Winzler. 1962. Comparative antigenicity of mature "desialized" orosomucoid in rabbits. Proc. Soc. Exp. Biol. Med., 3:353-354.

Babes, V. 1888. Sur l'hemoglobinuria bacterienne de boeufs. C. R. Acad. Sci. (Paris), 107:692-700.

Barnett, S. F. 1955. Mechanical transmission of East Coast fever. East African Veterinary Research Organization Annual Report (1955-1956), p. 20.

———— 1963. The biological race of the bovine *Theileria* and their host-parasite relationship. *In* Immunity to Protozoa. Garnham, P. C. C., Pierce, A. E., and Roitt, I., eds. Oxford, Blackwell Scientific Publications, pp. 180-195.

———— 1965. The *Theileria* of cattle in Africa. *In* Progress in Protozoology. II. International Conference on Protozoology, London. International Congress Series No. 91. Amsterdam, Excerpta Medica Foundation, p. 36.

———— 1968. Theileriosis. *In* Infectious Blood Diseases of Man and Animals, Vol. 2. Weinman, D., and Ristic, M., eds. New York, Academic Press Inc., pp. 269-328.

———— and D. W. Brocklesby. 1958. Immunization against E. C. F. with Aurofac. East African Veterinary Research Organization Annual Report (1956-1957), p. 47.

———— and D. W. Brocklesby. 1966. A mild form of E. C. F. (*T. parva*) with persistence of infection. Brit. Vet. J., 122:361.

Bennett, B., L. J. Old, and E. A. Boyse. 1963. Opsonization of cells by isoantibody *in vitro*. Nature (London), 198:10-12.

Bessis, M. C. 1962. Cytological basis of hemoglobin production. *In* The Harvey Lectures, Series 58, New York, Academic Press, Inc., pp. 125-156.

Brocklesby, D. W., K. P. Bailey, W. B. Martin, W. P. H. Jarrett, H. R. P. Miller, P. Nderito, and G. M. Urquhart. 1965. Experiments in immunity to East Coast fever. Vet. Rec., 77:512.

Brown, C. G. D., J. K. H. Wilde, and L. Hulliger. 1965. Hematological changes in experimental theileriosis. *In* Progress in Protozoology. II. International Conference on Protozoology, London. International Congress Series No. 91. Amsterdam, Excerpta Medica Foundation, p. 37.

———— J. K. H. Wilde, and L. Hulliger. 1966. Personal communication. Wellcome Research Laboratory, Kabete, Kenya.

Burnet, F. M., and S. G Anderson. 1946. Modification of human red cells by virus action. II. Agglutination of modified human red cells by sera from cases of infectious mononucleosis. Brit. J. Exp. Path., 27:236-244.

Cherry, W. B., M. Goldman, and T. R. Carski. 1960. Fluorescent antibody techniques in diagnosis of communicable diseases. U. S. Dept. of Health, Education, and Welfare, Public Health Service, Bureau of State Services, Communicable Disease Center, Atlanta, Georgia.

Cox, H. W., W. F. Schroeder, and M. Ristic. 1966. Hemagglutination and erythrophagocytosis associated with the anemia of *Plasmodium berghei* infections of rats. J. Protozool., 13:327-332.

D'Alesandro, P. A. 1963. Soluble parasite antigens in the serums of rats infected with *Trypanosoma lewisi*. J. Protozool., 10(Suppl.):22.

Dacie, J. V. 1962. The Haemolytic Anemias. II. Auto-immune Haemolytic Anemias. London, J. A. Churchill Ltd.

Daly, G. D., and W. T. K. Hall. 1955. A note on the susceptibility of British and some Zebu type cattle to tick fever (Babesiosis). Aust. Vet. J., 31:152.

Davies, S. F. M., L. P. Joyner, and S. B. Kendall. 1958. Studies on *Babesia divergens* (M'Fadyear and Stockman, 1911). Ann. Trop. Med. Parasit., 52:206-215.

Dennis, E. W. 1932. The life cycle of *Babesia bigemina* (Smith and Kilbourne) of Texas cattle fever in the tick *Margaropus annulatus* (Fay) with notes on the embryology of *Margaropus*. Univ. Calif. Publ. Zool., 36:263-298.

Dodd, M. C., C. S. Wright, J. A. Baxter, B. A. Bouroncle, A. E. Bunner, and H. J. Winn. 1953. The immunologic specificity of antiserum for trypsin-treated red blood cells and its reactions with normal and hemolytic anemia cells. Blood, 8:640-647.

Du Toit, P. J. 1928. Observations on immunity in East Coast fever. S. Afr. J. Sci., 25:282-287.

Fitzpatrick, J. E. P., C. C. Kennedy, M. G. McGeown, D. G. Oreopoulos, J. H. Robertson, and M. A. O. Soyannuva. 1968. Human case of piroplasmosis (babesiosis). Nature (London), 217:861-862.

Friedhoff, K., and E. Scholtyseck. 1968. Feinstrukturen von *Babesia Ovis* (Piroplasmidea) in *Rhipicephalus bursa* (Ixodoidea): Transformation sphäroider Formen zu Vermicula Formen. Z. Parasitenk., 30:347-359.

Garnham, P. C. C., and R. Bray. 1959. The susceptibility of the higher primates to piroplasms. J. Protozool., 6:361-366.

Gonder, R. 1910. The life cycle of *Theileria parva*, the cause of East Coast fever in South Africa. J. Comp. Path., 23:328-335.

Grogan, J. W. 1953. Piroplasmosis in a dog. J. Amer. Vet. Med. Ass., 123:123-124.

Hall, W. T. K. 1960. The immunity of calves to *Babesia argentina* infection. Aust. Vet. J., 36:361-366.

Healy, G. R., N. N. Gleason, and M. Schultz. 1969. The origin of "Gray" strain of human babesiosis. (Manuscript in preparation.)

Henningsen, K. 1949. A case of polyagglutinable human red cells. Acta Path. Microbiol. Scand., 26:339-344.

Hirato, K., N. Ninomiya, Y. Uwano, and T. Kutii. 1945. Studies on the complement fixation test reaction for equine piroplasmosis. Jap. J. Vet. Sci., 7:204-205.

Holbrook, A. A. 1965. Equine piroplasmosis and its diagnosis. *In* Proceedings of the 11th Annual Meeting of the American Association of Equine Practice, pp. 157-166.

Huff, C. G. 1957. Organ and tissue distribution of the exoerythrocytic stages of various avian malaria parasites. Exp. Parasit., 6:143-162.

Hulliger, L. 1965. Cultivation of three species of *Theileria* in lymphoid cells *in vitro*. J. Protozool., 12:649-655.

——— C. G. D. Brown, and J. K. H. Wilde. 1965. Theileriosis (*T. parva*) immune mechanisms investigated *in vitro*. *In* Progress in Protozoology. II. International Conference on Protozoology, London. International Congress Series No. 91. Amsterdam, Excerpta Medica Foundation, p. 37.

——— C. G. D. Brown, and J. K. H. Wilde. 1966. Transition of developmental stages of *Theileria parva in vitro* at high temperature. Nature (London), 211:328-329.

Jarret, W. F. H., S. Jennings, W. B. Martin, P. Nderito, G.M. Urquhart, D. W. Brocklesby and K. P. Bailey. 1964. The transition of East Coast fever using cells from infected animals. Proc. 1st Int. Congr. Parasit., Rome.

Kreier, J. P., M. Ristic, and W. F. Schroeder. 1964. Anaplasmosis. XVI. The pathogenesis of anemia produced by infection with *Anaplasma*. Amer. J. Vet. Res., 25:343-352.

——— M. Ristic, and A. M. Watrach. 1962. *Theileria* sp. in a deer in the United States. Amer. J. Vet. Res., 23:657-662.

Mabry, D. S., J. A. Bass, M. C. Dodd, J. H. Wallace, and C. S. Wright. 1956a Differential phagocytosis of normal, trypsinized and virus-treated human and rabbit erythrocytes by macrophages in tissue culture. J. Immun., 76:54-61.

——— J. H. Wallace, M. C. Dodd, and C. S. Wright. 1956b. Opsonic factors in normal and immune sera in the differential phagocytosis of normal, trypsinized and virus-treated human and rabbit erythrocytes by macrophages in tissue culture. J. Immun., 76:62-68.

Madden, P. A., and A. A. Holbrook. 1968. Equine piroplasmosis: Indirect fluorescent antibody test for *Babesia caballi*. Amer. J. Vet. Res., 29:117-123.

Maegraith, B. G., H. M. Giles, and K. Devakul. 1957. Pathological processes in *Babesia canis* infections. Z. Tropenmed. Parasit., 8:485-514.

Mahoney, D. F. 1962. Bovine babesiosis: Diagnosis of infection by a complement-fixation test. Aust. Vet. J., 38:48-52.

Mann, D. K., and M. Ristic. 1963a. Anaplasmosis. XIII. Studies concerning the nature of autoimmunity. Amer. J. Vet. Res., 24:703-708.

——— and M. Ristic. 1963b. Anaplasmosis. XIV. The isolation and characterization of an autohemagglutinin. Amer. J. Vet. Res., 24:709-712.

Maurer, D. F. 1962. Equine piroplasmosis—Another emerging disease. J. Amer. Vet. Med. Ass., 141:699-702.

Meissner, H. 1931. Piroplasmosen und Splenektomie. Arch. Wiss. Prakt. Turnek., 63:68-90 (Abstr.: Vet. Bull., 1931, 1:210).

Merenda, J. J. 1939. Piroplasmosis in a French poodle. J. Amer. Vet. Med. Ass., 95:98.

Morton, J., and M. M. Pickles. 1947. Use of trypsin in the detection of incomplete anti-Rh antibodies. Nature (London), 159:779-780.

—— and M. M. Pickles. 1951. The proteolytic enzyme test for detecting incomplete antibodies. J. Clin. Path., 4:189-199.

Neitz, W. O. 1953. Aureomycin in *Theileria parva* infection. Nature (London), 171:34-35.

—— 1956. Classification, transmission and biology of piroplasms of domestic animals. Ann. N. Y. Acad. Sci., 64:56-111.

—— 1957. Theileriosis, gonderioses and cytauxzoonoses: A review. Onderstepoort J. Vet. Res., 27:275-430.

—— 1959. Theilerioses. *In* Advances in Veterinary Science. Brandly, C. A., and Jungherr, E. L., eds., New York, Academic Press, Inc., Vol. 5, pp. 241-297.

—— 1964. Immunity in East Coast fever. J. S. Afr. Vet. Med. Ass., 35:5-6.

—— and B. C. Jansen. 1956. A discussion on the classification of the theilerioses. Onderstepoort J. Vet. Res., 27:7-18.

Oliver-Gonzales, J. 1944. Blood agglutinins in Blackwater Fever. Proc. Soc. Exp. Biol. Med., 57:25-26.

Perkins, E. H., and M. P. Leonard. 1963. Specificity of phagocytosis as it may relate to antibody formation. J. Immun., 90:228-237.

Rao, P. J., and M. Ristic. 1963. Serum sialic acid levels in experimental anaplasmosis. Proc. Soc. Exp. Biol. Med., 114:447-452.

Riek, R. F. 1963. Immunity to babesiosis. *In* Immunity to Protozoa. Garnham, P. C. C., Pierce, A. E., and Roitt, I., eds. Oxford, Blackwell Scientific Publications, pp. 160-179.

—— 1968. Babesiosis. *In* Infectious Blood Diseases of Man and Animals, Vol. 2. Weinman, D., and Ristic, M., eds. New York, Academic Press Inc., pp. 219-268.

Ristic, M. 1960. Anaplasmosis. *In* Advances in Veterinary Science. Brandly, C. A., and Jungherr, E. L., eds. New York, Academic Press, Inc., Vol. 6, pp. 111-192.

—— 1961. Studies in anaplasmosis. III. An autoantibody and symptomatic macrocytic anemia. Amer. J. Vet. Res., 22:871-876.

—— 1962. A capillary tube-agglutination test for anaplasmosis. A preliminary report. J. Amer. Vet. Med. Ass., 141:588-594.

—— and D. K. Mann. 1963. Anaplasmosis. IX. Immunoserologic properties of soluble *Anaplasma* antigens. Amer. J. Vet. Res., 24:478-482.

—— and S. Sibinovic. 1964. Equine babesiosis: Diagnosis by a precipitation test in gel and by a one-step fluorescent antibody inhibition test. Amer. J. Vet. Res., 25:1519-1526.

—— D. K. Mann, and R. Kodras. 1963. Anaplasmosis. VIII. Biochemical and biophysical characterization of soluble *Anaplasma* antigens. Amer. J. Vet. Res., 24:472-477.

—— J. Opperman, S. Sibinovic, and T. N. Phillips. 1964. Equine piroplasmosis—A mixed strain of *Piroplasma caballi* and *Piroplasma equi* isolated in Florida and studied by fluorescent-antibody technique. Amer. J. Vet. Res., 25:15-23.

—— D. Huxsoll, S. Siwe, and R. Weisiger. 1969a. A capillary tube-agglutination test for canine babesiosis. (Manuscript in preparation.)

—— S. Siwe, and G. R. Healey. 1969b. *Babesia* spp. from a human being isolated and studied in monkeys. (Manuscript in preparation.)

Robson, J. 1961. *Rhipicephalus appendiculatus* and East Coast fever in Tanganyika. The epidemiology of arthropod-borne diseases. E. Afr. Council Med. Res., Nairobi.

Sanders, D. A. 1937. Observations of canine babesiosis. J. Amer. Vet. Med. Ass., 90:27.

Schaeffler, W. F. 1962. *Theileria cervi* infection in white-tailed deer (*Dama virginiana*) in the United States. Ph.D. Thesis, Urbana, Illinois, University of Illinois.

—— 1963. Serologic tests for *Theileria cervi* in white-tailed deer and other species of *Theileria* in cattle and sheep. Amer. J. Vet. Res., 24:784-791.

Schindler, R., and H. K. Dennig. 1962a. Über eine Methode zum Nachweis von Antikörpern gegen intraerythrozytäre Protozoen. Berlin München. Tierärztl. Wschr., 75:111-112.

—— and H. K. Dennig. 1962b. Versuche zum Nachweis von Antikörpern gegen Babesien mit der Komplementbindung reaktion. Z. Tropenmed. Parasit., 13:480-488.

—— and R. Wokatsch. 1965. Versuche zur Differenzierung der Theilerienspezies des Rindes durch serologische Untersuchungen. Z. Tropenmed. Parasit., 16:17-23.

Scholtens, R. G., E. H. Braff, G. R. Healey, and N. Gleason. 1968. A case of babesiosis in man in the United States. Amer. J. Trop. Med. Hyg., 17:810-813.

Schroeder, W. F. 1966. Autoimmune processes associated with anemia of infections with *Babesia rodhaini, Plasmodium berghei* and *Anaplasma marginale*. Ph.D. Thesis, Urbana, Illinois, University of Illinois.
———— and M. Ristic. 1965. Anaplasmosis. XVII. The relation of autoimmune processes to anemia. Amer. J. Vet. Res., 26:239-245.
———— and M. Ristic. 1968. Autoimmune response and pathogenesis of blood parasite diseases. *In* Infectious Blood Diseases of Man and Animals, Vol. 1. Weinman, D., and Ristic, M., eds. New York, Academic Press, Inc., pp. 63-77.
———— H. W. Cox and M. Ristic. 1966. Anaemia, parasitemia, erythrophagocytosis and hemagglutinins in *Babesia rodhaini* infection. Ann. Trop. Med. Parasit., 60:31-38.
Seddon, H. R. 1952. Diseases of domestic animals in Australia. Part 4. Protozoan and viral diseases. Serv. Publ. Comm. Dept. Hlth. Aust., No. 8.
Seed, J. R., and D. Weinman. 1963. Characterization of antigens isolated from *Trypanosoma rhodesiense*. Nature (London), 198: 197-198.
Sibinovic, K. H. 1966. Immunogenic properties of purified antigens isolated from the serum of horses, dogs and rats with acute babesiosis. Ph.D. Thesis, Urbana, Illinois, University of Illinois.
———— M. Ristic, S. Sibinovic, and N. T. Phillips. 1965. *Equine babesiosis*: Isolation and serologic characterization of a blood serum antigen from acutely infected horses. Amer. J. Vet. Res., 26:147-153.
———— M. Ristic, S. Sibinovic, and J. O. Alberts. 1966. Bentonite agglutination test for transmissible gastroenteritis of swine. Amer. J. Vet. Res., 27:1339-1344.
———— R. MacLeod, M. Ristic, S. Sibinovic, and H. W. Cox. 1967a. A study of some physical, chemical, and serologic properties of antigens from sera of horses, dogs, and rats with acute babesiosis. J. Parasit., 53:919-923.
———— S. Sibinovic, M. Ristic, and H. W. Cox. 1967b. Immunogenic properties of babesial serum antigens. J. Parasit., 53:1121-1129.
Sibinovic, S., K. H. Sibinovic, M. Ristic, and H. W. Cox. 1966. Physical and serologic properties of an antigen prepared from infected erythrocytes of equines with babesiosis. J. Protozool., 13:551-552.
———— K. H. Sibinovic, and M. Ristic. 1969. *Equine babesiosis*: Diagnosis by the bentonite agglutination and passive hemagglutination tests. Amer. J. Vet. Res., 30:691-695.
Sippel, W. L., D. E. Cooperrider, J. H. Gainer, R. W. Allen, J. E. B. Mouw, and M. B. Teigland. 1962. Equine piroplasmosis in the United States. J. Amer. Vet. Med. Ass., 141:694-698.
Skrabalo, Z., and Z. Deanovic. 1957. Piroplasmosis in man. Report of a case. Soc. Med. Geogr. Trop., 9:11-6 (Abstr.: Vet. Bull., 1958, 28:125).
Smith, J. W., M. C. Dodd, C. S. Wright, and A. E. Bunner. 1954. Isoimmunization of rabbits with trypsinized erythrocytes. Fed. Proc., 13:512.
Smith, T., and F. L. Kilbourne. 1893. Investigation into the nature, causation and prevention of southern cattle fever. Bulletin of the U. S. Bureau of Animal Industry, No. 1, p. 177.
Splitter, E. J. 1950. *Theileria mutans* associated with bovine anaplasmosis in the United States. J. Amer. Vet. Med. Ass., 117:134.
Starcovici, C. 1893. Cited by Neitz, W. O., 1956.
Stone, W. H., and W. J. Miller. 1955. Alterations in the reactivity of cattle erythrocytes following treatment with enzymes. Genetics, 40:599.
Theiler, A. 1904. Rhodesian tick fever. Transvaal Agric. J., 2:421-438.
Todorovic, R., M. Ristic, and D. H. Ferris. 1967. A tube latex agglutination test for diagnosis of malaria. Trans. Roy. Soc. Trop. Med. Hyg., 62:58-68.
Tomsick, J., and J. B. Baumann-Grace. 1960. Action of proteolytic enzymes on the mononucleosis antigens in sheep and beef erythrocytes. Path. Microbiol. (Basel), 23:172-183.
Tsur, I., and S. Adler. 1965. Growth of lymphoid cells in *Theileria annulata* schizonts from bovine blood during the reaction period. *In* Progress in Protozoology. II. International Conference on Protozoology, London. International Congress Series No. 91. Amsterdam, Excerpta Medica Foundation, pp. 37-38.
Vaughan, R. B., and S. V. Boyden. 1964. Interactions of macrophages and erythrocytes. Immunology, 7:118-126.

Wallace, J. H., M. C. Dodd and C. S. Wright. 1955. Antigenic studies of virus and trypsin-treated erythrocytes. J. Immun., 74:89-95.
Western, K. A., G. D. Benson, N. N. Gleason, G. R. Healy, and M. G. Schultz.
1969. Babesiosis in a Massachusetts resident: First case in a patient with a spleen.
New Eng. J. Med. (In press.)
Wiener, A. S., and L. Klatz. 1951. Studies on the use of enzyme-treated red cells in
tests for R. A. sensitization. J. Immun., 66:51-66.
Wilde, J. K. H. 1966. Changes in bovine bone marrow during the course of East Coast
fever. Res. Vet. Sci., 7:213-224.
——— 1967. East Coast fever. *In* Advances in Veterinary Science. Brandly, C. A., and
Cornelius, C., eds. New York, Academic Press, Inc., Vol. 11, pp. 207-259.
Zuckerman, A. 1958. Blood loss and replacement in plasmodial infections. II. *Plasmodium vinckei* in untreated weanling and mature rats. J. Infect. Dis., 103:205-224.
——— 1960. Autoantibodies in rats with *Plasmodium berghei*. Nature (London),
185:189-190.
——— 1964. Autoimmunization and other types of indirect danger to host cells
as factors in certain protozoan diseases. Exp. Parasit., 15:138-183.

Toxoplasmosis and Coccidiosis in Mammalian Hosts

ZBIGNIEW KOZAR

Veterinary Faculty, Agricultural School, University of Wrocław, Wrocław, Poland

INTRODUCTION

The ultrastructures of certain organelles of *Toxoplasma gondii* trophozoites and of *Eimeria* merozoites have been shown by Scholtyseck and Piekarski (1965) to be somewhat similar. However, the existence of essential differences in the biology, epidemiology, and immunology of these parasitic infections has prompted us to treat them as two separate categories. Immunologic phenomena play a major role in both toxoplasmosis and coccidiosis, although the respective mechanisms seem to differ.

At present we are inclined to think of *Toxoplasma* as one species, *T. gondii*, which is common throughout the world in man, in numerous mammals, in birds, and perhaps in lower vertebrates. The organism's ability to adapt to a wide variety of hosts and to their various organs and tissues is remarkable for a protozoan. On the other hand, numerous species of coccidia are characterized by a great specificity in selecting hosts, organs, and occasionally tissues or even areas of the same organ, e.g., the intestine.

Toxoplasmosis is a common cause of pathology in man and some domestic animals (dogs, cats, and sheep), whereas coccidiosis is of great practical importance in fowl. Coccidiosis probably has a negligible pathologic effect in mammals, except in rabbits and perhaps in calves. In man the infection is very rare and rarely causes serious pathologic symptoms. In this connection, immunologic phenomena occurring in response to toxoplasmosis have been studied mostly in mammals, and in response to coccidiosis, mostly in birds. Therefore, the first part of this chapter concerns toxoplasmosis and is more extensive than the following part on coccidiosis, which is discussed in greater detail in the chapter on avian immunity to coccidia (*see* pp. 372-387).

TOXOPLASMOSIS

Historical survey: Past studies and present problems

As early as the period from 1908 to 1939, when *Toxoplasma gondii* was still poorly known and dealt with exclusively by protozoologists who primarily registered its incidence in various hosts, there were also some publications dealing with immunologic phenomena. Laveran and Marullaz (1913) noted a certain resistance to reinvasion in rabbits. Different conclusions were, however, drawn from the experiments of Sarrailhe (1914), who mixed live virulent *Toxoplasma* with sera from convalescent dogs and mice and injected these intraperitoneally in healthy mice. Both convalescent dog and mouse sera were compared with normal dog and mouse sera as controls, and no difference was observed between the normal and immune sera with regard to conferring protection in the infected (but previously unexposed) mice.

Levaditi et al. (1928, 1929), among others, found that as early as two hours after intracerebral administration of *Toxoplasma* to resistant rabbits, no parasites could be detected at the site of injection. Having failed to demonstrate *in vitro* toxoplasmodicidal properties of nervous tissue, the authors sought antibodies in the blood by mixing *Toxoplasma* with immune serum. After incubation for several hours at 37°C, the parasites were then injected intracerebrally or intraocularly into healthy rabbits, but they were unaltered in their pathogenicity. Since intravenous injection of sera from resistant rabbits also failed to protect animals after intracerebral infection, the authors concluded that immunity to toxoplasmosis is of cellular origin. We cannot contradict this hypothesis, though humoral immunity has long been considered to play a greater role than cellular.

The discovery that *T. gondii* may be the cause of a severe, even fatal, disease in man (Wolf and Cowen, 1938; Wolf et al., 1939) initiated a new period of intensive studies on toxoplasmosis. Though initially handicapped in Europe by the war, these studies have continued up to the present time with considerable interest, as indicated by the numerous publications appearing throughout the world. The bibliography on this subject covering the period from 1908 to 1962 amounts to 3,706 references (Galuzo and Zassuchin, 1963). Toxoplasmosis is the subject of several monographs, including one by the present author (Kozar, 1954) from which some data for this chapter were taken. Among the recent publications on toxoplasmosis are: the proceedings of the symposium devoted to ophthalmologic aspects of toxoplasmosis (Maumenee, 1962), chapters on the immunology and immunodiagnosis of toxoplasmosis by Beattie and Fulton, respectively (Garnham et al., 1963), a concise review of current information on toxoplasmosis by Beattie (1964), the proceedings of the 1964 symposium held in Italy, concerned mainly with aspects of ophthalmology and internal medicine (Bartorelli et al., 1964), a monograph on toxoplasmosis in animal hosts studied in Alma-Ata, U.S.S.R. (Galuzo, 1965), and monographs with contributions of several authors, published by Korovickij et al. (1966), and by Kirchoff et al. (1966). For some years the International Toxoplasma Sub-committee has been organizing meetings to discuss the standardization of diagnostic methods (Copenhagen, 1958), taxonomy, and other current problems (Rio de Janeiro, 1963; Rome, 1964; London, 1965).

Although a considerable literature dealing with toxoplasmosis has accumulated, a number of basic problems remain unsolved. In view of the presence of a micropyle, endodyogeny as a special form of schizogony, and other morphologic features, some investigators are inclined to place *Toxoplasma* among the sporozoa. There is also very little evidence concerning the full developmental cycle of the parasite and the parasite's mode of spread in nature; for instance, the means by which herbivores became infected.

Occasionally, over 50 percent of a sample human population demonstrates antibodies against or reacts positively to an intracutaneous test for toxoplasmosis, which indicates a history of infection. The pathogenicity of the parasite is not great, and most infections are asymptomatic or accompanied, as a rule, by negligible manifestations of disease. Only relatively few infections lead to clinical disease, which has a range of severity from mild lymphadenopathy to the grave, violent, and lethal syndromes of encephalomyelitis or of acute inflammatory states of various organs. Almost all medical disciplines, including pediatrics, internal medicine, gynecology, ophthalmology, psychiatry, and neurology, share an interest in toxoplasmosis.

A variety of clinical aspects which are hardly pathognomonic, as well as difficulties in detecting and recognizing the parasite in the host, have accounted for the wide use of indirect immunologic methods. Of greatest practical importance in the diagnosis of toxoplasmosis are the dye test

(Sabin and Feldman, 1948), the complement-fixation test (Nicolau and Ravelo, 1937; Warren and Sabin, 1942), and the skin test (Frenkel, 1948). Recently, fluorescent-antibody methods for toxoplasmosis, introduced by Goldman (1957), seem to be equally, if not more, efficient than the others and are being used with increasing frequency and with various modifications. Other methods, such as the skin protection test (Sabin and Olitzky, 1937), the hemagglutination test (Jacobs and Lunde, 1957), the precipitin test (O'Connor, 1957), the direct agglutination test (Fulton and Turk, 1959), and the flocculation tests with acrylic particles (Siim and Lind, 1960) or with latex particles (Bozděch and Jira, 1961), were either abandoned or never used in routine practice. However, the clinical diagnostic aspect is beyond the scope of this chapter; though immunodiagnostic problems have for years appealed to specialists, it was not until recently that the more general immunologic phenomena in toxoplasmosis have received attention.

Since immunologic phenomena are important in the pathogenesis of toxoplasmosis, they must be envisaged in a broader context, including general changes in the host-parasite relationship. Because the problems are highly complex, we will try to classify them roughly into two groups: (1) those involving factors dependent on the parasite, and (2) those related to the host; i.e., "the seed and soil," as Beattie (1963) put it. The distinction between these factors is not always feasible, as additional difficulties are fostered by ecologic conditions, including various environmental elements acting on the parasite through the host organism, or perhaps even directly. We must admit that our knowledge of immunity in toxoplasmosis is rather poor and fragmentary, and does not justify any general conclusions. Moreover, in spite of their importance, the known immunologic phenomena have not been utilized for practical purposes, apart from the above-mentioned immunodiagnostic procedures.

Parasite strain differences and virulence

In spite of the generally accepted theory postulating a single species of *Toxoplasma*, *T. gondii* (Nicolle and Manceaux, 1908), the existence of conspicuous differences among various samples warrants distinguishing numerous strains of the parasite. The variations consist mainly in the degree of virulence, both for the primary hosts from which they were isolated and for laboratory animals, usually mice, in which the strains are inoculated, maintained, and then examined in serial passages.

The best known strain, RH, is used mainly for experimental purposes and was isolated from the brain of a six-year-old boy who died with symptoms of encephalitis (Sabin, 1942). It is highly virulent, killing mice usually in 3 to 6 days, though nothing is known about its pathogenicity for man, which might have been lost as a result of hundreds of passages in laboratory animals. In spite of frequent contact with the parasite in laboratory practice and the attendant risk of infection, severe cases of laboratory infection are rare, as observed in our 16-year experience. However, other factors, which will be discussed, may be responsible in part for this low rate of laboratory infection.

In a number of laboratories, many strains of *T. gondii* have been isolated from people and animals, some of them being characterized by a high virulence, others by a weaker one, or even by the lack of pathogenicity. Naturally, only certain strains, now well-known, are being maintained in animals and are being utilized for experimental purposes. One strain, BK, isolated in Holland, is less virulent than RH. Among the avirulent strains, Bev, (Beverly, 1959), isolated in England from a rabbit, is often mentioned as causing no lethal infection in mice, but produces cysts rapidly. It persists in the host organism for many years and is even transmitted to future generations. Beverly noted nine murine generations with congenital infection due to this strain (Beattie, 1963).

In the developmental cycle of *Toxoplasma*, two phases can be distinguished: (1) extensive multiplication of the proliferative form, also referred to as trophozoites in almost all tissues and organs, and (2) cysts, previously misnamed pseudocysts, which contain numerous parasites enclosed in a thick capsule of parasite origin. In addition to slight differences in the shape, size, and number of cytoplasmic constituents (Wanko et al., 1962), another variation consists in a varying susceptibility of the parasites to physiologic factors. The parasites originating from the cysts are more resistant to the action of the gastric juice. This fact is used as a criterion for differentiating between encysted and proliferative forms (Jacobs et al., 1960; Jacobs and Melton, 1965). These parasites may, therefore, be regarded as durable forms and occur in the various organs of the host, especially in the brain, muscles, and the myocardium.

Within the host, *Toxoplasma* first multiplies in the lymph nodes and spreads through the organism by the blood and lymphatic vessels. Once established, a strain of trophozoites of high virulence may be encountered in relative abundance in various organs, as well as in the peritoneal exudate. With some host species, the host often dies of infection before cysts have been formed. But when infected by a strain of low virulence, the host, as a rule, survives the infection, and the number of parasites obtained from various organs and from the exudate is generally small. However, after a certain period (occasionally as early as 5 to 7 days after infection) cyst formation begins, mostly in the brain. The parasite divides rapidly within a growing membrane and there is a progressive increase in the dimensions of the cysts (from 7 to 300μ or greater) and in the number of toxoplasms contained in them (up to about 14,000 per cyst).

The differences in cyst formation constitute, therefore, another feature of different strains of *Toxoplasma*. The avirulent strains are thought to produce cysts rapidly, whereas more virulent ones persist in the host, mostly in the form of trophozoites which are sometimes detected after the cysts have been formed. There is no evidence thus far to suggest the existence of strains that fail to produce cysts. Cyst formation is usually related to the defense reaction of the host (Van der Waaij, 1959, 1964), though different opinions are advanced to explain this phenomenon (Stahl et al., 1965). At any rate, cyst formation coincides with the initial appearance of antibodies.

The higher virulence of certain strains cannot be accounted for by a higher degree of toxicity. Toxotoxin is not considered to play a pathogenic role. This substance was isolated from the parasites and affects some animals, but it does not seem to be a true toxin such as those produced by other micro-organisms (Weinman and Klatchko, 1950). However, a higher multiplication rate of virulent strains has been noted in tissue culture (Kaufman et al., 1959). Electron microscope studies revealed that in strains of high virulence (e.g., RH) the limiting membrane surrounding the vacuole within the host cytoplasm is thinner and bursts more frequently than in avirulent ones, e.g., Bev (Matsubayashi and Akao, 1963). These are apparently only manifestations of hitherto unidentified physiologic properties of the parasite, but they are of great practical interest in light of the recent studies on the metabolism of *Toxoplasma* (Fulton and Spooner, 1960; Tomita, 1960; Capella and Kaufman, 1964; Głowiński and Niebrój, 1965; Kishida and Kato, 1965; Gutierrez and Calero, 1966).

It appears that most strains occurring in nature are of low virulence; in humans as well as in animals infection is common, but clinical cases are comparatively rare. Strains of *T. gondii* isolated from humans showing slight clinical symptoms are also of low virulence for animals, in contrast to those obtained from severe or lethal human cases.

The criteria to be taken into consideration in the evaluation of virulence include the size of the inoculum leading to lethal infection, the survival time and/or the mortality rate of the hosts, the extent and character of pathologic symptoms, and so forth. The evaluation of virulence depends mainly upon the mortality rate of mice. It is probable that infection with any strain, even the least virulent, causes an enlargement of the host's spleen. Consequently, it seems unlikely that completely avirulent strains exist, and that in practice we deal with a greater or lesser degree of virulence.

Strangely enough, very little is known about the variations in the characteristics of *Toxoplasma* discussed above. Whether they are genetically determined and how they may be influenced are unknown. Although evidence suggests a longstanding virulence of certain strains (e.g., RH), we also know that strains progressively adapt to new hosts. When passaged from man to mouse, for instance, they are likely to be nonpathogenic in the first passages and are frequently difficult to detect. It is only in successive transfers that their virulence and invasiveness increase and give rise to symptoms occasionally leading to death.

Attempts to induce changes in the virulence of *T. gondii* have been few. Jacobs (1953) claims strain 113 is nonvirulent in chick embryos but becomes highly virulent following serial passage in mice. Gałuszka (1962) succeeded in reducing the virulence of RH strain after 20 passages in tissue culture. Lainson (1955) was able to enhance considerably the virulence of a strain for mice after he had passaged it through another host, *Rattus coucha*. Furthermore, this strain, when maintained in canaries, produced a lethal infection in only 50 percent of mice, but when transferred back to mice, it exhibited an increased virulence for this host. A similar procedure was applied by Roever-Bonnet (1964), who passaged a Burk strain of low virulence for mice and golden hamsters through young gerbils (*Meriones*), thus potentiating the virulence of the strains for mice (they died within 3 days), while the strain's effects on hamsters remained unchanged.

The small number of observations hardly warrants any definite conclusions. However, under some circumstances, such as a change of host species, the biologic properties of the particular strain may be changed. The nature of the host species is naturally of fundamental importance in the course of toxoplasmosis.

Natural immunity

Variations due to host species differences. Unlike many protozoan parasites, *Toxoplasma gondii* is characterized by an exceptional ability to develop in numerous host species. So far, no mammal or bird has been found to be fully resistant to experimental infection, and *Toxoplasma* is also known to survive in certain lower vertebrates and arthropods. However, the degree of host susceptibility varies, being conditioned by differences of species and by inherent individual factors. Among laboratory animals a considerable susceptibility is exhibited by the mouse, guinea pig, and rabbit, whereas the rat is by nature more resistant and survives even when challenged by highly virulent strains. The ground squirrel (*Citellus citellus*) is more susceptible than the mouse, and hence it serves well for isolation of slightly virulent strains (Simitch et al., 1960). Less susceptible are dogs and monkeys, which usually develop only subacute toxoplasmosis. Among birds, pigeons are thought to be susceptible, though chickens are comparatively resistant to infection.

The course of infection depends not only on the strain of parasite and host susceptibility, but also on the route of administration and the size of the inoculum. Infection by intracerebral and intraperitoneal routes kills the host more rapidly than that acquired by subcutaneous inoculation. Perhaps certain tissues vary in their immunologic roles, for instance, some may show a diminished natural resistance, and others, a more slowly acquired immunity, such as brain tissue. Certain strains (e.g., RH) show a greater affinity for central nervous system cells than for other tissues. Perhaps these strains of *Toxoplasma* develop at a higher rate in nerve cells because the concentration of antibodies there is negligible and/or there are other favorable growth conditions.

There is a fairly close correlation between the size of the inoculum and the time of death of animals. This can be determined by a linear regression analysis based on the logarithm of the number of free organisms injected (Eyles and Coleman, 1956). However, with highly virulent strains, the minimum lethal dose is similar in magnitude to the minimum infective dose.

No extensive information is available to explain the mechanism of the natural immunity of certain hosts to *Toxoplasma*. Feldman (1956) found substances with toxoplasmocidal properties in fresh sera of some laboratory animals. These substances were lacking in human and mouse sera. Similar natural substances with this protective effect against *Toxoplasma* were described by Jettmar (1962). They were present particularly in bovine serum and lacking in the sera of white mice, golden hamsters, and gerbils. These thermolabile substances, causing agglutination and lysis of parasites, and related to environmental factors such as climate, are regarded by Jettmar as a factor (or one of the factors) which determines variation in host susceptibility.

The presence of the so-called Jettmar factor in some rats and guinea pigs was confirmed by Metzger et al. (1963). Animals with a high content of the factor survived for 3 months after injection of 100 toxoplasms of RH strain per gram of body weight (though parasites were found at necropsy), whereas those with a small amount of the mentioned factor succumbed in 6 to 18 days. These aspects necessitate additional studies which might disclose the more complex nature of this protective reaction in view of differences in the host metabolism and the parasite strains.

In addition to species differences, variations related to the host race and the breeding conditions are conceivable. The latter is suggested by the results of Michael (unpublished), who infected Wistar rats obtained from two different laboratory animal breeders with a virulent strain (BK) and a slightly virulent strain (DX) of *Toxoplasma* (Piekarski, 1966). Each group was infected with both strains. He maintained experimental conditions carefully (i.e., similar body weights and same inocula) and invariably found high antibody titers in one group and consistently low ones in the other. Apart from immunologic differences in the host groups, variations in the parasites might account for the higher multiplication rate in animals which produced lower antibody titers.

Individual differences.   The course of toxoplasmosis also depends on individual characteristics of the host, such as age, general condition, and other features. Individual differences are practically a rule even among animals maintained under identical conditions.

Age.   Age of the host plays a pronounced role in *Toxoplasma* infections, since the greatest susceptibility to *Toxoplasma* is observed not only in fetuses lacking their own defenses, but also in infants and in children. Clinical cases are the most common in infants, and in them, the course of the infection is the most severe. Antibodies may be transferred passively from the mother and protect the fetus *in utero* to some degree, but after delivery there is a decline of protection until active immunity appears. These problems are discussed by Frenkel (1953), Jacobs (1953), and Kulasiri (1962).

Effect of Hormones.   Some differences in susceptibility to *Toxoplasma* occur regardless of age in adults. They are caused by variations in the physiologic state or by pathologic factors. Pregnancy and lactation are periods of increased susceptibility of the host. A certain significance may be attributed to hormones in this regard, as indicated by the results of experiments in rats, mice, and guinea pigs (Kozar and Soszka, 1956a,b). The strongest death-accelerating effect is exhibited by folliculin (estrone), gonadotropin exerting a weaker effect, and luteine (progesterone) almost none at all.

The adrenal and pituitary hormones, known to influence the course of infectious diseases, were also studied for their effects in toxoplasmosis. Erichsen and Harboe (1953) used cortisone to enhance the susceptibility of mice to a slightly virulent strain of *Toxoplasma* from chickens. The same method was then applied by Havlik and Zastěrà (1954) and other investigators. In these studies some difficulties were noted in evaluating the effects of cortisone on mice merely by LD_{50} determination. Though animals treated with higher doses of cortisone die more rapidly than controls, other effects of the drug, such as accelerating the activity of latent microorganisms, cannot be excluded (Havlik et al., 1955). At any rate, the authors failed to influence the virulence of a strain of *Toxoplasma* (CB) by six serial passages in cortisone-treated mice. A similar result was obtained by Swatek (1956), who showed that in spite of a greater multiplication rate of *Toxoplasma* and exacerbation of infection in RH-infected, ACTH-treated mice, the time of death could not be accelerated.

Cortisone and zymosan given to rats for 5 days after infection with RH strain were found by Metzger et al. (1963) to prolong the occurrence of parasites and to decrease to a considerable degree the ability to resist *Toxoplasma* infection. There was a decline of the Jettmar factor to 30 percent of its original level in 30 minutes, after which it gradually rose, reaching half of its original level in 24 hours, and returned to normal in 48 hours. Irradiation with x-rays did not affect the Jettmar factor.

The administration of steroids to rats (Giroud et al., 1962) was reported as resulting in potentiated virulence of some strains (e.g., Congolese B12), which previously had been almost avirulent for this host. In this case, however, a reduced resistance in the host is also possible.

Effect of Enzymes.   Little is known so far concerning the influence of enzymes on the course of toxoplasmosis. Hyaluronidase accelerated the deaths of RH-infected mice, though it was also found to have an adverse effect on the parasite which was apparently caused by inadequate purification of the compound (Kozar, 1958). The author also used hyaluronidase in an attempt to isolate strains from the brain and muscles of animals with latent infections and succeeded in obtaining a certain exacerbation of infection.

These observations are corroborated by Lycke et al. (1965), who have shown that hyaluronidase and lysozyme, which act on mucopolysaccharide-mucoprotein complexes by attacking the glucosidic linkages of amino sugars, have a protective effect on the penetration of toxoplasms into Hela cells. A synergistic effect of enzymes was also observed.

Stress.   The course of toxoplasmosis is also affected by physical and psychological stresses. Though no exact experimental data are available, certain observations are fairly convincing. It is probable that stress has contributed to the detection and description of *Toxoplasma* (Nicolle and Manceaux, 1909). The rodent, *Ctenodactylus gundi*, when captured in the wild exhibited no pathologic symptoms due to *Toxoplasma*, though they were already infected. However, in prolonged captivity, they developed an acute toxoplasmosis which was often fatal (Chatton and Blanc, 1917). Toxoplasmosis in hares observed in Denmark occurs more often in winter than in summer, which could be due to the effect of physical stress (Christiansen, 1948; Christiansen and Siim, 1951).

Concurrent disease.   A similar role may be attributed to various diseases sometimes concurrent with toxoplasmosis. The literature contains numerous reports of this kind, mentioning bartonellosis, malaria, tuberculous bacterial meningitis, reticulosarcoma, and others. Also to be considered are the effects of debilitation, generally reduced resistance of the host, and the existence of *loci minoris resistentiae*, or even mechanical damage to the cysts with the resulting liberation of toxoplasms. This is readily seen in the cerebral tissue, the usual site of cysts, and is exemplified by a case of *cysticercosis cerebri*, which complicated acute toxoplasmosis of the brain, taking a lethal course in a 47-year-old woman (Kozar et al., 1954). Intravital and postmortem studies showed that this case of toxoplasmosis was unusually acute for the age of the host.

Dogs are known to develop frequent complications of toxoplasmosis which are induced by distemper (Fankhauser, 1952; Campbell et al., 1955). Such complications should not be overlooked in considering the pathology of toxoplasmosis and natural immunity.

Antibody production and antigens

The demonstration of antibodies to *Toxoplasma* implies a history of infection. The serologic tests used routinely in toxoplasmosis are thought to be specific, particularly in the presence of high titers, in spite of antigens being shared with *Benoitia jellisoni* (Lunde and Jacobs, 1965). Only newborns possess antibodies without previous infection, which are acquired passively from the mother during fetal life. Their antibody level is then no higher than that of the mother. Antibodies of this kind usually disappear within 5 to 10 months after delivery.

In initial infections, antibodies usually appear in the serum 5 to 8 days after infection; their level gradually increases, followed by a subsequent slow decline and disappearance. Sometimes they persist for years (at low titer) after infection. The appearance of antibodies, their level, and their subsequent loss offer a characteristic pattern determined by various serologic methods and serve essentially as an index in the diagnosis of toxoplasmosis. Data thus obtained enable a distinction to be made between active and latent toxoplasmosis.

The absence of antibodies or the failure to detect them by means of routine tests does not necessarily mean the absence of infection. Some persons may react weakly or fail to produce detectable antibodies. Mentioned previously were the appreciable differences in the level of antibody produced by rats of the same breed but from various strains. In long-standing latent infections, the antibodies may vanish in spite of the presence of parasites in cysts. The literature cites cases in which *T. gondii* were isolated from individuals whose sera were negative in serologic tests. In some cases, the antibody production process is inhibited for a certain period. Jadin et al. (1965) injected rabbits intracutaneously with the C13 strain and succeeded in detecting parasites in resulting skin ulcerations. Nonetheless, the dye test (DT), which measures serum antibody level, was negative for two months, and four subcutaneous injections of formalin-treated suspension from the spleen of infected mice were required to stimulate the production of high-titer antibodies and the development of resistance to superinfection. This case is rather exceptional and puzzling if the possibility of technical errors is excluded. One should bear in mind the occurrence of the so-called prozone phenomenon, i.e., the period of DT-reaction inhibition at low concentrations of examined serum in spite of high-titer antibodies.

Ophthalmologic aspects of toxoplasmosis offer particular difficulties in serologic diagnosis. In spite of active processes in the eye, the serum antibody level may be low. However, local antibodies may be produced in the eye. Desmonts et al. (1960) correlated the antibody and globulin levels in the aqueous humor of the eye with those in serum.

Antigen preparation. Evidently both the production and the detection of antibody depend largely on the quality of the antigens involved. This is a crucial and hitherto unsolved problem in toxoplasmosis. The recovery of a pure antigen free of contaminating host or culture tissue materials presents great technical difficulties.

The antigenic structure of *Toxoplasma* was studied mostly by means of the dye test (DT) and complement-fixation test (CFT). The antigens involved were shown to be protein in nature (Hoak and Faber, 1957). As in the case of toxoplasmin used in the cutaneous test (Frenkel, 1948), activity is found in the protein fraction (Szurman and Szaflarski, 1964). By means of immunoelectrophoresis, Körting (1958) was able to demonstrate four components located in the α_1, α_2, and β_1 regions of the globulin fraction, and possibly a fifth component in the β to γ region. Chordi et al. (1964) studied *Toxoplasma* antigens by agar-gel diffusion methods and drew definite conclusions as to ways of increasing the specificity and sensitivity of immunologic tests. For instance, they described a method for preparing a suspension of pure *Toxoplasma* without previous washing, and they recommended the fractionation of sera in order to obtain the diagnostically essential α_1 and β_2 components. The peritoneal exudate from infected mice was used for antigen production, and after ultracentrifugation, extracts were taken from the sediment.

Some workers prefer to use *Toxoplasma* grown in tissue culture as the initial material for antigen production. It is to be noted, however, that the cell-free nontreated supernatant of the centrifuged peritoneal exudate contains as many precipitinogens as the frozen and thawed sediment of the same exudate (Strannegård, 1962). Further studies by this author show that ultrasonic treatment did not cause any alterations in the precipitation patterns. Some antigenic factors were lost at temperatures exceeding 60°C, but one factor resisted 100°C for 20 minutes. Jirovec and Jira (1961) have found that supernatants may be good skin-test antigens, and Körting (1960) demonstrated antigenic activity for CFT in cell-free supernatants.

Antibody types. Antibodies detected in toxoplasmosis are of varying types. It is thought that the DT and CFT demonstrate two different types of antibodies and that DT antibodies appear earlier and persist longer than CFT antibodies. Kass and Steen (1951) found DT antibodies in infected rabbits as early as 4 days after infection, with the highest titer, 1:81,920, being reached after 4 weeks. CFT antibody appeared by the second week, and by the fourth week its titer was only 1:384.

A correlation was found between the titer of DT antibodies and the number of precipitating antibody components demonstrated with double gel-diffusion methods (Strannegård, 1962). It is probable that DT antibodies are not identical with any of the precipitating antibodies demonstrated. A correlation between the CFT titers and the number of precipitating antibody components in human sera was apparent, but other differences indicated (as in the previous case) that the antibodies were not identical. In the sera of rabbits, the number of precipitin bands reached its maximum 12 weeks after infection, whereas the maximum titer of CFT and DT antibodies occurred 4 weeks after infection. In human sera, precipitating antibodies were demonstrated more than two years after the onset of the disease. These antibodies often seem to disappear at about the same time as the CFT antibodies, i.e., at a time when the DT titer is quite high.

Antibody levels. The level of antibodies produced seems to depend to some degree on the parasite strain used. Agglutinating antibodies appeared earlier and persisted longer in rats infected with the highly virulent RH strain than in rats infected with the slightly virulent 113 strain (Lunde and Jacobs, 1963). These authors found that the antibodies detected by hemagglutination were produced in rats regardless of the strain of *Toxoplasma* used, and were invariably lower in titer than antibodies demonstrated by DT. This suggested the presence in rat serum of hemagglutination-inhibiting substances. Likewise, in Strassmann's experiments, strains of relatively low virulence, in spite of higher infective doses, produced lower antibody titers in rats than did highly virulent ones (Piekarski, 1966).

The level of antibodies produced may also be related to the magnitude of immunizing doses and the mode of immunization (Bozdech et al., 1965). Small doses (300 organisms) of the RH strain stimulated the production of CFT antibodies in low titer in rats only after several inoculations. Higher doses (30,000 parasites) stimulated, as a rule, higher titers, though still lower than with heavy infective doses (3,000,000 parasites). In rabbits, better results were achieved by immunization at monthly intervals rather than at weekly intervals. The highest titer occurred about 10 days after the last immunizing dose was administered. CFT antibodies thus obtained persisted for at least 6 months. The immunization of animals other than rats, i.e., those with greater susceptibility to infection, is more difficult. Thus, various procedures are being applied to attenuate (mostly by heating) or to kill the parasites. The methods described sometimes fail to establish accurately whether the parasites have been killed or only attenuated.

Umiński and Toś-Luty (1959) used peritoneal exudates from mice previously infected with attenuated RH strain and heated these at 56°C for 60 minutes. The dried exudate failed to produce antibodies (CFT) or to protect animals against challenge, whereas inoculation with a suspension of fresh parasites from the liver of infected mice led to the premature death of experimental animals.

The developmental stage of parasites used for immunization seems to play no major role in antibody production. Mas Bakal (1965) obtained both low and high antibody titers (DT) in mice after administration of either proliferative or encysted, live or spiramycin-killed *Toxoplasma*.

It is noteworthy that killed parasites also stimulate the production of antibodies, though the level is generally lower than that observed after the administration of live organisms. Both DT and CFT antibodies develop in guinea pigs immunized with formalin-killed, ultrasonically disrupted parasites or with ammonium sulfate-precipitated *Toxoplasma* antigen (Cutchins and Warren, 1956; Hook and Faber, 1957; and others).

The use of killed *Toxoplasma* for repeated inoculations of a rabbit brought about a very weak antibody response (Strannegård, 1962). The DT-titer became moderately positive rather quickly, unlike the CFT which never became definitely positive. The precipitating antibody components (only one or two faintly visible lines) could not be demonstrated until after more than 3 months of repeated injections.

Serum protein changes. As in other infectious diseases, serum protein changes are observed which might be in part attributed to immunization processes. The hitherto obtained results are not invariably uniform, suggesting differences dependent on the host species.

Dobrzańska et al. (1958) demonstrated electrophoretically a decline in the albumin content and a rise in the total level of globulins, particularly in β_1, β_2, and γ fractions, in the serum of eleven patients with toxoplasmosis. In six rabbits examined between the 9th and 16th weeks of infection, there was a simultaneous increase in α- and β-globulin fractions. Likewise, Wildführ et al. (1958) found that in infected rats, an increase in the total level of protein occurs at 3 to 4 weeks of infection, with a fall in albumin and an elevation of γ-globulins.

Kulasiri (1960) fractionated immune rabbit serum by alcohol precipitation and found the highest DT antibody titers in the fractions containing γ-globulin. Körting (1958) demonstrated by immunoelectrophoresis that *Toxoplasma*-precipitating antibodies of rabbit sera migrated with the γ-globulin fraction. Strannegård (1962), using similar techniques, found the

Toxoplasma-precipitating antibodies of human sera to be γ-globulins or β-globulins. However, all three types of antibodies (DT, CFT, and precipitins) of rabbit sera, as well as the DT and CFT antibodies of human sera, had mobilities similar to human serum β_2-globulins.

In rats, the increase of DT antibodies at 4 to 5 days of infection was associated with the rise in γ-globulin concentration (Remington and Hackman, 1965). After some time, however, the level of the latter returned to normal, though high antibody titers persisted. By starch-block electrophoresis, these authors demonstrated that the DT antibody in rats was localized in the γ-globulin fraction; small amounts found in the α_2 and β fractions were apparently due to contamination. This is not in keeping with similar experiments in mice (Remington, 1964), for in these animals the essential changes in acute infection due to virulent or slightly virulent strains involved α- and β-globulin fractions. This author is inclined to assume a certain correlation between the serum protein variations found in mice and rats, and the susceptibility of these animals to toxoplasmosis. This aspect requires further study.

Acquired immunity

Acquired immunity involves both passive and active forms. In infectious diseases, the former is usually weaker than the latter, affording a partial and temporary protection to the host while active immunity develops. Both forms of immunity can be acquired under either natural or artificial conditions.

Passive immunity. Passively acquired immunity is exemplified in cases of newborns that acquire antibodies from their mother, though they were not infected in fetal life. The evaluation is more difficult to make in older humans and experimental animals, since we cannot exclude a congenital infection with a strain of low virulence which may take a latent course.

Levis and Markell (1958) demonstrated that young rats born of females with latent toxoplasmosis are more resistant to challenge than control animals of toxoplasmosis-free mothers. A still higher degree of resistance was found in sucklings of healthy mothers, but which were fed on milk of chronically infected females. The interpretation of these results is difficult. In the former case, there may be a light intrauterine infection, since we know from other experiments (Beverley, 1959) that in rats, for example, a slightly virulent strain is transmitted congenitally. This is, however, less likely in the latter case, in which the parasites are found in the milk of the chronically infected females.

The effect of immune sera on the host-parasite relationship during infection seems to be negligible. It was studied by Eichenwald (1949) in young mice infected *in utero*. Administration of antiserum to *Toxoplasma* along with sulfadiazine was more effective than either given separately. In further studies, Eichenwald (1952) demonstrated continued parasitemia following injection of potent specific antisera in chronic toxoplasmosis. Wildführ

(1957) administered to hamsters immune serum from rabbits 8 hours before or simultaneously with infectious organisms. All animals died in 16 to 23 days. However, those hamsters that received immune serum died 4.2 days later on the average than those that did not. In other similar experiments using mice, almost 50 percent of the animals immunized with rabbit or pig antiserum survived 3 weeks or more when the infective dose of RH strain of *Toxoplasma* (100 parasites) was small (Nakayama, 1965). With a higher dose (3,000 parasites) no difference was found between the treated group and the control animals.

Actively acquired immunity. Much better results were obtained with active immunization. The results of several studies indicate that in normally reacting mammals, *Toxoplasma* infection stimulates immunity to challenge or to superinfection (Weinman, 1943; Ruchman and Johansmann, 1948; Cutchins and Warren, 1956; Frenkel, 1956; Hahn and Alm, 1957; Beverley, 1958; Ueda, 1960; Sato, 1963; Nakayama, 1964; Stahl and Akao, 1964, and others). Such immunity has been reported as being neither absolute nor of very long duration.

Cutchins and Warren (1956) found that immunized guinea pigs after challenge with the same strain did not die, nor were as severely ill as the control animals. Simitch et al. (1960) immunized hamsters with strains of different virulence. The initial infection failed to afford absolute protection against superinfection with highly virulent heterologic strains. It is known, however, that slightly virulent strains also partially protect animals from infection with highly virulent strains (De Roever-Bonnet, 1963).

Immunity against *Toxoplasma* has also been reported as developing slowly and in some experiments, persisting for a rather long time. Stahl and Akao immunized mice with slightly virulent Bev strain and then challenged them at various intervals with the RH strain. Two weeks after initial infection, protection against challenge could be demonstrated, which reached its peak after one month and persisted for seven months. Those immune mice that did die after challenge exhibited symptoms more like those of hypersensitivity than of acute toxoplasmosis.

Immunity is frequently sufficient to protect against challenge with exceedingly high doses of a strain of virulent parasite. Guinea pigs infected with a strain of low virulence isolated from human lymph nodes died, as did the controls, following a heavy challenge dose (10,000 parasites) of a highly virulent laboratory strain, in spite of high DT and CFT antibody titers (Piekarski, 1966). However, when the challenge dose was reduced to 1,000 parasites, acquired immunity could be demonstrated and the animals survived and could be safely infected for the third time.

Role of antibodies. Though there is some evidence suggesting that the presence of antibodies does not necessarily protect or even suppress the parasite burden of the host after challenge (Verlinde and Makstenieks, 1950), a certain correlation is also demonstrable between the degree of host defense and the level of humoral antibodies. Rabbits with low or moderate antibody levels after natural infection (DT < 1250, CFT < 120) were not as resistant to challenge as were animals immunized with killed parasites, though the level of the latters' antibodies was occasionally as high (Huldt, 1965). On the other hand, a pronounced immunity was exhibited by rabbits possessing high antibody titers produced after natural infection. The authors found that only active infection protects animals from challenge and under these conditions there is a correlation existing between immunity and antibodies. Rabbits immunized with killed antigens showed an even stronger antibody response. It is of interest that these rabbits were negative in the cutaneous test with toxoplasmin, whereas all rabbits immunized by natural infection were toxoplasmin-positive. It follows that humoral immunity is not the only factor in the defense mechanism of animals to toxoplasmosis.

Effects on parasites. As immunity measured in terms of antibody increases, morphologic changes are noticeable in the parasite (Werner, 1963). These occur with the first appearance of antibodies at 4 to 5 days post-infection. At that time, toxoplasms are still alive and capable of further multiplication. At 5 to 6 days after infection when the DT titer reaches 1:256 to 1:4,000, the number of toxoplasms diminishes, they pick up stain more readily, and they do not detach one from another after division, frequently remaining grouped together. At a still higher titer (1:16,000 or more), and particularly with the appearance of CFT antibodies, two kinds of changes are observed. Some parasites disintegrate without being acted on by phagocytes, whereas others take the shape of cysts. Similar phenomena, which appeared earlier, were found by the author in animals with latent infection, and in those immunized with killed antigen.

Nakayama (1966) immunized mice with the slightly virulent Bev and the S-273 strain (isolated in Japan from a pig) and after 40 to 120 days injected intravenously 1,000 trophozoites of the RH strain. Within two minutes, the parasites were found in the lungs, liver, and spleen. At first they developed primarily in the cells of the pulmonary tissue as they did in the nonimmunized control animals. Three days later the tissues of the immunized animals showed fewer parasites than did those of the controls, and by the fourth and fifth day only very few organisms were detectable. This condition persisted for about two weeks, though at three to eight weeks after infection, some toxoplasms could still be found in the tissues of immunized animals. In control mice the infection was extremely severe and led to death within 10 days.

Such observations suggest that immunity inhibits the multiplication of parasites and thus protects animals against heavy infection and death; however, immunity is unable to suppress the infection entirely and (at least in some animals) it persists for a long time (De Roever-Bonnet, 1963).

It is generally thought that immunity in toxoplasmosis is of the premunition type, persisting as long as latent infection exists. The fact that antibodies are detected for long periods would suggest their continuous production owing to the presence of persistent and active antigenic stimuli. The toxoplasms contained in cysts seem to be sufficiently protected from the effects of host antibodies. In the vicinity of cysts, no cellular defense reaction is observed, and thus cysts may persist for a long time. Cysts occasionally burst due to various factors, and the released antigen, or the parasite itself, is a sufficient stimulus for the formation of new antibodies. Remington et al. (1961) occasionally found parasites in chronic infections in spite of the presence of high-titer antibodies. These antibodies mostly prevent the spread of the infection by acting on extracellular parasites and thus accelerate the formation of new cysts. This process may recur several times, supporting both the antibody level and to some extent the defense mechanism against reinfection for several years. These phenomena, however, are probably more complex than the explanations we have presented.

Artificially acquired immunity. Perhaps the acquired immunity demonstrated in toxoplasmosis could be utilized for practical purposes. It is conceivable that animals which are infected with a strain of low virulence thus become immunized against infection with a more virulent one. Beattie (1963) proposed that this procedure be applied to sheep in which abortions have been observed fairly frequently in the course of toxoplasmosis. Since our knowledge of the variability of strain virulence is so meager, the introduction of live parasites for vaccination purposes would be unsafe.

Huldt failed to immunize animals against toxoplasmosis with killed vaccines, as mentioned previously. Levaditi et al. (1929) first obtained almost negative results when immunizing animals with a heat-killed suspension of toxoplasms. Jacobs (1953), in making a vaccine, exposed toxoplasms to the action of antibodies and activator (a thermolabile substance, *see* p. 890) at 37°C and then inactivated them at 56°C. This vaccine administered with Freund's complete adjuvant also failed to afford protection against challenge with the highly virulent RH strain (Stahl and Akao, 1964). Nakayama (1965) administered a suspension of heat-killed toxoplasms four times, and only in one of five groups examined was he able to obtain a detectable degree of immunity. Here again the use of complete or incomplete adjuvants was ineffective.

Some differences in immunity were noted, however, and these depended on the host. Wildführ (1957) injected rabbits frequently, i.e., every 3 to 4 days, subcutaneously or intravenously, with the exudate from infected mice which had been inactivated by heating at 56°C for 30 minutes. Though some of these rabbits died in the course of the experiments, the author succeeded in obtaining in some animals, after about 16 injections, both a fairly high antibody level and an immunity to challenge. Similar experiments in hamsters failed; low antibody titers were obtained (DT to 1:100) and all the animals died after challenge. Senega (1957) was unable to prolong the survival time of mice through immunization, but he had more success using guinea pigs: three of six immunized animals survived challenge with *Toxoplasma* of the RH strain.

Many authors conclude that killed vaccines, although sometimes a sufficient stimulus for antibody production, hardly are efficient in protecting the host from challenge. Mas Bakal (1965) observed that in mice at one and six weeks after injection, DT titers of 1:125 and 1:32, respectively, followed a single parenteral injection of spiramycin-killed toxoplasms, and that titers of 1:4,096 and 1:128 after one and eight weeks, respectively, followed such injections.

Cutchins and Warren (1956) suggested that the antigen active in the production of immunity is associated with the whole parasite rather than with extracts. This is not in keeping with the data of Nakayama (1965), who found that neither soluble nor insoluble fractions of parasites disrupted by ultrasonic vibration produced a clear-cut defense reaction in the host.

The most encouraging experimental results so far obtained are those of Jadin et al. (1965), who found that after four injections of formalin-treated suspensions of *Toxoplasma* from infected mice, rabbits demonstrated both high antibody titers and immune reactions to challenge. It is of interest that a formalin-treated suspension of infected exudate, as well as formalin-treated and filtered emulsions from the spleen, were not effective to the same degree, and a phenol-treated emulsion from the spleen of infected mice proved to be of no value at all. After a first administration of the vaccine, antibodies were also found in the aqueous humor of the eye, as demonstrated by the fluorescent-antibody method.

These results on the effectiveness of vaccines are fairly promising and the reason for the recorded failures may reside in the mode of preparing the antigen.

Use of vaccines on human subjects should be mentioned, since they were undertaken mostly for therapeutic purposes or in order to stimulate antibody production (Paul and Schlanstedt, 1956; Fair, 1959). Tolentino and Bucalossi (1952) used a heat-killed *Toxoplasma* suspension which they injected seven times, first intravenously, then subcutaneously, into children at increasing concentrations of parasites. In nine of the ten children whose sera failed to react in the DT, the antibodies were found to occur at low titer (1:2 to 1:64).

Assuming that allergy plays a certain role in pathogenesis of toxoplasmosis, Jira et al. (1963) tried to desensitize some persons by repeated twice-weekly subcutaneous injections of toxoplasmin at gradually decreasing concentrations. Some cases showed transitory desensitization and clinical improvement was observed in almost 50 percent of treated patients. This was particularly true in cases with chronic relapsing ocular inflammation, in women with repeated chronic miscarriages or abortions, and in patients with the so-called neurasthenic symptom complex. These findings, interesting from the practical point of view, are yet to be confirmed.

An inherent risk of vaccination consists of post-vaccination encephalomyelitis, as observed by Kunert and Schleussing (1965). Many rabbits, immunized with a long series of injections of killed *Toxoplasma* (strain BK) and then inoculated with live parasites, were killed when the vaccines were inactivated at 56°C to 60°C rather than at 100°C.

Mechanisms of immunity

Though the cause of pathogenesis in toxoplasmosis has not yet been elucidated, the major factor is generally attributed to mechanical damage of the host cells during the development of the parasite in various organs and tissues. In later phases of infection, allergic processes are involved which presumably account for ocular lesions and other symptoms. Toxic substances contained in the parasites or produced by them have also been suggested as playing a role. Weimann and Klatchko (1950) described a toxotoxin which acted only on mice. Balducci and Tyrrel (1956) studied filtrates from infected tissue cultures. Though toxins comparable to those isolated from bacteria have not been isolated, the participation of toxic substances should not be rejected categorically. Acquired immunity is probably directed not only against live parasites but, at least in part, against toxic substances associated with infections. Intravenous injection of *Toxoplasma* lysates prepared from the exudate of infected mice are toxic for rabbits, leading to their death within 6 to 24 hours (Lunde and Jacobs, 1964), whereas animals with chronic toxoplasmosis are resistant not only to challenge but also to the lethal effect of lysate.

Humoral mechanisms: The action of antibody. It is not always feasible to separate the humoral from cellular aspects of immunity. As to the cellular effects in toxoplasmosis immunity, our knowledge is not as extensive as that of humoral effects.

The direct action of antibodies on toxoplasms has been studied *in vivo* and *in vitro* and the results obtained have served as a basis for a few diagnostic methods, e.g., the neutralization test in which toxoplasms are injected into rabbits intracutaneously (Sabin and Olitsky, 1937) or onto chorioallantoic membranes of chick embryos (McFarlane and Ruchman, 1948; McDonald, 1949). Physiologic changes in the parasite induced by antibodies may also be reflected by the respiratory inhibition test (Fulton and Spooner, 1960; Fulton, 1963). It has been found that immune sera of certain laboratory animals inhibit, to varying degrees, the respiration of parasites, and that this phenomenon is also accompanied by agglutination and lysis.

Of great interest is the dye test (DT) of Sabin and Feldman (1948), in which thermostable antibodies and a thermolabile activator (*see* p. 890) induce changes in the cytoplasm of *Toxoplasma* such that the organism is not stained by methylene blue in an alkaline environment. This phenomenon not only permits the detection of antibodies, but allows one to study their effect on the parasite *in vitro*, thus ruling out the possible intervention of hitherto unidentified factors of host origin (Hirschlerowa and Kozar, 1956). Changes in the shape and internal structure of the parasite damaged by antibodies may be observed prior to the addition of the dye indicator, which is not a critical component of the system. Microscopy is particularly useful for observing a cytoplasmic lysis similar to that occurring in Pfeiffer's phenomenon. This has prompted some authors to replace the term "dye test" with "cytoplasm modifying or lysing test" (Lelong and Desmonts, 1951, 1952; Desmonts, 1960).

The dye test was the subject of numerous studies including some by electron microscopy. Bringmann and Holz (1953) advanced an hypothesis that the clearing of the cytoplasm by antibody is due to the dissolution of cytoplasmic ribonucleic acid, which is not a specific phenomenon, also being obtainable by other means. This was supported by cytochemical findings of Kulasiri and Das Gupta (1959) which suggest that antigen-antibody reactions result in the mobilization of intracellular ribonuclease, and consequently the cytoplasm's ability to be stained.

Further studies by electron microscopy disclosed a number of morphologic details suggesting damage to the parasite as a result of antibody action (Braunsteiner et al., 1957; Thalhammer, 1960; Ludwig and Piekarski, 1961; Ludwig et al., 1963). They can be summarized as follows: antibodies penetrate the parasite apparently through the conoid and toxonemes, the cytoplasm becomes almost homogeneous, and the cell nucleus undergoes dissolution. The process begins at the pointed pole of the parasite and results in the subsequent disappearance of toxonemes and in the swelling and rounding of mitochondria. The cristae are to be seen on the external side of the membranes with their centers hollow in appearance. The cell membranes may also be involved, particularly their interior layer, and the external one shows numerous tiny granules accumulated all around the parasite.

The nature and function of activator.   In the dye test, an interesting phenomenon consists in the participation of the activator, a thermolabile substance occurring in the serum of some persons. This factor frequently causes considerable difficulties in the performance of the test. Roth (1953) found that the activator system contained at least three complement factors: C'_2, C'_3, and C'_4. On the other hand, Grönroos (1955) showed that properdin is an integral part of the so-called activator system, necessary for the action of antibodies to *Toxoplasma*. In the author's opinion, the activator is composed of the complement components C'_2, C'_3, C'_4, and Mg^{++}, along with properdin. Feldman (1956) confirmed these findings and showed that properdin *per se* had no antitoxoplasmic effect, but that the complement components C'_1, C'_2, C'_3, C'_4, and magnesium ions, i.e., the whole properdin system, were indispensable.

Various concepts are advanced to explain the action of properdin. Some consider it to be an antibody capable of reacting with zymosan, others believe that it is distinct from antibody, still others propose that it depends on the interaction of antigen with specific antibody. The exceptional position of *Toxoplasma* in this respect makes it possible to study this general phenomenon with greater accuracy.

The recent studies of Strannegård and Lycke (1966) indicate that properdin and immune antibodies are different entities. The hypothesis postulating that the action of properdin is dependent on the interaction of *Toxoplasma* with specific antibodies appears to be plausible. The antibody concentration necessary for this interaction may, however, be extremely small, being nondetectable by dye tests. Properdin sensitizes the parasites to the action of antibody. In addition to its activating effect, properdin seemed to be able to dissociate antibodies attached to reactive sites of the toxoplasms. Properdin in high concentrations inhibits antibody effects; the inhibition occurs independently of antibody concentration and could also be elicited when properdin was added to parasites after the addition of the antibody.

As suggested by these studies, antibodies exert an influence on *Toxoplasma* in the presence of the activator. Jacobs et al. (1959) demonstrated that the parasites damaged by this system are not pathogenic for mice. Lycke et al. (1965) showed, using a tissue culture system, that the penetration of toxoplasms into cells is inhibited not only by the action of immune serum and activator, but also by serum in which the thermolabile components of the activator were destroyed by heating. The effect of antibodies is evidently greater in the presence of all activator components, though it has been noted that the properdin system alone, in the absence of antibodies, is capable of producing a certain degree of inhibition of the penetration of parasites into the host cells. The effect of these factors, as observed in tissue culture, was discussed by Strannegård (1965), who took two criteria into consideration: (1) the ability of the parasites to penetrate host cells, and (2) morphologic alterations of toxoplasms under the effect of antibodies. The former phenomenon is seen somewhat earlier than the latter. In the mechanism by which the immune serum acts on the parasites, the author distinguishes two phases, the first involving the reaction between antibody, properdin, and parasites, and the second comprising an effect on the parasites evoked by antibodies, properdin, and complement in the presence of magnesium.

It appears that the mode of action of humoral antibodies involves only extracellular toxoplasms and not those within cells, particularly within cysts. Using the method of ferritin-conjugated antibody, Matsubayashi et al. (1964) found a great number of ferritin particles on the surface of extracellular parasites but not on the surface of intracellularly located toxoplasms. Assuming that the extracellular period of the parasites is of short duration (i.e., during parasitemia), the effect of humoral immunity seems to be fairly limited.

Cyst formation. The participation of antibodies in the formation of the cyst is another controversial point. Most authors believe that encystment is closely related to the appearance of immunity. Using fluorescent-antibody methods, Carver and Goldman (1959) demonstrated that the membrane of cysts is at least in part derived from the parasite. This process was studied in more detail with the electron microscope by Matsubayashi and Akao (1963, 1966), who found that particulate precipitates appear in host cell vacuoles containing parasites. These precipitates are deposited on the limiting membrane of the vacuole, forming a layer of granules which later fuse and develop into the compact, almost homogeneous cyst wall. Further observations of these authors (Matsubayashi et al., 1964, 1966), using ferritin-conjugated antibody staining, suggest that antigenic material of parasitic origin is retained on the limiting vacuolar membrane. Antibody was prevented from reaching the parasite by the limiting membrane, and this explains why toxoplasms in the host cell always remain negative to the Sabin-Feldman dye test. In other words, parasite material deposited on the limiting membrane of the vacuole contributes to the formation of the cyst wall, presumably with the participation of antibodies, which then cease to penetrate the cysts.

Van der Waaij (1960), assuming that lysine is necessary for γ-globulin synthesis, studied cyst formation in the brains of mice infected with a strain of *Toxoplasma* of low virulence after administration of a lysine-free diet. In these animals, the number of cysts was lower than in the controls, and the author attributed this to the lysine requirements of the parasite. However, it is also possible that the lack of γ-globulins causes a decreased antibody level or interferes with cyst formation.

This observation is, to some degree, contradicted by similar experiments done by Matsubayashi and Akao (1966) with the use of 6-mercaptopurine (6-MP) which is known to inhibit immune reactions in mice. When used in infected mice, the metabolic inhibitor allowed parasites to have a lethal effect on some of these animals in spite of the use of a strain of low virulence, and in survivors it inhibited the development of immunity to reinfection with a more virulent strain. Contrary to what was expected, cysts were formed in increased numbers and gathered in clusters earlier in the 6-MP treated mice than in controls. It is possible that besides inhibiting the immune reaction, the drug exerts some additional action.

Cellular mechanisms. There are often discrepancies in the available information on cellular immunity in toxoplasmosis. An important role for cells of the reticuloendothelial system (RES cells) is suggested by the studies of Glowinski et al. (1964, 1966). By injecting colloidal carbon into mice infected with *Toxoplasma* and counting carbon-containing histiocyte cells in various organs, an increased phagocytic activity could be demonstrated in the liver and lungs as early as 12 hours after infection. Twenty-four hours after infection, phagocytic activity was reduced two-fold in the lungs, whereas in the liver and spleen it was 2 to 3 times higher. This state persisted for 4 days, but 6 to 8 days after infection, just before death of the animals, the RES activity of examined organs was generally reduced, though an increase was sometimes noted in the lungs (probably related to the inflammatory process). The thymus was unaffected.

The authors also reported on cytochemical studies. Using the Gomori technique, they stained for acid phosphatase activity in the RES histiocytes of various organs, assuming this would reflect the total activity of the system. Up to the sixth day of infection, the results were consistent with previous findings, confirming an increase in activity of the RES. Only 8 days after infection was the number of cells capable of trapping colloidal carbon distinctly reduced as compared to the number of cells containing acid phosphatase. At this time the immunity of animals was markedly diminished. Although no definite conclusions are warranted by these experiments, it is almost certain that a significant role is played by cells of the RES, or the lymphoid-macrophage system (LMS). (The latter is a classification proposed by Taliaferro and Mulligan [1937] and was intended to replace Aschoff's RES [1924]; the LMS includes the RES and also lymphocytes, other lymphoid cells of mesodermal origin, and their intermediate forms.)

Cellular phenomena offer additional difficulties in studies of toxoplasmosis. The phagocytic activity of RES cells and their ability to digest foreign bodies may not apply in this infection since the *Toxoplasma* organism seems to have a great affinity for these cells, penetrating them and perhaps migrating in them from the blood (during parasitemia) to various organs. Multiplication of toxoplasms has been observed inside macrophages, often without adverse effects on the parasite.

Visher and Suter (1954) observed the multiplication of toxoplasms in macrophage culture. They noted that the development of the parasite was inhibited both by antisera and the addition of macrophages from a resistant animal. The greatest inhibiting effect was, however, achieved by the combination of both factors, suggesting a common action of humoral and cellular antibodies.

This is contradicted to some extent by the observations of Nakayama (1965), who inserted diffusion chambers into the peritoneal cavity of mice and noted that the macrophages of resistant hosts were more refractive to *Toxoplasma* invasion than those of normal animals. Similarly, a passive transfer of cells from the peritoneal exudate of resistant animals to susceptible ones neither protected nor prolonged the survival time after challenge with the RH strain.

Effects of splenectomy, cortisone, and x-irradiation. Experiments conducted in physiologically altered hosts might throw light on the mechanism of the immune processes, since results so far obtained are far from uniform. In Weinman's studies (1943), splenectomy failed to reactivate latent toxoplasmosis, and Jacobs (1953) also found that splenectomized mice were not more sensitive to challenge with a *Toxoplasma* strain of low virulence, strain 113, than control animals. X-irradiation, despite causing marked lymphoid destruction, did not reactivate toxoplasmosis or affect the immunity in mice; Frenkel et al. (1952) ascribed this to the slight role of cellular immunity to toxoplasmosis.

Different conclusions are prompted by the recent work of Stahl et al. (1966), who studied the immune phenomena in splenectomized mice and in those pretreated with cortisone. In both cases, infection with the slightly virulent Bev strain was followed by fatal encephalitis, prolonged persistence of trophozoites in the peritoneal exudate, somewhat early cyst formation in the brain, the accumulation of cysts in large clusters, strong inflammatory reactions in the neighborhood of cysts (particularly when arranged in clusters), and a failure to protect against reinvasion. Though these symptoms were slightly less severe in splenectomized than in cortisone-treated mice, the over-all consistency of the results indicates that the mechanism of action in both cases is comparable and can be ascribed to an inhibition or suppression of the immune response.

As noted above, cortisone administered to susceptible animals prior to infection with *Toxoplasma* promotes the development and multiplication of the parasites, leading to severe infections. Similarly, in rabbits immunized with killed toxoplasms, the intensity of infection is more pronounced when these animals have also been pretreated with cortisone (Huldt, 1965). It is of interest, however, that in rabbits naturally immunized by previous infection and showing a high level of antibodies, the administration of cortisone before challenge does not affect the degree of immunity.

X-irradiation also acts by impairing any ability of phagocytes to destroy the parasite but does not affect the Jettmar factor (*see* p. 878) (Metzger et al., 1963). A single whole body irradiation of 600 roentgens followed the next day by inoculation with the RH strain resulted in death of all the rats in a sample group in 14 to 22 days. All irradiated controls which did not receive *Toxoplasma* and those which received *Toxoplasma* but were not irradiated survived for more than 90 days.

Hypersensitivity.   In addition to antibody production, the *Toxoplasma* infection leads to delayed hypersensitivity of the host, a phenomenon utilized routinely in the cutaneous test (Frenkel, 1948; Kozar, 1953; Jirovec et al., 1957; Jirovec and Jira, 1961; Jira et al., 1963). Skin reactivity usually occurs after the time when humoral antibodies may be demonstrated, usually at about a month, and occasionally as late as one or two years after infection. It persists for a long time, frequently for life. Skin reactivity is an allergy associated with certain clinical symptoms, but may also indicate to some degree the existence of immunity, as suggested by the results of Huldt (1965).

Summary.   Although humoral antibodies in toxoplasmosis probably play a role in immunity, we also know that the mere presence of such antibodies is insufficient for host defense. Animals immunized with killed antigen are not resistant to challenge in spite of demonstrable antibody production. The contact of the animal with live parasites seems indispensable for maximum protection. The experiments of Nakayama (1965) suggest that the participation of cellular factors alone is also inadequate for protection. Though our knowledge of immune phenomena in toxoplasmosis is better than in some other parasitic diseases, many gaps in our understanding are yet to be filled.

COCCIDIOSIS

Coccidiosis may be defined as infections caused by protozoa belonging to members of the family Eimeriidae, order Coccidiida, class Sporozoa. We will deal exclusively with *Eimeria*, since other genera are only occasionally found in domestic animals (except in carnivores, which mostly harbor *Isospora*). Coccidiosis in fowl (mostly chickens and turkeys), rabbits, calves, and probably in pigs is of special interest because of its economic importance. In this section, we will deal primarily with coccidiosis in mammalian hosts, since coccidiosis in avian hosts is dealt with elsewhere in this volume (*see* chapter by Cuckler, pp. 372-387).

Species of *Eimeria* differ from one another in morphologic characteristics (mostly of their oocysts), the time to sporulation, developmental features, localization in the host, and degree of pathogenicity. A pronounced specificity of parasite species in relation to the host species and even particular tissues is an important feature of coccidiosis, though many details have remained unexplained.

Once swallowed by a mammalian host and liberated in the intestine, the sporozoites develop intracellularly, occasionally even intranuclearly as in the case of *E. alabamensis* in cattle. Most species of *Eimeria* develop in the epithelium or in deeper layers of the intestine; only some of them parasitize other organs such as the liver and kidneys. The schizonts of some species, having penetrated superficial epithelial cells of the intestine, are then transferred by macrophages into deeper layers. The life cycle of coccidia involves an alternation of multiplicative asexual generations reproducing by schizogony (sporozoite, schizonts, merozoites) and propagative sexual generations reproducing by gametogony (micro- and macrogametocytes, zygote, oocyst). Because coccidia cannot multiply indefinitely within a host, in the absence of reinfection the disease is not long-standing and strictly self-limiting.

The tissues invaded, the size of the parasites, and even the site of localization in a cell determine the degree of damage to a host and the pathogenicity of a parasite species. Occasionally, it is the second generation of schizonts, located deep in the submucosa, which causes the major clinical symptoms; in other cases these are ascribed to the sexual stages. Though toxic effects or other hitherto unidentified influences of the parasite's metabolic products may be involved in coccidiosis, the mechanical damage to cells and tissues caused by invasion is probably the major cause of pathogenesis, leading occasionally to death.

As with avian hosts, immune phenomena play a decisive part in the protective aspects of coccidiosis, and thus severe epizootics do not destroy all of the animals infected, especially since the duration of infection is self-limited. This has been observed both in practice and in experimental studies. Partial or even complete immunity after oral infection or direct injection was found by Smith (1910) with intestinal coccidiosis in rabbits, by Hall and Wigdor (1918) and Andrews (1926) in dogs and cats, by Biester and Schwarte (1932) in pigs, by Henry (1932) in guinea pigs, and by Becker et al. (1932) in rats. Bachman (1930b) showed that in rabbits, the immune response was highly specific with regard to the species of coccidia involved. Such specificity has also been demonstrated in avian hosts (*see* Cuckler's chapter, pp. 378-379).

Some research centers (Houghton Poultry Research Station, Weybridge Central Veterinary Laboratory, Liverpool School of Tropical Medicine) have been conducting intensive studies for several years now, which are showing an accumulation of new details. The animals used in these experiments are most often rabbits infected with *E. stiedae* (the only species parasitizing the bile duct of the host), chicks infected with *E. tenella* in the paired ceca, chicks infected with other intestinal species, turkeys infected with *E. meleagrimitis*, and calves infected with *E. bovis*. In these studies, no essential differences seem to exist among individual host and parasite species in respect to immune phenomena.

Natural immunity

Age resistance. It has been long known that coccidiosis mostly affects young animals. This was found, for instance, in rabbits by Wasielewski (1904), Kolpakoff (1926), Chapman (1929), and others, who ascribed the phenomenon to age susceptibility. In the experiments of Kotlán and Pellérdy (1935, 1937), young rabbits proved to be more sensitive to *E. stiedae* than older ones. Beyer (1961) could also confirm age resistance in rabbits infected with *E. intestinalis*. While four-month-old animals infected with 50,000 to 75,000 oocysts per animal showed clinical symptoms and numerous oocysts were present in their feces, one-year-old rabbits were free of symptoms and only a few oocysts could be detected. The author assumes that rabbits of neither group were ever exposed to natural infections with this species. Similar age susceptibility is found in avian hosts (*see* Cuckler's chapter, p. 378).

Infection and disease susceptibility may be distinguished in that older animals are known to be carriers, i.e., they excrete oocysts without displaying pathologic symptoms. For example, in *E. tenella* infections of the highly susceptible chicken, older birds show a lower degree of anemia when compared to young ones (Herrick et al., 1936). Ten-day-old chicks are more susceptible to *E. necatrix* infection than older ones (10 to 12 weeks), though judging by the fecal oocyst count, the invasion in older ones is stronger (Brackett and Bliznick, 1950). The occurrence of physiologic changes in animals with age is another explanation of age immunity. A general toughening process could be involved which makes it more difficult for parasites to enter cells and to develop in them. This is suggested by the observations of Augustin and Ridges (1963), who found age resistance in turkeys to *E. meleagrimitis*; the birds excreted large numbers of oocysts but showed no clinical symptoms. This is in contrast to the lack of oocyst production in solidly immune birds. Presumably, similar age-dependent phenomena occur in mammals, though this hypothesis lacks adequate confirmation.

Congenital and other factors. Apart from age, there are other factors partly responsible for the immunity or susceptibility of the host to coccidia. It appears that at least in birds there is some degree of congenital immunity (*see* p. 378) though Long and Rose (1962) studied the susceptibility to *E. tenella* infection in the progeny of resistant and nonresistant hens without finding any differences between them. These studies were designed to investigate whether congenital immunity was transferred from hen to chick via the yolk. It is not known whether congenital immunity to coccidiosis occurs in mammals. Some authors succeeded in demonstrating a genetically conditioned change in susceptibility of some host races to coccidioses, e.g., in rats to *E. miyairii* (Becker and Hall, 1933).

Like other diseases, coccidiosis depends on individual or conditional factors, such as general fitness, diet, intercurrent diseases, and so on. For instance, a milk diet was found to have a definite effect on the course of coccidiosis, apparently by changing the physiologic environment in the intestine. In tropical countries, frequent outbreaks of coccidiosis in cattle are observed following rinderpest vaccinations. Elevated temperature of lodgings is known to mitigate the course of the disease in chickens infected with *E. tenella*.

Acquired immunity

Acquisition of active immunity. It has been proved repeatedly that single or repeated infections with coccidia confer protection on the host against reinfection, i.e., there is an active acquired immunity. This immunity ranges from relative to absolute and depends on a variety of factors, e.g., the number of past infections, the size of immunizing dose, the parasite species, and so forth. Active acquired immunity may be expressed by the clinical condition of the host animals and by the number of oocysts excreted in their feces. With considerable immunity, clinical symptoms may be slight or absent, though the host excretes oocysts after reinfection. This is often observed under both natural and experimental conditions. Usually it is only the second or third infection that affords an absolute immunity with almost no oocysts in the feces (Biester and Schwarte, 1932; Jankiewicz and Scofield, 1934; Farr, 1943). Fully immune animals are then resistant not only to disease but to coccidial parasitism as well.

Even a slight infection of rabbits with *E. stiedae* confers immunity to challenge, the clinical symptoms on reinfection being milder and the fecal oocyst count comparatively low compared to previously uninfected rabbits. On the other hand, following a heavy, almost lethal, immunizing dose (5,000 oocysts per four-year-old rabbit), the animals remain in good health and few or no fecal oocysts are seen after challenge with a large oocyst dose (Rose, 1963).

In cattle, each successive dose of *E. bovis* produces fewer and less extensive symptoms, and by the fourth challenge with 20 million oocysts, hosts no longer have diarrhea or blood-stained feces (Senger et al., 1959).

Though Horton-Smith et al. (1963b) reported that sporozoites of *E. tenella* harvested from cecal mucosal washings of immune or susceptible chickens were infective when introduced into another susceptible chicken, Beyer (1961) was inclined to believe that the presence of immunity had a certain effect on the oocysts themselves. *E. intestinalis* oocysts, excreted by repeatedly immunized rabbits, were less resistant to maintenance in culture and were found to lose their invasiveness more rapidly than oocysts excreted after the first infection. Beyer confirmed the correlation existing between the degree of immunity and the number of immunizing doses and distinguished two phases in the development of immunity in rabbits: an antitoxic and an antiparasitic one. In the former (which follows a second infection), the host is resistant to the toxic action of the parasite, but it is not able to inhibit its development; in the latter stage (following the third infection), the developmental cycle of coccidia is fully blocked.

Effects of parasite species differences. It is well known that certain differences in the immunity of a single host species depend on the species of parasite involved (Tyzzer, 1929). Generally, more pronounced protection occurs with species in which the parasites penetrate deeply and tend to be retained in the tissues of the host. This is noticeable in chickens which harbor several species of coccidia in the alimentary tract. The immunity is stronger after infection with *E. maxima*, as compared with *E. mitis* which develops superficially in the intestinal epithelium. *E. tenella*, with its second generation of schizonts situated deeply in the subepithelial tissues, affords the stimulation of a stronger and more lasting immunity than *E. acervulina*, the parasitic forms of which are situated superficially. In cattle, the immunity to *E. alabamensis* is also less than to *E. bovis*, apparently because of the particular localization of the former in the nuclei of epithelial cells (Davis et al., 1955).

Kendall (1961) attributed a species-dependent degree of immunity to the developmental properties of the parasite. It is known that immunity to *E. tenella* occurs earlier and is more pronounced than in the case of *E. necatrix*. Development of the former is related to the cecum, i.e., the comparatively small tissue area accessible to the parasite. This might also account for the fact that schizogony in this species is limited to two generations. In contrast, *E. necatrix*, potentially infecting a large area of tissue, is capable of persisting for long periods, and for this reason tissue immunity to reinfection develops at a slower rate.

An important feature of immunity in coccidiosis is its great species specificity, a rather exceptional phenomenon for protozoan parasites. Rabbits resistant to *E. perforans* are fully susceptible to *E. stiedae* (Bachman, 1930b), as are *E. tenella*-resistant chickens to *E. acervulina* and *E. maxima* (Tyzzer, 1929).

Here again, some aspects of infection are obscure or unusual. Tyzzer (1929) noted that the development of immunity to *E. maxima* may be delayed in mixed infections of gallinaceous hosts. Birds infected exclusively with *E. maxima* develop a rapid and pronounced immunity, whereas in infection with three species, *E. acervulina*, *E. mitis*, and *E. maxima*, the immunity was weaker and invasion by all three species persisted for a longer time. It is not known whether such a reaction also occurs in mammals.

Duration. The duration of acquired immunity is difficult to assess because of accidental reinfection. Immunity of chickens to *E. maxima* is comparatively short-lived (3 to 10 weeks); that of other species seems to be of slightly longer duration (Long, 1962). Rabbits exhibited immunity for more than two months after a single heavy dose of *E. stiedae* oocysts, which might be explained by prolonged retention of antigenic material in the degenerated tissues of the liver. In cattle, the immunity to *E. bovis* develops at a comparatively higher rate, appearing 14 days after infection, and may persist for as long as 7 months, depending on the age of the immunized animals (Senger et al., 1959).

The duration of immunity depends on the size of the immunizing dose and the mode of immunization (Tyzzer, 1929; Horton-Smith, 1949). In calves, 50,000 occysts of *E. bovis* conferred greater immunity than 10,000 oocysts (Senger et al., 1959). No marked difference in immunity was observed when similar numbers of oocysts were given in a single dose or in divided doses administered on five subsequent days.

Antibodies. Early studies on the serum antibodies of mammals, as well as of birds, infected with or resistant to coccidia have yielded contradictory results. Blumenthal (1908) and Kuczyński (1920) found antibody to the Wasserman test antigen in infected rabbits, but Marcuse (1922) and Torres (1924) could not establish a correlation between *E. stiedae* infection and Wasserman serology. However, Kidd and Friedewald (1942) demonstrated that normal rabbit serum contained a reagin that reacted in the Wasserman test. Paterson (1923), using alcohol, carbonate-buffered saline, and unbuffered saline extracts of infected livers as antigens, obtained varying results in complement-fixation tests with sera of rabbits infected with *E. stiedae*. Similarly, Chapman (1929) in his experiments with extracts of rabbit intestine infected with *E. perforans* recorded slightly positive results in the CFT and in the skin test, and invariably negative ones in precipitin and agglutination tests with merozoites. Bachman (1930a) obtained invariably negative results in precipitation tests with sera from *E. stiedae*-infected rabbits, and only transiently positive ones with sera from artificially immunized animals. Somewhat better skin test results with antigen from powdered oocysts were achieved by Henry (1932) in guinea pigs infected with *E. caviae*.

It was not until recently that the studies of humoral immunity have progressed to the point where positive results are being obtained with increasing frequency. McDermott and Stauber (1954) could agglutinate *E. tenella* merozoites with sera of infected birds, as well as with sera of rabbits immunized with formalin-treated preparations of the parasite. Similar antibodies were demonstrated in rabbit serum by Itagaki and Tsubokura (1955), but Augustin and Ridges (1963) could not confirm this phenomenon with merozoites of *E. meleagrimitis* in the serum of resistant turkeys.

Significant studies by Rose (1959) demonstrated distinct complement-fixing and precipitating antibodies in the sera of rabbits infected with *E. stiedae*. Antigens prepared from the exudate of infected bile ducts, saline extracts of crushed oocysts, or a mixture of schizonts and gamonts yielded a complex of precipitin reactions by Ouchterlony testing. The number of bands increased in proportion to the development of the parasite. Similar results were obtained by Rose with sera of birds infected with *E. necatrix*, *E. tenella*, *E. maxima*, and *E. acervulina*, with their respective homologous antigens from oocysts or schizonts and sexual stages of the parasite. The time at which the maximal reaction appeared varied slightly in individual species. The reaction was the slowest to appear and the weakest in birds infected with *E. necatrix*. When infected with other species, some birds showed two bands of precipitation, indicating that at least two antigen-antibody reactions were involved.

Antibodies were found by CFT in sera of rabbits infected with *E. stiedae*. Their demonstration in chickens met some difficulties. but they were measurable at least after infection with *E. tenella* (Rose and Orlans, 1962). In rabbits, the CF antibodies appeared between the tenth to twentieth day, occasionally even by the fifth day of infection, reaching the peak titer between the twenty-second to fortieth day, with subsequent slow decline, but they were still detectable up to 165 days. Challenge, to which the animals were resistant, did not recall the antibodies; this was attributed to the infection being blocked early in the course, or to a reaction too slight to be detectable in the serum (Rose, 1961). The antibodies detected both in Ouchterlony plates and in CFT can also be elicited with nonviable antigenic materials such as tissue stages or oocysts (Rose, 1959).

In electrophoretic studies with sera of fowl infected with *E. tenella*, Pierce et al. (1962) found no quantitative differences between those of the experimental and the control groups, probably because of an increase in protein synthesis by the young chickens. They showed subsequently that in immune sera there were precipitins associated with the slowest migrating proteins, the gamma-globulin fraction.

Passive or artificially acquired active immunity. Repeated attempts at passive or artificial immunization of animals against coccidiosis by various routes have failed so far to give satisfactory results. Tyzzer (1929) did not succeed in protecting susceptible chicks by injecting them subcutaneously, intraperitoneally, or per rectum with whole blood or sera from immune birds. Nor could Bachman (1930b) immunize rabbits against *E. perforans* infection by injecting dried pulverized oocysts or sera which contained precipitating antibodies. In experiments using rats infected with *E. miyairii* and *E. separata* (Becker et al., 1932) immunity could not be transferred passively by the intravenous administration of citrated or defibrinated blood from resistant hosts (Becker and Hall, 1933). Negative results were also obtained by injecting rats with ground-up oocysts or infected intestines (Becker, 1935). It was thought that serum antibodies are of little or no significance in the protection of animals against reinfection (Chapman, 1929).

In recent years, the detection of distinct humoral antibodies has encouraged a renewal of immunization studies. Horton-Smith et al. (1963) injected young rabbits intravenously or intraperitoneally each day for 3 days with large amounts of serum globulin from rabbits resistant to *E. stiedae*, and on the next day infected them with a known number of oocysts. No differences were found in the degree of infection between experimental and control animals.

Renewed attempts to immunize rabbits actively by means of antigens from the exudate of infected bile ducts containing a mixture of schizonts and gametocytes of *E. stiedae* or chickens with schizonts of *E. tenella* were disappointing. These antigens were injected subcutaneously or intramuscularly, undiluted or precipitated with alum or Freund's adjuvant (Horton-

Smith et al., 1963). Despite the formation of precipitating antibodies (detected by the Ouchterlony agar diffusion test) and complement-fixing antibodies (in the case of rabbits) the differences observed after challenge in experimental and control animals were too small to justify the conclusion that acquired immunity has been secured in this way. Apparently, the antibodies detected were not protective, or their level was inadequate.

However, Long and Rose (1965) reported positive results in actively immunizing chickens against *E. tenella* sporozoites with schizont antigen (parenterally injected) and with serum globulin from immune chickens (injected intravenously or intraperitoneally). (*See* Cuckler's chapter, p. 383 for further discussion of this work.) The mechanisms involved in this reaction provide a subject for further study.

The above discussion suggests that a pronounced immunity is possible only after a normal infection. Attempts have been made to utilize this phenomenon for practical purposes. Several such attempts with avian hosts are discussed in Cuckler's chapter (*see* pp. 374-377). Experiments using x-ray attenuated oocysts or coccidiostatic drugs (such as sulfonamides) to confer immunity in birds are also discussed in that chapter (*see* pp. 375-376 and 380). However, no attempt to vaccinate potential mammalian hosts by any of these methods has been reported.

Mechanisms of immunity

The studies discussed above leave unexplained the mechanisms in immunity to coccidiosis. However, this is the subject of considerable experimental study and much still remains to be done. In view of the fairly complex development of the parasite in the host, it is important to establish when and how the immunity acts and which of the developmental stages of the parasite, if not all, are active in the production of immunity.

Developmental stages affected by immune mechanisms. Although, after challenge, sporozoites are liberated from the oocysts under the effect of gastric juice in rats resistant to *E. nieschultzi*, Moorehouse (1938) suggested that they are not able to penetrate the epithelial cells, being eventually eliminated with the feces. Pellérdy (1965) also showed that the resistance of the host does not inhibit the excystation of oocysts. When attempting to infect a resistant animal intragastrically with a suspension of crushed *E. stiedae* oocysts, i.e., with material containing both free sporocysts and sporozoites, he failed to produce infection, as judged by fecal oocyst examination and by necropsy three weeks later.

Other studies show that not only excystation but also the penetration of the host cells by parasites remains unaffected by host resistance. Which of the intracellular stages are affected by the immune mechanism and to what extent have yet to be determined.

A definite resistance of calves to *E. bovis* reinfection was demonstrated by Senger et al. (1959). At first, no appreciable differences could be seen in the number and size of schizonts in resistant and nonresistant animals examined 15 to 20 days after challenge, which might suggest that the schizonts are not particularly damaged by the immune response (Hammond et al., 1959). In another paper, Hammond et al. (1961) postulated that the immune reaction in some calves induces a decrease in the number of merozoites, this being more pronounced in animals immunized with heavy doses. The absence of this phenomenon in other calves suggested that immunity prevents merozoites from developing into gametocytes. In a more recent publication (Hammond et al., 1963) the authors abandoned their previous beliefs and stated that primarily schizont forms are affected by immune processes.

Other authors postulated that in resistant rabbits and birds, the excystation of the oocysts proceeds normally and the development of the parasites is blocked before schizogony occurs. Again, the developmental cycle of the parasite is interrupted by the immune response.

Sporozoites released in the intestine of resistant rabbits penetrate the epithelial cells lining the duodenum and are detectable at varying levels during the initial stage of the infection, but by the fourth day of infection they cannot be found there nor in the bile ducts, though they are present at these sites in nonresistant animals (Rose, 1959). This suggests that the early schizont stages prior to the first reproductive cycle are affected or that the early sporozoite stage of the parasite is stopped between the gut and the liver, supposedly in the mesenteric lymph glands. For further discussion of the relation of developmental stages of the parasite to the immune response in avian hosts, see Cuckler's chapter (pp. 380-381).

Cellular and humoral factors. Repeated failures to transfer immunity passively by means of antisera as well as the negative results of serologic and allergic tests suggest that the nature of immunity in coccidioses is a cellular and local one (Tyzzer, 1929; Bachman, 1930a,b; Becker et al., 1932; Becker and Hall, 1933). Other evidence, primarily from recent studies of immunity of chickens to coccidia, lends support to this hypothesis and is discussed in Cuckler's chapter (see pp. 386-387).

In connection with the cellular and local nature of immunity, Reyer (1941) developed a hypothesis that has not, so far, been supported by experimental data. He postulated the existence of two kinds of cells: those fully susceptible to infection, and those partially or entirely resistant. The number of the latter is pronouncedly increased during infection, and with subsequent immunizations all susceptible cells are replaced by resistant ones. This concept has been recently supported by Pellérdy (1965) who endeavors to explain, on this basis, a number of immune phenomena.

In *E. stiedae* infections of rabbits there is a great increase in lymphoid tissue, plasma cells, and eosinophils. The participation of these cells in the production of immunity in coccidiosis has not yet been elucidated. However, macrophages frequently transport sporozoites of *E. tenella* from epithelial cells of the villi to their final positions in the intestinal glands of Lieberkühn.

Though the possible role of hypersensitivity reactions in coccidioses has not as yet been investigated, Augustin and Ridges (1963) suggested a similar role for such reactions to that which occurs in nematode infections (in the so-called self-cure phenomenon).

The local nature of immunity in chickens is suggested by the experiments of Horton-Smith et al. (1963). When merozoites incubated in saline extracts of the ceca of resistant and nonresistant birds were injected intrarectally into susceptible hosts, certain, though inconclusive, differences in the course of infection could be observed. On the other hand, when sporozoites harvested from the contents of the ceca of resistant and nonresistant fowl were inoculated into the rectum of susceptible chicks, no differences were detected in the resulting infection, which suggests that no parasiticidal factors are secreted into the lumen of resistant ceca. Local immune reactions of mammals to coccidia have not, however, been adequately investigated, and it is not known whether analogous reactions to merozoites occur in these hosts.

Opinions among workers in the field differ as to the relative importance of humoral versus cellular factors in immunity to coccidiosis. Discussions of humoral factors, such as the lytic effects of avian immune sera, are presented in Cuckler's chapter (see pp. 384-385), as well as evidence supporting the view that immunity to coccidia is general rather than local in the case of chickens (see pp. 382-387). Even less is known about the relationships between these factors in mammals, though presumably they will be found to be similar to those found in avian hosts. However, this is an open field of investigation.

Little is known about the mode of immune action. Are parasites destroyed, or are they merely inhibited at the physiologic level by, e.g., the neutralization of enzymes which facilitate their penetration into host cells?

The influence of circulating antibodies could be demonstrated in vitro only when the parasites were subsequently injected by intravenous routes. This was true for sera from animals immunized both by infection and by nonliving antigens. Therefore, it may be presumed that antibodies could act on parasites in vivo, but their concentration at the actual site of parasitization by per oral infection may be too low to be effective.

According to Rose (1963), the concentration of antibody (or of antibody-producing cells) at the site of parasitization in immune animals is much higher than that detectable in the serum. The immune animals may already be locally sensitized by a previous infection, and the additional penetration of parasites increases the permeability of the mucosa to antibody. This local reaction to infection fails, however, to develop in animals unsensitized by previous infection, and for this reason the local concentration of antibodies, which may be available in the serum, is insufficient to secure their action against the parasites.

The role of humoral factors in immunity to coccidiosis remains most unclear. Some recently described experiments show that sera derived from resistant birds contains factors which act on sporozoites and merozoites at least in vitro. It seems, however, that the antibodies involved are different from those detected by precipitation and complement-fixation tests.

The outstanding argument against the humoral theory of antibody is based on the frequent failures to transfer it passively by means of immune sera. Further evidence against the theory is provided by the recent studies of Long (1965) and Pierce and Long (1965) with bursectomized and thymectomized chickens (see Cuckler's chapter, p. 387), which suggest that at least in birds, the immune phenomena are not related to the production of antibody which is detectable later in the blood. There may be local antibodies, but their role is still obscure.

Our knowledge about the mechanisms of immunity in coccidioses is obviously far from being complete, with many problems still to be solved. Most of the above-mentioned topics remain in the sphere of speculation. It is probable that immunity to coccidioses is a complex of humoral and cellular factors. Very little, if anything, is known about the activity of cells such as lymphocytes, plasma cells, and globular leukocytes which infiltrate the sites of infection.

REFERENCES

Andrews, J. M. 1926. Coccidiosis in mammals. Amer. J. Hyg., 6:784-798.
Aschoff, L. 1924. Das reticulo-endotheliale System. Ergebn. Inn. Med. Kinderheilk., 26:1-118.
Augustin, R., and A. P. Ridges. 1963. Immunity mechanisms in *Eimeria meleagrimitis*. *In* Immunity to Protozoa. Garnham, P. C. C., Pierce, A. E., and Roitt, I., eds. Oxford, Blackwell Scientific Publications, pp. 296-335.
Bachman, G. W. 1930a. Serological studies in experimental coccidiosis of rabbits. Amer. J. Hyg., 12:624-640.
———— 1930b. Immunity in experimental coccidiosis of rabbits. Amer. J. Hyg., 12:641-649.
Balducci, D., and D. Tyrrell. 1956. Quantitative studies of *Toxoplasma gondii* in culture of trypsin-dispersed mammalian cells. Brit. J. Exp. Path., 37:168-175.
Bartorelli, C., A. Berengo, A. Bencini, and R. Frezzotti. 1964. La toxoplasmosi (I. Medica; II. Oculistica). Atti dei Congr. della Soc. Ital. di Med. Intern. Roma. L. Pozzi, ed. pp. 1-354.
Beattie, C. P. 1963. Immunity to *Toxoplasma*. *In* Immunity to Protozoa. Garnham, P. C. C., Pierce, A. E., and Roitt, I., eds. Oxford, Blackwell Scientific Publications, pp. 253-258.
———— 1964. Toxoplasmosis. Roy. Coll. Phys. (Edinburgh), 1-64.
Becker, E. R. 1935. The mechanism of immunity in murine coccidiosis. Amer. J. Hyg., 21:389-404.
———— and P. R. Hall. 1933. Cross-immunity and correlation of oocysts production during immunization between *Eimeria miyairii* and *E. separata* in the rat. Amer. J. Hyg., 18:220.
———— P. R. Hall, and A. Hager. 1932. Quantitative, biometric and host-parasite studies on *Eimeria miyairii* and *E. separata* in rats. Iowa State College J. Sci., 6:299-316.
Beverley, J. K. A. 1958. A rational approach to the treatment of toxoplasmic uveitis. Trans. Ophthal. Soc., UK, 78:109-121.
———— 1959. Congenital transmission of toxoplasmosis through successive generations of mice. Nature (London), 183:1348.
Beyer, T. V. 1961. Immunity in experimental coccidiosis of the rabbit caused by heavy infective doses of *Eimeria intestinalis*. *In* Progress in Protozoology. Ludvick, J., Lom, J., and Vávra, J., eds. Prague, Czechoslovak Academy of Sciences, Publ., p. 448.
Biester, H. E., and L. H. Schwarte. 1932. Studies in infectious enteritis in swine. VI. Immunity in swine coccidiosis. J. Amer. Vet. Med. Ass., 81:358-375.

Blumenthal, F. 1908. Zur Serodiagnose der Syphilis. Diskussion (Wassermann Reaktion und Kokzidiose der Kaninchen). Berlin Klinische Wochenschrift, 45:618.

Bozděch, V., and J. Jira. 1961. Latex Agglutination Test mit dem *Toxoplasma* Antigen. Deutsch. Gesund., 16:2398-2400.

──── J. Jira, D. Princova, and R. Cee. 1965. Dynamika komplementfixacnich profilatek v laboratornich krys ve vztahu k častosti a veli kosti imunizačnich davek virulentniho kmene *Toxoplasma gondii.* Česk. Parazitologie, 12:111-124.

Brackett, S., and A. Bliznick. 1952. The reproductive potential of five species of coccidia of the chicken as demonstrated by oocyst production. J. Parasit., 38:133-139.

Braunsteiner, H., F. Pakesch, and D. Thalhammer. 1957. Elektronenmikroskopische Untersuchungen über die Morphologie des *Toxoplasma gondii* und das Wesen des Farbtestes nach Sabin-Feldman. Wien Z. Inn. Med., 38:16-27.

Bringmann, G., and J. Holz, 1953. Licht- und elektronenmikroskopische Untersuchungen zum Sero-Farbtest auf Toxoplasmose nach Sabin-Feldman. Z. Hyg. Infektionskr., 138:151-154.

Campbell, R. S. F., W. B. Martin, and E. D. Gordon. 1955. Toxoplasmosis as a complication of canine distemper. Vet. Rec. 67:708-715.

Capella, J. A., and H. E. Kaufman. 1964. Enzyme histochemistry of *Toxoplasma gondii.* Amer. J. Trop. Med., 5:664-666.

Carver, R. V., and M. Goldman. 1959. Staining *Toxoplasma gondii* with fluorescein-labeled antibody. III. The reaction in frozen and paraffin sections. Amer. J. Clin. Path., 32:159-164.

Chapman, M. J. 1929. A study of coccidiosis in an isolated rabbit colony. The clinical symptoms, pathology, immunology and therapy. Amer. J. Hyg., 9:389-429.

Chatton, E., and G. Blanc. 1917. Notes et réflexions sur le Toxoplasme et la toxoplasmose du gondi. Arch. Inst. Pasteur (Tunis), 10:1-40.

Chordi, A., K. W. Walls, and I. G. Kagan. 1964. Analysis of *Toxoplasma gondii* antigens by agar diffusion methods. J. Immun., 93, 6:1034-1044.

Christiansen, M. 1948. Toxoplasmose hos harer i Danmark. Medlemsblad for den danske Dyrlaegerforening, 31:93-105.

──── and J. C. Siim. 1951. Toxoplasmosis in hares in Denmark. Lancet, 1:1201-1206.

Cutchins, E. C., and J. Warren. 1956. Immunity patterns in the guinea pig following Toxoplasma infection and vaccination with killed Toxoplasma. Amer. J. Trop. Med., 5:197-209.

Davis, L. R., D. C. Boughton, and G. W. Bowman. 1955. Biology and pathogenicity of *Eimeria alabamensis* Christensen, 1941, an intranuclear coccidium of cattle. Amer. J. Vet. Res., 16:274-281.

Desmonts, G. 1960. Diagnostie sérologique de la toxoplasmose. Path. Biol. (Paris), 8:109-125.

──── A. Baron, G. Offret, J. Couvreur, M. Lelong, and L. Cousin. 1960. La production locale d'anticorps au cours des toxoplasmoses oculaires. Arch. Ophthal. (Paris), 2:137-145.

Dobrzańska, A., T. Mierzejewski, and J. Umiński. 1958. Badania elektroforetyczne bialek surowicy krwi w zakażeniu toksoplazmoza. (Electrophoretic studies of blood serum proteins in infections with Toxoplasma). Wiad. Parazyt., 4:401-403.

Eichenwald, H. 1949. Experimental toxoplasmosis. II. Effect of sulfadiazine and antiserum on congenital toxoplasmosis in mice. Proc. Soc. Exp. Biol. Med., 71:45-49.

──── 1952. New phenomenon: Production of recurrent parasitaemia in chronic toxoplasmosis by the injection of potent specific antisera and its inhibition by cortisotropin (ACTH) and cortisone. Amer. J. Dis. Child., 83:75.

Erichsen, S., and A. Harboe. 1953. Toxoplasmosis in chickens. I. An epidemic outbreak of toxoplasmosis in a chicken flock in south-eastern Norway. Acta Path. Microbiol. Scand., 33:56-71.

Eyles, D. E., and N. Coleman. 1956. Relationship of size of inoculum to time to death in mice infected with *Toxoplasma gondii.* J. Parasit., 3:272-276.

Fair, J. R. 1959. Stimulation of dye-test antibodies in human volunteers using heat killed Toxoplasma. Amer. J. Ophthal., 48:322-325.

Fankhauser, R. 1952. Toxoplasmose-Enzephalitis beim Hunde. Schweiz. Arch. Neurol. Neurochir. Psych., 69:391-397.

Farr, M. M. 1943. Resistance of chickens to cecal coccidiosis. Poult. Sci., 22:277-286.

Feldman, H. A. 1956. The relationship of *Toxoplasma* antibody activator to the serum-properdin system. Ann. N.Y. Acad. Sci., 66:263-267.

Frenkel, J. K. 1948. Dermal hypersensitivity to toxoplasma antigens (toxoplasmins). Proc. Soc. Exp. Biol. Med., 68:634-639.

——— 1953. Host, strain and treatment variation as factors in the pathogenesis of toxoplasmosis. Amer. J. Trop. Med., 2:390-415.

——— 1956. Pathogenesis of toxoplasmosis and of infections with organisms resembling toxoplasma. Ann. N.Y. Acad. Sci., 64:215-251.

——— L. Jacobs, and M. Melton. 1952. Effects of total body radiation on a chronic, latent infection in which immunity is not dependent on the spleen (toxoplasmosis). Amer. J. Path., 28:555-556.

Fulton, J. D. 1963. Serological tests in toxoplasmosis. In Immunity to Protozoa. Garnham, P. C. C., Pierce, A. E. and Roitt, I., eds. Oxford, Blackwell Scientific Publications pp. 259-272.

——— and D. F. Spooner. 1960. Metabolic studies on *Toxoplasma gondii*. Exp. Parasit., 9:293-301.

——— and J. L. Turk. 1959. Direct agglutination test for toxoplasmosis. Lancet, 2:1068-1069.

Galuzo, I. G., ed. 1965. Toksoplazmoz zhivotnych. Alma-Ata Izd. Nauka, pp. 1-523.

——— and D. N. Zassuchin. 1963. Toxoplasmosis of man and animals. Bibliography of the native and foreign literature 1908-1962. Alma-Ata Akad. Sci., Kazakh SSR, Publ. pp. 1-411.

Gałuszka, J. 1962. Observations on virulence of *Toxoplasma gondii* in cultures of trypsinized embryonic cells of guinea pigs. Acta Parasitologica Polonica, 10, 18:265-269.

Garnham, P. C. C., A. E. Pierce, and I. Roitt, eds. 1963. Immunity to Protozoa. Oxford, Blackwell Scientific Publications.

Giroud, T., M. Capponi, and N. Dumas. 1962. De la maladie inapparente à la maladie mortelle chez le rat blanc infecté par *Toxoplasma gondii* et traité aux stéroides synthétiques. Bull. Soc. Path. Exot., 3:335-339.

Głowiński, M., and T. K. Niebrój. 1965. Studies on *Toxoplasma gondii*. I. Distribution of unspecific phosphatases. II. Distribution of specific phosphatases and nucleases. III. Localization and activity of esterases and cathepsins. Acta Parasitologica Polonica, 13, 39-41:395-398, 399-402, 403-405.

——— Z. Steplezski, W. Waroński, and H. Wacławczyk. 1964. Das Retikuloendothelialsystem (RES) bei der experimentellen Toxoplasmose. I. Die phagozytische Aktivität des RES. Zbl. Gynäk., 86, 36:1273-1276.

——— Z. Steplezski, and W. Waroński. 1966. Das Retikuloendothelialsystem (RES) bei der experimentellen Toxoplasmose. II. Zytotopochemie der sauren Phosphatasen. Zbl. Gynäk., 88, 24:777.

Goldman, M. 1957. Staining *Toxoplasma* by fluorescein labeled antibody. II. A new serologic test for antibodies to *Toxoplasma* based upon inhibition to specific staining. J. Exp. Med., 105:557-573.

Grönroos, P. 1955. Studies on *Toxoplasma* and the serology of toxoplasmosis. Ann. Med. Exp. Biol. Fenn., 33(Suppl. 11):113.

Gutierrez, J. M., and J. del Rey Calero. 1966. Algunas consideraciones citochimicas sobre los acidos nucleicos in el *Toxoplasma gondii*. Rev. Iber. Parasit., 1:95-109.

Hahn, E., and L. Afrelius-Alm. 1957. Das Verhalten der neutralisierenden und komplementbindenden Antikörper bei der Toxoplasmose. Aertzl. Wschr., 12:953-956.

Hall, M. C., and M. Wigdor. 1918. Canine coccidiosis with a note regarding protozoan parasites from the dog. J. Amer. Vet. Med. Ass., 6:64-76.

Hammond, D. M., R. A. Heckman, M. L. Miner, C. M. Senger, and P. R. Fitzgerald. 1959. The life cycle stages of *Eimeria bovis* affected by the immune reaction in calves. Exp. Parasit., 8:574-580.

——— W. N. Clark, and M. L. Miner. 1961a. Observations on the life-cycle and pathogenicity of *Eimeria auburnensis* in calves. In Progress in Protozoology. Ludvick, J., Lom, J., and Vávra, J., eds. Prague, Czechoslovak Academy of Sciences, Publ., p. 437.

——— M. L. Miner, and F. L. Andersen. 1961b. The effect of the immune reaction on the number of merozoites of *Eimeria bovis* in calves. In Progress in Protozoology. Ludvick, J., Lom, J., and Vávra, J., eds. Prague, Czechoslovak Academy of Sciences, Publ., p. 438.

——— F. L. Andersen, and M. L. Miner. 1963. The site of the immune reaction against *Eimeria bovis* in calves. J. Parasit., 49: 415-424.

Havlik, O., and M. Zastĕra. 1954. Toxoplasmosa jako ohniskova nakaza. Česk. Epidem., 3:214.

—— J. Hübner, and M. Zastĕra. 1955. Vliv kortisonu na experimentalni toxoplasmosu bilych mysi. (The influence of cortisone in experimental toxoplasmosis in the white mouse). Česk. Parasit., 2:75-81.

Henry, D. P. 1932. Coccidiosis of the guinea pig. Univ. Calif. Publ. Zool., 37: 211-268.

Herrick, C. A., G. L. Ott, and C. E. Holmes. 1936. Age as factor in the development of resistance of the chicken to the effects of the protozoan parasite, Eimeria tenella. J. Parasit., 22:264-272.

Hirschlerowa, Z., and Z. Kozar. 1956. Sabin-Feldman test as an investigation method of the mechanism of immunity. Bull. Inst. Mar. Med. (Gdańsk). 7:145-155.

Hook, W. A., and J. E. Faber. 1957. Fractionation studies on the antigenic nature of Toxoplasma gondii. Exp. Parasit., 5:449-458.

Horton-Smith, C. 1949. Some factors influencing the course and origin of epidemics of coccidiosis in poultry. Ann. N.Y. Acad. Sci., 52:449-457.

—— 1958. Coccidiosis in domestic mammals. Vet. Rec., 70:1-7.

—— P. L. Long and A. E. Pierce. 1963a. Behaviour of invasive stages of Eimeria tenella in the immune fowl (Gallus domesticus). Exp. Parasit., 13:66-74.

—— P. L. Long, A. E. Pierce and M. E. Rose. 1963b. Immunity to coccidia in domestic animals. In Immunity to Protozoa. Garnham, P. C. C., Pierce, A. E., and Roitt, I., eds. Oxford, Blackwell Scientific Publications, pp. 273-295.

Huldt, G. 1965. Immunity in experimental toxoplasmosis. In Progress in Protozoology. Second International Conference on Protozoology, London. International Congress Series No. 91. Amsterdam, Excerpta Medica Foundation, p. 186.

Itagaki, K., and M. Tsubokura. 1955. Studies on coccidiosis in fowls. IV. On the agglutination by merozoites. Jap. J. Vet. Sci., 17:139.

Jacobs, L. 1953. The biology of Toxoplasma. Amer. J. Trop. Med., 2:365-389.

—— and M. N. Lunde. 1957. A haemagglutination test for toxoplasmosis. J Parasit., 43:308-314.

—— and M. L. Melton. 1963. Toxoplasma cysts in tissue culture. In Progress in Protozoology. Second International Conference on Protozoology, London. International Congress Series No. 91. Amsterdam, Excerpta Medica Foundation, pp. 187-188.

—— J. S. Remington, M. L. Melton, and M. N. Lunde. 1959. The relationship of Toxoplasma dye test and neutralizing antibodies. J. Parasit., 45(Suppl.):52.

—— J. S. Remington, and M. L. Melton. 1960. The resistance of the encysted form of Toxoplasma gondii. J. Parasit., 46:11-21.

Jadin, J., J. François, M. Wery, and J. Van de Casteele. 1955. L'immunité dans la toxoplasmose expérimentale. Ann. Soc. Belg. Méd. Trop., 2:161-168.

Jankiewicz, H. A., and R. H. Scofield. 1934. The administration of heated occysts of Eimeria tenella as a means of establishing resistance and immunity to coecal coccidiosis. J. Amer. Vet. Med. Ass., 84:507-526.

Jettmar, A. M. 1962. Cytolyse der Toxoplasmen durch Frischsera. Arch. Hyg. Bakt., 146,7:511-529.

Jira, J., O. Jirovec, F. Fencl, R. Blaha, and V. Bozdech. 1963. Desensibilisierungsversuche mit Toxoplasmin. Z. Aerztl. Fortbild. (Jena), 11:933-945.

Jirovec, O., and J. Jira. 1961. A contribution to the technique of intracutaneous testing with toxoplasmin. J. Clin. Path., 14:522-524.

—— J. Jira, V. Fuchs, and R. Peter. 1957. Studien mit dem Toxoplasmintest. Zbl. Bakt. [Orig.], 169:129-159.

Kass, E., and E. Steen. 1951. Serological investigations of rabbits experimentally infected with Toxoplasma gondii. Acta Path. Microbiol. Scand., 28,2:169-173.

Kaufman, H. E., M. L. Melton, J. S. Remington, and L. Jacobs. 1959. Strain differences of Toxoplasma gondii. J. Parasit., 45:189-190.

Kendall, B. S. 1961. Some aspects of the host-parasite relationship in species of Eimeria. In Progress in Protozoology. Ludvick, J., Lom, J., and Vávra, J., eds. Prague, Czechoslovak Academy of Sciences, Publ., pp. 435-436.

Kidd, J. G., and W. F. Friedewald. 1942. A natural antibody that reacts in vitro with a sedimentable constituent of normal tissue cells. J. Exp. Med., 76:543-546 and 557-578.

Kirchhoff, H., et al. 1966. Toxoplasmose. Praktische Fragen und Ergebnisse. Stuttgart, Georg Thieme Verlag.

Kishida, T., and S. Kato. 1965. Autoradiographic studies on intracytoplasmic multiplication of *Toxoplasma gondii* in FL cells. Biken J. (Osaka), 2:107-113.

Kolpakoff, T. A. 1926. Le rôle de suc gastrique dans l'immunité naturelle des lapins dans la coccidiose. Bull. Soc. Path. Exot., 19:266-268.

Korovickij, L. K., M. N. Melnik, A. E. Grigorachenko, and A. G Stankov. 1966. Toksoplazmoz: epidemiologia, klinika, terapia i profilaktika (In Russian). Kiev, Zdorovie, 2nd ed., pp. 1-288.

Kotlán, S., and L. Pellérdy. 1935. Kiserleti virsgaldtok a házinyúl májcoccidiosisáról. I. (Experimental studies on hepatic coccidiosis in domestic rabbits. I.). Közl. Osszehas. Kórtan, 26:11-12.

────── and L. Pellérdy. 1937. Kiserleti virsgaldtok a házinyúl májcoccidiosisáról. II. (Experimental studies on hepatic coccidiosis in domestic rabbits. II.). Közl. Osszehas. Kórtan, 28:105-120.

Kozar, Z. 1953. Wartość i znaczenie próby środskórnej dla rozpoznawania toksoplazmozy (Value and significance of the intradermal test for the diagnosis of toxoplasmosis). Acta Parasitologica Polonica, 1,8:159-229.

────── 1954. Toksoplazmoza. (In Polish). Warsaw, Państwowy Zaktad Wydawnictw Lekarskich, pp. 1-197.

────── 1958. Wpływ hialuronidazy na zakażenie Toxoplasma gondii u myszy (Action of hyaluronidase on infection with *Toxoplasma gondii* in mice). Wiad. Parazyt., 4,5:427-430.

────── and S. Soszka. 1956a. Czynniki hormonalne w rozwoju zakażenia toksoplazma. (Hormonal factors in the development of the *Toxoplasma* infection). Bull. Inst. Mar. Med. (Gdańsk). 7:165-168.

────── and S. Soszka. 1956b. Badania własne nad rola czynników hormonalnych w rozwoju zakażenia toksoplazma. Ginekologia Polska. Pam. Zjazdu Ginekol. Pol. w Lublinie, pp. 186-188.

────── L. Dłużewski, Z. Hirschlerowa, and Z. Jaroszewski. 1954. Przypadek toksoplazmozy powikłanej wagrzyca mózgu (A case of toxoplasmosis complicated by the cysticercosis of the brain in an adult). Bull. Inst. Mar. Med. (Gdańsk), 5:146-147, 1953; and Neurol. Neurochir. Psychiat Pol., 1:67-77, 1954.

Körting, H. J. 1958. Immunoelektrophoretische Untersuchungen bei der Toxoplasmose. Zbl. Bakt. [Orig.], 172:621-629.

────── 1960. Toxoplasmose Komplementbindungsreaktion mit ultraschallbehandelten Antigenen. Zbl. Bakt. [Orig.], 179:278-288.

Kuczyński, M. H. 1921. Über die Wassermannsche Reaktion beim Kaninchen. Berlin Klinische Wochenschrift, 58:125-126.

Kulasiri, C. 1960. The nature of the cytoplasm-modifying antibodies. Parasitology, 50:419-423.

────── 1962. The behaviour of suckling rats to oral and intraperitoneal infection with a virulent strain of *Toxoplasma gondii*. Parasitology, 52:193-198.

────── and B. Das Gupta. 1959. A cytochemical investigation of the Sabin-Feldman phenomenon in *Toxoplasma gondii* and an explanation of its mechanism on this basis. Parasitology, 49:586-593.

Kunert, A., and H. Schleussing. 1965. Experimentelle Untersuchungen zur Genese der postvakzinalen Enzephalomyelitis bei bestehender Toxoplasma-Infection. Arch. Hyg. Bakt., 149:133-153.

Lainson, R. 1955. Toxoplasmosis in England. II. Variation factors in the pathogenesis of *Toxoplasma* infections; the sudden increase in virulence of a strain after passage in multimammate rats and canaries. Ann. Trop. Med. Parasit., 49:397-416.

Laveran, A., and M. Marullaz. 1913. Recherches expérimentales sur le *Toxoplasma gondii*. Bull. Soc. Path. Exot., 6:460-468.

Lelong, M., and G. Desmonts. 1951. L'emploi du microscope à contraste de phase dans la réaction de Sabin-Feldman. C. R. Soc. Biol. (Paris), 145:1660-1661.

────── and G. Desmonts. 1952. Sur la nature du phénomène de Sabin et Feldman. C. R. Soc. Biol. (Paris), 146:207-209.

Levaditi, C., P. Lépine, and R. Schoen. 1928. L'immunité antitoxoplasmique. C. R. Soc. Biol. (Paris), 99:1130-1133.

────── P. Lépine, and R. Schoen. 1928. Mécanisme de l'immunité antitoxoplasmique du névraxe. C. R. Soc. Biol. (Paris), 99:1219-1222.

————— S. Sanchis-Bayarri, P. Lépine, and R. Schoen. 1929. Étude sur l'encéphalo-myélite provoquée par le *Toxoplasma cuniculi*. Ann. Inst. Pasteur (Paris), 43:1063-1080.

Levis, W. P., and E. K. Markell. 1958. Acquisition of immunity to toxoplasmosis by the newborn rat. Exp. Parasit., 7:463-467.

Long, P. L. 1962. Observations on the duration of the acquired immunity of chickens to *Eimeria maxima* Tyzzer, 1929. Parasitology, 52:89-93.

————— 1965. Immune mechanisms of the fowl in the mediation of acquired resistance to *Eimeria tenella*. Prog. Protozool. (London), p. 156.

————— and M. E. Rose. 1962. Attempted transfer of resistance to *Eimeria tenella* infections from domestic hens to their progeny. Exp. Parasit., 12:75-81.

————— and M. E. Rose. 1965. Active and passive immunization of chickens against intravenously induced infections of *Eimeria tenella*. Exp. Parasit., 16:1-7.

————— M. E. Rose, and A. E. Pierce. 1963. Effects of fowl sera on some stages in the life cycle of *Eimeria tenella*. Exp. Parasit., 14:210-217.

Ludwig, J., and G. Piekarski. 1961. Einfluss der Antikörper auf die Toxoplasma-Zellen in Elektronenmikroskop. *In* Progress in Protozoology. Ludvick, J., Lom, J., and Vávra, J., eds. Prague, Czechoslovak Academy of Sciences, Publ., p. 369.

————— J. C. Siim, and A. Birch-Andersen. 1963. The ultrastructure of *Toxoplasma gondii* after treatment with specific antibodies. International Congress of Tropical Medicine and Malaria. Rio de Janeiro, 2:351.

Lund, E. 1965. Respiratory enzymes in *Toxoplasma gondii*. *In* Progress in Protozoology. Second International Conference on Protozoology, London. International Congress Series No. 91. Amsterdam, Excerpta Medica Foundation, p. 188.

Lunde, M. N., and L. Jacobs. 1963. *Toxoplasma* hemagglutination and dye test antibodies in experimentally infected rats. J. Parasit., 6:932-936.

————— and L. Jacobs. 1964. Properties of toxoplasma lysates toxic to rabbits on intravenous injection. J. Parasit., 1:49-51.

————— and L. Jacobs. 1965. Antigenic relationship of *Toxoplasma gondi* and *Besnoita jeuisoni*. J. Parasit., 2:273-276.

Lycke, E., E. Lund, and O. Strannegård. 1965a. Enhancement by lysozyme and hyaluronidase of the penetration by *Toxoplasma gondii* into cultured host cells. Brit. J. Exp. Path., 2:189-199.

————— E. Lund, O. Strannegård, and E. Falsen. 1965b. The effect of immune serum and activator on the infectivity of *Toxoplasma gondii* for cell culture. Acta Path. Microbiol. Scand., 2:206-220.

Marcuse, K. 1922. Wassermannsche Reaktion und Kokzidiose beim Kaninchen. Zbl. Bakt. [Orig.], 355-362.

Mas Bakal, P. 1965. Interpretation of Sabin-Feldman dye-test titres. *In* Progress in Protozoology. Second International Conference on Protozoology, London. International Congress Series No. 91. Amsterdam, Excerpta Medica Foundation, p. 187.

Matsubayashi, H., and S. Akao. 1963. Morphological studies on the development of the *Toxoplasma* cyst. Amer. J. Trop. Med., 3:321-333.

————— and S. Akao. 1966. Immuno-electronmicroscopic studies on *Toxoplasma gondii*. Amer. J. Trop. Med., 15:486-491.

————— W. Stahl, and S. Akao. 1964. Immuno-electron microscopy in experimental Toxoplasmosis. Proceedings of the First International Congress of Parasitology, Rome.

Maumenee, A. E., ed. 1962. Toxoplasmosis, with special reference to uveitis. Baltimore, The Williams and Wilkins Co., pp. 699-972.

McDermott, J. J., and L. A. Stauber. 1954. Preparation and agglutination of merozoite suspensions of the chicken coccidium *Eimeria tenella*. J. Parasit., 40(suppl.):23.

McDonald, A. 1949. Serological diagnosis of human toxoplasmosis. Lancet, 1:950-953.

McFarlane, J. O., and I. Ruchman. 1948. Cultivation of *Toxoplasma* in the developing chick embryo. Proc. Soc. Exp. Biol. Med., 67:1-4.

Metzger, M., A. Przerwa-Tetmajer, and Z. Wojciechowski. 1963. The influence of zymosan, cortisone and X-rays on the course of experimental toxoplasmosis in white rats. Arch. Immun. Ther. Exp., 11:227-233.

Morehouse, N. F. 1938. The reaction of the immune intestinal epithelium of the rat to reinfection with *Eimeria nieschulzi*. J. Parasit., 24:311-317.

Nakayama, J. 1964. Persistence of the virulent RH strain of *Toxoplasma gondii* in the brains of immune mice. Keio J. Med., 1:7-12.

——— 1965. Effects of immunization procedures in experimental toxoplasmosis. Keio J. Med. 2:63-72.

——— 1966. On the survival of high virulent strain of *Toxoplasma gondii* inoculated intravenously into immune mice. Keio J. Med., 1:13-24.

Nicolau, S., and A. Ravelo. 1937. La réaction de fixation du complément dans le serum et dans des extraits d'organes d'animaux atteints de toxoplasmose expérimentale. Bull. Soc. Path. Exot., 66:855-859.

Nicolle, C., and L. Manceaux. 1908. Sur une infection à corps Leishman (ou organismes voisins) du gondi. C. R. Acad. Sci. (Paris), 147:763-766.

——— and L. Manceaux. 1909. Sur un protozoaire nouveau du gondi (Toxoplasma n. gen.). Arch. Inst. Pasteur (Tunis), 4:97-103.

O'Connor, R. G. 1957. Precipitating antibody to toxoplasma. A follow-up study on findings in the blood and aqueous humor. Amer. J. Ophthal., 44: 75-83.

Paterson, S. W. 1923. A complement fixation test in coccidiosis of the rabbit. Brit. J. Exp. Path., 4:1-4.

Paul, J. and R. Schlanstedt. 1956. Antikörperbildung nach Toxoplasma-Antigenzufuhr bei Kindern. Z. Immunitätsforsch., 113:1-14.

Pellérdy, L. P. 1965. Coccidia and Coccidiosis. Budapest, Akadémiai Kiadá, pp. 1-657.

Piekarski, G. 1966. Zur Deutung der Ergebnisse immunbiologischer Methoden bei der Toxoplasmose. *In* Toxoplasmose. Kirchhoff, H., et al., eds. Stuttgart, Georg Thieme Verlag, pp. 33-52.

Pierce, A. E., and P. L. Long. 1965. Studies on acquired immunity to coccidiosis in bursaless and thymectomized fowls. Immunology, 9:427-439.

——— P. L. Long, and C. Horton-Smith. 1962. Immunity to *Eimeria tenella* in young fowls (*Gallus domesticus*). Immunology, 5:129-152.

——— P. L. Long, and C. Horton-Smith. 1963. Attempts to induce a passive immunity to *Eimeria tenella* in young fowls (*Gallus domesticus*). Immunology, 6:37-47.

Remington, J. S. 1964. Studies on changes in serum proteins and immunity during acute and chronic toxoplasmosis. Proceedings of the First International Congress of Parasitology, Rome.

——— and R. Hackman. 1965. Changes in serum proteins of rats infected with *Toxoplasma gondii*. J. Parasit., 5:865-870.

——— M. L. Melton, and L. Jacobs. 1961. Induced and spontaneous recurrent parasitemia in chronic infections with avirulent strains of *Toxoplasma gondii*. J. Immun., 5:578-581.

Reyer, W. 1941. Zur Klärung der Resistenzerscheinungen bei den Darmcoccidiosen der Warmblüter. Zbl. Bakt. [Orig.], 146:305.

Roever-Bonnet, A. De. 1963. Mice and golden hamsters infected with an avirulent and a virulent *Toxoplasma* strain. Trap. Geogr. Med., 15:45-60.

——— 1964. *Toxoplasma* parasites in different organs of mice and hamsters infected with avirulent and virulent strains. Trop. Geogr. Med., 4:337-345.

Rose, M. E. 1959. Serological reactions in *Eimeria stiedae* infection in the rabbit. Immunology, 2:112-122.

——— 1961. The complement-fixation test in hepatic coccidiosis of rabbits. Immunology, 4:346-353.

——— 1963. Some aspects of immunity to *Eimeria* infections. Ann. N.Y. Acad. Sci., 113:383-399.

——— and E. Orlans. 1962. Fowl antibody. 3. Its haemolytic activity with complements of various species and some properties of fowl complement. Immunology, 5:633-641.

Roth, W. 1953. Zur Wirkungsweise des Aktivatorserums auf *Toxoplasma gondii*. Schweiz Allg. Path., 16:914-918.

Ruchman, I. and R. J. Johansmann. 1948. Biological properties of a strain of toxoplasma recovered from a fatal case of congenital toxoplasmosis. Amer. J. Trop. Med., 28:687-695.

Sabin, A. B. 1942. Toxoplasmosis. A recently recognized disease of human beings. Advances Pediat., 1:1-60.

——— and H. A. Feldman. 1948. Dyes as microchemical indicators of a new immunity phenomenon affecting a protozoon parasite (*Toxoplasma*). Science, 108: 660-663.

———— and P. K. Olitsky. 1937. *Toxoplasma* and obligate intracellular parasitism. Science, 85:336-338.

Sarrailhe, A. 1914. Notes sur la toxoplasmose expérimentale. Bull. Soc. Path. Exot., 7:232-240.

Sato, H. 1963. Animal and bacteria. *In* On the Immunity to Toxoplasmosis (In Japanese). Nankodo, pp. 124-130.

Scholtyseck, E., and G. Piekarski. 1965. Elektronenmikroskopische Untersuchungen on Merozoiten von Eimerien (*Eimeria perforans* und *E. stiedae*) und *Toxoplasma gondii*. Zur systematischen Stellung von *T. gondii*. Z. Parasitenk., 2:91-115.

Senaga, R. 1957. Studies on chronic toxoplasmosis I. An attempt to produce chronic *Toxoplasma* infection in guinea pigs and mice (In Japanese). Nissin Igaku, 44:429-435.

Senger, C. M., D. M. Hammond, J. L. Thorne, A. E. Johnson, and G. M. Wells. 1959. Resistance of calves to reinfection with *Eimeria bovis*. J. Protozool., 6:51-58.

Siim, J., and K. Lind. 1960. A toxoplasma flocculation test. Acta Path. Microbiol. Scand., 50:445-6.

Simitsch, T., B. Tomanovitsch, A. Bordjochski, Z. Petrovitch, and Z. Savin. 1960 Sensibilité comparée de *Citellus citellus* et de la souris blanche à l'infection avec la souche RH de *Toxoplasma gondii*. Arch. Inst. Pasteur d'Algérie, 3:377-385.

Smith, T. 1910. A protective reaction of the host in intestinal coccidiosis of the rabbit. J. Med. Res., 23:407-415.

Stahl, W., and S. Akao. 1964. Immunity in experimental toxoplasmosis. Keio J. Med., 1:1-6.

———— H. Matsubayashi, and S. Akao. 1965. Effects of 6-mercaptopurine on cyst development in experimental toxoplasmosis. Keio J. Med., 1:1-10.

———— H. Matsubayashi, and S. Akao. 1966. Experimental toxoplasmosis: Effects of suppression of the immune-response of mice by cortisone and splenectomy. Keio J. Med., 1:1-12.

Strannegård, O. 1962. Studies of *Toxoplasma* precipitinogens and their corresponding antibodies by means of diffusion-in-gel methods. Brit. J. Exp. Path., 6:600-613.

———— 1965. Kinetics of the *in vitro* inactivation of *Toxoplasma gondii* by specific antibodies. *In* Progress in Protozoology. Second International Conference on Protozoology, London. International Congress Series No. 91. Amsterdam, Excerpta Medica Foundation, p. 186.

———— and E. Lycke. 1966. Properdin and the antibody-effect on *Toxoplasma gondii*. Acta Path. Microbiol. Scand., 66:227-238.

Swatek, M. 1956. O wpływie ACTH na przebieg doświadczalnego zakażenia *Toxoplasma gondii* u białych myszek (About the influence of ACTH on the course of experimental infection of white mice with *Toxoplasma gondii*). Wiad. Parazyt., 2:153-159.

Szurman, J., and J. Szaflarski. 1964. Ein Beitrag zur chemischen Natur des Toxoplasmins. Angew. Parasit., 5:169-172.

Taliaferro, W. H., and H. W. Mulligan. The histopathology of malaria with special reference to the function and origin of macrophages in defence. Indian Medical Research Memoir, 29:1-138.

Thalhammer, O. 1960. Difficult and unsolved problems in the diagnosis of toxoplasmosis. *In* Human Toxoplasmosis. Siim, J., ed. Copenhagen, pp. 191-200.

Tolentino, P., and A. Bucalossi. 1952. Possibilita di ottenere una risposta anticorporale mediante vaccinazione con toxoplasmi uccisi. Boll. Soc. Ital. Biol. Sper., 12:2002-2003.

Tomita, T. 1960. A study on oxygen consumption in organs of *Toxoplasma*-infected mice. Osaka City Med. J., 9:1713-1729.

Torres, C. M. 1924. Coccidiose lésions de la moelle osseuse et réaction de Wassermann positive, non-spécifique, chez le lapin. C. R. Soc. Biol. (Paris), 91:986-987.

Tyzzer, E. E. 1929. Coccidiosis in gallinaceous birds. Amer. J. Hyg., 10:269-383.

Ueda, H. 1960. On the virulence and antigenic property of a cyst-producing strain of *Toxoplasma* (In Japanese). Keio J. Med., 37:1631-1638.

Umiński, J., and S. Toś-Luty. 1959. Dalsze próby otrzymywania toksoplazmowej surowicy odpornosiowej na królikach. Wiad. Parazyt., 5:245-248.

Van der Waaij, D. 1959. Formation, growth and multiplication of *Toxoplasma gondii* cysts in mouse brains. Trop. Geogr. Med., Amsterdam, 11,4:345-360.

———— 1960. The effect of a lysine-deficient diet on the course of a chronic toxoplasma infection. Trop. Geogr. Med., 2:180-182.

———— 1964. The transmission of toxoplasmosis after birth. Trop. Geogr. Med., 4:331-336.

Verlinde, J. D., and O. Makstenieks. 1950. Repeated isolation of *Toxoplasma* from the cerebrospinal fluid and from the blood, and the antibody response in four cases of congenital toxoplasmosis. Antonie van Leeuwenhoek J. Microbiol. Serol., 16:365-372.

Visher, W. A., and E. Suter. 1954. Intracellular multiplication of *Toxoplasma gondii* in adult mammalian macrophages cultured *in vitro*. Proc. Soc. Exp. Biol. Med., 86:413-419.

Wanko, T., L. Jacobs, and M. A. Gavin. 1962. Electron microscope study of toxoplasma cysts in mouse brain. J. Protozool., 9,2:235-242.

Warren, J., and A. B. Sabin. 1942. The complement fixation reaction in toxoplasmic infection. Proc. Soc. Exp. Biol. Med., 51:11-14.

Wasielewski, T. von. 1904. Studien und Mikrophotogramme zur Kenntnis der pathogenen Protozoen. I. Untersuchungen über den Bau, die Entwicklung and über die pathogene Bedeutung der Coccidien. Leipzig, J. A. Barth, Publishers.

Weinman, D. 1943. Chronic toxoplasmosis. J. Infect. Dis., 73:85-92.

———— and H. J. Klatchko. 1950. Description of toxin in toxoplasmosis. Yale J. Biol. Med., 22:323-326.

Werner, H. 1963. Über die Formvariabilität von *Toxoplasma gondii* unter dem Einfluss von Antikörpern. Zbl. Bakt. [Orig.], 4:497-510.

Wildführ, G. 1957. Tierexperimentelle Immunitätsversuche mit *Toxoplasma gondii*. Immunitätsforsch., 113:435-452.

———— G. Naumann, and J. Wilde. 1958. Elektrophoretische Untersuchungen von Rattenseren nach latenter Infektion mit *Toxoplasma gondii*. Z. Immunitätsforsch., 115:122-134.

Wolf, A., and D. Cowen. 1938. Granulomatous encephalomyelitis due to a protozoan (*Toxoplasma* or *Encephalitozoon*). II. Identification of a case from the literature. Bull. Neurol. Inst. N.Y., 7:266-290.

———— D. Cowen, and B. H. Paige. 1939. Toxoplasmic encephalomyelitis. III. A new case of granulomatous encephalomyelitis due to protozoon. Amer. J. Path., 15:657-694.

Direct-Infection Nematodes

RALPH E. THORSON

Department of Biology, University of Notre Dame, Notre Dame, Indiana

INTRODUCTION

Direct-infection nematodes are those roundworm parasites which gain access to the host without the intervention of an intermediate host or vector. Entry into the host is usually by the oral route or, less frequently, by skin penetration.

The interplay between direct-infecting nematode species and their hosts is an expression of two ecologic relationships: that of the helminth and the external environment before infection, and that of the helminth and the host (the internal environment). The delicacy of the latter relationship involves a multitude of physiologic factors on the part of both host and helminth, and in many instances the balance is weighed in favor of the host. This results in the development of an immune state against these parasites.

The sheer bulk of experimental data available on the immune response of hosts to direct-infection nematodes has resulted from a logarithmic rate of publication since World War II. The variety of exquisite new techniques and new study systems has contributed to this flood, and certainly our understanding of the basic mechanisms involved has improved. This is not to say that all is known and that further work is not required. Rather, it will be the purpose of this discussion to assess the status of our present knowledge and to point out potentially productive areas of research on the immune state to direct-infection nematodes.

Merely listing the publications since Culbertson's book, *Immunity against Animal Parasites*, in 1941 would fill the pages of this book, and thus, the present discussion is not intended to be all-inclusive. The major portion of the work on mechanisms of immunity to direct-infection nematodes has been done by the North American, Australian, and British parasitologists. The field of immunologic diagnostic testing has also received contributions from the Japanese, South American, and Eastern European workers. These tests will be discussed in a later chapter of this book.

The routes of infection of these nematodes and their subsequent contact with the tissues of the host play an important role in the level and potential effectiveness of resulting protective immunity. Metazoan parasites such as helminths have a large variety of tissues and thus a wide variety of antigens to stimulate antibody formation. However, it seems apparent that although the host is stimulated to produce antibodies to most of these antigens, all of them may not be protective in nature. Thus, when one discusses antibodies formed against helminths (or any metazoan infection), it is well to remember that some serve as protective antibodies and some as simple responses to antigenic stimulation.

NATURAL IMMUNITY

Physical and physiologic factors

Effect of age.   As one reviews the experimental work which has been performed to demonstrate the effect of age on natural immunity, the results are
so similar that one is prepared to suggest a biologic "law," i.e., as an animal
ages, its natural resistance to helminth infection increases. But, as in all
attempts to formulate such laws in biology, exceptions do occur. In infection
with directly infecting nematodes, such exceptions are quite rare.

One seldom sees, for instance, a clinical infection with *Ancylostoma caninum* in mature dogs. However, such infections do occur and a careful diagnostic follow-up usually demonstrates the presence of a coexisting infection
or pathologic state which has apparently interfered with the immune status
of the host and thus explains the increased susceptibility to the worm. On
the other hand, in certain areas of the United States, particularly the southeastern section, probably 100 percent of the puppies born are prenatally
infected with the dog hookworm. The absence of worms in adult dogs in
endemic areas, then, is due to an acquired immunity, and it is not apparent
that a natural immunity develops with age. This point should be carefully
considered in any laboratory or epidemiologic consideration of age immunity.
Fortunately, much of the work on age immunity has been done with laboratory animals whose prior history of exposure to direct-infection helminths is
well-known and controlled.

The classical studies by Herrick (1928) and by Sarles (1929) of hookworms and by Ackert and his co-workers (Ackert and Edgar, 1939) of *Ascaridia* (a bird form) demonstrated an increase of immunity with age and have
frequently been cited. The work with hookworms has particularly been open
to the criticism that it was unknown whether the dogs and cats had had
prior experience with hookworm. In the last 25 years, the additions to our
knowledge on natural immunity and age have been expanded by a somewhat
better understanding of the mechanism of such a relationship.

Certain variations in the level of age immunity depend on sex in certain
hosts. Discussion of this point will be deferred to the next section of this
chapter.

Miller (1965b) demonstrated quite conclusively that puppies 2 to 5
months old were much more susceptible to *Ancylostoma caninum* than were
adult dogs. This susceptibility of younger dogs continued until approximately 8 months of age, when certain differences in the susceptibility of
males and females were observed. However, at 11 months of age, both male
dogs and bitches showed a marked age resistance.

Larsh and Hendricks (1949) showed that there were no differences in
worm burdens of old and young (1 month) mice infected with *Trichinella*.
However, judging from other infections (Mathies, 1962), it would appear
that their experimental "young" mice were just approaching puberty.

With infections of *Aspiculuris tetraptera* in mice, a relationship similar to that seen by Miller was shown (Mathies, 1962). However, the susceptibility, though more marked in younger animals, disappeared and effective age resistance developed in about 5 to 6 weeks. This observation and that of Miller (1965b) illustrate that certainly the development of age resistance is associated with some as yet incompletely explained mechanism involved in the maturation of the host; the dog matures at about 8 to 10 months, whereas the mouse reaches puberty in 5 to 6 weeks.

An attempt to understand the mechanisms involved in the development of age immunity naturally includes such considerations as maturity and sex (which will be considered in the next section), but Lewert and Lee (1957) felt that at least in the case of skin-penetrating nematodes (*Strongyloides ratti*), the worms were prevented from entering the older host because of changes occurring in the basement membrane and ground substance of the skin. Studies of the histochemistry (Lewert and Lee, 1954) of the skin revealed that the penetrating larva must traverse the nonliving stratum corneum, the cellular layers of the epidermis, and the extracellular barriers presented by the basement membrane and ground substance of the dermal connective tissue. The acellular elements become more highly polymerized with age and resist the enzymes used by the larvae in penetration, thus effectively reducing their infectivity in older hosts. Most ingeniously, these authors recognized that in young hypophysectomized rats, the basement membrane becomes more highly polymerized and thus should become more resistant to larval penetration. The experimental test of this hypothesis showed that young animals so treated demonstrated a "natural age resistance" similar in nature to that of older animals.

At the present time, except for the theory that the goblet cells and/or globule leukocytes increase with age in host animals (Ackert and Edgar, 1939; Whur, 1966) and this coincides with the development of age immunity, no satisfactory mechanism of action has been developed for this type of immunity in animals infected orally by nematodes which do not migrate in the host.

In contrast to the almost unequivocal evidence that young animals are more susceptible to nematodes than older animals, Bass and Olson (1965) showed that with *Trichinella spiralis*, new-born mice were markedly more resistant to infection than 80-day-old animals. If, however, the mice are infected at 6 weeks (rather than just after birth) and compared with mice 5 months old, the typical young-to-old development of resistance occurs (Riedel, 1948). The resistance shown by new-born mice as opposed to those a few weeks older is difficult to explain, but physiologic differences in the gut are suggested by the present author.

Effect of sex differences. It is abundantly clear that the sex of the host may influence the qualitative and quantitative development of natural immunity. Roman (1951), in an epidemiologic study of natural infections with *Aspiculuris tetraptera* in rats, found 49 percent of the males infected as compared to 24 percent of the females. Mathies (1959a, b) showed that in experimental infections with the same worm in mice, males had twice as many worms as females and the females showed this resistance at first estrus. Males showed a gradually increasing resistance with age. Using *Nippostrongylus brasiliensis* in mice, Neafie and Haley (1962) found that until 2 to 3 weeks of age there was no difference in susceptibility of either sex, but that at 4 to 5 weeks, females contained about one-half as many worms as males. Puberty in mice occurs at about 5 weeks of age.

Miller (1965b) found that natural age resistance to *Ancylostoma caninum* appeared at an earlier age in the bitch than in the male dog. Again, this earlier appearance and qualitative response of the female was related to the onset of puberty (at approximately 11 months of age).

Using the data of these workers, a generalization may be made with respect to the effect of sex on the development of natural age immunity to worm infection. In the male the immunity develops gradually from shortly after birth to adulthood, whereas in the female the immunity develops similarly to that of the young male until just before the onset of puberty when there is a sudden and dramatic increase of resistance in the female (Fig. 1). It becomes apparent that the study of age immunity *per se* is best done with male animals, since the complications which may be partly due to female sex hormones would be avoided.

Effect of nutrition.   Since natural immunity exists and since it develops without apparent stimulus, it would seem to follow that well-nourished hosts would fare better than the malnourished. However, the evidence for the roles of proteins, carbohydrates, lipids, vitamins, or trace minerals in this relationship is meager. The important studies of Foster and Cort (1932) demonstrate the very real contribution of protein and iron to the development and maintenance of an acquired immunity to hookworm infections, but it does

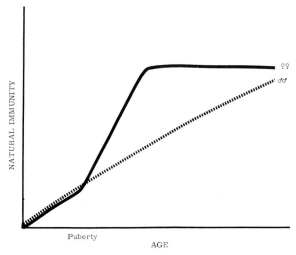

FIG. 1. The development of age immunity to direct-infection nematodes in male and female hosts.

not necessarily follow that the mechanisms are similar in natural immunity. In the latter it is difficult to demonstrate a humoral response, whereas in acquired immunity it is easy to show such a response.

In an abnormal host, the mouse, Rohrbacher et al. (1963) demonstrated that animals on a reduced dietary intake (1.5 g per day versus 3 to 4 g per day for controls) harbored greater numbers of larvae of *Ascaris suum* in their livers. Substitution in the commercial ration of 50 or 100 percent cornstarch or 50 percent casein did not decrease the number of worms in mice with the reduced intake.

Biochemical and physiologic factors. Natural immunity to helminths is an expression of the resistance to infection in hosts which have had no prior experience with the invader. The broadest interpretation of such resistance requires delineating all factors which play a role. This section will suggest some of these factors and hopefully will encourage further study of them.

The ecologic "fitness" of the host frequently requires the presence of several conditions for a given helminth to develop. The work of Rogers (1963), Rogers and Sommerville (1960, 1963), and Sommerville (1966) illustrates some of these factors. The transition of a helminth from an infective stage outside the host to a parasitic individual requires that the host have in its physiologic and biochemical make-up the stimuli and requisites for establishment and persistence of the parasite. Such physiologic responses of the parasite as molting, growth, and maturation are frequently initiated by host stimuli. Lacking these, the parasite is unable to complete its life cycle. The importance of proper pH, reducing agents, and especially carbon dioxide has been demonstrated in the reports cited above and in numerous other papers on the *in vitro* cultivation of nematodes (*see* Silverman, 1965, and Rogers, 1966).

The ingenious demonstration by Lewert and Lee (1956) that the acellular barrier of the skin changes with increasing age and thus inhibits infection by skin-penetrating helminths explains another factor. Host specificity also plays a role, since this barrier varies from host to host (consider the inability of *Ancylostoma brasiliense*, normally a parasite of cats and dogs, to penetrate past the stratum germinativum of man, thus causing creeping eruption rather than intestinal infection).

DeWitt and Weinstein (1964) demonstrated that such a simple device as a purified, synthetic diet would cause a reduction in the numbers of pinworms in mice. The effect of such diets on *Nematospiroides dubius*, a parasite of the upper small intestine, was similar but not as marked. Simple location of the worms in the host may dictate this response. The effect of diets reduced in quality and/or quantity on bacterial flora in various intestinal locations should also be considered.

The helminth must also have certain biochemical entities which respond to the host's stimuli. Certain enzymes required for the hatching of eggs reflect the suitability of the host. The evolutionary history of helminths and their hosts must certainly have developed in accordance with these physiologic and biochemical needs.

The role of genetic factors

In a consideration of genetic factors in helminth infections, the complexity of the system requires a careful analysis of both parties in the parasitic relationship. The delineation of these relationships will prove to be a most rewarding study for little is known about either side of this complex equilibrium.

The host may vary genetically in its susceptibility, thus contributing to the presence and degree of infection. But the most variable aspect of the relationship between the host and direct-infecting nematodes is the genetic constituency of the parasite itself. Little has been accomplished in developing genetically marked strains of helminths which are reasonably homozygous, and to date, little difference in such characteristics as infectivity or virulence among "strains" has been observed. Rats are quite susceptible to *Trichinella* and are frequently used in laboratory studies. However, a "strain" of *Trichinella* isolated from humans in Kenya displayed low infectivity when administered to rats (Forrester et al., 1961).*

Schad (1965) has demonstrated that *Trichinella* isolated from a civet cat in Calcutta was less well-adapted to rats than a Canadian strain. He suggested that the Indian strain is "genetically isolated from classical North Temperate forms." The Indian form is smaller, less fecund, and the female: male ratio is in favor of the females. Successive passages of the Indian strain in rats, however, yield results similar to the Canadian strain.

With regard to the host, some interesting observations have come to light which should lead to exciting new studies. Whitlock (1955, 1958) reported a strain of sheep which displayed heightened natural resistance to trichostrongyles. In these sheep there is a factor which appears to be a simple dominant whose allele in the homozygous recessive condition represents susceptibility. He called this the "violet factor." The phenotypic expression of this genetic factor depends on diet and pregnancy, among other things. The establishment of a breeding flock which was homozygous for the recessive allele and was more susceptible than sheep with the dominant expression illustrated the genetic nature of this character. The "resistant" expression of violet factor seemed to be contained in the gastric mucosa, since direct infection of isolated gastric pouches with larvae resulted in higher survival rate of worms in susceptible sheep.

Recently, Liu (1966), in a series of experiments with several genetically derived strains of mice and *Nematospiroides dubius*, reported some interesting observations and one puzzle. Using mice of C₃H, A, CF1, C57, and Webster strains, he determined that C₃H mice were most susceptible, with resistance increasing in the strains in the order listed; mice of the Webster strain were most resistant. Several factors were suggested as contributing to

*This report and one by Ozeretskovskaya (1968) suggest that laboratory studies with different strains might be possible. Single pair crosses between fourth stage males and females could be made, and the comparison of larval yields in the homologous and heterologous crosses may yield genetic data of value.

this. C₃H mice are congenitally handicapped by lower tissue resistance to the mechanical and chemical effects of larvae, and they also display lowered cytopoiesis of reticuloendothelial elements in healing. The puzzling observation was that in a cross-strain breeding experiment between the resistant Webster and the susceptible C₃H strain, the F_1 individuals showed a greater resistance than the already resistant Webster parents. This unexpected result certainly points the way to new experiments.

Ross et al. (1959) described a bull line of Nigerian Zebu cattle in which there was genetically controlled resistance to *Haemonchus*. Resistant progeny, after experimental infection, had comparatively lower parasite egg counts and a high immunologic response, whereas in susceptible animals the responses were reversed.

In humans, the very great susceptibility to hookworm of whites as compared with Negroes is another instance of genetic influence on resistance and susceptibility (Andrews, 1942).

Abnormal hosts as tools to study natural immunity

In an effort to determine the mechanisms which influence age immunity, abnormal hosts have been used which have a heightened resistance to various nematodes as compared to the normal hosts. Also, if the host animal is large and difficult to manage in large numbers in the laboratory, small animals such as the mouse, hamster, guinea pig, and rabbit have been useful in maintaining at least part of the life cycles of worms.

The incidence of infection and numbers of *Nippostrongylus* in hamsters, an abnormal host, showed a greater susceptibility of males (Haley, 1958). This increased susceptibility of the male paralleled in many ways the differences seen in natural immunity. The greatest differences in numbers of worms were seen when older females were compared to younger males or to males of a comparable age. It should be pointed out that hamsters infected with strains of *Nippostrongylus* which had been adapted to this host by continuous passage did not exhibit as great a difference in male and female susceptibility as was observed when normal rat strains were introduced into hamsters.

Ecologic factors in natural immunity

Since parasitism is a relationship marked by ecologic complexity and any consideration of immunity might be viewed as an ecologic study, certain interrelationships between host and parasite can be cited in this context. It has frequently been observed that stress in its many forms can trigger very complex reactions in animals, and parasites and their hosts, existing in a delicate relationship, are no exception. The effects of stress are marked on endocrine balance, and even concurrent infections can complicate the picture of developing natural immunity.

Effects of stress.   In an ingenious experiment, designed to determine the effect of stress on parasitism, Davis and Read (1958) infected two groups of wild male mice with *Trichinella spiralis*. In one group, each animal was placed in a separate jar, and at necropsy 15 days later each harbored only a few adult worms. The experimental mice were placed in separate jars, but from day 2 to 11 post-infection they were in groups of 6 for 3 hours each day in large cans. Severe fighting occurred immediately, and on the third day social rank was established. These mice harbored more worms than the isolated mice at necropsy. Crowding is known to lead to adrenal hypertrophy, and the sequelae of crowding or isolation are observable though not completely understood. At necropsy on the 15th day, there were insignificant differences in the adrenal weights of the isolated and grouped mice. However, necropsy of normal mice at 30 days revealed significant differences between their adrenal weights and those of the grouped mice, the latter having larger adrenals (means of 5.08 mg versus 4.24 mg). This illustrates the remarkable chain reaction that stress such as crowding may initiate in the natural immunity of a host to helminths. The ranking patterns in rodents in nature would presumably lead to stress and to different levels of infection.

Robinson (1961) demonstrated the deleterious effect of mild electrical stimulation, bright lights, and loud noise in "immunized" mice challenged with *Trichinella*.

Noble (1966) stressed ground squirrels (*Citellus armatus*) by removing bedding during the night and by placing blocks of ice in the cages. After two weeks of this treatment, the adrenal weights of the stressed animals were appreciably higher than those of the controls (110 versus 81 mg per kg body weight). Worm burdens (*Syphacia citelli*) were higher in the stressed animals as well.

Effects of hormones. As has been stated, stress may disturb endocrine relationships in a host animal, thus rendering it more susceptible to an initial infection by a helminth. There are abundant data on the effects of either the increase or decrease in various endocrine levels in host animals. In any consideration of such experiments, one must at all times keep in mind the rather circular effects that manipulation of endocrine glands or hormone levels may have. The interplay of various of the endocrine glands in the homeostatic state makes the isolation of particular cause and effect relationships most difficult. Certainly this area of investigation, though frustrating at times, will be fruitful.

Cortisone and cortisone derivatives have been used extensively in studies of acquired immunity, but their effects on natural immunity are not as well studied. The naturally occurring age immunity to many helminths can usually be weakened by subjection of the host to treatments with cortisone (Mathies, 1962; Briggs, 1965; Weinstein, 1955). Ritterson (1959) compared the susceptibility of two species of hamsters (Chinese and golden) to *Trichinella*. The Chinese hamster showed more natural resistance to the muscle-stage larvae than did the golden hamster. After treatment with cortisone, the reaction of the Chinese hamster more closely resembled that of the golden hamster. In untreated infections in the Chinese hamster, a heightened round cell response, which apparently resulted in a more efficient immune response,

was observed. This was not observed in the golden hamster. However, cortisone treatment depressed this round cell infiltration and permitted greater
survival of the muscle stages.

Mathies (1962) found that estradiol treatment of male mice reduced the
numbers of adults of *Aspiculuris*. This effect resembles that generally seen in
untreated females, which usually harbor fewer worms than do males. The
exact effects of testosterone and estrogen are not clearly understood, but
Katz (1963) demonstrated that in young animals which were gonadectomized
and treated with hormones, the host-parasite relationships were very complicated. Gonadectomy without hormone treatment caused the males and
females to become similar in their susceptibilities. If animals were gonadectomized and treated with either testosterone or estradiol, there were no
observed differences in susceptibility to *Aspiculuris*. However, gonadectomized animals always had more worms than sham-operated animals. One is
tempted to explain this difference in terms of the effects of estradiol, but
these experiments demonstrate that a rather intricate balance of hormones
may play a more important role than either of the sex hormones.

Dunn and Brown (1962) found that pregnancy had no effect on pinworm
infections in mice. One might anticipate some difference due to the changed
levels of certain of the hormones during pregnancy, but if the diagram in
Figure 1 is considered, the level of natural immunity is fairly well established
by puberty and the hormonal effect is not apparent.

One can only speculate on the effects of exact hormonal relationships on
natural immunity, but the later discussion of hormone influence on acquired
immunity may be relevant to certain of these points (*see* p. 944).

Effects of concurrent infection. Concurrent infections with viruses,
bacteria, or other helminths can apparently play a role in what we might
describe as natural immunity. Infections with viruses or bacteria may
decrease resistance to worms as a result of physical or physiologic effects; it
is highly unlikely that any immunologic cross-reactions would occur which
would increase it. However, with helminths, enhanced protection against
other helminth species occurs which might be due to immunologic cross-
reactions. If this latter effect is carefully studied, it may become apparent
that the "cross-reactions" are really physiologic or physical disturbances of
the ecologic niche by the presence of the other species.

With *Trichinella* infections, Kilham and Olivier (1961) found that concurrent infection with encephalomyocarditis virus (EMC) caused a much
higher rate of crippling and death than with either infection alone. It was
obvious that the virus could more easily reach and infect the skeletal muscles
containing trichina larvae. This is an example of the physiologic or physical
alteration of a niche and illustrates a nonimmunologic but ecologic alteration
in resistance.

Bacterial influences on helminth infections have been most definitive in
work with "germ-free" animals and this will be discussed in a later paragraph. However, Stefanski and Przyjalkowski (1966) studied the effect of
various bacteria on the intestinal establishment of *Trichinella*. To negate the

effect of the normal flora of the host, the test mice were "sterilized" with antibiotics. Interestingly, *Lactobacillus* sp. prevented development of adult worms, while *Escherichia, Proteus, Serratia, Pseudomonas*, and several other Gram-negative bacteria favored the development of worms in the intestine. The physiologic differences between the *Lactobacillus* and the Gram-negative organisms and the effect of these differences on the intestinal environment are areas for speculation and testing.

There are many examples of the effects of concurrent infections with helminths. Senterfit (1958), Weinmann (1960), and Jachowski and Anderson (1961) all worked with *Schistosoma mansoni* and *Trichinella*. They found a cross-protection and suggested that this was due to related antigenic substances. It is not unusual for *Trichinella* and *Schistosoma* to give cross-reactions in diagnostic testing.

Nematode-nematode infections have been the subject of several studies: Stewart and Gordon (1953) studied the effect of *Haemonchus* on *Trichostrongylus* infection; Cox (1952), the effect of *Ancylostoma caninum* on *Trichinella*; and more recently, Louch (1962) demonstrated an increased resistance in laboratory rats to *Trichinella* following an infection with *Nippostrongylus*. Stahl (1966) reported that prior infection with *Hymenolepis nana* had no effect on the susceptibility of mice to *Aspiculuris*, but that *Trichinella* or *Syphacia* infections caused an increased resistance to *Aspiculuris*. Here it would be unwise to suggest immunologic identity, since other less obvious but more practical solutions may be offered. It is entirely conceivable that an infection with one species of worm causes an inflammatory reaction in the intestine. This then creates an unsuitable environment, either physically or physiologically, for the developing worms of another infection. Exactly what factors are altered to cause this "resistance" is not as yet clear.

The intriguing use of gnotobiotic animals, i.e., animals reared in the absence of contact with bacteria, helminths, protozoa, and ectoparasites (for a review, *see* Luckey, 1963), seemed to offer a possible solution to the question of the effect of these invaders on helminth infections. Newton et al. (1959) observed that *Nippostrongylus* and *Nematospiroides dubius* developed to adulthood in germ-free guinea pigs but not in conventional ones. The guinea pig is considered to be an abnormal host for these worms. Westcott and Todd (1964) found that the normal bacterial flora favorably influenced the development of *Nippostrongylus* in conventional mice, as compared to a reduced development in germ-free mice. Doll and Franker (1963) and Franker and Doll (1964) studied the most interesting relationship of *Heterakis-Histomonas* and turkeys in a germ-free environment and found less histomoniasis in germ-free than in conventional turkeys. The exact reason is not too clear, but contamination of previously germ-free turkeys with certain species of bacteria enhanced the production of histomoniasis. It is interesting to speculate that the germ-free cecum of the turkeys was not a suitable environment for the worm, *Heterakis*, and thus there was inadequate opportunity for invasion by the histomonad organisms.

ACTIVELY ACQUIRED IMMUNITY

Immunity in the host to direct-infection nematodes may be acquired in two basic ways: actively and passively. The latter method will be discussed in the next section of this chapter.

A basic objection frequently cited in immunity studies with nematodes is that the protective immunity which is developed is not always complete, i.e., some worms usually remain in the immune host. The parasitologist need not be embarrassed by this objection, since we are usually able to see even one worm with ease whereas in other parasitic infections, remaining parasites may escape detection because of their smaller size. It is equally necessary to understand that because of the relatively large size of helminths, it should be possible to develop a better understanding of mechanisms of protective immunity than one can with bacteria, viruses, and protozoa (World Health Organization Expert Committee, 1965).

Methods of producing active immunity

Infection. The classical and still most effective method of producing active protective immunity in a host with direct-infection nematodes is by subjecting the host to actual infection. This is easily accomplished with such worms as *Nippostrongylus brasiliensis*. A single dose of 500 to 1,000 infective larvae in 4-week-old rats will run a course of maturation and egg deposition, but by 20 days post-infection, essentially all adult worms will be gone. Subsequent challenge infections are at best poorly established. The added early stimulus of tissue migration in subsequent infections develops a higher degree of protective immunity, but no adult worms develop. *Nippostrongylus* is frequently used in experimental studies because it is easily maintained in laboratory rats and mice and has a very short life cycle (14 days from egg to egg). However, similar examples of the development of protective immunity have been shown for *Trichinella, Ancylostoma caninum, Nematospiroides, Ascaris, Nematodirus, Trichostrongylus, Haemonchus, Toxocara, Heterakis,* and many other worms. In principle, it is quite easy to produce actively acquired protective immunity by infections with most worms. However, one also assumes the risk that the pathology caused by living worms may endanger the life of the host or in other ways disturb its physiology, e.g., causing poor feed economy and low meat production in domestic animals such as sheep, cattle, and swine.

Dead worms. Because of the above-mentioned risk, there have been many attempts to develop vaccines containing dead worms as has been done for vaccines with viruses and bacteria. An analysis of the comparative size and biologic complexity of helminths versus bacteria and viruses suggests that a vaccine with metazoan parasites would contain a very wide variety of potential antigens, and many of which would not stimulate protective immunity. The effective antigens may also exist in very low quantities with respect to the total bulk of injected vaccine. This, then, could dilute the effectiveness of the antibody-forming system of the host.

The experiences of most workers with vaccines which contain dead worms, though somewhat conflicting, generally confirm this hypothesis (see Thorson, 1953, for a review). Little or no protective immunity is developed against direct-infecting nematodes when they are killed before injection.

The argument raised above (i.e., that dead worms contribute too many useless antigens and thus dilute the efforts of the antibody-forming system) has been circumvented to a certain extent by other methods. Chief of these is the chemical extraction of various biochemical components; another important possibility is the dissection and chemical extraction of specific tissues rather than using the whole worm. The latter is simply a logical refinement of the former. It is tantamount to extracting insulin from the pancreas rather than from the whole cow.

Worm products—*Somatic.* Oliver-Gonzales (1943) and Kagan (1957) prepared somatic antigens from *Ascaris* from extractions of isolated tissues such as cuticle, muscle, pseudocoelomic fluid, and eggs. Thorson (1956a, b) extracted materials from various tissues of the dog hookworm, *Ancylostoma caninum*, and studied their physiologic activities. The esophagus extracts with wide physiologic activities were used to stimulate protective immunity in puppies against the hookworm. The protection was not of the level associated with natural infection, but it was easily demonstrable. Rose et al. (1964) isolated immunologically active substances from the excretory glands of *Stephanurus dentatus*, the swine kidney worm.

Melcher's method (1943) of extracting materials from whole worms, including delipidization, extraction of proteins, and separating acid-soluble and acid-insoluble proteins, has been commonly used by later workers. Campbell (1936) prepared an antigenically active polysaccharide fraction from *Ascaris* by repeated alcoholic precipitation of a borate-buffer extract of whole worms. These extracts have generally been more useful in serologic diagnosis than in stimulating protective immunity.

More recently, Kent (1963a, b) has used column chromatography with DEAE-cellulose for separation of antigens from aqueous extracts of *Ascaris* and *Trichinella*. The fractions are interesting in that all contain protein and some have variable quantities of carbohydrate. This matter will be discussed in greater detail in a later section (*see* p. 932). Further investigation of chromatographic techniques are dictated by the results achieved by Kent.

Excretion and secretion antigens. The classic work of Sarles (1938) and Taliaferro and Sarles (1939) suggested that antibodies were formed to certain substances which were secreted and/or excreted from the body openings (mouth, excretory pore, and anus) of *Nippostrongylus brasiliensis*. Precipitation of these substances was observed *in vitro* with larvae and adults in sera from rats repeatedly infected with the worm. Histologically, they also demonstrated comparable reactions to worms in the skin, lungs, and intestines of animals made hyperimmune by repeated infections. Similar reactions were observed by Oliver-Gonzalez (1940), Roth (1941), and Mauss (1941) with *Trichinella spiralis*; by Otto (1940) with *Ancylostoma caninum*; by Lawler (1940) with *Strongyloides ratti*; by Otto et al. (1942) with *Necator americanus*; by Oliver-Gonzalez (1943) with *Ascaris lumbricoides*; and by Smith (1946) with *Trichosomoides crassicauda*. Additional observations of this type have been recorded with certain avian nematodes as well. The Russian worker, Lejkina, adapted this test in 1948 for use in diagnosis of *Ascaris* infections (Lejkina, 1965). Numerous workers have since studied this reaction.

The first demonstration that collections of secretions and excretions (ES antigens) might be useful in stimulating protective immunity was that by Thorson (1953). Other workers have since observed this effect with additional worm infections (Table 1). It is apparent from this outline that *Trichinella* has been often used, and it is a good model system aside from the fact that the life cycle is a closed one with the infective forms remaining in the definitive host, thus making separation of adult and larval effects on acquired immunity difficult.

The actual details of collection and administration of ES antigens vary from study to study, so the original publications should be consulted. The practical use of such antigens as prophylactic vaccines will be considered in a later chapter by Dr. Silverman (*see* pp. 1169-1170). The theoretical relationships of such substances to active immunity will be discussed later in this chapter.

Attenuation of infective stages by irradiation. The principle that exposure to products of living worms produces a better protective immunity than to those of dead worms has been amplified by the use of various radiation sources to weaken the infective stages so that they will not complete their life cycle in the host but will remain sufficiently long to release ES antigens and stimulate a protective immunity. However, the radiation dose should not be so great as to prevent completely any development of larval stages in the host as well.

Infective larvae of *Trichinella* exposed to various doses of Co^{60} produced

Table 1
Production of Protective Immunity to Direct-Infection Nematodes with ES Antigens

Date	Author	Parasite	Source of ES Antigen
1953	Thorson	*Nippostrongylus brasiliensis*	Infective larvae
1955	Campbell	*Trichinella spiralis*	Infective larvae
1956	Chute	*Trichinella spiralis*	Infective larvae
1956a, b	Thorson	*Ancylostoma caninum*	Adult esophagus
1957	Chipman	*Trichinella spiralis*	Adults
1957	Soulsby	*Ascaris lumbricoides*	Infective larvae
1961	Ewert and Olson	*Trichinella spiralis*	Infective larvae
1962	Silverman et al.	*Dictyocaulus viviparus*	Fourth-stage larvae
		Trichostrongylus colubriformis	Fourth-stage larvae
		Strongyloides papillosus	Fourth-stage larvae
1965	Mills and Kent	*Trichinella spiralis*	Infective larvae

protection in rats against later challenge doses (Gomberg and Gould, 1953; Gould et al., 1955). There were few second generation infective larvae in the muscles since the radiation apparently sterilized the adults which developed from the initial infection. Controlled irradiation has been used to determine if immunity can be engendered by pre-adults, adults, and/or muscle larvae. It appears that pre-adults alone may produce a low degree of immunity, but that adults and pre-adults produce a more solid immunity. These experiments were done in rats, but Cabrera and Gould (1964) have induced similar resistance in swine by administration of irradiated larvae.

Larsh et al. (1959) and Zaiman et al. (1961) have also studied immunity produced with irradiated trichina larvae. Zaiman's very interesting studies with parabiotic rats demonstrate that the immunity developed with irradiated larvae of trichina is also present in the nonexposed parabiotic mate, indicating a generalized humoral immunity or antigenic stimulation which does not require the stimulation of pre-adult and adult residence in the intestinal wall of the nonexposed individual.

The Glasgow group (Urquhart, Jarrett, and Mulligan) has contributed much to the use of irradiated larvae as producers of protective immunity (*see* review by Urquhart et al., 1962), even to the development of a commercial vaccine composed of irradiated larvae for *Dictyocaulus* spp. (lung worms of cattle and sheep). The Yugoslavian workers, Sokolic et al. (1963), have also developed a vaccine for the sheep lung worm, *Dictyocaulus filaria*.

Miller (1965a,c) has studied the immunity engendered in dogs to irradiated infective larvae of *Ancylostoma caninum*. He has carefully studied dosage and routes of administration. Interestingly, the vaccination was even more effective if there was also a continued low level stimulus of natural infection, called a "trickle" infection. This clearly suggests a need for repeated stimulation much like that required for the immunity developed in dogs with natural infections. One very important factor to be considered in hookworm infection is that puppies in high endemic areas are practically all prenatally infected. The bitches, apparently immune, seem to concentrate the undeveloped larvae, and these are transferred to the fetal pups who have no appreciable immunity. This interpretation should be re-examined in light of the report of Stone and Girardeau (1968). They found that infection with hookworm occurred in the neonate and was transmitted to the puppies in the milk of bitches.

Using the classical and convenient *Nippostrongylus* infection, Ashley (1964) and Prochazka and Mulligan (1965) have been carefully studying the immune state caused by irradiated larvae. Their results clearly illustrate that too low a dose of radiation is not suitable to prevent complete development of larvae and too large a dose prevents good immunity from developing. It would also appear that the forms which migrate through the lungs and return to the intestine for a period will stimulate a higher degree of immunity than those reaching only the lungs. Here, contrary to the findings of Zaiman et al. (1954) with parabiotic rats and *Trichinella*, the intestinal phase seems to be necessary for a high degree of protection.

Chemically (therapeutically) abbreviated infections. The use of effective anthelmintics to remove worms before they mature is similar to the above-mentioned types of stimulation of protective immunity, i.e., the worms live long enough to produce ES antigens and possibly to stimulate or sensitize infected tissues. Practically, one would have to know with reasonable precision when the host was infected to use this method effectively. However, in laboratory helminth infections it has great utility in studies of immune mechanisms. Unfortunately, all anthelmintics are not equally effective against pre-adult stages of parasites. Thiabendazole is effective against these, and it has been used by Campbell et al. (1963) to remove pre-adults of *Trichinella* (after one day). They have been able to show substantial protection against challenge infections 30 days later. Campbell and Timinski (1965) also removed *Ascaris suum* before the lung phase (in rats), and these hosts were resistant to a challenge infection. Denham (1966), using *Trichinella* in mice, was able to terminate infections with methyridine. He found, however, that if the infection was terminated after 48 hours, no immunity developed, though termination after 3 to 4 days produced a good immunity. The fourth-stage larva undergoes its molt at this time. This is of interest in relation to the "self-cure" phenomenon to be discussed later (*see* pp. 937-939). The discrepancy in the results reported by Denham and by Campbell also needs to be explained.

Young lambs which were infected daily for 6 days (at 66 to 71 days of age) with *Haemonchus contortus* were treated on days 73 and 77 with thiabendazole (Christie and Brambell, 1966). On days 84 through 92, they were given eight additional doses of *Haemonchus*. Thiabendazole was used again on days 94 and 98. On their 108th day, the animals resisted a challenge of 50,000 *Haemonchus* quite effectively. It is apparent that a role was played by the repeated stimulus with molting fluid as the third stage larvae went to fourth stage. There will be further discussion of the molting fluid stimulus (*see* p. 933).

Transfer of immunologically competent cells. The transfer of immunologically competent cells from an immunized host to a susceptible host may be considered as a passive type of immunization. However, some of the transferred cells have the potencies of primitive cells. If they are stimulated properly, they may actively produce offspring which will be effective antibody-producers, utilizing the metabolic effort of the new host. This type of study is limited in direct-infection nematodes, but some work has been done on the subject and comment is necessary.

Typically, studies on transfer of immunologically competent cells in direct nematode infections have involved as yet poorly understood mechanisms, even in purified antigen-antibody systems. Hunter and Leigh (1961), using lymph node and spleen cells from *Nippostrongylus*-immunized mice, could not demonstrate a protective effect with transplanted cells. C. A. Crandall (1965) was unable to demonstrate adoptive immunity to *Ascaris* using either peritoneal exudate or spleen cells. Larsh et al. (1964) described an unsuccessful attempt to transfer immunity with lymph node cells from *Trichinella*-sensitized mice. However, two later publications (Larsh et al.,

1966a,b) establish the fact that peritoneal exudate cells from *Trichinella*-infected donor mice caused a significant loss of adult worms in a challenge infection in the recipient mice. They explained the results on the basis of serologic and histopathologic evidence as being due to delayed hypersensitivity. One important facet of these studies was the fact that the challenge infections were given 21 days after the inoculation of sensitized cells. If the immune response is to be considered strictly cellular, this fact implies a rather long lifetime for the cells.

Wagland and Dineen (1965) injected both sera and mesenteric lymph node cells from guinea pigs sensitized with *Trichostrongylus colubriformis* into an isogenic strain of normal guinea pigs. Cells alone and sera alone were likewise injected into additional guinea pigs. Sera plus sensitized cells and cells alone reduced the susceptibility of normal guinea pigs to infection with *Trichostrongylus*. One anomaly in this study was the fact that animals receiving both sera and sensitized cells had patent infections (although of much lower order than controls); the animals receiving only cells did not become patent. The time lag between cell transfer and challenge cited in the previous work was not a factor in these studies, since challenge occurred one day after transfer. However, the issue is obscured by the addition of sera to cells. The authors caution that since few animals were used, these experiments bear repeating. They concluded that "failure of susceptible guinea pigs to become infected with *T. colubriformis* was due to an immunological reaction in which cellular factors were more important than humoral antibodies." This conclusion seems unwarranted. Sensitized cells injected into the peritoneal cavity, if they have an effect, must operate through a humoral response to show any activity in the intestinal lumen. All the successful studies can be explained on the basis of Nossal's careful review (1962) of the cellular genetics of immune responses. Lymph nodes or peritoneal exudates contain a large number of cells, but even though a large percentage are already committed, there are usually a few primitive cells. Primitive lymphocytes are capable of tremendous proliferation so that a few of the transferred cells may develop a whole new "effector" population of plasma cells capable of specific antibody synthesis. As Nossal so carefully states, our knowledge of the cytology of antibody formation is in the same confused state that it was 15 or 20 years ago, particularly with respect to the primitive ancestors and intermediates of the plasma cells. The unsuccessful trials may be explained as a rejection of the inoculated and sensitized cells on the basis of genetic heterogeneity of the hosts. The positive trials discussed above used the usual graft criteria as evidence for isogenicity.

The possible role of macrophages serving as intermediaries in "activation" of antigens before lymphoid cells are stimulated, as suggested by Ada and Lang (1966), should be carefully considered in the above discussions.

Abnormal locations for living stages. The stimulation of protective immunity by placing living nematodes at various stages of their life cycle in abnormal locations in the host should be useful in a study of the mechanisms of such immunity. Soulsby (1957) and Berger and Wood (1964) studied the effects of subcutaneous inoculation of infective eggs of *Ascaris* into guinea pigs and rabbits, respectively. Both studies indicated a rather high degree of protective immunity. In rabbits, a host in which *Ascaris* will mature, Berger and Wood (1964) observed that though the infective eggs were placed in an abnormal location, the larvae hatched and went through a normal migration to the intestinal lumen.

It would appear to be essential that in such studies, no matter in what abnormal location the larval stages are placed, they should be restricted to that site. Crandall and Arean (1965) observed the effectiveness of second-stage larvae of *Ascaris* placed in diffusion chambers intraperitoneally. This produced an immune state equivalent to that produced by ES antigens but not as good as infection by the normal route. This has been also demonstrated by Despommier and Wostmann (1968), who placed larvae of *Trichinella* in intraperitoneally planted Millipore diffusion capsules in mice. Thus, there is an exchange of worm and host products in the milieu, and they have shown that a protective immunity (60 to 80 percent) is produced to challenge infection. One problem in all such implantation studies is that the host tissue reaction may, after some time, restrict diffusion of worm materials through the Millipore membranes.

Although such methods do not suggest practical immunization measures, they are most useful in analytical studies.

Problems in production of purified antigens. The production of purified antigens from direct-infection nematodes has been characterized by Tanner (1963) as "an art usually peculiar to the investigator proposing them." He makes a strong and legitimate plea for standardization so that other laboratories may duplicate the work.

Much of the work done in this particular area has centered on *Trichinella spiralis*, and one of the great difficulties is to isolate infective larvae which are free of the host substances. The studies with such forms as *Ancylostoma caninum* (the dog hookworm) and *Nippostrongylus brasiliensis* require that the infective larvae be separated from the bacteria in the usual feces-charcoal culture. Of course, *in vitro* cultivation should surmount some of these difficulties, but again the present culture media are sufficiently complex to present a similar problem, i.e., the media ingredients must also be separated from the worms and their products.

The production of large quantities of antigens capable of stimulating protective antibodies is also a very difficult problem. Silverman (1963) has reviewed the useful *in vitro* cultivation procedures. This approach seems the most potentially useful in production of adequate antigen. A much more rigorous control of chronologic development in culture is needed if there is, as will be discussed later (*see* pp. 931-933), a qualitative and quantitative difference in antigens elaborated by different stages of the parasites. When all the environmental and individual stimuli needed for this control are known, this goal will be reached. This emphasizes, however, the very great need for work on the ecology and physiology of these helminths so that the goal will be reached more quickly.

Methods of separation of specific antigens from helminths are fraught with difficulties. Kent (1963a) describes some interesting chromatographic techniques in the isolation of antigens, which should be consulted. Because of the great number and diversity of potential antigens in direct-infecting helminths, ever-increasing doses of ingenuity will be required.

One precaution which must be observed as much as possible is to avoid physicochemical changes in the antigens during fractionation. Tanner (1965) showed that saline extracts of *Trichinella* larvae, when treated with 2-mercaptoethanol to cleave disulfide bridges and then alkylated to insure the integrity of the split, produced an antigen which resembled normal human serum albumin in double diffusion studies. This illustrates the necessity of gentle treatment of any antigenic preparation from direct-infection helminths.

Antigenic components of helminths

The sheer size and complexity of direct-infecting helminths increase enormously the number of possible antigenic components which can be isolated. Any molecule of sufficient size to be antigenically stimulatory and which can in some way be introduced into the hosts' antibody-forming system will, if sufficiently different from the materials of the host, cause the production of an antibody to it. Organisms with digestive, nervous, excretory, muscular, and exoskeletal systems are characterized by large numbers of what we will call somatic antigens (structural antigens). In addition, each of these systems contains large numbers of molecules which play a role in the physiologic maintenance of the system and the ultimate life of the worm in the host. These, we will characterize as physiologic antigens.

Also, though less well-studied, there is the group of antigens which can be called host-parasite antigens, i.e., substances from worm and host which in combination are sufficiently unique to be recognized as "non-host" materials by the hosts' antibody-forming centers. This category includes the possibly antigenic antigen-antibody complexes which have been formed in the host undergoing immunization. The qualitative and quantitative responses of the host to these compounds may be quite different from those to the antigen alone (*see* Harshman and Najjar, 1963).

Somatic antigens. Somatic antigens may be prepared in a number of ways. Whole worms may be ground up and used as suspensions or for preparing saline extracts. Ground-up worms may be extracted with aqueous or polar solvents and fractionated in several ways so that various biochemical fractions are obtained. If the worms are sufficiently large, such as *Ascaris* or *Ancylostoma*, isolated tissues, such as cuticle, muscle, intestine, or coelomic fluid, may be extracted. It should be recognized that in extracts of worms for somatic antigens, there will also be limited quantities of physiologic antigens present.

One of the most commonly used systems has been that developed by

Melcher (1943) for *Trichinella* antigens. This method consists of delipidization with ether, extraction of the residue with buffered saline, precipitation of the acid-insoluble components, and harvesting of acid-soluble components from the supernate. The acid-insoluble components are albumin-like; the acid-soluble components are globulin-like. Campbell (1936) also isolated an antigenically active polysaccharide fraction from *Ascaris* by repeated precipitations of a borate-buffer extract with cold alcohol.

Oliver-Gonzalez (1943) and Kagan (1957) used, instead of whole worms (*Ascaris*), isolated tissues, such as cuticle, muscle, enteric fluid, and eggs, to demonstrate various antigens. As might be expected, even these more selective isolations produced a broad mosaic of antigens. In most instances the isolation procedures were such that the antigens were predominantly proteins.

Until recently, the methods of extraction and characterization of somatic antigens has lacked precision, particularly with respect to complexes of proteins with lipids and polysaccharides. Defatted whole-worm extracts (*Ascaris, Trichinella*) have been separated into several well-characterized antigens by DEAE-Sephadex column fractionation (Kent 1960, 1963a, b). As an example, five fractions from an aqueous extract of *Ascaris* were obtained by elution with NaCl solutions of increasing normality. Interestingly, the first fraction eluted contained 80 percent protein and 20 percent carbohydrate; the second fraction, 86 percent protein and 14 percent carbohydrate; the third fraction, 99.5 percent protein and no carbohydrate; the fourth fraction, 23 percent protein and 76 percent carbohydrate; and the fifth fraction, 37 percent protein and 65 percent carbohydrate. All the fractions are apparently single compounds and are antigenically active. However, the third fraction (all protein) was much less antigenic than the other fractions, all of which contained some polysaccharide. This illustrates the necessity for using extraction methods which preserve protein-polysaccharide complexes. Additional studies using column chromatography for the extraction of complement-fixing antigens from *Trichinella* should be consulted (Sleeman, 1961; Sleeman and Muschel, 1961).

Only recently have proper and more sophisticated techniques been used to isolate and characterize biochemically the somatic antigens of direct-infection nematodes. Much yet needs to be done.

Physiologic antigens.   Here again, the study of substances with physiologic activities isolated from direct-infection nematodes is still in its infancy. Thorson (1953) demonstrated that ES antigens prepared from infective larvae of *Nippostrongylus* showed lipolytic activity. These preparations were far from pure, but they contained enzymatic activity and produced protective immunity in rats. In addition, sera from rats made resistant to *Nippostrongylus* by repeated infections inhibited the lipolytic activity of these preparations. Another example of antigens with physiologic activity is provided by the work of Rhodes et al. (1964, 1965, 1966), who isolated purified malic dehydrogenase and aminopeptidase from whole worms (*Ascaris suum*). They used these preparations as antigens and demonstrated rather appreciable protection in pigs.

Similarly, Thorson (1956a,b) demonstrated proteolytic activity in extracts of the esophagus of the dog hookworm, *Ancylostoma caninum*. These extracts, when injected into young puppies, produced a low degree of active immunity as evidenced by reduced worm burdens and smaller worms in challenge infections. Subsequently, Thorson (1963) reported that there was similar activity in esophagus and intestinal extracts of *Ascaris lumbricoides* and *Toxocara canis*. Peptidase and lipolytic activities were also noted in all of these extracts.

This type of study is very rewarding and further work along these lines is necessary to substantiate some of the theories of functional mechanisms in immunity, which will be discussed later (*see* pp. 947-953).

Other substances which play an important role in stimulating of protective immunity are the so-called hatching fluids and molting or exsheathing fluids. These have been investigated in several direct-infection nematodes. Soulsby showed in 1961 that the effective stimulation of immunity in the host to *Ascaris* infection was most marked when the parasite was going through a molt. This was presumably due to the release of appreciable quantities of molting fluid. Further studies by Stewart (1953), Soulsby et al. 1959), and Soulsby and Stewart (1960) showed that the molt from the third to fourth larval stage of *Haemonchus* was the essential stimulus for the termination of an infection.

Sommerville (1957) and Rogers and Sommerville (1960) studied the nature of the exsheathing fluid of *Haemonchus* and found that its release was stimulated by low oxygen tensions (i.e. high CO_2 tensions). This fluid contains protein and a low molecular weight cofactor. Rogers (1963) has shown that the hatching fluid of *Ascaris* contains substances with chitinase and esterase activities. Exsheathing fluid of *Haemonchus* contains a leucine aminopeptidase. Needless to say, much study needs to be done with these substances, and the preparation of large samples is necessary for a proper characterization of their physiologic and immunologic functions in nematode-host relations. Silverman et al. (1962) described the collection of such materials and their use to produce protective immunity in laboratory animals. They used larval stages of *Dictyocaulus viviparus*, *Trichostrongylus colubriformis*, and *Strongyloides papillosus*.

It is apparent that molting or exsheathing fluids serve as antigenic stimuli and they possess physiologic activity. This area deserves concentrated attention since it is entirely conceivable that other substances with physiologic activity, such as hormones, may be present in such preparations of *Trichinella* (Thorson et al., 1968).

Humoral versus cellular acquired immunity

Historically, there has been a controversy between those who felt that humoral antibodies were most important in acquired immunity and those who felt that certain cellular elements were the chief instruments of protection. For the most part, this reflected a lack of understanding of the mediation of cellular elements stimulated by antibody. It is now recognized that there are humoral reactions between antigens and antibodies and that cells also play a role in the defense mechanisms of the host. Frequently, the role of cells in these reactions was established by studying histologic reactions in tissues of affected organs in immunized hosts. The chronology of such reactions was poorly understood. The initiation of a cellular lesion around a worm might well have been due to an initial reaction between an antigen from the worm and antibody from the host, assuming prior experience of the host with that particular parasite. The accumulation of cellular elements might be mediated by the antibody, as might the opportunity for cells to gather around the helminth. In the nonimmune host, the worm is probably able to move at will and thus there is no opportunity for cells to collect.

Types of antibodies. Helminthologists engaged in studies of immunity have for the most part not adopted the classification of antibodies proposed by immunologists for the immunoglobulins. In addition, little work has been done to determine which of the immunoglobulins are involved in humoral immunity to direct-infection helminths. It is likely that γM (19S) antibodies appear after initial stimulation by an antigen and are followed by the production of γG (7S) antibodies, at which time production of γM usually ceases or proceeds at a slower rate. This is generally the case, and it probably is true of immunity to helminths (Soulsby, 1965).

One of the greatest deterrents to careful and accurate identification of the exact nature of immunoglobulins in direct-infection nematode immunity has been the lack of a clearly isolated antigen-antibody system.

Rose et al. (1964) assumed from ultracentrifugal fractionation of sera taken from pigs infected with *Stephanurus dentatus* that the antibodies were 7S globulins (i.e., γG). This seems reasonable, but it does not negate the possibility that γM antibodies had also been present, since the sera were taken from swine infected for 2.5 months. Sera taken earlier in the course of infection may have revealed the heavier antibodies.

Mauss (1941) ingeniously demonstrated that the protective effect of anti-*Trichinella* serum and the antibodies capable of precipitating secretions and excretions of larvae *in vitro* were both (if not identical) in the γ-globulin fraction which was isolated by ammonium sulfate fractionation. Whether the antibodies were γG or γM was not determined, since these differences in antibodies were unknown at that time.

A most interesting observation is that of Douvres 1962), who isolated antibodies from various extracts of tissues (cecum and colon) of cattle, which precipitated secretions and excretions of *Oesophagostomum*. However, sera from the same animals did not cause a similar precipitation. This anomalous result can be explained in two possible ways: 1. The antibodies were formed and acted in a localized area, or 2. The presence of worms in these tissues marshalled all the specific antibodies from the sera in these tissues. The wealth of data on the presence of such precipitating antibodies in serum in other nematode infections makes the latter explanation probably more valid.

With the exquisite and useful technique of immunoelectrophoresis developed by Grabar and co-workers (*see* Grabar and Burtin, 1964), it should be now possible to follow the formation of various types of antibody chronologically through the course of an infection with a direct-infecting nematode.

Ogilvie (1967) has drawn attention to the fact that antibodies resembling human reagins are produced in rats infected with *Nippostrongylus brasiliensis*. These antibodies are not detectable by ordinary *in vitro* methods, but they have the ability to sensitize the skin of normal individuals passively. In this host-parasite relationship, the "reagins" are rather long-lived and are detectable up to 7 months after a single infection.

Types of cells. The role of cells in immunity to direct-infection helminths is not completely understood. One must differentiate between a cellular function in antibody production and a direct effect of cells on the infection. The antibody-forming function has been discussed in an earlier section (*see* pp. 928-929).

Ackert and Edgar (1939) suggested the possible role of goblet cells (secretory cells in the intestinal epithelium) in age and natural resistance. For the most part, their work was with *Ascaridia galli*. Whur (1966) has discussed the relationship of the globular leukocytes to infections with sheep gastrointestinal nematodes and *Nippostrongylus* in rats. These leukocytes are characterized (in stained sections) by strongly acidophilic intracytoplasmic globules which are spherical and usually 10 to 20 in number. The nucleus is peripheral and resembles that of a plasmocyte. In worm-free sheep, the average number of these cells per sq mm of gastric mucosa is less than one. In sheep experimentally infected with *Ostertagia circumcincta*, there were 25 and 93 cells per sq mm. Animals naturally infected with the lung worms *Muellerius* and *Dictyocaulus* had 24 to 26 globule leukocytes per sq mm.

In a careful study of experimental infections with *Nippostrongylus brasiliensis*, Whur found the following:

Day after infection	Number of worms*	Number of globule leukocytes/sq mm in intestinal mucosa
2	36	0
4	892	0
6	207	0
8	1,225	0
10	266	0
12	15	116
14	15	154
16	1	582
18	0	600
20	0	153

* Infecting dose = 3,500 larvae. At each sampling time one rat was necropsied. From Whur, P. 1966. *J. Comp. Path.*, 76:57-65.

Whur feels that the worms are responsible for the presence of the globule leukocytes because the numbers of leukocytes are greatest at the infection sites. In addition, the increase in the number of cells to the maximum on day

18 also coincides with the time of "self-cure." The actual function of these cells was not suggested. Dobson (1966), using the direct fluorescent-antibody test, has demonstrated that the globules of these leukocytes contain condensed globulins. In addition, he suggests that similar globules are found in plasma cells, indicating a possible relationship between plasma cells, known to be antibody producers, and the globule leukocytes, which also may produce antibodies.

In a clever demonstration of the interdependence of cellular and humoral factors, R. B. Crandall (1965) showed that a positive chemotaxis of polymorphonuclear leukocytes was observable when antigenically complex ES or saline extracts of *Trichinella* were incubated in anti-*Trichinella* immune sera or immune gamma-globulin from rats or rabbits. He also showed that *Ascaris suum* extracts were chemotactic for leukocytes in normal serum which was not inactivated. A labile serum component seemed to be necessary for this effect. These observations may help to explain the heavier infiltration of cellular elements around parasites of second, third, and later infections.

It has been demonstrated that mast cells with a suitably adsorbed antibody can be disrupted very quickly by the injection of a helminth antigen (Goldgraber and Lewert, 1965; Briggs, 1963a,b). This disruption of cells is known to release pharmacologically active substances (histamine, 5-hydroxytryptamine, and bradykinin). These substances may act on susceptible tissues at the site of infection by nematodes or at more distant points. Mast cells and their products will be discussed more fully in the section on anaphylaxis (*see* pp. 950-951).

Larsh et al. (1966a,b) reported that transplants of peritoneal exudate cells from *Trichinella*-infected donors to noninfected recipients caused a significant loss of adult worms of the challenge infection in these recipients. Since the actual quantitative and qualitative composition of the exudate is unclear, it is difficult to say whether the delayed hypersensitivity was due to cellular action alone or to intervention by antibody-forming cells. Further clarification is necessary to answer this question.

Wagland and Dineen (1965) state categorically that the transfer of mesenteric lymph node cells from resistant to susceptible guinea pigs is responsible for protection against *Trichostrongylus colubriformis* in the latter and is due to "an immunological reaction in which cellular factors are more important than humoral antibodies." Their data, however, are subject to other explanations, since the cells were transplanted intraperitoneally and the worms develop within the intestine. Also, immune serum was injected with the cells in some of the experimental animals.

Dual (or multiple) basis of antibody formation

Much speculation and experimental work have been directed at the possible delineation of qualitatively different antibodies directed at various stages of a helminth parasite in a host. An example of an infection in which this has been studied intensively is *Trichinella*. All the stages of the life cycle occur in the same host; the ingested infected meat introduces first-stage larvae which rapidly go through four molts to become adults. The adult female worms deposit rudimentary larvae (called a pre-larva by Khan, 1966) in the intestinal mucosa, which migrate to the muscles, develop into first-stage larvae, and are encysted. Oliver-Gonzalez (1941) first suggested that there was a dual antibody basis for acquired immunity in trichinosis and that some of the antibodies against the tissue larvae were not identical to those against the adults.

Some workers have felt that the antibodies to larvae and adults are similar and that the antigens of the two stages differ only quantitatively (Ross, 1952; Chute, 1956; Jackson, 1959). Certainly, there probably are quantitative differences, but Oliver-Gonzalez (1941), Hendricks (1952), and Ivey (1965) felt that qualitative differences exist between the antigens of larvae and adults. This view has given rise to the dual antibody theory. Actually "dual" may be a misnomer, since if the theory is valid, there may be more than two stages elaborating qualitatively different antigens and thus stimulating more than two types of antibody. Oliver-Gonzalez and Levine (1962) showed differences in the number of bands produced in gel-diffusion plates (three bands against larval antigens and two against adult antigens). One must interpret this difference cautiously because low concentrations of antigens in gel-diffusion studies may cause the loss of single bands.

A more adequate comparison of the ES antigens from adults and larvae of *Trichinella* is suggested by the writer. Each can be prepared according to the methods of Campbell (1955) or Chute (1956) for the larvae and of Chipman (1957) for adults. Recent techniques for isolating large numbers of adult *Trichinella* may facilitate this study (McCue and Thorson, 1963). Standardization and equilibration of the two antigens is a necessity. The results of Chipman and of Campbell illustrate that from the protective standpoint, the ES antigens from both adults and larvae stimulated immunity against all stages.

The important findings regarding hatching and/or exsheathing or molting fluids should lead to further productive research along these lines.

Self-cure and premunition

Self-cure and premunition are two commonly used words in the study of helminth immunity. The latter term, premunition, is a state of relative immunity in which low numbers of parasites persist in the host and stimulate the immune state. As stated in the World Health Organization Expert Committee Report on immunology and parasitic diseases (1965), premunition is not a special immunologic phenomenon needing new concepts for its explanation. Although, by its definition, it can describe the immune state in some helminth infections, the excessive vocabulary which has arisen may dictate the word's demise.

Self-cure as a functional term was introduced by Stoll (1929) to describe the marked rapid loss of *Haemonchus contortus* by sheep and their subsequent immunity to further infection. Self-cure has been studied carefully by many workers, but it again, as with premunition, can be explained by conventional immunologic terms.

Stewart (1953) found that in sheep infected with *Haemonchus* and properly sensitized, a challenge dose of *Haemonchus* infective larvae would cause a sudden and dramatic loss of the adult worms. Serologic studies illustrated that the titer of complement-fixing (CF) antibodies rose immediately after the challenge, but Stewart felt they played no role in the self-cure. The relation of the test antigen and resulting antibody with protective systems has not been clarified. One might suggest that in the sensitized host the sudden rise in antibody is an anamnestic response similar to those seen in bacterial immunizations.

Blood histamine levels rose at the same time as the CF antibody titers. This could possibly be explained as the effect of an antibody-cell conjugate and subsequent lysis of mast cells by antigen exposure (*see* pp. 950-951). This pharmacologically active substance may cause increased gastrointestinal motility and marked edema, and both factors could well make the abomasum an unsuitable parasitic environment. The histamine rise occurs between the second and fourth days of superinfection and is contemporaneous with the molt of the third-stage larva to the fourth stage (Soulsby et al., 1959; Soulsby and Stewart, 1960). It is suspected that the antigenic stimulus comes from the exsheathing fluid released by the larvae during molting. After the initial rapid loss of worms, the animals remain immune for a period of time. The persistent immunity after self-cure is seen to decline, and the serologic response in agar-gel diffusion plates indicates a loss of lines which react with exsheathing fluid (Soulsby, 1960). Much of this work has been done with experimental infections in lambs, but it is also important in natural infections since lambs with a naturally acquired burden of worms show a self-cure reaction at the time when the populations of infective larvae on the pasture are highest. The self-cure has been described by Stewart (1950) as a violent hypersensitive reaction.

It should be emphasized that the self-cure reaction is not restricted to *Haemonchus* in sheep, but it also occurs in infections with other gastrointestinal nematodes. Mulligan et al. (1965) and Barth et al. (1966) studied the mechanism of self-cure in infections with *Nippostrongylus brasiliensis*. This phenomenon is not exactly identical to that of *Haemonchus* since in the latter it is quite apparent that a challenge infection with infective larvae, which molt from third to fourth stage, is the stimulus. All who have worked with *Nippostrongylus* in the laboratory rat recognize that after an initial infection with 500 or more infective larvae, there is maturation, egg laying, and towards the end of the second week of infection, there is a sudden drop in egg production followed by a rapid expulsion of the worms.* It will be seen

---

*Unawareness of this fact has led to the loss of many laboratory strains of *Nippostrongylus*.

that this self-cure is unlike that described for *Haemonchus* in that an additional challenging dose of infective larvae is not needed. The stimulus apparently comes from the initial infection. Actually, in preparing hyperimmune sera in rats by multiple infection, there may be a basis for a *Haemonchus*-type of self-cure, but this has not been studied in detail with *Nippostrongylus*. In an effort to delineate the mechanism of the *Nippostrongylus* self-cure reaction, Mulligan et al. (1965) and Barth et al. (1966) proposed three hypotheses:

1. The antibody acts directly on the worm;
2. The antibody does not act directly on the worm but creates a state of hypersensitivity in the intestine by, for example, fixed antibody and antigen from the worm reacting to produce a local anaphylactic response and thus creating an unsuitable environment in the intestine for the worm;
3. Increased permeability of the capillaries associated with the local anaphylactic reaction might permit significant extravascular leakage of plasma into the subepithelial spaces of the villi or intestinal lumen.

To test this last hypothesis, these workers sensitized rats to ovalbumin, transferred adult worms into the intestine of these rats, and two days later intraperitoneally injected a dose of hyperimmune serum to *Nippostrongylus*. Eighteen hours after the serum treatment the rats were shocked with ovalbumin. Necropsy 18 hours after shock and subsequent worm enumeration demonstrated that hosts receiving hyperimmune serum and shock harbored fewer worms than rats receiving hyperimmune serum alone, shock alone, or normal serum. The pathology of the intestinal location of worms showed large fluid filled spaces between the blood vessels and epithelium of the villi, and these permitted extravascular leakage into villi and lumen. These lesions are marked and occur as early as four days after infection with larvae and two days after transplants of adult worms. At the time of self-cure they are most pronounced. The lesions can be produced in other systems, e.g., by an ovalbumin-pertussis shocking system, but worm removal will not result unless hyperimmune serum to the parasite is present. These authors concluded that a leak lesion and contact of antiworm antibodies with the worms are necessary for self-cure.

It is apparent that much remains to be clarified in these two types of self-cure reactions, but the work of the past 10 years has added much to our ideas.

Role of hypersensitivity

Hypersensitivity may be classified in various ways, but Osler (1963) gives a very useful outline. Hypersensitivity can be divided basically into reactions mediated by serum antibody, the immediate or anaphylactic type, and into reactions mediated by cell-associated reactants, i.e., delayed hypersensitivity.

Much effort has been devoted to skin reactions in helminth infections which are dependent on a hypersensitive state. This effort may lead to the development of precise diagnostic antigens. The aim of the present discussion is to consider whether hypersensitivity *per se* plays a role in active acquired immunity. The discussion in the previous section on self-cure would suggest that such is the case. It is very difficult to derive clearcut cause and effect relationships in this regard, but recent work by Olson and his co-workers (1961, 1963) and Briggs (1963a,b) has helped clarify this issue considerably. Anaphylactic shock has been produced to direct-infection nematodes such as *Ascaris*, *Trichinella*, and *Toxocara* (Oliver-Gonzalez, 1946; Sprent and Chen, 1949; Sprent, 1949, 1950, 1951; Werle and Ringler, 1951; Matsumura et al., 1955; Matsumura, 1963; Sharp and Olson, 1962). Thus, there is ample evidence that sensitization of hosts to nematodes can occur. Anaphylactic shock is, however, a violent reaction characterized by an overwhelming shocking dose of antigen and by severe side effects. Except in rare instances, this would not be the usual useful mode of action of hypersensitivity if the latter contributes to mechanisms of active immunity in infection. It is possible to demonstrate increased contractility of smooth muscle in the intestine of sensitized animals when the tissues are exposed to very small doses of antigen (Sharp and Olson, 1962). This conceivably could hasten the intestinal emptying time (as in the previously cited work on self-cure) and cause a loss of worms of an early or later infection.

In tests of hypersensitivity (Schultz-Dale reactions and passive cutaneous anaphylaxis) with *Toxocara*, *Trichinella*, and *Ascaris*, Ivey (1965) and Sharp and Olson (1962) observed some antigenic cross-reactions in guinea pigs, but the reactions were always stronger with homologous than with heterologous antigens. This points up again the very great need for using species-specific antigens. Of note is Ivey's statement that "though variable, there were striking quantitative differences between stage-specific and heterologous antigens." There was marked correlation between Schultz-Dale and passive cutaneous anaphylaxis reactions but poor correlation with hemagglutination and gel-diffusion tests, indicating qualitative differences in the antigen-antibody systems mediating each.

The effect of antigen on mast cells in sensitized hosts has been studied in *Trichinella* infections (Briggs 1963a,b) and in *Strongyloides ratti* infection by Goldgraber and Lewert (1965). This reaction is an extremely sensitive tool for observing the hypersensitive state. It also is one of the best ways of showing in passive transfers that serum contains sensitizing antibody. This reaction will be discussed later in this chapter (*see* pp. 950-951).

Eosinophilia, which so commonly accompanies helminth infections and especially those with nematodes, is certainly bound up in an as yet unclear way with hypersensitivity. Loeffler's syndrome (or similar conditions characterized by a transient eosinophilia) and radiologic changes in the lungs are of interest (Danaraj and Schacher, 1957). These conditions must be separated from the condition of eosinophilic lung which Danaraj and Schacher feel may be due to exposure to filarial worms. Epidemiologically, conditions similar or identical to Loeffler's syndrome occur often in nonfilarial areas. For example,

Gelpi and Mustafa (1967) have reported a high incidence of a pneumonic condition characterized by high eosinophilia in Saudi Arabians. This occurs in the spring after the winter rains when eggs of nematodes would have a reasonable chance of surviving the vicissitudes of the desert elements and of becoming infective. At the same time, dust storms are quite prevalent. Third-stage infective larvae of *Ascaris* have been isolated from the sputum of these patients. It is tempting to speculate that the eosinophilia and pulmonary symptoms are due to the inhabitants of these areas having been sensitized at an earlier time by infections with adults of *Ascaris*. Interestingly, the winter of 1965-1966 was essentially rain free and no cases of the seasonal Loeffler's syndrome were seen.

Ivey and Slanga (1965) evaluated passive cutaneous anaphylaxis (PCA) as a tool for the study of *Trichinella* and *Toxocara* antigen-antibody systems and found some cross-reactions. Again, the writer suggests that antigens are not sufficiently specific. The exquisite sensitivity of PCA in detecting minute amounts of antigen and antibody (Osler, 1963) place this test in the foreground of techniques to be further studied.

Larsh et al. (1964, 1966a,b) were unable to demonstrate delayed or cellular hypersensitivity to *Trichinella* in mice by transfer of lymph node cells, but transfer of peritoneal exudate cells, the latter stimulated by an injection of warm mineral oil, caused an acceleration in the rate of casting off of adult worms of a challenge infection. Kim (1966), in a careful study, outlined the requisites of delayed hypersensitivity and was able to demonstrate that all were fulfilled in guinea pigs infected with *Trichinella*. He found that his results were more consistent if all of his sensitization injections were in Freund's complete adjuvant. The requisites were: (1) the detection of positive skin test after several hours, (2) peak intensity of the skin reaction at 18 to 24 hours, (3) primarily mononuclear cell infiltration into the skin test site, (4) no detectable circulating antibody, and (5) the transfer of hypersensitivity by cells. In his system all of these requirements were fulfilled, giving unequivocal evidence of delayed hypersensitivity in a *Trichinella*-guinea pig system.

Physical and physiologic factors

Effect of nutrition. As stated earlier, the effect of nutrition on natural immunity is not so easily demonstrated. However, the classic work of Foster and Cort (1932) with *Ancylostoma caninum* and that of Donaldson and Otto (1946) with *Nippostrongylus* (*see also* Cort and Otto, 1940) must be cited. Both of these studies gave similar results. If one attempts to stimulate immunity in a host by repeated infection with the helminth, it was observed that the protection engendered was much more marked in hosts with a good nutritional level than in those with deficient diets (particularly those deficient in protein). Also, in well-nourished hosts which have been immunized, one may demonstrate a loss of the immunity by placing the host on a protein-deficient diet (and in hookworm infections, an iron-deficient diet). Most interesting is the fact that when an adequate diet is restored, the lost immunity is recovered. Therefore, adequate protein in the diet plays a role in the acquisition and maintenance of acquired immunity to helminth infections. The importance of this fact in the hookworm infections of man is obvious. Geographically, hookworm is most commonly found in tropical areas and in epidemic proportions in areas where protein deficiency is a characteristic of life.

Stewart and Gordon (1953) found that sheep which had previously experienced infection with *Trichostrongylus colubriformis* and were then placed on a protein-deficient diet developed more severe infections than similarly experienced controls on an adequate ration. However, if worm-free lambs experiencing their first infection were placed on a protein-deficient diet, there was little difference between them and previously worm-free lambs on a good diet.

With the increasing knowledge of antibody structure and synthesis and with the sophisticated techniques for aminoacid analysis, a study of the necessary aminoacids for antibody synthesis in response to helminth infections would be fruitful.

Larsh and Kent (1949) demonstrated that alcohol will interfere with the development of immunity to *Trichinella* in mice. The exact mechanisms involved are unknown, but drainage of vitamins, particularly vitamin A, from liver stores and other tissues by the alcohol was suspected. Larsh and Gilchrist (1950) were, however, unable to demonstrate any effect of prolonged feeding of vitamin A-deficient diets on acquired immunity.

Effect of stress. It is difficult to explain precisely what constitutes stress, but the factors of stress as usually defined play a role in acquired immunity. Malnutrition, as mentioned in the previous section, is certainly a stress factor and its effect on acquired immunity is obvious. Various types of irradiation can affect immunity, as will be discussed in the next section. However, irradiation is usually a highly artificial laboratory method of stressing animals, and probably no such counterpart exists in naturally exposed hosts.

The presence of worms and their induced pathology in addition to the hosts' response to the worms can cause marked weight loss in mice infected with *Trichinella*. It is of interest that this effect is less marked in immunized animals. The explanation of the weight loss seems to be reduced food intake and possible interference with protein digestion caused by local pathology in the intestine. In immunized mice, the weight loss occurs earlier but weight is recovered more quickly than in nonimmunized mice. This is presumably due to a heightened and accelerated inflammatory response (Yarinsky, 1962) and consequent earlier worm loss.

The sociopsychologic stress of crowding (Davis and Read, 1958) and the effect of intermittent stresses, such as mild electrical stimulation, bright lights, and loud noise (Robinson, 1961) have been cited previously.

Effect of host irradiation. Irradiating the host with increasing dosages affects the acquisition and persistence of acquired immunity. There are two obvious effects of whole body irradiation. First, the usual disturbance and sloughing of intestinal mucosa which occurs in irradiated animals cannot fail to have an effect on the intestinal parasites since their environment is so radically changed. Second, the effect of irradiation on hemopoiesis can hamper development of the antibody-forming cells and the cells active in the inflammatory response.

Low radiation doses, although causing disturbances in white cell numbers and general condition, do not seem to have any marked effect on the immunity of rats to *Trichinella* (Moskwa et al., 1958).

Stoner and Hale (1952) showed that all mice immunized with *Trichinella* prior to exposure to a reasonably heavy dose of radiation (γ-radiation source of Co^{60}) died when challenged with a rather large dose of infective larvae (1,500). Immunized but nonirradiated controls had a high survival rate (74 percent). All nonimmunized mice died as a result of the challenge dose. Precipitin titers in immunized mice remained the same, indicating that the already present antibody was not affected by irradiation. (This statement depends on the fact that the serologic test determined effective protective antibody.) In these experiments, it would appear that the radiation dose (750 rad) was too high and the immunizing doses were too infrequent (once) with too few larvae (100).

Yarinsky (1962) demonstrated that the time between irradiation and infection had much to do with whether there was an interference with the immune response to *Trichinella* in mice when x-ray dosages of 50, 250, 450, and 650 r were used. Antibody titers (hemagglutinating antibody) were not greatly affected, but this is a reflection of an often cited problem about what antibodies are being measured in an *in vitro* test. However, if the complete immune response is involved, one would expect marked differences in all antibodies at high radiation dosages.

It has been suggested that radiation interference with the development of protective immunity in *Trichinella* infections primarily causes damage to the hemopoietic system and there are simply not enough cellular elements to participate in the cellular response (Yarinsky, 1962). It is also conceivable that the damage caused greatly affects antibody-forming cells.

Most of the irradiation studies have been done with mice and it should be pointed out that although there is no evidence that preformed antibody is affected by irradiation, there is a strong possibility that the lifetime of antibody molecules in mice is different from that of antibody molecules in man. Antibody halflife in the mouse is 1 to 2 days, and in man, 14 to 21 days (Talmadge, 1955). If indeed the radiation affects antibody-forming cells whose antibodies mediate a hypersensitivity reaction, the inflammation factors may well be disturbed if the antibody is short-lived.

It would seem advisable to consider the effects of whole body irradiation on other host-parasite systems in which the entire life cycle is not contained in a single host, e.g., on *Nippostrongylus* or *Nematospiroides dubius* infections. With these infections, especially the former, a strong immunity is developed quickly with a single infection. Some of the puzzles which have arisen in the *Trichinella* work may be clarified.

Effect of hormones. Certain hormones, such as cortisone and adrenocorticotropic hormone (ACTH), are known to suppress hypersensitive and inflammatory reactions. It was obvious, then, to determine whether such a characteristic suppression of the cellular response in immune hosts might permit increased development of larvae of direct-infection nematodes.

The classical laboratory infection, *Nippostrongylus* in the rat, seemed an ideal choice for endocrinologic studies of this kind because the nature of this animal's immunity to the parasite is so well-known. Weinstein (1955), using well-immunized rats, demonstrated that cortisone treatment suppressed markedly the usual cellular response in the skin of two groups of treated rats. These groups were: (1) those receiving cortisone throughout the immunizing process and (2) those receiving cortisone starting five days prior to the challenge exposure. The rats of the first group had significantly higher numbers of worms than the nontreated immunized controls; those of the second group were not different from the nontreated immunized controls, indicating that the period of immunization prior to cortisone treatment (25 days) had permitted the development of a high degree of immunity. The *in vitro* precipitate test of Sarles (1938) was positive in all groups. It may be seen from these experiments that cortisone at high dosages can lead to a partial breakdown of the immune response.

Ogilvie (1965), using daily treatments of a cortisone derivative, prednisolone, suppressed the initiation of acquired resistance to *Nippostrongylus*.

PASSIVE IMMUNITY

Humoral passive immunity

There have been many attempts to immunize hosts passively against direct-infection nematodes by injection of immune serum. Sarles (1938) reported success with *Nippostrongylus* in rats, as did Lawler (1940) with *Strongyloides ratti*. However, there were many attempts which were unsuccessful. Even when it was known that the serum was from an animal refractory to infection, there frequently was no demonstrable protection. It can be suggested that in the case of helminth infections, the level of protective antibodies which are present is extremely low though effective in the actively immunized host, and that passive transfer dilutes these antibodies to less than effective levels in the recipient animal.

Jarrett et al. (1955), in an effort to circumvent this possibility, obtained immune sera from six recovered cases of parasitic bronchitis caused by the cattle lung worm, *Dictyocaulus viviparus*. In order to stimulate a high level of protective antibody, they had challenged these calves before bleeding with rather large doses of infective larvae. When the complement-fixing antibodies were at their highest level, the animals were bled and 23 liters of serum were processed. The globulins were separated, and five young calves were treated with globulins equivalent to 500 ml of serum daily for 3 days. Two days later, they were challenged with infective larvae. At necropsy 30 days later, there were fewer worms in the lungs of the passively immunized calves than in the controls. In addition, the pathology usually caused by these worms was markedly reduced in the immunized animals. The amounts of serum used in this carefully executed experiment indicate the feasibility of the above proposal that high concentrations of antibodies are required to create passive immunity.

Rubin and Weber (1955), using whole serum in *Dictyocaulus* infection, showed decreased pathology of passively immunized calves compared to controls. After serious challenge, two of the animals receiving 5 ml serum per pound of body weight survived, whereas all controls died.

It may be concluded that in general, attempts to transfer immunity passively are not consistently successful.

There is, however, another useful method to demonstrate presence of protective antibodies. Several workers (Mauss, 1941; Thorson, 1954a,b; Mills and Kent, 1965) have demonstrated that exposing larvae of nematodes to immune serum for a period of time before feeding or injecting them into the host causes a marked reduction in worm burdens of hosts as compared to those shown by hosts receiving worms exposed to normal serum. Mauss (1941) actually fractionated the serum to recover gamma-globulins which displayed protection. This test has been used in *Nippostrongylus* infections to show absorption of protective antibodies by ES antigens (Thorson, 1954b). A simplification of the test is possible with such worms as *Nippostrongylus*, since their infective larvae are usually inoculated subcutaneously. Simply suspending the larvae in immune serum with no incubation period will result in reduced worm burdens if the serum has protective antibodies present. With *Trichinella* this is not as easy, since the infective larvae are usually given orally and the serum is exposed to proteolytic enzymes in both the stomach and intestine. With this infection, an incubation period is recommended. Mills and Kent (1965) exposed larvae to serum for 15 hours and tested the infectivity of the larvae to normal hosts. They followed the production of protective antibodies in rats undergoing immunization to *Trichinella* in this way. These results seem to suggest that given adequate contact with serum containing protective antibodies, a modified "neutralization" test will demonstrate passive immunity.

Cellular passive immunity

The transplantation of immunologically competent and active cells can represent another type of passive immunity. Transplantation of cells which are in the process of becoming but are not yet plasma cells and which have the ability to produce antibody against a parasite through the mediation of the host's metabolic pool would not, in the writer's opinion, be considered a passive transfer. The transfer of cells capable of playing a part in the inflammatory response and in hypersensitivity was discussed above (*see* p. 936). If these cells play this role actively, there is evidence for such passive transfer in *Trichinella* infections. Larsh et al. (1966a,b) and Wagland and Dineen (1965) felt that they had transferred cellular immunity to *Trichinella* in the mouse and to *Trichostrongylus colubriformis* in the guinea pig, respectively. C. A. Crandall (1965), working with *Ascaris suum* in mice, was able to transfer immunity by parabiosis but not by cells.

Zaiman and his colleagues (1954, 1955a,b), using parabiotic rats, a most useful tool, may have demonstrated passive transfer of immunity. However, if the noninfected parabiotic twin has any circulatory involvement with its mate, the more probable explanation is that there was a passive transfer of antigens to a ready and willing antibody-forming system. This seems likely, since they demonstrated that the immunity is "transferred" from the other parabiont.

In this same vein, although not directly related, is the fact that certain of the biochemical entities in worms are similar to host substances. Dineen (1963) has suggested that in the evolution of a host-parasite system, the active immunologic response may put selective pressure on the parasite to favor the genetic variants which show reduced antigenic disparity with the host. This leads to a situation in which worm burdens are maintained at a subliminal level, giving a threshold level of tolerance (Donald et al., 1964; Dineen et al., 1965).

Damian (1962) has suggested a similar theory on the basis of "immuno-selection" pressures in evolutionary development for eclipsed antigens, i.e., antigens of helminths which by their similarity or "selfness" to the substances of the host are no longer antigenic, thus permitting continued development of the helminth in the host.

As a corollary of this, Tanner (1965) found that saline extracts of *Trichinella* if treated with reducing agents (2-mercaptoethanol) would result in antigenic materials with reduced disulfide bridges. One of the substances so produced was similar or identical to normal serum albumin. A similar electrophoretic mobility does not prove identity, but since there was an immuno-electrophoretic reaction with an antiserum to serum albumin, the similarity must be great. The importance of this finding is that in a responding host, there are ample opportunities for reduction of the disulfide bridges of an invading parasite's antigens. This would have the effect of reducing the total impact of the parasite on the host's immune response. Further experimentation and discussion of these stimulating ideas are warranted.

Schad (1966) describes a similar mechanism for nonreciprocal cross-immunity developing from an evolutionary adaptation of the parasite to its host environment, which limits populations of competing parasitic species. Further discussion of this point may be found in Dineen et al. (1965) and Damian (1964).

MECHANISMS IN IMMUNITY

It has been stated earlier that the complexity of direct-infection nematodes provides a mosaic of potential antigens which challenge the host's protective system. This complexity, as well as other factors, makes a simple explanation of the mechanisms of protective immunity impossible. Some of the mechanisms in the immune state are not as yet explainable in terms of simple antigen-antibody relationships. However, certain hypotheses have been steadily receiving more confirmation by experimental results. Frequently we have to rely on *in vitro* data which are extrapolated to *in vivo* actions, and this may lead to over-generalization. The complexity and size of the helminths however, is such, that if adequate data can be developed, interesting generalizations may be made about immunity in general.

In many mechanisms operative in protective immunity to helminths, we see only the end result. The mediating physiologic mechanisms are obscure. They may be categorized as gross, i.e., those seen indirectly only as an end result, and specific, i.e., those seen at the actual level of operation.

Antienzymatic functions of antibodies

Chandler (1932) first suggested that the antibodies formed to substances from helminths would interfere in some way with the metabolism of these worms or worms of later infections. Thorson (1953, 1954b), on the basis of studies demonstrating lipolytic activity in ES preparations from *Nippostrongylus* and the inhibition of this activity by serum from rats made immune to the worm by repeated infections with larvae, suggested that at least part of the protective immunity to nematodes arose as a result of an enzyme-antienzyme relationship. In this case, enzymes used by the worm to maintain itself in the host were absorbed by the host and served as antigens. The antibodies created to these enzymes then reacted with them in such a way as to cause inhibition of the parasites. This inhibition made the continued presence of the worms of the present or a later infection difficult, and they would be cast off.

Unfortunately, it is not possible to determine with certainty the source of the enzymes in ES antigens, so a compromise was effected. By dissection, the esophagus was removed from *Ancylostoma caninum*. It was found that proteolytic activity was present in extracts of these tissues (Thorson, 1956a,b). Later, other enzymatic activities (peptidase and lipolytic) were also determined (Thorson, 1963). Sera from dogs made immune to *Ancylostoma* by repeated infections almost completely inhibited these activities. Since the dog hookworm spends much time sucking blood, there is ample opportunity for the antibodies formed against these substances to be ingested and to inhibit these activities in the esophagus. In addition, the injection of extracts of thousands of esophagi will stimulate a measurable degree of immunity to a challenge of infective larvae in puppies.

Rhodes et al. (1964, 1965), using purified preparations of malic dehydrogenase (MDH) from *Ascaris suum*, demonstrated the production of specific antibodies in guinea pigs, which inhibited the activity of these enzymes. Precipitins were also present in the sera. Serum fractionation demonstrated that the two activities occurred in different serum fractions. The precipitin activity occurred in the gamma-globulin fraction, whereas the enzyme inhibitor was eluted along with beta-globulins. Although guinea pigs are not a normal host, development does occur through the lung stage. These authors immunized guinea pigs with embryonated eggs or purified MDH. After challenge, the resulting lung lesions due to helminth-induced hemorrhagic pneumonia were very marked in the controls and greatly reduced in the two immunized groups (Fig. 2).

As stated earlier, the enzyme-antienzyme (antigen-antibody) hypothesis has only recently begun to be substantiated by experimental studies. Much more work needs to be done, since the multiplicity of the enzyme mosaic in nematodes is great, and it is possible that many are unable to play a role in protective immunity because of their lack of contact with and consequent lack of stimulation of the host's antibody-forming system.

This is an example of an immune mechanism which can be observed at the specific level.

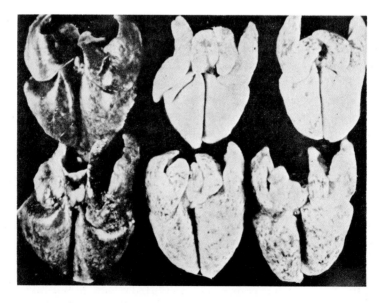

FIG. 2.   Lungs of guinea pigs infected with eggs of *Ascaris suum*. Left, control. Middle, immunized with eggs. Right, immunized with malic dehydrogenase (MDH) from *Ascaris*. Note the hemorrhagic pneumonia in the control lungs and the relatively fewer localized hemorrhagic spots on the lungs of animals immunized with eggs and MDH. (Courtesy of Dr. M. B. Rhodes and Academic Press, Inc.)

Inhibition of reproduction by antibodies

The effect of antibody in reducing production of eggs or larvae of a parasitic worm in an immune host has much experimental support. Chandler (1936) observed this with *Nippostrongylus*, and many later studies have confirmed this (e.g., Barth et al., 1966). As the host becomes immune, there is a precipitous drop in egg production. Chandler showed that this was a real immune effect instead of senescence by transplanting non-egg-laying adult worms from an immune host into a non-immune host. The worms resumed egg-laying at pre-immune levels.

There is ample evidence that a similar situation applies in the case of *Trichinella* infection (Campbell, 1955; Chute, 1956; Chipman, 1957; Mills and Kent, 1965). All of these studies used the criterion of reduced numbers of larvae in the muscles of the host as compared to controls as evidence for the stimulation of protective immunity.

This is an example of a gross mechanism of immunity, since it is hardly possible that the effect is mechanical. We can only speculate whether the effect of the antibody is to deplete the nutritional status of the worm or whether it has a direct effect on the reproductive system, causing lowered oogenesis or spermatogenesis. The former possibility seems more likely, but until helminth cultivation is more fully developed, the study of this *in vivo* effect will not be observable *in vitro*. Nonetheless, this is an important and readily recognizable immune mechanism. Its effect in most infections with direct-infection nematodes (except *Trichinella*, an infection with all stages in one host) has less influence on the current infection of the host than on future ones in the same and in different hosts. The net epidemiologic result is to reduce the numbers of potential infective forms outside the host.

Inhibition of parasite development

Chandler (1936) was one of the earliest observers of the fact that in immune hosts, worms did not grow to their full size. Again, by transplantation experiments he demonstrated that the worms could realize their potential growth, thus illustrating that the effect noted was an immune phenomenon.

Immunizing young puppies with extracts of esophagus from *Ancylostoma caninum* produced a very definite stunting of worms in a challenge infection (Thorson, 1956b). In this case, the stunting was produced by antibodies to extracts of isolated tissues in which at least some of the physiologic activities of these tissues were known. Sprent and Chen (1949) used inhibition of larval growth as a criterion of an immune state in *Ascaris* infections in rodents. Similarly, Soulsby (1961) observed stunting with *Ascaris* in guinea pigs. However, he found that there was no effect on the growth until the 4th or 5th day of infection. This is when the first parasitic molt takes place. Crandall and Arean (1964) placed second-stage larvae of *Ascaris suum* in Millipore diffusion chambers into the peritoneal cavity of immune and non-immune mice. Certain technical difficulties, such as host cellular reaction, were considered as slightly abnormal and possibly limiting. However, there was definite stunting of larvae in the immune mice. When chambers in which stunting had occurred were placed into nonimmune mice, parasite growth was resumed readily.

This stunting is again a gross effect and the exact mechanism is unclear. One would suspect that an improper nutritional intake by the larvae might be responsible, which suggests the possibility of an enzyme-antienzyme mechanism. However, another possibility is that simple mechanical blockage of the digestive tract, as suggested by Taliaferro and Sarles (1939), occurs. *In vitro* study of the effect of antibody on developing worms would be useful, but until cultivation methods are better standardized, this will be difficult.

Difference in the effectiveness of various stages to stimulate immunity

The earlier discussion of the dual (or multiple) antibody basis of immunity (*see* pp. 936-937) has raised this point in the case of some infections. Also, the effect of molting fluids in the expression of immunity as a hypersensitive state in *Haemonchus* and in *Ascaris* infections has been discussed in detail (*see* p. 933). These latter studies have, for the most part, demonstrated very real specificity for the first parasitic molt. The actual mechanism has been studied as a gross effect until now, but it is in great need of study at the physiologic level. Among the known components of molting fluid are enzymes which actually have already performed their function in the life of the worm so that their inhibition at this time would be of little use as a protective mechanism. However, the succeeding parasitic molts may be affected. It is also entirely conceivable that other substances with physiologic activity are present, and the release of rather large quantities at molting stimulate an anamnestic response in antibody level, causing the inhibition discussed earlier. The effect of these substances in creating a hypersensitive state and in possibly creating a completely unsuitable parasite environment is at the moment only conjectural. The definitive identification of all of the components in these fluids is necessary.

Effect of antigens on mast-cell release of pharmacologically active substances

Briggs (1963a,b) and Goldgraber and Lewert (1965) have demonstrated appreciable injury to mast cells in *Trichinella* and *Strongyloides ratti* infections, respectively. These cells are known to be cellular depots of pharmacologically active amines (histamine, 5-hydroxytryptamine, and others). The damage to these cells is accentuated in actively or passively immunized hosts. The release of these amines or other unknown products can be triggered by somatic or ES antigens. These substances seem to confer a degree of immunity against these organisms.

Briggs (1963a) showed that injection of histamine or serotonin (5-hydroxytryptamine) produced limited effects against infections with *Tri-*

chinella, but of the two, the latter is suspected to play a more important role than histamine in murine anaphylaxis. Interestingly, injection of 5-hydroxytryptophan increased resistance of mice to primary infections. Serotonin was less effective. This is consistent with the theory that exogenous serotonin is excreted very rapidly, and thus the 5-hydroxytryptophan, a natural precursor of serotonin, is actively metabolized to serotonin in the host. This then would lead to an increased level of circulating serotonin.

One of the pharmacologic properties of serotonin is the stimulation of contraction of smooth muscle (intestinal). Presumably, increased peristalsis would lead to diarrhea and hence to an inhospitable environment for intestinal worms.

Apparently, the increase in mast cell rupture is mediated by a lytic system consisting of cells, specific antibody, and its antigen. Whether complement is needed is not known. This effect of the immune state is different from the enzyme-antienzyme theory previously discussed, and merits much further investigation. Of the two categories of mechanisms, gross and specific, mast cell rupture falls in the latter, although it is not as yet completely understood.

Encapsulation as an immune mechanism

It is well-known that worms will be encapsulated by the host in *Trichinella* infections. Since the worms would not go on to develop to adults in the same host, this form of encapsulation is probably nothing more than the host reaction to foreign matter. It presumably would seal off the host from harmful products of the larvae, but it is doubtful that such is the case since the larvae are able to live in the capsules for many years. During this time, a certain amount of physiologic exchange must occur.

Encapsulation is not unknown in other worm infections. Some of the work of Taliaferro and Sarles (1939) on the histology of *Nippostrongylus* infections in immune and nonimmune hosts indicates a heightened cellular response in immune hosts. A rapid infiltration of macrophages, neutrophils, and eosinophils surrounds and eventually walls off and destroys the worms in the skin and lungs. This is probably a secondary effect, however, since it is inconceivable to the writer that the cells are capable of mechanically slowing down or stopping the invading larvae. The effect, mediated in some as yet unknown manner, is to demonstrate a heightened cellular response and subsequent destruction of the worms in the immune as opposed to the nonimmune host. This may be related to an *in vitro* phenomenon, immune adherence, which will be discussed below.

The role of the cuticle and immune adherence

One of the most puzzling questions in the study of mechanisms of immunity to direct-nematode infections is whether the cuticle plays a role in stimulating protective immunity. It has been adequately demonstrated that cuticle can stimulate antibody formation by itself, but the evidence for these antibodies serving a protective function is scanty.

Jackson (1959, 1960) in two excellent studies was unable to demonstrate that fluorescent antibodies from either *Trichinella*- or *Nippostrongylus*-infected rats reacted with the cuticle. He did show, however, that there was a rather considerable degree of fluorescence between the old and new cuticle of the fourth-stage larvae of *Nippostrongylus*. This must be considered as related to molting fluids and other excretions and secretions which collect there. Sadun (1963), using the fluorescent-antibody test in diagnosis of *Trichinella*, found that considerable fluorescence occurred around the cuticle. It must be remembered that in this test dead larvae were used. He felt that the fluorescence was not due to a cuticle-antibody reaction, but rather it was due to a seepage of antigens through the fixed cuticle.

The evidence for immune fluorescence arising from the combination of fluorescein-tagged antibody with cuticular antigenic sites is not all negative. Sulzer (1965), using isolated cuticle and an indirect fluorescent-antibody test, showed fluorescence of the cuticle, and he suggested that there are active cuticular sites. One might ask if these sites are not simply material retained from the rest of the worm, since enzymatic digestion was used to remove the rest of the worms' bodies. A similar observation was made with larvae of *Ascaris suum* by Crandall et al. (1963) and Taffs and Voller (1962). The latter study, however, described cuticular precipitates which fluoresced. Jackson (1959, 1960) demonstrated such precipitates, but he felt that they are related to antibody reacting with excretions and secretions and that some of these fluorescent antigen-antibody precipitates are displaced from oral, excretory, and anal openings. The three positive studies all suggest that there are actively antigenic sites on the cuticle.

It is obvious that the role of the cuticle in protective immunity is unclear. It has been suggested that certain of these reactions may be due to a reaction of antibody, complement, and cuticle which causes an increase in permeability of the cuticle to substances from within and outside the worms (Soulsby, 1962). Jamuar (1966), in his elegant electron microscope study of the cuticle of *Nippostrongylus*, suggested that the use of ferritin-labeled antiserum might be useful in determining how the cuticle is involved in such reactions.

Despommier et al. (1967), using ferritin-tagged gamma-globulin, demonstrated collections of the antibody on the cuticle of *Trichinella* with electron micrographs. They feel that the cuticle is itself active, and the inhibition of exchange of materials from inside and outside the worm may be the functional mechanism involved. Just what exchanged materials are involved is still unknown.

It is difficult for the writer to accept the concept that the cuticle plays a major role in inducing protective immunity to direct-infection nematodes. When worms are captured in tissue, the cuticle remains long after the rest of the worm has been destroyed by host reaction.

Another phenomenon which is cuticle-related is the immune adherence reaction demonstrated by Soulsby (1963). This has been observed for numerous bacterial infections as well, and in this case, consists of a reaction between complement and larvae of *Ascaris* exposed to immune globulin plus red blood cells. The red cells adhere in large numbers to the outside of the larvae; there is likewise an adhesion of white cells to larvae in the presence of immune serum, which is complement-independent. It is remarkable that in the latter test, eosinophils and other pyroninophilic cells were most prominent in the adhesion phenomenon, although a mixture of cells was present in the samples obtained from the peritoneal cavity of a rabbit.

R. B. Crandall (1965) demonstrated that *in vitro*, polymorphonuclear leukocytes from rat and rabbit exudates reacted chemotactically to saline extracts or ES antigens of *Trichinella* in the presence of immune serum or globulins, but not in the presence of normal serum. In contrast, *Ascaris* extracts in inactivated normal serum were attractive to leukocytes. This attraction required a heat-labile substance, presumably complement.

All of these results point out the confused state of our knowledge with respect to these mechanisms and offer fruitful fields for investigations.

Other gross effects

Schwabe (1957) observed that the respiration of free-living infective and parasitic stages of *Nippostrongylus* was inhibited by immune serum. Such results indicate a rather basic interference with essential functions of the worms. At what stage of the oxidative cycle this interference occurs is not known, but it introduces very interesting experimental problems.

Nippostrongylus adults, when placed in a thermal gradient, display a positive thermotaxis (McCue and Thorson, 1965). Worms of a given age migrate at roughly similar rates, but worms of a young infection (7 days) migrate much faster than those of a 17-day infection (about the time "self-cure" begins to operate, *see* pp. 937-939). If worms of a 17-day infection are transplanted into a previously uninfected rat, they migrate at the same rate as worms of a 7-day infection. This illustrates that the host, as it becomes immune, inhibits gross characteristics such as movement. These experiments should be considered along with Chandler's work on renewal of growth and egg production in transplanted *Nippostrongylus* (Chandler, 1936).

CONCLUSION

Since 1941, there have been literally thousands of studies on immunity to direct-infection nematodes and it may be anticipated that there will be many more in the future. The direct-infection nematodes, in contrast to helminths utilizing vectors or other intermediate hosts, are better suited for this type of study because of their independence from these intermediate hosts.

The techniques and tools of immunology increase daily, and the advances in *in vitro* cultivation of helminths presage even greater activity. We have suggested certain areas which will lead to a better understanding not only of immunity to direct-infection nematodes but to all parasitic forms. If the discussions of this chapter lead others to follow these suggestions, our effort will be well rewarded.

REFERENCES

Ackert, J. E., and S. A. Edgar. 1939. Goblet cells and age resistance of animals to parasitism. Trans. Amer. Micr. Soc., 58:81–89.

Ada, G. L., and P. G. Lang. 1966. Antigen in tissues. II. State of antigen in lymph node of rats given isotopically-labelled flagellin, haemocyanin or serum albumin. Immunology, 10:431–443.

Andrews, J. 1942. New methods of hookworm disease investigation and control. Amer. J. Public Health, 32:282-288.

Ashley, W., Jr. 1964. Development of irradiated *Nippostrongylus brasiliensis* larvae and the immunogenic effect produced in rats. J. Parasit., 50(Suppl.):27.

Barth, E. E. E., W. F. H. Jarrett, and G. M. Urquhart. 1966. Studies on the mechanism of the self-cure reaction in rats infected with *Nippostrongylus brasiliensis*. Immunology, 10:459–464.

Bass, G. K., and L. J. Olson. 1965. *Trichinella spiralis* in newborn mice: Course of infection and effect on resistance to challenge. J. Parasit., 51:640–644.

Berger, H., and I. B. Wood. 1964. Immunological studies with *Ascaris suum* in rabbits with observations on natural and artificially acquired immunity. J. Parasit., 50(Suppl.):25–26.

Briggs, N. T. 1963a. Hypersensitivity in murine trichinosis: Some responses of *Trichinella* infected mice to antigen and 5-hydroxytryptophan. Ann. N. Y. Acad. Sci., 113:456–466.

———— 1963b. Immunological injury of mast cells in mice actively and passively sensitized to antigens from *Trichinella spiralis*. J. Infect. Dis., 113:22–32.

———— 1965. Inhibitory effect of cortisone on the sensitivities of *Trichinella*-infected mice to specific antigen and serotonin. J. Parasit., 51(Suppl.):37.

Cabrera, P. D., and S. E. Gould. 1964. Resistance to trichinosis in swine induced by administration of irradiated larvae. J. Parasit., 50:681–684.

Campbell, C. H. 1955. The antigenic role of the excretions and secretions of *Trichinella spiralis* in the production of immunity in mice. J. Parasit., 41:483–491.

Campbell, D. H. 1936. An antigenic polysaccharide fraction of *Ascaris lumbricoides* (from hog). J. Infect. Dis., 59:266–280.

Campbell, W. C., and S. F. Timinski. 1965. Immunization of rats against *Ascaris suum* by means of non-pulmonary larval infections. J. Parasit., 51:712–716.

———— R. K. Hartman, and A. C. Cuckler. 1963. Induction of immunity to trichinosis in mice by means of chemically abbreviated infections. Exp. Parasit., 14:29–36.

Chandler, A. C. 1932. Susceptibility and resistance to helminth infections. J. Parasit., 18:135–152.

———— 1936. Studies on the nature of immunity to intestinal helminths. 3. Renewal of growth and egg production in *Nippostrongylus* after transfer from immune to non-immune rats. Amer. J. Hyg., 23:1–16.

Chipman, P. B. 1957. The antigenic role of the excretions and secretions of adult *Trichinella spiralis* in the production of immunity in mice. J. Parasit., 43:593–598.

Christie, M. G., and M. R. Brambell. 1966. Acquired resistance to *Haemonchus contortus* in young lambs. J. Comp. Path., 76:207–216.

Chute, R. M. 1956. The dual antibody response to experimental trichiniasis. Proc. Helminth. Soc. (Washington), 23:49–58.

Cort, W. W., and G. F. Otto. 1940. Immunity in hookworm disease. Rev. Gastroent. 7:2–11.

Cox, H. W. 1952. The effect of concurrent infection with the dog hookworm. *Ancylo-*

stoma caninum, on the natural and acquired resistance of mice to *Trichinella spiralis.* J. Elisha Mitchell Sci. Soc., 68:222–235.

Crandall, C. A. 1965. Studies on the transfer of immunity to *Ascaris suum* in mice by serum, parabiotic union, and cells. J. Parasit., 51:405–408.

—— and V. M. Arean. 1964. *In vivo* studies of *Ascaris suum* larvae planted in diffusion chambers in immune and non-immune mice. J. Parasit., 50:685–688.

—— and V. M. Arean. 1965. The protective effect of viable and nonviable *Ascaris suum* larvae and egg preparations in mice. Amer. J. Trop. Med. Hyg., 14:765–769.

—— R. Echevarria, and V. M. Arean. 1963. Localization of antibody binding sites in the larva of *Ascaris lumbricoides* var. *suum* by means of fluorescent techniques. Exp. Parasit., 14:296–303.

Crandall, R. B. 1965. Chemotactic response of polymorphonuclear leukocytes to *Trichinella spiralis* and *Ascaris suum* extracts. J. Parasit., 51:397–404.

Culbertson, J. T. 1941. Immunity against Animal Parasites. New York, Columbia University Press.

Damian, R. T. 1962. A theory of immuno-selection for eclipsed antigens of parasites and its implications for the problem of antigenic polymorphism in man. J. Parasit., 48(Suppl.):16.

—— 1964. Molecular mimicry: antigen sharing by parasite and host and its consequences. Amer. Natur., 98:129–149.

Danaraj, T. J., and J. F. Schacher. 1957. Eosinophilic lung (tropical eosinophilia) and its relation to filariasis. Proceedings of the 9th Pacific Science Congress, 17:377–385.

Davis, D. E., and C. P. Read. 1958. Effect of behavior on development of resistance in trichinosis. Proc. Soc. Exp. Biol. Med., 99:269–272.

Denham, D. A. 1966. Immunity to *Trichinella spiralis*. I. The immunity produced by mice to the first four days of the intestinal phase of the infection. Parasitology, 56:325–327.

Despommier, D. D., and B. S. Wostmann. 1968. Diffusion chambers for inducing immunity to *Trichinella spiralis* in mice. Exp. Parasit., 23:228-233.

—— M. Kajima, and B. S. Wostmann. 1967. Ferritin conjugated antibody studies on the larvae of *Trichinella spiralis*. J. Parasit., 53:618–624.

DeWitt, W. B., and P. P. Weinstein. 1964. Elimination of intestinal helminths of mice by feeding purified diets. J. Parasit., 50:429–434.

Dineen, J. K. 1963. Immunological aspects of parasitism. Nature (London), 197:268–269.

—— A. D. Donald, B. M. Wagland, and J. H. Turner. 1965. The dynamics of the host-parasite relationship. II. The response of sheep to primary and secondary infection with *Nematodirus spathiger*. Parasitology., 55:163–171.

Dobson, C. 1966. Immunofluorescent staining of globule leucocytes in the colon of the sheep. Nature (London), 211:875.

Doll, J. P., and C. K. Franker. 1963. Experimental histomoniasis in gnotobiotic turkeys. I. Infection and histopathology of the bacteria free host. J. Parasit., 49:411–414.

Donald, A. D., J. K. Dineen, J. H. Turner, and B. M. Wagland. 1964. The dynamics of the host-parasite relationship. I. *Nematodirus spathiger* infection in sheep. Parasitology, 54:527–544.

Donaldson, A. W., and G. F. Otto. 1946. Effect of protein-deficient diets on immunity to a nematode (*Nippostrongylus muris*) infection. Amer. J. Hyg., 44:384–400.

Douvres, F. W. 1962. The *in vitro* cultivation of *Oesophagostomum radiatum*, the nodular worm of cattle. II. The use of this technique to study immune responses of host tissue extracts against the developing nematode. J. Parasit., 48:852–864.

Dunn, M. C., and H. W. Brown. 1962. Effect of pregnancy on pinworm infections in albino mice. J. Parasit., 48:32–33.

Ewert, A., and L. J. Olson. 1961. The use of a mouse oral LD50 to evaluate the immunogenicity of *Trichinella* metabolic antigens. Texas Rep. Biol. Med., 19:580–584.

Forrester, A. T. T., G. S. Nelson, and G. Sander. 1961. The first record of an outbreak of trichinosis in Africa south of the Sahara. Trans. Roy. Soc. Trop. Med. Hyg., 55:503–513.

Foster, A. O., and W. W. Cort. 1932. The relation of diet to the susceptibility of dogs to *Ancylostoma caninum*. Amer. J. Hyg., 16:582–601.

Franker, C. K., and J. P. Doll. 1964. Experimental histomoniasis in gnotobiotic turkeys. II. Effects of some cecal bacteria on pathogenesis. J. Parasit., 50:636–640.

Gelpi, A. P., and A. Mustafa. 1967. Seasonal pneumonitis with eosinophilia. Amer. J. Trop. Med. Hyg., 16:646–657.

Goldgraber, M. B., and R. M. Lewert. 1965. Immunological injury of mast cells and connective tissue in mice infected with *Strongyloides ratti*. J. Parasit., 51:169–174.

Gomberg, H. J., and S. E. Gould. 1953. Effect of irradiation with cobalt-60 on trichina larvae. Science, 118:75–77.

Gould, S. E., H. J. Gomberg, F. H. Bethell, J. B. Villella, and C. S. Hertz. 1955. Studies on *Trichinella spiralis*. I–V. Amer. J. Path. 31:933–963.

Grabar, P., and P. Burtin, eds. 1964. Immuno-electrophoretic analysis; applications to human biological fluids. Amsterdam, Elsevier Publishing Co.

Haley, A. J. 1958. Sex difference in the resistance of hamsters to infection with the rat nematode, *Nippostrongylus muris*. Exp. Parasit., 7:338–348.

Harshman, S., and V. A. Najjar. 1963. The theory of subcomplementarity as it pertains to the mechanism of antibody-antigen reaction. *In* Immunodiagnosis of Helminthic Infections. Jackowski, L. A. Jr., ed. Amer. J. Hyg. Monog. Ser. No. 22.

Hendricks, J. R. 1952. Studies in mice on the dual antibody basis of acquired resistance to *Trichinella spiralis*. J. Elisha Mitchell Sci. Soc., 68:12–26.

Herrick, C. A. 1928. A quantitative study of infections with *Ancylostoma* in dogs. Amer. J. Hyg., 8:125–157.

Hunter, G. C., and L. C. Leigh. 1961. Studies on the resistance of rats to the nematode *Nippostrongylus muris* (Yokogawa, 1920). II. Attempts to transfer immunity adoptively. Parasitology, 51:357–366.

Ivey, M. H. 1965. Immediate hypersensitivity and serological responses in guinea pigs infected with *Toxocara canis* or *Trichinella spiralis*. Amer. J. Trop. Med. Hyg., 14:1044–1051.

————— and R. Slanga. 1965. An evaluation of passive cutaneous anaphylactic reactions with *Trichinella* and *Toxocara* antibody-antigen systems. Amer. J. Trop. Med. Hyg., 14:1052..4-1056.

Jachowski, L. A., and R. I. Anderson. 1961. Evaluation of some laboratory procedures in diagnosing infections with *Schistosoma mansoni*. Bull. W.H.O., 25:675–693.

Jackson, G. J. 1959. Fluorescent antibody studies of *Trichinella spiralis* infections. J. Infect. Dis., 105:97–117.

————— 1960. Fluorescent antibody studies of *Nippostrongylus muris* infections. J. Infect. Dis., 106:20–36.

Jamuar, M. P. 1966. Electron microscope studies on the body wall of the nematode *Nippostrongylus brasiliensis*. J. Parasit., 52:209–232.

Jarrett, W. F. H., F. W. Jennings, W. I. M. McIntyre, W. Mulligan, and G. M. Urquhart. 1955. Immunological studies on *Dictyocaulus viviparus* infection. Passive immunization. Vet. Rec., 67:291–296.

Kagan, I. G. 1957. Serum-agar double diffusion studies with *Ascaris* antigens. J. Infect. Dis., 101:11–19.

Katz, F. F. 1963. Testosterone and estrogen treatments of gonadectomized rats in experiments on the host sex difference in *Strongyloides ratti* intestinal burdens. J. Parasit., 49(Suppl.):52.

Kent, N. H. 1960. Isolation of specific antigens from *Ascaris lumbricoides* (var. *suum*). Exp. Parasit., 10:313–323.

————— 1963a. Seminar on immunity to parasitic helminths. V. Antigens. Exp. Parasit. 13:45–56.

————— 1963b. Fractionation, isolation and definition of antigens from parasitic helminths. *In* Immunodiagnosis of Helminthic Infections. Jackowski, L. A. Jr., ed. Amer. J. Hyg. Monogr. Ser. No. 22.

Khan, Z. A. 1966. The postembryonic development of *Trichinella spiralis* with special reference to ecdysis. J. Parasit., 52:248–259.

Kilham, L., and L. J. Olivier. 1961. The effect of *Trichinella* infection on encephalomyocarditis (EMC) virus infections in rats. J. Parasit., 47(Suppl.):17.

Kim, C. W. 1966. Delayed hypersensitivity to larval antigens of *Trichinella spiralis*. J. Infect. Dis., 116:208–214.

Larsh, J. E., and J. R. Hendricks. 1949. The probable explanation for the difference in the localization of adult *Trichinella spiralis* in young and old mice. J. Parasit., 35:101–106.

————— and D. E. Kent. 1949. The effect of alcohol on natural and acquired immunity of mice to infection with *Trichinella spiralis*. J. Parasit., 35:45–53.

———— and H. B. Gilchrist. 1950. The effect of a vitamin A deficient diet on the natural and acquired resistance of mice to infection with *Trichinella spiralis*. J. Elisha Mitchell Sci. Soc., 66:76–83.

———— G. J. Race, and H. T. Goulson. 1959. A histopathologic study of mice immunized with irradiated larvae of *Trichinella spiralis*. J. Infect. Dis., 104:156–163.

———— H. T. Goulson, and N. F. Weatherly. 1964. Studies on delayed (cellular) hypersensitivity in mice infected with *Trichinella spiralis*. I. Transfer of lymph node cells. J. Elisha Mitchell Sci. Soc., 80:133–135.

———— H. T. Goulson, and N. F. Weatherly. 1966a. Studies on delayed (cellular) hypersensitivity in mice infected with *Trichinella spiralis*. II. Transfer of peritoneal exudate cells. J. Parasit., 50:496–498.

———— G. J. Race, H. T. Goulson, and N. F. Weatherly. 1966b. Studies on delayed (cellular) hypersensitivity in mice infected with *Trichinella spiralis*. III. Serologic and histopathologic findings in recipients given peritoneal exudate cells. J. Parasit., 52:146–156.

Lawler, J. J. 1940. Passive transfer of immunity to the nematode, *Strongyloides ratti*. Amer. J. Hyg., 31(Sect. D):28–31.

Lejkina, E. S. 1965. Research on ascariasis immunity and immunity diagnosis. Bull. W.H.O., 32:699–708.

Lewert, R. M., and C. L. Lee. 1954. Studies on the passage of helminth larvae through host tissues. I. Histochemical studies on extracellular changes caused by penetrating larvae. II. Enzymatic activity of larvae *in vitro* and *in vivo*. J. Infect. Dis., 95:13–51.

———— and C. L. Lee. 1956. Quantitative studies of the collagenase-like enzymes of cercariae of *Schistosoma mansoni* and the larvae of *Strongyloides ratti*. J. Infect. Dis., 99:1–14.

———— and C. L. Lee. 1957. The collagenase enzymes of skin-penetrating helminths. Amer. J. Trop. Med. Hyg., 6:473–477.

Liu, S. 1966. Genetic influence on resistance of mice to *Nematospiroides dubius*. Exp. Parasit., 18:311–319.

Louch, C. D. 1962. Increased resistance to *Trichinella spiralis* in the laboratory rat following infection with *Nippostrongylus muris*. J. Parasit., 48:24–26.

Luckey, T. D. 1963. Germfree Life and Gnotobiology. New York, Academic Press, Inc.

Mathies, A. W., Jr. 1959a. Certain aspects of the host-parasite relationship of *Aspiculuris tetraptera*, a mouse pinworm. I. Host specificity and age resistance. Exp. Parasit., 8:31–38.

———— 1959b. Certain aspects of the host-parasite relationship of *Aspiculuris tetraptera*, a mouse pinworm. II. Sex resistance. Exp. Parasit., 8:39–45.

———— 1962. Certain aspects of the host-parasite relationship of *Aspiculuris tetraptera*. III. Effect of cortisone. J. Parasit., 48:244–248.

Matsumura, T. 1963. Ascaris allergy. Gunma J. Med. Sci., 12:186–226.

———— S. Yugami, T. Hosoya, T. Suzuki, K. Uchida, and H. Tadokoro. 1955. Studies on ascaris allergy. Gunma J. Med. Sci., 4:170–171.

Mauss, E. A. 1941. The serum fraction with which anti-trichinella (*Trichinella spiralis*) antibody is associated. Amer. J. Hyg., 34(Sect. D):73–80.

McCue, J. F., and R. E. Thorson. 1963. A rapid method for collecting large numbers of intestinal helminths. J. Parasit., 49:997.

———— and R. E. Thorson. 1965. Host effects on the migration of *Nippostrongylus brasiliensis* in a thermal gradient. J. Parasit., 51:414–417.

Melcher, L. R. 1943. An antigenic analysis of *Trichinella spiralis*. J. Infect. Dis., 73:31–39.

Miller, T. A. 1965a. Effect of route of administration of vaccine and challenge on the immunogenic efficiency of double vaccination with irradiated *Ancylostoma caninum* larvae. J. Parasit., 51:200–206.

———— 1965b. Influence of age and sex on susceptibility of dogs to primary infection with *Ancylostoma caninum*. J. Parasit., 51:701–704.

———— 1965c. Persistence of immunity following double vaccination of pigs with x-irradiated *Ancylostoma caninum* larvae. J. Parasit., 51:705–711.

Mills, C. K., and N. H. Kent. 1965. Excretions and secretions of *Trichinella spiralis* and their role in immunity. Exp. Parasit., 16:300–310.

Moskwa, W., W. Stephan, and B. Urzula. 1958. Przebieg wlosnicy u białych szczurow naswietlauych promieniami roentgena (Trichinellosis development in white x-rayed rats). Wiad. Parazyt., 4:373–375.

Mulligan, W., G. M. Urquhart, F. W. Jennings, and J. T. M. Neilson. 1965. Immunological studies on *Nippostrongylus brasiliensis* infection in the rat: The "self-cure" phenomenon. Exp. Parasit., 16:341–347.

Neafie, R. C., and A. J. Haley. 1962. Sex difference in resistance of the mouse, *Mus musculus*, to infection with the rat nematode, *Nippostrongylus brasiliensis* (Travassos, 1914). J. Parasit., 48:151.

Newton, W. L., P. P. Weinstein, and M. F. Jones. 1959. A comparison of the development of some rat and mouse helminths in germfree and conventional guinea pigs. Ann. N. Y. Acad. Sci., 78:290–307.

Noble, G. A. 1966. Stress and parasitism. III. Reduced night temperature and the effect on pinworms of ground squirrels. Exp. Parasit., 18:61–62.

Nossal, G. J. V. 1962. Cellular genetics of immune responses. *In* Advances in Immunology, Vol. 2. Taliaferro, W. H., and Humphrey, J. H., eds. New York, Academic Press, Inc.

Ogilvie, B. M. 1965. Use of cortisone derivatives to inhibit resistance to *Nippostrongylus brasiliensis* and to study the fate of parasites in resistant hosts. Parasitology, 55:723–730.

——— 1967. Reagin-like antibodies in rats infected with the nematode parasite *Nippostrongylus brasiliensis*. Immunology, 12:113–132.

Oliver-Gonzalez, J. 1940. The *in vitro* action of immune serum on the larvae and adults of *Trichinella spiralis*. J. Infect. Dis., 67:292–300.

——— 1941. The dual antibody basis of acquired immunity in trichinosis. J. Infect. Dis., 69:254–270.

——— 1943. Antigenic analysis of the isolated tissues and body fluids of the roundworm, *Ascaris lumbricoides* var. *suum*. J. Infect. Dis., 72:202–212.

——— 1946. Functional antigens in helminths. J. Infect. Dis., 78:232–237.

——— and D. M. Levine. 1962. Stage specific antibodies in experimental trichinosis. Amer. J. Trop. Med. Hyg., 11:241–244.

Olson, L. J. and A. Ewert. 1961. Further studies on immunological tolerance with mice and *Trichinella*. Texas Rep. Biol. Med., 19:866–868.

——— and C. W. Schultz. 1963. Nematode induced hypersensitivity reactions in guinea pigs: Onset of eosinophilia and positive Schultz-Dale reactions following graded infections with *Toxocara canis*. Ann. N. Y. Acad. Sci., 113:440–455.

Osler, A. G. 1963. Skin reactions of the immediate and delayed types of hypersensitivity: some aspects of their mechanism. In Immunodiagnosis of Helminth Infections. Jachowski, L. A., Jr., ed. Amer. J. Hyg. Monogr. Ser. No. 22.

Otto, G. F. 1940. A serum antibody in dogs actively immunized against the hookworm, *Ancylostoma caninum*. Amer. J. Hyg., 31 (Sect. D):23–27.

——— N. J. Schugam, and M. E. Groover. 1942. A precipitin reaction resulting from *Necator americanus* larvae in sera from hookworm-infected individuals. Proc. Helminth Soc. (Washington), 9:25–26.

Ozeretskovskaya, N. N. 1968. Peculiarities of trichinosis outbreaks borne by strains from different geographical regions of the U.S.S.R. Eighth International Congress of Tropical Medicine and Malaria, Abstracts and Reviews, pp. 228–230.

Prochazka, Z., and W. Mulligan. 1965. Immunological studies on *Nippostrongylus brasiliensis* infection in the rat: Experiments with irradiated larvae. Exp. Parasit., 17:51–56.

Rhodes, M. B., C. L. March, and G. W. Kelley, Jr. 1964. Studies on helminth enzymology. III. Malic dehydrogenases from *Ascaris suum*. Exp. Parasit., 15:403–409.

——— D. P. Nayak, G. W. Kelley, Jr., and C. L. Marsh. 1965. Studies in helminth enzymology. IV. Immune response to malic dehydrogenase from *Ascaris suum*. Exp. Parasit., 16:373–381.

——— C. L. Marsh, and L. C. Payne. 1966. LNA-hydrolyzing aminopeptidases of *Ascaris suum*. Fed. Proc., 25:642.

Riedel, B. B. 1948. Age resistance of mice to the nematode *Trichinella spiralis*. Trans. Amer. Micr. Soc., 67:268–271.

Ritterson, A. L. 1959. Innate resistance of species of hamsters to *Trichinella spiralis* and its reversal by cortisone. J. Infect. Dis., 105:253–266.

Robinson, E. J., Jr. 1961. Survival of *Trichinella* in stressed hosts. J. Parasit., 47(Suppl):16–17.

Rogers, W. P. 1963. Physiology of infection with nematodes: Some effects of the host stimulus on infective stages. Ann. N. Y. Acad. Sci., 113:208–216.

——— 1966. The reversible inhibition of exsheathment in some parasitic nematodes. Comp. Biochem. Physio., 17:1103–1110.

——— and R. I. Sommerville. 1960. The physiology of the second ecdysis of parasitic nematodes. Parasitology, 50:329–348.

——— and R. I. Sommerville. 1963. The infective stage of nematode parasites and its significance in parasitism. *In* Advances in Parasitology, Vol. 1. Dawes, B., ed. New York, Academic Press, Inc., pp. 109–177.

Rohrbacher, G. H., Jr., S. Occhipinti, and E. Waletzky. 1963. Inhibition of development of *Ascaris suum* larvae in rodents fed a restricted diet. J. Parasit., 49(Suppl.):52.

Roman, E. 1951. Étude écologique et morphologique sur les acanthocephales et les nematodes parasites des rats de la région lyonnaise. Mém. Mus. Nat. Hist., Ser. A. Zool., 2:49–268.

Rose, J. E., L. A. Baisden, and F. G. Tromba. 1964. Ultracentrifugal fractionation of reactants in a gel-diffusion precipitin technique in stephanuriasis. J. Parasit., 50:504–508.

Ross, J. G., R. P. Lee, and J. Armour. 1959. Haemonchosis in Nigerian Zebu cattle: the influence of genetical factors in resistance. Vet. Rec., 71:27–31.

Ross, W. M. 1952. A preliminary comparative study of test antigens prepared from adult and larval forms of *Trichinella spiralis*. Canad. J. Med. Sci., 30:534–542.

Roth, H. 1941. The *in vitro* action of trichina larva in immune serum—a new precipitin test in trichinosis. Acta Path. Microbiol. Scand., 18:160–167.

Rubin, R., and T. B. Weber. 1955. The effect of immune serum on *Dictyocaulus viviparus* in calves. Preliminary report. Proc. Helminth. Soc. (Washington), 22:124–129.

Sadun, E. H. 1963. Seminar in immunity to parasitic helminths. VII. Fluorescent antibody technique for helminth infections. Exp. Parasit., 13:72–82.

Sarles, M. P. 1929. Quantitative studies on the dog and cat hookworm, *Ancylostoma brasiliense*, with special emphasis on age resistance. Amer. J. Hyg., 10:453–475.

——— 1938. The *in vitro* action of immune rat serum on the nematode, *Nippostrongylus muris*. J. Infect. Dis., 62:337–348.

Schad, G. A. 1965. Ann. Rep. Johns Hopkins CMRT 1964–1965.

——— 1966. Immunity, competition and natural regulation of helminth populations. Amer. Natur., 100:359–364.

Schwabe, C. 1957. Effects of normal and immune rat sera upon the respiration of free-living and parasitic *Nippostrongylus muris* larvae. Amer. J. Hyg., 65:338–343.

Senterfit, L. B. 1958. Immobilization of the miracidia of *Schistosoma mansoni* by immune sera. I. The nature of the reaction as studied in hamster sera. Amer. J. Hyg., 68:140–147.

Sharp, A. D., and L. J. Olson. 1962. Hypersensitivity responses in *Toxocara-*, *Ascaris-*, and *Trichinella-*infected guinea pigs to homologous and heterologous challenge. J. Parasit., 48:362–367.

Silverman, P. H. 1963. *In vitro* cultivation and serological techniques in parasitology. *In* Techniques in Parasitology. Taylor, A. E., ed., Oxford, Blackwell Scientific Publications.

——— 1965. *In vitro* cultivation procedures for parasitic helminths. *In* Advances in Parasitology, Vol. 3. Dawes, B., ed. New York, Academic Press, Inc.

——— D. Poynter, and K. R. Podger. 1962. Studies on larval antigens derived by cultivation of some parasitic nematodes in simple media: protection tests in laboratory animals. J. Parasit., 48:562–571.

Sleeman, H. K. 1961. Studies on complement fixing antigens isolated from *Trichinella spiralis* larvae. II. Chemical analysis. Amer. J. Trop. Med. Hyg., 10:834–838.

——— and L. H. Muschel. 1961. Studies on complement fixing antigens isolated from *Trichinella spiralis* larvae. I. Isolation, purification and evaluation as diagnostic agents. Amer. J. Trop. Med. Hyg., 10:821–833.

Smith, V. S. 1946. Studies on reactions of rat serum to eggs of *Trichosomoides crassicauda*, a nematode of the urinary bladder. J. Parasit, 32:136–141.

Sokolic, A., M. Jovanovic, K. Cuperlovic, and M. Movsesijan. 1963. Inhibition of development of *Dictyocaulus filaria* as an expression of immunity attained in sheep. J. Parasit., 49:612–616.

Sommerville, R. I. 1957. The exsheathing mechanism of nematode infective larvae. Exp. Parasit., 6:18–30.

——— 1966. The development of *Haemonchus contortus* to the fourth stage *in vitro*. J. Parasit., 52:127–136.

Soulsby, E. J. L. 1957. Immunization against *Ascaris lumbricoides* in the guinea pig. Nature (London), 179:783–784.

——— 1960. Immunity to helminths—Recent advances. Vet. Rec., 72:322–327.

——— 1961. Some aspects of the mechanism of immunity to helminths. J. Amer. Vet. Med. Ass., 138:355–362.

——— 1962. Antigen-antibody reactions in helminth infections. *In* Advances in Immunology, Vol. 2. Taliaferro, W. H., and Humphrey, J. H., eds. New York, Academic Press, Inc.

——— 1963. The nature and origin of functional antigens in helminth infections. Ann. N. Y. Acad. Sci., 113:492–509.

——— 1965. Differential maternal transfer of antibodies to gastro-intestinal nematodes of sheep. J. Parasit., 51(Suppl.):39.

——— and D. F. Stewart. 1960. Serological studies of the self-cure reaction in sheep infected with *Haemonchus contortus*. Aust. J. Agric. Res., 11:595–603.

——— R. I. Sommerville, and D. F. Stewart. 1959. Antigenic stimulus of exsheathing fluid in self-cure of sheep infected with *Haemonchus contortus*. Nature (London), 183:553–554.

Sprent, J. F. A. 1949. On the toxic and allergic manifestations produced by the tissues and fluids of *Ascaris*. I. Effect of different tissues. J. Infect. Dis., 84:221–229.

——— 1950. On the toxic and allergic manifestations produced by the tissues and fluids of *Ascaris*. II. Effect of different chemical fractions on worm-free, infected and sensitized guinea pigs. J. Infect. Dis., 86:146–158.

——— 1951. On the toxic and allergic manifestations produced by the tissues and fluids of *Ascaris*. III. Hypersensitivity through infection in the guinea pig. J. Infect. Dis., 88:168–177.

——— and H. H. Chen. 1949. Immunological studies in mice infected with the larvae of *Ascaris lumbricoides*. I. Criteria of immunity and immunizing effect of isolated worm tissues. J. Infect. Dis., 84:111–124.

Stahl, W. 1966. Experimental aspiculuriasis. II. Effects of concurrent helminth infection. Exp. Parasit., 18:116–123.

Stefanski, W., and Z. Przyjalkowski. 1966. Effect of alimentary tract micro-organisms on the development of *Trichinella spiralis* in mice. Part II. Exp. Parasit., 18:92–98.

Stewart, D. F. 1950. Studies on resistance of sheep to infestation with *Haemonchus contortus* and *Trichostrongylus* spp. and on the immunological reactions of sheep exposed to infestation. IV. The antibody response to natural infestation in grazing sheep and the "self-cure" phenomenon. Aust. J. Agric. Res., 1:427–439.

——— 1953. Studies on resistance of sheep to infestation with *Haemonchus contortus* and *Trichostrongylus* spp. and on the immunological reactions of sheep exposed to infection. V. The nature of the "self-cure" phenomenon. Aust. J. Agric. Res., 4:100–117.

——— and H. M. Gordon. 1953. Studies on resistance of sheep to infestation with *Haemonchus contortus* and *Trichostrongylus* spp. and on the immunological reactions of sheep exposed to infestation. VI. The influence of age and nutrition on resistance to *Trichostrongylus colubriformis*. Aust. J. Agric. Res., 4:340–348.

Stoll, N. R. 1929. Studies with the strongyloid nematode, *Haemonchus contortus*. I. Acquired resistance of hosts under natural reinfection conditions out-of-doors. Amer. J. Hyg., 10:384–418.

Stone, W. M., and M. Girardeau. 1968. Transmammary passage of *Ancylostoma caninum* larvae in dogs. J. Parasit. 54:426–429.

Stoner, R. D., and W. M. Hale. 1952. Effect of cobalt⁶⁰ gamma radiation on susceptibility and immunity to trichinosis. Proc. Soc. Exp. Biol. Med. 80:510–512.

Sulzer, A. J. 1965. Indirect fluorescent antibody tests for parasitic diseases. I. Preparation of a stable antigen from larvae of *Trichinella spiralis* J. Parasit., 51:717–721.

Taffs, L. F., and A. Voller. 1962. Fluorescent antibody studies *in vitro* on *Ascaris suum*, Goeze, 1782. J. Helminth. 36:339–346.

Taliaferro, W. H., and M. P. Sarles. 1939. The cellular reactions in the skin, lungs and intestine of normal and immune rats after infection with *Nippostrongylus muris*. J. Infect. Dis., 64:157–192.

Talmadge, D. W. 1955. Effect of ionizing radiation on resistance and infection. Ann. Rev. Microbiol. 9:335–346.

Tanner, C. E. 1963. Formal discussion of paper by Kent, *In* Immunodiagnosis of Helminthic Infections. Jachowski, L. A., Jr., ed. Amer. J. Hyg. Monog. Ser. 22

—— 1965. Identification of a host antigen in extracts of *Trichinella spiralis* larvae. J. Parasit., 51 (Suppl.): 37.

Thorson, R. E. 1953. Studies on the mechanism of immunity in the rat to the nematode, *Nippostrongylus muris*. Amer. J. Hyg., 58: 1–15.

—— 1954a. Effect of immune serum from rats on infective larvae of *Nippostrongylus muris*. Exp. Parasit., 3: 9–15.

—— 1954b. Absorption of the protective antibodies from serum of rats immune to the nematode, *Nippostrongylus muris*. J. Parasit., 40: 300–303.

—— 1956a. Proteolytic activity in extracts of the esophagus of adults of *Ancylostoma caninum* and the effect of immune serum on this activity. J. Parasit., 42: 21–25.

—— 1956b. The stimulation of acquired immunity in dogs by injections of extracts of the esophagus of adult hookworms. J. Parasit., 42: 501–504.

—— 1963. Seminar on immunity to parasitic helminths. II. Physiology of immunity to helminth infections. Exp. Parasit., 13: 3–12.

—— G. A. Digenis, A. Berntzen, and A. Konyzalian. 1968. Biological activities of various lipid fractions from *Echinococcus granulosus* scolices on in vitro cultures of *Hymenolepis diminuta*. J. Parasit., 54: 970–973.

Urquhart, G. M., W. F. H. Jarrett, and W. Mulligan. 1962. Helminth immunity. *In* Advances in Veterinary Science, Vol. 7. Brandley, C. S., and Jungherr, E. L., eds. New York, Academic Press, Inc.

Wagland, B. M., and J. K. Dineen. 1965. The cellular transfer of immunity to *Trichostrongylus colubriformis* in an isogenic strain of guinea pig. Aust. J. Exp. Biol. Med. Sci., 42: 429–438.

Weinmann, C. J. 1960. Studies on schistosomiasis. XV. Resistance to *Schistosoma mansoni* in mice immunized with *Trichinella spiralis*. J. Parasit., 46 (Suppl.): 37.

Weinstein, P. P. 1955. The effect of cortisone on the immune response of the white rat to *Nippostrongylus muris*. Amer. J. Trop. Med. Hyg., 4: 61–74.

Werle, E., and W. Ringler. 1951. Über die Wirkung des Colonsaftes von Askariden nach intravenoser Injektion beim Hund. Z. Immunität. Exp. Therap. 109: 60–65.

Westcott, R. B., and A. C. Todd. 1964. A comparison of the development of *Nippostrongylus brasiliensis* in germ-free and conventional mice. J. Parasit., 50: 138-143.

Whitlock, J. H. 1955. A study of inheritance of resistance to trichostrongylidosis in sheep. Cornell Vet., 45: 422–439.

—— 1958. The inheritance of resistance to trichostrongylidosis in sheep. I. Demonstration of the validity of the phenomena. Cornell Vet., 48: 127–133.

Whur, P. 1966. Relationship of globule leucocytes to gastrointestinal nematodes in the sheep, and *Nippostrongylus brasiliensis* and *Hymenolepis nana* infections in rats. J. Comp. Path, 76: 57–65.

World Health Organization Expert Committee Report. 1965. Immunology and Parasitic Diseases. W.H.O. Tech. Rep. Ser. No. 315, pp. 1–64.

Yarinsky, A. 1962. The influence of x-irradiation on the immunity of mice to infection with *Trichinella spiralis*. J. Elisha Mitchell Sci. Soc., 78: 29–43.

Zaiman, H., J. D. Wilson, J. Rubel, and J. M. Stoney. 1954. Studies on the nature of immunity to *Trichinella spiralis* in parabiotic rats. III. The immune response in "uninfected" parabiotic rats surgically separated from the mates 2, 3, 4, and 5 days after the latter received an immunizing infection. Amer. J. Hyg., 59: 39–51.

—— J. M. Stoney, J. Rubel, and N. C. Headley. 1955a. Studies on the nature of immunity to *Trichinella spiralis* in parabiotic rats. VII. The immune response of the "uninfected" twin one month after its mate received an immunizing dose of irradiated (x-ray) larvae. Amer. J. Hyg., 61: 5–14.

—— J. M. Stoney, and N. C. Headley. 1955b. Studies on the nature of immunity to *Trichinella spiralis* in parabiotic rats. VIII. The duration of the immune response in the "uninfected" parabiotic rat following infection of one twin with *Trichinella spiralis*. Amer. J. Hyg., 61: 15–23.

—— R. G. Howard, and C. J. Miller. 1961. Immune response in rats infected with *Trichinella spiralis* larvae subjected to roentgen radiation. Amer. J. Trop. Med. Hyg., 10: 215–219.

Insect-Borne Nematodes

GILBERT F. OTTO

Department of Zoology, University of Maryland, College Park, Maryland

INTRODUCTION

Relatively few of the nematodes which require arthropods as intermediate hosts have been colonized in experimental laboratories. Furthermore, such colonization as has taken place is quite recent, and most of the studies have been and are currently being directed primarily towards elucidating various aspects of the basic life cycles. Only a limited amount of exploratory work on protective immunity is undertaken in these laboratory controlled systems. Thus, although few data have been developed on protective immunity against insect-borne nematode infections, such studies have produced evidence of some immune response. The more extensive studies on immunodiagnosis of filariasis during the past 40 years have clearly demonstrated that experimental animals respond immunologically to injection of emulsion extracts or fractions of the filarioids. Similarily it has been shown that the infected host responds immunologically.

Much of the work on immunodiagnosis of insect-borne nematode infections has been concerned with the diagnosis of the several filarioid infections, most commonly *Wuchereria bancrofti*. The subject has been thoroughly reviewed by Kagan (1963), and there would be little gained by an additional analysis now. In any event, immunodiagnosis *per se* is not the subject of this review. Although there has been continuing improvement in the specificity and sensitivity of the several serologic tests developed, in general they fall short of the accuracy desired as a laboratory aid to clinical diagnosis. Their most useful role is as an additional epidemiologic parameter. Even here, the question of specificity has to be considered in any evaluation of the data. The intradermal test appears to have little specificity. However, for the purpose of our present discussion, the important consideration is the unquestioned evidence that infection stimulates the production of antibodies which may be detected by intradermal tests and by the several serologic tests with antigens from either microfilariae or adult filariae of several species. Furthermore, in several different studies, these antigens have been injected into rabbits to produce antibodies against them. The antigens may be conveniently referred to as somatic antigens (Thorson, 1963), since they were derived from the tissues and fluids of worms, particular tissues or organs of the worms, or extracts or fractions thereof. There is no evidence, despite their antigenicity, that they are involved in protective immunity. It would be easy to assume, then, that any protective immunity against the filarioids does not involve a circulating antibody, and some of the early workers apparently come to this conclusion. However, as Taliaferro (1940) has pointed out, even though the serum antibody level does not bear a direct relation to the presence or absence of protective immunity, one is not justified, on that evidence alone, in concluding that there is not a serologic basis for immunity. We may add that any such negative evidence does not justify the assumption that protective immunity does not occur.

Since it has been shown that enzymes in the metabolic products (excretions and secretions) of intestinal nematodes are antigenic (*see* below), there have been attempts to use these metabolic products as diagnostic antigens both for schistosomes as well as for some of the intestinal nematodes. So far as I am aware, there has not been any attempt to utilize such metabolic products for detecting infections with arthropod-borne nematodes. However, the results with this method have not been such as to encourage further exploration for purely diagnostic purposes. Nevertheless, exploration in this area may provide more significant evidence on the level and the nature of protective immunity against insect-borne nematode infections.

EXPERIMENTAL STUDIES ON PROTECTIVE IMMUNITY

Attempts to confer protective immunity

The first attempt to confer protective immunity with an insect-borne nematode infection appears to be that of Feng (1937) with the dog heart worm, *Dirofilaria immitis*. Feng gave one dog a series of subcutaneous injections of an emulsion of pulverized male worms totaling 2.0 mg of dried worms. On subsequent challenge, the same number of worms was recovered seven months later from the heart of the injected dog as from the heart of the uninjected control. A third dog similarly given an even larger total amount of pulverized female worms (3.9 mg of dried worms) had no worms in the heart when it died less than three months after challenge (the cause of death was not recorded). However, no significance can be attached to the failure to find worms in the heart in less than three months after infection, since the available evidence indicates that the developing heart worms require three to four months after infection to reach the heart (Kume and Itagaki, 1955; Orihel, 1961). Using a somewhat different approach, Murata (1939) found that injection of extracts of *D. immitis* into infected dogs did not alter the number, activity, or appearance of microfilariae in the peripheral circulation. When rabbits were immunized by similar injections of extracts of *D. immitis* and subsequently transfused with blood from a *D. immitis*-infected dog, there was no reduction in activity of the microfilariae although they disappeared from the blood a little sooner than from the blood of nonimmunized rabbits.

More recently, Worms (1967) states that: "The second course [of *D. immitis* infection in the dog] is radically modified by the immune response of the host which limits the duration and magnitude of the microfilaraemia but had little effect upon the longevity and fecundity of the adult worm." No details are given.

Although Feng (1937) and Murata (1939) failed to produce demonstrable immunity with injections of pulverized worms, this cannot be interpreted as evidence that the phenomenon is not operative in this mosquito-borne filaria infection. It should be noted that Feng himself does not so interpret his results. Subsequent studies by a number of different authors have been concerned with this phenomenon in infections with nematodes which have direct life cycles, i.e., which do not utilize intermediate hosts. These studies are reviewed in Dr. Thorson's chapter, to which the reader is referred for detailed coverage. In brief, it has been demonstrated that a highly protective immunity will be induced by previous infection against *Nippostrongylus brasiliensis*, *Strongyloides ratti*, *Ancylostoma caninum*, and *Necator americanus*, to mention only a few. However, attempts to induce such protective immunity with dead whole larvae or pulverized larvae have been singularly unsuccessful. The conspicuous exception to this was the immunization of rats against *Strongyloides ratti* by 13 subcutaneous injections of heat-killed larvae at 3-day intervals, for a total of 16,000 such larvae. The resulting immunity was almost as great as that resulting from a single infection of only 1,000 living larvae. So far as I am aware, no other attempt to immunize animals by injection of dead worms, either whole, macerated, or powdered, has yielded comparable results. Sheldon (1937) did not obtain such results with heat-killed *S. stercoralis* larvae, although living larvae produced essentially complete immunity.

The contrast in immunity produced by injections of living and dead larvae is sharply illustrated by the immune phenomenon in canine hookworm infections. It has been demonstrated that an initial infection with 1,200 to 1,400 larvae of *Ancylostoma caninum* will protect a puppy from a challenge infection with 50,000 larvae four to five months later. In sharp contrast, the injection of several hundred thousand heat-killed larvae two to three times a week for five months (a total of 8 to 10 million larvae) produced only a slight reduction in worms established from the challenge infection (Otto, 1948). The quantitative aspects are further illustrated by immunization with living larvae. While 1,200 to 1,400 living hookworm larvae will immunize a puppy to a challenge dose of 50,000 larvae, no such protection is afforded by an initial dose of 300 to 600 living larvae (Otto, 1941, 1948).

Where it has been sought, an antigenic enzyme has been found in the metabolic products (excretions and secretions) of nematodes. All the available evidence indicates that such an antigen induces protective immunity (*see* Thorson's chapter, pp. 925-926; 947). The amount of such an antigen in the larvae at any given time would be extremely low, and it is probably wholly or partially denatured by the heat necessary to kill the larvae. Thus, in attempting to evaluate any studies on immunity to arthropod-borne nematode infections, consideration must be given to both the quantitative aspects of the phenomenon and the nature of the as yet unidentified antigen.

Immune reactions to living worms and larvae

More recently, Wong (1964a,b) has experimentally studied the possibility of immunity to *D. immitis* infection by using the number of microfilariae as the indicator of immunity and, in part at least, using the microfilariae to stimulate immunity. She transfused large numbers of microfilariae into (1) a normal filariae-free dog, (2) a splenectomized filariae-free dog, (3) an otherwise normal dog into whose heart an adult female *D. immitis* had been previously introduced, and (4) two *D. immitis*-infected dogs. The microfilariae remained detectable in the circulation of the normal dog for 7 weeks, in the splenectomized dog for 4 weeks, but in the dog with the surgically introduced female worm, only for 2 weeks. In the two infected dogs, the increased microfilariae were evident for a few days, but the number returned to the preinoculation level in less than two weeks. It remained at that level in one of the two dogs, but in the other, there was thereafter a gradual increase, presumably due to the established female worms rather than to the inoculated microfilariae. The results are suggestive but ambiguous, and they need to be repeated before any interpretations are justified.

In additional experiments, she demonstrated that microfilariae decreased in number and disappeared from the circulation (instead of increasing) as repeated intravenous injections of concentrated microfilariae (over 1,000,000 microfilariae in each injection) were given over a period of several weeks to uninfected dogs. The antimicrofilarial action of the sera of such dogs was tested in dogs with established infections. The injection of 2 to 4 ml per kg body weight, with few exceptions, produced an immediate and dramatic reduction in the number of circulating microfilariae in these infected animals. The decrease in number of microfilariae lasted from a few days to a week or more, and it was repeatable with additional injections of sera. Although Wong demonstrated agglutination of microfilariae in such animals, the relation of such agglutination to specific protective immunity is obscure. Mundt et al. (1965) have demonstrated *in vivo* agglutination of microfilariae in infected dogs during extracorporeal circulation and hypothermy. Furthermore, they found that when blood containing microfilariae was refrigerated and then administered intravenously to normal (i.e., uninfected) dogs, extensive *in vivo* agglutination occurred. They cite unpublished studies by Jachowski demonstrating *in vitro* agglutination in autologous serum following cooling of the blood below body temperature. It occurred readily at body temperature if the autologous serum or normal serum (i.e. from uninfected dogs) was previously cooled. The extent of the agglutination was directly related to the degree of cooling down to 4°C. Whether or not such *in vivo* agglutination removed microfilariae from the circulation of Wong's experimental dogs is not known. Again, her experiments are highly suggestive, but there are some possible ambiguities which are still to be resolved.

The only arthropod-borne nematode for which the question of protective immunity has been studied in a continuing program is *Litomosoides carinii*. This filarioid occurs naturally in the cotton rat (*Sigmodon hispidus*) and has been established in several experimental laboratories both in the cotton rat and in the white rat. Unlike most other filarioids whose life cycles are known, it is not transmitted by an insect but by a mite, *Ornithonyssus (Bdellonyssus) bacoti.* Nevertheless, the results of these studies are appropriately included here.

In one of the first studies reported, Bertram (1953) introduced uninfected cotton rats and mites into nests containing one or more cotton rats with established infections. They were left together for varying periods up to five months. The available evidence suggests that continuing reinfection (or superinfection) occurred, but the most impressive evidence is that there was no great accumulation of adult worms over that which occurs with a single infection. In fact, there were on the average fewer worms. Bertram notes that in his experience, 500 or more worms can be acquired in a single day under the same exposure conditions. In this series of continuing exposure, only one animal had over 500 worms (552), one had 346, two had 200 to 300, while six had less than 200. Evidently, there had been continued acquisition of infection. Either continued loss of worms at an increasing rate, the failure of some of the newly acquired larvae to develop, or some combination of these produced a net reduction in the number of living worms by the end of the experimental period. That some worms had died and been absorbed seems evident from the fact that encapsulated masses of worms were seen in various stages of destruction, including some calcified fragments. On the average, the living worms, particularly the females, were smaller than those developed from a single infection. There was evidence throughout the experimental period of reduced microfilaria production. Thus, in this attempt to reproduce experimentally the natural epizootiology of cotton rat filariasis and simulate the natural epidemiology of human filariasis, there is undeniable evidence that the host response alone, i.e., the immunologic response, exerted some measure of control over the infection. At the same time, the host did not escape some adverse effects since on the average, these cotton rats weighed less than uninfected rats of the same age or than rats with an even heavier primary infection.

Scott and his co-workers have attempted a more direct measure of the immunologic response to *L. carinii* in a series of tightly controlled experimental infections. They established evidence (Macdonald and Scott, 1958) that a series of light individual infections totaling about 200 or more infective larvae (173 to 434) produced a measurable adverse effect upon a challenge infection of 23 to 65 infective larvae administered 44 to 64 days later. The obvious effect was the significantly retarded growth, including conspicuous delay in molting and evidently permanent stunting of the female worms. There was even some suggestion that fewer worms developed in the immunized animals than in the previously uninfected controls. Much smaller immunizing infections (30 to 46 larvae) produced a less pronounced but still detectable retardation in the growth and development of the females, including a delay in molting to the next stage. Furthermore, there was no evidence that the injection of four times as many dead (frozen) larvae had any adverse effect upon the subsequent challenge infection. The subcutaneous or intraperitoneal introduction of 22 to 100 dead adult worms also had no clear-cut adverse effect upon subsequent challenge infection. The similarity between these results and those with nematodes which develop directly is further illustrated by Scott's (1952) finding *in vitro* oral precipitates on infective larvae in sera from infected cotton rats, although earlier, McFadzean (1953) had not succeeded in detecting such precipitates either in the sera of infected animals or in sera from rabbits which had been injected with dead worms. Jachowski (personal communication) reports oral precipitates on infective larvae of *W. bancrofti* incubated in the sera of monkeys (*Macacus irus*) which had been exposed previously to infective larvae of the same parasite.

In subsequent studies (Scott et al., 1958a; Scott and Macdonald, 1958), these workers reconfirmed the delay in development and molting with apparently ultimate reduction in size of both male and female worms from a challenge infection after immunizing infections of 200 or more larvae. With lower immunizing infections the results were variable, but in one experiment as few as 69 to 80 adult worms in an immunizing infection produced some reduction in numbers of worms developing, as well as delayed development of those that did establish. Furthermore, the intraperitoneal implant of 69 to 207 living adult worms appeared to delay the development of worms from a subsequent challenge with infective larvae, but the effect was not as pronounced as that produced by immunization with infective larvae in the same experiment. They also found that the immunity to challenge infection as seen in the reduced size and delayed molting was effective as long as 12 to 22 months after immunization with infective larvae (Macdonald and Scott, 1958). Evidence showed that the effect of the immunity expressed itself primarily, if not exclusively, against the very young stages, apparently against the penetrating and migrating third-stage (infective) larvae. Seven-day-old larvae (i.e., those before the third molt) taken from a primary infection (i.e., from a nonimmune animal) and transferred to either immune or nonimmune animals were able to develop normally in both (Scott, 1958b). Conversely, seven-day-old larvae from the immunized rat did not develop normally when transferred to nonimmune (i.e., previously uninfected) animals. Thus, the exposure in the immune environment during the first seven days of life adversely affected the subsequent growth and development even in a favorable environment. Both males and females resulting from larvae which had spent the first seven days in immune hosts were smaller and had a markedly reduced molting rate during the subsequent 17 days of growth in nonimmune hosts as compared with those which had never been in an immune host, i.e., which had been transferred at seven days from one nonimmune host to another. There was, however, no evidence in this series that any fewer worms established after seven days in the immune environment than did those which had never been in an immune environment.

It is probable that retardations in growth, molting, and reproductive potential are more delicate indices of immunologic pressures than is percentage development. If such is the case, one would expect fatal effects upon the worms to occur consistently as the animals become much more highly immunized by greater exposure to invading larvae, perhaps over a longer period of time. It would appear that this is exactly what happened in Bertram's long-term natural exposure of cotton rats to infection in the laboratory (Bertram, 1953). The animals were continuously exposed over many months, and from Bertram's observation of a single day's exposure under such conditions, it is evident that the potential severity of infection was far greater than in Scott's series of quantitatively identified exposures. The biologic effect of this exposure is seen both in the maintenance of a fairly constant or reduced number of worms, certainly no greatly increasing accumulation, and in the continuing pathologic strain on the host.

Working with *Loa loa*, Duke (1960) found evidence of marked microfilarial suppression on repeated experimental infections in drills or mandrills (*Mandrillus leucophaeus*), as they are variously named. When the microfilariae from a primary infection had disappeared from the peripheral circulation, two of the drills were reinfected and at the same time a previously uninfected drill was infected. The approximate maximum number of microfilariae in a cubic millimeter of blood (read from the microfilaria curves) were as follows:

Control animals, primary infection	300	980
Immunized animals, second infection	15	50

In a second series, the microfilaremia in the primary infection was compared with that resulting from subsequent infections in the same animals:

Primary infections	50	300
Subsequent infections	10	25

Furthermore, splenectomy was found to reverse the gradual (i.e., normal) diminution in the number of microfilariae in a primary infection. The relative numbers of adult worms produced in the primary and secondary infections are unknown. Nevertheless, it is obvious that the infected host responds to relatively few worms and at least limits their reproductive potential. Whether this evidence of acquired immunity results from the establishment of fewer worms from the second infection, from reduction in reproductive capacity of the established worms, from rapid destruction of microfilariae, or from a combination of these is also unknown.

In an interesting study on the chemotherapeutic prevention of *Loa loa* in human volunteers, Duke (1957) found that 5.0 mg per kg of body weight of drug daily (diethylcarbamazine) were required to prevent the maturation and microfilaria production of a primary infection. However, in subsequent reinfections no more than 2.5 mg per kg and as little as 1.0 mg per kg of body weight was required to accomplish the same effect. Duke concluded that the difference in doses required was directly associated with the presence or absence of immunity and the relative level of the immunity. Since his primary concern was the establishment of the necessary drug level to protect all elements of the population, he did not pursue in depth or greater detail the relationship to protective immunity.

EVIDENCE FROM NATURALLY OCCURRING INFECTIONS

Epidemiologic studies

Most of the epidemiologic data on arthropod-borne nematode infections in nature have been obtained from mosquito-borne filarial infections of man. The interpretation of microfilaria prevalence rates for various ages and the two sexes poses some difficult problems. The question of comparative exposure risk of the two sexes and of the several age groups is an important and often unknown factor in interpreting the underlying reasons for different microfilaria rates with regard to age and sex. Even more ill-defined in general is the question of hormonal effect on the susceptibility of males and females and perhaps even on the comparative susceptibility of children, young adults, and older adults. Although this latter question has not been resolved, it appears to offer few complications (other than differential exposure risks) in attempts to separate the various factors which influence the dynamics of the infection in a community.

One conspicuous example of the probable influence of exposure risk is reflected in the host age-specific microfilaria rates of periodic and nonperiodic *Wuchereria bancrofti* infections. In the Virgin Islands, where transmission is by the highly domestic *Culex fatigans* in the houses, and in Guyana, where transmission is also by highly domestic mosquitoes (*Culex fatigans* and *Anopheles darlingi*) in the houses, there is a very rapid rise in the microfilaria rate during the first decade of life to essentially the maximum level achieved. The early development of parasitemia is the same for both sexes and is apparently due to the equal exposure risks in the house (Anderson et al., 1923; Hughens, 1927; Jachowski and Otto, 1955). Nevertheless, the maximum rate at which the microfilaremia in females leveled off was slightly lower (30 to 35 percent) than that of the males (35 to 40 percent). Furthermore, while the male rates continued through all succeeding age groups without any appreciable change, the female rates declined after age 40. Whether the lower adult female rates and the further decline after age 40 is a function of lower exposure risks or a function of differential hormonal effect on resistance (i.e., sex effect on immunity) is difficult to say. Both have been suggested.

In areas of the South Pacific where transmission is primarily or exclusively in a sylvan environment by such forms as *Aedes polynesiensis* which rarely enter houses or venture into clearings, there is essentially no microfilaremia in children under five and the microfilaria rate thereafter rises slowly to reach a maximum at age 20 to 30. The maximum male adult rate is consistently higher, sometimes nearly double, the female rate. This appears to be directly related to the exposure risk (Jachowski and Otto, 1955), but it has also been suggested that there is a differential susceptibility of the mature males and females. The possibility of mature males being more susceptible than females or male castrates to other nematode infections has been shown in experimental animals (Solomon, 1966). Many other examples could be cited but these will serve to illustrate the problems involved in trying to evaluate the precise role of the several controlling factors from the basis of epidemiologic data.

Nevertheless, there appears to be very convincing evidence that the host responds immunologically to continuous or repeated exposure to infection and reinfection. In the various epidemiologic studies with *Brugia malayi* (Senoo and Lincicome, 1951; Wilson, 1961; Rozeboom and Cabrera, 1965; Cabrera and Tamondong, 1966; and others), with aperiodic *Wuchereria bancrofti* on South Pacific Islands, (Bahr, 1912; Buxton, 1928; Murray, 1948; Jachowski and Otto, 1955; Rosen, 1955; and others), and with periodic *W. bancrofti* (Anderson et al., 1923; Hughens, 1927; Cabrera and Tamondong, 1966; and others), there is one consistent and impressive fact: Regardless of whether the maximum microfilaria prevalence rate is reached at ten years of age or in the 20- to 30-year-old age group, such a maximum is reached relatively early in infections and thereafter remains fairly constant. This maximum rate varies with the several areas under study, and it is apparently heavily dependent upon the abundance of mosquitoes. But regardless of whether this maximum prevalence is 10 percent or 40 percent of the population, it levels off early and remains relatively constant thereafter. This is true of the rates for both males and for females. Admittedly, there are examples in which there is some apparent increase in the microfilaria rate in those over 60 years of age. However, the rates in the upper age groups are necessarily always derived from a conspicuously smaller sample than the rates in younger people. More often the percentage of microfilaria positives declines in the terminal age groups, though again this is based on a disproportionately small sample.

If we assume (1) no intrinsic host pressure adversely affects the penetration of the infective larvae; the migration, development or reproduction of the worms; or the activity and distribution of the resulting microfilariae in the body (specifically with respect to the occurrence of microfilariae in the peripheral circulation), and (2) there is random distribution of those being bitten by infected mosquitoes, i.e., no selection of any kind occurs, in any given age group and between age groups, then some very interesting base lines develop. The total microfilariae in the population would be the summation of the total microfilariae in each age group. Each age group would be expected to add approximately the same additional number of microfilariae to the population. If each group contained the same number of people, the total number of microfilariae per each age group would be represented by a straight line from the new-born to the elderly. Relatively few data have been developed on the number of microfilariae in the several age groups.

Buxton (1928) and Rosen (1955) have provided such data from Polynesia, where aperiodic *W. bancrofti* occurs. As is usual, the populations sampled from the several age groups are far from uniform. Whether or not the same proportion of each age group was sampled is not known, but it seems unlikely that any serious bias was created by the sampling. Therefore, using the samples as roughly representative of the population, it is at once evident that the greatest population, at least the greatest sample, is among the young adults. Therefore, any attempt to convert the microfilaria counts into total numbers of microfilariae for each age group produces an unrealistic concentration of the total microfilariae in these age groups and suggests a rapid rise in total microfilariae in 20- to 40-year-old age groups with an almost equally rapid decline thereafter. Using the mean number of microfilariae per positive in each group, which both Buxton and Rosen present in their tables, produces the same bias but a little less pronounced. Accordingly, I have converted these into the average of the total sampled in each age group. This is depicted in Figure 1. This is also the nearest approach to depicting a steady build-up in total number of microfilariae with increasing age. Rosen's data for the females, with their generally lower microfilaremia, actually suggests such a steady build-up. However, neither Rosen's data on the males nor Buxton's data (which only include data on males) fits this concept. Obviously, more data are needed, but this analysis comes closer than any of the other analyses used to show a steady build-up in numbers with increasing age. Unfortunately, it fails to offer convincing evidence that this occurs. Thus, the data on the number of microfilariae in each age group contain at least the suggestion that some intrinsic host factor is depressing microfilaremia with increasing exposure to infection, which may be exaggerated or partially hidden by the inevitable sampling errors, differences in exposure risk, and possible sex differences in susceptibility.

It seems profitable, then, to return to the picture set forth by the age-

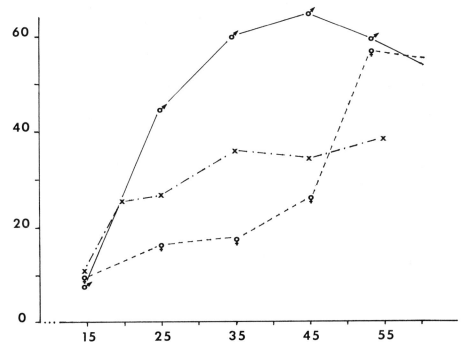

FIG. 1. The average number of microfilariae (in 20 cu mm of blood) in various age groups in Polynesia: ♂ males and ♀ females (Rosen, 1955) and × males (Buxton, 1928). The average number of microfilariae are shown on the ordinate and the ages of the population on the abscissa.

specific prevalence rates. On the basis of the same two above-stated assumptions, the percentage of microfilariae would not increase in a straight line but at gradually decreasing increments as the percentage of positives increases. The resulting curve would be a function of the infection potential and the resulting cumulative infection rates in each successive age group. Death would remove both infected and uninfected hosts, whereas births would provide a continuing supply of a noninfected (susceptible) segment of the population. Both the birth rate and death rate would modify the curve slightly. Since we do not have a direct measure of the transmission potential and do know either the birth rate or the death rate in the populations, the several extremes can be shown most readily by plotting a series of curves based on specific rates of acquisition. In Figure 2 are shown the curves resulting from exposure risks that would produce 5, 10, 20 and 30 percent microfilaremia in the youngest age groups. At the lowest exposure risk, whether the age group is either 5 or 10 years (the common units used in reporting microfilaremia), it is evident that there would be an essentially straight line increase with little evidence of the curvilinear relationship during the normal life expectancy. On the other hand, with an exposure risk which would produce 20 to 30 percent microfilaremia in the first age group, the curvilinear relationship is seen immediately. Although the microfilaremia

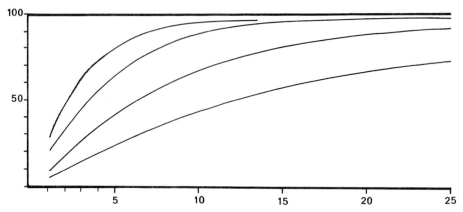

FIG. 2. Theoretical increase in microfilaria prevalence rates assuming uniform exposure and uniform susceptibility for four different levels of exposure risk which would produce 5, 10, 20, and 30 percent microfilaremia, respectively, in the first age group. The percentage of microfilaremia is shown on the ordinate and the age groups on the abscissa.

increases at a readily discernible declining increment, the actual increase is very rapid in the first few age groups. Thus, if the initial 20 to 30 percent is in the first decade of life, we would anticipate 60 to 80 percent by age 40 and 70 to 90 percent by age 60. One would scarcely expect 100 percent microfilaremia at any age group during the normal life expectancy, but one would expect figures in excess of 90 percent and approaching 100 percent in the older age groups.

In contrast to this, as already pointed out, in areas of high endemicity with transmission in households by anthropophilic mosquitoes, the microfilaria rate in males commonly rises to 20 to 40 percent in the first decade of life and essentially levels off thereafter. In the vicinity of Belem, Brazil, scarcely a highly endemic area, the microfilaremia rate rose more gradually to 10 percent at age 19 and thereafter leveled off (Causey et al., 1945). Where transmission is in a sylvan setting, as with aperiodic *W. bancrofti* and *B. malayi* in which exposure risk is less uniform, little transmission takes place in the first five years of life, but microfilaremia rates in males commonly reach a peak in the 20- to 30-year-old age group and thereafter level off. The female microfilaremia rates follow the same basic pattern, but the peak is usually at a lower level. In part, this appears to be due to reduced exposure risk, but it is impossible to escape the indications that there may be a hormonal effect rendering the males more susceptible than the females. However, in both males and females the microfilaria rates esentially level off after maturity.

Thus, neither the total increase in microfilariae nor the increase in the microfilaria prevalence rates follows the anticipated course if there were random distribution in the mosquito biting (i.e., equal exposure risk) and no intrinsic host factor to reduce the resulting microfilaremia. To only a limited degree can these differences be associated with known or suspected differences in exposure risk. There is even less evidence of a specific sex difference in susceptibility. Thus, we are left with the impression that there is an intrinsic host factor in both males and females that manifests itself with increasing exposure to infection both by reduction in the microfilaria prevalence rates in the older age groups and by reduction in the number of microfilariae in the older population.

Possible host factors

To complete the picture, we must consider the conspicuous physical and pathologic evidence of immunity to mosquito-borne filariasis in man, namely, the effect of elephantiasis. Manson (1898) was probably the first to call attention to the fact that elephantiasis was most prevalent where the total community prevalence of microfilaremia is highest, but that the individuals with elephantiasis have a negative correlation with microfilaremia. This has been brought out by many others (Low, 1908; Iyengar, 1938; Kessel, 1957; Wilson, 1961; and others). Manson believed that the reaction in the lymphatics blocked the escape of the microfilariae. Certainly, the work of Drinker and Homans (1934) and Drinker et al. (1935) suggests that a simple foreign-body reaction or local chemical reaction or both would block the lymphatics. These workers found that the intralymphatic injection of quinine solution or a suspension of silicone would provoke sufficient tissue reaction in the lymphatics to occlude them completely. Furthermore, such blocked lymph channels would provide the opportunity for local bacterial infection, i.e., they would prevent or retard the normal lymph node function of removing the bacteria. It would be easy enough, then, to assume that the reaction to the presence of filariae was simply a foreign-body reaction intensified by continued or intermittent presence of the worms and further aggravated by secondary bacterial infection. It will be recalled that Grace (1943), while recognizing that the worms were the precipitating cause, appeared to be convinced that the total reaction was predominantly due to the secondary bacterial invaders.

This appears to be an unfortunate oversimplification. Napier (1944) suggests that it is more logical to visualize the reaction as an allergic or antibody function. O'Connor and Hulse (1932) were impressed with the evidence that there is a specific response to the dead worms which exceeds that of a simple foreign-body response. They are further impressed with the "fragility" of the worms, since recovery of dead worms from hosts exceeded that of living worms in studies in endemic areas. Since we have found that microfilariae will remain in an infected individual for about a decade after leaving an endemic area (Jachowski et al., 1951), the possibility exists that in the presence of continuing reinfection the antigenic stimulus may have a lethal effect upon the worms. While recognizing that many of the lesions are complicated by bacterial infection, Lichtenberg (1957) stresses the allergic nature of many of the lesions, as do Schacher and Sahyoun (1967). The recurrent evidence of tissue eosinophilia in connection with adult filariae in man and experimental animals appears to set these lesions apart from purely inert foreign-body reactions. It certainly suggests an allergic state. Furthermore, Schacher and Sahyoun (1967) have found evidence of intensified reaction associated with molting *Brugia* in experimental animals. Such molting would release exsheathing fluid or other metabolic products and suggests a situation very comparable to that seen with intestinal nematodes. Oral precipitates are also reported.

One wonders about the relation between the initial worm infections and subsequent reinfections. The experience with U. S. military personnel in the Pacific suggests that a severe allergic reaction and tissue response occurs early. Nevertheless, these men were exposed on a continuing basis until clinical manifestations occurred. There is nothing to suggest that they had acquired only a single infection. This is of significance in interpreting the data. It has been shown (Andrews, 1939) that with the nodular worm of sheep (*Cooperia curticei*), nodules were not formed with the primary infection but only on reinfection. Does this bear any relationship to the tissue response to filariae in the lymphatics? I think so.

In the course of investigating acute fatal heart-worm diseases (Jackson et al., 1962), we developed some interesting data on the distribution of heart worms in dogs of different ages (Jackson et al., 1966). We found that with massive infections, young dogs with no previous history of heart disease or other debilitating disease would collapse with acute hepatic syndrome and die shortly thereafter (*see* Table 1). Most were young dogs 3 to 5 years old, and half of them were no more than 3 years old.

Table 1

Average Number of Adult *Dirofilaria immitis* Recovered on Postmortem Examination of Infected Dogs in Florida

Symptom Group	Age	No. of Dogs	Average No. of Worms
Asymptomatic	all ages	50	25
Moderately ill	all ages	11	47
Chronic heart-worm disease	old	32	58
Acute hepatic syndrome	young	24	101

The asymptomatic dogs and the moderately ill dogs were mainly pound dogs but included some accident cases. The chronic heart-worm dogs included both these sources and debilitated dogs brought to the clinic for euthanasia. The last group (those with acute hepatic syndrome) included only dogs brought to the clinic because they were acutely ill. There was no history of recent treatment of any of them. Furthermore, in our earlier studies of asymptomatic and chronic heart-worm dogs from this area of Florida before modern therapy was available, we found that dogs of all ages rarely harbored more than 35 to 40 worms and usually fewer.

It would appear, then, that the massive infections may be acquired at one time or over a short period of time by young dogs. These can be fatal just as massive hookworm infections can be fatal. It would also appear that older dogs do not continue to build up a continuing increase in the number of worms. On the contrary, any young dogs which acquired nonfatal massive infections appeared to have lost many of the worms while in the enzootic area and continuously exposed to reinfection. We have no precise information on the number of microfilariae in the peripheral blood of these dogs, but in other studies in the same area we have found no correlation between the number of microfilariae in the circulation and the number of adult worms found on post-mortem examination. It would appear that with increasing numbers of worms, there is decreasing microfilaria production per worm. Regardless of the number of circulating microfilariae, it would appear that large numbers of adult heart worms may be acquired by young dogs early in their exposure to infection. Whether these represent unusual and accidental infections which are usually fatal, or whether such heavy nonfatal infections occur is unknown. However, it is clear that these massive infections do not routinely occur in old dogs with long continued exposure to infection. On the contrary, long continued exposure to infection, despite its debilitating effect, appears to result in progressively fewer adult heart worms.

CONCLUSION

The available data on the natural occurrence of *Wuchereria bancrofti* and *Brugia malayi* in man and *Dirofilaria immitis* in dogs suggest that there is an intrinsic host factor which adversely affects the worms on continued exposure to reinfection. In man this is seen in declining microfilaria prevalence rates and declining numbers of microfilariae in the older age groups. Whether there is a similar reduction in numbers of adult worms, a reduction in fecundity of female worms, a direct destruction of microfilariae, or a combination of these is unknown. Apparently, there has been no attempt to determine the total number of adult worms in the relatively few post-mortem cases of older subjects with filariasis. Even less is known about the number of worms in the younger age groups in the same endemic areas. However, routine post-mortem examination of dogs of various ages suggests that continued exposure to heart-worm infection directly limits and in fact reduces the number of worms which survive.

Explorations of the phenomenon of acquired immunity in arthropod-borne nematode infections in the laboratory have not revealed any evidence of a highly protective immunity. Sometimes the results have been entirely negative, sometimes they have been suggestive but inconclusive, and the most carefully controlled studies with *Litomosoides carinii* have indicated only some stunting of worms and some reduction in reproduction. The experimental studies with laboratory infections suggest that there may be a significant reduction in the number of adult worms as a result of continuing exposure to reinfection.

It appears that the situation is very comparable to that of 30 to 40 years ago with the intestinal helminths. The most detailed epidemiologic studies, notably on hookworm disease, made it amply clear that the total picture was not revealed by the summation of the several factors involved in the exposure risk. Intrinsic host factors seemed to be involved. However, probing experiments in the laboratory developed equivocal and ambiguous information. It was not until the development of the concept of repeated infection ("hyperimmunization") followed by challenge with otherwise lethal infections that it was discovered that even the severely pathogenic hookworm of man or dog could produce a powerful and highly protective immunity. Only after this was demonstrated was it reasonable to consider the quantitative relations between immunity and challenge and to evaluate other factors such as the role of nutrition (Otto, 1948).

The rather limited number of worms used by Scott and his co-workers in attempts to immunize cotton rats against *Litomosoides carinii* is reminiscent of the limited numbers of worms used in the early and inconclusive studies on possible immunity to hookworm, strongyloides, and other intestinal nematodes. It is of more than passing interest that the only experimental study that suggests a reduction in the number of arthropod-borne nematodes due to reinfection is that of Bertram, who used much heavier exposures than did Scott in his more rigidly controlled studies.

As Scott (1960) points out, "the evidence for protective immunity to *Wuchereria* infection is quite unsatisfactory." Nevertheless, it does seem evident that the same immunologic phenomena are operative in insect-borne nematode infections as have been demonstrated with direct-cycle intestinal nematodes. Whether or not they are potentially as powerful and as fully protective is yet to be demonstrated, and whether or not the phenomena can be controlled for practical use can be determined only when we know the nature of the antigen involved in the stimulation of protective immunity. The W.H.O. Expert Committee on Filariasis (1967) has indicated that basic studies on immunity are needed. One approach would be to follow the experience with other nematode infections—namely, to increase experimentally the antigenic stimulus by more frequent and heavier exposure to infection with known numbers of infective larvae and to challenge the resulting immunity with infections that would overwhelm the nonimmune animal. If this is successful in demonstrating protective immunity, it should thereafter be easier to detect and to determine the nature of the antigen or antigens involved. The use of actual infection to produce protective immunity does not appear to have any practical application in either man or lower animals. Synthesis of the antigen would appear to offer one possible approach. However, such an approach must await the detection and identification of the naturally occurring antigen.

REFERENCES

Anderson, J., M. Khalil, C. U. Lee, and R. T. Leiper. 1923. A filaria survey in British Guiana, 1921. J. Helminth., 1:215–226.

Andrews, J. S. 1939. Life cycle of the nematode *Cooperia curticei* and development in resistant sheep. J. Agric. Res., 58:771–786.

Bahr, P. H. 1912. Filariasis and elephantiasis in Fiji. Research Memoirs of the London School of Tropical Medicine, 1:1–198.

Bertram, D. S. 1953. Laboratory studies on filariasis in the cotton-rat. Trans. Roy. Soc. Trop. Med. Hyg., 47:85–106.

Buxton, P. A. 1928. Researches in Polynesia and Melanesia. An account of investigations in Samoa, Tonga, The Ellice Group, and the New Hebrides, in 1924, 1925. Parts V–VII (Relating to human diseases and welfare). Research Memoirs of the London School of Hygiene and Tropical Medicine, 2:1–139.

Cabrera, B. D., and C. T. Tamondong. 1966. Bancroftian and Malayan filariasis in Palawan. Extent and distribution. Acta Med. Philipp., 3:20–36.

Causey, O. R., M. P. Deane, O. da Costa, and L. M. Deane. 1945. Studies on the incidence and transmission of filaria, *Wuchereria bancrofti*, in Belem, Brazil. Amer. J. Hyg., 41:143–149.

Drinker, C. K. and J. Homans. 1934. The experimental production of edema and elephantiasis as a result of lymphatic obstruction. Amer. J. Physiol., 108:509–520.

———— M. E. Field, and H. K. Ward. 1935. Increased susceptibility to local infections following blockage of the lymph drainage. Amer. J. Physiol., 112:74–.

Duke, B O. L. 1957. Studies on the chemotherapy of loiasis. II. Observations on diethylcarbamazine citrate (Banocide) as a prophylactic in man. Ann. Trop. Med. Parasit., 57:82–96.

———— 1960. Studies on loiasis in monkeys. II. The population dynamics of the microfilariae of *Loa loa* in experimentally infected drills (*Mandrillus leucophaeus*). Ann. Trop. Med. Parasit., 54:15–31.

Feng, L. C. 1937. Attempt to immunize dogs against infection with *Dirofilaria immitis* Leidy 1856. Festschrift Nockt, pp. 140–142.

Grace, A. W. 1943. Tropical lymphangitis and abscesses. J.A.M.A.. 123:462–466.

Hughens, H. V. 1927. Filariasis. Report on 1,742 person observed in St. Croix, Virgin Islands. U. S. Naval Med. Bull., 25:111–117.

Iyengar, M. O. T. 1938. Studies on the epidemiology of filariasis in Travancore. Indian Med. Res. Mem., 30:1–179.

Jachowski, L. A. 1967. Personal communication.

———— and G. F. Otto. 1955. Filariasis in American Samoa. IV. Prevalence of microfilaremia in the human population. Amer. J. Hyg., 61:334–348.

———— G. F. Otto, and J. D. Wharton. 1951. Filariasis in American Samoa. I. Loss of microfilariae in the absence of continued reinfection. Proc. Helminth Soc. (Washington), 18:25–28.

Jackson, R. F., F. von Lichtenberg, and G. F. Otto. 1962. Occurrence of adult heartworms in the venae cavae of dogs. J. Amer. Vet. Med. Ass., 141:117–121.

———— G. F. Otto, P. M. Baumon, F. Peacock, W. L. Hinricks, and J. H. Maltby. 1966. Distribution of heartworms in the right side of the heart and adjacent vessels of the dog. J. Amer. Vet. Med. Ass., 149:515–518.

Kagan, I. G. 1963. A review of immunologic methods for the diagnosis of filariasis. J. Parasit., 49:773–798.

Kessell, J. F. 1957. Disabling effects and control of filariasis. Amer. J. Trop. Med. Hyg., 6:402–414.

Kume, S., and S. Itagaki. 1955. On the life cycle of *Dirofilaria immitis* in the dog as the final host. Brit. Vet. J. 111:16–24.

Lichtenberg, F. 1957. The early phase of endemic bancroftian filariasis in the male. J. Mount Sinai Hosp. N.Y., 24:983–1000.

Low, G. C. 1908. The unequal distribution of filariasis in the tropics. Lancet, 1:279–281.

Macdonald, E. M., and J. A. Scott. 1958. The persistence of acquired immunity to the filarial worm of the cotton rat. Amer. J. Trop. Med. Hyg., 7:419–422.

Manson, P. 1898. A Manual of Diseases of Warm Climates. London, 607 pp.

McFadzean, J. A. 1953. Immunity in filariasis of experimental animals. Amer. J. Trop. Med. Hyg., 2:85–94.

Mundt, E. D., Y. G. Jacobson, D. M. Long, A. J. Defalco, L. A. Jachowski, and J. E. McClenathan. 1965. Systemic pathology in dogs undergoing extracorporeal circulation as a result of *Dirofilaria immitis* (heart-worm) infection or the use of microfilaria positive donor blood. J. Surg. Res., 5:437–442.

Murata, H. 1939. Immunologische Studien über *Dirofilaria immitis*. Fukuoka Acta Med., 32:945–972.

Murray, W. D. 1948. Filariasis studies in American Samoa. U.S. Naval Med. Bull., 48(2):327–341.

Napier, L. E. 1944. Filariasis due to *Wuchereria bancrofti.* Medicine, 23:149–179.

O'Connor, F. W., and C. R. Hulse. 1932. Some pathological changes associated with *Wuchereria (Filaria) bancrofti* infection. Trans. Roy. Soc. Trop. Med. Hyg., 25:445–454.

Orihel, T. C. 1961. Morphology of the larval stages of *Dirofilaria immitis* in the dog. J. Parasit., 47:251–262.

Otto, G. F. 1941. Further observations on the immunity induced in dogs by repeated infections with the hookworm, *Ancylostomum caninum.* Amer. J. Hyg., 33:39–57.

———— 1948. Immunity against canine hookworm disease. Vet. Med., 43:180–191.

Rosen, L. 1955. Observations on the epidemiology of human filariasis in French Oceania. Amer. J. Hyg., 61:219–248.

Rozeboom, L. E., and B. D. Cabrera. 1965. Filariasis caused by *Brugia malayi* in the republic of the Philipines. Amer. J. Epidem., 81:200–215.

Schacher, J. F., and P. F. Sahyoun. 1967. A chronological study of the histopathology of filarial disease in cats and dogs caused by *Brugia pahangi* (Buckley and Edeson, 1956). Trans. Roy. Soc. Trop. Med. Hyg., 61:234–243.

Scott, J. A. 1952. Studies on the mechanism of immunity to filarial worms in the cotton rat. J. Parasit., 38:18.

———— 1960. Immunity to infection with *Wuchereria.* Indian J. Malar., 14:575–583.

———— and E. M. Macdonald. 1958. Immunity to challenging infections of *Litomosoides carinii* produced by transfer of developing worms. J. Parasit., 44:187–191.

———— E. M. Macdonald, and L. J. Olson. 1958a. Attempts to produce immunity against filarial worms of cotton rats by transfer of developing worms. Amer. J. Trop. Med. Hyg., 7:70–73.

———— E. M. Macdonald, and L. J. Olson. 1958b. Early induction in cotton rats of immunity to their filarial worms. J. Parasit., 44:507–511.

Senoo, T., and D. R. Lincicome. 1951. Malayan filariasis. U S. Armed Forces Med. J., 2:1483–1489.

Sheldon, A. J. 1937. Studies on active acquired resistance, natural and artificial, in the rat to infection with *Strongyloides ratti.* Amer. J. Hyg., 25:53–65.

Solomon, G. B. 1966. The development of *Nippostrongylus brasiliensis* in gonadectomized and hormone-treated hamsters. Exp. Parasit., 18:374–396.

Taliaferro, W. H. 1940. The mechanism of acquired immunity in infections with parasitic worms. Physiol. Rev., 20:469–492.

Thorson, R. E. 1963. Immunodiagnosis of helminth infections. V. The use of metabolic and somatic antigens in the diagnosis of helminth infections. Amer. J. Hyg. Monogr. Ser., 22:60–67.

Wilson, T. 1961. Filariasis in Malaya. A General Review. Trans. Roy. Soc. Trop. Med. Hyg., 55:107–129.

Wong, M. M. 1964a. Studies on microfilaremia in dogs. I. A search for the mechanisms that stabilize the level of microfilaremia. Amer. J. Trop. Med. Hyg., 13:57–65.

———— 1964b. Studies on microfilaremia in dogs. II. Levels of microfilaremia in relation to immunologic responses of the host. Amer. J. Trop. Med. Hyg., 13:66–77.

World Health Organization Expert Committee, Second Report. 1967. Filariasis *Wuchereria* and *Brugia* Infections. W.H.O. Tech. Rep. Ser. No. 359, pp. 3–47.

Worms, M. J. 1967. WHO/Fil/67.71.

Schistosomes

ROBERT M. LEWERT

Department of Microbiology, The University of Chicago, Chicago, Illinois

INTRODUCTION

Immunity and resistance to infection with the schistosomes has occupied the attention of investigators in parasitology and in tropical medicine from the very beginnings of our discovery and understanding of these organisms and the diseases they produce. With the proliferation of immunologic techniques and immunodiagnostic methodology of the last twenty years, the literature on the serology of schistosomal infections has proportionately increased. Because of the importance of human schistosomiasis, this has been, in a sense, disproportionate to the literature in other areas of parasitic infection and disease. Additionally, it has had a disproportionate share of attention because of the uniquely varied and prolonged nature of the host-parasite contact in schistosomal infections.

The host initially has a brief exposure to secretions of the infecting cercariae as they penetrate the skin and enter the dermis. This is followed by exposure to antigenic substances derived from those vitiated and dying decaudicated cercariae which are unable to migrate past the superficial tissues. The host is then subjected to the secretions, excretions, and somatic substances of the developing schistosomula, some of which may die in the process of maturation. The host is subsequently subject to the constant stimulus of antigenic secretions and excretions of the adult worm over a period of many years, as well as to the secretions and excretions of the embryonated eggs which are trapped in its tissues. The latter die or are destroyed by the host, giving a continuous stimulation to its various immune mechanisms. The relative ease with which some of the antigens associated with this parasitic infection may be obtained, as well as the fact that substances from all stages of the parasite are shown to have serologic reactivity in infection or in artificially immunized animals, have stimulated many investigators to pursue the will-o-the-wisp of an antigen or antigen complex which might evoke the production of protective immunity.

In recent years there have been a number of reviews covering various aspects of immunity to schistosomal infections (Kagan, 1958, 1966; Soulsby, 1962; Smithers, 1962a; Stirewalt, 1963; Sadun, 1965; von Lichtenberg, 1967a; Smithers and Terry, 1969). In addition, we are fortunate in having an excellent series of bibliographies devoted exclusively to the subject of schistosomiasis and covering, up to recent times, all aspects of parasitism and disease by this group (Khalil, 1931; Bouillon, 1949; World Health Organization, 1960; Warren and Newill, 1967). Because of the ready availability of most of this material, this chapter on immunity to schistosome infections is deliberately selective. A completely comprehensive chapter would, if only a brief note were to be included on each of the pertinent works, be so lengthy as to necessitate an entire volume on this subject.

EARLY STUDIES OF IMMUNITY TO SCHISTOSOMIASIS

The literature on schistosomiasis begins with the discovery of adults of *Schistosoma hematobium* by Bilharz and his association of the organism to disease in 1852 (Bilharz, 1852a,b). In the half century following these observations, came the recognition that schistosome species are important in contributing to pathogenesis of disease in man. A clear elucidation of the life cycle of the parasite evaded investigators until the first two decades of the twentieth century, culminating in such excellent monographs as that of Faust and Meleney (1924) on *Schistosoma japonicum* and the collected series of papers by various authors published in the Puerto Rican Journal of Tropical Medicine from 1933 to 1937. The history of the various early discoveries of this period is covered best by Girgis (1934) in his monograph on schistosomiasis. In spite of the lack of detailed information on the life history of these parasites and on all aspects of their pathogenicity, there evolved during this period concepts of immunity to schistosomal infection, which were based on clinical and epidemiologic evidence in human infections with all three major species (Faust and Meleney, 1924; Puerto Rican J. Public Health Trop. Med., 1933-1937; Girgis, 1934; Dixon, 1934; Fisher, 1934).

Experimental studies with animals in attempts to confer immunity were undertaken in the early part of the twentieth century. Investigators of *Schistosoma japonicum* were probably the first to discuss immunity in man, to use immunodiagnostic techniques in this infection, and to attempt artificial immunization. As early as 1910, a complement-fixing reaction was described by Yoshimoto Fujinami (1916a,b), and Fujinami and Sueyasu (1917, 1918) indicated that animals which recovered from infection with *Schistosoma japonicum* were resistant to subsequent infection. These investigators also claimed to have produced a degree of immunity by the injection of *Schistosoma japonicum* antigens, as well as claiming passive transfer of immunity using sera of heavily infected animals. Kawamura (1928) was one of the investigators who believed that immunity to *Schistosoma* infection occurred in natives of endemic areas who, initially infected as youths, gradually become refractory to reinfection, and he also noted that immigrants to the endemic area may suffer severely from the disease. He also claimed that in passive transfer of serum or in animals immunized with extracts of the schistosomes, the pathology produced was less and there was an interference with the normal development of the worm. Additional observations on resistance to reinfection were made by Ozawa (1930), who reported that dogs infected with *Schistosoma japonicum* and subsequently cured by chemotherapy were found to be partially or completely refractory to further infection.

The relationship of hypersensitivity and allergic responses to schistosome infections was suggested as early as 1910 by Houghton, and Lambert (1911a,b) related urticaria and eosinophilia to *Schistosoma japonicum* infection of man. The possibility that hypersensitivity reactions were related to immunity was also considered, and it was speculated that during the early hypersensitivity responses to infection, hosts were refractory to further infection. Observations on dermatitis and skin eruptions (possibly associated with the penetration of cercariae) made in areas of Japan where schistosomiasis is endemic led to the assumption by some that this condition, called "Kabure," was a manifestation of infection with *Schistosoma japonicum* (Miyagawa, 1913). Since this was later found in areas of Japan where schistosomiasis was not endemic, it was recognized that the condition was probably a reaction due to penetration of cercariae, or schistosomes normally parasitizing animals other than man. As early as 1914, Lanning reported no dermatitis in initial infections of humans with *Schistosoma japonicum*. The findings at this time were confused, since experiments with laboratory animals in some cases produced an initial dermatitis with cercarial penetration.

Some changes in serum proteins in schistosome infections of man were observed as early as 1922 by Patterson and Libbey, using a globulin precipi-

tin test devised at that time for the diagnosis of kala-azar. Faust and Meleney (1924) indicated that the serum globulins were as much as twice the
normal level in infection with *Schistosoma japonicum.*

Studies on immunity to other schistosomes gathered impetus slowly. Fairley (1919), Fairley and Williams (1927), and Fairley et al. (1930) investigated the complement-fixation reaction in *Schistosoma mansoni* and *S.
hematobium* infections, and they described the possibility of using intradermal tests for diagnosis. Fairley introduced the use of antigens from *S. spindale,* a cattle schistosome, from the "liver" of the parasitized snail intermediate host for immunodiagnosis of human infections. Further studies of *S. spindale* in the macaque were conducted, and spontaneous cure with the production of immunity was reported, as well as the relationship of hypersensitivity
to infection. Taliaferro et al. (1928) investigated the utility of precipitin
tests in humans infected with *Schistosoma mansoni.* They noted that a variety of schistosome-derived antigens would give positive reactions and that a
positive reaction persisted for years after apparently successful treatment.
This led them to state that the precipitin test had limited use as a diagnostic
tool in schistosome infection. Taliaferro and Taliaferro (1931), using the
Prausnitz-Küstner reaction, demonstrated passive cutaneous hypersensitivity in man with sera from *S. mansoni* infections, and they mentioned the
presence of cell-bound or reaginic antibody.

RESISTANCE AND IMMUNITY IN THE SNAIL INTERMEDIATE HOST

A relatively high degree of intermediate host specificity is recognized in
many of the digenetic trematode life cycles. The susceptibility of certain
mollusc species (or alternatively, the natural resistance) to infection is variable (McQuay, 1953). This variability is not necessarily species oriented, as
it has been shown that certain strains of a single species of suitable
intermediate host are more susceptible to infection than are others. This is,
however, made more complex by the fact that parasite strains of a single
schistosome species also vary with respect to the success with which they
infect a particular snail strain. Consequently, we find some instances of
almost total incompatibility between the intermediate host and parasite originating from different endemic areas. It has been found, for example, that
Australorbis glabratus from Puerto Rico, completely susceptible to strains of
Schistosoma mansoni from Puerto Rico, Venezuela, and Brazil, is relatively
resistant to an Egyptian strain of *Schistosoma mansoni.* On the other hand,
Australorbis from Brazil are found to be susceptible to both Brazilian and
Puerto Rican strains of the parasite, but not to parasites originating from
Venezuela or Egypt (Files, 1951; Files and Cram, 1949). Evidence of a simi-
lar nature is reported for the susceptibility of *Biomphalaria boissyi* to strains
of *Schistosoma mansoni* (Abdel-Malik, 1950). Differences in the susceptibil-

ity of snail vectors to various strains of *Schistosoma japonicum* are also well-documented (Moose, 1963; Moose and Williams, 1963a,b; Hsü, H.F., 1950). One result of findings of this nature have led to the general concept that snails of one endemic area are often or even usually refractory to infections with parasites from other endemic areas. Although this appears to be true in some instances, it is not a valid generalization. We can cite, for example, *Tricula chuii* (*Oncomelania formosana chuii*), a strain not serving as a schistosome vector in an endemic area, but highly susceptible to infection with all strains of *Schistosoma japonicum*, as well as being a suitable intermediate host for *Paragonimus westermanii* (Chui, 1965).

Although the resistance of various snail species to a particular parasite may be athreptic, other reasons for the variations in susceptibility of a host species must be sought. One factor shown to be of importance is the age of the snail at the time of exposure to infection, and numerous instances of this relationship have been recorded (Abdel-Malik, 1950; McQuay, 1953). It is more pertinent to the present discussion, however, to consider the possibility that the snail intermediate host acquires resistance to infection by virtue of previous exposure. We have little direct evidence to support this in schistosomes, although there is some suggestion of acquired resistance to the strigeid, *Cotylurus flabelliformis*, for which it has been shown that *Lymnea* parasitized with sporocysts exhibited an immunity to the penetration of the cercariae and subsequent development of the metacercariae of the same species (Winfield, 1932; Nolf and Cort, 1933). Negative results have been obtained in attempts to demonstrate increased resistance in *Biomphalaria boissyi* first exposed to miracidia of a Puerto Rican strain of *Schistosoma mansoni*, to which they are resistant, and later exposed to the Egyptian strain to which they are highly susceptible (Abdel-Malik, 1950). It has also been shown that snails which have recovered from an infection of *Schistosoma mansoni* may be readily reinfected with the same parasite, although there was some indication of enhanced cellular response to the penetrating miracidia of the challenging infection (Simões Barbosa and Vasconcellos Coelho, 1956) and to *Schistosoma hematobium* in *Bulinus truncatus* (Wadji, 1966).

It is possible that innate and acquired resistance to infection in molluscs have both cellular and humoral aspects. Abnormal snail hosts may respond with cellular amoebocytic infiltration about degenerating parasite sporocysts (Newton, 1952). Variations within a strain of susceptible host with regard to the degree of cellular response occur, and more normal hosts respond slightly if at all, to the presence of the parasite, whereas a less suitable host strain has a cellular response comparable to that of non-host snails (Simões Barbosa and Vasconcellos Coelho, 1956). This reaction and degree of susceptibility is considered on the basis of crossing experiments to be an inherited characteristic (Newton, 1954). Although we have some knowledge of cellular responses of molluscs and, in particular, the tissue responses of *Australorbis glabratus* (Tripp, 1963; Pan, 1963), we have very little information on the nature of the humoral changes taking place in the infected mollusc, or whether these are of significance in the production of an immunity to subsequent infection.

The possibility that a humoral response to infection occurs in molluscs in a manner in some degree analogous to antibody production has been considered by several investigators. Bénex and Lamy (1959) observed the immobilization of *Schistosoma mansoni* miracidia in extracts of those planorbids which were not natural hosts of the parasite. Dusanic and Lewert (1963) reported that the motility of *Schistosoma mansoni* is affected by hemolymph taken from snails shortly after their exposure to miracidia of the same species. Proteins and free aminoacids of the hemolymph were analyzed at intervals following exposure to infection by miracidia, and changes in the ratio of the faster to slower moving protein components were found to occur almost immediately following penetration by miracidia. Changes in free aminoacid composition also occur. However, both of these changes were transient and not apparent beyond a 20-hour period after exposure to miracidia. Michelson (1963) has also studied the production and specificity of the miracidial immobilizing substances in extracts of *Australorbis glabratus*. It has been suggested that these substances may play a role in the immunity of snails to subsequent infection. With the relatively minor amount of investigation to date, there is no wholly convincing evidence at present that an effective resistance to reinfection occurs in the snail as far as the schistosome species are concerned. Our conclusions on this aspect of the host-parasite relationship must be deferred until more definitive experiments are devised and performed.*

INNATE RESISTANCE AND IMMUNITY

Immunity to the schistosomes must be considered in its relation to the innate resistance of the definitive host, not only as this pertains to the individual, whose status in this respect may change, but also as it is related to the spectra of species and genetic strains of hosts available to the parasite. The relative importance of this innate resistance in the subsequent development of acquired resistance in the susceptible host has yet to be adequately delineated. Its importance should not be underestimated, as it may be that similar mechanisms operate in both acquired resistance and innate resistance, and that to some degree, a protective immunity is the result of an enhanced innate resistance to infection.

As in the case of the intermediate host, investigators have usually described innate resistance as the condition in which the host does not allow the maturation of infection and the production of viable eggs, or does so transiently, or to such a low degree that no permanent pathology is produced. This concept of innate resistance has been applied to the rat, which is

*For a further discussion of snail immunity, see Vol. 1, Part 3, pp. 149-171.

a host unsuitable for maintenance of *S. mansoni* infection. It is, nevertheless, highly susceptible to invasion, and many of the invading cercariae complete the early stages of development and reach near-adult condition. This would thus lead us to question whether or not the rat in this instance is really innately immune, or rapidly develops an immunity as a result of infection, eliminating the infection before the worms have a chance to mature and cause extensive disease. It is difficult to recognize or to isolate the effect of single factors in this dynamic situation. It is unfortunate that we have little basis for a unifying principle here, since each of the species of blood flukes studied differs in invasive capabilities, and thus the innate resistance of animals to these infections appears to differ. We have more experimental evidence concerning resistance to *S. mansoni* than to other species of schistosomes, and we can be relatively sure that the innate resistance to this form varies with the strain of parasite with which we are concerned, as well as with the strain and species of mammalian host. As with other infecting organisms, we may accept the concept that more and less virulent strains of each species of the schistosomes exist. It is unfortunate that in many investigations, these variables, i.e., the strain of host and the strain of parasite, are not taken into account. As a consequence of this, comparison of experiments from different laboratories or from different areas of the world must be made with care, and generalizations are difficult to make with any assurance.

Of the various species of schistosomes, little innate resistance or immunity appears to be found in mammals with respect to *S. japonicum*. All primates tested, as well as a large number of ungulates and rodents, allow the invasion and maturation of the parasite. From experimental studies, one has the impression that the individual cercaria is a relatively successful invader and a high percentage of these invading cercariae do in fact mature. Even in this species, however, strain differences of parasites are recognized. The Formosan variety, although capable of maturing in rodents and various carnivores, does not apparently have the capacity to parasitize man or other primates successfully and to develop to the point where viable eggs are produced (Hsü, H.F., and Hsü, S. Y. Li, 1956, 1960a,b, 1962; Hsü, S. Y. Li, et al., 1962).

Innate resistance to *S. mansoni* is pronounced in many mammalian hosts used experimentally if we use the relative ability of the helminths to mature and produce viable eggs as a criterion of resistance. The reports in the literature are, however, clouded by the fact that the same innate resistance or host spectrum is not found for the different strains of *S. mansoni* available for experimentation. Puerto Rican strains maintained in the laboratory for many years will not mature in guinea pigs or in dogs, whereas some of the South American schistosome strains of the same species are reported to infect both readily. As we have mentioned, rats are generally considered to be poor hosts for the species. Nevertheless, a high percentage of the cercariae applied to the skin penetrate, very few mature, and infection is transient, self-limiting, and results in spontaneous cure. *Schistosoma hematobium* has been studied less than the other species in this respect, and it does not appear to be widely distributed in mammals other than man under natural conditions. However, rodents and some of the primates may be readily infected. The range of susceptible species and the indications of innate resistance, as defined here, are summarized in several investigations (Fairley, 1938; Kuntz, 1955; Newsome, 1956; Sadun and Bruce, 1964a; Stirewalt, 1963).

The characteristics outlined depend to a great extent on the genetic make-ups of the parasite and of the host that determine their degree of compatibility. This innate immunity, which may vary with genetic strain of host, may have physical aspects, such as the thickness of the skin or resistance of membranes through which the cercariae must pass; chemical aspects, such as the unsuitability of substrates with respect to the penetration enzymes of the cercariae; humoral aspects, such as naturally occurring cercariacidal substances in serum of an unsuitable host; or other nonspecific activities. These various aspects may act in concert to prevent successful invasion. It has been shown that the nature of the surface of the skin is important in penetration, and that a strain of hairless mice is relatively insusceptible to penetration by *S. mansoni* in comparison with the normal strains of mice (Stirewalt, 1963). The thickness of the stratum corneum alone may cause the cercariae to exhaust their gland contents before reaching the dermis. Immunoglobulins and other substances possibly inimical to cercariae may be present in surface secretions and in the skin of sweating animals (Tomasi et al., 1965; Heremans et al., 1966; Page and Remington, 1967), and in fact small changes in the presence or amounts of metallic ions in the immediate environment of cercariae greatly influence success of initial penetration (Lewert et al., 1966). Once the organism has passed the epidermis, the structure of the acellular elements of the connective tissue of the dermis and the degree of their polymerization also play a role in the success of parasitic invasion (Lewert and Lee, 1954). Using a single strain of mice, it has been shown that age-related increases in innate resistance to infection with *S. mansoni* are the result o fthe state of organization of the acellular elements of the connective tissue and, in particular, the polysaccharide-protein complexes that form the subepithelial basement membranes, ground substance, and the intercellular cement (Lewert and Mandlowitz, 1963). These acellular connective tissue substances vary in their density and resistance to enzymatic alteration. Schistosome cercariae can more readily penetrate the skin and migrate through the tissue of those animals whose acellular elements of the dermal connective tissue are least resistant to enzymatic alteration, e.g., in youth and in certain genetic strains, in those aged individuals which retain the youthful connective tissue state, and in animals exposed to certain stresses, such as radiation or certain nutritional deficiencies that alter connective tissue. On the other hand, in those animals whose connective tissue elements are more highly polymerized and less readily altered by enzymatic digestion, penetration is less rapid and fewer organisms are able to reach sites where they are capable of continuing development.

ACQUIRED RESISTANCE AND IMMUNITY

Experimental evidence of acquired immunity in laboratory animals

The experimental evidence for acquired immunity in schistosomiasis has been adequately and recently reviewed (Stirewalt, 1963; Kagan, 1966; Sadun, 1963; Thompson, 1954). Experimentation has been very extensive, but it is sometimes difficult to make comparisons or generalizations because of the lack of uniformity in hosts, parasite strain, and methodology used in the various laboratories.

By far the most common host-parasite system investigated has been the white mouse and *Schistosoma mansoni*. In the homologous system, using living or nonliving antigen, some investigators find no significant evidence of immunity developing to challenge infection, no matter the nature, quantity, timing, or route used for the administration of the immunizing antigen (Thompson, 1954; Ritchie et al., 1962). Other investigators find adequate, statistically significant evidence of increased resistance to infection in essentially similar experiments (Sadun, 1963). The mouse infected with *Schistosoma mansoni* (or the other schistosomes to which it is susceptible) ultimately succumbs to the initial infection. Subsequently invading organisms may be delayed in migration, slightly reduced in number, or stunted in size in comparison with controls, but no clearly effective protective immunity is developed. Also, very little effective immunity is conferred to mice subjected to repeated small cercarial exposures or produced in mice exposed and treated chemotherapeutically to terminate mature infection and later challenged (Cheever et al., 1965).

The mouse and the hamster, as highly susceptible hosts to schistosomes, are clearly not the most desirable model systems for investigations of immunity to these parasites. Using these hosts, there is no instance in which a substantially protective immunity has been demonstrated. Nevertheless, from the numerous studies made, evidence is incontrovertible that an increased resistance or statistically demonstrable immunity may be obtained. Whether or not lessened numbers of parasites are able to survive as a second infection in the mouse, the initial infection stimulates this host to react to a second group of invading larvae. Using isotopically labeled cercariae, it can be shown that although the number of cercariae penetrating is not substantially decreased, the rates of migration through the tissue and of passage through the lungs are markedly slower than in previously uninfected controls (Lewert and Para, 1970).

In contrast to the study of highly susceptible hosts, experiments of a different nature with initially refractory hosts have also been performed in an attempt to show an increase in natural resistance to infection. Rats and guinea pigs, in which the usual laboratory strains of *Schistosoma mansoni* will not completely mature and in which the infection is self-limiting with destruction of the worms, remain susceptible to repeated invasion and partial maturation of the helminths. Although there is some evidence that smaller numbers are able to survive in these previously "immunized" animals or survive for shorter periods of time (Sadun, 1963), other investigators dispute the claim that any significant enhancement of resistance occurs (Thompson, 1954).

The lower primates as hosts of the schistosomes appear in some cases to exhibit an immunity that is in many respects similar to that of man. A very substantial protective immunity to challenge by S. mansoni or S. japonicum develops in the rhesus monkey as a result of prior infection with the homologous species (Vogel and Minning, 1953; Naimark et al., 1960; Liu and Bang, 1950; Meleney and Moore, 1954; Sadun, 1963). It has generally been assumed that an extended period of infection is necessary to confer this protective immunity in primates (Vogel and Minning, 1953). This has led to the concepts that continuous stimulation by metabolic products of the adult worm is critical, or that the eggs trapped in the tissues supply antigen necessary for the stimulation of the protective immunity (Vogel and Minning, 1953; Naimark et al., 1960; Smithers, 1962a,b). In Schistosoma japonicum, and to a lesser degree, in Schistosoma mansoni, unisexual male infection will confer protection in the rhesus monkey (Sadun, 1963; Vogel and Minning, 1953). Injections of viable eggs do not increase resistance, nor does the introduction of living adults in ectopic sites such as the peritoneal cavity (Sadun, 1963; Smithers, 1962a, b). The concept that long-term or intense infections are necessary for the production of immunity has been challenged by the work of Smithers and Terry (1967). They found that a single exposure of the rhesus monkey to as few as 25 cercariae of S. mansoni will induce a high degree of resistance when the host is challenged even within 17 weeks. The studies with rhesus monkeys indicate that resistance to reinfection may be complete, and the worms of the challenging infection do not mature and are destroyed. In the challenged monkey, as far as S. mansoni infection is concerned, the initial infection is ultimately terminated as well. The rhesus monkey is not to be considered representative of the rest of the primates, since considerable variation in the susceptibility of different genera of primates has been found (Sadun et al., 1966b). Some of the lower primates are insusceptible to infection and do not allow Schistosoma mansoni to mature, while others, such as Cercopithecus (the African green monkey), appear to be highly susceptible and do not develop protective immunity (Ritchie et al., 1967). The baboon (Papio hamadryas), on the other hand, may present a picture closer to that found in man. Infections with Schistosoma mansoni persist for years, and in the presence of current infection the baboon is protected from otherwise lethal doses of a cercariae (Newsome, 1956). Since a high level of resistance and immunity can be demonstrated in the rhesus monkey, it might be supposed that this resistance could be induced by the injection of worm products or of various antigens derived from the schistosomes. In spite of numerous attempts to induce immunity with nonliving adults, eggs, or cercariae, with or without adjuvants, no clear-cut resistance against reinfection has been obtained (Smithers, 1962a,b; Smithers and Terry, 1967; Sadun et al., 1966b).

The possibility that living cercariae attenuated by radiation might be used as an effective vaccine was considered by a number of investigators as a result of the success of using nematodes attenuated by radiation to immunize against the cattle lung worm (Jarrett et al., 1960). Cercariae of *S. mansoni* were exposed to gamma radiation from a cobalt-60 source, and mice exposed to such cercariae exhibited a degree of resistance to challenge (Villella et al., 1961). *S. mansoni* cercariae have also been attenuated by exposure to x-rays by various investigators (Sadun, 1963; Smithers, 1962c; Perlowagora-Szumlewicz, 1964; Erickson and Caldwell, 1965). Depending on the dose of radiation received by the cercariae, schistosomula may survive up to 6 weeks without producing viable eggs. With higher radiation levels, cercariae may still be capable of penetrating the skin, but the schistosomula die after reaching the liver during the second to fourth week after penetration. Some studies indicate that mice and hamsters stimulated by cercariae treated in this way have a slight or partial protection similar to that conferred by previous infection or extensive immunizations with nonliving antigen. Other investigators did not find significant changes in the course of the challenging infection, except for a lengthened tissue migration and development (Perlowagora-Szumlewicz, 1964). Thus, as far as mice are concerned, the results are no more encouraging than those obtained in attempts to enhance resistance by exposure to cercariae by other means.

It has been shown by Frick et al. (1965) that intraperitoneal injection of viable cercariae increases resistance in white mice to a greater extent than exposure by the normal route of skin penetration. Fewer worms of the initial infection survive to maturity when infection is via this route, and it might be assumed that the antigenic stimulation of the host is greater due to those organisms which are not able to survive. However, in another way the ectopic introduction of viable cercariae has been shown not to increase resistance materially. Cercariae of *S. mansoni* do not ordinarily survive intravenous inoculation, and weekly inoculations over a period of 5 weeks do not confer a significant increased resistance in mice (Lewert and Mandlowitz, unpublished data).

In monkeys exposed to x-irradiated cercariae of *S. mansoni*, a substantial increase in resistance to subsequent infection has been obtained (Smithers, 1962a; Sadun, 1963), and a more substantial but incomplete protection has been obtained in rhesus monkeys following exposure to irradiated cercariae of *S. japonicum* (Hsü, H. F., et al., 1962, 1963). However, mice exposed to irradiated cercariae of *S. japonicum* are not protected (Hsü, S. Y. Li, et al., 1965). From the results of these various experiments, it can be stated that a partial resistance to challenge, and in some cases protection from otherwise fatal infection, can be produced in monkeys vaccinated with irradiated cercariae. The level of the irradiation of the cercariae and the numbers administered are of importance. The resistance produced, however, is not, with respect to *Schistosoma mansoni* in the rhesus monkey, sufficient to produce a fully protective immunity.

Another type of "vaccination" utilizing the transfer of living adult worms to a previously unparasitized host has yielded provocative results (Smithers and Terry, 1967). Adult worms obtained from monkeys, hamsters, or mice were transferred surgically to the hepatic portal system of normal monkeys. When challenged 8 to 14 weeks later, some individuals were almost completely resistant to infection; others were less resistant but exhibited less severe disease than control animals. Worms cut in two and immediately introduced into the hepatic portal system also induced resistance. However, worms killed by freezing and then introduced intravenously did not confer any protection. No correlation was found between egg production of the transferred worms (or non-egg production in the case of portions of worms) and the degree of resistance induced. It may be concluded that in the rhesus monkey at least, stimulation of protective immunity may be related to the secretory and excretory products of the adult worm. Thus, in *S. mansoni* infections there is no completely convincing evidence for the necessity of stimulation by antigens of eggs, cercariae, or schistosomulae for the development of protective immunity in the rhesus monkey.

Immunity acquired by previous exposure to related or heterologous parasites

There have been a number of essentially unsuccessful attempts to confer immunity to one species of schistosome by previous exposure to other or related species of parasites (Hsü, H. F., et al., 1964; Hsü, S. Y. Li, et al., 1966; Hunter et al., 1961; Kagan, 1953). It has been reported that monkeys resistant to *Schistosoma japonicum*, when challenged by *Schistosoma mansoni* cercariae, had an extended prepatent period with the production of lesser numbers of eggs than expected from exposure to 1,500 cercariae (Vogel and Minning, 1953). Partial protection to *S. mansoni* was also shown in a rhesus monkey already resistant to *Schistosoma hematobium* (Meleney and Moore, 1954). A degree of increased resistance to *S. japonicum* has been reported in monkeys previously exposed to *Schistosomatium douthitti* (Hsü, H. F., et al., 1964), and a slight increase in resistance to *Schistosoma hematobium* in monkeys has been obtained by administration of the cercariae of *Schistosoma bovis* (Hsü, S. Y. Li, et al., 1966). A nonreciprocal but slight cross-resistance has been described between *Schistosoma mansoni* and *Schistosomatium douthitti* in mice (Hunter et al., 1961).

More significant is the relatively high degree of protection, and in some instances almost complete immunity, resulting when rhesus monkeys are first exposed to cercariae of the Formosan strain of *Schistosoma japonicum* and later challenged with highly pathogenic strains of the same species (Sadun, 1963; Hsü, S. Y. Li, and Hsü, H. F., 1961, 1963). The Formosan strain is a non-human strain which will naturally terminate its infection, presumably in the schistosomulal state in man, and which produces no detectable permanent pathology. The rhesus monkey, like man, is not susceptible to infection with this strain—or to be more precise, although it becomes infected, the worms do not mature, and since eggs are not produced, the pathology is so slight as to be inconsequential (Hsü, S. Y. Li, et al., 1962).

Acquired resistance by man to schistosomes

Based largely on circumstantial evidence, investigators in areas where schistosomiasis is endemic have been convinced that acquired resistance to infection occurs and is expressed as a relatively high degree of protection for the majority of those adults who are repeatedly exposed to reinfection. Fujinami was probably the first to express this observation relative to man and domestic animals (Fujinami, 1916 a, b; Fujinami and Sueyasu, 1917, 1918). Within those endemic areas having relatively stable populations, it is observed that the disease state caused by schistosomiasis is most severe in childhood and that older survivors, although most certainly exposed to reinfection on numerous occasions, have less severe disease. Older members of the community may be completely free of the usual physical signs of infection. To some, this has been interpreted as an age-dependent resistance. In areas where schistosomiasis might be considered hyperendemic for *Schistosoma intercalatum*, Dixon (1934) was unable to diagnose infection in individuals over 40 years of age. In the same year, Fisher (1934) also noted that in one hyperendemic area, adults over the age of 35 were uninfected with *S. intercalatum*, although a 96 percent incidence was to be found in children. In a different area where a lower incidence was described in the children (40 percent), the percentage of infection of adults of all ages was at a similar level (40 percent). If we are able to assume that these findings are not reflections of genetic variation or differences in the behavior patterns of these two groups, it may be inferred that in man, continually repeated cercarial exposure is necessary for the development of a protective immunity. It is true, however, that there are reports from other locales of high percentages of infection with schistosomes found in all age groups in both sexes (De Morais, 1962). All of these observations suggest that the total pattern of infection, including intensity and frequency of contact, is a major factor in whether or not an individual or a population becomes immune.

Fisher (1934) in his study also demonstrated the presence of a truly protective immunity in individuals from his "hyperendemic" area in the Congo. Six individuals over 35 years of age, who as fishermen would in the course of their ordinary activities be exposed to infection, voluntarily exposed their arms to water containing several hundred cercariae. Cercariae from the same pool were used successfully to infect mice, and penetration of the human subjects' skin was accompanied by a dermatitis. None of the six individuals exhibited clinical evidence of infection during the 8 months following exposure. No infection could be demonstrated at 6 months, while at 8 months three of the six volunteers had small numbers of eggs in their feces. Eggs could not be demonstrated after this period, and no symptomology attributable to schistosomiasis resulted.

No adequate controlled experiments involving challenge of man after known exposure to cercariae of other species have been reported. There is one claim of immunization to *S. hematobium* being acquired by Gothe after 16 exposures of himself to cercariae of *S. hematobium* which had been attenuated by exposure to a 1:10,000 suspension of wettable DDT (Gothe, 1963). It is also claimed that exposure of man to several thousand cercariae of *S. matthei* which were shown to be infective for a baboon conferred protection to an individual who subsequently had repeated exposure to cercariae of both *S. mansoni* and *S. capense* under natural field conditions (Clarke, 1966). Another person similarly "immunized" became infected at a later date with *S. mansoni* as a result of exposure on a field collecting trip (Clarke, 1966). The zoophilic strain of *Schistosoma japonicum* which is found in Formosa and which has been used experimentally to immunize monkeys against virulent human strains of *Schistosoma japonicum* has also been used in a single experiment in which no maturation of the zoophilic strain was found to occur in humans exposed to their cercariae (Hsü, S. Y. Li, et al., 1962). These individuals were not subsequently exposed to strains which might develop in man, so we do not know whether any degree of protective immunity resulted.

A number of other authors have made observations giving additional indirect evidence of human resistance (Vogel and Minning, 1953; Schwetz, 1956; Gerber, 1952a, b). Of these, the study by Gerber is of considerable interest since the incidence and intensity of infection by *Schistosoma hematobium* was studied in two groups of individuals having differing natural exposures to infection. One of these was presumed to have regular re-exposure to infection, and the other was only occasionally or sporadically exposed to cercarial reinfection. His study suggests that a protective immunity in man is most often produced with a light or moderate initial infection followed by regular subsequent exposures, probably minimally at annual intervals. A heavy initial infection followed by further heavy infections was not favorable for the development of protective immunity. In some of the villages studied in Sierra Leone, he found the older age groups had an increase in the rate of infection compared to immediately younger age groups. This he interpreted as indicating that although these individuals may have had a protective immunity earlier in their lives, death of the worms and lack of re-exposure resulted in a loss of immunity, and that continuing protective immunity was dependent on survival of some adult worms.

Observations made in the hyperendemic areas in the Philippines by Lewert and Yogore (unpublished data) also are indicative of a strong protective immunity, especially in young adult males in this area. A study has been made of some 50 individuals native to Leyte who were without clinical symptoms attributable to schistosomiasis but who had serologic indications of infection or were sporadically passing small numbers of eggs in their feces. At various times over the course of 3 years, by virtue of the work activity of this group, known exposures to infective cercariae occurred. This was adequately documented by the simultaneous exposure of mice to the water in which the men were working. During this 3-year period, no increase in severity of infection was observed, as evidenced by quantitative stool examinations or by the development of physical symptoms attributable to schistosomiasis.

At the present time, there is little question in the minds of serious investigators that a highly protective resistance may develop in man. The factors related to the development or nondevelopment of this, however, remain speculative in the absence of definitive experiments or long-term observations of the natural exposures of specific individuals in endemic areas.

SERUM PROTEINS AND RESISTANCE TO SCHISTOSOME INFECTION

In the introduction of this chapter it was pointed out that in the normal course of infection with schistosomes, the host is exposed to antigens derived not only from the infective larval stages, but also to those of the adult and its products, and to the eggs trapped in the tissues and their products. In contrast to viral and bacterial infections, there is a multiplicity of antigens, some unique to each stage and others shared by the various stages, as well as being shared by the various schistosome species. For example, it can be shown that more than 20 separate precipitin lines against adult antigens can be visualized using immunoelectrophoretic techniques in sera derived from infections (Capron et al., 1966, 1967). In fact, as many as 16 antigen-antibody complexes related to different enzymatic activities of adult schistosomes have been described (Tran Van Ky et al., 1967).

The appearance of precipitins in schistosome infections accompanies the marked increase in gamma-globulins (Sadun and Walton, 1958; Hsü, S. Y. Li, and Hsü, H. F., 1964; Jachowski et al., 1963; Hillyer and Ritchie, 1967) which generally occurs 4 to 6 weeks after exposure of animals to cercariae. In rhesus monkeys infected with *S. mansoni*, total immunoglobulins usually increase markedly within 4 to 8 weeks after exposure. Early in infection, increases in gamma-globulins may occur in the absence of increased macroglobulins (Hsü, S. Y. Li, and Hsü, H. F., 1964; Jachowski et al., 1963; Smithers, 1962b). It has been suggested that the increase in α_2-globulins, which occurs simultaneously with the tissue damage caused by egg deposition, is a direct result of this damage, while the macroglobulin increase found in chronic schistosomiasis is possibly a result of the concomitant splenomegaly. It has been shown that of the gamma-globulins produced during infection, most are nonspecific, and only a relatively small portion can be shown to be directed at schistosome-produced antigens (Jachowski et al., 1963). Hypergammaglobulinemia cannot, in general, be equated with resistance in schistosome infection, since increased resistance has been demonstrated in rhesus monkeys without quantitative changes in immunoglobulins (Jachowski et al., 1963).

Antibodies have been demonstrated not only by immunoelectrophoretic techniques, but also by a large variety of reactions around living stages of schistosomes *in vitro,* including the circumoval precipitin test (COP), the Cercarien-hüllen reaction (CHR), and cercarial or miracidial agglutination and immobilization techniques. Fluorescent-antibody methods, indirect hemagglutination, and flocculation of substances coated with schistosome antigens have also been used to demonstrate the antibodies produced. Sera taken from man infected with *Schistosoma mansoni* has been separated electrophoretically, and various fractions having different mobilities have been shown to have differing specific activities, such as miracidial immobilization, cercariacidal activities, complement fixation, cercarial agglutinins, and circumoval precipitins (Lee and Lewert, 1960). It has also been shown that sera from infections of man have increased ability to inhibit cercarial penetration enzymes, and that this is a stable factor in comparison with a heat-labile enzyme inhibitor normally found in serum (Lewert et al., 1959). Additional evidence of the possible direct effect of human immune serum on the parasite has been shown in that sera from individuals infected with *Schistosoma japonicum* are capable of altering the surface of miracidia, thus causing structural changes as well as immobilizing the organism (Jamuar and Lewert, 1967).

These various reactions may be utilized as methods of immunodiagnosis, are useful as an index of the status of infection, and may even be used to give some indication of the relative success of chemotherapy (Lewert and Yogore, 1966). Nevertheless, none of these serum protein changes can be directly correlated to resistance or immunity of the host (Jachowski et al., 1963; Smithers, 1962a; Hsü, S. Y. Li, and Hsü, H. F., 1966; Vogel and Minning, 1953). This has been recently shown, for example, in *Schistosoma mansoni* infections in which the green monkey and rhesus have been qualitatively and quantitatively compared with respect to precipitins. The rhesus, as we have mentioned, may be highly immune, whereas the green monkey remains fully susceptible to reinfection (Ritchie et al., 1967; Hillyer and Ritchie, 1967). In humans who appear to be immune and who under field conditions have had known re-exposure to *Schistosoma japonicum* infection, neither quantitative nor qualitative changes in precipitating antibody follows such re-exposure (Lewert and Yogore, unpublished data). In fact, in the population of the endemic area of the Philippines, those with the most severe pathology exhibit higher antibody levels and have both qualitatively and quantitatively more precipitins against *Schistosoma japonicum* adults and eggs. Complement-fixing antibody and antibodies detectable through indirect hemagglutination techniques for *Schistosoma mansoni* and *Schistosoma japonicum* are also high, but neither appear to be indicators of the severity of the disease, of intensity of infection, or of immunity to reinfection (Jachowski et al., 1963; Hsü, S. Y. Li, and Hsü, H. F., 1966).

The attempts at passive transfer of immunity in schistosomiasis have not been notably successful. In some of the earliest studies of *Schistosoma japonicum,* claims were made of success in protecting dogs with sera of animals previously immunized (Yoshimoto, 1910; Fujinami, 1916a,b; Fujinami and Sueyasu, 1917, 1918). Attempts to repeat this have been unsuccessful (Sadun and Lin, 1959). The transfer of high titer heterologous sera in an attempt to confer immunity passively from rabbit to rat or mouse with *Schistosoma mansoni* and *Schistosoma japonicum* has been done, and a degree of increased resistance has been claimed for the latter system (Sadun and Lin, 1959). However, even in a homologous system with the transfer of large amounts of immune blood from an immune to a susceptible monkey, negative results have been obtained (Meisenhelder et al., 1960). A high level of success could not be expected in most of these experiments, since with the exception of the monkey none of the donor animals used develop more than a partial immunity or slightly increased resistance to reinfection.

This anomaly of humoral antibody reacting with the numerous antigens of the schistosomes without having any discernible function in immunity to reinfection has stimulated various investigators to explore the possibility that other mechanisms are more important or must work in concert with these reactions to produce the functionally immune state. Foremost among these are recent investigations related to hypersensitivity responses.

In many helminthic infections and in the schistosomes in particular, hypersensitivity reactions are prominent features of infection in man and account not only for the extent of damage to the host, but also have proved to be useful as diagnostic procedures. The Prausnitz-Küstner reaction (PK) and the presence of reagin-like antibodies were noted by some of the earliest investigators (Taliaferro, W. H., and Taliaferro, L. G., 1931; Guerra et al., 1945; Coker and Oliver-Gonzalez, 1956; Mendes and Amato Neto, 1963). The possibility that such hypersensitivity responses and reagins, in particular, might be directly related to the immune state in helminth infections has been suggested by Ogilvie (1964, 1967). Reagin-like antibodies in rats and monkeys infected with *Schistosoma mansoni* were first demonstrated by means of a passive cutaneous anaphylaxis reaction with fixation and persistence for 3 days or longer of the heat-labile reaginic antibody in tissues. In rats, reagins were first demonstrated 4 weeks after infection by cercariae and disappeared by 12 weeks (Ogilvie et al., 1966). In monkeys infected with *S. mansoni*, they were first demonstrated 1½ to 4 months after exposure, disappearing some weeks after their first appearance. Although passive transfer of this reagin-containing serum failed to elicit resistance to challenge, the same serum injected intradermally, followed by application of cercariae to the same site 3 days later, produced resistance to challenge infection.

Reagin-like antibody in rhesus monkeys immune to *Schistosoma japonicum* has been studied by H. F. Hsü and S. Y. Li Hsü (1966). They concluded that the reagin-like antibody of immune monkeys as demonstrated by the PCA reaction did not bear a direct relationship to resistance or protective immunity. In their experiments, intracutaneous passive transfer of such sera did not confer any protective effect against challenge by the application of cercariae to the site where reagins were fixed in the skin of susceptible monkeys. Sadun et al. (1966a) have noted that reaginic antibodies are present in chimpanzees infected with *Schistosoma mansoni* and persisted throughout a 7-month infection. Using passive cutaneous anaphylaxis in the rhesus monkey, they demonstrated that similar antibodies occurred in human infections with *Schistosoma mansoni*. Using the same technique, reaginic antibodies have been demonstrated in humans infected with *Schistosoma japonicum*, although in children and some young adults with severe pathology they may be absent (Lewert and Yogore, unpublished data). It should be pointed out that it is perhaps insufficient to measure reagin present in the circulation, since reagin passively fixed to cells may persist and be detectable even 2 months after injection. In the individual producing reagins, it might be assumed that effective quantities might persist within tissues for a considerable period after they could no longer be detected in serum by using a passive cutaneous anaphylaxis technique (Augustin, 1967).

The direct involvement of reagins as truly antiparasitic substances does not seem likely. However, their role may be of fundamental importance by virtue of their triggering the release of histamine or other substances. These substances might immobilize the parasite and/or summon cells which actively destroy the invading organisms. It is thought by some that histamine release transforms endothelial cells into reticuloendothelial phagocytes, and as an activator of phagocytosis, plays a major role in inflammatory processes and in defense reactions (Jansció, 1947). In this way these immediate hypersensitivity reactions may be of great consequence in delaying and in indirectly effecting the destruction of schistosomulae in the skin or in the lungs of the sensitized host.

CELLULAR ASPECTS OF PROTECTIVE IMMUNITY

It is probable that the actual death as well as physical elimination of all stages of the schistosomes is due to invading cells. The cellular attack of the host on the adults and eggs precedes the death of these stages of the schistosome, and it may be mediated by humoral antibody. In the case of the schistosomes, and very possibly other helminths, it seems probable that even though adequate levels of antibody are available, cellular defensive mechanisms are ineffective unless the mobility of the parasite is first impaired.

Newsome (1962) has shown that *in vitro*, schistosomes incubated in immune serum plus leukocytes are rapidly killed. In various mixtures involving *Schistosoma mansoni* adults, blood, serum, leukocytes, and saline at 37°C, the movement of the worms is slowed, leukocytes adhere to their surfaces, and the helminths die. This adherence phenomenon, which is attributed to an opsonin in the serum, does not occur if the cells and organisms are kept in motion (Newsome, 1962). He has suggested that this reaction potentiates chemotherapy and that the success of chemotherapy would in a large sense be dependent on the presence of antibody with this type of activity. This would be of great consequence in explaining the apparent variation of the *in vivo* activity of those compounds which inhibit motor functions of the helminths but which are not in themselves parasiticidal at the levels reached during therapy. Such drugs as the organophosphorous compounds which inhibit cholinesterases and others influencing the mobility of the parasite are worthy of mention in this connection.

Other evidence supporting the hypothesis that immobilization allows destruction of the adults, and in fact any stage of the parasite, in the mammal has been derived from hibernating animals. Shortly after induction of hibernation by hypothermia of the host, the immobilized adults are found in the liver where they are invaded by leukocytes and rapidly destroyed (Lewert and Cahill, unpublished data). Within a very short time after the parasites are immobilized at 5°C *in vivo*, leukocyte sheaths and accumulations are found that appear to be identical to those described by Newsome *in vitro*.

Although not related to protective immunity, the pseudotubercle or granulomatous lesion arising about the schistosome egg in the host tissue is a cellular reaction basic to the pathology produced by the schistosomes. It is a manifestation of delayed hypersensitivity that may be reduced by immunosuppressive drugs or thymectomy (Von Lichtenberg, 1967b; Domingo and Warren, 1966; Domingo et al., 1967).

TOLERANCE AND HYPERSENSITIVITY IN SCHISTOSOME INFECTIONS OF MAN

The most remarkable feature of the host-parasite relationship in schistosomiasis is the extraordinary tolerance of the mammalian host for these intravascular intruders. The adult schistosome may live for decades continuously bathed in antibodies prepared by the host against its antigens, and it appears not to be inconvenienced by contact with these or with the host leukocytes. The reasons for this tolerance have not been adequately investigated and are as yet unexplained. The parasite shares but few antigens (Capron et al., 1965; Damian, 1967) with the host, and from the relatively large number of antigen-antibody reactions that have been demonstrated, it is clear that the host recognizes the foreign nature of the parasite and its products. Perhaps when initial infection by cercarial invasion occurs, this relatively small number of foreign cells "sneaks through," being essentially unperceived by the immune mechanism until a stage of growth or metabolism is reached where the parasite is relatively invulnerable. Later or secondary infections might, however, be challenged earlier by the host and destroyed by the more alert "prepared" immune mechanisms before the worms become "invulnerable" adults.

It is interesting to speculate on the possibility that these adult worms escape host damage in a process of "immunologic enhancement." Even a relatively heavy infection with adult worms does not represent a large foreign antigenic surface in comparison with the amounts of specific antibody protein the mammalian host can produce. In a strongly antigenic system with relatively few and nondividing organisms, humoral antibody might be stimulated at the expense of cell-mediated responses. The surface of the worm may indeed be "coated" by antibody in such a way that its leukocyte-vulnerable antigenic sites are excluded from contact with these cells. Also, such a coating might conceivably protect the organism from nonglobulin cytotoxic agents. Since there is no convincing evidence at present that any direct relationship exists between production of precipitating antibody and protective immunity in the schistosomes, it would be curious if survival of the parasite was indeed enhanced by such protein production.

Since making this speculation, Smithers et al. (1969) have presented evidence that there is incorporation of host antigens by the schistosome worm surface. These are host-species specific and do not confer protection to the adult worm if it is transferred surgically to the vascular system of another host species.

The intensity of the pathology of schistosomiasis in the individual is undoubtedly influenced by the type and degree of immune response. It has been well-demonstrated in animal experiments that hypersensitivity reactions are greater in the less natural host. This is demonstrated by the greater size of granulomas about the eggs in tissues. Von Lichtenberg et al. (1962) have, in fact, described a series of such examples in various species of mammals, which relates size and intensity of reaction to the suitability of the host. Such granulomas are shown to be minimal in thymectomized animals (Domingo and Warren, 1966) or those in which antibody production has been chemically decreased (Domingo et al., 1967).

As mentioned previously, cercarial dermatitis is another hypersensitivity reaction most commonly seen in hosts not normal to the penetrating parasite. These phenomena and more general systemic hypersensitivity reactions have interesting implications in human infection, and they allow us to speculate on the basis of variation in certain characteristic pathology observed in man. It is well-established that in an endemic area, the indigenous population does not exhibit the intense and fulminating type of infection accompanied by marked hypersensitivity found in new immigrants (Yoshimoto, 1910; Fujinami and Sueyasu, 1918; Kawamura, 1928). This has been particularly well-documented when Caucasians come into contact with *Schistosoma japonicum*, as described by Lambert (1911a, b) and Mühlens (1937). This type of response has been described as the "Katayama syndrome" and is thought by some to be preceded by Kabure itch due to cercarial penetration. Similar fulminating infections occur in endemic areas of the Philippines, such as Mindanao, with immigrants arriving from nonendemic areas. This is not, however, limited to *Schistosoma japonicum*, and a similar Katayama syndrome and Kabure itch are found in South Africa in Europeans moving to areas where *Schistosoma mansoni* and *Schistosoma hematobium* are endemic (Gelfand et al., 1964b).

This leads one to the curious conclusion that the individual or population with the greatest chance of repeated exposure develops the least hypersensitivity. They are, nevertheless, from the standpoint of disease, less vulnerable and very likely may be protected from superinfection or may be immune. Two explanations of this seem possible. Perhaps the most obvious is that in an old well-established endemic area these parasites (as is the case in malaria) may have been a factor in selecting a population tolerating the infection. Another possible explanation is that the individual, by virtue of being born in an infected population in an endemic area, has an immune mechanism which has been conditioned not to respond to those antigens responsible for the hypersensitivity reactions of this infection. Excretory and secretory products of the adult worms are present in the circulation and have been also reported in urine of the host. These have been detected by immunoprecipitation techniques (Okabe and Ono, 1961; Sherif, 1962; Berggren and Weller, 1967). It seems possible that antigenic, secretory and execretory products of the worms in the circulation of an infected mother might cross the placental barrier. The developing competent cells of the embryonic immune mechanism may in this way be conditioned *in utero* not to recognize certain of these antigenic substances as non-self materials. Thus, after birth, if they were exposed to infection, they would not exhibit the hypersensitive state of individuals born of mothers not infected with schistosomiasis. We have experimental evidence that such a tolerance may be induced in mice when impregnation of the mothers takes place after maturation of infection with *Schistosoma mansoni*. Delayed hypersensitivity, as expressed by granuloma formation about schistosome eggs, is greatly decreased in such offspring as compared to controls from uninfected mothers (Lewert and Mandlowitz, 1969). If a similar induction of tolerance occurs in man, it could well explain many of the observed differences in reactions to infection discussed above. The congenital transfer of circulating antigens is not necessarily limited to those small molecules found by Berggren and Weller (1967). Transplacental passage of such large molecules as specific antibody has been shown to occur in schistosomiasis (Gelfand et al., 1964a; Hillyer et al., 1970). In this regard, it is unlikely that the presence of the antibody in the newborn has any significance in protective immunity since passive transfer experiments have been essentially unsuccessful, antibody levels are not high in the offspring, and the degradation of antibody would proceed at such a rate that it is probable that little would remain at the time of initial exposure of the individual infant.

CONCLUSION

In spite of the extensive research of the last decade, we still have not achieved full elucidation of the basic mechanisms involved in acquired resistance and immunity in schistosome infections. On the positive side, we have acquired much fundamental information and have also come to the realization that we cannot readily correlate immunity in these infections with levels of precipitating antibody and other commonly demonstrated serologic responses. There has been a gradual evolution in our thinking which has led a number of investigators to consider new concepts and reopen consideration of concepts and observations of earlier students of helminth immunity. The possible interplay of humoral and cellular responses, a concept advanced by Taliaferro (1940) in a number of his basic investigations of immunity to parasites, is again receiving attention, with the role of cellular mechanisms in immunity being further examined by von Lichtenberg and others (von Lichtenberg and Sadun, 1963). We have also become aware of a series of nonprecipitating antigen-antibody reactions occurring in schistosome infections (Dusanic and Lewert, 1966). Although some hypersensitivity reactions may be of no consequence, the possible role of reagins in immunity has been advanced by Ogilvie (1964) with the result that other hypersensitivity responses are also being more fully investigated for their possible role in protective immunity. Although the mouse and hamster have provided excellent material for experimentation as schistosome hosts, their suitability as models for development of immunity in man is now recognized to be limited. The use of less suitable hosts to study mechanisms of innate immunity, as has been done by Sadun and Bruce (1964b), may be expected to yield further important information, as will the increased utilization of primates as models more closely approximating infection of man. It is unfortunate that the lack of fully reliable and relatively innocuous chemotherapeutic agents still militates against the performance of safe and well-controlled experiments in man.

REFERENCES

Abdel-Malek, E. T. 1950. Susceptibility of the snail *Biophalaria boissyi* to infection with certain strains of *Schistosoma mansoni*. Amer. J. Trop. Med., 30:887–894.

Augustin, R. 1967. Demonstration of reagins in the serum of allergic subjects. *In* Handbook of Experimental Immunology. Weir, D. M., ed. Philadelphia, F. A. Davis Co., pp. 1076–1151.

Bénex, J. and L. Lamy. 1959. Immobilisation des miracidium de *Schistosoma mansoni* par des extraits de planorbes. Bull. Soc. Path. Exot., 52:188–193.

Berggren, W. L., and T. H. Weller. 1967. Immunoelectrophoretic demonstration of specific circulating antigen in animals infected with *Schistosoma mansoni*. Amer. J. Trop. Med. Hyg., 16:606–612.

Bilharz, T. 1852a. Ein Beitrag zur Helminthographia humana des Bilharz in Cairo nebst Bemerkungen von Prof. C. Th. v. Siebold in Breslau. Z. Wiss. Zool., 4:53–72.

———— 1852b. Fernere Beobachtungen über die Pfortader des Menschen bewohnende *Distomum haematobium* und sein Verhältniss zu gewissen pathologischen Bildungen (aus brieflichen Mitteilungen an Professor v. Siegold vom 29. März 1852). Z. Wiss. Zool., 4:72–76.

Bouillon, A. 1949. Bibliographie des schistosomes et des schistosomiasis (bilharzioses) humaines et animales de 1931 à 1948. Memoires de l'Institut Royal Colonial Belge, 1949. pp. 7–141.

Capron, A., J. Biguet, F. Rose, and A. Vernes. 1965. Les antigènes de *Schistosoma mansoni*. II. Étude immunoélectrophoretique comparée de divers stades larvaires et des adultes des deux sexes. Aspects immunologiques des relations hôte-parasite de la cercaire et de l'adulte de *S. mansoni*. Ann. Inst. Pasteur (Paris), 109:798–810.

———— A. Vernes, J. Biguet, and F. Rose, with A. Clay and L. Adenis. 1966. Les précipitines sériques dans les bilharzioses humaines et expérimentales à *Schistosoma mansoni, S. haematobium* et *S. japonicum*. Ann. Parasit. Hum. Comp., 41:123–187.

—— A. Vernes, J. Biguet, and P. Tran Van Ky. 1967. Apport de l'immunoélectrophorèse à l'étude immunologique des bilharzioses (Essai de synthèse). Ann. Soc. Belg. Med. Trop., 47:127–142.

Cheever, A. W., W. B. DeWitt, and K. S. Warren. 1965. Repeated infection and treatment of mice with *Schistosoma mansoni*: Functional, anatomic and immunologic observations. Amer. J. Trop. Med. Hyg., 14:239–253.

Chui, J. K. 1965. *Tricula chuii*: A new snail host for Formosan strain of *Schistosoma japonicum*. J. Parasit., 51:206.

Clarke, H. V. de V. 1966. Evidence of the development in man of acquired resistance to infection of *Schistosoma* spp. Cent. Afr. J. Med., 12:1–3.

Coker, C. M., and J. Oliver-Gonzalez. 1956. Studies on immunity to schistosomiasis—passive transfer of anti-egg antibody in humans. Amer. J. Trop. Med. Hyg., 5:385.

Damian, R. T. 1967. Common antigens between adult *Schistosoma mansoni* and the laboratory mouse. J. Parasit., 53:60–64.

DeMorais, T. 1962. Frontiers in research in parasitism. I. Cellular and humoral reactions in experimental schistosomiasis. Lincicome, D. R., ed. Exp. Parasit., 12:238.

Dixon, P. K. 1934. Age incidence of schistosome infection and species of malaria parasites in Katanga. Trans. Roy. Soc. Trop. Med. Hyg., 27:505–506.

Domingo, E O. and K. S. Warren 1966. The effect of thymectomy on granuloma formation around schistosome eggs. Presented to the 15th Annual Meeting, Amer. Soc. Trop. Med., San Juan, Puerto Rico.

—— R. B. T. Cowan, and K. S. Warren. 1967. The inhibition of granuloma formation around *Schistosoma mansoni* eggs. I. Immunosuppressive drugs. Amer. J. Trop. Med. (in press)

Dusanic D. G., and R. M. Lewert. 1963. Alterations of proteins and free amino acids of *Australorbis glabratus* hemolymph after exposure to *Schistosoma mansoni* miracidia. J. Infect. Dis., 112:243–246.

—— and R. M. Lewert. 1966. Electrophoretic studies of the antigen-antibody complexes of *Trichinella Spiralis* and *Schistosoma mansoni*. J. Infect. Dis., 116:270–284.

Erickson, D. G., and W. L. Caldwell. 1965. Acquired resistance in mice and rats after exposure to gamma-irradiated cercariae. Amer. J. Trop. Med. Hyg., 14:566–573.

Fairley, N. H. 1919. A preliminary report on the investigation of the immunity reactions in Egyptian bilharziasis. J. Roy. Army Med. Corps, 32:243–267.

—— 1938. Discussion on immunity to animal parasites. Metazoal immunity. Proc. Roy. Soc. Med., 31:1291–1298.

—— and F. E. Williams. 1927. A preliminary report on an intradermal reaction in schistosomiasis. Med. J. Aust., 2:811–818.

—— F. P. Mackie, and F. Jasudasan. 1930. Studies in *Schistosoma spindale*. Parts I–VI. Indian Med. Res. Mem., 17:180.

Faust, E. C., and H. E. Meleney. 1924. Studies on schistosomiasis japonica with a supplement on molluscan hosts of the human blood fluke in China and Japan and species liable to be confused with them, by Nelson Annandale. Amer. J. Hyg. Monogr. Ser. No. 3, pp. 1–339.

Files, V. S. 1951. A study of the vector-parasite relationships in *Schistosoma mansoni*. Parasitology, 41:264–269.

—— and E. B. Cram. 1949. A study on the comparative susceptibility of snail vectors to strains of *Schistosoma mansoni*. J. Parasit., 35:555–560.

Fisher, K. C. 1934. A study of the schistosomes of the Stanleyville district of the Belgium Congo. Trans. Roy. Soc. Trop. Med. Hyg., 28:277–306.

Frick, L. P., L. S. Ritchie, W. B. Knight, and J. H. Tauber. 1965. Enhancement of acquired resistance against *Schistosoma mansoni* in albino mice by intraperitoneal immunizing exposures. J. Parasit., 51:230–234.

Fujinami, A. 1916a. Immunity to disease due to macroparasites. Kyoto Igakai Zasshi (J. Kyoto Med. Ass.), 13:454–463.

—— 1916b. Supplement to "Immunity to disease due to macroparasites". Kyoto Igakai Zasshi (J. Kyoto Med. Ass.), 13:464–465.

—— and H. Sueyasu. 1917. Über die Hautinvasion des *Schistosomum japonicum* und Beitrag zur Kenntnis der natürlichen Immunität der Schistosomum-Krankheit (Abstrakt). Verh. Japan. Path. Ges., 7:137–138.

—— and H. Sueyasu. 1918. Eindringen der Schistosomum-Cerkarien sowohl in immune Tiere als auch in Fremdkörper. Verh. Japan. Path. Ges., 8:159.

Gelfand, M., V. de V. Clarke, and C. Turnbull. 1964a. The detection of antibodies to *Schistosoma* spp. in newly born infants of mothers having the same antibodies. J. Trop. Med. Hyg., 67:254.

——— V. de V. Clarke, and C. Turnbull. 1964b. The hypersensitive response of the European to schistosomiasis. J. Trop. Med. Hyg., 67:255–256.

Gerber, J. H. 1952a. Bilharzia in Baojibu. Part I. J. Trop. Med. Hyg., 55:52–58.

——— 1952b. Bilharzia in Baojibu. Part II. The human population. J. Trop. Med. Hyg., 55:79–93.

Girgis, R. 1934. Schistosomiasis (Bilharziasis). London, John Bale Sons & Danielson, Ltd, pp. 1–527.

Gothe, K. M. 1963. Beobachtungen über die Immunität bei *Schistosoma haematobium*-Infektionen. Z. Tropenmed. Parasit., 14:512–518.

Guerra, P., M. Mayer, and J. Di Prisco. 1945. la especificidad de las intradermorreacciónes con antigenos de *Schistosoma mansoni* y *Fasciola hepatica* por el método de Prausnitz-Küestner. Revista Sanidad Assistencia Social (Venezuela), 10:51–63.

Heremans, J. F., P. A. Crabbe, and P. L. Masson. 1966. Biological significance of exocrine gamma-A-immunoglobulin. Acta Med. Scand., 179(Suppl. 455):84–88.

Hillyer, G. V., and L. S. Ritchie. 1967. Immunoprecipitins in *Schistosoma mansoni* infections: II. *Cercopithecus sabaeus* and *Macacca mulatta* monkeys. Exp. Parasit., 20:326–333.

——— R. Menedez-Corrada, R. Lluberes, and F. Hernandez-Morales. 1970. Evidence of transplacental passage of specific antibody in *Schistosomiasis mansoni* in man. Amer. J. Trop. Med. Hyg., 19:289–291.

Houghton, H. G. 1910. Notes on infection with *Schistosomum japonicum*. J. Trop. Med. Hyg., 13:185–187.

Hsü, Hsi-Fan. 1950. A preliminary study on the bionomics of *Oncomelania* snails, intermediate hosts of *Schistosoma japonicum*, in Kiangsu and Chekiang provinces, China. Amer. J. Trop. Med., 30:397–410.

——— and S. Y. Li Hsü. 1956. On the infectivity of the Formosan strain *Schistosoma japonicum* in *Homo sapiens*. Amer. J. Trop. Med. Hyg., 5:521–528.

——— and S. Y. Li Hsü. 1960a. The infectivity of four geographic strains of *Schistosoma japonicum* in the rhesus monkey. J. Parasit., 46:228.

——— and S. Y. Li Hsü. 1960b. Susceptibility of albino mice to different geographic strains of *Schistosoma japonicum*. Trans. Roy. Soc. Trop. Med. Hyg., 54:466–468.

——— and S. Y. Li Hsü. 1962. *Schistosoma japonicum* in Formosa: A critical review. Exp. Parasit., 12:459–465.

———S. Y. Li Hsü. 1966. Reagin-like antibody in rhesus monkeys immune to *Schistosoma japonicum*. Z. Tropenmed. Parasit., 17:166–176.

——— Y. L. Hsü and J. W. Osborne. 1962. Immunization against *Schistosoma japonicum* in rhesus monkeys produced by irradiated cercariae. Nature (London), 194:98–99.

——— S. Y. Li Hsü, and J. W. Osborne. 1963. Further studies on rhesus monkeys immunized against *Schistosoma japonicum* by administration of X-irradiated cercariae. Z. Tropenmed. Parasit., 14:402–412.

——— S. Y. Li Hsü, and C. T. Tsai. 1964. Immunization against *Schistosoma japonicum* in rhesus monkeys by administration of cercariae of *Schistosomatium douthitti*. Z. Tropenmed. Parasit., 15:435–440.

Hsü, S. Y. Li, and H. F. Hsü. 1961. New approach to immunization against *Schistosoma japonicum*. Science, 133:766.

——— and H. F. Hsü. 1963. Further studies on rhesus monkeys immunized against *Schistosoma japonicum* by administration of cercariae of the Formosan strain. Z. Tropenmed. Parasit., 14:506–512.

——— and H. F. Hsü. 1964. Serum protein changes in rhesus monkeys during immunization and following challenge by *Schistosoma japonicum*. Z. Tropenmed. Parasit., 15:43–56.

——— and H. F. Hsü. 1966. Complement fixation reaction in rhesus monkeys infected with *Schistosoma japonicum*. Z. Tropenmed. Parasit., 17:264–278.

——— J. R. Davis, and H. F. Hsü. 1962. Pathology in rhesus monkeys infected with the Formosan strain of *Schistosoma japonicum*. Z. Tropenmed. Parasit., 13:341–356.

——— H. F. Hsü, and J. W. Osborne. 1965. Immunizing effect of X-irradiated cercariae of *Schistosoma japonicum* in albino mice. Z. Tropenmed. Parasit., 16:83–89.

———— H. F. Hsü, K. Y. Chu, C. T. Tsai, and V. K. Eveland. 1966. Immunization against *Schistosoma haematobium* in rhesus monkeys by administration of cercariae of *Schistosoma bovis*. Z. Tropenmed. Parasit., 17:407–412.

Hunter, G. W., III, C. J. Weinmann, and R. G. Hoffmann. 1961. Studies on schistosomiasis XVII. Non-reciprocal acquired resistance between *Schistosoma mansoni* and *Schistosomatium douthitti* in mice. Exp. Parasit., 11:133–140.

Jachowski, L. A., R. I. Anderson, and E. H. Sadun. 1963. Serologic reactions to *Schistosoma mansoni*. I. Quantitative studies on experimentally infected monkeys (*Macaca mulatta*). Amer. J. Hyg., 77:137–145.

Jamuar, M. P., and R. M. Lewert. 1967. Effect of immune serum on the miracidial surface of *Schistosoma japonicum*. J. Parasit., 53:220–221.

Janscó, M. 1947. Histamin: a reticulo-endothelialis sejtrendszer élettani aktivátora. Orvosak Japja (Budapest), 3:1025–1030.

Jarrett, W. F. H., F. W. Jennings, W. I. M. McIntyre, W. Mulligan, and G. M. Urquhart. 1960. Immunological studies on *Dictyocaulus viviparus* infection. Immunity produced by the administration of irradiated larvae. Immunology, 3:145–151.

Kagan, I. G. 1953. Experimental infections of rhesus monkeys with *Schistosomatium douthitti* (Cort 1914). J. Infect. Dis., 93:200–206.

———— 1958. Contributions to the immunology and serology of schistosomiasis. Rice Institute Pamphlet No. 45, pp. 151–183.

———— 1966. Mechanisms of immunity in trematode infection. *In* Biology of Parasites. Soulsby, E. J. L., ed. New York, Academic Press, Inc., pp. 277–299.

Kawamura, R. 1928. The recent researches in schistosomiasis japonica in Japan. C. R. Congr. Int. Med. Trop. Med. Hyg. Cairo, 4:311–319.

Khalil, M. B. 1931. The bibliography of schistosomiasis (bilharziasis), zoological, clinical and prophylactic. Cairo, Egyptian University, The Faculty of Medicine Pub. No. 1, pp. 1–506.

Kuntz, R. E. 1955. Biology of the schistosome complexes. Amer. J. Trop. Med. Hyg., 4:383–413.

Lambert, A. C. 1911a. Schistosomiasis (Jap.) and so-called urticarial fevers. Their identity. China Med. J., 25:308–312.

———— 1911b. Fevers with urticaria and eosinophilia and their relation to infection with *Schistosomum japonicum*. Trans. Roy. Soc. Trop. Med. Hyg., 5:38–45.

Lanning, R. H. 1914. Schistosomiasis on the Yangtze river with report of cases. U. S. Naval Med. Bull., 8:16–36.

Lee, C. L., and R. M. Lewert. 1960. The distribution of various reactants in human anti-*Schistosoma mansoni* serums fractionated by starch electrophoresis. J. Infect. Dis., 106:69–76.

Lewert, R. M., and C. L. Lee. 1954. Studies on the passage of helminth larvae through host tissues. I. Histochemical studies on extracellular changes caused by penetrating larvae. II. Enzymatic activity of larvae in vitro and in vivo. J. Infect. Dis., 95:13–51.

———— and J. Cahill. 1968. Unpublished data.

———— and S. Mandlowitz. 1963. Innate immunity to *S. mansoni* relative to the state of connective tissue. Ann. N. Y. Acad. Sci., 113:54–62.

———— and S. Mandlowitz. 1969. Unpublished data.

———— and S. Mandlowitz. 1969. Schistosomiasis: Prenatal induction of tolerance to antigens. Nature (London), 224:1029–1030.

———— and B. J. Para. 1969. The migration of isotopically labeled cercariae in mice previously exposed to *S. mansoni*. (In preparation)

———— and M. G. Yogore, Jr. 1966. Alterations in immunoelectrophoretic reactions following chemotherapy of human schistosomiasis japonica. Proc. 11th Pacific Sci. Congr., Tokyo. Vol. 8, Symposium No. 34 (Abstract).

———— and M. G. Yogore, Jr. Unpublished data.

———— C. L. Lee, S. Mandlowitz, and D. Dusanic. 1959. Inhibition of the collagenase-like enzymes of cercariae of *Schistosoma mansoni* by serums and serum fractions. J. Infect Dis., 105:180–187.

———— D. R. Hopkins, and S. Mandlowitz. 1966. The role of calcium and magnesium ions in invasiveness of schistosome cercariae. Amer. J. Trop. Med. Hyg., 15:314–323.

Liu, C., and F. B. Bang. 1950. The natural course of a light experimental infection of schistosomiasis japonica in monkeys. Bull. Hopkins Hosp., 86:215–233.

McQuay, R. M. 1953. Studies on variability in the susceptibility of a North American snail *Tropicorbis havenensis*, to infection with the Puerto Rican strain of *Schistosoma mansoni*. Trans. Roy. Soc. Trop. Med. Hyg., 47:56.

Meisenhelder, J. E., B. Olszewski, and P. E. Thompson. 1960. Observations on therapeutic and prophylactic effects by homologous immune blood against *Schistosoma mansoni* in rhesus monkeys. J. Parasit., 46:645–647.

Meleney, H. E., and D. V. Moore. 1954. Observations on immunity to superinfection with *Schistosoma mansoni* and *S. haematobium* in monkeys. Exp. Parasit., 3:128–139.

Mendes, E., and V. Amato Neto. 1963. Alguns aspéctos imunólogicos relativos à esquistossomiase mansônica: Prova da transferência passiva de anticorpos e prova das precipitinas. Hospital (Rio de Janeiro), 64:1289–1293.

Michelson, E. H. 1963. Development and specificity of miracidial immobilizing substances in extracts of the snail *Australorbis glabratus* exposed to various agents. Ann. N. Y. Acad. Sci., 113:486–491.

Miyagawa, Y. 1913. Beziehungen zwischen Schistosomiasis japonica und der Dermatitis, und Berücksichtigung der Methode der Auffindung von Parasiteneiern in den Faeces, und Beiträge zur Kenntnis des Schistosomum-Infektion. Zbl. Bakt. [Orig.], 69:132–142.

Moose, J. W. 1963. Susceptibility of young and old *Oncomelania nosophora* to infection with *Schistosoma japonicum*. J. Parasit., 49:813.

——— and J. E. Williams. 1963a. Infectivity of hybrid snails obtained from the reciprocal cross of *Oncomelania nosophora* and *O. formosana* to the Japanese strain of *Schistosoma japonicum*. J. Parasit., 49:284.

——— and J. E. Williams. 1963b. Susceptibility of *Oncomelania formosana* from three different areas of Taiwan to infection with Formosan strain of *Schistosoma japonicum*. J. Parasit., 49:702–703.

Mühlens, P. 1937. Yangtse-Fieber—Erkrankungen (Schistosomiasis japonica) an Bord eines deutschen Handelsschiffes. Archiv für Schiffs- und Tropen-Hygiene, Deutsche Tropenmedizinische Monatsschrift, 41:308–317.

Naimark, D. H., A. S. Benenson, J. Oliver-González, D. B. McMullen, and L. S. Ritchie. 1960. Studies on schistosomiasis in primates: Observations on acquired resistance (Progress report). Amer. J. Trop. Med. Hyg., 9:430–435.

Newsome, J. 1956. Problems of fluke immunity: With special reference to schistosomiasis. Trans. Roy. Soc. Trop. Med. Hyg., 50:258–274.

——— 1962. Immune opsonins in schistosoma infestations. Nature (London), 195:1175–1179.

Newton, W. L. 1952. The comparative tissue reaction of two strains of *Australorbis glabratus* to infection with *Schistosoma mansoni*. J. Parasit., 38:362–366.

——— 1954. Tissue response to *Schistosoma mansoni* in second generation snails from a cross between two strains of *Australorbis glabratus*. J. Parasit., 40:352–355.

Nolf, L. W., and W. W. Cort. 1933. On the immunity reactions of snails to the penetration of the cercariae of the strigeid trematode, *Cotylurus flabelliformis* (Faust). J. Parasit., 20:38–48.

Ogilvie, B. M. 1964. Reagin-like antibodies in animals immune to helminth parasites. Nature (London), 204:91–92.

——— 1967. Reagin-like antibodies in rats infected with a nematode parasite *Nippostrongylus brasiliensis*. Immunology, 12:113–131.

——— S. R. Smithers, and R. J. Terry. 1966. Reagin-like antibodies in experimental infections of *Schistosoma mansoni* and the passive transfer of resistance. Nature (London), 209:1221–1223.

Okabe, K., and N. Ono. 1961. Some additions to the urine precipitin reaction for schistosomiasis japonica. Kurume Med. J., 8:95–99.

Ozawa, M. 1930. Experimental studies on acquired immunity to schistosomiasis japonica. Japan J. Exp. Med., 8:79–84.

Page, C. O., and J. S. Remington. 1967. Immunologic studies in normal human sweat. J. Lab. Clin. Med., 69:634–650.

Pan, Chia-Tung. 1963. Generalized and focal tissue responses in the snail, *Australorbis glabratus*, infected with *Schistosoma mansoni*. Ann. N. Y., Acad. Sci., 113:475–485.

Patterson, J. L. H., and W. E. Libbey. 1922. Unpublished. (Quoted in Faust, E. C., and H. E. Meleney, 1924.)

Perlowagora-Szumlewicz, A. 1964. Studies on acquired resistance to *Schistosoma mansoni* in mice exposed to X-irradiated cercariae. Bull. W. H. O., 30:401–412.

Puerto Rican J. Public Health Trop. Med. 1933–1937. Studies on *S. mansoni* in Puerto Rico. Puerto Rican J. Public Health Trop. Med., 9:154–168, 9:228–282, through 13:171–254.

Ritchie, L. S., S. Garson, and D. G. Erickson. 1962. Attempts to induce resistance against *Schistosoma mansoni* by injections, cercarial, adult worm, and egg homogenates in sequence. J. Parasit., 48: 233–236.

———— W. B. Knight, J. Oliver-Gonzalez, L. P. Frick, J. M. Morris, and W. L. Crocker. 1967. *Schistosoma mansoni* infections in *Cercopithecus sabeus* monkeys. J. Parasit., 53: 1217–1224.

Sadun, E. H. 1963. Immunization in schistosomiasis by previous exposure to homologous and heterologous cercariae, by inoculation of preparations from schistosomes, and by exposure to irradiated cercariae. Ann. N. Y. Acad. Sci., 113: 418–439.

———— 1965. Trichinosis, hydatid diseases, schistosomiasis, and ascariasis. *In* Immunological Diseases. Samter, D., and Alexander, H. L., eds. Boston, Little, Brown and Co., pp. 469–484.

———— and J. I. Bruce. 1964a. Natural history of infection with *Schistosoma mansoni* in different species of monkeys. J. Parasit., 50: 22.

———— and J. I. Bruce. 1964b. Resistance induced in rats by previous exposure to and by vaccination with fresh homogenates of *Schistosoma mansoni*. Exp. Parasit., 15: 32–43.

———— and S. S. Lin. 1959. Studies on the host-parasite relationships to *Schistosoma japonicum*. IV. Resistance acquired by infection, by vaccination, and by the injection of immune serum, in monkeys, rabbits and mice. J. Parasit., 45: 543–548.

———— and B. C. Walton. 1958. Studies on the host-parasite relationships to *Schistosoma japonicum*. II. Quantitative changes in the concentration of serum proteins in humans and rabbits. Amer. J. Trop. Med., 7: 500–504.

———— F. von Lichtenberg, R. L. Hickman, J. I. Bruce, J. H. Smith, and M. J. Schoenbechler. 1966a. Schistosomiasis mansoni in the chimpanzee: parasitologic, clinical, serologic, pathologic and radiologic observations. Amer. J. Trop. Med. Hyg., 15: 496–506.

———— F. von Lichtenberg, and J. I. Bruce. 1966b. Susceptibility and comparative pathology of ten species of primates exposed to infection with *Schistosoma mansoni*. Amer. J. Trop. Med. Hyg., 15: 705–718.

Schwetz, J. 1956. Sur l'immunité clinique dans les bilharzioese humaines. Bull. Soc. Path. Exot. 49: 52–56.

Sherif, A. F. 1962. Schistosomal metabolic products in the diagnosis of bilharziasis. *In* Bilharziasis. Ciba Foundation Symposium. Boston, Little, Brown and Co., pp. 226–238.

Simoes Barbosa, F. A., and M. Vasconcellos Coelho. 1956. Pesquisa de imunidade adquirida homóloga em *Australorbis glabratus*, nas infestações por *Schistosoma mansoni*. Rev. Brasil. Malar., 8: 49–56.

Smithers, S. R. 1962a. Acquired resistance to bilharziasis. *In* Bilharziasis. Ciba Foundation Symposium. Boston, Little, Brown and Co., pp. 239–265.

———— 1962b. Stimulation of acquired resistance to *Schistosoma mansoni* in monkeys: Role of eggs and worms. Exp. Parasit., 12: 263–273.

———— 1962c. Immunizing effect of irradiated cercariae of *Schistosoma mansoni* in rhesus monkeys. Nature (London), 194: 1146–1147.

———— 1967. The induction and nature of antibody response to parasites. *In* Immunologic Aspects of Parasitic Infections. Pan American Health Organization Scientific Publication No. 150, pp. 43–49.

———— and R. J. Terry. 1966. The nature of the antibody response in schistosomiasis. Proc. 1st Int. Congr. Parasit. Corradetti, A., ed. Vol. 1, p. 139.

———— and R. J. Terry. 1967. Resistance to experimental infection with *Schistosoma mansoni* in rhesus monkeys induced by the transfer of adult worms. Trans. Roy. Soc. Trop. Med. Hyg., 61: 517–533.

———— and R. J. Terry. 1969. The immunology of schistosomiasis. *In* Advances in Parasitology, Vol. 7. Dawes, B., ed. New York, Academic Press, Inc., pp. 41–93.

———— R. J. Terry, and D. J. Hockley. 1969. Host antigens in schistosomiasis. Proc. Roy. Soc., Series B, 171: 483–494.

Soulsby, E. J. L. 1962. Antigen-antibody reactions in helminth infections. Advances Immun., 2: 265–308.

Stirewalt, M. A. 1963. Seminar on immunity to parasitic helminths. IV. Schistosome infections. Exp. Parasit., 13: 18–44.

Taliaferro, W. H. 1940. The mechanisms of acquired immunity in infections with parasitic worms. Physiol. Rev., 20: 469–492.

———— and L. G. Taliaferro. 1931. Skin reactions in persons infected with *Schistosoma mansoni*. Puerto Rico J. Public Health Trop., Med., 7: 23–35.

———— W. A. Hoffman, and D. H. Cook. 1928. A precipitin test in intestinal schistosomiasis (*S. mansoni*). J. Prevent. Med., 2:395–414.

Thompson, J. H., Jr. 1954. Host-parasite relationships of *Schistosoma mansoni*. Exp. Parasit., 3:140–160.

Tomasi, T. B., E. M. Tan, A. Solomon, and R. A. Prendergast. 1965. Characteristics of an immune system common to certain external secretions. J. Exp. Med., 121:101–124.

Tran Van Ky, P., T. Vaucell, A. Capron, and J. Biguet. 1967. Caractérisation des types d'activités enzymatiques dans les broyats de *Schistosoma mansoni* adultes après immunoélectrophorèse en agarose. Ann. Inst. Pasteur (Paris), 112:763–771.

Tripp, M. R. 1963. Cellular responses of mollusks. Ann. N. Y. Acad. Sci., 113:467–474.

Villella, J. B., H. J. Gomberg, and S. E. Gould. 1961. Immunization to *Schistosoma mansoni* in mice inoculated with radiated cercariae. Science, 134:1073–1074.

Vogel, H., and W. Minning. 1953. Über die erworbene Resistanz von *Macacus rhesus* gegenüber *Schistosoma japonicum*. Z. Tropenmed. Parasit., 4:418–505.

Von Lichtenberg, F. 1967a. Mechanisms of schistosome immunity. *In* Bilharziasis. Mostofi, F. K., ed. New York, Springer-Verlag New York Inc., pp. 286–300.

———— 1967b. The bilharzial pseudo-tubercle: A model of the immunopathology of granuloma formation. *In* Immunologic Aspects of Parasitic Infections. Pan American Health Organization Scientific Publication No. 150, pp. 107–127.

———— and E. H. Sadun. 1963. Parasite migration and host reaction in mice exposed to irradiated cercariae of *Schistosoma mansoni*. Exp. Parasit., 13:256–265.

———— E. H. Sadun, and J. I. Bruce. 1962. Tissue responses and mechanisms of resistance in schistosomiasis mansoni in abnormal hosts. Amer. J. Trop. Med. Hyg., 11:347–356.

Wadji, N. 1966. Immunity to *Schistosoma haematobium* in *Bulinus truncatus*. Trans. Roy. Soc. Trop. Med. Hyg., 60:774–776.

Warren, K. S., and V. A. Newill. 1967. Schistosomiasis: A Bibliography of the World's Literature from 1852–1962. Cleveland, The Press of Western Reserve University, Vols. 1 and 2, pp. 1–1984.

Winfield, G. F. 1932. On the immunity of snails infested with sporocysts of the strigeid, *Cotylurus flabelliformis*, to the penetration of its cercariae. J. Parasit., 19:130–133.

World Health Organization. 1960. Bibliography on Bilharziasis, 1949–1959. Geneva, World Health Organization, pp. 7–158.

Yoshimoto, S. 1910. Über die Komplementbindungs-reaktion bei Schistosomum-Krankheit in Japan. Z. Immunitäts. Exp. Ther., 5:438–445.

Trematodes of the Liver and Lung

EDWARD G. PLATZER
.The Rockefeller University, New York, New York

INTRODUCTION

The immunology of trematodes other than schistosomes has received comparatively little attention. Most trematode immunology other than of blood flukes has been confined to *Clonorchis sinensis*, *Fasciola hepatica*, and *Paragonimus westermani*, primarily in relation to the diagnosis of human infections by serologic means. Associated with the serologic studies, there have been some extensive attempts at purification of trematode antigens to improve the specificity and sensitivity of the serologic tests. Protective immunity has been investigated mainly in *F. hepatica* infections. Reviews of clonorchiasis (Komiya, 1966), fascioliasis (Dawes and Hughes, 1964; Pantelouris, 1965; Sinclair, 1967), paragonimiasis (Yokogawa et al., 1960; Yokogawa, 1965), and their serology (Kent, 1963) have thoroughly surveyed the early literature; therefore, this chapter will survey only selected older publications as a background to recent investigations.

Before discussing the immunology, it is appropriate to consider briefly the particular host-parasite relationships—especially the mode of infection and the migrations of the parasites. This may give some insight into how parasite antigens stimulate the host's immune response. Infection of the mammalian hosts with *C. sinensis*, *F. hepatica*, and *P. westermani* takes place by the gastric route. The metacercariae escape from the metacercarial cysts in the duodenum, and this phase presumably constitutes the first exposure of the host to the parasites' antigenic materials, i.e., its secretory and excretory products. *C. sinensis* is generally thought to lack a tissue phase (Komiya, 1966; Sun et al., 1968), but Wykoff and Lepěs (1957) reported that young flukes were found in the liver bile ducts even when the common bile duct was ligated and cut. This finding suggested that early circulating antibodies may result from a tissue migration of the young flukes. Further antigenic stimulation of the host presumably occurs during the flukes' residence in and feeding on secretions of the bile ductules (Komiya, 1966).

In contrast, both *F. hepatica* and *P. westermani* have tissue migration stages which are initiated by penetration of the intestinal wall, followed by a period of wandering in the abdominal cavity. *F. hepatica* penetrates the liver capsule and burrows into parenchyma, at which time the maximal mechanical damage occurs (Sinclair, 1967). Subsequently, the flukes move into the bile ducts where they feed on bile duct epithelium (Dawes and Hughes, 1964). The migration of *P. westermani* may involve the penetration of abdominal organs and a short period of development in the abdominal wall before the flukes finally penetrate the diaphragm and burrow into the surface of the lungs (Yokogawa, 1965). Here, sometimes in pairs, the worms are partially encapsulated by a host fibrotic response. The mode of feeding has not been described, but the fluke probably obtains nutrients from the cyst fluid.

CLONORCHIASIS

As early as 1921, several Japanese workers attempted serologic diagnosis of clonorchiasis (Komiya, 1966). An alcohol extract of *C. sinensis*-infected rabbit liver was utilized as the antigen for complement fixation, but subsequent egg counts showed that the serologic tests failed to identify light infections. Subsequent investigators used saline extracts, homogenates, and crude antigen preparations from adult worms. However, these early attempts at immunodiagnosis were considered equivocal.

Sadun et al. (1959b) prepared Melcher antigen fractions from adult worms recovered from rabbits. They reported that the acid-soluble protein fraction of lyophilized worms was reliable for intradermal tests. Some cross-reactivity with *P. westermani* infections occurred, but the homologous infection could be distinguished on the basis of wheal size. These results were confirmed by another study in the Republic of Korea (Walton and Chyu, 1959). Subsequently, Pacheco et al. (1960) developed an indirect hemagglutination test with two antigen fractions of adult worms. One, a defatted fraction, had high specificity with sera from human and rabbit clonorchiasis. Sun and Gibson (1969) reported that only 14 percent of infected humans gave precipitin lines with whole worm antigen on gel diffusion, and 97 percent of the positives occurred in patients with concurrent liver disease. It appeared that liver dysfunction facilitated precipitin formation against *C. sinensis* antigens.

Sawada et al. (1965) have carried out the most extensive work on antigen isolation and purification from *C. sinensis* in an effort to eliminate the ambiguity resulting from using crude antigen preparations. They subjected a whole-worm preparation to gel filtration and ion-exchange chromatography and monitored the major fractions by complement-fixation and precipitin tests. One fraction, which contained 91 percent polyglucose at the end of the fractionation, was active in complement-fixation tests but not in precipitin tests. No reaction occurred with Folin reagent. The possibilities of cross-reactions were not studied.

The antibody response to *C. clonorchis* infections has been studied experimentally in rabbits, guinea pigs, and rats. Circulating antibody could be detected by complement-fixation (Sadun et al., 1959b; Wykoff, 1959) and indirect hemagglutination (Pacheco et al., 1960) tests four weeks after infection in rabbits. These antibodies decreased 16 to 25 weeks after infection. Precipitating antibodies were detectable in rabbits five weeks after infection and persisted for 21 weeks (Sun and Gibson, 1969). The main precipitation line in human, rabbit, guinea pig, and rat antisera was with metabolic products; however, precipitins for eggs were not found in natural infections. Artificial immunization of rabbits with lipid-free worm fractions or alkali-soluble protein fractions gave low complement-fixation titers when immune sera were tested with the alkali-soluble protein fraction (Wykoff, 1959). Sun and Gibson (1969) injected rabbits with somatic antigen, metabolic products, and eggs. Anti-metabolite and anti-egg sera did not cross-react, whereas cross-reactions occurred in anti-metabolite and anti-adult fluke sera. There were no cross-reactions with antigen preparations from *Schistosoma japonicum* or *P. westermani*.

Absence of protective immunity in *C. sinensis* infections of animals has been reported (Sun et al., 1968; Sun and Gibson, 1969). Adult worms were killed *in vitro* by sera from naturally infected animals, but artificially immunized animals were infected as readily as nonimmunized animals, and the worm burdens were equivalent.

FASCIOLIASIS

Many serologic tests have been utilized in the effort to find a sensitive and efficient means of diagnosing fascioliasis. Complement fixation has been used in conjunction with alcohol extracts of whole worms to diagnose fascioliasis in sheep, but the reliability of complement fixation has not been fully established (Kent, 1963; Pantelouris, 1965). Complement fixation did not distinguish between *F. hepatica* and *Dicrocoelium dendriticum* infections in sheep (Bénex et al., 1959). In contrast, intradermal tests have proven to be more successful for *F. hepatica* (Soulsby, 1954; Pantelouris, 1965) and *Fasciola gigantica* (Patnaik and Das, 1961). Commercial antigens are available for *F. hepatica*. Wikerhauser (1961) developed a microprecipitin test with live excysted metacercariae. Precipitates formed at the mouth and excretory pore of the metacercaria in sera from infected animals; however, the test was nonspecific since a high percentage of sera from uninfected cattle also formed the same precipitates. Soulsby (1957) found that sera from both uninfected and infected sheep had lethal effects on *F. hepatica* miracidia, and therefore this reaction was not a satisfactory technique for serology. Immunoelectrophoresis has been advanced as a fast and specific method for the detection of human infection (Teodorovič et al., 1963). Human fascioliasis has been diagnosed with a slide agglutination technique involving delipidized antigen adsorbed on latex particles (Bénex, 1964). The results were equivalent to those obtained with complement fixation. Serologic diagnosis by hemagglutination gave very high titers, but comparable titers were not found with complement fixation (Biguet et al., 1965).

The immunology of the host-parasite relationship has been studied with the fluorescent-antibody technique. Thorpe (1965) labelled globulin from infected rats and found that the fluorescence was localized in the cecal lining, excretory ducts, and cuticle of *F. hepatica*, both *in situ* and in isolated parasites. Positive staining of phagocytic cells occurred in fluke burrows through the liver, showing an initial process of antigen uptake by host cells during migration of the parasite.

In experimental infections, there have been extensive investigations of the antibody response. Sewell (1964) reported that the circulating antibody response in cattle was at a maximum 10 to 14 days after infection with *F. gigantica*. He also reported that the protein antigens of *F. hepatica* and *F. gigantica* did not show species-specific reactions with antisera. In addition, he was not able to stimulate an antibody response in rabbits or mice by injecting crude antigen or worm metabolic products. *F. hepatica* antisera from mice gave up to three precipitin bands with the metabolic products of *F. gigantica*. Capron et al. (1965) detected circulating antibody in rabbits two weeks after infection with *F. hepatica*. Dawes and Hughes (1964) obtained a circulating antibody response both in infected rabbits and rabbits injected with *F. hepatica* antigen. Lyophilized fluke eggs showed a precipitin line with sera from artificially immunized rabbits, but not with naturally infected rabbit sera.

A considerable amount of investigation has been concentrated on the isolation, purification, and characterization of *F. hepatica* antigens in order to provide a specific and sensitive antigen for immunodiagnosis. Protein, lipid, and carbohydrate fractions have been prepared from adult worms, but these fractions were not as effective antigenically as alcohol extracts of whole worms (Pantelouris, 1965).

Maekawa et al. (1954) crystallized a protein fraction which was active in intradermal tests. On further investigation, they found two more fractions, one phenol soluble (P4) and the other phenol insoluble (C5), which were also active in intradermal tests (Maekawa and Kushibe, 1961a). These fractions were purified until they were homogeneous in the analytical ultracentrifuge and on electrophoresis. Moreover, fractions C5 and P4 were active in the intradermal test at a dilution of 1:100,000. Both fractions contained ribonucleic acid. Fraction P4 was 95 percent ribonucleic acid and 4.6 percent peptide (Maekawa and Kushibe, 1961b). Subsequent studies showed that P4 could be dinitrophenylated without loss of biologic activity, and that the peptide was linked to adenosine-3'-phosphate in the ribonucleic acid portion of the antigen (Maekawa and Kushibe, 1964).

Lyophilization of worm material is commonly employed prior to fractionation of antigens. Korach (1966) found that lyophilization destroyed a major lipoprotein antigen in *F. hepatica*. This lipoprotein made up 2 percent of the worm dry weight. It was a homogeneous material, as shown by ultracentrifugation and by free boundary and zone electrophoresis (Korach, 1966; Korach and Bénex, 1966a). The antigen contained 47 percent lipid, 51 percent protein, and small amounts of glucose and iron. Immunoelectrophoresis showed only one arc of precipitation with infected rabbit or human sera (Korach and Bénex, 1966b). The lipid moiety alone fixed complement, but it was only a hapten since the protein portion was necessary to prepare a specific antiserum in rabbits. Since the lipoprotein could not be isolated from the bile surrounding the worms, it was probably not a secretory substance.

Lipid-free extracts, protein, and polysaccharide fractions have been prepared from *F. gigantica* by solvent extraction, ammonium sulfate precipitation, enzyme digestion, and paper electrophoresis (Rifaat and Abdel-Aal, 1968a,b; Rifaat et al., 1968). The fractions were tested in the intradermal test which the authors had developed for *Schistosoma haematobium*, and the protein fraction was found to be the most active. Large quantities of *F. gigantica* can be obtained, and this development has practical advantages since *S. haematobium* is difficult to obtain in quantities sufficient for diagnostic purposes. However, no control sera were tested for other possible heterologous reactions.

Field studies of *F. hepatica* infections in goats and sheep have given no indications of acquired immunity (Pantelouris, 1965). Cattle develop a nonspecific resistance because bile duct calcification occurs in response to infection (Sinclair, 1967).

Acquired immunity to *F. hepatica* has been difficult to show experimentally. Ross (1966) found that previously infected rabbits, when given a challenge infection, had worm burdens lower than those of controls, but the results were so variable in individual animals that they were not statistically significant. Ross (1967) later reported a reduction in the numbers of challenge worms in previously infected cattle, but there was the possibility of a nonspecific response of the bile ducts. Kendall et al. (1967) reported that when rabbits were infected, reinfected 12 weeks later, and killed 20 weeks from the time of the first infection, the number of flukes recovered was smaller than that expected on the basis of primary and secondary infection controls. However, the authors attributed the apparent decrease in worm burden to competitive inhibition of fluke establishment and development and to technical difficulties in recovering very small flukes, rather than postulating acquired resistance. This thorough analysis illustrated the disadvantages of immunologic experiments designed to show protective immunity through data gathered from primary and challenge infection controls. The sum of the primary and challenge infections, as shown by Kendall et al. (1967), does not necessarily represent the physiologic situation in the animals receiving both infections.

The experiments by Lang (1967) suggested that acquired immunity could be stimulated in mice infected with *F. hepatica*. After mice had received two stimulating infections with two metacercariae per infection, Lang reported that there was a reduction in the number of challenge worms reaching the common bile duct. In addition, there was an earlier migration of the challenge worms into the common bile duct, which Lang suggests may have been induced by the altered biochemical environment of the liver parenchyma. Earlier host response to the challenge occurred, as evidenced by loss of body weight, increase in total leukocyte numbers, and liver histopathology. Lang suggested that delayed hypersensitivity was responsible for the decreased worm numbers in the challenge infection. This was based on his observations that lymphocytes appeared earlier in the liver in challenged animals, which elicited a nonspecific inflammatory reaction. Lang (1968) also found that challenge worms were damaged at 17 days after infection since they could not establish themselves in the bile ducts of normal mice, as could 17-day-old primary worms in surgical transfer experiments.

Earlier attempts at passive immunization of animals with sera from *F. hepatica*-infected animals were unsuccessful (Dawes and Hughes, 1964). However, Lang et al. (1967) recently reported that peritoneal exudate cells from infected isologous donors, when injected into normal mice, transferred immunity to challenge infections with *F. hepatica* 21 days later. As in the natural infections, the immunized mice showed a more rapid response to infection, and significantly fewer worms became established.

Attempts at artificial immunization with worm tissue, excretion products, and x-irradiated cercariae have been generally unsuccessful in *F. hepatica* infections. Kerr and Petkovitch (1935) reported that protective immunity developed in rabbits injected with saline extracts of dried worms. However, subsequent investigators (Urquhart et al., 1954; Healy, 1955; Dawes and Hughes, 1964) were unable to confirm these results in rabbits or sheep, although slight effects on worm development and worm nitrogen content were observed (Urquhart et al., 1954; Healy, 1955). The work with x-irradiated cercariae is conflicting. Thorpe and Broome (1962) reported that rats infected with x-irradiated cercariae developed lower worm burdens on challenge infection than did controls. However, their method is subject to the possible errors discussed by Kendall et al. (1967), since the results were based only on worm recoveries. In contrast, x-irradiated cercariae elicited no protective immunity in sheep, rabbits, and mice, though there was a serologic response in the last two groups (Hughes, 1962; Dawes and Hughes, 1964). The failure of x-irradiated cercariae to stimulate acquired immunity may be due to their limited survival, since Lang (1968) suggested that the 8- to 17-day-old worms were responsible for the immune effects in mice.

PARAGONIMIASIS

Development of serologic tests for paragonimiasis has been expedited by the difficulties inherent in finding eggs of *P. westermani* in sputum and stool samples. Complement fixation was first used in 1917 by Ando with saline or alcohol extracts of adult worms; however, false positives occurred with tuberculosis and syphilis (Yokogawa et al., 1960; Yokagawa, 1965). Numerous serologic tests have been applied since then with varying degrees of success (Kent, 1963). Intradermal tests appear to be the most efficient and sensitive method of serodiagnosis. Antigen prepared by extraction of worm material with veronal-buffered saline or saline gave good results (Yokogawa, 1965). Sadun et al. (1959a) reported that an acid-soluble protein fraction from adult worms worked well for intradermal tests, whereas the acid-insoluble but alkali-soluble protein fraction was best for complement fixation. Walton and Chyu (1959) found that an acid-soluble protein fraction functioned well in intradermal tests, and the slight cross-reaction with *C. sinensis* infections could be distinguished by the larger wheal size with the homologous antigen. Capron et al. (1965) reported that immunoelectrophoresis gave good results, but some cross-reactions with other human flukes were found.

Partial fractionation of adult worm antigens was reported by Sawada et al. (1964a). They used starch-block electrophoresis to prepare three protein fractions. Cathodic and nonmigrating proteins containing carbohydrate gave the highest precipitin titers. Subsequently, the anodic material was found to be very active in intradermal tests, giving no false positives (Sawada et al., 1964b). Fractionation of crude lipid-free antigen by ion-exchange chromatography yielded a highly active fraction which did not cross-react in the intradermal test with other human helminth infections (Sawada et al., 1964b). The authors suggested that this preparation would be appropriate for field diagnosis of paragonimiasis.

Experimental infections with *P. westermani* have shown some indications of protective immunity; however, further and better controlled experiments are required (Yokogawa et al., 1960; Yokogawa, 1965). Others have studied the circulating antibody response in infected animals. Sadun et al. (1959a) found by complement fixation that circulating antibodies appeared in cats 30 days after infection and persisted for 100 days. Since eggs did not appear until 60 days, complement fixation was suggested as useful for early diagnosis of paragonimiasis. Immunodiffusion studies demonstrated the presence of precipitating antibodies to whole-worm extracts and metabolic products in both human and cat sera (Yogore et al., 1965). This suggested that secretory and excretory products of the encysted worms entered the circulatory system.

The immunologic responses in other species of *Paragonimus* have been studied. Seed et al. (1966) have studied *P. kellicotti* in cats. Infected cat sera contained low titers of complement-fixing and precipitating antibodies, but did not immobilize miracidia nor show the Cercariah-hüllen, cercarial immobilization, or agglutination reactions. Intradermal tests were negative, and only one of six anaphylactic tests was positive. Up to five precipitin bands were found in agar-gel diffusion tests. Two precipitin bands formed with cyst fluid and suggested the presence of metabolic antigens.

Infections of *P. miyazakii* in rats were studied by Tada (1967). Precipitin bands appeared 10 to 21 days after infection, and the number of precipitin bands formed decreased 90 days after infection. Early precipitin band formation was associated with migration, and Tada suggested that the decrease in precipitin bands may have been related to a quantitive reduction in the amount of worm metabolic products reaching the host circulation because of worm encapsulation.

CONCLUSION

Compared with that of schistosomiasis, our knowledge of immunology of non-blood-dwelling trematodes is in its infancy. Only three species, *Clonorchis sinensis*, *Fasciola hepatica*, and *Paragonimus westermani*, have been extensively investigated, and these have been studied because of their medical and economic importance. Serologic diagnoses for these species are relatively reliable compared with diagnosis by the detection of eggs. Intradermal testing appears to be the most sensitive and efficient method, although complement fixation might be better for detection of prepatent infections of *C. sinensis*. A number of antigen fractions have been highly purified and have proved effective in serologic tests; however, partially fractionated antigens are easier to prepare and, in general, show few cross-reactions with heterologous infections.

The functional importance of the antibodies found in the hosts has not been determined. Protective immunity to *C. sinensis* was absent in rabbits even though precipitating antibody titers were high. Protective immunity has been reported for *F. hepatica* infections in mice and was attributed to delayed hypersensitivity. No protective immunity in other host species for *F. hepatica* has been shown unequivocally, even though high titers of circulating antibody were present. The circulating antibodies undoubtedly represent a host response to foreign material, but they are ineffective because of their lack of access to the parasites or because they are not directed towards essential antigens. Insufficient data are available for assessment of possible protective immunity in *P. westermani* infections.

REFERENCES

Bénex, J. 1964. Le diagnostic sérologique pratique de la distomatose. 1. Une méthode d'agglutination sur lame à l'aide d'antigène absorbé sur des particules de latex. Bull. Soc. Path. Exot., 57:495-502.

———— L. Lamy, and J. Glebel. 1959. Étude de la réaction de fixation du complément à l'antigen distomien chez le mouton. Bull. Soc. Path. Exot., 52:83–87.

Biguet, J., G. Rosé, and A. Capron. 1965. Le diagnostic de la distomatose à *Fasciola hepatica* par la réaction d'hémagglutination. Comparaison avec les résultats de l'immunoélectrophorèse et de la réaction d'hémolyse. Bull. Soc. Path. Exot., 58:866-878.

Capron, A., M. Yokogawa, J. Biquet, M. Tsuji, and G. Luffau. 1965. Diagnostic immunologique de la paragonimose humaine. Mise en évidence d'anticorps sériques spécifiques par immunoélectrophorèse. Bull. Soc. Path. Exot., 58:474-487.

Dawes, B., and D. L. Hughes. 1964. Fascioliasis: The invasive stages of *Fasciola hepatica* in mammalian hosts. Advances Parasit., 2:97-168.

Healy, G. R. 1955. Studies on immunity to *Fasciola hepatica* in rabbits. J. Parasit., 41 (Suppl.):25.

Hughes, D. L. 1962. Observations on the immunology of *Fasciola hepatica* infections in mice and rabbits. Parasitology, 52:4P.

Kendall, S. B., N. Herbert, J. W. Parfitt, and M. A. Pierce. 1967. Resistance to reinfection with *Fasciola hepatica* in rabbits. Exp. Parasit., 20:242-247.

Kent, J. F. 1963. Current and potential value of immunodiagnostic tests employing soluble antigens. Amer. J. Hyg. Monograph. Series, 22:68–90.

Kerr, K. B., and O. L. Petkovich. 1935. Active immunity in rabbits to the liver fluke, *Fasciola hepatica*. J. Parasit., 21:319-320.

Komiya, Y. 1966. *Clonorchis* and clonorchiasis. Advances Parasit., 4:53-106.

Korach, S. 1966. Isolement et propriétés d'une lipoprotéine soluble de *Fasciola hepatica*. Biochim. Biophys. Acta, 125:335-351.

———— and J. Bénex. 1966a. A lipoprotein antigen in *Fasciola hepatica*. I. Isolation, physical and chemical data. Exp. Parasit., 19:193-198.

———— and J. Bénex. 1966b. A lipoprotein antigen in *Fasciola hepatica*. II. Immunological and immunochemical properties. Exp. Parasit., 19:199-205.

Lang, B. Z. 1967. Host-parasite relationships of *Fasciola hepatica* in the white mouse. II. Studies on acquired immunity. J. Parasit., 53:21-30.

———— 1968. Acquired immunity to *Fasciola hepatica* in the laboratory white mouse. Amer. J. Trop. Med. Hyg., 17:561-567.

———— J. E. Larsh, Jr., N. F. Weatherly, and H. T. Goulson. 1967. Demonstration of immunity to *Fasciola hepatica* in recipient mice given peritoneal exudate cells. J. Parasit., 53:208-209.

Maekawa, K., and M. Kushibe. 1961a. Studies on allergen of *Fasciola hepatica*. Part III. Separation of allergenic substances (C5 and P4). Agric. Biol. Chem., 25:542-549.

———— and M. Kushibe. 1961b. Studies on allergen of *Fasciola hepatica*. Part IV. Composition of allergen P4. Agric. Biol. Chem., 25:550-552.

———— and M. Kushibe. 1964. Studies on allergen of *Fasciola hepatica*. Part V. Constitution of allergen P4. Agric. Biol. Chem., 28:382-387.

———— K. Kitazawa, and M. Kushibe. 1954. Purification et cristallisation de l'antigène pour la dermo-réaction allergique vis-à-vis de *Fasciola hepatica*. C. R. Soc. Biol., (Paris), 148:763-765.

Pacheco, G., D. E. Wykoff, and R. C. Jung. 1960. Trial of an indirect hemagglutination test for the diagnosis of infections with *Clonorchis sinensis*. Amer. J. Trop. Med. Hyg., 9:367-370.

Pantelouris, E. M. 1965. The Common Liver Fluke, *Fasciola hepatica* L. Oxford, Pergamon Press.

Patnaik, B., and K. M. Das. 1961. Diagnosis of fascioliasis in cattle by intradermal allergic test. Cornell Vet., 51:113-123.

Rifaat, M. A., and T. M. Abdel-Aal. 1968a. I. Protein and polysaccharide content of *Fasciola gigantica* skin test antigens and their reactivity in the diagnosis of bilharziasis. J. Trop. Med. Hyg., 71:302-304.

——— and T. M. Abdel-Aal. 1968b. II. Fractionation of the antigens of *Fasciola gigantica* by salting out with reference to the use of the isolated fractions as skin test antigens in cases of urinary schistosomiasis. J. Trop. Med. Hyg., 71:304-305.

——— H. G. Osman, I. R. Shimi, and T. M. Abdel-Aal. 1968. III. Fractionation of the antigen of *Fasciola gigantica* by electrophoresis and the use of the fractions in the intradermal test for diagnosing bilharziasis. J. Trop. Med. Hyg., 71:306-312.

Ross, J. G. 1966. Studies of immunity to *Fasciola hepatica*. Naturally acquired immunity in rabbits. Brit. Vet. J., 122:209-211.

——— 1967. Experimental infections of cattle with *Fasciola hepatica*: The production of an acquired self cure by challenge infection. J. Helminth., 41:223-228.

Sadun, E. H., A. A. Buck, and B. C. Walton. 1959a. The diagnosis of paragonimiasis westermani using purified antigens in intradermal and complement fixation tests. Milit. Med., 124:187-195.

——— B. C. Walton, A. A. Buck, and B. K. Lee. 1959b. The use of purified antigens in the diagnosis of clonorchiasis sinensis by means of intradermal and complement fixation tests. J. Parasit., 45:129-134.

Sawada, T., K. Takei, and K. Yoneyama. 1964a. Studies on the immunodiagnosis of paragonimiasis. I. The precipitin reaction with crude and fractionated antigens. J. Infect. Dis., 114:311-314.

——— K. Takei and K. Yoneyama. 1964b. Studies on the immunodiagnosis of paragonimiasis. II. Intradermal tests with fractionated antigens. J. Infect. Dis., 114:315-320.

——— K. Takei, J. E. Williams, and J. W. Moose. 1965. Isolation and purification of antigen from adult *Clonorchis sinensis* for complement fixation and precipitin tests. Exp. Parasit., 17:340-349.

Seed, J. R., F. Sogandares-Bernal, and R. R. Mills. 1966. Studies on American paragonimiasis. II. Serological observations of infected cats. J. Parasit., 52:358-362.

Sewell, M. M. H. 1964. The immunology of fascioliasis. II. Qualitative studies on the precipitin reaction. Immunology, 7:671-680.

Sinclair, K. B. 1967. Pathogenesis of *Fasciola* and other liver-flukes. Helminth. Abstr., 36:115-134.

Soulsby, E. J. L. 1954. Skin hypersensitivity in cattle infested with *Fasciola hepatica*. J. Comp. Path., 64:267-274.

——— 1957. An antagonistic action of sheep serum on the miracidia of *Fasciola hepatica*. J. Helminth., 31:161-170.

Sun, T., S. T. Chou, and J. B. Gibson. 1968. Route of entry of *Clonorchis sinensis* to the mammalian liver. Exp. Parasit., 22:346-351.

——— and J. B. Gibson. 1969. Antigens of *Clonorchis sinensis* in experimental and human infections. An analysis by gel-diffusion technique. Amer. J. Trop. Med. Hyg., 18:241-252.

Tada, I. 1967. Physiological and serological studies of *Paragonimus miyazakii* infection in rats. J. Parasit., 53:292-297.

Teodorovič, D., I. Berkeš, and M. Milovanovič. 1963. Diagnosis of liver fluke (*Fasciola hepatica*) infection in human beings by means of immunoelectrophoresis. Nature (London), 198:204.

Thorpe, E. 1965. An immunocytochemical study with *Fasciola hepatica*. Parasitology, 55:209-214.

——— and A. W. J. Broome. 1962. Immunity to *Fasciola hepatica* infection in albino rats vaccinated with irradiated metacercariae. Vet. Rec., 74:755-756.

Urquhart, G. M., W. Mulligan, and F. W. Jennings. 1954. Artificial immunity to *Fasciola hepatica* in rabbits. I. Some studies with protein antigens of *F. hepatica*. J. Infect. Dis., 94:126-133.

Walton, B. C., and Chyu, I. 1959. Clonorchiasis and paragonimiasis in the Republic of Korea. Report on a prevalence survey using intradermal tests. Bull. W.H.O., 21:721-726.

Wikerhauser, T. 1961. Immunobiologic diagnosis of fascioliasis. II. The in vitro action of immune serum on the young parasitic stage of *F. hepatica*—a new precipitin test for fascioliasis. Vet. Arh., 31:71-80. (Reviewed in Sinclair, 1967).

Wykoff, D. E. 1959. Studies on *Clonorchis sinensis*. II. Development of an antigen for complement fixation studies on the antibody response in infected rabbits. Exp. Parasit., 8:51-57.

———— and T. J. Lepěs. 1957. Studies on *Clonorchis sinensis*. I. Observations on the route of migration in the definitive host. Amer. J. Trop. Med. Hyg., 6:1061-1065.

Yogore, M. G., Jr., R. M. Lewert, and E. D. Madraso. 1965. Immunodiffusion studies on paragonimiasis. Amer. J. Trop. Med. Hyg., 14:586-591.

Yokogawa, M. 1965. *Paragonimus* and paragonimiasis. Advances Parasit., 3:99-158.

Yokogawa, S., W. W. Cort, and M. Yokogawa. 1960. *Paragonimus* and paragonimiasis. Exp. Parasit., 10:81-205.

Cestodes and Acanthocephala

CLARENCE J. WEINMANN

Department of Entomology and Parasitology, University of California, Berkeley, California

INTRODUCTION

It has often been said that tapeworms, along with the closely related acantho-cephalans, are more completely committed to parasitism than any other group of metazoan parasites (e.g., Read and Simmons, 1963). As stated by Baer (1951), "Tapeworms are by far the most highly specialized parasites known and although their origin from some distant platyhelminth stock is obvious, all traces of any direct affinities have disappeared." They parasitize all classes of vertebrates, living as adults almost exclusively in the lumen of the small intestine. Their life cycles are complex: in the more primitive groups, marine arthropods and fish are involved, and in the more recent cyclophyllidean families, a wide range of terrestrial invertebrates and vertebrates serve as hosts. In the most specialized, e.g., the taenioid parasites of mammals, the invertebrate host has been lost and vertebrates serve as intermediate and definitive hosts. Morphologic and life cycle data suggest that cestodes are descended from parasites of arthropods before the appearance of fishes, and that vertebrate hosts were gradually acquired through food chains as these unfolded during evolution (Stunkard, 1967).

The organization, ontogeny, and orientation of the Cestoda have been discussed by Stunkard (1962), and the biology of cestode life-cycles has been surveyed by Smyth (1963) and Voge (1967). Advances in cestode physiology and biochemistry have recently been reviewed (Read and Simmons, 1963; von Brand, 1966; Agosin, 1968), as have aspects of pathogenesis in cestode infections (Rees, 1967).

As long-established, successful parasites, cestodes have in various ways achieved the necessary balance between unbridled growth and reproduction within a host and exclusion from the host. Given favorable physiologic and ecologic circumstances for reaching a nutritionally suitable host, cestodes have adjusted to host defenses that tend to restrict their activities or to expel them. The role of these host defenses as selective pressures during parasitic evolution is discussed in the first chapter of Volume 1.

Although central to an understanding of tapeworm biology, interactions between these parasites and host defenses have not yet been extensively investigated. Although some of the earliest experimental work on metazoan immunity was done with cestodes (e.g., Miller, 1931a), research on immunity in tapeworm infections, apart from that applicable to diagnostics, has lagged behind that carried out with other groups of helminths. This has mainly been due to the greater economic and medical importance of other metazoans and not to shortcomings in intrinsic interest or to unsuitability of these organisms for basic biologic research.

One of the objectives of this chapter will be to emphasize some advantages of using cestodes in immunologic studies. Since information concerning immunity in cestode infections has been recently reviewed (Urquhart et al., 1962; Euzéby, 1965; Weinmann, 1966; Gemmell and Soulsby, 1968) this account will focus on those observations and experiments that indicate or suggest immune mechanisms in the interactions between host and tapeworm. An effort has been made to summarize the current status of knowledge in this field, but references, though selective, often had to be arbitrarily chosen. Much less is known concerning immunity in acanthocephalan infections and this is reflected in the brief summary account presented at the end of this chapter.

NATURAL RESISTANCE TO CESTODES

Once entry into a host has been gained (almost invariably via the digestive tract), many diverse factors may deleteriously affect the establishment and/or the survival of cestodes. Factors independent of prior conditioning by the parasite or its antigens constitute the natural or innate immunity of the host. Natural resistance factors may be viewed as the reciprocal of adaptations by parasites during evolution of the host-parasite complex. They reflect preadaptive and adaptive responses of a living environment (i.e., the host) to the presence of a foreign invader. Although for the most part they are not well-defined, these factors constitute the dominant or determining features of the environment for the parasite, along with the intrinsic nutritional suitability of the host.

Host specificity

Host specificity has been one important consequence of adaptive and counteradaptive interactions during evolutionary history, and cestodes have been favorite subjects for comment and speculation on this subject (e.g., Baer, 1955; Dollfus, 1957; Smyth, 1968; Yamashita, 1968). In general, each order of mammals and birds possesses its characteristic cestodes. A number of experiments have been carried out with various cestodes to determine growth patterns in ranges of host species or strains, and the literature abounds with observations on natural infections of various hosts by particular parasites (Shults and Bondareva, 1935; Archer and Hopkins, 1958; Hutchison, 1959; Schiller, 1959; Bondareva et al., 1960; Webster and Cameron, 1961). For the most part, these studies have indicated a relatively narrow range of tolerance for optimum establishment and growth by tapeworms, which is sometimes evident even between inbred strains of the same host species (Curtis et al., 1933; Yamashita et al., 1958; Olivier, 1962a; Lubinsky, 1964). Ecologic partitioning may contribute to the relatively high degree of specificity of tapeworms for their final vertebrate hosts, but much apparently depends upon the phylogenetic relationships of the hosts themselves.

A possible explanation for this lies in the isolation in which these hermaphroditic organisms frequently live, with reduced, or often nonexistent opportunities for cross-fertilization. A proclivity for inbreeding would eventually result in comparatively uniform populations of worms, genetically speaking, against which selective pressures would be great (Smyth, 1964a). The frequency of morphologic anomalies and of but-once-reported species or rare species among cestodes has been attributed to their isolation in small populations with consequent enhancement of the opportunity for change through genetic drift (Jones, 1948). Thus, to a greater extent than with most helminths, the host presents a highly selective environment to these essentially homozygous parasites. Although cross-fertilization probably occurs whenever possible, one study has indicated that *Hymenolepis nana*, individually isolated for five generations, were not significantly different in morphologic variability or in infectivity from those reared in mice in groups averaging 20 worms (Rogers and Ulmer, 1962). While close adaptation to particular host strains or races, or even to individual hosts, may at times compound experimental difficulties in replicating results of research with these organisms, it may also offer unique opportunities for investigations concerned with genetic components in the associations between vertebrates and their metazoan parasites. In addition, certain cestodes (e.g., *Echinococcus*) may present experimental opportunities for studies requiring an abundance of parasites with identical genotypes, since larval reproduction may produce numerous offspring derived from a single fertilized egg (Smyth et al., 1966).

Factors involved in parasite development

Upon entering the mammalian host's body, the tapeworm must be activated and released from enclosing membranes if it is to become established in its new environment. The factors involved in these processes represent important aspects of natural resistance, and there are indications that they may play a large role in determining host specificity, at least with some species. Knowledge concerning these factors has been reviewed recently (Smyth, 1963, 1964b; Read and Simmons, 1963).

Larvae of pseudophyllidean cestodes may or may not be enclosed by host reaction products at the time of ingestion by warm-blooded vertebrates, but the higher temperature of the latter is apparently the principal "trigger" promoting the change from a plerocercoid to an adult growth pattern and for the establishment of residency in the small intestine (Sinha and Hopkins, 1967). Relatively little is known concerning the selectivity of stimuli affecting larvae during initial phases of establishment in a vertebrate, but it appears to be minimal judging from the frequency with which plerocercoids invade beyond the intestine in paratenic and abnormal hosts. Among cyclophyllidean cestodes, the factors involved in hatching and activation of oncospheres in vertebrates are known primarily from studies with taenioid cestodes and the dwarf tapeworm, *Hymenolepis nana*. The cement substance which binds the keratin-like embryophoric blocks surrounding the taenioid embryo (Morseth, 1966) is probably variable in composition in different tapeworm species, and differences in reactivity to stimuli affecting hatching have been experimentally shown (Silverman, 1954; Laws, 1968).

Observations on the hatching *in vitro* of *Echinococcus* eggs in the presence of digestive fluids from various host species have indicated a correlation with the natural susceptibility of these hosts (Berberian, 1957). It has been suggested (Smyth, 1963) that selective intestinal factors may operate in two ways: by hatching and activating eggs in favorable hosts only or by destroying those oncospheres that do succeed in hatching in unfavorable hosts. Although Meymarian (1961) observed dissolution of embryophores of *Echinococcus* in strong alkaline solutions, oncospheres were not activated without the aid of intestinal enzymes, and bile salts or whole bile enhanced the activating effect. A few observations have tentatively suggested that intestinal fluids may not be essential for the activation and hatching of at least some tapeworm eggs. *Echinococcus* has been reported to develop after eggs were introduced into the trachea of a squirrel (Dévé, 1907), and Borrie et al. (1965) obtained cyst development in the lungs of lambs following the instillation of intact eggs into surgically isolated regions of the lung. Although *H. nana* eggs may be activated and hatched by appropriate treatment with digestive enzymes or insect extracts (Berntzen and Voge, 1962), it was consistently observed in this laboratory that some eggs developed to cysticercoids following subcutaneous injection of intact eggs into mice (DiConza, 1966, unpublished observations). In comparing the hatching responses of four species of *Hymenolepis*, Berntzen and Voge (1965) found differences with respect to optimal hatching conditions. The *in vitro* stimulus for oncosphere activation was thought to be related to the presence of dissociated sodium bicarbonate and free carbon dioxide, but external enzyme action was necessary for optimal hatching and a varying pH was apparently also critical.

Responses to given combinations of hatching stimuli may vary widely, not only between cestodes of different taxa, but between individuals of the same species or between batches of eggs from the same worm. For example, Huffman and Jones (1962) found marked variability in the hatching of eggs from different specimens of *H. taeniaeformis* and from different proglottids of the same specimen, and Silverman (1954) observed that *T. saginata* egg maturation was sometimes independent of the chronologic order of proglottids. It has been suggested that variable hatching rates may have selective value in increasing the dissemination of eggs (Jones et al., 1960). This variation may at times pose difficulties for experiments requiring eggs of comparable infectivity at different time intervals or from more than one source. Variations in hatching rates in different hosts undoubtedly complicate assessments of natural resistance based on numbers of worms established from known egg doses. The finding of unusually susceptible hosts to tapeworm eggs in a large series of animals is not uncommon in infection experiments, and enhanced egg hatching may be involved.

Infective larval stages of cestodes are usually enclosed by cystic structures of one sort or another, and the contained larvae (e.g., cysticercoids, cysticerci) generally have invaginated scolices upon arrival in the vertebrate digestive tract. To become established, larvae must free themselves from enclosing membranes and the scolices must become evaginated for attachment. The various stimuli producing these effects have been associated with digestive secretions of the host (Rothman, 1959). With most cyclophyllidean cestodes, the cystic membranes are weakened by pepsin and finally digested by trypsin in the presence of bile salts. Species differences exist with regard to the responses to these stimuli, and it has been suggested that bile salts may serve as selective chemical agents determining host specificity in many, and perhaps all, cestodes of vertebrates (Smyth, 1963).

Excystation apparently involves a complex of processes which generally results in the release and evagination of the scolex in appropriate sites in the proper host. In addition to quantitative and qualitative differences among hosts in hatching or excystation stimuli, the duration of exposure to these stimuli may be critical and can be expected to vary with host species and with the physiologic state of the host. Rothman (1959) observed that *Oochoristica symmetrica* was sensitive *in vitro* to a pepsin-HCl solution, many being killed in a short time, and the suggestion was made that this species might not survive in hosts with prolonged gastric emptying time or with a strongly acid gastric secretion. Decreased intestinal emptying time has been associated with increased establishment of *Hymenolepis nana* (Larsh, 1947) and *H. diminuta* in mice (Read and Voge, 1954), presumably through enhancement of hatching or excystment. Digestive fluids may influence host specificity in other ways, e.g., the "urea barrier" in elasmobranchs bars parasitism by all but certain specialized groups of tapeworms that not only tolerate high concentrations of urea in the intestine but apparently require it for permeability control and osmotic regulation (Read et al., 1959).

Once free in the intestinal lumen, the cestode encounters fluid movements that propel it posteriorly. It must soon attach or penetrate into the intestinal wall if it is to establish itself. Invasion by oncospheres occurs rapidly (Hunninen, 1935; Silverman and Maneely, 1955), and it has been suggested that even short delays in penetration probably result in the loss of free oncospheres (Gemmell, 1962a). Relatively little is known concerning the mechanisms of penetration among cestodes. Glandular structures have been described from oncospheres of various species (Enigk and Sticinsky, 1957; Ogren, 1961), and it has been presumed that they function as "penetration glands" (Reid, 1948). Silverman and Maneely (1955) furnished supporting evidence for this by showing that secretions from oncospheres of *Taenia saginata* and *T. pisiformis* acted on the ground substance of the intestinal mucosa and exerted a cytolytic effect. The secretory material positive for the periodic acid-Schiff reaction was found to be absent within such glands following host penetration, further indicating an invasive function (Sawada, 1961). Lewert and Lee(1955) found that infection of rats by *Hydatigera taeniaeformis* was accompanied by alterations in the state of glycoprotein in areas of the liver adjacent to the parasites. These alterations were encountered during the first 20 days when the parasites were growing rapidly and displacing the surrounding tissue and before inflammatory changes led to complete enclosure by connective tissue. It has been suggested that collagenase-like enzymes may be released from growing larvae, as has been postulated for skin-penetrating helminths, and that such material might act to soften intercellular substances and basement membranes, allowing cells to be displaced more readily to accommodate the rapidly growing larvae, and perhaps also enhancing nutrient uptake through changes in membrane character

(Lewert, 1958). Progress in understanding certain aspects of immunity to larval cestodes awaits further elucidation of the invasive properties of these parasites.

Host cellular and humoral reactions

The cellular reactions elicited by invasion with tapeworms presumably represent a major component of the host's natural defenses, as in other parasitic infections. A number of histopathologic accounts of such reactions may be found in the literature (*see* Rees, 1967). Although differences in host susceptibility have been correlated with the intensity or type of cellular reaction produced, e.g., in *Echinococcus* in mice (Schwabe et al., 1959) and *Hydatigera* in various mouse strains (Orihara, 1962), it has generally not been possible to evaluate separately the protective function of cellular responses. In this laboratory, *Hymenolepis nana* larvae apparently developed normally when introduced into preformed granulomatous lesions in extraintestinal sites in mice (DiConza, 1966, unpublished data) or in acute inflammatory sites in the intestine (Weinmann, 1964). A sequestering function has often been postulated for the chronic inflammatory changes elicited by tissue-invading cestodes. For example, the growth rate of *H. taeniaeformis* in lightly infected rats has been shown to decrease sharply at about the time the parasites are completely enclosed by host-derived connective tissue (Hutchison, 1958). While cellular responses might play a restrictive role, e.g., in limiting the entry of metabolites into parasites, humoral elements and other factors undoubtedly are also involved. The encapsulation of various cestode larvae by host reaction products has also been described (Berezantsev, 1962).

Intensified cellular (and humoral) reactions usually accompany the administration of higher egg doses, and this has been correlated with decreased parasite growth. For example, Hinz (1962) found an inverse relationship between *H. taeniaeformis* egg dosages and the numbers of parasites developing in the livers of mice. A comparable dosage effect has been observed with *H. taeniaeformis* in this laboratory (Weinmann, 1965, unpublished data), and it has been regarded as most probably being a manifestation of rapidly elicited acquired immunity. Similar dosage effects have been observed in trematode and nematode infections (e.g., World Health Organization Expert Committee, 1965), but the relatively slow growth of cestode larvae in vertebrates may make them especially vulnerable to acquired immune responses.

Treatment of hosts with cortisone has been accompanied by increased susceptibility to primary infection by larval cestodes (Roman, 1958a; Weinmann, 1960; Esch, 1964, 1967). However, the manifold effects of such drugs have not permitted assessment of the relative importance of cellular defenses in cestode infections.

Little is known about the effects on cestodes of substances in mammalian body fluids that are known to have protective activity against microorganisms and other parasites (e.g., "natural antibody," the complement-properdin complex, lysozyme, interferon, and so forth). Bacterial endotoxins have been found to exert little or no effect on the natural resistance of mice to subsequent infection with eggs of *Hymenolepis nana* (Weinmann, 1965), although such substances rapidly stimulate nonspecific resistance to infection with immunologically unrelated microorganisms (Landy and Pillemer, 1956). Some larval cestodes are capable of development in a much wider range of vertebrate host than indicated by feeding experiments if the eggs are artificially hatched and introduced parenterally. This has been shown for taenioid cestodes (Froyd and Round, 1960; Gemmell, 1964) and *Hymenolepis nana* (Weinmann, 1965, unpublished observations), the latter developing to cysticercoids in animals of at least several of the vertebrate classes. This suggests broad compatibility upon primary contact between larval cestodes and vertebrate body fluids.

Lack of vertebrate host specificity is well-known for pseudophyllidean larvae, but exceptions occur. Plerocercoids of *Spirometra mansonoides* survived and grew in all vertebrate classes except fish, and when surgically introduced into the muscles or body cavities of fish, they were destroyed by elements denuding the cuticle (Mueller, 1966). When incubated *in vitro* in sera from different species of fish, they were unaffected by some sera yet died in others. Some species of fish whose sera were without effect in these tests were, nevertheless, the most active in killing surgically implanted plerocercoids (Mueller, 1960). Plerocercoids of *Schistocephalus* regularly survived surgical implantation into their normal fish hosts, but they were rapidly destroyed in abnormal hosts, even when sealed in diffusion chambers (Braten, 1966).

Factors affecting natural resistance

Host age. As with many parasites, susceptibility of the host to primary infection may be greatly modified by host age, usually for reasons which are poorly understood but which are assumed to involve maturation processes when ecologic factors can be excluded. Increased resistance with age has commonly been encountered in cestode infections (Nosik, 1953; Sinha and Srivastava, 1958; Ronzhina, 1961; Kireev, 1965), but in at least some instances acquired immunity may also be involved. For example, although *Moniezia expansa* is primarily a parasite of young sheep (Potemkina, 1959), there is evidence that it may elicit a protective immune response (Seddon, 1931; Stoll, 1938; Hansen et al., 1951) which would contribute to the host age-resistance pattern seen so often with this parasite.

There have been many reports of a distinct age immunity in various strains of rodents infected with *Hydatigera taeniaeformis* (Greenfield, 1942; Dow and Jarrett, 1960; Rhode, 1960; Olivier, 1962a; Orihara, 1962; Hinz, 1965; Ohbayashi and Sakamoto, 1966). Young mice, but not rats, have been shown to be highly resistant to infection with eggs of *Hymenolepis nana* if exposed prior to weaning (Shorb, 1933). Hunninen (1935) suggested that this was probably due to the more rapid passage of eggs through the young mouse intestine and to the relatively small size of its intestinal villi. Larsh (1943) tested this hypothesis by experimentally increasing the length of the small intestine of young mice through the administration of prolactin and thereby enhanced susceptibility to infection. A correlation was shown between the rate at which *H. nana* eggs passed through the host's intestine and parasite establishment (Larsh, 1947).

Although increased resistance to *H. nana* has often been observed with advancing age (Woodland, 1924; Shorb, 1933; Hunninen, 1935; Larsh, 1944b; Bailenger et al., 1961), this pattern has not always been found in the various strains of rodents and parasites that have been tested (Heyneman, 1962a). Also, certain conditions, such as splenectomy, alcoholism, and treatment with thyroid extracts, have been reported to interfere with age resistance (*see* Larsh, 1951). An observation suggesting senile loss of age resistance has been reported (Hunninen, 1935).

Host sex and hormonal effects. As with most parasites, cestodes are closely attuned to the homeostatic "machinery" of the host and can be markedly affected by hormonal changes and imbalances. It seems probable, therefore, that hormones controlling seasonal and other periodic fluctuations in host physiology would directly or indirectly influence susceptibility to cestode infection. Something of this nature might explain the failure of *Proteocephalus filicollis* to mature in its fish host except during early summer months, even though worms could establish themselves following experimental exposure during other seasons (Hopkins, 1959).

In view of the manifold factors that may produce variation in responses to hormonal changes, it is not surprising that there are conflicting reports concerning the influence of host sex upon cestode infections. Several investigators have found little or no difference in the susceptibility of male and female rodents to *H. taeniaeformis* (Dow and Jarrett, 1960; Olivier, 1962a; Hinz, 1965), whereas other reports have indicated that males are much better hosts for this parasite (Curtis et al., 1933; Campbell, 1939; Campbell and Melcher, 1940), and the results of one study suggested that females may be more susceptible (Fortuyn and Feng, 1940). Recently, Ohbayashi and Sakamoto (1966) observed marked differences among strains of mice in natural resistance to experimental infection with *Echinococcus multilocularis*. However, sex related differences were absent or marginal in rabbits infected with larval taenioids (Bull, 1964).

Mammalian sex hormones have been shown experimentally to affect worm loads in the intestine. Addis (1946) reported that castration caused stunting of *Hymenolepis diminuta* in male rats and that normal growth could be restored by the injection of testosterone. Spaying of female rats did not have a similar effect. However, Landt and Goodchild (1962) found no sex-related differences in *H. diminuta* in gonadectomized rats and attributed the different results to host diets and methods of measuring worms. Beck (1952) demonstrated that egg production by *H. diminuta* decreased in castrated male rats, but it could be returned to normal by administration of testosterone. A similar observation has been made with *Diphyllobothrium sebago* in male hamsters (Meyer and Valleau, 1967). Treatment of normal male mice with testosterone was found to lower resistance to *H. nana*, while treatment of normal females with estrogens enhanced host resistance as measured by the size and numbers of parasites (Bailenger et al., 1964). Estrogens have recently been shown to have an adjuvant effect on the primary immune response in mice (Nicol et al., 1966).

Although helminth surveys have often revealed changes in worm burdens during host breeding seasons (*see* Dogiel, 1962), few experimental observations have been made on the relationship of pregnancy and lactation to resistance to infection. Addis (1946) observed normal growth of *Hymenolepis diminuta* in pregnant rats, even when on a vitamin-deficient diet which produced stunted worms in normal females. Progesterone acted like testosterone in stimulating worm growth in gonadectomized females as well as in gonadectomized males. However, progesterone treatment of normal female rats on a vitamin-deficient diet failed to bring about normal worm growth, indicating a more complex hormonal interrelationship during pregnancy. Hunninen (1935) observed that pregnant female mice lost their *H. nana* burdens shortly after parturition, and he postulated that a sudden dietary change, such as the ingestion of afterbirth, might have been involved. However, Kevorkov (1946) did not observe any loss of this worm after pregnancy in humans or rodents. Larsh (1949) infected pregnant mice with eggs of *H. nana* and found twice as many parasites in them as in controls.

Alterations in host thyroid activity have been associated with changes in resistance to helminths (Todd, 1949), but few experiments have been carried out with cestodes. Larsh (1950a) found that mild depression or elevation of thyroid activity produced by thiouracil and thyroid extract, respectively, had no effect on natural resistance of mice to *H. nana*, although thiouracil interfered with normal weight gains. Higher doses of thyroid extract abolished age immunity in older mice. Landt and Goodchild (1962) observed significant increases in the size of *H. diminuta* in mice and female rats that had undergone both gonadectomy and thyroidectomy. But either operation alone had no effect on worms in male rats, suggesting a synergistic effect between the testes and thyroid. In females, thyroidectomy alone caused significant increases in worm weights, and these increased further when both operations were performed.

Corticosteroid hormones have also been shown to have some effect on natural resistance in tapeworm infections. Rodents showing age immunity or being otherwise refractory to infection have been rendered more susceptible to *H. nana* by treatment with cortisone acetate (Roman, 1958a; Pinto, 1960; Bailenger et al., 1964). Cortisone treatment for one week depressed the natural resistance of mice to *H. nana*, but daily treatment for two and three weeks before infection permitted recovery of natural resistance (Weinmann, 1960). Relatively low doses of cortisone had a marked effect on the survival of *H. taeniaeformis* in mice and made refractory hosts highly susceptible (Olivier, 1962b). In addition to producing significant increases in the number of *Multiceps serialis* established in mice, cortisone was found to influence parasite distribution in superficial and central nervous tissues (Esch, 1964, 1967).

The endocrine changes associated with various types of physical and psychologic stress probably have some influence on natural resistance to cestodes, but little experimental data is available. Social stresses (e.g., fighting), which were sufficient to increase adrenal sizes significantly, reduced resistance to *H. nana* in mice (Weinmann and Rothman, 1967). Trauma (e.g., surgery) may also lower resistance to this parasite (Hearin, 1941), as may a reduction in body temperature (Larsh, 1945).

Splenectomy of adults and neonatal thymectomy had no effect on the natural immunity of mice to *H. nana* (Weinmann, 1968). Larsh (1944b) also found that splenectomy of young adult mice was without immediate effect on resistance to this parasite. However, an anemia developed in older mice which were splenectomized while young, and these mice showed reduced resistance to primary infection. Hoeppli (1941) reported data which suggested that splenectomy slightly enhanced the susceptibility of a strain of mouse which was unfavorable for *H. taeniaeformis*.

Host diet. Host diet and feeding habits may directly affect worms in the intestine, and effects may be produced indirectly through any of a multiplicity of changes in host physiology that may be set in motion by dietary alterations. Establishment, growth, maturation, reproduction, or longevity of tapeworms can be markedly influenced by what the host ingests. Many tapeworms require carbohydrate in the host diet for normal development and fecundity, but they have a limited capacity for utilization of different kinds of carbohydrate (*see* Read, 1959). *H. diminuta* grown in rats on diets lacking carbohydrate were reduced in size and numbers, and female parts of the reproductive system were defective (Roberts and Platzer, 1967). Host diets deficient in protein or in vitamins have had little or no effect on this parasite (Chandler, 1943; Mettrick and Munro, 1965), but recent studies have indicated a dependence upon dietary fatty acids (Ginger and Fairbairn, 1966). Mettrick (1967, 1968) found that the addition of aminoacid supplements to the diet of rats markedly influenced the growth of *H. diminuta*, but Hopkins and Young (1967) reported that aminoacid imbalances in the diet had no effect on this parasite.

Reduced food intake or starvation has been shown to dramatically effect a loss of tapeworms in the intestines of poultry (Levine, 1938; Reid, 1942), though starvation may significantly increase the establishment of *Multiceps serialis* in the tissues of mice (Esch, 1964). Direct effects undoubtedly account for the former, and various indirect effects may have been involved in the latter (e.g., reduced intestinal motility). Short periods of starvation before infection with *H. taeniaeformis* had no effect on the establishment of this parasite in rats (Hinz, 1965). Avitaminosis in mice has been reported to enhance establishment of *H. nana*, presumably through effects on intestinal physiology (Vailova, 1946, cited in Dogiel, 1962; Larsh, 1951).

Non-nutrient factors in the host diet may also affect cestodes in various ways. Roughage-free diets apparently caused a loss of *H. nana* in mice (DeWitt and Weinstein, 1964); however, smaller *H. diminuta* were produced in rats on a high roughage diet than in hosts on low roughage or roughage-free diets (Roberts and Platzer, 1967).

Interactions between organisms within a host. In their definitive hosts, tapeworms undergo development in close association with a wide range of intestinal organisms, from viruses and bacteria to other members of the same parasite species. The complexities of these relationships are compounded by interactions with the host. Although scarely defined, one result of this interplay has been the formation of numerous microhabitats within the intestine, each with a characteristic or usual flora and fauna. Certain niches may favor optimal growth of one cestode and not another, while nearby the reverse may obtain.

Maximal growth, fecundity, and even establishment may thus depend upon occupancy of favored microhabitats (*see* Stefansky, 1965). The observation of Newton et al. (1959) that *Hymenolepis nana* grew into mature adults in germ-free guinea pigs but not in conventional guinea pigs has suggested that the microflora may play a role in rendering hosts less suitable for tapeworms. These worms grow poorly in the intestinal lumen of normal guinea pigs (Ransom, 1921; Hunninen, 1935). However, *Raillietina cesticillus* in gnotobiotic chicks (Reid and Botero, 1967) and *H. diminuta* in gnotobiotic rats (Houser and Burns, 1968) apparently grew normally. At minimum, the normal microbial flora and fauna exert an indirect effect on host resistance to cestodes in that they are mainly responsible for inciting the development of mucosal structures in the small intestine that are undoubtedly involved in defense against invasion, namely a thickened lamina propria, abundant lymphoid elements, and a capacity for more rapid renewal of epithelium than in germ-free animals (Abrams et al., 1963)

Alterations in the normal flora by antibiotics variably influenced the establishment and growth of *H. diminuta* in the rat (Beaudoin, 1965). Certain antibiotics (i.e., neomycin, streptomycin, or polymixin B) were either without effect or brought about a reduced number of worms established and reduced growth, whereas others (i.e., bacitracin) promoted tapeworm growth. The latter observation suggested that bacitracin-sensitive bacteria may inhibit or compete with *H. diminuta*. Coleman et al. (1967a) found a significant decrease in the survival time of x-irradiated mice infected with *H. nana* in the absence, but not the presence, of streptomycin, and they suggested that there may be a synergistic relationship between the worms and intestinal flora. Przyjalkowski (1962) found that the microorganisms occurring in or on intestinal helminths, including *Taenia saginata* and *Moniezia expansa*, were the same as those in the host's intestine. A significant reduction in size of *H. Diminuta* has been reported in rats heavily infected with *Trypanosoma lewisi* (Rigby and Chobotar, 1966).

Competition between helminths within a host can be as influential in determining the fate of tapeworms as host resistance factors. One of the earliest reports of interspecific competition between helminths was that of Cross (1934), who observed an inverse relationship between the numbers of *Proteocephalus exigus* and an acanthocephalan in the gastrointestinal tract of their fish host. Larsh and Donaldson (1944) found that subcutaneous injections of *Nippostrongylus brasiliensis* larvae just prior to exposure to *H. nana* enhanced resistance to the latter. Similarly, the simultaneous exposure of mice to *Trichinella spiralis* and *H. nana* produced lower tapeworm yields (Larsh and Campbell, 1952). It has been suggested that these effects may have been occasioned by acute physiologic changes due to stresses during and shortly after infection (Weinmann, 1964). When the interval of time between infections was extended, prior infection with *Capillaria hepatica*, *Ascaris lumbricoides*, and *T. spiralis* either had no effect or produced only transient changes in host reactivity to challenge with *H. nana*. Froyd (1960b) reported interference between *E. granulosus* and *Fasciola gigantica* in the livers of cattle; the presence of one parasite, presumably the first arrival, restricted the other. *Echinococcus* in the lungs had no effect on *Fasciola* in the liver. Holmes (1961) observed that when *Hymenolepis diminuta* and the acanthocephalan, *Moniliformis dubius*, were grown together in rats, the tapeworms showed greater size reductions than the acanthocephalans and were displaced posteriorly in the intestine from positions they occupied in rats with tapeworms only. *Moniliformis* was displaced somewhat anteriorly from its normal position in the rat, and the worms were also smaller. A reduction in worm numbers was not observed with either species. Read and Phifer (1959) showed that when a hamster was infected with a single *H. diminuta* and a single *H. citelli*, there was a reduction in the size attained by both worms. In hamsters on a low carbohydrate diet, *H. diminuta* was reduced in size to a greater extent in the presence of *H. citelli* than in its absence, but the extent of size reduction in *H. citelli* was the same in the presence or absence of *H. diminuta*. Lang (1967) observed displacement of *H. microstoma* from its optimal site of attachment in the common bile duct of the mouse by the subsequent invasion of this region by *Fasciola hepatica*.

A common observation in cestode infections is that the size of individual worms bears an inverse relationship to the number of worms present (Mueller, 1938; Wisniewski et al., 1958). This crowding effect has been studied mainly with *Diphyllobothrium latum* (Pavlovskii and Gnezdilov, 1949, 1953), *Raillietina cesticillus* (Reid, 1942), and *Hymenolepis diminuta* and *H. nana* (Woodland, 1924; Shorb, 1933; Hunninen, 1935; Chandler, 1939; Hager, 1941; Read, 1951; Roberts, 1961, 1966). Evidence has been obtained indicating that competition for utilizable carbohydrate is an important limiting factor in tapeworm growth and is involved in the crowding effect (*see* Read and Simmons, 1963). Similarities in the developmental characteristics of worms from crowded infections and those from hosts with suboptimal carbohydrate diets have further indicated the importance of competition for host dietary carbohydrate (Roberts, 1966).

ACQUIRED IMMUNITY TO CESTODES

Active immunity acquired by infection

Research on this aspect of cestode biology has focused mainly on the relatively few tapeworms with a mammalian tissue phase during larval development. Most of these have been found to be highly immunogenic; few larvae are required to elicit a strong and durable resistance to reinfection, sometimes bordering on absolute immunity.

Although brief statements and preliminary experimentation concerning immunity to reinfection with cestodes may be found in the early literature (see Joyeux, 1920), critical experimental demonstration of acquired immunity began when Miller (1931a) showed that the presence of a few cysts of *Hydatigera taeniaeformis* in rats was sufficient to prevent the development of additional parasites when the rats were challenged with this organism. The development of strong reinfection immunity was subsequently shown in rabbits infected with *Taenia pisiformis* (Solomon, 1934; Kerr, 1935), in rodents infected with *Hymenolepis nana* (Hunninen, 1935; Hearin, 1941; Kevorkov and Shleikher, 1944), in cattle harboring *T. saginata* (Penfold et al., 1936; Urquhart, 1958; Froyd, 1964a), and in sheep with *T. hydatigena* (Sweatman, 1957). Although high levels of acquired immunity have been reported for sheep infected with *Echinococcus granulosus* (Ulyanov and Baidaliev, 1963), uncertainties exist regarding the methods used in this study to assess immunity. The observations of Sweatman et al. (1963) indicate that sheep develop only moderate levels of acquired immunity to this parasite, even after primary exposure to large egg doses.

Although *H. nana* has often been reported to elicit virtually absolute immunity following a primary egg infection (Larsh, 1951), other studies have shown or suggested low but fairly consistent reinfection rates (Shorb, 1933; Bailenger et al., 1961; Heyneman, 1962b), and there are a few reports claiming relatively weak and transitory immunity to reinfection with this parasite (Astafiev, 1966). Reinfection immunity has been shown to develop rapidly following primary exposure to eggs of *H. nana* (Hearin, 1941; Badalyan, 1958; Weinmann, 1958; Heyneman, 1962c) and *H. taeniaeformis* (Weinmann, 1964), occurring in one or two days (or less, depending upon dosage). A low threshold for immunization by infection seems to obtain with these parasites, and single exposures to low egg doses are sometimes sufficient to stimulate high levels of protective immunity (Heyneman, 1962a).

The persistence of strong infection immunity long after the removal or loss of the parasites is uncommon among helminths, but it apparently occurs in some cestode infections, e.g., *H. taeniaeformis* (Miller and Massie, 1932) and *H. nana* (Hearin, 1941). Potentially, this is of considerable interest, for the mechanism of immunologic memory is a major unresolved problem. Heyneman (1962a) has reported that acquired immunity to the short-lived

H. nana may remain strong for almost the life span of the mouse host. However, the availability of *H. nana* for immunologic stimulation may have to be extended in view of its potential for extraintestinal development (Astafiev, 1966). Immunity to *T. saginata* is also generally regarded as life-long (Urquhart, 1961). Recently, it has been found that cysticerci of this parasite survive somewhat longer in bovine tissues than it was previously thought (Dewhirst et al., 1963; Froyd, 1964b; Urquhart and Brocklesby, 1965; van der Heever, 1967), and there is some indication that parasite survival may be extended in cattle exposed to light infections when young. Although immunologic tolerance may be involved in the latter case (Soulsby, 1963), an accelerated immune response due to dosage effects may account for reduced survival, much as has been postulated to occur with *H. taeniaeformis* in rats (Hinz, 1962). Re-exposure of infected calves to oncospheres of *T. saginata* has been reported to shorten the life span of primary cysticeri (Leikina et al., 1964).

Epidemiologic data on larval cestode infections tend to support experimental observations. The incidence of *Echinococcus* in sheep and cattle has been reported to increase with host age (Pullar and Marshall, 1958; Froyd, 1960a; Gemmell, 1961), a finding inconsistent with an unusually strong and durable immunity. On the other hand, observations of natural infections with *T. hydatigena*, *T. saginata*, and *T. pisiformis* indicate that acquired immunity is a major factor in limiting the abundance of these parasites in their hosts (Froyd, 1960a; Peel, 1961; Gemmell, 1961; Urquhart et al., 1961; Bull, 1964).

In contrast to the marked immunogenicity of cestode larvae in mammalian tissues, tapeworms living exclusively in the intestinal lumen of their vertebrate hosts have been widely regarded as poorly immunogenic (Culbertson, 1941; Joyeux, 1948; Heyneman, 1963). A number of observations based on infection experiments with various cestodes have indicated that adult tapeworms do not stimulate protective immunity in their hosts—for example, *H. taeniaeformis* in cats (Miller, 1932a); *Raillietina cesticillus* in chickens (Luttermoser, 1938; Sinha and Srivastava, 1958); *Diphyllobothrium erinacei* (Joyeux and Baer, 1939), *Multiceps glomeratus* (Clapham, 1940), and *T. hydatigena* (Vukovic, 1949) in dogs; and *H. diminuta* in rodents (Heyneman, 1962b). Chandler (1939) presented data on *H. diminuta* in rats clearly showing that factors other than acquired immunity may influence the fate of superimposed cestodes. It was observed that inhibitory effects on challenge cestodes were correlated with the primary worm mass and that removal or reduction of the latter relieved these effects. Rats could readily be reinfected with normally developing worms if the primary worms were removed.

Competition between parasites, host nutrition, and natural resistance factors have in recent years been considered sufficient to account for most instances of apparent acquired resistance with adult tapeworms. The persistence for years of large, actively growing tapeworms (e.g., *T. saginata* and *T. solium* in man and *H. diminuta* in rats) has not seemed consistent with the development of protective immunity. On the other hand, a number of observations point to the involvement of protective immunity in at least some adult cestode infections. This protective immunity was postulated by Brumpt (1913), who observed that *T. saginata* usually occurred singly in man, even in Ethiopia where opportunity for reinfection was common).

Worms residing in the intestinal lumen are not immunologically inert; they abundantly secrete antigens (Coleman, 1963; Coleman et al., 1967b) which may be taken up sufficiently to elicit antibodies detectable by serologic or intradermal tests (Hacig et al., 1959; Bredikhina, 1959; Hutchins, 1961; Chordi et al., 1962; Coleman and deSa, 1964; Foster and Hanson, 1965). Adult worm infections have changed host reactivity to challenge with the eggs of other cestodes, even after loss of the primary worms (Weinmann, 1964). Intestinal tapeworms may be inhibited in growth and longevity by the immunity evoked through prior infection with homologous or heterologous cestode larvae (Yutuc, 1951; Heyneman, 1962b). Lumen-dwelling species of *Hymenolepis* (i.e., *H. citelli, H. diminuta*, and *H. microstoma*) were shown to be capable of stimulating in mice a protective immunity to homologous challenge, provided sufficient time and continuous or repeated infections were involved (Weinmann, 1964, 1966). Recently, Tan and Jones (1967, 1968) demonstrated a protective immunity against *H. microstoma* through the use of irradiated primary worms, and Movsesijan et al. (1968) protected dogs against *Echinococcus granulosus* by prior infection with irradiated larval worms. The possibility of immunologic interference has been suggested to account in part for the poor development of *Spirometra mansonoides* in cats infected with *H. taeniaeformis* (Mueller, 1966), and for the difficulty in establishing superimposed infection with *Diphyllobothrium latum* in dogs (Wardle et al., 1937). Sima (1937) expressed the opinion that the presence of *T. pisiformis* in dogs protected them against *T. hydatigena*. Sequential changes (with time after initial infection) in reactivity to challenge with lumen stages of *H. nana* have been observed in mice immunized by egg infection (Weinmann and Rothman, 1962, unpublished data). Initially no effects on the challenge worms could be detected, then a stunting and early loss of many worms occurred, and eventually, after weeks of exposure, challenge worms failed to survive more than a few hours in immune hosts.

It is well-known that *H. nana* is a short-lived parasite, with a mean longevity recorded variously as being from 12 to 35 days in definitive hosts (Joyeux, 1920; Woodland, 1924; Saeki, 1925; Shorb, 1933; Schiller, 1959). Host immune factors may well contribute to its short life span. Worm losses, while somewhat irregular following egg infections, have been found to occur mainly after the host serum acquires maximal potency in passive transfer tests (Weinmann, 1964, unpublished data). The same strain of *H. nana* has been maintained *in vitro*, and the worms have survived, in good growing condition, for at least several times their usual life span in a host (Berntzen, 1965). The relatively short-lived *Moniezia expansa* in sheep may prove to be another example of the effect of host factors on life span, for there is some evidence that it may be markedly affected by immune reactions (Seddon, 1931; Stoll, 1938; Hansen et al., 1951).

While the contribution of immunologic events to changes in the intestinal environment of infected hosts may be decisive with some species, other tapeworms may manifest detrimental effects only during periods of maximum vulnerability, such as during the early phases of establishment and the period of rapid growth which follows (Roberts, 1961). Evidence for the latter type of effect has been reported by Roberts and Mong (1968), who observed suppression of growth and establishment rates in *H. diminuta* when superimposed on primary infections with this parasite in rats. This aspect of cestode biology clearly requires additional investigation.

Artificial active immunity

Although an extensive literature has accumulated on antigen-antibody systems in cestode infections, mainly dealing with problems of diagnosis (Kent, 1963; Froyd, 1963; Machnicka-Roguska, 1965; Chordi and Kagan, 1965; Hariri et al., 1965; Proctor et al., 1966; Norman et al., 1966; Kagan, 1968; Kagan and Agosin, 1968; Fischman, 1968), relatively few investigations have been concerned with immunization against infection using nonviable antigens. Several studies have shown that repeated injections of antigens extracted from larval or adult worm tissues may stimulate significant levels of immunity to challenge with the tissue-invading larvae of *H. taeniaeformis* (Miller, 1931b; Campbell, 1936), *Multiceps multiceps* (Pukhov et al., 1953), and *H. nana* (Larsh, 1944a; Bailenger et al., 1961; Coleman et al., 1968). Failures to achieve a protective response by such means have also been recorded, e.g., in rabbits or lambs challenged with *Echinococcus granulosus* (Dévé, 1927; Moya and Blood, 1964).

Although the establishment and growth of *H. diminuta* was not influenced by the injection of nonviable antigens (Chandler, 1940), several reports indicate that artificial immunization may have some effect against intestinal tapeworms. Partial protection against *Echinococcus granulosus* in dogs has apparently been achieved by vaccination with hydatid fluid, membranes, or scolices (Turner et al., 1936; Matov and Vasilev, 1955; Frošek and Rukavina, 1959). Gemmell (1962b) observed that the inhibition of establishment and growth of *E. granulosus* was somewhat greater in dogs vaccinated with adult worm material than in those vaccinated with a crude preparation from hydatid scolices.

Living antigens introduced parenterally in the form of eggs, larvae, or adult worms have generally been found to stimulate a greater degree of protective immunity than nonviable antigens (Miller, 1932b, 1935a). In a series of cross-infection experiments with taenioid larvae in sheep and rabbits, Gemmell (1964, 1965a, 1966) observed that the intramuscular injection of active, artifically hatched oncospheres usually evoked a stronger protective immunity than viable, unhatched eggs, and that the latter were in this respect superior to dead eggs similarly injected. Protection was strongest against challenge with the homologous parasite. Though cross-protection was marked between *T. hydatigena* and *T. ovis* (presumably because they shared antigens functional in stimulating protective immunity), it was lacking between these species and *T. pisiformis* and *E. granulosus*. Gemmell (1967) has reported additional evidence, based on cross-infection data, suggesting that free oncospheres of taenioid species have common functional antigens, whereas the intact eggs contain species-specific antigens. The former antigen complex was thought to exert an effect on both the establishment and survival of challenge parasites, while the latter induced resistance only to growing challenge larvae. Actively growing cysticerci of *T. solium* produced higher complement-fixing antibody titers in rabbits than did intact eggs when these were introduced intracerebrally (Kepski et al., 1963).

Prior infection of mice with several cestode species was shown to vary in enhancing resistance to *H. nana*, with the greatest effect being produced by *H. taeniaeformis* egg infections in contrast to cyst infections with *T. crassiceps*, *H. microstoma*, and *H. citelli* (Weinmann, 1964). The strongest immunity elicited, however, was not comparable to that evoked by even a light primary infection with *H. nana*, which suggests that a species-specific factor was also involved. Group antigens among cestodes have long been known from serologic and intradermal tests (Wharton, 1930; Eisenbrandt, 1938; Wilhelmi, 1940; Culbertson and Rose, 1941; Vogel, 1953; Hadano, 1959; Lamy et al., 1959; Maddison et al., 1961; Coleman et al., 1968). There is also evidence of sharing of some antigens between the adults and the eggs or cysts of *H. nana* (Coleman et al., 1967b).

The immunization of mice by infection *per os* with x-irradiated eggs of *H. taeniaeformis* has been accomplished, and high levels of immunity were induced (Dow et al., 1962). In addition, a preliminary report has indicated that calves may be similarly protected through infection with attenuated *T. saginata* eggs (Urquhart et al., 1963).

The antigenicity of various regions of adult tapeworms has been shown by the localization of fluorescent antibody in the case of *H. nana* (Coleman and Fotorny, 1962) and *Moniezia expansa* (Duwe, 1967).

In general, observations with living material have indicated that the antigens most functional in eliciting protective immunity are associated with the more actively metabolizing stages, including the active oncosphere. Although functional antigens remain to be characterized, it has recently been shown that some of the antigens produced by immature and adult *H. nana* exhibited esterase activity which was not, however, inactivated by the antibodies they engendered in rabbits (Coleman et al., 1967b). The diversity of antigens, living and dead, that have been shown to stimulate a degree of functional immunity suggests qualitative as well as quantitative requirements for the development of a full measure of acquired immunity in cestode infections (Weinmann, 1966).

The route of immunization with living antigens may be of considerable importance in larval cestode infections. Leonard and Leonard (1941) reported that about the same number of *T. pisiformis* cysticerci developed in the livers of nonimmune rabbits whether a standard egg dose was given *per os* or by inoculation into a mesenteric vein following artificial hatching. But in passively immunized rabbits, it was claimed that far fewer larvae developed in the liver after challenge *per os* than following intravenous challenge.

The intestinal tract was regarded as the most likely site where the invading parasites were arrested, and it was postulated that acquired immunity involved two distinct phases, one parenteral and the other intestinal. A similar conclusion was reached by Bailey (1951) after observing very few *H. nana* in histologic sections of the intestinal wall of immune mice just 12 hours after a heavy challenge with eggs. It was concluded that the great majority of oncospheres were unable to invade the intestinal mucosa of previously infected animals. The few larvae that succeeded in entering the immune mucosa were met by an accelerated host tissue response. Weinmann (1963) found a 10-fold reduction in *H. nana* larvae within the intestinal tissues of immune mice at both 4 and 12 hours after massive egg challenge. The larvae that managed to invade the immune intestinal mucosa failed to develop into cysticercoids. Additional evidence that larval cestodes encounter an "intestinal barrier" in immune hosts was presented by Froyd and Round (1960), who were able to infect immune calves by subcutaneous or intramuscular inoculation of artificially hatched eggs of *T. saginata*, even though these animals were highly resistant to oral challenge. It was postulated that the intestinal phase of immunity had been by-passed. Dow et al., (1962) found that a distinct intestinal phase was less evident in rats immunized against *H. taeniaeformis* by infection with eggs attenuated by x-irradiation. Histologic examination of livers following challenge with normal eggs indicated that fewer challenge larvae reached the liver, and these were trapped and destroyed in the portal tracts.

Although a pattern of two phases in the immune response (i.e., intestinal and parenteral) seems to obtain generally in larval cestode infections, it remains to be determined whether or not this distinction reflects anything more fundamental than indicating the main site at which immunity is effected. There is evidence that it does. The rapidity with which acquired immunity develops in *H. nana* direct-cycle infections has suggested a stimulation of local immunocytes in the intestinal wall (Heyneman, 1962c), and greater anticestode activity (to *H. nana*) has been found in intestinal extracts than in spleen extracts or the sera of immune mice (Weinmann, 1966; Coleman et al., 1967b). Mice have been strongly immunized against oral challenge with *H. nana* by prior subcutaneous inoculation with activated oncospheres, but the immunity thus induced was slower in developing and of a lower level than that engendered with low egg doses administered orally (Weinmann, 1965, unpublished data). However, the separation of intestinal and extra-intestinal infections with *H. nana* is more complicated than previously thought (Price, 1930; Mahon, 1954; Garkavi, 1956; Garkavi and Glebova, 1957; Astafiev, 1966).

Passive immunity

There is evidence that a measure of protective immunity may be passively transferred from infected mothers to offspring in the case of *H. taeniaeformis* in rats (Miller, 1935b) and *H. nana* in mice (Larsh, 1942). With *H. nana*, protection was obtained through substances transferred *in utero* and in the milk, the latter providing a greater degree of protection for a longer time. Sima (1937) was unable to show parenteral transfer of immunity with *T. pisiformis*, and Urquhart (1961) observed that the colostrum of immune dams did not confer a significant protection against *T. saginata* in calves.

Humoral involvement in cestode immunity has been indicated most directly by the protective effects of sera from infected hosts following injection into normal recipients. Passive transfer of immunity has been demonstrated against several larval tapeworms: *H. taeniaeformis* in rats (Miller and Gardner, 1932, 1934; Campbell, 1938a; Kraut, 1956), *T. pisiformis* in rabbits (Kerr, 1935; Liebmann and Boch, 1960), *H. nana* in mice (Hearin, 1941; Weinmann, 1966), and *T. hydatigena* and *T. ovis* in sheep (Blundell et al., 1968). An unsuccessful attempt at passive immunization against *T. saginata* in calves has been reported (Froyd, 1964c).

The studies of Campbell (1938a, b, c) have indicated that the protective properties of immune rabbit and rat sera change during the course of donor infection. Serum taken during the second week of infection or artificial immunization with *T. pisiformis* and *H. taeniaeformis* was protective, and its primary effect was against the establishment of challenge parasites. Protective potency could be removed from the serum by adsorption *in vitro* with larval and adult worm tissues. Serum taken several weeks after infection was also protective, but its main effects were thought to be associated with a marked increase in the destruction of established larvae. Artificial immunization did not produce this effect, and the protective qualities of late serum were not adsorbed *in vitro* by larval and adult worm tissues. Campbell suggested that two types of protective antibody were formed during infection, and that "late immunity" was probably stimulated by antigens released from growing larvae.

Sera from mice infected with *H. nana* were reported to have variable protective potency against oral challenges (Weinmann, 1966), but recent results have shown such sera to contain 7S gamma-globulins with strong antiparasitic activity against ectopically growing *H. nana* larvae (DiConza, 1967, unpublished data). Passively administered antibody has been observed to affect established tapeworm larvae adversely (Miller and Gardiner, 1934; Campbell, 1938b; Liebmann and Boch, 1960), but in the case of *H. nana*, immune serum had no effect if administered after infections were established (Weinmann, 1966).

Since immune serum appeared to exert its protective effect only during the initial phases of infection, Weinmann suggested that the active oncosphere was inhibited, probably at the mucosal surface. Gemmell (1964) made a similar suggestion after observing *in vitro* a fairly rapid destruction of hatched oncospheres by intestinal enzymes, which is the probable fate of oncospheres whose penetration is delayed by immune mechanisms. Interference with egg hatching in immune hosts was regarded as improbable, and hatching in immune serum has been observed *in vitro* (Collings and Hutchins, 1965). Silverman (1955) has described several types of reactions about the activated oncospheres in immune serum. In contrast, Chen (1950) was unable to observe any effect on intact eggs by sera having antilarval activity.

Heyneman and Welsh (1959), using antiserum from artificially immunized rabbits, showed that serum antibodies *in vitro* can adversely affect all stages of *H. nana*, including the intact egg. Some of the effects seen were: precipitate formation within or about eggs, cysticercoids, and adults; a tendency for eggs to agglutinate; increased motility of adults in immune serum; and a marked decrease in the infectivity of eggs and cysticercoids when fed to mice after incubation. These effects, however, were not observed in immune sera from mice infected with *H. nana* (Weinmann, 1966). An immunoelectrophoretic comparison of sera from infected mice and from rabbits artificially immunized with adult *H. nana* homogenates revealed different reactive systems (Coleman and Fotorny, 1962). Precipitates have been observed to form about other larval cestodes on incubation in immune serum (Mueller, 1961). In addition, reduced motility was observed with *Echinococcus* scolices when incubated in immune serum (Shults and Ismagilova, 1962, 1963).

No correlation was found between serum potency in passive protection tests and the serum protein changes revealed by electrophoresis during the course of infection with *H. taeniaeformis* (Kraut, 1956). Also, no significant change in serum protein patterns was seen after artificial immunization, although rats showed some protection against infection. Changes in serum protein patterns have also been reported for infections with *T. pisiformis*, *E. granulosus*, and *M. multiceps*, but these were not directly correlated with infection immunity or the protective capacity of serum (Liebmann and Boch, 1960; Katsova, 1963; Shults et al., 1963; Sweatman et al., 1963).

Serum antibody has been shown to reach levels detectable by serologic means rapidly; it is found within 24 hours in the case of implanted adult *H. nana* in mice (Coleman and deSa, 1964) and within 72 hours after intracerebral inoculation of *T. solium* cysticerci into rabbits (Kepski et al., 1963).

It has been suggested (Weinmann, 1966) that passively transferred antibody may be adsorbed or "fixed" to host tissues, since there is some evidence that relatively small amounts of immune serum may provide protection for days (Campbell, 1938c) and certain immunoglobulins are known to bind to host tissues (Ovary et al., 1963; Crabbé et al., 1965). The observation that extracts of intestinal mucosa from immune mice had greater antiparasitic activity against *H. nana* than their sera (Weinmann, 1966) and the finding of higher concentrations of antiesterase antibody in intestinal tissues than in spleen or serum (Coleman et al., 1967b) further suggest involvement of localized immune factors.

Recent investigations of the properties of the immunoglobulin, IgA, suggest that it is an important line of defense at mucous surfaces, and selective transport to such surfaces appears to occur in recipients of passively transferred serum (Tomasi and Zigelbaum, 1963; South et al., 1966). The relationship of the various immunoglobulins and their activities to immunity in cestode infections remains to be investigated.

Passive immunization against cestodes by the transfer of immunologically competent cells has only recently been studied. Friedberg et al. (1967a) transplanted spleen cells from mice immune to *H. nana* into irradiated nonimmune recipients and later observed that the latter mice were somewhat more resistant to an egg challenge than were controls with spleen cells from nonimmune donors.

Cellular aspects of acquired immunity

Although many descriptive accounts of histopathology are available, relatively little is known concerning the mechanisms of direct cellular action against cestodes. Monkeys immunized against *Spirometra mansonoides* were observed to wall off challenge spargana in tough cysts, whereas the parasites were free in controls (Mueller and Chapman, 1937). Leonard (1940) reported accelerated cellular reactions in the livers of passively immunized rabbits following challenge with *T. pisiformis* eggs. In rodents immune to *H. nana*, challenge oncospheres encounter heightened host tissue reactions (Bailey, 1951), and adult worms have been observed living adjacent to mucosal areas with high concentrations of "globule leucocytes" (Whur, 1966). The number of mast cells has been shown to increase in mice infected with *H. nana* (Fernex and Fernex, 1962).

Intestinal tissues of immune and nonimmune mice examined histologically soon after challenge with heavy egg doses showed no marked differences with respect to sloughing of mucosal epithelium or to goblet cell content (Weinmann and Lee, 1964). Nor was a difference seen in the rate of egg passage through the intestine, which would have been one possibility had an anaphylactic reaction been prominent in the intestine. *H. nana* larvae have been observed developing in sites of acute inflammation (Weinmann, 1964) and in established granulomatous lesions in ectopic sites in mice (DiConza, 1966, unpublished data).

Host resistance to secondary echinococcosis (i.e., following injection of scolices or rupture of the parent cyst) was regarded as dependent on the rapid destruction of scolices by cellular reactions (Schwabe et al., 1959). Silverman and Hullard (1961) also observed an apparent association between the intensity of cellular reactions around *T. saginata* cysticerci and reduced growth. Freeman (1964) noted a correlation between the rate at which eosinophilia developed and the destruction of *T. crassiceps* cysticerci in mice. Lewert and Lee (1955) described cellular changes occurring in the livers of rats infected with *H. taeniaeformis*, and they observed that changes in hepatic cells and the acellular matrix were more pronounced during early phases of infection when parasites were growing rapidly. A marked reduction in certain metabolic activities and in growth coincided with the formation of well-defined connective tissue capsules around the parasites. They suggested that the "early immunity" proposed by Campbell (1938a) might be directed against the production of "collagenase-like enzymes" by young larvae, thus impairing their invasiveness and/or development.

The mammalian intestinal mucosa is abundantly supplied with potential immunocytes and is the logical site for immunologic activity directed against invasion from the intestinal lumen. However, local antibody formation in the intestinal mucosa has not yet been clearly demonstrated, and the immunologic competence of lymphoid elements in the mucosa and their role in immunity to enteric organisms remain largely speculative. Evidence has been obtained indicating that antibody-producing cells remain localized in the intestine and in the local draining mesenteric lymph nodes after stimulation by antigen injected directly into Peyer's patches (Cooper and Turner, 1967). In a recent study on cholera toxin neutralization, Felsenfeld et al. (1967) found more antibody-producing cells in the mesenteric lymph nodes than in the spleen or other lymphoid tissues. It may be significant that invasion of mesenteric lymph nodes occurs in a high percentage of mice exposed to eggs of *H. nana* (Garkavi, 1956).

Evidence against at least certain kinds of antibody production in the intestine was obtained by Coleman et al. (1965) working with *H. nana* in mice. While whole-body irradiation inhibited immune responses, direct irradiation of surgically isolated intestine prior to implantation of adult *H. nana* produced no inhibition of the hemagglutination titer, provided the rest of the body was shielded. When mice were irradiated (whole body) after the loss of their primary *H. nana* infection, it was observed that bone marrow cells from nonimmune syngeneic donors (i.e., donors of the same inbred strain) apparently promoted persistence of acquired immunity (Neas et al., 1966; Friedberg et al., 1967b). It was suggested that syngeneic marrow cells might function in this fashion either by supplying a factor needed to stimulate immunologically committed cells injured by radiation or by becoming immunologically committed themselves through contact with persisting antigen.

The question of persisting immunity in some larval cestode infections in the apparent absence of living antigens is particularly interesting. If the evidence for this is critically substantiated, these cestodes may be valuable subjects for research on broader problems concerning immunologic memory. The instructional theory of antibody formation would require that antigen persist somewhere in the body, whereas clonal selection theories would require that there be continued proliferation and persistence of immunologically committed cells. Small lymphocytes of the lymph nodes are known to be long-lived and have recently been shown to be relatively resistant to radiation, as is apparently also true of immunologic memory (Miller and Cole, 1967). Certain of the lymphocytes of the intestinal wall also form self-perpetuating cell lines with low rates of cell division and low rates of loss (Darlington and Rogers, 1966).

Other immunologic reactions

Hypersensitivity in cestode infections has been studied almost exclusively from the viewpoint of diagnostics and the clinical problems that it may present (*see* Soulsby, 1962, for early references). The common occurrence of skin-sensitizing antibodies in infected patients has been exploited by numerous intradermal tests, and clinicians are familiar with the danger of anaphylactic shock following rupture of *Echinococcus* cysts. Arthus' reactions have often been observed in experimental situations after repeated vaccinations with tapeworm antigens, and eosinophilia frequently accompanies larval cestode infections. Skin reactivity typical of delayed hypersensitivity is known to occur in some patients infected with *Echinococcus* (e.g., following an immediate response in the Casoni test).

The development of immunologic tolerance to cestode antigens has been demonstrated. Soulsby (1963) observed a difference in immunologic responsiveness between calves initially infected with *T. saginata* when 4 to 6 months of age and those infected neonatally. Animals infected at birth showed poor antibody responses as indicated by weekly serologic tests, and this was coupled with an inability to resist reinfection when challenged at 9 months. In contrast, calves infected when immunologically competent showed good serologically measured antibody levels, and they were completely immune to reinfection. Moriarty (1966) rendered rats tolerant to antigens in the cyst fluids of *E. granulosus* and *T. hydatigena* by neonatal injections of this material. Unresponsiveness to the two helminth fluids was reciprocal, as determined by an indirect hemagglutination test. Tolerance was shown to be of short duration, and there was evidence that unresponsiveness was dependent on the continued presence of antigen.

Factors affecting acquired immunity

Effects of irradiation. Studies on the sensitivity of cestode immunity to radiation effects are few. Acquired immunity to *H. taeniaeformis* in rats has been reported as lowered following whole-body exposure to gamma-radiation from cobalt-60 sources (Ciordia and Jones, 1955; Wyant et al., 1959). Coleman et al. (1965) reported suppression of antibody responses to implanted *H. nana* in mice following whole-body x-irradiation, with or without shielding of surgically sequestered intestines. No suppression of the immune response occurred when only the intestines were exposed to radiation, indicating that reactive antibodies were produced at other sites. Whole-body x-irradiation markedly lowered the survival time of mice infected with *H. nana* (Coleman et al., 1967a). Neas et al. (1966) observed that immunity to *H. nana* acquired before irradiation persisted longer in x-irradiated mice treated with bone marrow from nonimmune mice of the same inbred strain than in similarly irradiated mice implanted with rat marrow. Acquired immunity was not rapidly lost even in rat-mouse chimeras, which suggested the involvement of pre-existing antibody or radioresistant committed immunocytes. Friedberg et al. (1967b) showed that increasing amounts of syngeneic marrow enhanced persistence of acquired immunity to *H. nana*.

Effects of hormones. Acquired immunity to *H. nana* responds to hormonal imbalances caused by treatment with cortisone acetate (Roman,

1958b; Weinmann, 1960). Immune mice were readily reinfected with eggs if treated with cortisone during or after induction of infection immunity. Massive autoinfection regularly occurred in treated mice harboring adult worms, although higher cortisone doses were needed to produce this effect after the first few weeks of infection (Weinmann, 1961, unpublished data).

When intense fighting among mice occurred during the induction period of immunity to *H. nana*, the development of acquired immunity was inhibited in all but the dominant animal (Weinmann and Rothman, 1967). But prolonged and intense fighting was needed to increase reinfection rates in mice with well-developed acquired immunity. Reinfection rates were also raised when immune mice were repeatedly stressed by forced associations with strange groups of mice. An endocrine influence was indicated by increased adrenal weights in stressed mice. It was suggested that stress responses which may play a role in murine population regulation (Christian and Davis, 1964), may also contribute to the perpetuation of this short-lived and highly immunogenic parasite.

Host diet and metabolism. Several factors related to host diet and metabolism have been shown to influence acquired immunity to cestodes. Alcoholism produced a retarding effect on the development of immunity to *H. nana* in mice (Larsh, 1946a), and some interference with immunization to this parasite was reported for mice on a protein-deficient diet (Larsh, 1950b). The susceptibility of mice with newly acquired immunity to *H. nana* was increased by severe nutritional stress (Weinmann and Rothman, 1967).

The administration to mice of the antimetabolite, 6-mercaptopurine, lowered their resistance to *H. nana* and depressed antibody formation, as indicated by serologic responses (Coleman and Fotorny, 1963). When administration was initiated at the time of parasite inoculation, there was also a stunting of worms. A complete suppression of antibody detectable by hemagglutination was observed in *H. nana*-infected mice treated with vinblastine sulfate, a mitotic inhibitor like colchicine (deSa and Coleman, 1964).

Acquired immunity to *H. nana* was retained by ground squirrels during the period of winter hibernation, even though immunizing infections were spontaneously lost (Simitch and Petrovitch, 1953).

Concurrent infection. Aside from the examples of cross-immunity already discussed, few interactions between cestodes and other parasites have been reported as having an effect on acquired immunity. Brumpt (1933) described a massive infection with *H. nana* in a mouse already heavily parasitized with *Strongyloides ratti* and suggested that the latter interfered with immunity to the tapeworm. Hunninen (1936) found no evidence of autoinfection in healthy mice infected with *H. nana*, but heavy autoinfection occurred in several animals suffering from a bacterial infection, probably *Salmonella typhimurium*. Suslov (1958) debilitated mice immune to *H. nana* by spleen removal and a staphylococcal infection and observed a high percentage of autoinfection.

Splenectomy and thymectomy. Removal of the spleen of adult mice did not interfere with a subsequent rapid acquisition of acquired immunity to *H.*

nana, and thymectomy of newborn mice did not abolish or substantially reduce the capacity to develop resistance to this parasite (Weinmann, 1968). Acquired immunity was delayed somewhat in thymectomized animals. It was suggested that immunologic competence may not be primarily thymus-directed in the case of intestinal parasites such as *Hymenolepis*. Good et al. (1966) have postulated that peripheral lymphoid tissues in the mammal (e.g., Peyer's patches in the intestine) may function in a capacity comparable to the bursa of Fabricius of birds. However, Okamoto (1968) has reported a marked depression of acquired immunity to *H. nana* in mice thymectomized at birth. The effects of neonatal thymectomy on cestode infections must therefore be regarded as uncertain.

ACANTHOCEPHALA

Adult acanthocephalans, or "thorny-headed worms," are parasitic in the intestinal tract of various aquatic and terrestrial vertebrates, primarily fish, birds, and mammals. Their life cycle requires an arthropod intermediate host, generally an insect, isopod, or amphipod. Unique morphologic features have long posed difficulties concerning the systematic position of these organisms, and a generally accepted solution has been to place them in a separate phylum. A diagnostic feature of the phylum is the organ of attachment, a spiny retractable proboscis at the anterior end. Mouth, anus, and digestive tube are completely lacking; nutrients and waste products are exchanged through the body surface. A peculiar system of channels in the body wall, the lacunar system, is believed to function in these exchanges. The sexes are separate, and reproductive organs occupy most of the body cavity. The genital pore is the only body opening in most forms. Various aspects of acanthocephalan biology have been summarized (*see* Hyman, 1951; Van Cleave, 1952; Petrochenko, 1956; Oshmarin, 1959; Baer, 1961; Golvan, 1962; Yamaguti, 1963; Nicholas, 1967).

Relatively little, beyond descriptive aspects, is known about these organisms, although a few (mainly *Moniliformis dubius*) have proved in recent years to be valuable subjects for physiologic research (*see* von Brand, 1966). Accounts of some of the pathologic effects of acanthocephalan infection in vertebrates have recently been presented (Bullock, 1963; Crompton, 1963). Problems of immunity to infection in vertebrates have received little experimental attention, apart from the studies of Burlingame and Chandler (1941) and Holmes (1961, 1962a) on *Moniliformis* in the laboratory rat. The question of host specificity among the Acanthocephala has been reviewed (Golvan, 1957).

Infection of the vertebrate host occurs after ingestion of an arthropod harboring cystacanths, the infective resting stage. Release of the cystacanth from its enclosing membranes is apparently effected by the activities of the parasite rather than by host digestive enzymes (Graff and Kitzman, 1965).

Bile salts were found to be important for activation of *Moniliformis dubius*, and carbon dioxide enhanced activation *in vitro*. Cystacanths were unable to establish themselves in rats with bile ducts cannulated to the cecum.

Burlingame and Chandler (1941) observed that this parasite became established and grew optimally only in certain regions of the rat intestine. A "crowding effect" occurred in these areas when the worms were abundant and had grown to sufficient size. Worms from challenge exposures which succeeded in establishing themselves in preferred zones grew as well as primary parasites, but those attaching behind this region either did not become established or were lost soon thereafter. It was concluded that immunologic events were not involved, and that competition between worms for a habitat within the host was sufficient to account for observed reductions in the size and number of challenge worms. Fasting of the host for two days caused a large number of worms to be expelled. Holmes (1961) also observed that *M. dubius* had a limited capacity for extending its distribution in the rat intestine under conditions of crowding. When in direct competition with *Hymenolepis diminuta*, the acanthocephalans showed fewer effects from crowding than the tapeworm but were forced into the anterior part of their range in the intestine.

Cross (1934) found an inverse relationship between the numbers of tapeworms and acanthocephalans in the gastrointestinal tract of fish, even though they occupied different regions of the alimentary tract. Serologic cross-reactivity with antigens from other helminths has been reported, particularly with antigens from *Macrocanthrorhynchus hirudinaceus* (Eisenbrandt, 1938; Oliver-Gonzalez, 1946).

REFERENCES

Abrams, G. D., H. Bauer, and H. Sprinz. 1963. Influence of the normal flora on mucosal morphology and cellular renewal in the ileum. Lab. Invest., 12:355–364.

Addis, C. J. 1946. Experiments on the relation between sex hormones and the growth of tapeworms (*Hymenolepis diminuta*) in rats. J. Parasit., 32:574–580.

Agosin, M. 1968. Biochemistry and physiology of *Echinococcus*. Bull. W.H.O., 39:115–120.

Archer, D. M., and C. A. Hopkins. 1958. Studies on cestode metabolism. III. Growth pattern of *Diphyllobothrium* sp. in a definitive host. Exp. Parasit., 7:125–144.

Astafiev, B. A. 1966. Some regularities in the development of superinvasion in hymenolepidosis in white mice (In Russian). Med. Parazit. (Moskva), 35:705–712.

Badalyan, A. L. 1958. Resistance of white mice to experimental superinfection with *Hymenolepis* (In Russian). Papers on helminthology presented to Academician K. I. Skrjabin on his 80th birthday. Moscow, Izdatelstvo Akademii Nauk SSSR, pp. 50–54.

Baer, J. G. 1951. Ecology of Animal Parasites., Urbana, Illinois, University of Illinois Press.

——— 1955. Incidence de la spécificité parasitaire sur la taxinomie. Problèmes d'évolution chez les cestodes cyclophyllidiens. Bull. Soc. Zool. France, 80:275–287.

——— 1961. Embranchment des acanthocéphales. *In* Traité de Zoologie, Vol. 4. Grassi, P., ed. Paris, Masson et Cie, pp. 731–782.

Bailenger, J., M. Baudoin, and R. Pautrizel. 1961. Étude de l'immunité des rongeurs à l'égard d'*Hymenolepis nana* (Von Siebold 1852, Blanchard 1891). Ann. Parasit., 36:595–611.

—— G. Roger, and R. Pautrizel. 1964. Étude de l'immunité des rongeurs à l'égard d'*Hymenolepis nana*. II. Facteurs spécifiques et aspécifiques. Ann. Parasit., 39:33–52.

Bailey, W. S. 1951. Host-tissue reactions to initial and superimposed infections with *Hymenolepis nana* var. *fraterna*. J. Parasit., 37:440–444.

Beaudoin, R. L. 1965. Action of selected antibiotics on *Hymenolepis diminuta* in the rat host. J. Parasit., 51(Sec. 2):34.

Beck, J. W. 1952. Effect of gonadectomy and gonadal hormones on singly established *Hymenolepis diminuta* in rats. Exp. Parasit., 1:109–117.

Berberian, D. A. 1957. Host specificity and the effect of digestive juices on ova of *Echinococcus granulosus*. In Tenth Annual Report, Orient Hospital, Beirut, pp. 33–43.

Berezantsev, Y. A. 1962. Encystment of cestode larvae in the tissues of the intermediate host (In Hungarian). Acta Vet. Hungaria, 12:87–98.

Berntzen, A. K. 1965. Personal communication.

—— and M. Voge. 1962. *In vitro* hatching of oncospheres of *Hymenolepis nana* and *Hymenolepis citelli* (Cestoda: Cyclophyllidea). J. Parasit., 48:110–119.

—— and M. Voge. 1965. *In vitro* hatching of oncospheres of four Hymenolepidid cestodes. J. Parasit., 51:235–242.

Blundell, S. K., Gemmell, M. A., and F. N. MacNamara. 1968. Immunological responses of the mammalian host against tapeworm infections. VI. Demonstration of humoral immunity in sheep induced by the activated embryos of *Taenia hydatigena* and *T. ovis*. Exp. Parasit., 23:79–82.

Bondareva, V. I., S. N. Boev, and I. B. Sokolova. 1960. Comparative susceptibility of domestic and wild animals to *Coenurus* infection (In Russian). Helminthologia (Bratislava), 2:224–234.

Borrie, J., M. A. Gemmell, and B. W. Manktelow. 1965. An experimental approach to evaluate the potential risk of hydatid disease from inhalation of *Echinococcus* ova. Brit. J. Surg., 52:876–878.

Bråten, T. 1966. Host specificity in *Schistocephalus solidus*. Parasitology, 56:657–664.

Bredikhina, V. I. 1959. New methods of immunological diagnosis of *Moniezia* infections in sheep (In Russian). Trudy Vsesoyuznogo Instituta Gelmintologii im K. I. Skryabina, 7:146–184.

Brumpt, E. 1913. Précis de Parasitologie, Paris, Masson et Cie.

—— 1933. Évolution d'*Hymenolepis nana* var. *fraterna*. Arch. Zool. Exp. Gen., 75:235–246.

Bull, P. C. 1964. Ecology of helminth parasites of the wild rabbit *Oryctolagus cuniculus* (L.) in New Zealand. New Zeal. Sci. Indust. Res. Bull. No. 158, pp. 1–147.

Bullock, W. L. 1963. Intestinal histology of some salmonid fishes with particular reference to the histopathology of acanthocephalan infections. J. Morph., 112:23–44.

Burlingame, P. L., and A. C. Chandler. 1941. Host-parasite relations of *Moniliformis dubius* (Acanthocephala) in albino rats and the environmental nature of the resistance to single and superimposed infections with this parasite. Amer. J. Hyg., 33:1–21.

Campbell, D. H. 1936. Active immunization of albino rats with protein fractions from *Taenia taeniaeformis* and its larval form *Cysticercus fasciolaris*. Amer. J. Hyg., 23:104–113.

—— 1938a. The specific protective property of serum from rats infected with *Cysticercus crassicollis*. J. Immun., 35:195–204.

—— 1938b. The specific absorbability of protective antibodies against *Cysticercus crassicollis* in rats and *Cysticercus pisiformis* in rabbits from infected and artificially immunized animals. J. Immun., 35:205–216.

—— 1938c. Further studies on the "non-absorbable" protective property in serum from rats infected with *Cysticercus crassicollis*. J. Immun., 35:465–476.

—— 1939. The effect of sex hormones on the normal resistance of rats to *Cysticercus crassicollis*. Science, 89:415–416.

—— and L. R. Melcher. 1940. Relationship of sex factors to resistance against *Cysticercus crassicollis* in rats. J. Infect. Dis., 66:184–188.

Chandler, A. C. 1939. The effects of number and age of worms on development of primary and secondary infections with *Hymenolepis diminuta* in rats, and an investigation into the true nature of "premunition" in tapeworm infections. Amer. J. Hyg., 29:105–114.

—— 1940. Failure of artificial immunization to influence *Hymenolepis diminuta* infections in rats. Amer. J. Hyg., 31:17–22.

————— 1943. Studies on the nutrition of tapeworms. Amer. J. Hyg., 37:121–130.

Chen, H. T. 1950. The *in vitro* action of rat immune serum on the larvae of *Taenia taeniaeformis*. J. Infect. Dis., 86:205–213.

Chordi, A., and I. G. Kagan. 1965. Identification and characterization of antigenic components of sheep hydatid fluid by immunoelectrophoresis. J. Parasit., 51:63–71.

————— J. González-Castro, and J. Tormo. 1962. Aportación al estudio de las helmintiasis intestinales en los perros. II. Resultados de la prueba de floculación con "Benthid" y de la de fijación de complemento en perros con *Echinococcus granulosus*. Rev. Iber. Parasit., 22:285–290.

Christian, J. J., and D. E. Davis. 1964. Endocrines, behavior, and population. Science, 146:1550–1560.

Ciordia, H., and A. W. Jones. 1955. Immunity to *Hydatigera taeniaeformis* affected by radiation of the host. J. Parasit., 41 (Sec. 2):29.

Clapham, P. 1940. Studies on *Coenurus glomeratus*. J. Helminth., 18:45–52.

Coleman, R. M. 1963. Antigenicity of viable hymenolepids maintained *in vitro*. J. Parasit., 49 (Sec. 2):37.

————— and L. M. deSa. 1964. Host response to implanted adult *Hymenolepis nana*. J. Parasit., 50 (Sec. 2):17.

————— and N. M. Fotorny. 1962. *In vivo* isolation of *Hymenolepis nana* and antibody binding sites. Nature (London), 195:920–921.

————— and N. M. Fotorny. 1963. Effect of 6-mercaptopurine administered during infection of mice with *Hymenolepis nana*. J. Parasit., 49 (Sec. 2):18.

————— W. J. Fimian, and L. M. deSa. 1965. Effect of ionizing radiation on the immune response to implanted dwarf tapeworms. J. Parasit., 51 (Sec. 2):64.

————— J. M. Carty, and W. J. Fimian 1967. Effect of X-irradiation on host resistance to the dwarf tapeworm. Proc. Soc. Exp. Biol. Med., 126:371–374.

————— F. X. Venuta, and W. J. Fimian, Jr. 1967b. Secretion and immunogenicity of dwarf tapeworm esterases. Nature (London), 214:593.

————— J. M. Carty, and W. D. Graziadei. 1968. Immunogenicity and phylogenetic relationship of tapeworm antigens produced by *Hymenolepis nana* and *Hymenolepis diminuta*. Immunology, 15:297–304.

Collings, S. B., and C. P. Hutchins. 1965. Motility and hatching of *Hymenolepis microstoma* oncospheres in sera, beetle extracts, and salines. Exp. Parasit., 16:53–56.

Cooper, G. N., and K. Turner. 1967. Immunological responses in rats following antigenic stimulation of Peyer's patches I. Characteristics of the primary response. Aust. J. Exp. Biol. Med. Sci., 45:363–378.

Crabbé, P. A., A. O. Carbonana, and J. F. Hekemans. 1965. The normal human intestinal mucosa as a major source of plasma cells containing γ-A immunoglobulin. Lab. Invest., 14:235–249.

Crompton, D. W. T. 1963. Morphological and histochemical observations on *Polymorphus minutus* (Goeze, 1782) with special reference to the body wall. Parasitology, 53:663–685.

Cross, S. X. 1934. A probable case of non-specific immunity between two parasites of ciscoes of the Trout Lake region of northern Wisconsin. J. Parasit., 20:244–245.

Culbertson, J. T. 1941. Immunity against Animal Parasites. New York, Columbia University Press.

————— and H. M. Rose. 1941. Further observations on skin reactions to antigens from heterologous cestodes in echinococcus disease. J. Clin. Invest., 20:249–254.

Curtis, M. R., W. F. Dunning, and F. R. Bullock. 1933. Genetic factors in relation to the etiology of malignant tumors. Amer. J. Cancer, 17:894–923.

Darlington, D., and A. W. Rogers. 1966. Epithelial lymphocytes in the small intestine of the mouse. J. Anat., 100:813–830.

deSa, L. M., and R. M. Coleman. 1964. Effect of an indole-indoline alkaloid on the immune response to *Hymenolepis nana*. J. Parasit., 50 (Sec. 2):20–21.

Dévé, F. 1907. L'action des sucs digestifs n'est pas indispensable pour la mise en liberté de l'embryon hexacanthe échinoccique. C. R. Soc. Biol. (Paris), 63:332–334.

————— 1927. Essai de vaccination antiechinococcique par de sable hydatique tyndalisè. C. R. Soc. Biol. (Paris), 97:1130–1131.

Dewhirst, L. W., J. D. Cramer, and W. J. Pistor. 1963. Bovine cysticercosis. I. Longevity of cysticerci of *Taenia saginata*. J. Parasit., 49:297–300.

DeWitt, W. B., and P. P. Weinstein. 1964. Elimination of intestinal helminths of mice by feeding purified diets. J. Parasit., 50:429–434.

Dogiel, V. A. 1962. General Parasitology, 3rd Ed. London, Oliver and Boyd, Ltd.

Dollfus, R. P. 1957. Que savons-nous sur la spécificité-parasitaire des Tétrahynques? *In* Premier symposium sur la spécificité parasitaire des parasites de vertébrés. International Union of Biological Sciences, Sér. B, No. 32, pp. 255–258.

Dow, C., and W. F. H. Jarrett. 1960. Age, strain and sex differences in susceptibility to *Cysticercus fasciolaris* in the mouse. Exp. Parasit., 10:72–74.

——— W. F. H. Jarrett, F. W. Jennings, W. I. M. McIntyre, and W. Mulligan. 1962. The production of immunity to *Cysticercus fasciolaris*, using X-irradiated oncospheres. Amer. J. Vet. Res., 23:146–149.

Duwe, A. E. 1967. Antigens of *Moniezia expansa*: fluorescent antibody localization. Trans. Amer. Micr. Soc., 86:126–132

Eisenbrandt, L. L. 1938. On the serological relationship of some helminths. Amer. J. Hyg., 27:117–141.

Enigk, K., and E. Sticinsky. 1957. Über die Bohrdüsen der Onkosphäre von *Davainea proglottina* (Cestoidea). Z. Parasitenk., 18:48–54.

Esch, G. W. 1964. The effects of cortisone and pre-infection starvation in the establishment of larval *Multiceps serialis* in mice. J. Elisha Mitchell Sci. Soc., 80:114–120.

——— 1967. Some effects of cortisone and sex on the biology of coenuriasis in laboratory mice and jackrabbits. Parasitology, 57:175–180.

Euzéby, J. 1965. L'immunologie des helminthoses. Rev. Méd. Vét., 116:435–473.

Felsenfeld, O., W. E. Greer, and A. D. Felsenfeld. 1967. Cholera toxin neutralization and some cellular sites of immune globulin formation in *Cercopithecus aethiops*. Nature (London), 213:1249–1250.

Fernex, M., and P. Fernex. 1962. Increased number of mast cells and helminthic diseases. Experimental mastocytosis in mice. Acta Trop. (Basel), 19:248–251.

Fischman, A. 1968. A new whole-scolex complement-fixation test for Hydatid disease. Bull. W.H.O., 39:39–43.

Foršek, Z., and J. Rukavina. 1959. Eksperimentalna imunizacija pasa protiv *Echinococcus granulosus*. I. Prva zapazanja. Veterinaria (Sarajevo), 8:479–482.

Fortuyn, A. B. D., and L. C. Feng. 1940. Inheritance in mice of the resistance against infection with eggs of *Taenia taeniaeformis*, Peking Nat. Hist. Bull., 15:139–145.

Foster, W. B., and W. L. Hanson. 1965. Antibodies in mice infected with *Hymenolepis microstoma* against freshly excysted cysticercoids as demonstrated by the fluorescent antibody technique. J. Parasit., 51(Sec. 2):62.

Freeman, R. S. 1964. Studies on responses of intermediate hosts to infection with *Taenia crassiceps* (Zeder, 1800) (Cestoda). Canad. J. Zool., 42:367–385.

Friedberg, W., B. R. Neas, D. N. Faulkner, and M. N. Friedberg. 1967a. Immunity to *Hymenolepis nana*: transfer by spleen cells. J. Parasit., 53:895–896.

——— B. R. Neas, M. H. Friedberg, and D. N. Faulkner. 1967b. Syngeneic marrow graft: effect on persistence of pre-irradiation immunity to *Hymenolepis nana* in mice. Proc. Soc. Exp. Biol. Med., 124:792–793.

Froyd, G. 1960a. Cysticercosis and hydatid disease of cattle in Kenya. J. Parasit., 46:491–496.

——— 1960b. The incidence of liver flukes (*Fasciola gigantica*) and hydatid cysts (*Echinococcus granulosus*) in Kenya cattle. J. Parasit., 46:659–662.

——— 1963. Intradermal tests in the diagnosis of bovine cysticercosis. Bull. Epizoot. Dis. Afr., 11:303–306.

——— 1964a. The artificial oral infection of cattle with *Taenia saginata* eggs. Res. Vet. Sci., 5:434–440.

——— 1964b. The longevity of *Cysticercus bovis* in bovine tissues. Brit. Vet. J., 120:205–211.

——— 1964c. The effect of post-infection serum on the infectability of calves with *Taenia* eggs. Brit. Vet. J., 120:162–168.

——— and M. C. Round. 1960. The artificial infection of adult cattle with *Cysticercus bovis*. Res. Vet. Sci., 1:275–282.

Garkavi, B. L. 1956. The ability of *Hymenolepis fraterna* (Stiles, 1906) to develop in mesenteric lymph nodes (In Russian). Dokl. Akad. Nauk SSSR, 111:240–241.

——— and I. Y. Glebova. 1957. Development of *Hymenolepis fraterna* (Stiles, 1906) and *Hymenolepis nana* (Siebold, 1852) in the organs of white mice. Zool. Zh., 36:986–991.

Gemmell, M. A. 1961. Some observations on the differences in incidences between

Echinococcus granulosus and *Taenia hydatigena* in the livers of sheep in New Zealand. New Zeal. Vet. J., 9:40–41.

——— 1962a. Natural and acquired immunity factors inhibiting penetration of some hexacanth embryos through the intestinal barrier. Nature (London), 194:701–702.

——— 1962b. Natural and acquired immunity factors interfering with development during the rapid growth phase of *Echinococcus granulosus* in dogs. Immunology, 5:496–503.

——— 1964. Immunological responses of the mammalian host against tapeworm infections. I. Species specificity of hexacanth embryos in protecting sheep against *Taenia hydatigena*. Immunology, 7:489–499.

——— 1965a. Immunological responses of the mammalian host against tapeworm infections. II. Species specificity of hexacanth embryos in protecting rabbits against *Taenia pisiformis*. Immunology, 8:270–280.

——— 1965b. Immunological responses of the mammalian host against tapeworm infections. III. Species specificity of hexacanth embryos in protecting sheep against *Taenia ovis*. Immunology, 8:281–290.

——— 1966. Immunological responses of the mammalian host against tapeworm infections. IV. Species specificity of hexacanth embryos in protecting against *Echinococcus granulosus*. Immunology, 11:325–336.

——— 1967. Species specific and cross-protective functional antigens of the tapeworm embryo. Nature (London), 213:500.

——— and E. J. L. Soulsby. 1968. The development of acquired immunity to tapeworms and progress towards active immunization, with special reference to *Echinococcus* spp. Bull. W.H.O., 39:45–50.

Ginger, C. D., and D. Fairbairn. 1966. Lipid metabolism in helminth parasites. II. The major origins of the lipids of *Hymenolepis diminuta* (Cestoda). J. Parasit., 52:1097–1107.

Golvan, Y. J. 1957. La spécificité parasitaire chez les acanthocéphales. *In* Premier symposium sur la spécificité parasitaire des parasites de vertébrés. International Union of Biological Sciences, Sér. B., No. 32, pp. 244–254.

——— 1962. Le phylum des Acanthocephals (Quatrième note). La Classe des Archiacanthocephala (A. Meyer 1931). Ann. Parasit. Hum. Comp., 37:1–72.

Good, R. A., A. E. Gabrielsen, M. D. Cooper, and R. D. A. Peterson. 1966. The role of the thymus and Bursa of Fabricius in the development of effector mechanisms. Ann. N. Y. Acad. Sci., 129:130–154.

Graff, D. J., and W. B. Kitzman. 1965. Factors influencing the activation of acanthocephalon cystacanths. J. Parasit., 51:424–429.

Greenfield, S. H. 1942. Age resistance of the albino rat to *Cysticercus fasciolaris*. J. Parasit., 28:207–211.

Hacig, A., P. Solomon, and R. Weinbach. 1959. Recherches sérologiques sur l'hyménolépidose. L'étude d'un antigène d'*Hymenolepis diminuta* dans les réactions antigène-anticorps *in vivo* et *in vitro*. Arch. Roumaines Path. Exp. Microbiol., 18:611–625.

Hadano, N. 1959. Studies on tapeworm antigens (In Japanese). Acta Scholae Medicinalis (Gifu), 7:808–821.

Hager, A. 1941. Effects of dietary modifications of host rats on the tapeworm, *Hymenolepis diminuta*. Iowa State Coll. J. Sci., 15:127–153.

Hansen, M. F., A. C. Todd, G. W. Kelley, and M. Cawein. 1951. Effects of a pure infection of the tapeworm *Moniezia expansa* on lambs. Kentucky Agric. Exp. Sta. Bull., 556:1–11.

Hariri, M. N., C. W. Schwabe, and M. Koussa. 1965. Host-parasite relationships in echinococcosis. XI. The antigen of the indirect hemagglutination test for hydatid disease. Amer. J. Trop. Med. Hyg., 14:592–604.

Hearin, J. T. 1941. Studies on acquired immunity to the dwarf tapeworm, *Hymenolepis nana* var. *fraterna*, in the mouse host. Amer. J. Hyg., 33:71–87.

Heyneman, D. 1962a. Studies on helminth immunity. I. Comparison between lumenal and tissue phases of infection in the white mouse by *Hymenolepis nana* (Cestoda: Hymenolepididae). Amer. J. Trop. Med. Hyg., 11:46–63.

——— 1962b. Studies on helminth immunity. II. Influence of *Hymenolepis nana* (Cestoda: Hymenolepididae) in dual infections with *H. diminuta* in white mice and rats. Exp. Parasit., 12:7–18.

——— 1962c. Studies on helminth immunity. IV. Rapid onset of resistance by the white

1052 IMMUNITY IN MAMMALIAN HOSTS

mouse against a challenging infection with eggs of *Hymenolepis nana* (Cestoda: Hymenolepididae). J. Immun., 88:217–220.

——— 1963. Host-parasite resistance patterns—Some implications from experimental studies with helminths. Ann. N. Y. Acad. Sci., 113:114–129.

——— and J. F. Welsh. 1959. Action of homologous antiserum *in vitro* against life cycle stages of *Hymenolepis nana*, the dwarf mouse tapeworm. Exp. Parasit., 8:119–128.

Hinz, E. 1962. Vergleichende Untersuchungen an der experimentellen Zystizerkose von Ratte and Maus. Z. Tropenmed. Parasit., 13:182–194.

——— 1965. Beitrag zur Standardisierung der experimentellen Zystizerkose der Maus als Modellversuch zur Testierung finnenwirksamer Substanzen. Z. Tropenmed. Parasit., 16:322–331.

Hoeppli, R. 1941. Influence of splenectomy on susceptibility of mice to infection with *Taenia taeniaeformis* eggs. Proc. Soc. Exp. Biol. Med., 46:29–31.

Holmes, J. C. 1961. Effects of concurrent infections on *Hymenolepis diminuta* (Cestoda) and *Moniliformis dubius* (Acanthocephala). I. General effects and comparison with crowding. J. Parasit., 47:209–216.

——— 1962a. Effects of concurrent infections on *Hymenolepis diminuta* (Cestoda) and *Moniliformis dubius* (Acanthocephala). II. Effects on growth. J. Parasit., 48:87–96.

——— 1962b. Effects of concurrent infections on *Hymenolepis diminuta* (Cestoda) and *Moniliformis dubius* (Acanthocephala). III. Effects in hamsters. J. Parasit., 48:97–100.

Hopkins, C. A. 1959. Seasonal variations in the incidence and development of the cestode *Proteocephalus filicollis* (Rud. 1810) in *Gasterosteus aculeatus* (L. 1766). Parasitology, 49:529–542.

——— and R. A. L. Young. 1967. The effect of dietary amino acids on the growth of *Hymenolepis diminuta*. Parasitology, 57:705–718.

Houser, B. B., and W. C. Burns. 1968. Experimental infection of gnotobiotic *Tenebrio molitor* and white rats with *Hymenolepis diminuta* (Cestoda: Cyclophyllidea). J. Parasit., 54:69–73.

Huffman, J. L. and A. W. Jones. 1962. Hatchability, viability and infectivity of *Hydatigera taeniaeformis* eggs. Exp. Parasit., 12:120–124.

Hunninen, A. V. 1935. Studies on the life history and host-parasite relations of *Hymenolepis fraterna* (*H. nana* var. *fraterna* Stiles) in white mice. Amer. J. Hyg., 22:414–443.

——— 1936. An experimental study of internal autoinfection with *Hymenolepis fraterna* in white mice. J. Parasit., 22:84–87.

Hutchins, C. P. 1961. Immunological studies on *Hymenolepis microstoma* Dujardin. Bull. Ass. Southeastern Biol., 8:21.

Hutchison, W. M. 1958. Studies on *Hydatigera taeniaeformis*. I. Growth of the larval stage. J. Parasit., 44:574–582.

——— 1959. Studies on *Hydatigera* (*Taenia*) *taeniaeformis*. II. Growth of the adult phase. Exp. Parasit., 8:557–567.

Hyman, L. H. 1951. The Invertebrates: Acanthocephala, Aschelminthes and Ectoprocta, Vol. 3. New York, McGraw-Hill, Inc.

Jones, A. W. 1948. Speciation in the cestoda. J. Parasit., 34(Sec. 2):16–17.

——— J. M. Segarra, and K. D. Wyant. 1960. Growth and hatching of taeniid eggs. J. Parasit., 46:170–174.

Joyeux, C. 1920. Cycle évolutif de quelques cestodes. Recherches expérimentales. Bull. Biol. France Belg. (Suppl. II), p. 219.

——— 1948. Les phénomènes d'immunologie dans les helminthiases considérés chez les cestodes de l'homme. Med. Trop. (Marseilles), 8:463–470.

——— and J. G. Baer. 1939. Recherches biologiques sur quelques cestodes Pseudophyllidae. Vol. Jubilee pro Prof. Sadao Yoshida, 2:203–210.

Kagan, I. G. 1968. A review of serological tests for the diagnosis of hydatid disease. Bull. W.H.O., 39:25–38.

——— and M. Agosin. 1968. *Echinococcus* antigens. Bull. W.H.O., 39:13–24.

Katsova, L. B. 1963. The blood serum protein picture in sheep with *Coenurus* infections (In Russian). Trudy Kazanskogo Nauchno-Issledovatelskogo Veterinarnogo Instituto, 11:326–335.

Kent, J. F. 1963. Current and potential value of immunodiagnostic tests employing soluble antigens. Amer. J. Hyg., Monogr. Ser. No. 22:68–90.

Kepski, A., Z. Szlaminski, and W. Zapart. 1963. Serological tests in experimental cerebral cysticercosis in rabbits. Acta Parasitologica Polonica, 11:133–143.

Kerr, K. B. 1935. Immunity against a cestode parasite, *Cysticercus pisiformis*. Amer. J. Hyg., 22:169–182.

Kevorkov, N. P. 1946. Influence of gravidity and sex on the infection by *Hymenolepis nana* and *Hymenolepis fraterna* (In Russian). Gel'mintol Sbornik posv. Skrjabinu-Moske-Leningrad. pp. 142–145.

——— and E. I. Shleikker. 1944. Immunity to superinvasion in hymenolepidosis (In Russian). Med. Parazit. (Moskva), 13:26–30.

Kireev, N. A. 1965. Age susceptibility of turkeys to *Raillietina* infection (In Russian). Veterinariya, 42:60–62.

Kraut, N. 1956. An electrophoretic study of sera from rats artificially infected with and immunized against the larval cestode *Cysticercus fasciolaris*. J. Parasit., 42:109–121.

Lamy, L., J. Bénex, and J. Gledel. 1959. Étude de la réaction de fixation du complément à divers antigènes de cestodes chez le mouton. Deuxième note. Bull. Soc. Path. Exot., 52:193–198.

Landt, J. F. and C. G. Goodchild. 1962. Host endocrine effects on helminth parasites. I. Influence of castration and thyroidectomy of rats on physical measurements of *Hymenolepis diminuta* (Rudolphi, 1819). J. Parasit., 48:763–766.

Landy, M., and L. Pillemer. 1956. Elevation of properdin levels in mice following administration of bacterial lipopolysaccharides. J. Exp. Med., 103:823–833.

Lang, B. Z. 1967. *Fasciola hepatica* and *Hymenolepis microstoma* in the laboratory mouse. J. Parasit., 53:213–214.

Larsh, J. E., Jr. 1942. Transmission from mother to offspring of immunity against the mouse cestode, *Hymenolepis nana* var. *fraterna*. Amer. J. Hyg., 36:187–194.

——— 1943. The relationship between the intestinal size of young mice and their susceptibility to infection with the cestode, *Hymenolepis nana* var. *fraterna*. J. Parasit., 29:61–64.

——— 1944a. Studies on the artificial immunization of mice against infection with the dwarf tapeworm, *Hymenolepis nana* var. *fraterna*. Amer. J. Hyg., 39:129–132.

——— 1944b. The relation between splenectomy and the resistance of old mice to infection with *Hymenolepis nana* var. *fraterna*. Amer. J. Hyg., 39:133–137.

——— 1945. Effects of alcohol on natural resistance to the dwarf tapeworm in mice. J. Parasit., 31:291–300.

——— 1946a. The effect of alcohol on the development of acquired immunity to *Hymenolepis* in mice. J. Parasit., 32:72–78.

——— 1946b. A comparative study of *Hymenolepis* in white mice and golden hamsters. J. Parasit., 32:477–479.

——— 1947. The relationship in mice of intestinal emptying time and natural resistance to *Hymenolepis*. J. Parasit., 33:79–84.

——— 1949. The effect of pregnancy on the natural resistance of mice to *Hymenolepis* infection. J. Parasit., 35(Sec. 2):37.

——— 1950a. The effect of thiouracil and thyroid extract on the natural resistance of mice to *Hymenolepis* infection. J. Parasit., 36:473–478.

——— 1950b. The effects of a protein deficient diet on resistance of mice to *Hymenolepis* infection. J. Parasit., 36(Sec. 2):45–46.

——— 1951. Host-parasite relationships in cestode infections, with emphasis on host resistance. J. Parasit., 37:343–352.

——— and A. S. Donaldson. 1944. The effect of concurrent infection with *Nippostrongylus* on the development of *Hymenolepis* in mice. J. Parasit., 30:18–20.

——— and C. H. Campbell. 1952. The effect on the natural resistance of mice to *Hymenolepis nana* var. *fraterna* of a simultaneous infection with *Trichinella spiralis*. J. Parasit., 38(Sec. 2):20–21.

Laws, G. F. 1968. The hatching of taeniid eggs. Exp. Parasit., 23:1–10.

Leikina, E. S., S. N Moskvin, O. M. Sokolovskaya, and O. G. Poletaeva. 1964. Life span of *Cysticercus bovis* and development of immunity in cysticerciasis (In Russian) Med. Parazit. (Moskva), 33:694–700.

Leonard, A. B. 1940. The accelerated tissue response to *Cysticercus pisiformis* in passively immunized rabbits. Amer. J. Hyg., 32:117–120.

——— and A. E. Leonard. 1941. The intestinal phase of resistance of rabbits to larvae of *Taenia pisiformis*. J. Parasit., 27:375–378.

Levine, P. P. 1938. Observations on the biology of the poultry cestode *Davainea proglottina* in the intestine of the host. J. Parasit., 24:423–431.

Lewert, R. M. 1958. Invasiveness of helminth larvae. Rice Institute Pamphlet, No. 45, pp. 97–113.

———— and C. L. Lee. 1955. Studies on the passage of helminth larvae through host tissues. III. The effects of *Taenia taeniaeformis* on the rat liver as shown by histochemical techniques. J. Infect. Dis., 97:177–186.

Liebmann, H., and J. Boch. 1960. Untersuchungen an *Cysticercus pisiformis*-befallnen Kaninchen. Berlin. München. Tierärztl. Wschr., 73:123–125.

Lubinsky, G. 1964. Growth of the vegetatively propagated strain of larval *Echinococcus multilocularis* in some strains of Jackson mice and in their hybrids. Canad. J. Zool., 42:1099–1103.

Luttermoser, G. W. 1938. Susceptibility of chickens to reinfection with *Raillietina cesticillus* as determined by the presence of the original terminal segment. J. Parasit., 24(Sec. 2):14–15.

Machnicka-Roguska, B. 1965. Preparation of *Taenia saginata* antigens and chemical analysis of antigenic fractions. Acta Parasitologica Polonica, 13:337–347.

Maddison, S. E., H. Whittle, and R. Elsdon-Dew. 1961. The antigens of tapeworms. Preliminary note. S. Afr. J. Sci., 57:273–277.

Mahon, J. 1954. Observations on the abnormal occurrence of *Hymenolepis nana fraterna* cysticercoids in the liver of a rodent. Proc. Zool. Soc. London, 124:527–529.

Matov, K., and I. D. Vasilev. 1955. Active immunization of dogs against intestinal *Echinococcus* (In Bulgarian). Izvestiya na Tsentralnata Khelmintologichna Laboratoriya (Sofia), 1:111–125.

Mettrick, D. F. 1967. Effect of Zein diets on nitrogen content of *Hymenolepis diminuta* and on rat liver protein nitrogen. J. Parasit., 53:688–691.

———— 1968. Studies on the protein metabolism of cestodes. 2. Effect of free dietary amino acid supplements on the growth of *Hymenolepis diminuta*. Parasitology, 58:37–45.

———— and H. N. Munro. 1965. Studies on the protein metabolism of cestodes. 1. Effect of host dietary constituents on the growth of *Hymenolepis diminuta*. Parasitology, 55:453–466.

Meyer, M. C., and W. G. Valleau. 1967. The effect of gonadectomy and hormone therapy in male hamsters upon the egg output by the pseudophyllidean *Diphyllobothrium sebago*. Proc. Helminth. Soc. (Washington), 34:41–43.

Meymarian, E. 1961. Host-parasite relationships in Echinococcosis. VI. Hatching and activation of *Echinococcus granulosus* ova *in vitro*. Amer. J. Trop. Med. Hyg., 10:719–726.

Miller, H. M., Jr. 1931a. Immunity of the albino rat to superinfestation with *Cysticercus fasciolaris*. J. Prevent. Med., 5:453–464.

———— 1931b. The production of artificial immunity in the albino rat to a metazoan parasite. J. Prevent. Med., 5:429–452.

———— 1932a. Superinfection of cats with *Taenia taeniaeformis*. J. Prevent. Med., 6:17–29.

———— 1932b. Acquired immunity against a metazoan parasite by use of non-specific worm materials. Proc. Soc. Exp. Biol. Med., 29:1125–1126.

———— 1935a. Experiments on acquired immunity to a metazoan parasite by use of non-specific worm material. Amer. J. Hyg., 21:27–34.

———— 1935b. Transmission to offspring of immunity against infection with a metazoan (cestode) parasite. Amer. J. Hyg., 21:456–461.

———— and M. L. Gardiner. 1932. Passive immunity to infection with a metazoan parasite (*Cysticercus fasciolaris*) in the albino rat. J. Prevent. Med., 6:479–496.

———— and M. L. Gardiner. 1934. Further studies on passive immunity to a metazoan parasite, *Cysticercus fasciolaris*. Amer. J. Hyg., 20:424–431.

———— and E. Massie. 1932. Persistence of acquired immunity to *Cysticercus fasciolaris* after removal of the worms. J. Prevent. Med., 6:31–36.

Miller, J. J., III, and L. J. Cole. 1967. The radiation resistance of long-lived lymphocytes and plasma cells in mouse and rat lymph nodes. J. Immun., 98:982–990.

Moriarty, K. M. 1966. Immunological unresponsiveness in the rat to cestode antigens. Exp. Parasit., 19:25–33.

Morseth, D. J. 1966. Chemical composition of embryophoric blocks of *Taenia hydatigena*, *Taenia ovis*, and *Taenia pisiformis* eggs. Exp. Parasit., 18:347–354.

Movsesijan, M., A. Sokolić, and Z. Mladenović. 1968. Studies on the immunological potentiality of irradiated *Echinococcus granulosus* forms: immunization experiments in dogs. Brit. Vet. J., 124:425–432.

Moya, V., and B. D. Blood. 1964. Actividad immunogénica de un producto biòlógico ensayado como vacuna contra la hidatidosis ovina. Bol. Chile. Parasit., 19:7–10.

Mueller, J. F. 1938. Studies on *Sparganum mansonoides* and *Sparganum proliferum*. Amer. J. Trop. Med., 18:303–328.

——— 1960. The immunologic basis of host specificity in the sparganum larva of *Spirometra mansonoides*. Libro Homenaje al Dr. Eduardo Caballero y Caballero, Jubileo 1930–1960, pp. 435–442.

——— 1961. The laboratory propagation of *Spirometra mansonoides* as an experimental tool. V. Behavior of the sparganum in and out of the mouse host, and formation of immune precipitates. J. Parasit., 47:879–883.

——— 1966. Host-parasite relationships as illustrated by the cestode *Spirometra mansonoides*. In Host-Parasite Relationships. McCauley, J. E., ed. Corvallis, Oregon State University Press, pp. 15–58.

——— and O. D. Chapman. 1937. Resistance and immunity reactions in infections with *Sparganum mansonoides*. J. Parasit., 23:561–562.

Neas, B. R., W. Friedberg, and J. T. Self. 1966. Loss of pre-irradiation immunity to *Hymenolepis nana* in the rat-mouse chimera. Int. J. Radiat. Biol., 11:349–356.

Newton, W. L., P. P. Weinstein, and M. F. Jones. 1959. A comparison of the development of some rat and mouse helminths in germfree and conventional guinea pigs. Ann. N. Y. Acad. Sci., 78:290–307.

Nicholas, W. L. 1967. The biology of the Acanthocephala. In Advances in Parasitology, Vol. 5. Dawes, B., ed. New York, Academic Press, Inc., pp. 205–246.

Nicol, T., D. C. Quantock, and B. Vernon-Roberts. 1966. Stimulation of phagocytosis in relation to the mechanism of action of adjuvants. Nature (London), 209:1142.

Norman, L., I. G. Kagan, and D. S. Allain. 1966. Preparation and evaluation of antigens for use in the serologic diagnosis of human hydatid disease. II. Isolation and characterization from extracts of cysts of *Echinococcus multilocularis* of serologically reactive elements found in hydatid fluid of *Echinococcus granulosus*. J. Immun., 96:822–828.

Nosik, A. F. 1953. Immunity in some helminth diseases (In Russian). In Papers on helminthology presented to Academician K. I. Skrjabin on his 75th birthday. Moscow, Izdatelstvo Akademii Nauk SSSR, pp. 445–451.

Ogren, R. E. 1961. The mature oncosphere of *Hymenolepis diminuta*. J. Parasit., 47:197–204.

Ohbayashi, M., and T. Sakamoto. 1966. Studies on echinococcosis. XVII. Sex differences in resistance to infection with *Echinococcus multilocularis* in uniform strains of mice. Jap. J. Vet. Res., 14:65–70.

Okamoto, K. 1968. Effect of neonatal thymectomy on acquired resistence to *Hymenolepis nana* in mice. Jap. J. Parasit., 17:53–59.

Oliver-Gonzalez, J. 1946. Immunological relationships among polysaccharides from various infectious organisms. J. Infect. Dis., 79:221–225.

Olivier, L. 1962a. Studies on natural resistance to *Taenia taeniaeformis*. I. Strain differences in susceptibility of rodents. J. Parasit., 48:373–378.

——— 1962b. Studies on natural resistance to *Taenia taeniaeformis*. II. The effect of cortisone. J. Parasit., 48:758–762.

Orihara, M. 1962. Studies on *Cysticercus fasciolaris*, especially on differences of susceptibility among uniform strains of the mouse. Jap. J. Vet. Res., 10:37–55.

Oshmarin, P. G. 1959. Promorphology of Acanthocephala (In Russian). Acta Veterinaria (Budapest), 9:109–116.

Ovary, Z., B. Benacerraf, and K. J. Bloch. 1963. Properties of guinea pig 7S antibodies. II. Identification of antibodies in passive cutaneous and systemic anaphylaxis. J. Exp. Med., 117:951–964.

Pavlovskii, E. N., and V. G. Gnezdilov. 1949. The factor of intensity in experimental infection with the broad tapeworm (In Russian). Dokl. Akad. Nauk SSSR, 6:755–758.

——— and V. G. Gnezdilov. 1953. Intraspecific and interspecific relations among the component species in parasitic cenosis of the host intestine (In Russian). Zool. Zh., 32:165–174.

Peel, C. 1961. The influence of the age factor in *Cysticercus bovis* infestations in West African N'Dama cattle. J. Trop. Med. Hyg., 64:239–242.

Penfold, W. J., H. B. Penfold, and M. Phillips. 1936. Acquired active immunity in the ox to *Cysticercus bovis*. Med. J. Aust., 1:417–423.

Petrochenko, V. I. 1956. Acanthocephala of Domestic and Wild Animals (In Russian), Vol. I. Moscow, Izdatelstvo Akademii Nauk SSSR, pp. 1–435.

Pinto, M. I. M. 1960. Estudos sobre epidemiologia experimental. I. Acção da cortisona na infestação do rato albino pelo céstodo *Hymenolepis nana*, tipo "M." An. Inst. Med. Trop. (Liboa), 17:83–97.

Potemkina, V. A. 1959. Study of the reinfection and age susceptibility of sheep to *Moniezia* (In Russian). Byulleten'Nauchno-Tehnicheskoi Informatsii Vsesoyuznogo Instituta Gel'mintologii im K. I. Skrjabina, 5:78–82.

Price, E. W. 1930. *In* Proceedings of the Helminthological Society of Washington, J. Parasit., 17:17.

Proctor, E. M., S. J. Powell, and R. Elsdon-Dew. 1966. The serological diagnosis of cysticercosis. Ann. Trop. Med. Parasit., 60:146–151.

Przyjalkowski, Z. 1962. Investigations on antibacterial properties of parasitic worms. Acta Parasitologica Polonica, 10:77–96.

Pukhov, V. I., I. I. Zinichenko, and N. I. Chernobaev. 1953. Experimental immunization of lambs against *Coenurus* (In Russian). *In* Papers on helminthology presented to Academician K. I. Skrjabin on his 75th birthday. Moscow, Izdatelstvo Akademii Nauk SSSR, pp. 567–571.

Pullar, C. P., and W. K. Marshall. 1958. The incidence of hydatids in Victorian cattle. Aust. Vet. J., 34:193–201.

Ransom, B. H. 1921. Guinea pig as host for *Hymenolepis nana*. J. Parasit., 7:188.

Read, C. P. 1951. The "crowding effect" in tapeworm infections. J. Parasit., 37:174–178.

———— 1959. The role of carbohydrates in the biology of cestodes. VIII. Some conclusions and hypotheses. Exp. Parasit., 8:365–382.

———— and M. Voge. 1954. The size attained by *Hymenolepis diminuta* in different host species. J. Parasit., 40:88–89.

———— and K. Phifer. 1959. The role of carbohydrates in the biology of cestodes. VII. Interactions between individual tapeworms of the same and different species. Exp. Parasit., 8:46–50.

———— and J. E. Simmons, Jr. 1963. Biochemistry and physiology of tapeworms. Physiol. Rev., 43:263–305.

———— L. T. Douglas, and J. E. Simmons, Jr. 1959. Urea and osmotic properties of tapeworms from elasmobranchs. Exp. Parasit., 8:58–75.

Rees, G. 1967. Pathogenesis of adult cestodes. Helminth. Abstr., 36:1–23.

Reid, W. M. 1942. Certain nutritional requirements of the fowl cestode *Raillietina cesticillus* (Molin) as demonstrated by short periods of starvation of the host. J. Parasit., 28:319–340.

———— 1948. Penetration glands in cyclophyllidean onchospheres. Trans. Amer. Micr. Soc., 67:177–182.

———— and H. Botero. 1967. Growth of the cestode *Raillietina cesticillus* in bacteria-free chickens. Exp. Parasit., 21:149–153.

Rigby, D. W., and B. Chobotar. 1966. The effects of *Trypanosoma lewisi* on the development of *Hymenolepis diminuta* in concurrently infected white rats. J. Parasit., 52:389–394.

Roberts, L. S. 1961. The influence of population density on patterns and physiology of growth in *Hymenolepis diminuta* (Cestoda: Cyclophyllidea) in the definitive host. Exp. Parasit., 11:332–371.

———— 1966. Develomental physiology of cestodes. I. Host dietary carbohydrate and the "crowding effect" in *Hymenolepis diminuta*. Exp. Parasit., 18:305–310.

———— and E. G. Platzer. 1967. Developmental physiology of cestodes. II. Effects of changes in host dietary carbohydrate and roughage on previously established *Hymenolepis diminuta*. J. Parasit., 53:85–93.

———— and F. N. Mong. 1968. Developmental physiology of cestodes. III. Development of *Hymenolepis diminuta* in superinfections. J. Parasit., 54:55–62.

Rogers, W. A., and M. J. Ulmer. 1962. Effects of continued selfing on *Hymenolepis nana* (Cestoda). Proc. Iowa Acad. Sci., 69:557–571.

Rohde, K. 1960. Quantitative Infektion von weissen Ratten mit Eiern der Katzenbandwurmes (*Taenia taeniaeformis*) und deren Entwicklung zur Finne (*Cysticercus fasciolaris*). Tropenmed. Parasit., 11:43–50.

ACESTODES AND ACANTHOCEPHALA

Roman, E. 1958a. Possibilité d'infestation par *Hymenolepis nana fraterna* des rongeurs adultes traités par la cortisone. C. R. Soc. Biol. (Paris), 152:105–107.

———— 1958b. La cortisone peut inhiber la résistance à la reinfestation des souris parasitées par des *Hymenolepis nana fraterna* adultes. C. R. Acad. Sci. [D] (Paris), 246:1468–1470.

Ronzhina, G. I. 1961. Study of immunity after primary and secondary infections with *Coenurus* (In Russian). Trudy Saratovskogo Zoovetinstituta, 10:273–279.

Rothman, A. H. 1959. Studies on the excystment of tapeworms. Exp. Parasit., 8:336–364.

Saeki, Y. 1925. An experimental study on the development of the dwarf tapeworm. Ann. Trop. Med. Parasit., 19:305–308.

Sawada, I. 1961. Penetration glands in the oncospheres of *Raillietina cesticillus*. Exp. Parasit., 11:141–146.

Schiller, E. L. 1959. Experimental studies on morphological variation in the cestode genus *Hymenolepis*. II. Growth, development, and reproduction of the strobilate phase of *H. nana* in different mammalian host species. Exp. Parasit., 8:215–235.

Schwabe, C. W., L. A. Schinazi, and A. Kilejian. 1959. Host-parasite relationships in echinococcosis. II. Age resistance to secondary echinococcosis in the white mouse. Amer. J. Trop. Med. Hyg., 8:29–36.

Seddon, H. R. 1931. The development in sheep of immunity to *Moniezia expansa*. Ann. Trop. Med. Parasit., 25:431–435.

Shorb, D. A. 1933. Host-parasite relations of *Hymenolepis fraterna* in the rat and the mouse. Amer. J. Hyg., 18:74–113.

Shults, R. S., and V. Bondareva. 1935. On the primary (natural) immunity in coenurosis and other larval cestodoses (In Russian). Trudy Instituta Veterinarii, Akademiya Nauk Kazakhskoi SSR (Alma-Ata), 7:208–224.

———— and R. G. Ismagilova. 1962. A new immunological reaction (In Russian). Vestnik Selskokhozyaistvennoi Nauki (Alma-Ata), 6:45–49.

———— and R. G. Ismagilova. 1963. "Scolexo-precipitation reaction" in the diagnosis of hydatidosis (In Russian). Med. Parazit. (Moskva), 32:678–682.

———— V. M. Krasov, R. G. Ismagilova, A. S. Malishevskaya, and L. B. Kashchova. 1963. Changes in the albumin fraction of blood serum in experimental cysticerciasis of rabbits (In Russian) Trudy Kazanskogo Nauchno-Issledovatelskogo Veterinarnogo Instituta, 11:170–178.

Silverman, P. H. 1954. Studies on the biology of some tapeworms of the genus *Taenia*. I. Factors affecting hatching and activation of taeniid ova, and some criteria of their viability. Ann. Trop. Med. Parasit., 48:207–215.

———— 1955. A technique for studying the *in vitro* effect of serum on activated taeniid hexacanth embryos. Nature (London), 176:598–599.

———— and R. B. Maneely. 1955. Studies on the biology of some tapeworms of the genus *Taenia*. III. The role of the secreting gland of the hexacanth embryo in the penetration of the intestinal mucosa of the intermediate host, and some of its histochemical reactions. Ann. Trop. Med. Parasit., 49:326–330.

———— and T. J. Hullard. 1961. Histological observations on bovine cysticercosis. Res. Vet. Sci., 2:248–252.

Sima, I. A. 1937. A *Taenia* és *Cysticercus pisiformis* elleni immunitas. Allatorvosi Lapok., 60:1–4.

Simitch, T., and Z. Petrovitch. 1953. La reinfestation de *Citellus citellus* par *Hymenolepis nana* après le sommeil hibernal: Est-elle possible? Arch. Inst. Pasteur (Algerie), 31:397–399.

Sinha, D. P., and C. A. Hopkins. 1967. Studies on *Schistocephalus solidus*. 4. The effect of temperature on growth and maturation *in vitro*. Parasitology, 57:555–566.

Sinha, P. K., and H. D. Srivastava. 1958. Studies on the age resistance and resistance to superinfection of poultry against *Raillietina cesticillus* (Molin), with some observations on the host specificity of the parasite. Indian Vet. J., 35:288–291.

Smyth, J. D. 1963. The Biology of Cestode Life-Cycles. Commonwealth Bureau of Helminthology Technical Communication No. 34, Commonwealth Agricultural Bureau, Farnharm Royal, England, pp. 1–38.

———— 1964a. Genetical aspects of speciation in trematodes and cestodes: some speculations. Proc. 1st Int. Congr. Parasit., Rome, 1964, 1:473–474.

———— 1964b. The biology of Hydatid organisms. *In* Advances in Parasitology, Vol. 2. Dawes, B. ed. New York, Academic Press, Inc., pp. 169–219.

—— 1968. *In vitro* studies and host-specificity in *Echinococcus*. Bull. W.H.O., 39:5–12.
—— A. B. Howkins, and M. Barton. 1966. Factors controlling the differentiation of the hydatid organism, *Echinococcus granulosus*, into cystic or strobilar stages in vitro. Nature (London), 211:1374–1377.

Solomon, G. 1934. Some points in the early development of *Cysticercus pisiformis* (Bloch, 1780). J. Helminth, 12: 197–204.

Soulsby, E. J. L. 1962. Antigen-antibody reactions in helminth infections. *In* Advances in Immunology, Vol. 2, Taliaferro, W. H., and Humphrey, J. H., eds. New York, Academic Press, pp. 265–308.
—— 1963. Immunological unresponsiveness to helminth infections in animals. Proc. 17th World Vet. Congr., 1:761–767.

South, M. A., M. D. Cooper, F. A. Wollheim, R. Hong, and R. A. Good. 1966. The IgA system. I. Studies on the transport and immunochemistry of IgA in the saliva. J. Exp. Med., 123:615–627.

Stefansky, W. 1965. Bacterial flora as one of the ecological factors affecting the establishment of parasites in the intestines of their hosts. Acta Parasitologica Polonica, 13:1–6.

Stoll, N. R. 1938. Tapeworm studies. VII. Variations in pasture infestation with *Moniezia expansa*. J. Parasit., 24:527–545.

Stunkard, H. 1962. The organization, ontogeny, and orientation of the Cestoda. Quart. Rev. Biol., 37:23–34.
—— 1967. Platyhelminthic parasites of invertebrates. J. Parasit., 53:673–682.

Suslov, I. M. 1958. On the biology of *Hymenolepis nana* (dwarf tapeworm) (In Russian). Med. Parazit. (Moskva), 27:573–575.

Sweatman, G. K. 1957. Acquired immunity in lambs infected with *Taenia hydatigena*. Canad. J. Comp. Med. Vet. Sci., 21:65–70.
—— R. J. Williams, K. M. Moriarty, and T. C. Henshall. 1963. On acquired immunity to *Echinococcus granulosus* in sheep. Res. Vet. Sci., 4:187–198.

Tan, B. D., and A. W. Jones. 1967. Autoelimination by means of X-rays: Distinguishing the crowding factor from others in premunition caused by the mouse bile duct cestode, *Hymenolepis microstoma*. Exp. Parasit., 20:147–155.
—— and A. W. Jones. 1968. Resistance of mice to reinfection with the bile-duct cestode, *Hymenolepis microstoma*. Exp. Parasit., 22:250–255.

Todd, A. C. 1949. Thyroid condition of chickens and development of parasitic nematodes. J. Parasit., 35:255–260.

Tomasi, T. B., and S. Zigelbaum. 1963. The selective occurrence of γA globulins in certain body fluids. J. Clin. Invest., 42:1552–1560.

Turner, E. L., D. A. Berberian, and E. W. Dennis. 1936. The production of artificial immunity in dogs against *Echinococcus granulosus*. J. Parasit., 22:14–28.

Ulyanov, S. D., and A. B. Baidaliev. 1963. Study of immunity in sheep with hydatidosis (In Russian). Trudy Kazanskogo Nauchno-Issledovatelskogo Veterinarnogo Instituta, 11:165–169.

Urquhart, G. M. 1958. The production of experimental cysticercosis in calves in Kenya. Bull. Epizoot. Dis. Afr., 6:385–393.
—— 1961. Epizootiological and experimental studies on bovine cysticercosis in East Africa. J. Parasit., 47:857–869.
—— and D. W. Brocklesby. 1965. Longevity of *Cysticercus bovis*. J. Parasit., 51:349.
—— W. F. H. Jarrett, and W. Mulligan. 1962. Helminth immunity. *In* Advances in Veterinary Science, Vol. 7. Brandley, C. A., and Jungherr, E. J., eds. New York, Academic Press, Inc., pp. 87–129.
—— W. I. M. McIntyre, W. Mulligan, W. F. H. Jarrett, and N. C. C. Sharp. 1963. Vaccination against helminth disease. Proc. 17th World Vet. Congr., 1:769–774.

Van Cleave, H. J. 1952. Some host-parasite relationships of the Acanthocephala, with special reference to the organs of attachment. Exp. Parasit., 1:305–330.

Van der Heever, L. W. 1967. On the longevity of *Cysticercus bovis* in various organs in a bovine. J. Parasit., 53:1168.

Voge, M. 1967. The post-embryonic developmental stages of cestodes. *In* Advances in Parasitology, Vol. 5. Dawes, B., ed. New York, Academic Press, Inc., pp. 247–297.

Vogel, H. 1953. A serological study of some helminth reactions. J. Immun., 70:503–506.

Von Brand, T. 1966. Biochemistry of Parasites. New York, Academic Press, Inc.

Vukovic, V. 1949. L'infection et surinfection du chien par *Taenia hydatigena*. Arch. Sci. Biol. (Belgrade), 1:258–261.

Wardle, R. A., M. J. Gotschall, and L. J. Horder. 1937. The influence of *Diphyllobothrium latum* infestation upon dogs. Trans. Roy. Soc. Canad., 31:59–69.

Webster, G. A., and T. W. M. Cameron. 1961. Observations on experimental infections with *Echinococcus* in rodents. Canad. J. Zool., 39:877–891.

Weinmann, C. J. 1958. Rate of development of acquired immunity to *Hymenolepis nana* var. *fraterna*. J. Parasit., 44(Sec. 2):16.

———— 1960. Cortisone and resistance to infection with *Hymenolepis nana*. Bull. Ass. Southeastern Biol., 7:40.

———— 1963. Factors in host resistance to the dwarf tapeworm, *Hymenolepis nana*. Proc. 16th Int. Congr. Zool., Washington, D.C., 1963, 1:135.

———— 1964. Host resistance to *Hymenolepis nana*. II. Specificity of resistance to reinfection in the direct cycle. Exp. Parasit., 15:514–526.

———— 1965. Bacterial endotoxin and host resistance to *Hymenolepis nana*. J. Parasit., 54:560.

———— 1966. Immunity mechanisms in cestode infections. *In* The Biology of Parasites. Soulsby, E. J. L., ed. New York, Academic Press, Inc., pp. 301–320.

———— 1968. Effects of splenectomy and neonatal thymectomy on acquired immunity to the dwarf tapeworm, *Hymenolepis nana*. Exp. Parasit., 22:68–72.

———— and D. L. Lee. 1964. Intestinal reactions of immune and normal mice after massive challenge with eggs of *Hymenolepis nana*. J. Parasit., 50(Sec. 2):17.

———— and A. H. Rothman. 1967. Effects of stress upon acquired immunity to the dwarf tapeworm, *Hymenolepis nana*. Exp. Parasit., 20:61–67.

Wharton, D. R. A. 1930. Immunological studies with tapeworm antigens. Amer. J. Hyg., 12:511–536.

Whur, P. 1966. Relationship of globule leucocytes to gastrointestinal nematodes in the sheep, and *Nippostrongylus brasiliensis* and *Hymenolepis nana* infections in rats. J. Comp. Path., 76:57–67.

Wilhelmi, R. W. 1940. Serological reactions and species specificity of some helminths. Biol. Bull., 79:64–90.

Wisniewski, W. L., K. Szymanik, and K. Bazánska. 1958. The formation of a structure in tapeworm populations. Česk. Parasit., 5:195–212.

Woodland, W. N. F. 1924. On the life-cycle of *Hymenolepis fraterna* (*H. nana* var. *fraterna* Stiles) of the white mouse. Parasitology, 16:69–83.

World Health Organization Expert Committee. 1965. Immunology and parasitic diseases. W.H.O. Tech. Rep. Ser. No. 315, pp. 1–64.

Wyant, K. D., H. K. Lee, and A. W. Jones. 1959. The effect of Cobalt-60 gamma radiation on the development of acquired immunity in the rat to larval *Hydatigera taeniaeformis*. Bull. Ass. Southeastern Biol., 6:34.

Yamaguti, S. 1963. Systema Helminthum, Vol. V. Acanthocephala, New York, Interscience Publishers, Inc.

Yamashita, J. 1968. Natural resistance to echinococcosis and the biological factors responsible. Bull. W.H.O., 39:121–122.

———— M. Ohbayashi, Y. Kitamura, K. Suzuki, and M. Okugi. 1958. Studies on echinococcosis. VIII. Experimental echinococcosis multilocularis in various rodents; especially on the differences of susceptibility among uniform strains of the mouse. Jap. J. Vet. Res., 6:135–155.

Yutuc, L. M. 1951. Observations on Manson's tapeworm, *Diphyllobothrium erinacei* (Rudolphi, 1819), in the Philippines. Philippine J. Sci., 80:33–51.

Immunity to Arthropods

E. BENJAMINI

Laboratory of Medical Entomology, Kaiser Foundation Research Institute,
San Francisco, California

BEN F. FEINGOLD

Department of Allergy, Kaiser Foundation Hospital,
San Francisco, California

INTRODUCTION

It is estimated that in the phylum Arthropoda, the class Insecta alone
embraces from 625,000 to 1,500,000 species comprising approximately 8 per-

cent of all known animal species (Sabrosky, 1952). Through this tremendous diversification, arthropod life can be found almost anywhere on earth, so the contact of man and other animals with arthropods is virtually unavoidable. Throughout the centuries man and animals have been plagued by arthropods which consume enormous quantities of food and which are responsible for numerous pathologic conditions either by serving as vectors of etiologic agents of disease or by being themselves the causative agents. This chapter is mainly concerned with this latter category.

Apart from adverse psychologic reactions to arthropods (entomophobia) and the consequences of such reactions, arthropods may be the direct cause of pathologic conditions in man and other mammals by: (1) bites (e.g., spi- into the body by arthropods (e.g., venoms of scorpions, spiders, bees, and wasps), (3) invasion into tissues (certain mites and dipterous larvae), (4) contact (e.g., various stages of some Lepidoptera, blister beetles), (5) inges- tion (e.g., shrimp, lobsters, crayfish, and certain dipterous larvae), and (6) inhalation (many arthropods and arthropod fragments). In the latter three categories, even dead arthropods may be the cause of disease.

As in cases of attack by other pathogenic organisms, mammals are capa- ble of exhibiting both native and acquired immunity to arthropods. Im- munity can be developed not only to parasitic arthropods but also to pre- datory arthropods or arthropod fragments. These aspects of immunity are frequently neglected. Therefore, the discussion which follows will deal with the cellular and humoral responses of mammals to arthropods and to arthro- pod fragments or parts, and with the acquired immunity to these agents.

It will become apparent throughout the discussion that acquired immu- nity to arthropods may be roughly divided into three major categories: (1) immunity associated with the neutralization of toxic substances introduced into the body by arthropods (e.g., venoms of scorpions, spiders, bees, and wasps), (2) hypersensitivity to antigens of arthropod origin (e.g., reactions to arthropod bites, stings, urticating hairs and spines, allergy induced by inhaled arthropod fragments, and allergy induced by ingested arthropods), and (3) immunity to infestation or invasion by arthropods (e.g., infestation by certain ticks and invasion by certain myiasis-producing dipterous larvae). This division, although of practical value, is nevertheless arbitrary since these categories are not necessarily mutually exclusive. It will be shown later, for example, that while immunity in response to a bee sting is associated with antibodies to some toxic components of the bee venom, death resulting from a bee sting is caused by an anaphylactic reaction to antigenic compo- nents of the venom rather than by its toxicity. In the same vein, the acquired hypersensitive response of the host to bites of certain ticks is apparently responsible for host immunity to infestation by these ticks. Moreover, as will be discussed, there also exists the possibility that acquired immunity in mammals to the direct effect of some arthropods may influence the suscepti- bility of the host to microorganisms for which the arthropods serve as vectors, thus perhaps participating in the infective mechanisms underlying diseases caused by arthropod-borne pathogens.

There are thousands of communications dealing with various aspects of immunity to arthropods; many, if not most, are confined to descriptions of case histories, and others report on the quest for better understanding of the basic mechanisms associated with the immunity. This chapter is not intended to be a review of these reports, nor is it intended to recommend measures for specific problems associated with attacks by arthropods. Instead, it deals with some of the fundamental aspects of immunity to arthropods in order to point out that despite the tremendous diversity of arthropods, many common denominators may be found for the mechanisms underlying immunity to these animals. It also serves to emphasize that these mechanisms are the same as those operating in immunity to other organisms.

Finally, many reports have not been included in the present chapter. This was not due to any intention of minimizing their significance but rather to the almost unavoidable necessity to limit, for the sake of clarity, the examples chosen for the elucidation of the general principles of immunity to arthropods.

IMMUNITY TO ARTHROPOD BITES

Since the introduction of antigenic materials by the biting arthropods involves their mouth parts, the groups most pertinent to the discussion which follows are the hematophagous arthropods which feed on warm-blooded animals. Nevertheless, immunity to severe reactions caused by some other biting arthropods, such as spiders, is quite common and will, therefore, be included.

Classical medical entomologic research has been primarily concerned with disease transmission and with the control of the arthropods involved. The early discoveries that hematophagous arthropods serve as vectors of diseases such as malaria, typhus, plague, and yellow fever greatly intensified research on their role in the transmission of many other diseases affecting man and animals. But apart from disease transmission, the manner in which the hematophagous arthropods obtain their blood meal more often than not triggers a reaction by the host. This reaction may not only be unpleasant; it may actually result in severe manifestations ranging from pruritus and generalized urticaria to systemic anaphylaxis and death. It is this aspect of parasitism, i.e., the host's reaction to the bite of the hematophagous arthropod, which has been neglected. Actually it is of great importance, both from the standpoint of the host-parasite relationship and from the standpoint of its possible role in disease transmission. By virtue of dependence on the host for survival, the degree of reactivity of the host to the bite of the arthropod may, to a certain extent, play a role in the host-parasite interrelationship. Also, the reaction of the host to the bite of a disease vector may affect infectivity with pathogens and their survival in the host. In view of such considerations, it is surprising that so little attention has been devoted to the bite reaction, and that most of the reports dealing with the subject of immunity to bites are confined to descriptions of case histories, rather than to discussions of the more fundamental aspects of the problem.

All hematophagous arthropods appear to obtain their blood meal by essentially the same mechanism: They pierce the skin of the host with their mouth parts and feed either directly in a capillary or from a pool of extravasated blood. The evolution of the blood-sucking type of mouth parts from the primitive chewing type is rather complex, and large variations in mouth parts can be found among the various hematophagous arthropods. This variation makes it possible to classify medically important arthropods on the basis of mouthpart structure (Herms and James, 1961). For detailed descriptions and a discussion on insect mouth parts, the reader is referred to a monograph by Snodgrass (1944). Some hematophagous arthropods use their blade-like mandibles to slash the host's skin and capillaries; they then feed on the extravasated blood pool on the surface of the host's skin. This type of feeding, exemplified by that of the stable fly *Stomoxys calcitrans*, is very painful to the host. Some other arthropods such as the mosquito, *Anopheles maculipennis*, insert their needle-like mouth parts through the skin into the tissue and capillaries of the host. In general, the bites of mosquitoes are in fact so benign that they are hardly noticed. These two examples are brought forth by Herms and James (1961) with respect to the possible relationship between disease transmission and host reactions to the bite. These authors pointed out that insects which inflict painful bites are seldom vectors of diseases, whereas insects with benign bites are commonly potent vectors. The authors postulated that perhaps in order to be a successful vector of disease, the arthropod must have a reduced severity of its bite. True as this may be, there are several factors (such as the development of hypersensitivity to substances present in the saliva of arthropods) which may contribute to severe reactions to bites of a normally mildly biting arthropod such as the *Anopheles* mosquito.

Until relatively recently, the mechanical process involved in hematophagous arthropod feeding was studied from histologic sections of the host's skin containing the mouth parts of the arthropod (reviewed by Lavoipierre et al., 1959). Results of such "static" studies, however correct, are at best conjectural, since the dynamics of the feeding process had to be inferred from the position of the mouth parts in the skin. It was not until Gordon and his collaborators (Gordon and Lumsden, 1939; Gordon and Crew, 1948; Griffiths and Gordon, 1952; Lavoipierre et al., 1959; Dickerson and Lavoipierre, 1959) devised an apparatus which enabled them to view *in vivo* the movements of the mosquito mouth parts in the tissue of a live host, that the actual feeding process of a hematophagous insect was elucidated. Observations made on some of the deep-feeding insects revealed that the mandibles and maxillae cut the skin of the host, and that the needle-like proboscis, consisting of the labrum, hypopharynx, mandibles, and maxillae, is thrust through the opening. The mandibles and maxillae continue to cut the tissue, allowing for the deeper penetration of the entire fascicle. The distal portion of the fascicle is flexible and can curve, which thus allows penetration in almost any direction. Blood is then withdrawn either from a pool resulting from the severed capillaries, or directly from the capillary, or from both.

The mouth parts of arachnids (spiders, ticks, and mites) are basically different from those of the hematophagous insects in that those of the former do not have true mandibles. Instead, the arachnids possess a pair of chelicerae (pincers) which serve for grasping the food source, and a highly developed sucking apparatus which serves for the intake of the liquid meal. During the bite of hematophagous arachnids (mites and ticks), the chelicerae, the distal portions of which are provided with recurved teeth, are inserted into the integument of the host. The pool of blood originating from ruptured capillaries is then sucked up. (For an excellent description of arachnid mouth parts, the reader is referred to a monograph by Snodgrass, 1948.) Several types of apparatus have been used for observations of the actual biting process of various arachnids (Lavoipierre and Riek, 1955; Gregson, 1960).

The trauma caused by the mechanical action of the mouth parts during the bite varies in magnitude depending both on the arthropod's mode of feeding and on the host. In general, the trauma resulting from arthropods which lacerate the skin with their blade-like mandibles (e. g., deer flies, black flies, stable flies, and tsetse flies) is more severe and noticeable by the host than is the trauma caused by those possessing piercing mouth parts (e.g., mosquitoes and fleas). Also, the magnitude of the trauma is affected by the size of the arthropod and by the duration of feeding. Several attempts have been made to elucidate the cellular response to trauma caused by the insertion of the mouth parts (Gordon and Crew, 1948; Goldman et al., 1952; and Larrivee et al., 1964). Such studies, however, must be carefully evaluated in view of the possibility that the witnessed response is not necessarily due to the action of the mouth parts only. It may be complicated by the introduction of various injurious chemicals present in the oral secretion of the arthropod and by a possible hypersensitive response of the host to these agents.

In addition to the mechanical process of the bite, other processes are involved in the acquisition of the blood meal. One such important process is the injection of oral secretions into the host's tissue. (Since more often than not the origin of materials present in the oral secretion of arthropods is obscure, the term "oral secretion" is used in this discussion to denote materials exuded from the arthropod's mouth, except in cases where the origin of the secretion has been ascertained.) Little is known about the mechanism which triggers the output of oral secretion of hematophagous arthropods; it would, however, be expected to be under nervous control similar to that inferred for some phytophagous arthropods (Day and Waterhouse, 1953).

The composition and function of the oral secretion of hematophagous arthropods vary depending on the food source, diet, and feeding habits. Studies revealed remarkable correlations among function, composition, and mode of feeding. It has been observed by A. Hudson et al. (1960) that bites of the mosquito, *Aedes stimulans*, from which the salivary glands have been surgically removed, were more painful than the bites of the normal mosquito.

This observation suggested the presence of an anesthetic component in the saliva of this mosquito, which undoubtedly would have a survival value in rendering the bite imperceptible to the host. The oral secretion of the slow-feeding tick, *Dermacentor andersoni*, contains substances, presumably originating in the salivary glands, which harden into a latex-like material which moulds itself around the mouth parts of the tick and the skin of the host, thus enabling the tick to attach itself firmly to the host for a prolonged period (Gregson, 1960). The oral secretion of the cat flea, *Ctenocephalides felis felis*, has been found to contain a powerful spreading factor (Feingold and Benjamini, 1961), which probably plays a role in the softening and the spreading of the host's dermal tissue, thus enabling the flea easier access to the blood source.

Other compounds which undoubtedly play an important role in the feeding process are the anticoagulants which were demonstrated in the oral secretions of several hematophagous arthropods (Cornwall and Patton, 1914; Yorke and MacFie, 1924; de Buck, 1937; Metcalf, 1945). Although their presence is not universal, anticoagulatory substances are particularly important when the arthropod feeds on a pool of blood rather than directly from the host's capillary. The oral secretions of hematophagous arthropods contain numerous other compounds (hemagglutinins, toxins, sugars, aminoacids, peptides, proteins, phenolic compounds, and many others), the origin, exact chemical composition, and function of which are obscure. Many substances undoubtedly play a role in the conditioning of the host's tissue for penetration and in the conditioning of the host's blood before or perhaps even after ingestion. However, some of the substances may be relics from times when arthropods fed on nutrients other than blood and which now may have no function (DeMeillon, 1949).

In addition to bites by hematophagous arthropods, numerous reports of bites by nonhematophagous arthropods of man and animals are encountered in the literature (Herms and James, 1961). However, in general these bites constitute part of a defense reaction by these arthropods, rather than contributing to the acquisition of nutrients. The black widow spider, *Latrodectus mactans*, is an example of an arthropod which does not normally feed on mammals but whose bites may inflict severe reactions and sometimes death. The diet of this spider consists largely of insects and other small arthropods which are killed by extremely potent toxins present in its oral secretion. Occasionally, however, especially when disturbed, the female spider will bite a mammal.

Whatever the nature of the substances in the oral secretions of arthropods may be, their deposition into the host is of paramount importance from the standpoint of local and systemic reactions of the host to the bites and of the development of hypersensitive host reactions to these substances. Also, as will be discussed later, the nature of substances in the oral secretion of hematophagous arthropods and the immune response of the host to their deposition may affect the fate of pathogens in the case of disease vectors, and may perhaps constitute a bridge for a relationship between hypersensitivity and infectivity (Fairbairn and Williamson, 1956; Williamson, 1956; Geigy and Huber, 1959; Kartman, 1964, 1965).

The response of the host to the bite of the arthropod varies, depending primarily on the nature of the arthropod's oral secretion and on the sensitivity of the host. An individual who may react severely to the bite of one species may not react to bites of other species. Similarly, a given species of arthropod may elicit severe reactions in some individuals but not in others. In addition to variations in the severity of reactions, there also exist variations in the time of appearance and in the duration of the reactions following the bite. Nevertheless, attempts have been directed toward the orderly classification of reactions both in terms of causal agents and in terms of immune phenomena with which reactions may be associated. Thus, apart from the trauma inflicted on the host by the mouth parts of an arthropod during the process of feeding, reactions of the host to the bite may be attributed to one of three factors present in the oral secretion: (1) antigenic or allergenic substances, (2) irritating or toxic substances, or (3) substances which are both antigenic and toxic. It is often difficult to determine by observation alone which of the above factors is responsible for the elicitation of a given reaction; however, several criteria may be used for the classification of the etiologic agent. These criteria will become apparent in the discussions which follow.

No attempt will be made here to evaluate the importance, with respect to incidence or severity, of reactions elicited by the above factors—each factor may contribute not only to discomfort of the bitten individual, but may actually inflict serious disability or even death.

Hypersensitivity to arthropod bites

Reactions to bites. It is common knowledge that different individuals react in different ways to the bites of arthropods. Numerous clinical surveys show that the response of some individuals may be in the form of a skin reaction which appears some 10 to 15 minutes following the bite and which disappears within a few hours. This type of reaction, termed an "immediate reaction," normally consists of erythema and edema at the bite site, and is usually accompanied by intense pruritus. In some individuals the appearance of a skin reaction is delayed until some 15 to 24 hours following the bite. This delayed reaction usually consists of erythema accompanied by papulation which within a day or two may become necrotic. This reaction may not disappear for several days, and frequently it may persist for several weeks. During the first few days, the individual may experience intense pruritus which, through scratching, may lead to secondary infection at the bite site. Still other individuals may manifest an immediate reaction which may or may not disappear within a few hours, and which later will be supplanted by delayed skin reactivity.

Several attempts have been made to discover whether or not a relationship exists between the immediate and delayed types of skin reactivity elicited in response to arthropod bites. These attempts utilized both humans and experimental animals which were subjected to repeated bites over long periods of time. Observations made by Kemper (1929) on his own reactions to bed bug bites during 11 months of repeated exposures revealed that at the beginning of the experiment, only delayed-type reactions occurred. As exposures to 30 bites at 2-day intervals continued, the time interval decreased from 24 hours between the bite and the appearance of skin reactions to the appearance of lesions immediately following the bite. Finally, at the end of the 11-month period, the bites failed to elicit skin reactivity. Theodor (1935) observed that in human subjects exposed to bites of the sand fly, *Phlebotomus papatasii*, the first skin reactions were delayed-type. However, after 2 to 4 months of further exposures, the delayed reactions were sometimes preceded by immediate reactions which appeared 20 to 30 minutes following the bite and disappeared completely within an hour.

In another study, Mellanby (1946) showed that human subjects who had no previous exposure to bites of the mosquito *Aedes aegypti* did not react to the first few bites by this mosquito. On further exposures, the subjects exhibited delayed skin reactions which appeared some 20 to 24 hours following the bites. The subjects were further bitten by *Aedes aegypti* on several occasions for about a month, at the end of which period the challenging bites elicited immediate reactions (which completely disappeared within a short time) and delayed reactions which appeared within 20 to 24 hours. After a further period of exposure, the subjects had immediate reactions, and the delayed reaction became gradually less severe, finally failing to appear. These subjects never lost their immediate reactivity, but in other individuals who were repeatedly exposed to thousands of bites from the *Aedes* mosquito, Mellanby noticed that the immediate reactions finally disappeared.

In addition to the above examples, other reports may be found in the literature which imply that on repeated exposures to bites of a given arthropod, the subject's skin reactivity changes. It was first postulated by Mellanby, and later confirmed by McKiel (1955), Benjamini et al. (1961), and Larrivee et al. (1964), that there is a definite sequence of events in the skin reactivity in response to arthropod bites. The sequence is summarized in Table 1.

The entire sequence of the skin reactivity with its various stages has been demonstrated by Benjamini et al. (1961) by exposing guinea pigs to bites of

Table 1

Stages of Skin Reactivity in Response to
Repeated Exposures to Arthropod Bites

Stage	Immediate Reactions	Delayed Reactions
I	−	−
II	−	+
III	+	+
IV	+	−
V	−	−

the cat flea *Ctenocephalides felis felis*. In these experiments, animals were first exposed daily to bites; after 10 days they were exposed to bites approximately twice a week for a total period of several months. For the first 4 days the animals did not react to the bites. Between the 5th and 9th day following the initial exposure, the majority of animals exhibited delayed skin reactions which appeared some 18 to 24 hours following the bite. Between the 9th and the 60th day, the majority of animals reacted with both immediate and delayed reactions, and between the 60th and 90th day most animals reacted with immediate reactions only. At the end of 90 days, most animals became refractory and showed no reactions to bites. The distinction between the stages was not clear-cut; the transition from stage to stage was gradual with respect to the numbers of reacting animals, but the trend toward the sequence as proposed in Table 1 is shown by the data in Table 2.

There are numerous excellent reports which describe the host's reactions in response to arthropod bites (Moore and Hirschfelder, 1919; Goldman et al., 1925; Wood, 1942; Allen, 1948; Goldman, et al., 1952; Rockwell and Johnson, 1952; Arean and Fox, 1955; Goldman, 1956; Jones, 1961; Perlman, 1962; Goldman, 1963). It would be difficult to compile these data in order to establish whether or not a correlation exists between the gross visual appearance of the reactions and the accompanying histopathologic situation. The data were obtained from numerous insect species, and most of the individuals tested had an unknown history of previous exposure.

Larrivee et al. (1964) attempted to evaluate skin reactivity in terms of histopathologic changes. These workers demonstrated that the sequence of events in the skin reactivity of guinea pigs in response to repeated exposures to bites of cat fleas could be characterized histopathologically on the basis of cellular responses to the bites. The results of these investigations are summarized in Table 3.

The occurrence of a definite sequence in skin reactivity in response to arthropod bites provides some clues to the mechanisms involved in this phenomenon. As mentioned above, the oral secretion of arthropods may contain substances which are antigenic, toxic, or both. The fact that a sequence exists indicates that the secretory materials associated with this sequence are antigenic in nature, and that the sequence is a manifestation of an immune response. If the bite reactions associated with the sequence were due to a toxic or irritating substance, skin reactivity would be normally expected to occur whenever a bite is administered, regardless of whether or not the animal had been bitten previously and regardless of the time and number of bites which follow the initial exposure. This, however, is not the case. In actuality, it appears that the type of reaction elicited by the bite definitely depends on the number of bites and on the time interval between the initial exposure and challenge. Furthermore, the fact that repeated exposures not only change the type of skin reactivity, but ultimately may result in a state of nonreactivity, points to some sort of immunity or hyposensitization of the individual. It is, therefore, logical to conclude that the sequence of events in skin reactivity is a manifestation of an immune mechanism.

Table 2

Stages of Skin Reactivity of Guinea Pigs in Response to Repeated Exposures to Flea Bites

Stage	Type of Predominant Reactions	Observed Reactions (Percent of Animals Reacting*)				Days from Initial Exposure	Approximate Duration of Stage
		Delayed	Immediate and Delayed	Immediate	No Reactions		
I	No reactions	12	1	0	87	4	4
II	Delayed	65	14	0	21	5	5
III	Immediate and delayed	36	37	9	18	9	50
IV	Immediate	2	5	71	22	60	30
V	No reactions	1	0	5	94	90	150

* The figures are based on averages obtained from numerous challenges given at various time intervals following the initial exposure. Thus, some animals challenged towards the end of each stage exhibited some reactions characteristic to the ensuing stage, and animals challenged at the beginning of a stage exhibited reactions characteristic to the preceding stage.

Table 3

The Sequence of Events in Terms of Cellular Responses in
the Skin Reactivity of Guinea Pigs in Response to Flea Bites

Stage	Skin Reactivity	Cellular Response at Bite Site	
		20 Minutes after Bite	24 Hours after Bite
I	No reactivity	No cellular abnormalities	No cellular abnormalities
II	Delayed	No cellular abnormalities	Intense monocytic and lymphocytic dermal infiltration
III	Immediate and delayed	Eosinophilic infiltration	Intense monocytic and lymphocytic dermal infiltration
IV	Immediate	Eosinophilic infiltration	Very mild, if any, monocytic and lymphocytic infiltration
V	No reactivity	No cellular abnormalities	No cellular abnormalities

Further evidence for this view is provided by the fact that a similar sequence of events in response to administration of protein antigens has been demonstrated. Repeated intracutaneous injections of ovalbumin into humans at first produced no reaction, but later elicited delayed reactions, and still later elicited delayed reactions which were preceded by immediate reactions (Tezner, 1934; Simon and Rackman, 1934). The "Jones-Mote" type of hypersensitivity in response to injections of humans and animals with foreign sera is also characterized by a similar sequence (Jones and Mote, 1934; Mote and Jones, 1936). These workers further demonstrated that when injections were discontinued, a reversal of the sequence shown in Table 1 took place. (For an excellent discussion of the "Jones-Mote" type of hypersensitivity, the reader is referred to Raffel, 1961.)

The sequence of events in the skin reactivity associated with arthropod bites may be interpreted in terms of the immune response as follows: The first exposure to the bite constitutes the initial antigenic stimulus which initiates the synthesis of antibodies against antigenic materials present in the oral secretion of the arthropod. Thus, the first stage, i.e., the stage in which the individual still does not respond to challenging bites, is the induction stage during which the immune response has been triggered and is being developed. It is, therefore, not surprising that during this stage the presence of antibodies, whether circulating or cellular, cannot be demonstrated. The next stage is that of delayed reactions only. These reactions, which are characterized by their time of appearance following the challenging bite, may also be characterized histopathologically by the dermal infiltration of monocytes and lymphocytes. This cellular response is closely analogous to that which

Dienes and Mallory (1932) and Kaplan and Dienes (1958) showed to be associated with delayed reactions to protein antigens. They showed that delayed reactions appeared within 4 to 5 days following sensitization and were characterized by the predominance of mononuclear over polymorphonuclear cellular infiltrations.

One criterion often used in the immunologic characterization of delayed-type hypersensitivity is the transfer of hypersensitivity from the sensitized animal to a nonsensitized animal via leukocytes of the sensitized individuals. Recently, leukocyte transfer of delayed-type hypersensitivity to mosquito bites was demonstrated by Allen (1964) and by Allen and West (1964). In these experiments, the investigators harvested leukocytes from guinea pigs which showed delayed reactions to mosquito bites following sensitization of the animals with oral secretions of mosquitoes. The leukocytes were then injected intraperitoneally into recipient guinea pigs, which showed delayed skin reactions in response to subsequent challenges with mosquito bites. Similar results were obtained by Allen with leukocyte transfer of delayed hypersensitivity from rabbits to guinea pigs, but not from rabbits to rabbits.

The immediate-type skin reactivity in response to arthropod bites has been the subject of numerous investigations, both with respect to the possibility that the reaction may be in response to toxic substances present in the oral secretion, and with respect to an immediate skin reactivity associated with an antigen-antibody interaction. The fact that the oral secretions of some biting arthropods are indeed toxic is well-established, as will be discussed later. However, it is also well-documented that the immediate reactions caused by bites of most of the hematophagous arthropods are not due to toxicity of the oral secretion, but rather to an antigen-antibody interaction.

It has been shown by many workers that immediate skin reactivity to the bites of arthropods is elicited only following prior sensitization, that the reactivity exhibits a certain degree of specificity to a given arthropod, and that during the stage in which the individual exhibits immediate reactivity, specific circulating humoral antibodies can be demonstrated. The existence of a sequence of events in the skin reactivity in response to repeated bites of arthropods adds support to the association of an immune mechanism with immediate skin reactivity, as mentioned above.

The immediate skin reaction may be characterized not only by the appearance of erythema and edema some 20 minutes following the bite, but also histopathologically by an eosinophilic response (see Table 3). The eosinophilic response is characteristic of immediate-type skin reactivity in response to various antigens, as has been demonstrated by many workers (Dienes and Mallory, 1932; Campbell et al., 1935; Samter, 1949; Raffel, 1951; Weiser, 1957; Kaplan and Dienes, 1958; Gell, 1959; Oda and Puck, 1961). Kaplan and Dienes (1958), for example, who worked with skin reactions elicited by protein antigens, characterized the immediate skin reactivity as edema and an infiltration of eosinophils, occasionally accompanied by focal accumulation of mononuclear cells.

If the thesis is accepted that the described responses to arthropod bites are associated with hypersensitivity, then the terminal stage (Stage V) in the sequence of skin reactivity represents a stage of hyposensitization. Stages of nonreactivity, presumably results of repeated exposures to bites of various arthropods, have been reported by many workers and will be discussed in a later section of this chapter (*see* pp. 1083-1085).

The occurrence of both delayed and immediate types of hypersensitive response to bites of arthropods raises the inevitable question: Are these reactions caused by the same antigen or do they constitute distinct responses to two or more antigens? Although a multiplicity of antigens related to arthropod-bite sensitivity has been indicated by several workers (Benson, 1936; DeMeillon, 1949), the involvement of more than one antigenic component in the two types of reactions is not at all certain. Since the antigen or antigens involved in arthropod-bite hypersensitivity have not been isolated or characterized, the answer to this question may be suggested by systems which involve both types of skin reactivities elicited in response to defined antigens. Even here, however, various workers still disagree as to the causes of these responses. There are those who propose that the antigens responsible for each type of reactivity are distinct. This hypothesis is based on experiments utilizing systems consisting of haptens conjugated to protein carriers. These experiments (summarized and discussed by Benacerraf and Gell, 1962) indicated that delayed hypersensitivity was associated with cellular antibodies directed against the protein carrier, whereas immediate hypersensitivity was associated with circulating antibodies directed against the hapten, thus implying that the immediate and delayed responses were distinct processes directed against different antigens. On the other hand, there are those who propose that the two reactions are immunologically related, that they may be associated with the same antigen, and that the delayed response constitutes an early stage of the immune process which ultimately will turn into an immediate response accompanied by demonstrable circulating antibodies (Salvin, 1958; Feingold et al., 1964). It is not within the scope of this chapter to delve into these hypotheses. The latter hypothesis, however, can best accommodate data on the immune response to arthropod bites. These data show that the early response, manifested by delayed skin reactions and associated with cellular antibodies, can gradually change, as sensitization progresses, into an immediate-type hypersensitivity with demonstrable circulating antibodies.

In view of the preceding considerations, it becomes apparent that much caution has to be exercised when reactions to arthropod bites are used as criteria for evaluating whether or not an individual is sensitive to bites of a given arthropod. The conclusion that an individual is not sensitive because he failed to react within an hour may be erroneous, since a delayed reaction may develop 24 hours after the bite. Also, the failure to react does not mean that the individual is a "nonreactor." The same individual may exhibit violent delayed skin reactions when challenged a week or so later, since the first bite may constitute sensitization. Also, the various types of skin reactivity may well explain the wide variety in results obtained from testing a given population with bites of an arthropod.

The foregoing discussion on the sequence of events in the skin reactivity of individuals in response to arthropod bites and the association of the response with the immune mechanism was presented with the awareness that it represents, at best, an idealized picture. Duration of reactivity stages and transitions from one stage to another depend on many factors, such as the arthropod, the frequency and quantity of the bite, and, of course, the host itself.

Antigens. During the past 50 years several attempts have been directed toward the elucidation of antigens involved in arthropod-bite hypersensitivity. Although these efforts have not yet been rewarded with the chemical identification of even one antigen, several antigens have been isolated and have been characterized immunochemically.

Antigens related to arthropod-bite hypersensitivity have been prepared from extracts of whole arthropods, from extracts of defined areas of the arthropod's body, and from the actual oral secretion of arthropods. The immunologic activity of these preparations, as it is related to arthropod-bite hypersensitivity, has been assayed by several methods, which include skin tests, sensitizations to bites, serologic tests, and hyposensitizations to bites.

Many workers have demonstrated that extracts of the whole arthropod body contain the antigen or antigens involved in arthropod-bite hypersensitivity. This conclusion has been based on the findings that:

1. The intradermal injections of such extracts elicit skin reactions in individuals who also react to the bite (Rockwell and Johnson, 1952; Fox and Berman, 1960; McKiel and Clunie, 1960; Feingold and Benjamini, 1961; and others);
2. The extract can sensitize individuals to bites of the arthropod (Dubin et al., 1948; McKiel and Clunie, 1960; Benjamini et al., 1960a; and others);
3. The extract exhibits typical serologic reactions with sera obtained from bite-reactive individuals (Wilson and Clements, 1965).

Extracts of the whole arthropod contain a multitude of components, the majority of which are not involved in the bite reaction. Consequently, attempts have been made to purify and isolate from these extracts the antigens specific to the bite reaction. McKiel and Clunie (1960) fractionated mosquito extract by chromatography, and they obtained a purified fraction which exhibited a high skin reactivity related to mosquito-bite hypersensitivity. Further fractionation showed that the skin-reactive material found in the extract of the mosquito *A. aegypti* was composed of at least four active fractions. In extracts of whole mosquitoes, the presence of more than one antigenic component involved in the bite reaction was also shown by Wilson and Clements (1965) by gel-diffusion reactions between the extract and sera obtained from mosquito-bite sensitive rabbits. There were other attempts to purify and isolate allergenic components from extracts of whole arthropods;

however, these attempts faced the obvious biochemical difficulties involved in isolating small amounts of material from overwhelmingly heterogeneous mixtures. More successful results have been obtained with extracts of limited regions of the arthropod's body, such as the salivary glands, and primarily with the actual oral secretion of the arthropod.

Early work with mosquitoes led to the hypothesis that the bite reaction was due to regurgitation of substances from the esophageal diverticula of the arthropods (Schaudinn, 1904; Hindle, 1914; Roxburgh, 1927). This hypothesis, however, was found to be erroneous in view of work by Hecht (1928), Pawlowsky and Shtein (1928), Manalang (1931), Gordon and Crewe (1948), McKiel (1959), and others. This later work suggested that the arthropod salivary secretion was the responsible etiologic agent. It was shown by Lester and Lloyd (1928) and by Gordon and Crewe (1948) that no reaction was elicited by the bite of a tsetse fly from which the salivary glands had been removed, although the insect did engorge itself on an individual who was extremely sensitive to the bite of a normal fly. A. Hudson et al. (1960) also showed that the bite of a mosquito from which the salivary glands had been removed did not produce a bite reaction when it fed on a sensitive individual. Other experiments utilizing skin tests with emulsions and extracts of salivary glands of mosquitoes (Cornwall and Patton, 1914; Metcalf, 1945; Rockwell and Johnson, 1952) suggested that the bite-reaction substances originated in the salivary glands.

This suggestion led several workers to collect the oral secretions of several arthropods and to characterize these secretions by immunochemical and chemical methods. Benjamini and associates succeeded in collecting a large amount of oral secretion from cat fleas by allowing the fleas to feed through membranes on distilled water. They showed that the intradermal inoculation of the oral secretion elicted reactions in guinea pigs which had been previously sensitized to flea bites (either by exposures to the bites of fleas or by injections with extracts of whole fleas), thus implicating the oral secretion in the bite reaction (Benjamini et al., 1960b, 1963a; and Benjamini, 1964). Attempts by these workers to sensitize guinea pigs by injections of the oral secretion in saline failed: The injected animals did not react to challenges given with flea bites, nor did they react to intradermal tests given with the collected oral secretion. However, when guinea pigs were injected with the collected oral secretion incorporated in Freund's complete adjuvant, they were sensitized to flea bites as well as to the oral secretion. Since the substance (or substances) responsible for the sensitizing activity was stable to heat and to acid hydrolysis and was of relatively low molecular weight (Benjamini, 1964; Michaeli et al., 1965a), it was postulated to be haptenic in nature rather than a complete antigen. (These data may perhaps explain unpublished findings by these same workers that the allergenic activity of extracts of whole fleas was stable to heat and to acid hydrolysis.) Young et al. (1963) fractionated the oral secretion of cat fleas by chromatography and electrophoresis, obtained purified active components, and indicated that activity was associated with more than one material. It should be recalled that several antigenically active fractions were obtained by McKiel and Clunie (1960) from extracts of whole mosquito bodies, and that antigenic activity related to mosquito-bite hypersensitivity was demonstrated to be associated with extracts obtained from several body regions of the mosquito. Also, more than one antigenic component was implicated by the gel-diffusion experiments performed by Wilson and Clements (1965) which were mentioned earlier.

Finding more than one compound associated with activity may mean that activity is due to a multiplicity of antigenic components present in the oral secretion of the arthropods. This was suggested by histochemical findings which showed that salivary glands of *Aedes aegypti* contain conjugated mucopolysaccharides, carbohydrate-protein complexes, proteins, and mucin, all of which are potentially antigenic (Orr et al., 1961). However, in the case of flea-bite hypersensitivity, there is also the possibility that the hapten involved may be associated with different peptides or other chemicals, which due to their different chromatographic and electrophoretic properties can be separated from each other, each still carrying the hapten and, therefore, exhibiting activity. The latter possibility becomes especially plausible in view of Michaeli's unpublished experiments (1967) which showed that an isolated crystalline fraction obtained from chromatographically purified oral secretions of fleas could completely inhibit passive cutaneous anaphylaxis elicited in guinea pigs either by sera obtained from flea-bite sensitive rabbits or by various antigens related to flea-bite hypersensitivity. In addition, studies on flea saliva by polyacrylamide-gel filtration revealed that the activity associated with a given peak could be totally transferred, under certain conditions, to a different peak, implying that the same hapten may be associated with different carriers. These findings suggest the presence of an antigenic determinant common to all the active fractions found by Young et al.

Collection and immunochemical studies of oral secretions of the mosquito *Aedes aegypti* were recently performed by Allen (1964), who showed that the oral secretion could elicit skin reactions when inoculated intradermally into humans or rabbits reactive to the bite of the mosquito. Also, the injection of the oral secretion, either in saline or in combination with Freund's complete adjuvant, into nonreacting guinea pigs sensitized them to the bites of the mosquito. Allen demonstrated that the principle responsible for the skin reactivity of this oral secretion was nondialyzable and thermostable. Furthermore, though it was stable to treatment with lysozyme and α-amylase, it lost activity following treatment with papain or trypsin, which indicated that a protein or a peptide was associated with activity. Allen concluded, however, that the skin-reactive component required a structurally intact protein or peptide in order to remain active, but that the antigenic determinant was not necessarily part of the protein or peptide molecule. This conclusion by Allen may imply that a hapten or haptens may be associated with the reactivity related to mosquito-bite sensitivity. Although this possibility is exciting in view of the finding that flea-bite hypersensitivity was found to be associated with a hapten, there is, of course, no basis for an assumption that all hypersensitivities to arthropod bites involve similar haptenic components.

It is widely believed that the injection of a hapten normally does not result in the production of antibodies, unless it is conjugated to relatively larger molecular weight carriers (Eisen, 1959; Raffel, 1961). Recently, it was shown that conjugation to a carrier was not always essential and that antibodies to low molecular weight compounds could also be produced by injections of the compounds mixed with large molecular weight substances (Plescia et al., 1966). Accepting the assumption that the immunochemical properties of the collected oral secretions of cat fleas are similar to those of the oral secretion deposited by the flea during the actual bite, the mechanism of sensitization by the flea hapten was further investigated. From preliminary experiments by Benjamini et al. (1963a), it appeared that whereas the collected oral secretion was nonimmunogenic when injected in saline, it became immunogenic, with respect to flea-bite hypersensitivity, following irreversible association with fibrous proteins. This finding led to the hypothesis that elements of the host's skin may play a role in sensitization by the flea hapten. This hypothesis was further supported by experiments in which injections of extracts of skin biopsies taken from guinea pigs following exposures to bites sensitized recipient guinea pigs to bites of fleas (Benjamini et al., 1963b). Sensitization was apparently achieved by a hapten-carrier association since it was induced by injections of the nondialyzable portions of the extract without addition of adjuvants, whereas the activity of the collected oral secretion was dialyzable and could be demonstrated only when injected with adjuvants.

Subsequent work confirmed these findings and elucidated the nature of the host components with which the hapten is associated. Michaeli et al. (1965b) showed that following bites of guinea pigs by cat fleas, the flea hapten was associated with both salt-soluble and acid-soluble collagens. These conclusions were based on the findings that injections, without adjuvants, of acid-soluble collagen (isolated from skin biopsies obtained from guinea pigs following exposure to bites) sensitized recipient guinea pigs to the bites of fleas. Furthermore, the salt-soluble collagen isolated from such biopsies was also capable of sensitization, but only when injected in combination with adjuvants or when injected in saline following in vitro polymerization. They concluded that the collagen served as a carrier for the flea hapten, and that the immunogenicity, related to flea-bite hypersensitivity, of the collagen-hapten complex increased with increasing polymerization of collagen. It is interesting to note that these workers were unable to demonstrate the association of the flea hapten with skin proteins other than collagen.

The association of the hapten with collagen could be demonstrated not only in biopsies following bites, but also by the in vitro reaction of collagen with collected oral secretion of fleas. Michaeli et al. (1966) further showed that the association resulting in the formation of an immunogenic complex occurred at both acidic and basic pH, but, curiously enough, did not take place at neutral pH. The fact that the product of the reaction at neutral pH was not immunogenic is perhaps related to earlier findings which showed that the intradermal injection of oral secretion of cat fleas, in neutral saline, into guinea pigs failed to sensitize the animals to bites of fleas, or for that matter, to the oral secretion itself (Benjamini et al., 1960b, 1963a). The ability of the flea hapten to associate with collagen at basic or acidic pH was interpreted by Michaeli and co-workers as indicating that the flea hapten contains more than one group capable of reacting with collagen (one or more reacting only at acidic pH and others reacting only at basic pH), or that the reaction with collagen is with a group or groups which may react at either basic or acidic pH. (The nonassociation of the hapten with collagen at neutral pH is somewhat puzzling. This interesting phenomenon will hopefully be elucidated when information becomes availale about the pH of the oral secretion of cat fleas during the actual bite and about its chemical composition.) From *in vitro* experiments, it appears that once association occurs, it is irreversible between pH 3 and 11 (Michaeli et al., 1966).

These findings can perhaps explain the phenomenon observed by B. W. Hudson et al. (1960a) that when animals become reactive due to sensitization by being bitten by fleas, sites of previously nonreactive bites flared up. If the allergen is indeed associated with the skin, then when sufficient hypersensitivity is finally induced, the presence of antigen at previously nonreacting bitten sites constitutes a challenge which results in the elicitation of a skin reaction. Perhaps this phenomenon is connected with summer eczema and flea-allergy dermatitis in dogs (Kissileff, 1938, 1962; Muller, 1961), and with observations by Theodor (1935), Heilesen (1949), and others of the flaring up of old sites of various arthropod bites which is triggered by new bites. It may also be associated with the generalized urticaria occasionally witnessed when individuals are infested with hematophagous arthropods. It should be emphasized, however, that these proposed explanations are strictly speculative and remain to be proved experimentally.

Antibodies. The presence of antibodies associated with hypersensitivity to arthropod bites and their participation in the skin reaction have been pointed out. It is widely accepted that delayed-type hypersensitivity to protein antigens is associated with cellular antibodies. It is, therefore, of significance that cellular antibodies associated with delayed skin reactivity to mosquito bites have been demonstrated by the successful transfer of this reactivity via cells of lymphoid origin (Allen, 1964). In view of these results, it is reasonable to expect that delayed hypersensitivity associated with other biting arthropods also involves cellular antibodies, and that these will be demonstrated in the future.

Circulating antibodies in arthropod-bite hypersensitivity have been demonstrated numerous times by showing that sera from humans sensitized to bites of a particular arthropod, when injected intradermally into nonsensitive humans, is able to sensitize the injected site so that challenge bites of that arthropod elicit immediate skin reactivity. Such successful passive transfers of immediate skin reactivity from humans to humans were demonstrated by Hecht (1929), Brown et al. (1938), and Rockwell and Johnson (1952) for mosquito bites; by Hecht for bed bug bites (reviewed by Hecht, 1943b); and by Feingold and Hudson (1960) for flea bites. Transfer of immediate-type skin reactivity from sensitized laboratory animals to normal animals has been demonstrated by Wilson and Clements (1965) and by Allen (1964) for mosquito bites, and by Michaeli (1967) for flea bites.

The fact that sera obtained from sensitive individuals sensitize the skin of nonreactive recipients could indicate the presence of skin-sensitizing, heat-labile, reaginic antibodies in the sensitive sera. The presence of this class of immunoglobulins in mosquito-bite sensitive serum was suggested by experiments by Rockwell and Johnson (1952), who further suggested that desensitization to the bite reaction was effected through blocking antibodies. The latter was based on the observation that when mosquito extract mixed with serum from a person who had been desensitized by repeated exposures to bites was injected intradermally, it elicited only a minor response compared to that elicited by the injection of the extract without the serum.

The ability of antibodies to sensitize the skin of recipients is not confined to reagins alone. In fact the technique of passive cutaneous anaphylaxis, which was developed by Ovary (1958) for the demonstration of circulating antibodies, is based on the ability of antibodies other than reagins to sensitize animal skin. However, whereas reaginic antibodies are capable of sensitizing skin for a relatively long period, nonreaginic skin-sensitizing antibodies can remain fixed to skin for short periods only, ranging from a few hours to one or two days, depending on the species from which the serum was derived and depending on the recipient species. Therefore, serum transfer of arthropod-bite sensitivity from humans to humans does not necessarily imply the presence of reagins, but it may actually be caused by other antibodies capable of remaining fixed to the skin for the time interval (in most cases 24 hours) between transfer and challenge. Also, the fact that hypersensitivity to bites of mosquitoes and fleas could be transferred by serum from one animal species to another (Allen, 1964; Wilson and Clements, 1965), and the finding that flea-bite hypersensitivity could be transferred from humans to guinea pigs (Michaeli, 1967), imply that antibodies other than reagins may be involved. This implication is based on the fact that, to date, it has not been demonstrated that human reaginic serum can sensitize skin of animals other than primates.

In addition to the demonstration by serum transfer that circulating antibodies are involved in arthropod-bite hypersensitivity, recent experiments demonstrated the presence of precipitating antibodies (although in relatively low titers) in sera of mosquito-bite and flea-bite sensitive rabbits (Allen, 1964; Wilson and Clements, 1965; Michaeli, 1967).

In general, information on antibodies involved in arthropod-bite hypersensitivity is meager, and almost nothing is known about their physicochemical and biologic properties.

Cross-reactivity.   An interesting aspect of hypersensitivity to arthropod bites is that of the specificity of the reaction, i.e., the question of whether or not an individual who is already sensitive (or is being sensitized) to bites of a given arthropod species might react or become sensitive to bites of other species. In addition to its clinical importance, specificity (or cross-reactivity) is of interest because it may be related to arthropod phylogenetics.

Since the hypersensitive response to arthropod bites may be manifested by either delayed or immediate (or by both) types of skin reactivity, the term "cross-reactivity" used herein refers to the elicitation of either of the above responses, unless otherwise specified. It should, however, be noted that often when cross-reactivity between two or more arthropod species exists, differences in the type of reactions may be observed (Hecht, 1933; Heilesen, 1949).

A high degree of specificity in hypersensitivity to bed bug bites was reported by Hase (1916), who observed that a human subject, while showing strong immediate reactions to the bites of *Cimex lectularius*, did not react to bites of *Cimex rotundatus*. Usinger (1966), who for three years regularly fed *Cimex lectularius* on himself, tested his reactivity to bites of *Cimex pilosellus*, *Hesperocimex sonorensis*, and *Leptocimex duplicatus*. The two species of *Cimex* showed cross-reactivity, the distantly related *Hesperocimex* also showed cross-reactivity with *Cimex* (except that the immediate reaction elicited by *Hesperocimex* was different in appearance from that elicited by *Cimex*), whereas *Leptocimex* showed no cross-reactivity with *Cimex*. Usinger noted that these reactions corresponded in a general way to the taxonomic relationship of the bugs.

In studying hypersensitivity to bites of fleas, Boycott (1913) reported that a human subject sensitive to *Pulex irritans* did not react to bites of *Xenopsylla cheopis*, and that another subject, sensitive to bites of *Ctenocephalides felis*, did not react to bites of *Nosopsyllus fasciatus*. Subsequent exposures of the subjects to *X. cheopis* and to *N. fasciatus*, respectively, induced sensitization to each of the corresponding species. Furthermore, when thus sensitized, the first subject also reacted to *N. fasciatus* and the second subject also reacted to *X. cheopis*, which indicated cross-reactivity between the latter two species.

Cross-reactivity between bites of *C. felis*, *P. irritans*, and *P. simulans* was demonstrated by B. W. Hudson et al. in man (1960b) and in experimental animals (1960a). Also, guinea pigs sensitized to bites of *C. felis* reacted to challenges given with *X. cheopis*, as well as with *C. felis* (Benjamini, 1967). Since cross-reactivity in guinea pigs was established between *C. felis* and *P. irritans*, cross-reactivity between *C. felis*, *X. cheopis*, and *P. irritans* would be expected (although Boycott's early experiments on humans did not establish cross-reactivity between the latter two species). Dealing with flea bites on humans, Hecht (1943a) demonstrated that although the magnitude of the reactions differed, cross-reactivity existed between *Rhopalopsyllus bohlsi* and *X. cheopis*. From the above data, it appears that cross-reactivity extends not only between species and genera, but even between families of the order Siphonaptera. This cross-reactivity is confined to Siphonaptera, since flea-bite sensitive individuals did not react to the bites of mosquitoes or of bed bugs (Benjamini, unpublished).

Various species of mosquitoes show cross-reactivity with respect to bite reactions (Gordon and Crewe, 1948; Heilesen, 1949; A. Hudson et al., 1958; and others). Though some reports show that the cross-reactivity is confined within species of a given subfamily in the family Culicidae (Heilesen, 1949), other reports extend the cross-reactivity between subfamilies (Hecht, 1933; Brown et al., 1938; McKiel, 1959). In this connection, however, it is interesting to note a case in which a person who was equally sensitive to bites of *Aedes aegypti* and *Culex molestus* lost his reactivity to the bites of *A. aegypti* following repeated exposures to this mosquito, but he did not lose his reactivity to *Culex* (Gordon and Crewe, 1948).

It is apparent that cross-reactivity with respect to bite reactions exists between heterologous species within an order, family, or genus. It is also apparent that cross-reactivity may be expressed either by the elicitation of the same type of reaction (i.e., immediate, delayed, or both) or by the elicitation of different types or magnitudes of reactions. Although differences in size and intensity of reactions may be due to differences in quantity of allergens injected into the host during the bites of the various species, the reasons for differences in the type of reactivity are obscure. A. Hudson et al. (1958) suggested that at least with mosquito bites, specificity may be lost with increases in the duration of sensitization by a given species. The fact that cross-reactivity to bite reactions exists between various arthropod species indicates that the oral secretions of the cross-reacting species contain common or immunologically cross-reacting substances. Perhaps the differences in reactivities observed between cross-reacting species can be explained by the participation in the bite-reaction phenomena of several allergenic substances, some of which are species-specific for a given reaction while others are not.

Cross-reactivity can be demonstrated not only by sensitization and tests given with bites, but also by antigens prepared from various arthropods. It has already been pointed out that individuals can be sensitized to the bites of a given arthropod by injections of various extracts of the arthropod, demonstrating that the extracts contain the allergenic substances involved in the bite reaction. Often, sensitization with extracts of a given arthropod may render the animal sensitive to bites of heterologous species. For example, injections of extracts of the cat flea *C. felis* sensitized guinea pigs not only to bites of *C. felis*, but also to bites of *P. irritans*, *P. simulans*, and *X. cheopis* (Benjamini, 1962). Injecting rabbits with extracts of the mosquito *A. atropalpus* sensitized them to the bites of *A. aegypti* as well as to the bites of the homologous species; injections of extracts of *A. aegypti* sensitized some rabbits to *A. atropalpus*, *A. excrucians*, and *A. flavescens*, but not to *A. campestris*, *A. canadensis*, *A. fitchii*, *A. hexodontus*, *A. nearcticus*, *A. nigripes*, *A. vexans*, *Mansonia perturbans*, or *Culex pipiens* (McKiel, 1959). The latter results could not be correlated on the basis of the taxonomic relationships among these mosquitoes, and they show some degree of species-specificity. Examples of apparent extensive cross-reactivity between species, genera, and families of biting arthropods have been demonstrated in many cases by intradermal tests given with antigens prepared from extracts of a particular arthropod, which elicited skin reactions in animals sensitized with extracts of other arthropods. Also, sera obtained from animals so sensitized reacted with extracts of heterologous species (e.g., Lawlor, 1949; Fox et al., 1963). These experiments indicate that the arthropods tested contained common antigenic components, but they do not necessarily show that these components are actually involved in the bite reaction. The complete absorption of antiserum produced against one species by antigens prepared from another species may suggest that these species also cross-react with respect to allergens involved in the bite reaction (Fox et al., 1963). However, nonprecipitating antibodies may be involved in the bite reactions, so two species may cross-react with respect to bites, although complete absorption will not be achieved.

Cross-reactivity may exist between various developmental stages of the same arthropod species or between its hematophagous and nonhematophagous forms. For example, McKiel (1959) showed that injections of extracts of eggs, larvae, or young pupae of the mosquito *A. aegypti* could not sensitize guinea pigs to bites of the adult female mosquito. However, extracts of older pupae induced sensitization, indicating that the sensitizing substance developed during the late stages of metamorphosis. McKiel also showed that the injections of extracts of the nonhematophagous male mosquito sensitized rabbits to the bites of the female. On the other hand, it was demonstrated that passive cutaneous anaphylaxis could be elicited in guinea pigs which were injected intradermally with serum obtained from a flea-bite sensitive rabbit (sensitized to bites by repeated exposures to the cat flea *C. felis*) and then challenged intravenously with extracts of larvae of this flea (Michaeli, 1967). Similarly, guinea pigs could be sensitized to bites of *C. felis* by injections of extracts of whole larvae or pupae of the flea (Benjamini, 1967). These findings indicate that the immature stages of the flea contain at least one antigenic component in common with the oral secretion of the adult. Unfortunately, in the absence of immunochemical characterization of the allergens present in whole extracts of the insects, it is difficult to relate their immunogenicity with that of the hapten involved in the bite reaction of the adult flea (Benjamini, et al., 1963a; Young et al., 1963). The cross-reactivity witnessed between the various developmental stages of the flea may be associated with this hapten. It should be emphasized, however, that this possibility is strictly speculative and should be investigated experimentally.

Cross-reactivity might also be expressed through the hyposensitization by one species to the bites of another species. Although concrete evidence for hyposensitization to bites of one species by repeated exposures to bites of another species is lacking, it is theoretically conceivable in cases where cross-reactivity to bites of the heterologous species has been demonstrated. Hyposensitization to bites of a given species by injections of extracts prepared from heterologous species have been reported by Benson (1936), Hecht (1943b), and Rockwell and Johnson (1952).

It is difficult to draw precise conclusions or to generalize about the data on cross-reactivity between bites of various species of arthropods. However, it seems that whereas hypersensitivity to the bites of some species is specific, there can be significant cross-reactivity at the species level, which becomes much less notable between genera. The elucidation of the allergens involved and of the type of antibodies associated with the bite reaction will contribute much to our understanding of the mechanisms underlying cross-reactivity and will provide an immunologic basis for understanding the phylogenetic relationships between the species involved.

Hyposensitization. Hyposensitization of man and animals to arthropod bites is of great importance from the clinical point of view. It was pointed out above that individuals can become nonreactive following repeated bites of an arthropod (*see* Tables 1–3, pp. 1068-1071). Loss of host reactivity due to repeated and prolonged exposures to bites has been reported for the body louse (Hase, 1916), for sand flies (Theodor, 1935), for bed bugs (Kemper, 1929), for mosquitoes (Morse, 1897; Mellanby, 1946; Gordon and Crewe, 1948; McKiel, 1955; McKiel and West, 1961b; Allen, 1964; and others), and for fleas (Feingold and Benjamini, 1961). These reports, together with subjective experiences of the loss of reactivity after prolonged residence and repeated exposures to bites of an endemic arthropod in a certain area, point to the inescapable conclusion that some sort of a hyposensitization takes place. A number of subjective reports from veterinarians in the San Francisco Bay area appear to show that the allergic dermatitis of dogs and cats, which is attributed to flea-bite hypersensitivity (Kissileff, 1938, 1962; Muller, 1961), is usually seen in dogs which are hosts to minimal numbers of fleas and which are frequently defleaed, but it is seldom encountered in stray dogs or cats heavily infested with fleas. The twice-weekly exposure of five flea-bite sensitive dogs to cat fleas (200 to 300 fleas) resulted in the induction of a state of nonreactivity in four of the dogs within 2 to 3 months (Benjamini, 1967). Data in Table 2 (*see* p. 1070) show that guinea pigs could be made refractory to bites by repeated exposures to fleas. In this experiment, the state of nonreactivity in some of the guinea pigs lasted for over one year, and it was specific to fleas, since these animals could be sensitized to bites of the mosquito *Aedes aegypti* (Benjamini, 1967).

From a clinical standpoint, hyposensitization by repeated exposure to bites is, of course, impractical. For this reason, numerous workers have attempted hyposensitization via injections of extracts of whole arthropods or extracts derived from various parts of the arthropod. Results of such attempts vary; some workers enthusiastically claim success while others report poor results. Working with patients hypersensitive to flea bites, Cherney et al. (1939) and McIvor and Cherney (1941, 1943) utilized injections of whole extracts of fleas for hyposensitization with seemingly successful results, since the great majority of the patients were relieved. Similar success was reported by Hatoff (1946). In contrast to these results are those of Hartman (1946) and of Feingold and Benjamini (1961), who reported that injections of extracts, even over long periods of time, failed to hyposensitize, and that in some cases the injections even intensified the reactions to bites of fleas. In cases of mosquito-bite hypersensitive humans, injections of mosquito extracts resulted in decreased delayed reactivity but with no change in immediate reactivity (Benson, 1936) or resulted in some temporary relief (Brown et al., 1938; Heilesen, 1949). The most notable feature of the reports on desensitization with extracts is their conflicting claims (McKiel and West, 1961a). This may be due to the fact that in most cases, conclusions were based on subjective reports of patients rather than on controlled tests in which the treated individuals were allowed to be bitten by the arthropod. Such tests are particularly essential for evaluating treatment efficacy in cases of hypersensitivity to arthropods which show seasonal variations in their population density (B. W. Hudson et al., 1960b). Perhaps the enthusiastic reports by the patients of the absence of reactivity is due to the disappearance of the offending arthropod rather than to the efficacy of the treatment.

Data on hyposensitization experiments with laboratory animals indicate that whole extracts may temporarily hyposensitize bite-sensitive animals. Subcutaneous injections of mosquito extracts into bite-sensitive rabbits failed to hyposensitize (Dubin et al., 1948; McKiel and West, 1961b), but intravenous injections of the extract resulted in the nonreactivity of rabbits to bites of the mosquito (McKiel and West, 1961b). Although the state of nonreactivity lasted for 5 days at most, the results of these experiments suggested that the extract contained the antigens necessary to neutralize the antibodies involved in the skin reaction. The latter experiments also showed that hyposensitization to *Aedes aegypti* bites was effected not only with extracts of the homologous species, but also with extracts of some other species of mosquitoes. Similarly, Rockwell and Johnson (1952) reported that a patient was hyposensitized to bites of *Culex pipiens* by injections of *Aedes aegypti* extract.

Speculation about the mechanisms involved in hyposensitization may lead to the hypothesis that it is caused by the neutralization of antibodies with antigens. Hyposensitization following the neutralization of antibodies by antigens is not unique to arthropod bites. However, as with other antigens, the effect is only temporary. Also, the possibility of anaphylaxis must be considered, since McKiel and West (1961b) observed that the injections of antigen resulted in the death of an animal from anaphylactic shock.

It was mentioned earlier (p. 1075) that the haptenic allergenic components found in the oral secretion of cat fleas were stable to heat and to acid hydrolysis. Attempts were made to hyposensitize flea-bite sensitive guinea pigs and dogs by injections of large dosages of collected oral secretion of fleas. Intradermal injections of oral secretion collected from thousands of fleas induced a state of nonreactivity in flea-bite sensitive dogs which lasted for several weeks and, in some cases, for several months (Feingold and Benjamini, 1961; Feingold, 1964; Benjamini, 1967). Similar success was encountered by these workers with flea-bite sensitive guinea pigs. Furthermore, whereas attempts failed to hyposensitize flea-bite sensitive guinea pigs by subcutaneous or intradermal injections of nondialyzable portions of whole extracts of fleas (in fact, sensitivity to bites was intensified), injections over a period of a few weeks of acid hydrolysate of the extract (6 N HCl for 24 hours at 110°C) induced hyposensitization lasting several weeks (Michaeli, 1967). These results of hyposensitization with haptenic portions are encouraging, especially in view of the fact that the injections of haptens were incapable of sensitizing animals to bites (unless, of course, these haptens were conjugated or associated with proteins) and they did not elicit reactions in the sensitive animals. Whether or not similar hyposensitization would be possible in cases of hypersensitivity to other arthropods remains to be investigated.

Hyposensitization by injections of massive dosages of antigens or haptens is probably achieved through neutralization of antibodies, a mechanism different from that associated with blocking antibodies which neutralize antigen. It is conceivable that the successful results which were reported by McIvor and Cherney (1941, 1943), Hatoff (1946), and others on hyposensitization by injections of relatively minute amounts of antigen prepared from the arthropod (*see* p. 1083) may have been achieved through blocking antibodies which neutralize the antigen prior to its reacting with skin-sensitizing antibodies. However, except for the example given earlier (p. 1079) in which the presence of blocking antibodies was implicated in serum of an individual who was hyposensitized by repeated exposures to bites (Rockwell and Johnson, 1952), the involvement of blocking antibodies in hyposensitization to arthropod bites has not been demonstrated.

The area of hyposensitization to arthropod bites provides fertile ground for investigation. This, however, is hampered by the lack of information on the antigens and antibodies which are involved in the hypersensitive reaction. The elucidation of these factors will greatly facilitate an intelligent approach to hyposensitization. The study of cross-reactivities in response to bites of several arthropods, as discussed earlier (pp. 1079-1083), will perhaps result in defining common antigenic determinants. Then, hyposensitization to bites of one arthropod species by administration of immunologically active components from other species might be achieved.

Hypersensitivity to arthropod bites and its possible
    relation to arthropod-borne infections

It is well-established that hematophagous arthropods serve as vectors of numerous diseases and that one of the most important routes for the introduction of pathogens into the host is via the oral secretion of the arthropod. It is evident from the preceding discussion that the deposition of oral secretion into the host may result in local and systemic reactions which may be due to toxic and/or allergenic substances. Of primary interest to the present discussion is the fact that a variety of cellular local responses may be elicited by the bites of a given arthropod and that such reactions are the manifestation of hypersensitivity to the bites, the response more or less corresponding

Table 4

Arthropod Vectors of Human and Animal Pathogens
and the Allergic Responses in the Vertebrate Host

Arthropod Vectors	Pathogen Transmitted					Histopathology			
	Virus	Rick-ettsia	Proto-zoa	Bac-teria	Hel-minth	Hemor-rhage	Edema	Vasodi-lation	Ne-crosis
Culicidae	+	−	+	−	+	+	+	+	−
Phlebotomus	+	−	+	+	−	+	+	−	−
Simulidae	−	−	+	−	+	+	+	+	−
Tabanidae	−	−	−	+	+	+	+	−	−
Glossina	−	−	+	−	−	+	+	+	−
Pediculus	−	+	−	+	−	−	+	+	−
Triatominae	−	−	+	−	−	+	+	−	−
Siphonaptera	−	+	+	+	+	−	+	+	−
Acarina	+	+	+	+	+	+	+	+	+

Adapted from Kartman. 1965. *Zoonoses Research*, 4.

to the state of sensitivity of the individual. Thus, the bite of an arthropod may have a dual function: It may infect the host with pathogens which will be deposited into the bite area, from where they will then be disseminated, and it can produce cellular responses at the vicinity of the bite area. These two functions may not be related; the vector may deposit pathogens into a host which has never before been exposed to its bites, or a noninfected arthropod may bite the host, which, if sensitive, will react to the bite as previously described. On the other hand, an infective vector may bite a host having sensitivity to bites induced by previous exposures. This new bite will result in the deposition of pathogens into the bite area and in the manifestation of a response to allergenic materials in the oral secretion. Such a bite may, therefore, result in the deposition of pathogens into a cellular milieu that immediately becomes different from that into which pathogens are introduced when a non-bite-sensitive host is infected.

On theoretical grounds, the question may be asked as to what effect the cellular differences will have on the introduced pathogen. These differences may not have an effect, in which case infectivity and dissemination will proceed in the same manner as it would in the non-bite-sensitive host. However, the cellular milieu may have a profound effect on the pathogen's further development and dissemination, creating the possibility of a relationship between hypersensitivity and disease transmission. Such a relationship, if it exists, may be of fundamental importance from the standpoint of a host-parasite relationship, since its effect may influence the survival and virulence of the pathogen.

The hypothesis that a relation exists between bite-hypersensitivity and disease transmission has been proposed by some workers, notably Gordon and Crewe (1948), and has recently been given attention by Kartman (1964,

Table 4

Arthropod Vectors of Human and Animal Pathogens
and the Allergic Responses in the Vertebrate Host

Cutaneous Response of Host to Injected Saliva

Histopathology			Symptoms								
Poly-morphs	Lym-pho-cytes	Histio-cytes	Wheal	Papule	Eryth-ema	Bulla	Lym-phad-enitis	Fever, local	Fever, general	Ana-phy-laxis	Paral-ysis
+	+	+	+	+	+	+	−	+	−	+	−
+	−	−	+	+	+	+	+	+	−	−	−
+	−	−	+	−	+	+	−	−	−	−	−
−	−	+	+	−	+	−	−	−	−	−	−
+	+	−	+	+	+	+	−	−	+	+	−
−	−	−	+	+	+	+	+	−	+	+	−
−	−	−	+	+	+	+	−	−	−	+	−
+	+	+	+	+	+	+	+	+	+	−	+

Adapted from Kartman. 1965. *Zoonoses Research*, 4.

1965). Although it is still a tentative hypothesis awaiting confirmation, it is felt that there is enough suggestive evidence for it to merit discussion.

The gross symptomatology and histopathology in the hypersensitive response to bites of several arthropods, together with pathogens which may be transmitted by these arthropods, is shown in Table 4, from which several examples to illustrate the possible relationship between hypersensitivity and infectivity will be taken.

An excellent example given by Kartman (1965) is that of the flea-rodent relationship in the epidemiology of plague. As mentioned earlier, there is a definite sequence in the skin reactivity of guinea pigs in response to repeated exposures to bites of fleas, and that different stages in this sequence are attended by a variety of cellular infiltrations in the vicinity of the bite area. Depending on the state of reactivity of the animal, the bites may elicit no skin reactions (either because the animal had not been sensitized or because it was hyposensitized), they may cause an intense monocytic dermal infiltration (as in delayed reactions), or they may result in an eosinophilic infiltration (immediate reactions). It has long been thought that a major factor in host reaction to the introduction of *Pasteurella pestis* via a flea is the cellular response at the bite site. The work of Cavanaugh and Randall (1959) on the role of mononuclear phagocytes in the pathogenesis of plague demonstrated that virulent *P. pestis* bacilli transmitted by blocked fleas are of the noncapsulated, phagocytosis-sensitive type. The bacilli which escape ingestion and destruction by neutrophils find a favorable environment and multiply within mononuclear phagocytes. Upon their release from ruptured monocytes, the bacilli are encapsulated and are then phagocytosis-resistant. More recent work showed that although resistance to phagocytosis is not necessarily the sole factor determining the virulence of *P. pestis*, the most critical factor in virulence is the intracellular survival and multiplication of the bacilli after phagocytosis (Janssen et al., 1963).

From the above descriptions, it is apparent that two seemingly distinct phenomena, i.e., that of the hypersensitive response to the bite and that of infectivity, may be operating concurrently. *P. pestis* may be inoculated into a cellular milieu which may be governed by the degree of hypersensitivity of the host to allergenic components in the oral secretion of the flea.

It has been shown (United States Public Health Service, 1966) that some *P. pestis* organisms may be found localized at the deposition site for as long as several days following injection. These organisms will be surrounded within 12 to 24 hours by an intense monocytic dermal infiltration associated with the delayed hypersensitivity to the bite. The effect of monocytes on *P. pestis* is particularly likely in cases where the blocked flea feeds from a pool of blood (which favors the localization of pathogens at the bite site) rather than directly from a capillary (which favors their introduction into the blood stream). When *P. pestis* is inoculated into a host showing immediate-type skin reactivity to the bite, the organism will be encountered within minutes by eosinophils, which predominate during this type of skin response. The effect of eosinophils on *P. pestis*, or for that matter the function of eosinophils in general, is still debatable. Although years ago eosinophils were reported to be able to phagocytize microorganisms (Weinberg and Sequin, 1914), recent experiments suggest that their possible role in the immune response is to be attracted to and to phagocytize antigen-antibody complexes (*see* Samter, 1965; Litt, 1964 for reviews). It is known, however, that during an immediate reaction caused by the interaction of antigen and antibody, there are many chemical changes which take place (e.g., the release of histamine). It is totally unknown what effects, if any, these changes have on the pathogen's development.

Another example of a possible relationship between hypersensitivity and infectivity given by Kartman (1965) is that of the cellular responses elicited by mosquitoes and the transmission of malaria by these hematophagous insects. From Rockwell and Johnson's (1952) evaluation of the reactions of humans sensitive to mosquito bites (both immediate and delayed skin reactions), it appears that a variety of cells are associated with the bite reaction. Skin sections taken following the bite showed perivascular infiltration of neutrophils, eosinophils, lymphocytes, and plasma cells. Biopsies taken 6 hours, 24 hours, 2 days, and 5 days following the bite showed a progressive increase in the proportion of lymphocytes and histiocytes, with some neutrophils and eosinophils. Regarding the infectivity of avian malaria parasites, several workers have shown that these are dependent on cells of lymphoid origin for development (Bray, 1957; Kikuth and Mudrow, 1939a, b). Thus, when the vector bites a reactive individual, the presence of various cellular components may affect the development and survival of the parasites, as compared to their fate when introduced by bites on a nonreactive host.

The reaction of allergic individuals to bites of hematophagous arthropods is not only manifested by cellular responses, but also by scratching, rubbing, biting, and so forth. Kartman (1965) points out that these latter responses may aid in causing infectivity by pathogens which are released when the body of the vector is crushed against the skin of the host or when pathogens are deposited on the surface of the skin.

Another example given by Kartman (1965) is the acquired immunity of animals to ticks. Trager (1939a, b, 1940) reported that animals can become immune to tick infestation either by exposures to the arthropods or by injections of extracts. This immunity depends on the presence of circulating antibodies that accelerate local cellular invasions, which in turn wall off the tick larvae from normal feeding (see p. 1112). The fact that animals could thus become immune to infestation is of particular importance from an epidemiologic point of view, when infestation by infected arthropods may result in zoonoses. It is possible that the immunity of the host to the vector arthropod may account in part for the absence of infection or disease in certain animals in areas abounding with an infected vector.

The preceding were but a few examples providing circumstantial evidence for the possible relation between infectivity and the immune response to the bites of arthropod vectors. Other examples can be found which suggest that a correlation may exist between hypersensitivity to bites of an arthropod vector and the transmission by the vector of rickettsial, protozoan, bacterial, or other infectious agents. The hypothesis was presented here with the hope that it will stimulate medical entomologic research in this direction. A connection between infectivity and hypersensitivity, if it indeed exists, may be of tremendous medical importance.

Immunity to toxic substances deposited during the bite

Unless it is complicated by hypersensitivity, the injury caused by the mechanical action of the mouth parts during arthropod bites is minor, and the deposition of oral secretion into a nonsensitive host does not usually elicit reactions. There are, however, certain arthropods, nonparasitic on mammals, which may occasionally bite mammals, primarily in self-defense and frequently with disastrous results to the bitten individual. Such biting arthropods, e.g., some spiders, are normally predators on other arthropods. They contain chemicals in their oral secretion which are used for paralyzing or killing their prey and for its partial digestion prior to ingestion.

The oral secretion of spiders is complex and contains a multiplicity of compounds, some of which have been implicated in its venomous activity (see Welsh, 1964, for a review). Many nonproteinaceous materials, such as histamine and tertiary ammonium compounds, which are present in venoms of numerous arthropods, are probably also present in the venoms of spiders. Such compounds are assumed to have a defensive role, since they are powerful pain producers. Serotonin, which occurs in secretions of many invertebrates, was found in the venom of five species of spiders (Welsh, 1964). No evidence exists that serotonin contributes directly to the toxicity of the venom; indirectly, however, serotonin may contribute to the overall effect of the venom by increasing capillary permeability and blood flow, thereby facilitating the spread of neurotoxic and cytotoxic components of the venom.

Of the numerous species of spiders, only a few are known to cause reactions in man and other mammals. Of these, the more familiar are the black widow spider and related species belonging to the genus *Latrodectus*, and the recluse spider and related species belonging to the genus *Loxosceles*. Other spiders associated with poisonous effects include members of the genera *Atrax, Phoneutria, Chiracanthium,* and *Lycosa* (Herms and James, 1961). Recently, the species *Steatoda paykulliana* has been found to be poisonous to mammals (Maretić et al., 1964).

Spider venoms may produce a dual reaction, i.e., cytotoxic and neurotoxic. Although a distinction according to this basis cannot be absolute, the venoms are usually classified by their dominant effect (Horen, 1963).

Latrodectus **venom.** The action of the venom of *Latrodectus* is primarily neurotoxic. The rapidity with which this venom is distributed throughout the body of the victim was demonstrated by Maretić and Stanic (1954) and by Lebez et al. (1965). Using P^{32}-labeled venom, the latter workers showed that within 3 minutes the venom spread throughout the body with significant amounts of it present in the cerebellum and peripheral nerves. The venom primarily affects the spinal cord, and a variety of symptoms, such as rigidity and muscle spasm, may be induced. Other symptoms may include a rise in body temperature, increase in blood pressure, leukocytosis, increase in pressure of spinal fluid, profuse perspiration, and nausea. Mortality ranges from 4 to 5 percent in diagnosed cases (Herms and James, 1961). Pathologic studies revealed the involvement of the liver, kidneys, spleen, lymph nodes, thymus, and adrenals. For descriptions of the clinical and pathologic effects of *Latrodectus* venom, the reader is directed to articles by Marzan (1955), D'Amour et al. (1936), Macchiavello (1947a, b), Sampayo (1943), Pirosky and Abalos (1963), Maretić and Stanic (1954), and Wiener (1961d).

Great variations exist in the susceptibility of mammals to the venom of *Latrodectus* (Maretić and Stanic, 1954). The most sensitive laboratory animal is the mouse, which can be killed by a single bite within 10 to 20 minutes; guinea pigs may be killed within 1 to 2 hours, rats and kittens within 24 hours. Rabbits are fairly resistant and can be killed only by several bites, dying several days after the bites. Dogs are quite resistant, since four to six spider bites caused no mortality in four dogs tested. Turtles and lizards are also resistant to large doses of the venom.

The potency of *Latrodectus* venom can be influenced by a variety of factors. Differences were reported for *Latrodectus* venom collected in the western United States during July and during October (D'Amour et al., 1936). Seasonal variation in toxicity to white mice has been demonstrated by Keegan et al. (1960), who found that the highest toxicity (as indicated by a fraction of cephalothorax required for LD_{50}) was exhibited in November (LD_{50} caused by 0.33 and 0.23 cephalothoraces), whereas the lowest toxicity (LD_{50} caused by 3.29 and 2.45 cephalothoraces) was exhibited during the months of April and May. Vellard (1936) reported changes in the pH of the venom with temperature. At temperatures above 25°C, it is alkaline and more toxic, whereas at lower temperatures it is acidic and less toxic. Drying the venom greatly reduces its toxicity, and incubation for 7 days at 36 to 37°C in the presence of 0.1 percent formalin causes inactivation (Maksianovich, 1939).

Work on the identification of the toxicants contained in *Latrodectus* venom has been reviewed by Welsh (1964) and by Frontali and Grasso (1964). Recent findings by the latter revealed that the toxicity of the venom to the housefly and to the guinea pig was approximately the same when expressed in terms of LD_{50} per unit body weight. Using electrophoresis and chromatography, Frontali and Grasso were able to separate three proteinaceous components from extracts of poison glands: one producing quick paralysis in the housefly (LV_1), one producing slow paralysis in the fly (LV_2), and one (LV_3) which produced in guinea pigs the characteristic symptoms of *Latrodectus* poisoning. The first two proteins $(LV_1$ and $LV_2)$ were relatively labile to heat (26°C cause 50 percent inactivation within 6 hours), whereas the third protein (LV_3) was stable at 26°C for at least 24 hours. The size of all three proteins, as estimated by gel filtration, was similar to that of hemoglobin (molecular weight 67,000). Neither LV_1 nor LV_2 seemed to depend on metallic ions for function, and both apparently needed several intact sulfhydryl bonds for their activity, since their inactivation by heat could be protected by 2 to 4×10^{-4} M mercaptoethanol; 5×10^{-3} M mercaptoethanol, however, almost completely abolished their activity. The physicochemical characterization of the LV_3 fraction, which apparently is the important fraction with respect to mammalian toxicity, awaits elucidation. However, from this report and from earlier reports by D'Amour et al. (1936), Sampayo (1943), and others, it is apparent that the substance or substances responsible for mammalian toxicity of *Latrodectus* venom are proteinaceous.

The proteinaceous nature of the venom of various species of *Latrodectus* has enabled many workers to obtain, from various animals, antibodies capable of neutralizing the toxic action of the venom. This neutralizing activity is generally standardized on the basis of the number of lethal dosages of venom for a given animal which a given volume of antiserum can neutralize. This has been further standardized in terms of antivenom units, each unit defined as the amount of antivenom able to neutralize one average, usually lethal dose when the antivenom and venom are injected simultaneously into the mouse. Another standard for the neutralizing potency of the antiserum is the number of milligrams of venom which can be neutralized by 1 ml of antiserum. This standardization depends on the specific activity of the venom (LD_{50} per mg), which must always be considered since several methods are employed for the preparation of venom and its potency has been shown to vary.

The activity of different anti-*Latrodectus* sera obtained by various workers from various animals was compared by Sampayo (1943). From this comparison it appears that whereas the neutralizing activity of antisera obtained by early workers was relatively low, those obtained by Pirosky et al. (1942) and by Sampayo (1943) were active to the extent that 1 ml of antiserum protected 50 percent of white mice against 3,000 minimal lethal doses of *L. mactans*.

The preparation of antigen for the production of antiserum to *Latrodectus* venom and the immunization procedures vary. A procedure employed by Maksianovich (1939), utilized saline extract of the poison glands of *L. tredecimguttatus*. The toxic activity of the extract was inactivated by incubation for seven days at 37°C in the presence of 0.1 percent formalin. The antiserum produced by the injection of the preparation was capable of neutralizing the toxic action of the venom. The antigenic properties of this anatoxin were fully retained even after a year's storage in the refrigerator.

Pirosky et al. (1942) used suspensions of the cephalothorax of *Latrodectus mactans* as antigen. The antiserum obtained from an immunized horse was fractionated by precipitation with sodium sulfate and by digestion with pepsin. The resulting preparation had a high neutralizing capacity. This was confirmed by Sampayo (1943) and by Finlayson and Hollow (1945).

A potent antigen which induced neutralizing antibodies within a relatively short period of immunization was produced by Wiener (1956), who adsorbed *Latrodectus hasseltii* venom onto aluminum phosphate and used the complex for injection. Venom obtained from a relatively small number of spiders, when thus adsorbed, produced potent antivenom. The efficacy of this antivenom was shown by Wiener and Fraser (1956) in a case of a human bitten by *Latrodectus hasseltii*: Forty-eight hours after the bite, when the patient suffered severe pain and showed symptoms of toxicity, 1 ml of the antivenom administered intramuscularly caused the complete disappearance of pain with no recurrence. Wiener (1961b) later reported results on anti-*Latrodectus hasseltii* horse serum which, following fractionation and digestion with pepsin, exhibited the high neutralizing activity of 3,900 units (one unit, as defined by Wiener, being the amount of serum required to neutralize 0.01 mg of venom). Since, according to Wiener, the mean weight of venom obtained from the venom glands of one spider is 0.12 mg and in 99 out of 100 spiders the venom yield per spider is not expected to exceed 0.29 mg, the specific activity of the horse antiserum which was produced (sufficient to neutralize 39 mg of venom) should be more than sufficient to neutralize the venom introduced by one bite.

Successful treatment of patients with anti-*Latrodectus* serum has been accomplished numerous times with antivenom produced and available in most parts of the world (Keegan, 1956).

Venoms obtained from different species of *Latrodectus* share common antigenic determinants, thus antiserum against the venom of one species can neutralize the toxic action of the venoms of other species. This cross-reactivity does not necessarily mean that the venoms of the cross-reacting species are identical, but it does point to similarities, at least with respect to the antigenic toxins. The immunologic cross-reactivity, or paraspecificity, was first demonstrated by Finlayson (1936), who showed that anti-*L. indis-*

tinctus also neutralized the venom of *L. geometricus*. Subsequently, it was shown that anti-*L. mactans* neutralized the venom of *L. indistinctus* (Finlayson and Hollow, 1945), and that anti-*L. tredecimguttatus* neutralized venoms of *L. mactans* and of *L. hasseltii* (Keegan, 1955). Further work by McCrone and Netzloff (1965) showed immunologic cross-reactivity among *L. mactans*, *L. variolus*, *L. bishopi*, and *L. geometricus*—immunodiffusion between anti-*L. mactans* and *L. variolus* showed antigenic determinants common to all the species tested, and the antiserum neutralized the venoms of these species. From a therapeutic standpoint, it is fortunate that cross-reactivity with respect to venom neutralization has been demonstrated among all the *Latrodectus* species thus far tested.

Loxosceles venom. The action of the venom of various species of *Loxosceles* is primarily cytotoxic, leading to necrosis and, in more severe cases, to leukopenia and hemolytic anemia. Local reactions include severe pain, bleb formation, erythema, ecchymosis, necrosis, and ulceration. Although the action of this venom is more localized than that of *Latrodectus*, systemic reactions may occur, which include fever, nausea, malaise, and thrombocytopenia. This type of arachnidism, also called necrotic arachnidism or loxoscelism, may result in extremely severe reactions, and in some cases, particularly in children, it may be fatal. For excellent descriptions of reactions to *Loxosceles*, the reader is referred to articles by Atkins et al. (1958), Dillaha et al. (1963, 1964), Mackinnon and Witkind (1953), Macchiavello (1947a, b), Schenone and Prats (1961), and Lessenden and Zimmer (1960). The species of *Loxosceles* associated with cutaneous arachnidism are *L. laeta* in South America and *L. reclusus* in the United States.

There is very little reported work on the isolation and physicochemical characterization of the venom of *Loxosceles*. Experiments by Macchiavello (1947b) showed that the glandular poison of *L. laeta* was not hemolytic for rabbit or guinea pig erythrocytes, whereas extract of the cephalothorax of the same species exhibited such activity. Experiments by Denny et al. (1964) demonstrated that extract of the poison glands of *L. reclusus* or pure venom (obtained directly from the spider after electrical stimulation) exhibited a marked hemolytic action. These authors suggested that this action may be enzymatic in nature and similar to the hemolytic nature of lecithinase-A activity of snake venom. Preliminary experiments by these authors indicated that the venom of the spider could cleave lecithin into two fractions and that the activity of the venom was lost by heating, which suggest that activity is associated with proteinaceous enzymatic action.

Although antibodies have not yet been demonstrated in human victims of loxoscelism, they have been demonstrated in experimental animals following exposures to bites or following injections of venom. Antiserum prepared by hyperimmunization of a rabbit with multiple subcutaneous injections of the venom was able to inhibit the *in vitro* hemolytic action of the venom (Denny et al., 1964). Also, the lethal effect of the venom on mice could be neutralized with immune serum. Mackinnon and Witkind (1953) reported that a rabbit became immunized to *Loxosceles laeta* after 6 to 14 bites, and that the rabbit antisera protected mice against at least one minimal lethal dose of venom, whereas sera prepared against venoms of *Lycosa*, *Phoneutria*, or *Latrodectus* had no protective effect against the venom of *Loxosceles*.

Neutralization of the venom by antibodies can be achieved by the association of the antibodies with the active site (or sites) of the molecule, in which case these sites must contain antigenic determinants. On the other hand, neutralization may be achieved through the association of antibodies with antigenic areas other than these sites, in which case neutralization may be conferred either through steric hindrance by the antibody between the active molecule and receptor, or through conformational changes of the molecule following association with antibody.

Atrax venom. There is, however, a case of resistance, or immunity, to a spider bite which is probably not through neutralizing antibodies, since the venom of the particular spider is nonproteinaceous and nonantigenic, and since neutralizing antibodies have never been demonstrable. The case in point is the resistance to the venom of *Atrax* spiders.

The medical problems caused by the bites of *Atrax robustus* in Australia and work on the effects of the venom and on its chemistry have been reviewed by Wiener (1961c, 1963). Attempts by Wiener to produce neutralizing antibodies in several animal species failed. Subsequent work (Wiener, 1961d) demonstrated that the majority of the toxic components of the venom possessed the properties of decomposition products of proteins, such as proteoses, peptones, and polypeptides. Moreover, some of the toxic components did not even contain aminoacids and others had the properties of organic acids. The toxicity of the venom was heat-stable, dialyzable, and resistant to the action of acid and pepsin, but it was reduced when the venom was heated in the presence of 0.1 N NaOH, or when treated with trypsin. It was destroyed by potassium permanganate, iodine, or hydrogen peroxide.

Injections of the venom into a horse, sheep, rabbits, and guinea pigs did not result in the production of neutralizing antibodies. Some precipitating (but not neutralizing) antibodies which were witnessed in several instances were probably directed against some nontoxic components of the venom. Nevertheless, guinea pigs which were injected several times with increasing dosages of the venom could tolerate approximately twice as much venom as those which were never injected (10.5 mg and 6 mg, respectively), but no neutralizing antibodies could be detected in the sera of the more resistant animals (Wiener, 1963). A similar type of resistance was shown to occur in the horse following repeated injections of increasing amounts of venom and again no detectable neutralizing antibodies were found (Wiener, 1963). These results point to some sort of resistance which is perhaps not mediated by an antibody response. The nature of this resistance is open for speculation. Wiener points out that it may be due to the development of tolerance by normally susceptible cells, or due to the elaboration of an enzyme (or enzymes) capable of detoxifying the venom to a limited extent.

An interesting aspect connected with *Atrax* venom is its neutralization by the hemolymph of the spider (the neutralization of other spider venoms by their own hemolymph has been demonstrated by Vellard, 1936). One-half milliliter of hemolymph incubated at 37°C for 30 minutes with 2, 4, and 8 mouse-LD_{50} dosages of spider venom completely neutralized the toxic action in mice. However, such neutralization could be achieved only following *in vitro* incubation; the injections of more than 20 times the amount of hemo-lymph capable of neutralizing *in vitro* a given dose of venom failed to protect a mouse from the lethal effect of a similar amount of venom (Wiener, 1961a). The hemolymph was not toxic to mice. The neutralizing activity was heat-labile, which suggested to Wiener that it could be due to an enzyme. Al-though no neutralizing effect could be demonstrated *in vivo*, Wiener points out the necessity for further studies on the *in vitro* neutralizing activity, which may lead to isolation and concentration of a neutralizing factor and ultimately to its potential use for the *in vivo* neutralization of the apparently nonantigenic *Atrax* venom.

IMMUNITY TO ARTHROPOD STINGS

Stinging arthropods are those belonging to Class Insecta, Order Hyme-noptera (bees, wasps, ants), and to Class Arachnida, Order Scorpionidae (scorpions). These stinging animals include parasites, predators, and some phytophagous arthropods. They possess powerful venoms which serve to par-alyze the host, to kill the prey, and/or to inflict painful stings in self-defense. This section is concerned primarily with the response and immunity of mam-mals to the stings of these arthropods. The responses of invertebrates to such stings have recently been reviewed by Beard (1963).

Generally, the venoms are ineffectual unless they are injected into the animal. Scorpions and the females of some Hymenoptera species have an aculeus or stinger for the injection of venom. The stinger of the Hymenop-tera consists of a modified ovipositor situated in the caudal segments of the arthropod. It consists of a piercing apparatus with its appendages, the venom glands, and the venom sac. The apex of the stinger in some Hymenoptera (honeybees, for example) is barbed so that following a sting, the stinger and the venom sac are forcibly detached from the insect's body and remain in the victim. This generally causes the death of the insect, and accounts for the fact that honeybees can ordinarily sting only once. In other Hymenoptera (wasps, hornets, ants, and some bees) the apex of the stinger is smooth and can easily be withdrawn after a sting, hence multiple consecutive stings can be administered. Those Hymenoptera which kill their prey by stinging pos-sess two poison glands: an acid gland and an alkaline gland, which secrete acidic and basic substances, respectively, the mixed product constituting the active venom. Hymenopterous insects which sting in order to paralyze the prey possess only acid glands.

The stinger of scorpions is situated in the terminal segment of the body.

It contains a pair of venom glands which, through fine ducts, empty at the apex of the stinger. During the actual stinging process, the stinger curves upward and is thrust forward over and beyond the scorpion's body and head. Details on the morphology and action of the stinging apparatus of Hymenoptera and scorpions are given by Herms and James (1961), Savory (1964), Cloudsley-Thompson (1958), Stahnke (1966), and others.

Immunity to stings of scorpions is normally due to neutralization of the toxic action of the venom, whereas immunity to stinging Hymenoptera is normally due to the development of hypersensitivity to chemicals introduced during the sting. For this reason, immunity to Hymenoptera stings and immunity to scorpion stings will be treated separately.

Hymenoptera stings

It has been long-known that the venoms of hymenopterous insects contain various substances which exhibit pharmacologic activity in both invertebrates and vertebrates. The effects of the venom on invertebrates have recently been reviewed by Beard (1963). Most of the studies on hymenopteran venom, however, have been concerned with its effect on mammals. The venoms studied were chiefly those of the honeybee (*Apis mellifera*), wasps (e.g., yellowjackets, hornets, and paper wasps, belonging to the genera *Vespula*, *Vespa*, *Polistes*, *Sceliphron*, and *Dolichovespula*), and stinging ants (primarily those belonging to the genus *Selenopsis*). Results of these investigations have been the subject of numerous communications and review articles, such as those by Hodgson (1955), Kaiser and Michl (1958), Pavan (1958), Beard (1963), and Haberman (1965).

There have been many studies on the composition and activity of bee and wasp venoms. These have been reviewed by Schachter and Thain, 1954; Jaques and Schachter, 1954; Holdstock et al., 1957; Mathias and Schachter, 1958; Pavan, 1958; Bhoola et al., 1961; Mohammed and Zaki, 1961; O'Connor and Rosenbrook, 1963; O'Connor et al., 1964; Rosenbrook and O'Connor, 1964; Langlois et al., 1965a; Shulman et al., 1966a; and others. It appears that some, but not all, of the pharmacologically active substances are shared by bees and wasps. The venoms of the honeybee *A. mellifera* and of the wasps *Vespa vulgaris* and *Vespa crabro* have been studied extensively by Haberman, Neumann, and co-workers, and these studies have been recently summarized by Haberman (1965). It has been found that the venom of all three groups contains histamine. In addition to histamine, the venom of both *V. vulgaris* and *V. crabro* contains serotonin and that of *V. crabro* also contains acetylcholine. All three venoms contain phospholipase-A, the wasps' venoms contain phospholipase-B, and the venoms of *Apis* and *V. vulgaris* contain hyaluronidase. In addition to these enzymatic proteins, pharmacologically active peptides are found in the venoms: that of the bee contains melittin and apamin, whereas those of the wasps contain kinins. From the chromatographic studies reported by Haberman (1965), it appears that these chemicals constitute the major portion of the venom peptides and proteins. The presence of lipase in bee venom has also been implicated (Vazquez-Colon and Elliott, 1966). Since histamine, serotonin, and some tertiary amines are commonly found in animal venom (Buckley and Porges, 1956; Welsh, 1964), it is not very surprising that they have been discovered in the venoms of a variety of arthropods.

The pharmacologic properties of the hymenopteran venom peptides and proteins are summarized by Haberman (1965). Melittin, which seems to be the major component (by weight) of bee venom, causes local pain and inflammation. It is a powerful hemolysin, and it liberates histamine and serotonin from mast cells and thrombocytes, respectively. Melittin increases capillary permeability and blocks synaptic transmission; it causes smooth muscle contraction and may affect oxidative phosphorylation. Thus, melittin appears to have broad pharmacologic activity. The LD_{50} of melittin in mice is 3 to 4 mg per kg of body weight. Investigations of the physicochemical properties of melittin revealed that it is a slowly dialyzing, basic peptide having a molecular weight of approximately 3,000, but it apparently exists in solution as the tetramer (Haberman and Jentsch, 1966).

Apamin, a minor component (by weight) of bee venom increases vascular permeability of the rat cutis and affects the central nervous system in mice, rats, and rabbits. The LD_{50} of apamin is approximately 4 mg per kg of body weight in mice and 2 mg per kg in rats. Death is preceded by extreme hyperexcitation and convulsions. Gel-filtration studies revealed that apamin is of relatively low molecular weight (lower than that of melittin). Like melittin, apamin is strongly basic (Haberman, 1965).

Phospholipase-A, a slowly dialyzable enzyme, is present in many animal venoms. It is again not surprising to find this enzyme in the venoms of bees and wasps. Phospholipase-A is hemolytic, lowers blood pressure, excites smooth muscles, increases capillary permeability, and inhibits succinic dehydrogenase and oxidative phosphorylation. The hemolytic effect of the enzyme is based on the conversion of lecithin to lysolecithin, a powerfully hemolytic substance. Whereas phospholipase-A removes the unsaturated fatty acids, phospholipase-B hydrolyzes both unsaturated and saturated acids from lecithin.

Like phospholipase-A, hyaluronidase is present in many venoms of animals (Favilli, 1956; Jacques. 1956). Apparently, this enzyme facilitates the spreading of other pharmacologically active components of the venom by the break-down of hyaluronic acid in the tissue.

The kinins present in wasps' venoms are pharmacologically active polypeptides which are slowly dialyzable. (Schachter and Thain, 1954). Unlike histamine, serotonin, or acetylcholine (which elicit rapid contractions of smooth muscles), the kinins produce a characteristic delayed slow contraction. The characterization of kinins of some hymenopteran venoms is reviewed by Schachter (1963). From physicochemical characterizations, it appears that kinins obtained from different wasps are chemically, and perhaps also pharmacologically, different. For example, kinin obtained from *V.*

crabro is resistant to inactivation by trypsin, and is less active than the trypsin-susceptible kinin of *V. vulgaris* (Schachter, 1963).

Recent work by O'Connor and Rosenbrook (1963) on the characterization of the venom of the mud-dauber wasp *Sceliphron caementarium* (which was obtained by electrical excitation of the insect) revealed an unexpected relatively low protein content, and the absence of histamine, serotonin, and acetylcholine. The author correlated the absence of these chemicals with the small pain produced by the stings of mud-dauber wasps. Subsequent work by Rosenbrook and O'Connor (1964) revealed 17 nonprotein constituents, including histidine, methionine, pipecolic acid, and a lecithin-like compound. In view of the presence of such large numbers of compounds in the venom, these authors suggested that venom activity is perhaps based on the cooperative or synergistic effect of all or most of these components.

Information on the venoms of stinging ants is rather meager. There are, however, a few reports on the physicochemical and pharmacologic properties of venoms from several species of ants. Reports by Blum and co-workers (1958, 1960) on the properties of the venom of the fire ant *Solenopsis saevissima* indicated that unlike the venom of other stinging insects, the venom of this ant is insoluble in water but soluble in most organic solvents. It is nonproteinaceous, but it does contain nitrogen. Its light-absorption spectrum has no peak in the ultraviolet region, hence it is nonaromatic. Infrared analyses indicated that it contains aliphatic hydrocarbons with methyl or methylene groups, and possibly ether linkages. The venom exhibits antibiotic and insecticidal activity, the latter being at least as powerful as DDT. Studies by Caro et al. (1957) indicated that the venom contains a necrotizing factor. A hemolytic component of the venom was isolated by Adrouny et al. (1959) and was shown to be an amine. Recent work by Blum (1963) on the venom of the ant *Pseudomyrmex pallidus* revealed that it is an alkaloidal colorless liquid which solidifies on exposure to air, methanol, chloroform, hexane, or ether. The venom of *Myrmecia gulosa* was characterized by Cavili et al. (1964). Unlike that of the fire ant, the venom of this stinging ant is proteinaceous, and it contains hyaluronidase, a hemolytic factor, kinin, and histamine. The composition of this venom seems to have the general chemical characteristics of the venoms of bees and wasps.

Reaction to stings. Unless complicated by hypersensitivity, local reactions to the stings of Hymenoptera are not severe. The mechanical action of the sting itself is rather mild, and the pain experienced with the sting is due to the introduced venom. Local reactions of man to Hymenoptera stings have been described by many workers. The description of Marshall (1957) may serve as an example: The sting may produce a sharp pain lasting for a few minutes; it is usually slight but can occasionally be severe. Erythema, edema, and some pruritus may ensue, but these symptoms usually disappear within 24 hours. However, if the sting is inflicted in the region of the mouth or throat, edema may cause a blockage of the air passage, which in turn may be fatal unless tracheotomy is performed. Stings of scavenger wasps may result in secondary infections. Histologic studies of lesions produced 1 hour, 24 hours, and 48 hours following honeybee stings of guinea pigs revealed edema, cellular infiltration, and muscle necrosis, with patches of cytolysis, which were followed by a walling-off of the damaged tissue by a palisade of mononuclear inflammatory cells (Crewe and Gordon, 1949). An interesting observation was that 1 hour after the sting, the severity of reaction varied at different points along the track of the wound: The most marked reaction occurring midway, rather than at the tip of the sting. This suggested to the authors that most of the venom had been introduced during the act of forcing the stinger through the tissue.

Local reactions to stings of the fire ant *Selenopsis* spp. have been described by Caro et al. (1957): Almost immediately following the sting, erythema and edema appeared and persisted for about an hour. Vesiculation took place about 4 hours later. Twenty-four hours after the sting, pruritic pustules were present at the sting sites. Reactions to fire ant stings may persist for days, and since the ant generally inflicts multiple stings, the afflicted individual may experience considerable discomfort. Histologic studies on biopsies taken from human volunteers at different time intervals ranging from 6 minutes to 72 hours after the sting showed that the features peculiar to these sting reactions consisted of the early appearance of intercellular edema in the epidermis, early necrosis in the upper corium, development of pustules at the sting sites, and necrosis deep beneath the pustules.

Unless complicated by hypersensitivity, systemic toxic reactions to hymenopteran stings are usually mild compared to those elicited by stings of some scorpions or by bites of some spiders. This is primarily due to the small amount of venom which is introduced during a single sting. The honeybee, for example, yields between 0.1 to 0.3 mg of venom, a quantity approximately one to two orders of magnitude less than the LD_{50} per kg of body weight. Systemic poisoning may occur in the case of concurrent multiple stings, such as when an individual is attacked by a swarm of bees (Marshall, 1957). Reports of multiple stings by bees and wasps are, however, quite uncommon. Systemic reactions of humans due to multiple stings by ants are described by Caro et al. (1957). These reactions are generally complicated by a previously obtained hypersensitivity to the sting, and therefore it is difficult to attribute the observed systemic reactions to the venomous effect of the sting.

Hypersensitivity to antigens introduced during the sting of Hymenoptera, rather than the toxic action of the venom, is the important medical problem. The reactions of hypersensitive individuals have been described by numerous workers (Prince and Secrest, 1939; Leclercq, 1950, 1961, 1963, 1965; Mueller and Hill, 1953; Miller, 1956; Ordman, 1958; Brock, 1961; Jensen, 1962; Mueller, 1965; and others). The reaction can be summarized as follows: some individuals exhibit local swelling and irritation; more sensitive individuals exhibit systemic symptoms suggestive of anaphylactic shock. In some cases the shock is expressed by pyrexia, diarrhea, polyuria, and dyspnea, while in more severe cases there is also cyanosis, with loss of consciousness. Extremely sensitive individuals react to a single sting with anaphylactic shock leading to death within a few minutes. For excellent detailed descriptions of reactions of allergic individuals to hymenopteran stings, the reader is referred to articles by Marshall (1957), by Jensen (1962), and to a recent publication by the Insect Allergy Committee of the American Academy of Allergy (1965). Analyses of autopsies performed in some cases of death by anaphylactic shock are summarized and reviewed by Jensen (1962) and by the Insect Allergy Committee Report (1966).

There are thousands of reports of severe reactions and deaths caused by stinging Hymenoptera. Analyses by Parrish (1963) of human deaths caused by venomous animals in the United States during the ten-year period (1950 to 1959, inclusive) showed that of the total recorded deaths (460) from all venomous animals, 229 (49.8 percent) were caused by hymenopterous insects. This is not surprising, considering the greater contact of man with these insects than with other venomous animals. The highest number of deaths was caused by bees (124 cases), followed by those caused by wasps, yellowjackets, and hornets (101 cases), and by ants (4 cases). The age distribution of the Hymenoptera victims showed that only 26 deaths occurred at ages up to 29 years, with 146 at ages 30 to 59, and 57 at ages over 60. These latter figures are in general accord with those reported by the Insect Allergy Committee (1965), which showed a sharp rise in the proportion of serious reactions after age 30. According to Parrish's survey, the sting suddenly kills the allergic patient: 80 percent died in less than 1 hour and 92 percent died within 5 hours following the sting. The incidence of fatalities from stings may be much higher than the above figures indicate, since many fatalities due to stings are mistakenly diagnosed as coronary attacks (Loveless, 1960). It is probably safe to say that fatalities caused by allergic reactions to hymenopterous insects are higher than those caused by any other single allergic disorder.

Antigens. Over fifty years ago, Waterhouse reported sensitivity to bee stings among beekeepers and described a case showing severe reactions within a few minutes following the sting, which he attributed to an anaphylactic hypersensitive response (Waterhouse, 1914). Since that time, many workers have tried to characterize the allergens involved in sensitivity to Hymenoptera stings. The probability that hypersensitivity was due to pollen carried by bees was minimized by the classical work of Benson and Semenov (1930), who attributed the hypersensitive reaction to allergens contained in the bee's body. During the last 35 years, attempts have been made to determine the origin and nature of the allergens of hymenopterous insects, the mode of sensitization, and means of desensitization.

A logical approach to the study of allergens involved in the sting reaction would be to define the antigens or allergens present in the venom of the insects and to correlate these to antibodies present in individuals who have had histories of stings. In fact, antibodies to phospholipase-A and to hyaluronidase were found in sera of animals actively immunized with bee venom (Haberman and El-Karemi, 1956), and anti-phospholipase-A was found in sera of beekeepers (Mohammed and El Karemi, 1961). However, the early experiments of Benson and Semenov (1930), which were subsequently confirmed by several workers (reviewed by Shulman, 1967), indicated that the allergens were not confined to the venom alone, but they were also present in extracts of bees from which the stingers were removed. This led to tremendous complications in the isolation and characterization of hymenopterous allergens.

Many conclusions have been based on a correlation between the degree of skin reactions elicited by various fractions and the sensitivity of the individual to stings. However, several reports indicate the absence of such correlation. A report by Bernton and Brown (1965) on the intradermal testing of 200 "normal" clinically nonsensitive individuals revealed that 37.5 percent gave positive reactions to three preparations of whole-body bee extracts. Schwartz (1965) similarly failed to correlate skin reactivity with clinical hypersensitivity to hymenopteran stings. In these experiments, serial skin testing was carried out with a mixture of bee, wasp, and yellowjacket whole-body extracts on three groups of patients: those who were hypersensitive to hymenopteran stings (as determined by case histories), those who were "non-insect sensitive" but who were atopic (i.e., patients who were under treatment for allergic rhinitis or asthma or both, but who had no history of insect-sting sensitivity), and patients who were generally healthy (but who were under treatment for various venereal diseases). Assuming the criteria used for the above grouping were valid, test results revealed no significant differences in the reactivity among these groups. These results suggest that the diagnoses of sting hypersensitivity must be based on case histories rather than on direct skin testing. Extreme care must be exercised when direct skin tests alone are employed in characterizing allergens.

More comprehensive knowledge on antigenicity and allergenicity associated with Hymenoptera-sting hypersensitivity was derived from experiments utilizing a variety of immunologic techniques in addition to direct skin tests. These included precipitin reactions, hemagglutination, immunodiffusion, and immunoelectrophoresis. This work has been the subject of several reviews (Brock, 1961; Loveless, 1966; Shulman, 1967).

An excellent example of work on the elucidation of allergens and antigenic components of bees is that of Langolis et al. (1965a), who combined a variety of immunologic techniques for this purpose. Sera collected from patients sensitive to bee stings (as determined by past histories of immediate sensitivity to stings, as well as by skin reactions elicited by direct skin testing with extracts) exhibited hemagglutinating properties with extracts of bees, which were derived from whole bodies, sacless bodies, and venom sacs. Also, the presence of antibodies in the sera was demonstrated by the fact that the intradermal inoculation of these sera to nonsensitive individuals, followed by challenge with extracts 24 to 48 hours later, elicited positive skin reactions. Although there was no direct correlation between the latter skin-sensitizing antibodies and hemagglutination titers, sera which had hemagglutination titers usually also transferred sensitivity. Passive transfer experiments utilizing venom-sac and sacless-body extracts revealed that both antigenic preparations were equally potent in reacting with skin-sensitizing antibodies, thus confirming the early reports of Benson and Semenov (1930) that allergenicity was found in the entire body of the bee and was not limited to venom. However, subsequent work by Langlois et al. (1965b), using rabbit antisera to the antigens in whole-bee bodies, sacless bodies, and venom sacs, revealed that the cross-reactivity between venom-sac extracts and sacless-body extracts was limited. These experiments showed that although antivenom-sac serum hemagglutinated in the presence of sacless-body extract and vice versa, the sacless-body extract inhibited (but only to a limited degree) hemagglutination by anti-venom-sac extract, thus indicating that the sac extract contained specific antigens. This was confirmed by gel-diffusion and absorption experiments which showed antigens specific to venom-sac extract.

Further work by Shulman et al. (1966a) on the immunochemical characterization of whole-bee bodies, sacless bodies, venom sacs, and pure venom indicated that in rabbits, antigenicity specific to the venom sac could be attributed to the venom content of the sac. Results of these experiments showed that the venom contained only one prominent antigenic component, since antivenom serum produced only one prominent band in gel-diffusion tests with venom. According to the authors, this component was specific for venom, since it could not be found in the sacless body of the insect. Antiserum to sacless-body extracts did not react with venom, hence the venom was characterized as a tissue-specific antigen. The experiments of Shulman and co-workers also revealed that whereas the venom-sac extracts contained body antigens (that is, the extracts could inhibit the reaction between whole-body extracts and antiserum to whole-body extracts), the pure venom did not react with antiserum to sacless bodies. However, immunization with pure venom elicited antiserum which recognized body antigens, since it reacted with sacless bodies. It thus appears that the venom contained trace amounts of body antigens which could not be detected when reacted with antiserum to sacless bodies. These antigens, however, could be demonstrated, following immunization with venom, by the reaction between the resulting antiserum and sacless-body extract. The source of body components in the venom is still unclear. The authors point out that it may be inherent in the venom, or that it may be the result of deposition of excreta or other body debris during the stinging process.

The foregoing results on the characterization of various bee antigens were obtained with rabbit antiserum, and the authors correctly point out that these results do not necessarily mean that the antigens and allergens involved in human hypersensitivity to stings are the same. Shulman et al. (1966b) reported on experiments dealing with passive transfers of sting-sensitive patients' and beekeepers' sera which indicated that skin-sensitizing antibodies against venom were more frequent in sting-sensitive patients, whereas antibodies against bee bodies were frequent in the sera of beekeepers. These findings suggest that different antigens (and perhaps also different antibodies) are involved in the sensitivities of these two groups to bee stings. Perhaps the frequent contact (not necessarily by stings) of bee-keepers with bees is responsible for their tendency to react to body allergens, whereas the accidental sting of persons who are not normally intimately associated with bees is responsible for the elicitation of antibodies directed mostly against the venom. However, the sting, which was shown to deposit antigens capable of inducing antibodies that can cross-react with sacless bodies (Shulman et al., 1966a), may also elicit antibodies (in humans) capable of reacting with sacless-body extracts. This is especially probable in the case of a honeybee sting, in which the stinger and the venom sac are forcibly torn out of the bee's body immediately after stinging and remain emebdded in the stung area until removed. It is not surprising, then, that allergenicity related to bee sting hypersensitivity has been demonstrated to be associated with the body of the bee as well as with the venom.

Investigations of the allergens and antigens of the wasp *Polistes exclamans* and the yellowjacket *Vespula pennsylvanica* indicated that as with bees, although many allergens and antigens are shared between whole bodies, sacless bodies, and venom sacs, there nevertheless exist antigens specific to venom-sac extracts (Langlois et al., 1965b).

There is much room for fertile research on the immunology of hypersensitivity to Hymenoptera. For example, little is known about the allergens involved in hypersensitivity to ant stings, and the immunochemical characterization of bee and wasp allergens is still incomplete. The antigenic components which are associated with human hypersensitivity to these insects are also still unknown.

Antibodies. The association of antibodies with hypersensitivity to hymenopteran stings is well-established. Beekeepers' sera have been shown to form precipitins with bee venom (Thompson, 1933). Circulating antibodies have been demonstrated numerous times in sera of sensitive humans and experimental animals by passive transfer tests (*see* Loveless, 1966, for review). Serum obtained post-mortem from a person who died 15 minutes after a sting by the wasp *Polistes fuscatus* contained antibodies which reacted with wasp extract and with bee extract (McCormick, 1963).

Various attempts have been made to characterize antigens to which the antibodies are directed, as well as the type of immunoglobulins involved. Haberman and El-Karemi (1956) demonstrated conclusively that injections of bee venom into rabbits elicited production of antibodies which were directed against phospholipase-A and hyaluronidase and which were capable of neutralizing the activity of these two enzymes. Anti-phospholipase-A was also demonstrated in sera of beekeepers (Mohammed and El Karemi, 1961). However, the pharmacologic properties of the venom on isolated guinea pig gut or uterus, its systemic toxicity in white mice, and its hemolytic effect on human erythrocytes were not diminished by the rabbit antiserum. The authors concluded that whereas the enzymatic components of the venom elicited the production of neutralizing antibodies, the nonenzymatic (but pharmacologically active) components were nonantigenic. From the multiplicity of bands obtained by gel diffusion, it is fairly certain that antibodies other than those against hyaluronidase and phospholipase may be present in sera of immunized animals and of sensitive humans. Such antibodies are most probably directed against various body constituents of the insects which have not yet been characterized physicochemically.

It is apparent that antibodies associated with Hymenoptera-sting hypersensitivity belong to several classes of immunoglobulins possessing different physicochemical and biologic properties, since precipitating, hemagglutinating, skin-sensitizing, and blocking antibodies have been demonstrated (see Loveless, 1966, for a review). The role of these various antibodies in the hypersensitive reaction to the insects is, however, still unclear. As has already been pointed out, in many instances no correlation could be found between a given type of antibody and clinical symptoms.

Positive passive transfers of skin sensitivity were successful with sera of only some sensitive patients, and were not necessarily demonstrable with sera obtained from patients who had responded to direct skin tests given with high dilutions of antigens (Mueller, 1965). Sera of some sensitive patients failed to show formation of precipitins by gel diffusion, and although antibodies were demonstrated in some sera by passive cutaneous anaphylaxis, no correlation was found between the presence of these antibodies, the severity of clinical symptoms, or the insects themselves which presumably were responsible for the clinical reaction (Terr and McLean, 1964). Even less understood are the changes in the composition and relative concentrations of various types of antibodies following treatments of sensitive patients with whole-body extracts or with venom sacs.

As with antigens, the type of antibodies involved in the clinical reactivity to hymenopteran stings remains a subject for further elucidation.

Cross-reactivity.   Considerable interest and work have been devoted to determine whether or not individuals sensitive to stings of a given Hymenoptera species are also sensitive to stings of other hymenopterous insects, and to determine whether or not antigens and allergens derived from one species show immunologic cross-reactivity with those derived from heterologous species. Apart from academic interest, the establishment of cross-reactivity between stings of hymenopterous insects is of great practical value. Often the identity of the stinging insect is obscure, but if cross-reactivity exists, hyposensitization can be achieved with preparations of other Hymenoptera species. In addition, the scarcity of many species for antigen preparation would not constitute a problem if antigens from more readily available species could be used.

Many reports of cross-reactivity among various Hymenoptera species can be found in the literature. Most conclusions, however, are based on direct intradermal skin tests performed on sting-sensitive individuals, using extracts of whole insects as allergens. The inadequacy of direct skin testing for this purpose has already been pointed out. Considerably more validity may be attributed to studies in which skin tests are performed in sites passively sensitized with sera of sensitive individuals, especially when these are combined with antibody neutralization experiments which employ passive transfer of sera mixed with heterologous antigens. Using these methods,

Loveless and Fackler (1956) demonstrated that yellowjackets (*Vespula maculifrons*), bold-faced hornets (*Vespula maculata*), paper wasps (*Polistes* spp.), honeybees (*Apis mellifera*), and bumblebees (*Bombus* spp.) possessed common allergens, and in addition, that each species contained an allergen or allergens specific for the species. The three wasps were closely related allergenically, and the honeybee was more closely related to the three wasps than was the bumblebee.

Langlois et al. (1965a) examined cross-reactivity among honeybees, wasps (*Polistes* spp.), and yellowjackets (*Vespula pennsylvanica*) by passive serum transfer, by tanned-cell hemagglutination, and by *in vivo* neutralization of passive serum transfer. These workers found that whereas some Hymenoptera-sensitive patients reacted to one type of insect only, another group reacted to two or three different insects. Also, sera of patients under treatment (by injections of unspecified hymenopteran extracts) for Hymenoptera-sting sensitivity showed hemagglutination titers for several types of stinging insects more frequently than did those of untreated patients. The interpretation of these results is difficult, since the cross-reactivity could have been the result of previous sensitization by stings of the different species. However, neutralization tests of passive transfers showed that whereas yellowjacket antigen also neutralized antibodies to bees and wasps, antibodies to yellowjackets could not be completely neutralized by bee or wasp antigens. In addition, bee antigen could not neutralize wasp antibodies, and vice versa. These results suggested to the authors that yellowjackets share a common allergen with wasps and another with bees, that there is an antigen specific to yellowjackets alone, but that there was no allergen in common to bees and wasps.

Antigenic cross-reactivity among several Hymenoptera species has been investigated by Foubert and Stier (1958). These workers immunized rabbits with whole-body extracts of wasps (*Polistes fuscatus*), yellow hornets (*Dolichovespula arenaria*), black hornets (*D. maculata*), yellowjackets (*Vespula pennsylvanica*), and the German honeybee (*Apis mellifica*). Gel diffusion studies with rabbit antisera and anaphylaxis studies in guinea pigs indicated that insects of each species contained antigens specific for the individual genus in addition to common antigens shared by all these insects, and that the bee antigen demonstrated the least degree of cross-reactivity. Arbesman et al. (1965) demonstrated a common antigen between bees and wasps and between bees and yellowjackets; the common antigen, however, was present in the bodies of the respective insects, not in the venom sacs. Cross-reactivity involving two antigens was also demonstrated by these workers between wasps and yellowjackets, one antigen present in the venom sacs and one present in the bodies.

In addition to the above examples, immunologic cross-reactivity, as well as some species-specificity among various Hymenoptera, has been demonstrated by other workers (Terr and McLean, 1964; O'Connor et al., 1964; and others). It is clear that various tests demonstrate cross-reactivity to varying degrees.

Hyposensitization. In view of the severe, sometimes fatal, hypersensitive reactions to Hymenoptera stings, numerous attempts have been made to hyposensitize sting-sensitive individuals. It appears that the severity of reactions may decrease in some individuals even without hyposensitization therapy, presumably due to the gradual decrease of sensitizing antibody titers in the absence of newly acquired stings. Since the correlation between reactions to live stings and results of various serologic tests is inadequate, it is almost impossible to predict on the basis of serologic tests whether or not sensitivity to stings has decreased. The procedure of determining sensitivity either by direct challenge with a live insect or by skin testing with extracts involves the risk of inducing sensitization and sometimes the risk of anaphylaxis.

Numerous clinical reports dealing with attempts to reduce sensitivity by means of injections of various extracts prepared from Hymenoptera indicate that in most cases hyposensitization is effective, although to varying degrees. Many of these reports have been summarized and reviewed by Marshal (1957), Brock (1961), Loveless (1966), and others. A large-scale study on the efficacy of hyposensitization to hymenopteran stings has been undertaken by the Committee on Insect Allergy of the American Academy of Allergy (see Kailin, 1965, for summary). The study, which was conducted over a period of several years, showed that of 647 persons who were injected with various dosages of extracts, only 26 (4 percent) had reactions of increased severity to stings, the reactions of 41 patients (6.3 percent) were unchanged, whereas 580 patients (89.6 percent) demonstrated improvement over their pretreatment state. In comparison, out of 763 sting-sensitive but untreated patients, 492 (65 percent) experienced reactions of increased severity, 199 (26 percent) reported the reactions unchanged, and 72 (9 percent) reported reactions of less severity. In a number of treated patients, hyposensitization was effective for a year, in one case for 10 years, and in another case for 18 years. In most cases protection was lost in less than a year (Kailin, 1965).

Numerous preparations, some of which are available commercially, are used for injections. Most of these consist of extracts of whole insects containing the venom sacs. Loveless and Fackler (1956) reported experiments on hyposensitization utilizing injections of crushed venom sacs freshly dissected out of live Hymenoptera. Challenges given with stings of live insects indicated the efficacy of the treatment. Subsequent reports by Loveless (1962, 1966) and by Loveless and Nall (1965) claimed that successful hyposensitization lasted about a year with a single injection of an emulsion of venom sacs in light mineral oil with Arlacel-A (mannide mono-oleate). In spite of this success, there is considerable hesitancy on the part of many clinicians to practice emulsion therapy in view of the potential risk arising from the possibility of introduction of large amounts (several sacs) of venom antigens in one injection.

Regarding hyposensitization to stings of one Hymenoptera species with preparations from other species, it has been pointed out that if the insect causing a severe reaction is unknown, or if there is a possibility of sensitivity to several stinging insects, hyposensitization with a mixture of antigens may be advisable (Foubert and Stier, 1958). However, if the stinging insect is known, hyposensitization with materials from heterologous species should be avoided in order to avert possible new sensitization to stings of hitherto untroublesome species. Also, in view of the findings that venom sacs of different Hymenoptera species contain antigens specific to the venoms, the advisability and efficacy of injections with preparations consisting of mixtures of antigens derived from several species are questionable.

Very little is known about the mechanisms involved in hyposensitization to hymenopteran stings. This is understandable in view of the meager knowledge of the antigens involved in hypersensitivity and of the sensitizing antibody. A review of the mechanisms involved in hyposensitization to Hymenoptera (Loveless, 1966) suggested that in the course of hyposensitization, blocking antibodies may be formed which presumably compete with sensitizing antibodies for antigen. A recent statement by Brown (cited by Loveless, 1966) indicated that whereas the sera of most Hymenoptera-sensitive individuals exhibited precipitins before treatment, the precipitins were not found after treatment (or in some cases, in untreated patients). The explanation of this phenomenon, according to Loveless, might be the formation, due to treatment, of blocking antibodies which compete with sensitizing antibodies.

Scorpion stings

Although scorpions are mostly found in warmer areas, they are also prevalent in all climatic regions except those in which there is continuous cold weather. Scorpions are nocturnal creatures, usually feeding upon insects, spiders, and millipedes. During the day they hide beneath loose stones, lumber, leaves and other debris. Some of these arachnids bury themselves in sand or loose earth; during rainy seasons they may invade human habitations. To feed, they seize and sting their prey, and the sting paralyzes or kills the victim. All scorpions are venomous, but there is considerable variation in the toxicity of scorpion venoms so that not all of them are dangerous to man. The relatively high incidence of contact with man and the high toxicity of their venom render certain species of the family Buthidae extremely dangerous.

Members of the genera *Centruroides* (found in Mexico and the southwestern United States); *Androctonus*, *Buthus*, and *Buthacus* (in North Africa); *Prionurus* (in the Middle East); and *Tityus* and *Parabuthus* (in South America) are considered to be the most dangerous scorpions and constitute an important public health problem (Herms and James, 1961). In the United States during the years 1950 to 1959, of the total of 229 mortalities caused by all varieties of venomous animals, eight deaths were due to scorpions (Parrish, 1963). This figure is not very impressive compared to that reported by Mazzotti and Bravo-Becherelle (1963) from Mexico, where in a 12-year period (between 1940 and 1949, and 1957 and 1958), a total of 20,352 persons were killed by scorpion stings (whereas 2,068 died from snake bites, 274 from spider bites, and 1,933 from stings by other venomous animals). A survey conducted by these workers showed that during these years the average annual death rate due to scorpion stings in 31 Mexican municipalities was higher than 100 per 100,000 inhabitants, i.e., over 0.1 percent. Although a downward trend has since been witnessed, the total number of deaths in Mexico due to scorpion stings is still more than 1,000 per year.

Stings of scorpions other than those of the above genera, although usually not lethal, can cause local reactions varying in severity from a slight swelling to severe painful swelling and ecchymosis (Stahnke, 1966). There is considerable variation in toxicity of the venom not only among different scorpion species, but even within a single species. The reasons for these variations are not clear (Schottler, 1954).

Scorpion venom. There is a fair amount of agreement in the descriptions of the systemic reactions resulting from stings of several genera of scorpions (Del Pozo, 1956). The symptomatology includes salivation, nausea, vomiting, temporary blindness, muscular contraction, mydriasis, and respiratory distress which may culminate in respiratory paralysis. The symptoms indicate that the venom acts on the parasympathetic nervous system. (For excellent descriptions of scorpion poisoning, the reader is referred to articles by Waterman, 1938, and by Stahnke, 1950.) Bertke and Atkins (1964) studied the pathologic effect of *Centruroides* venom on white rats and found that the effect is neither consistent nor marked. Only a few morphologic changes were observed in the tissue of the envenomized animals. In several animals, varying degrees of degeneration and necrosis were seen in the parenchymatous organs, especially in the liver, kidneys, and heart. Some petechiae and edema were also found in these organs. Lungs were sometimes congested, foci of hemorrhages were present, and the adrenal glands were affected. Macroscopic examination of dissected mice following envenomization by *Tityus* did not reveal visible alterations that might have been caused by the venom. Local symptoms at the sites of subcutaneous venom injections could not be found (Schottler, 1954).

Several excellent studies have been performed on the physiologic and pharmacologic action of scorpion venoms (Mohammed, 1950; Mohammed et al., 1954; Del Pozo, 1956; Diniz and Goncalves, 1956; Adam and Weiss, 1958, 1959; Patterson, 1960, 1962; Miranda et al., 1960, 1961, 1966a, b; Miranda and Lissitzky, 1961; Master et al., 1963). Venoms have been found to possess cholinergic and adrenergic activity. Some exert a slow-acting noncholinergic activity on smooth muscles; some contain serotonin. It should, however, be emphasized that venoms of different species show certain differences, as well as similarities, with respect to action and chemical composition.

Attempts to characterize the chemical nature of the venom of several varieties of scorpions have been made. Adam and Weiss (1959) showed that the activity of the venom of *Leiurus quinquestriatus* was nondialyzable, heatlabile (30 minutes at 100°C), and destroyed by trypsin or chymotrypsin.

Work by Diniz and Goncalves (1956) with the venom of *Tityus bahiensis* and *T. serrulatus* indicated that the principal toxic component was a thermostable substance of low molecular weight, and that in the natural venom the substance was probably bound to protein. The neurotoxic activity of the venoms of *Androctonus australis* and *Buthus occitanus* was attributed to two proteins of relatively low molecular weight (12,000), which were stable upon storage and stable to denaturing agents (Miranda and Lissitzky, 1961). Venoms of *Buthus tamulus* and *Palamneous gravemanus* contained protease, but not phospholipase-A, cholinesterase, or L-aminoacid oxidase (which are usually present in snake venoms). The venom of *B. tamulus* contained phosphodiesterase. It had two toxins, one producing increased breathing rates and another producing stiffening of the hind portions of injected mice. That of *P. gravimanus* contained 5-nucleotidase and a factor which caused ileum contractions in guinea pigs (Master et al., 1963).

Variation in composition and activity of the venoms of different scorpion species is further corroborated by Johnson and Stahnke (1960) and by Nitzan and Shulov (1966). Some of these differences are probably expressed in the immunochemical differences which were found by comparing the antigenicity of different venoms.

Scorpion antivenoms. Immunochemical evaluation of venoms of eight scorpion species (some lethal and some nonlethal) has been performed by Potter and Northey (1962). This was achieved by preparation of rabbit antisera and the evaluation of gel-diffusion patterns obtained with homologous and heterologous venoms. Band patterns produced by venoms and homologous antisera revealed that the venoms of various species differed in the number of bands formed, as well as in their immunogenicity (i.e., their ability to elicit antibody response). Venoms of species belonging to the genus *Centruroides* had the largest number of antigenic components as judged by the number of bands produced. The venom of *Androctonus australis*, on the other hand, had only two bands, thus showing that the number of bands is not related to venom lethality, since both genera possess highly potent venoms.

Experiments on the immunologic cross-reactivity among the venoms of these eight scorpion species revealed some interesting phenomena: The venoms of *Centruroides sculpturatus* and of *C. gertschi*, although forming the greatest number of bands with their homologous antisera, were incapable of forming bands with antisera to the venoms of other species. On the other hand, the venom of *Androctonus australis*, although producing only 2 bands with homologous antiserum, produced 4 and 3 bands with anti-*C. gertschi* and anti-*C. sculpturatus* respectively, 1 band with anti-*Leiurus quinquestriatus* (all of the family Buthidae), as well as 1 band with anti-*Vejovis spinigerus* (of the family Vejovidae). Furthermore, venom of *Hadrurus arizonensis*, a nonlethal variety of the family Vejovidae, produced 5 bands with homologous antiserum, as well as 5 bands and 2 bands with anti-*Leiurus quinquestriatus* and anti-*C. gertschi*, respectively, both belonging to the family Buthidae, although the venom did not produce bands with antisera to the venoms of *Vejovis flavus* and *V. spinigerus* (of the family Vejovidae). The venom of

Buthus occitanus, which produced 5 bands with homologous antiserum, did not react with antisera to venoms of other scorpions belonging to the family Buthidae, but did react with anti-*H. arizonensis* (5 bands), with anti-*V. flavus* (2 bands), and with anti-*V. spinigerus* (2 bands), all of the family Vejovidae. The venom of *Leiurus quinquestriatus* (family Buthidae) produced 6 bands with homologous antiserum, 1 band with anti-*C. gertschi* venom (family Buthidae), and 1 band with anti-*V. spinigerus* (family Vejovidae). Venom of *Vejovis flavus* produced 3 bands with homologous antiserum, and reacted with antiserum to *V. spinigerus* (4 bands), antiserum to *Hadrurus arizonensis* (1 band), and also with antiserum to the venoms of *Buthus occitanus* and *B. gertschi* (of the Buthidae family). Venom of *Vejovis spinigerus*, yielding 5 bands with homologous antiserum, reacted only with antiserum to *Vejovis flavus* (3 bands).

These results point to differences as well as similarities in the antigenicity and in the immunogenicity of the various venoms tested. They also indicate the poor correlation between the immunochemical properties of the venoms and the taxonomic classifications of the scorpions. More important, however, is the implication these results have for the feasibility of producing polyvalent antigens for the preparation of antivenoms capable of neutralizing the toxic effects of several scorpion venoms. Intergeneric antigenic relationships among several scorpion venoms have also been reported by Glenn and Whittemore (1962).

Antisera to venoms of several lethal scorpion species have been produced by many workers (Sergent, 1936; Shulov, 1939; Magalhães, 1947; Goren, 1950; Balozet, 1956; Vermeil, 1959; Shulov et al., 1960; Tulga, 1960; Whittemore et al., 1961; Glenn and Whittemore, 1962; and others). From studies on the neutralization of the toxic effects of various venoms by antivenom, it appears that in general, scorpion venoms are poor antigens, requiring several months of immunization before an adequate titer of neutralizing antibodies can be obtained (Balozet, 1956). It is also apparent that the power of antiserum to neutralize various venoms varies greatly. Balozet (1956) reported that in order to immunize horses against several species of North African scorpions, at least eight months were required before adequate neutralizing antibody titers were obtained. Not all horses produced sera of satisfactory titers, and certain physiologic actions of the venom were never suppressed in horses, although the animals were immunized for several years.

Studies by Whittemore et al. (1961) on the neutralization of venoms of several scorpion species by homologous and heterologous antisera revealed several instances of cross-protection, and, more interestingly, in several tests heterologous antivenom was more effective in neutralization than was homologous antivenom. For example, the venom of *Androctonus australis* was neutralized more effectively by anti-*Androctonus crassicauda* serum. This same serum was also as effective in neutralizing the venoms of *Buthus occitanus*, *Tityus serrulatus*, and *Tityus bahiensis* as the homologous antisera. Similarly, antivenom to *Centruroides* was as effective in neutralizing the venom of *Tityus bahiensis* and *Buthus occitanus* as was the homologous antiserum, and it could also neutralize the venom of *Tityus serrulatus*. However, the venom of *Androctonus crassicauda* was neutralized only by homologous antiserum. The comparison was based on the number of mouse-LD_{50} of a given venom which could be neutralized by 1 ml of antivenom.

The correlation of antigenic cross-reactivity of venom components with neutralization of toxic activity by antibodies points to the feasibility of producing antisera capable of neutralizing the toxic action of venoms of several species of scorpions. From the antigenic characterization of venom components performed by Potter and Northey (1962), it appears that antisera to venom of *Centruroides gertchi* and of *Vejovis spinigerus* will contain antibodies which will react with venoms of *C. gertschi*, *C. sculpturatus*, *Androctonus australis*, *Hadrurus arizonensis*, *Buthus occitanus*, *Leiurus quinquestriatus*, and *Vejovis spinigerus*. Whether or not this reaction will cause the neutralization of these venoms remains to be elucidated. It is important to point out that large variations exist in the potency of venoms (LD_{50} per mg) and in the yield of venom (mg per scorpion) of different scorpion species (Whittemore and Keegan, 1963). Therefore, antigenic cross-reactivity does not necessarily assure that practical neutralization of cross-reacting venoms can be achieved by antiserum to a given venom.

The therapeutic effect of antisera for scorpion stings has been reported by many workers (Cervera, 1936; Efrati, 1949, Sergent, 1949; Stahnke, 1950; Mazzotti and Bravo-Becherelle, 1963; and others). The availability and sources of antisera to venoms of many scorpions and the species whose venom they neutralize have been summarized by Keegan (1956).

The diversity of the chemical, pharmacologic, and immunologic properties of venoms of different scorpion species makes it impractical to deal with each species in sufficient detail in this chapter. For specific information on these aspects of any particular species, the reader should consult the references mentioned.

IMMUNITY TO INFESTATIONS AND INVASIONS BY ARTHROPODS

Hematophagous arachnids

An interesting aspect of immunity to arthropods was reported by Trager: The exposure of several laboratory animals to ixodid ticks resulted, within approximately two weeks, in the acquisition of immunity which was manifested by the inability of subsequent groups of larvae to engorge (Trager, 1939a). This type of immunity could also be produced by injections of extracts of tick larvae, and it was shown to be transferrable to nonimmune animals by sera from immunized animals, thus indicating dependence on circulating antibodies. Further experiments by Trager (1939b) demonstrated that the immunogens were present in the ticks' digestive tract, in the cephalic glands of partly engorged ticks, in the salivary glands of fed and unfed ticks, and in extracts of whole larval ticks. Moreover, sera of rabbits previously infested with *Dermacentor variabilis* specifically fixed complement with antigens prepared from larval tick extract.

According to Trager, this acquired immunity depends on the reaction of circulating antibodies with antigenic materials deposited in the host during the bite. The antigen-antibody reaction accelerates local cellular reactions, which, in turn, wall off the tick larvae from their food supply. This type of immunity could best be demonstrated with ticks of the family Ixodidae, which take one large blood meal at each of their three stages of life cycle and remain attached to the host at each meal for a relatively long period, ranging from several days to two weeks. The long feeding period is an important factor in the expression of this type of immunity, which requires a certain length of time to wall off effectively the tick larvae from their blood supply. Infestation of chickens with the tick *Argas persicus*, which normally requires a relatively short feeding period (a few minutes to a few hours), did not confer immunity against subsequent feeding by nymphs or adults of this tick. A low degree of immunity was conferred to subsequent infestation with larvae, but injections of extracts of *Argas persicus* did not produce immunity to larvae, nymphs, or adults. Similarly, no immunity was conferred upon guinea pigs against the feeding of larvae of *Ornithodoros venezuelensis* by previous infestations of animals with this tick (Trager, 1940).

A similar type of immunity was demonstrated by Riek in infestations of animals with the tick *Hemaphysalis bispinosa*. Riek (1958) succeeded in sensitizing mice and guinea pigs by daily subcutaneous injections for 3 to 5 days with antigens prepared from extracts of eggs of this tick. The sensitized animals became protected against the attachment of the larval ticks, and sensitization was transferrable to normal animals via sera from sensitized animals. The activity of the immune serum was attributed to a skin-sensitizing antibody, characterized as a β-globulin, which was destroyed by heating at 56°C for 4 hours. Riek also reported that the intravenous injections of the egg extracts once or twice per week for 3 weeks resulted in the formation of complement-fixing and precipitating antibodies which were able to neutralize the toxic activity of the extract, but did not afford protection against larval infestation. These antibodies were not destroyed by heating at 56°C for 4 hours and were principally γ-globulins. Riek (1959) showed that egg extract and larval extract contained closely related components, and that immunization with larval extract resulted in the formation of antibodies capable of neutralizing the toxic effect of egg extract. Further immunochemical studies, however, suggested that the principal antigen responsible for hypersensitivity in laboratory animals was distinct from the antigen responsible for the production of neutralizing antibodies. The extension of these investigations to infestations of cattle with *Boophilus microplus* (Riek, 1962) revealed a similar acquired resistance to infestation which was associated with hypersensitivity to the salivary secretion of the tick.

The work of Trager and of Riek with ixodid ticks indicates that acquired immunity can be developed to infestations of slow-feeding ticks. The immunity is associated with circulating antibodies that probably accelerate local cellular reactions which, in turn, result in the prevention of the arthropod from obtaining its blood meal.

Nelson and Bainborough (1963) described resistance of sheep to the ked (sheep tick) *Melophagus ovinus*, which developed following infestations. Histopathologic studies of skin sections obtained from resistant sheep showed arteriolar vasoconstriction. The subepidermal layer of the section biopsied from resistant sheep was edematous and showed eosinophilic and lymphocytic cellular infiltrations. The upper dermis of resistant sheep showed a preponderance of empty capillaries, in contrast to susceptible sheep whose capillaries were filled with erythrocytes. The authors concluded that acquired resistance to the ked was caused by cutaneous arteriolar vasoconstriction which cut off the capillary blood flow to the upper dermis, thus preventing the keds from obtaining their blood meal. Despite the possibility that the nonspecific Shwartzman phenomenon may contribute to the vasospasm, the results suggest that the resistance phenomenon involves the acquisition of hypersensitivity. For a discussion of the Shwartzman phenomenon, the reader is referred to Raffel (1961).

From the preceding reports, it appears that acquired immunity to infestations with several species of hematophagous arthropods can be developed. Antibodies are probably directed against antigens in the oral secretion of the arthropod, and the interaction of these antigens with antibodies leads to histopathologic changes which eventually result in blocking the blood supply to the arthropod. It is questionable, however, that a similar type of immunity can be developed against parasitic arthropods which obtain their blood meal within short periods.

Tissue-invading arthropods

Another interesting aspect of immunity to arthropods is that which is associated with tissue-invading arthropods such as myiasis-producing dipterous larvae and sarcoptoid and demodicoid mites.

The classical work of Blacklock and Thompson (1923), Blacklock and Gordon (1927), and Blacklock et al. (1930) on the response of the host to the myiasis-producing larvae of *Cordylobia anthropophaga* illustrates the development of immunity to tissue-invading arthropods. Observations on the incidence of infection indicated that young animals, including children, were more susceptible to infection than were old animals, and that the relatively higher resistance of older animals could not be attributed to the failure of larvae to penetrate the skin (Blacklock and Thompson, 1923). The authors concluded that resistance was due to acquired immunity as a result of previous attack by the larvae. This hypothesis was confirmed by the fact that in man, dogs, monkeys, and guinea pigs, immunity against larvae was developed experimentally by previous infection with them. The immunity was demonstrated by the fact that larvae introduced by the second infection were usually dead within six days. Later work by Blacklock and Gordon (1927) on the experimental production of immunity to *Cordylobia anthropophaga* in guinea pigs established that the acquired immunity was a skin immunity, confined at first to areas of the skin into which the parasite had previously invaded or which had been injected (subcutaneously) with emulsions of larvae. The immunity was found to spread later, so that areas which had never been infected ultimately became immune. Immunity lasted for at least three months. Utilizing an interesting experimental procedure, these workers showed that immunity could be demonstrated in new skin which grew on an abraded immune area, and that it could be transferred, via skin transplantation, to a nonimmune animal. However, immunity could not be demonstrated in a biopsy of skin from an immune area which was kept *in vitro*. Subsequent work (Blacklock et al., 1930) demonstrated that sera of previously infected animals contained antibodies which formed precipitins with the hemocoel fluid or excreta of third-instar larvae (but not with antigens derived from ground first-instar larvae or from the cuticle, salivary glands, or gut of third-instar larvae). The authors suggested that the death of larvae in the immune animals was due to the reaction between the gut content of the larvae and the serum of the immune animal.

Experiments on the development of immunity in guinea pigs to infection with the larvae of *Cochliomyia americana* (primary screw worm) were performed by Borgstrom (1938). He demonstrated that guinea pigs which had been reinfected with these larvae 20 days following a first invasion were able to survive the injurious effects of a dose of larvae which proved lethal to normal guinea pigs within 5 days. The immunity was shown to be confined to previously infected areas only, since infection of previously noninfected areas, opposite infected ones, resulted in mortality from dosages of larvae which were lethal to normal animals. The duration of the immunity was 20 to 40 days. Attempts by Borgstrom to immunize guinea pigs by subcutaneous and intraperitoneal injections of suspensions of dried and pulverized larvae were unsuccessful, except that some local immunity was produced by the subcutaneous injections and was sufficient to delay death for several days in animals which were subsequently infected in the injected area. However, the exudate from *C. americana* lesions had immunizing properties: Animals wounded and smeared with the exudate from infected lesions for 5 days showed the same ability as previously infected animals to survive a normal lethal dose of larvae after a 20-day interval. The author suggested that immunity to *C. americana* was not caused by the interference with nutrition (as is probably the case in immunity to *Cordylobia* and to some helminthic parasites), but that it was perhaps related to the presence of a species of bacteria which was associated with *C. americana* lesions. Perhaps, the author postulated, the proteolytic activity of the bacteria was somehow connected with immunity, although local and systemic injections of the bacteria alone did not confer immunity to infection and death by larvae.

There is some suggestive, although incomplete, evidence of immunity to the myiasis-producing *Hypoderma bovis*, *Gastrophilus equi*, and *G. haemor-*

rhoidalis. Sera obtained from cattle and horses infected with *Hypoderma* and with *Gastrophilus*, respectively, exhibited precipitating antibodies when tested with antigens prepared from the corresponding larvae. Furthermore, sera from uninfected calves borne by infected mothers also exhibited precipitating antibodies (implying *in utero* transfer). There was immunologic cross-reactivity between the two species of *Gastrophilus* and also (but to a lesser degree) between *Gastrophilus* and *Hypoderma*; the sera also reacted somewhat with extracts prepared from flies, fly larvae, and lice (Koegel, 1924). The above demonstration of antibodies may imply immunity to infection with *Gastrophilus* and *Hypoderma*. Attempts by Rouband and Perard (quoted by Blacklock and Gordon, 1927) to immunize rabbits against *Hypoderma bovis* by intravenous injections of glycerinated extracts of larvae were unfortunately inconclusive.

Considering the amount of research on immunity to other metazoan parasites, it is surprising that only few efforts have been devoted to study immunity to myiasis-producing organisms.

Another aspect of immunity to tissue burrowers should be mentioned, namely immunity to burrowing mites. At first, the invasion and the burrowing by the scabies-causing mites are tolerated by the host. After approximately a month, presumably due to the development of hypersensitivity to some antigens associated with scabies, the invaded areas become edematous and pruritic. The edema, pruritus, and pyodermia are detrimental to the mites (Mellanby, 1944). The reinvasion by scabies mites of individuals who had previously suffered from scabies brings about the pruritic and edematous reaction within 24 hours of invasion (Swellengrebel and Sterman, 1961). The existence of hypersensitivity in scabies was demonstrated by Prakken and Van Vloten (quoted by Swellengrebel and Sterman, 1961), who showed that intradermal injections of antigens prepared from scales of the skin obtained from a case of Norwegian scabies elicited positive responses in individuals who were suffering, or who had suffered, from this disease. Sensitivity could be passively transferred with sera from these individuals to normal individuals.

Whether or not hypersensitivity is associated with pruritic reactions to other sarcoptoid or demodicoid mites is still unclear.

IMMUNITY TO URTICATING HAIRS AND SPINES

Caterpillars, cocoons, and adult forms of many species of insects belonging to the order Lepidoptera may elicit local and systemic reactions in man by skin contact with urticating hair and spines of these insects. There are at least 10 families and more than 50 species of Lepidoptera larvae possessing urticating hair. From some of the more important urticating species of Lepidoptera, the reader is referred to a list by Herms and James (1961). In the United States the most troublesome species are the puss caterpillar (*Megalopyge opercu-*

laris), the flannel moth (*M. crispata* and *M. pyxidifera*), the saddleback caterpillar (*Sibine stimulea*), the brown-tail moth (*Euproctis phaeorroea*), and
the Io moth larva (*Automeris io*) (Jones and Miller, 1959). In the Far East
the troublesome caterpillars belong to the genera *Euproctis* (*E. flava, E.
flavociliate*, and *E. funeralis*), *Dendrolimus*, and *Suana*. An outbreak of dermatitis due to dead larvae and cocoons of the genus *Thaumatopoea* has been
reported from the Middle East by Ziprkowsky et al. (1959). Medical problems and outbreaks of caterpillar dermatitis have been reviewed by Gilmer
(1924), by Weidner (1937), and by Keegan (1963).

According to Keegan (1963), the venom is carried in modified hairs and
spines which occur singly or in clusters on the body of the caterpillar. The
venom glands are believed to consist of single cells located at the base of the
hair or the spine or in the spine itself. Upon contact with skin, the venom
may be liberated through an opening at the tip of the hair or through a
break in the hair or the spine. The venom is not a secretion—it is the proto-
plasm of the venom gland.

For some time it was believed that the urticaria caused by hairs and
spines was due to their mechanical action rather than to actual toxic components (Kemper, 1958). However, it is now fairly clear that the urticaria is
induced by chemicals. Almost nothing is known about the nature of these
chemicals, and generalizations on the basis of the presence of a chemical or
chemicals in a given species are conjectural. Histamine was found in *Dirphia*
species and in *Megalopyge* species by Valle et al. (1954). On the other hand,
investigations by Goldman et al. (1960) failed to correlate venomous activity
of several other species with dialyzable materials. The presence of a proteinaceous substance or substances responsible for the venomous activity of hairs
and spines of several caterpillars has been indicated by Foot (1922), Bishopp
(1923), Valle et al. (1954), and Goldman et al. (1960).

The clinical response to contact with urticating hairs or spines of Lepidoptera has been described by several workers (Bishopp, 1923; Micks, 1952;
Randel and Doan, 1956; Ziprkowsky et al., 1959; Goldman et al., 1960;
McGovern et al., 1961; and others). From these reports, it appears that the
local response to contact with different species of Lepidoptera is similar. It
may consist of erythema, edema, urticaria, swelling, burning pain, vesiculation, hemorrhage, and occasional necrosis. Sometimes, especially in very sensitive individuals, systemic reactions may occur. These may take the form of
fever, shock and paralysis. Hairs which may be blown by wind or are rubbed
into the eyes may cause eye reactions ranging from catarrhal conjunctivitis
and keratitis to iridocyclitis, and even to complete eye loss (Goldman et al.,
1960). Ingestion and inhalation of hairs may cause serious internal disturbances (Herms and James, 1961).

The histopathology of dermatitis caused by several caterpillars has been
studied extensively by Jones and Miller (1959) and by Goldman et al.
(1960). Jones and Miller reported that the lesion produced by contact with
Automeris io showed the formation of an immediate erythematous wheal,
with a rapid formation of edema of the corium and subcutaneous tissue.
However, no necrosis or vesicle formation was observed. Also, there was no

local increase in eosinophils. The reaction witnessed by these workers lasted approximately 6 hours. On the other hand, in histopathologic studies, Goldman et al. (1960) found edema with perivascular lymphocytic infiltration and eosinophilia in reactions to contact with several other species of caterpillars. Increase in eosinophils was also indicated by the studies of Randel and Doan (1956), who demonstrated that following contact with *Megalopyge lanata*, the differential blood count of a patient showed 28 percent neutrophils, 46 percent lymphocytes, 4 percent monocytes, and 22 percent eosinophils (out of a total leukocyte count of 13,000 per ml). Delayed reactions (as long as 48 hours after contact) consisting of marked perivascular lymphocytic infiltrations with some eosinophilic infiltration were reported by Goldman et al. (1960).

The involvement of allergic hypersensitivity in lepidopteran dermatitis is still uncertain. It is well-established that the severity of reactions varies, and that it may depend on the species involved, on the site of contact, and on the susceptibility of the individual (Randel and Doan, 1956). The study by Goldman et al. (1960) suggested that in general, reactivity was greater in atopic than in nonatopic individuals, although both groups responded to contact with skin reactions. Perhaps the differences in the results obtained from the histopathologic studies of Jones and Miller (1959) and those obtained by Goldman et al. (1960) and by Randel and Doan (1956) rest on differences in the susceptibility of the reacting subjects, and those used in the latter studies were more sensitive. Attempts by Ziprkowsky et al. (1959) to cause passive sensitivity by transfer of sera from sensitive individuals into nonsensitive individuals, followed by exposure of the injected areas to dead larvae or by challenges with larval extracts, failed to demonstrate skin-sensitizing antibodies.

Until the involvement of specific antibodies is established, the question of the participation of allergic hypersensitivity in caterpillar dermatitis will remain unanswered.

IMMUNITY TO INGESTED ARTHROPODS

A variety of arthropods, including lobsters, crayfish, shrimps, prawns, crabs and some insects, serve as food for man. Sometimes, as with other foodstuff, the ingestion of these arthropods may evoke severe allergic disorders which are not confined to the gastrointestinal tract only, but which may also be manifested by a variety of systemic disorders and even anaphylaxis.

In general, the allergic response to food may appear within an hour following ingestion, or it may be prolonged up to 24 hours or more (Chobot, 1947). It is recognized that the ingestion of foods to which an individual is sensitive may trigger a variety of disorders including asthma, allergic rhinitis, urticaria, angioedema, eczema, migraine, gastrointestinal disorders, and other syndromes (Markow, 1960).

It is not within the scope of this chapter to deal with food allergy. It is sufficient to say that the ingestion of arthropods has been implicated in severe allergic disorders. Several cases of anaphylactic reactions from shrimp, lobster, and crabmeat have been reported by Coleman and Derbes (1964). One case involved an individual who developed an anaphylactic reaction (nausea, vomiting, generalized urticaria, low blood pressure, irregular pulse, and angioneurotic edema) one hour following the ingestion of sea food consisting of oysters, shrimp, trout, and scallops. His reactivity to lobster and shrimp was correlated with positive skin tests to antigens prepared from these arthropods. It is interesting that this individual had no previous history of allergy except that a month prior to the anaphylactic episode, he experienced swelling of the lip following the ingestion of shrimp. Another case was that of an individual who developed acute urticaria, low blood pressure, and lost consciousness in 20 minutes following the ingestion of crabmeat. This individual had a previous history of reactions following the ingestion of crabmeat. A third case was that of an individual who developed an anaphylactic shock (dyspnea, wheezing, urticaria, cyanosis, and an unobtainable blood pressure) 10 minutes following the ingestion of crabmeat. This individual had previously exhibited a mild anaphylactic reaction after smelling fumes of cooking crabmeat.

Since the food is digested and metabolized following ingestion, characterization of antigens responsible for sensitization or of allergens responsible for the onset of symptoms has not been accomplished. This also accounts for the uncertainty of diagnoses by direct skin tests or by passive transfer tests, since the allergens used in testing are not necessarily those which are involved in the reaction following ingestion. For these obvious reasons, desensitization to food allergy is generally not attempted, and the elimination of food known from previous history to elicit allergic disorders is the present practice for avoiding allergic episodes.

IMMUNITY TO INHALANT ARTHROPODS

The most important and widely encountered problems in clinical allergy are attributed to antigens and allergens which gain access into the body by inhalation. The occurrence of asthma and hay fever due to inhalation of pollen or dust is common knowledge. However, as evident from numerous clinical reports, arthropods and arthropod fragments seem to play an important part in respiratory allergic disorders. In fact, the number of substantiated clinical reports on the role of arthropods in asthma and hay fever merits a wider recognition of these etiologic agents than is currently encountered in clinical medicine.

Wilson (1913) first mentioned insects as a factor in inhalant allergy, reporting that the May fly (*Ephemera*) was a cause of asthma. Following Parlato's studies (1929, 1930, 1932) on the caddis fly (Order Trichoptera), the role of insects and insect parts as etiologic agents in respiratory allergy gained wider recognition.

Soon, increased numbers of reports appeared in the literature, which implicated in addition to the above insects a wide variety of others, including members of the orders Diptera, Hemiptera, Orthoptera, Lepidoptera, Coleoptera, and Hymenoptera. These reports have been the subject of several reviews (Brown, 1944; Feinberg et al., 1956; Perlman, 1958, 1961, 1964; Wiseman et al., 1959; Brock, 1961; Shulman, 1967; and others).

In most instances the reports were concerned with a single species as the etiologic agent of either allergic rhinitis, hay fever, or asthma. The diagnosis was usually aided by skin tests, by ophthalmic tests, and by passive transfer tests with the patients' sera, using extracts of the insect as antigens. Reactions to these tests indicated that the offending allergen was present in the extracts. In most instances the extracts for both testing and treatment of patients were prepared from the whole body of the insect. In several cases, insect parts or even excreta were used for the preparation of extracts. The seasonal increase in the number of insects, at times even in swarms (as exemplified by the caddis fly and May fly), served as additional support for the clinical reports of seasonal hay fever and asthma attributed to arthropods. This was particularly significant when other seasonal factors, such as pollens, could not be incriminated as the etiologic agents.

Although the clinical evidence for insect inhalant allergy is quite convincing, the tremendous number of insect species (625,000 to 1,500,000, according to Sabrosky, 1952) makes specific identification of the causative insect a formidable task. The process of identification and characterization of the specific insect allergen is confronted with the same obstacles encountered in the immunologic and the immunochemical investigations of any other inhaled allergens, such as pollens or dusts.

To reduce the complexities presented by the large number of arthropod species which may serve as a source of antigenic material, Perlman (1961) has proposed that skin tests with insect material be prepared with a reasonably small number of arthropod orders which embrace 96 percent of the known species. These include the orders Coleoptera (beetles, weevils), Lepidoptera (moths and butterflies), Hymenoptera (honeybees, hornets, yellowjackets), Diptera (flies, mosquitoes), Orthoptera (grasshoppers, locusts, cockroaches), Hemiptera (box-elder bugs, squash bugs), and Homoptera (aphids, leafhoppers, cicadas, scales) all of which are of the class Hexapoda (Insecta). From the class Arachnida, they include the orders Aranea (spiders) and Acarina (mites and ticks), and from the class Crustacea, they include the orders Isopoda (sowbugs) and Branchiopoda (Daphnia, fairy shrimp). Perlman also proposed an additional list of several orders for testing cases involved in specific regional problems and with less common arthropods. These include the orders Ephemeroptera (May flies), Trichoptera (caddis flies), Neuroptera (lacewings), Thysanura (silverfish), all being of the class Hexapoda, as well as Chilopoda (centipedes) and Diplopoda (millipedes) of the class Myriapoda and Copepoda (plankton shrimp) of the class Crustacea. This author recommended that following tests with the above, a more detailed testing program with various families, genera, or even species should be undertaken.

Perlman's program is based on the premise that insects within a given class or family will cross-react. This assumption is based upon the observation that multiple sensitivities to hay fever-causing plants and to mammalian danders are usually exhibited by a reactive patient. Therefore, it is assumed that different families of insects will manifest multiple reactions in testing. The vulnerability of this assumption is recognized by the author; it should, however, not detract from the practical value of his testing program.

There are many studies based on skin testing which attempt to demonstrate common allergens among insect species. Wiseman et al. (1959) prepared extracts from 27 species embracing the orders Orthoptera, Neuroptera, Ephemerida, Odonata, Homoptera, Hemiptera, Coleoptera, Lepidoptera, Diptera, and Hymenoptera. Antigens were made from both the larvae and the adults of several species and the pupae and the adult of one species. Altogether, 33 different extracts were prepared. The extracts were dialyzed and then standardized for skin testing by determination of protein nitrogen units. The authors reported that the study had two purposes: (1) to learn whether common antigens were present in different orders of the class Insecta as well as among members of the same order, and (2) to determine if there were common antigens present in the various stages of the life cycle of the same insect. Results of the test showed that pollen-sensitive individuals exhibited a high degree of reactivity to the extracts, whereas the majority of the non-pollen-sensitive individuals exhibited low or no reactivity. The results also indicated cross-reactivity among species within the order Coleoptera and cross-reactivity among various stages of metamorphosis of caterpillars and of yellowjackets.

MacLaren et al. (1960) performed skin tests in 200 "allergic" individuals and 150 nonallergic controls, using extracts of bees, houseflies, moths, ants, aphids, yellowjackets, mosquitoes, and wasps to compare skin reactivity. A significantly higher incidence of reactivity was exhibited by the allergic group than by the nonallergic group.

A number of authors reporting on various insects have associated the causative agent with various insect parts or products. In Parlato's case report on the caddis fly, he claimed (although he did not demonstrate) that the symptoms were caused by the hairs and scaly epithelim which were thrown into the air by the fly from its rapidly beating wings (Parlato, 1929). Randolph (1934), reporting on the New Mexican range moth caterpillar, attributed the cause of hay fever and asthma in his patients to their contact with egg-shell dust and larvae. Jamieson (1938) attributed nasal allergy to wings of the house fly *Musca domestica*. A small fragment of wing produced a positive ophthalmic test, and half a wing brushed inside one nostril caused sneezing immediately and rhinorrhea within a few minutes. Scratch, intracutaneous, and passive transfer tests with an extract of fly wings were positive. Frankland (1953) observed allergic rhinitis and asthma in laboratory workers in close contact with locusts. A locust extract gave strong reactions on skin testing, and locust feces produced the most marked skin reactions.

Because proteins, carbohydrates, and sulfur-containing compounds are found in the exoskeleton, this portion of the arthropod's body has been considered the source of allergens. However, unless their allergenicity can be specifically demonstrated, the presence of these substances does not necessarily mean that they serve as allergens. The antigenicity of silk in animals has been well demonstrated by the studies of Cebra (1961). It is conceivable that silk could serve as an inhalant allergen. In view of its widespread distribution throughout the insect world, and because of its common application in everyday living, silk is a substance that deserves serious consideration in inhalant insect allergy.

With the presence of millions of arthropods per acre of surface soil, one would expect soil dust to contain substances of insect origin which could serve as allergens. Feinberg et al. (1956) failed to demonstrate positive skin tests in insect-sensitive patients using acetone-precipitated fractions of some samples of soil. The authors felt that these negative results may have been due to a faulty method of antigen preparation, rather than to the lack of insect allergens in the soil. However, in a group of 130 patients who gave positive skin tests to insect antigens, 69 percent were also positive to house dust, which implied (for these authors) the presence of insect fragments in house dust.

Immunologically active components of the caddis fly have been investigated by Rapp et al. (1962), by Shulman et al. (1962, 1963), and by Langlois et al. (1963a, b). These workers demonstrated that prolonged defatting during the preparation of caddis-fly extract decreased the allergenic activity of the extract when compared to extracts obtained from nondefatted insects (Rapp et al., 1962). Fractionation of the extract by zone electrophoresis yielded a fraction that contained most (but not all) of the allergenic activity found in the initial extract. Direct skin tests and passive transfers were employed for assay of allergenicity (Shulman et al., 1962). Subsequent work by Shulman et al. (1963) on the physicochemical characterization of the allergens showed that the electrophoretically purified fraction contained a peptide or a glycopeptide allergen with a molecular weight of approximately 3,000. This fraction failed to give positive immunologic reactions with anti-caddis-fly rabbit serum, which implied that this fraction is not antigenic in rabbits, although it had been shown to be a very potent allergen by skin-testing procedures in humans (Langlois et al., 1963a).

Several studies employing immunologic and immunochemical techniques for both the identification of the allergen and the demonstration of cross-reactivity among insects have been reported. The studies of Langlois et al. (1963b) are particularly noteworthy. Using rabbit antisera and employing tanned-cell hemagglutination and gel-diffusion techniques, these authors showed cross-reactions among the caddis fly, the field cricket (*Acheta assimilis*), the short-horned grasshopper (*Melanoplus bivittatus*), the monarch butterfly (*Danaus plexippus*), and the sphinx moth (*Phlegathontius quinquemaculata*). Very little cross-reaction was observed between the caddis fly and the grasshopper. These authors reported the interesting observation that the caddis fly showed the greatest cross-reactivity with the cricket, although these two insects are taxonomically distant, whereas the more closely related Lepidoptera showed less cross-reactivity.

Pruzansky et al. (1958) investigated the antigenicity in rabbits of extracts of the May fly, the fly *Phormia regina*, the cockroach, the cricket, and silk pupa by hemagglutination and agar-gel precipitation techniques. These investigators demonstrated the presence of specific antigens in each extract, as well as antigens common to one or more of the other extracts. They reported that their studies indicated an antigen common to the May fly, fly, roach, and cricket; one common to the fly, roach, and cricket; another one common to the fly and roach; and another to the cricket and roach. Although these data indicate common antigens in the insects themselves, the authors raise the possibility of common bacterial associates as a source of common antigens. This possibility has also been raised by Feinberg et al. (1956).

The possibility of the presence of contaminants in insect extracts warrants further consideration. The method for obtaining the insect material can be a very important determining factor. Most studies were conducted with wild insects. It is conceivable that many elements in the environment could serve to contaminate the extracts, either through coating the individual insects or through the ingestion of environmental material by the insects. In the case of a biting insect such as the bed bug, which has been reported as a source of inhalant allergens (Sternberg, 1929), the blood meal could be a contaminating factor. In the case of inhalant allergy caused by the mushroom fly *Aphiochaeta agarici*, reported by Kern (1938), it would be important to consider manure as a source of contamination. The house fly, which was reported by Jamieson (1938) to cause allergy, could certainly carry with it many contaminants. The Indian meal moth *Plodia interpunctella*, which was implicated by Wittich (1940a) as a cause of allergy, may have been contaminated with the mill dust in which it lives, and in his reports (1940b) on allergy to the Mexican bean weevil *Zabrotes subfasciatus*, bean dust as a possible contaminant must be considered. Almost every report suggests some possible environmental contaminant which could serve to explain the wide range of cross-reactivity to arthropod extracts demonstrated by skin testing and by other immunologic techniques. It would be of value to conduct simultaneous tests with extracts of some of the insect's environmental media.

In interpreting results of skin tests and other immunologic procedures, one must bear in mind that in inhalant allergy of any type, whether due to pollens, dust, or insect material, the reaction is usually identified with reaginic antibodies which are nonprecipitating humoral antibodies having strong affinity for skin. This type of antibody has so far not been demonstrated by *in vitro* immunologic procedures. For this reason, one cannot correlate inhalant allergic disease with antibodies titrated by various *in vitro* studies. In addition, it must be recognized that antibodies other than reagins can be skin-sensitizing. In this case, these antibodies differ from reagins in that they remain attached to skin for only brief periods (usually less than 24 hours) and in their relative stability to heat. Reagins lose their activity when heated at 56°C for periods of 1 to 10 hours, depending on the serum (Sehon and Gyenes, 1966). An immediate skin reaction does not necessarily indicate the presence of reagin. In the interpretation of passive transfer tests, it is important that more than 24 hours have elapsed after injection of the test site with serum and that an aliquot of the serum was heat-treated in order to demonstrate the thermolability of reagins, if present.

The considerable material on insect inhalant allergy, although still mainly speculative, serves as very strong circumstantial evidence to support the hypothesis that insects or their parts may serve as allergens to produce allergic respiratory disease. In the absence of other procedures for the identification of reagins, one must resort to skin testing and passive transfer tests as means for demonstrating the presence of reagins, while keeping in mind the characteristics of reagins as opposed to nonreaginic skin-sensitizing antibodies. One must also bear in mind possible reactions due to contaminants (unless the source of the insect material is well controlled, e.g., by artificial rearing of the insects). The inability to titrate reagins *in vitro* makes the task of identifying the allergen a more formidable one. Yet in view of the progress in immunochemical techniques, the prospects for the characterizations of allergens involved in reactions to inhaled arthopods and arthropod parts are promising.

REFERENCES

Adam, K. R., and C. Weiss. 1958. The occurrence of 5-hydroxytryptamine in scorpion venom. J. Exp. Biol., 35:39–42.
———— and C. Weiss. 1959. Action of scorpion venom on skeletal muscle. Brit. J. Pharmacol, 14:334–339.
Adrouny, G. A., V. J. Derbes, and R. C. Jung. 1959. Isolation of a hemolytic component of fire ant venom. Science, 130:449.
Allen, A. C. 1948. Persistent "insect bites" (dermal eosinophilic granulomas) simulating lymphoblastomas, histiocytoses, and squamous cell carcinomas. Amer. J. Path., 24:367–387.
Allen, J. R. 1964. Some properties of oral secretion of mosquitoes. Ph.D. Thesis, Queen's University, Kingston, Ontario.
———— and A. S. West. 1964. Recent advances in studies on reactions to mosquito bites. *In* Proceedings of the First International Congress of Parasitology, Vol. 2. Corradetti, A., ed. Oxford, Pergamon Press, pp. 1091–1092.
Arbesman, C. E., C. Langlois, and S. Shulman. 1965. The allergic response to stinging insects. IV. Cross-reactions between bee, wasp, and yellow jacket. J. Allerg. 36:147–157.
Arean, V. M., and I. Fox. 1955. Dermal alterations in severe reactions to the bites of the sandfly *Culicoides furens*. Amer. J. Clin. Path., 25:1359–1366.
Atkins, J. A., C. W. Wingo, W. A. Sodeman, and J. E. Flynn. 1958. Necrotic arachnidism. Amer. J. Trop. Med. Hyg., 7:165–184.
Balozet, L. 1956. Scorpion venoms and antiscorpion serum. *In* Venoms. Buckley, E. E., and Porges, N., eds. Washington, D.C., Amer. Ass. Advance Sci. Publ. No. 44, pp. 141–144.
Beard, R. L. 1963. Insect toxins and venoms. *In* Annual Review of Entomology. Smith, R. F. and Mittler, T. E., eds. Palo Alto, California., Annual Reviews Inc., pp. 1–18.
Benacerraf, B., and P. G. H. Gell. 1962. Immunological specificity of delayed and immediate hypersensitivity reactions. Mechanism of cell and tissue damage produced

by immune reactions. *In* Second International Symposium on Immunopathology, Brook Lodge, Michigan, 1961. Grabar, P., and Miescher, P., eds. Basel, Benno Schwabe and Co., pp. 136–145.

Benjamini, E. 1964. The immunochemistry of flea bite hypersensitivity. *In* Proceedings of the First International Congress of Parasitology, Vol. 2. Corradetti, A., ed. Oxford, Pergamon Press, p. 1090.

———— 1967. Unpublished data.

———— Ben F. Feingold, and L. Kartman. 1960a. Allergy to flea bites. III. The experimental induction of flea bite sensitivity in guinea pigs by exposure to flea bites and by antigen prepared from whole flea extracts of *Ctenocephalides felis felis*. Exp. Parasit., 10:214–222.

———— Ben F. Feingold, and L. Kartman. 1960b. Antigenic property of the oral secretion of fleas. Nature (London), 188:959–960.

———— Ben F. Feingold, and L. Kartman. 1961. Skin reactivity in guina pigs sensitized to flea bites. The sequence of reactions. Proc. Soc. Exp. Biol. Med., 108:700–702.

———— Ben F. Feingold, J. D. Young, L. Kartman, and M. Shimizu. 1963a. Allergy to flea bites. IV. *In vitro* collection and antigenic properties of the oral secretion of the cat flea. *Ctenocephalides felis felis* (Bouché). Exp. Parasit., 13:143–154.

———— Ben F. Feingold, and L. Kartman. 1963b. The physiological and biochemical role of the host's skin in the induction of flea-bite hypersensitivity. I. Preliminary studies with guinea pig skin following exposure to bites of cat fleas. Exp. Parasit., 14:75–80.

Benson, R. L. 1936. Diagnosis and treatment of sensitization to mosquitoes. J. Allerg., 8:47–57.

———— and H. Semenov. 1930. Allergy in its relation to bee sting. J. Allerg., 1:105–116.

Bernton, H. S., and H. Brown. 1965. Studies on hymenoptera. I. Skin reactions of normal persons to honeybee (*Apis mellifera*) extract. J. Allerg., 36:315–320.

Bertke, E. M., and J. H. Atkins. 1964. Effect of *Centruroides sculpturatus* venom upon rat tissue: A histopathologic study. Toxicon, 2:205–209.

Bhoola, K. D., J. Calle, and M. Schacter, 1961. Identification of acetylcholine, 5-hydroxytryptamine, histamine and a new kinin in hornet venom (*Vespa crabro*). J. Physiol., 159:167–182.

Bishopp, F. C. 1923. The puss caterpillar and the effects of its sting on man. U.S. Dept. Agric. Circular No. 288.

Blacklock, D. B., and M. G. Thompson. 1923. A study of the tumble-fly *Cordylobia anthropophaga* Grunberg, in Sierra Leone. Ann. J. Trop. Med. Parasit., 7:443–510.

———— and R. M. Gordon. 1927. The experimental production of immunity against metazoan parasites and an investigation of its nature. Ann. Trop. Med. Parasit., 21:181–224.

———— R M. Gordon, and J. Fine. 1930. Metazoan immunity: A report on recent investigations. Ann. Trop. Med. Parasit., 24:5–54.

Blum, M. S. 1963. The venom and poison glands of *Pseudomyrmex pallidus*. Psyche, 70:60–74.

———— and P. S. Callahan. 1960. Chemical and biological properties of the venom of the imported fire ant (*Solenopsis saevissima* var. *richteri* Forel) and the isolation of the insecticidal component. *In* Proceedings of the 11th International Congress of Entomology, Vienna, 1960, Vol. 3. Strouhal, H., and Beier, M., eds. Vienna, C. Reisser, pp. 290–293.

———— J. R. Walker, P. S. Callahan, and P. S. Novak. 1958. Chemical, insecticidal and antibiotic properties of fire ant venom. Science, 128:306–307.

Borgstrom, F. A. 1938. Studies on experimental *Cochliomyia americana* infestations with special reference to the bacterial flora and the development of immunity. Amer. J. Trop. Med., 18:395–411.

Boycott, A. E. 1913. The reaction of flea-bites. J. Path. Bact. 17:110.

Bray, R. S. 1957. Studies on the exo-erythrocytic cycle in the genus Plasmodium. Memoirs of the London School of Hygiene and Tropical Medicine, 12:24–26.

Brock, T. 1961. Résumé of insect allergy. Ann. Allerg. 19:288–297.

Brown, A., T. H. D. Griffiths, S. Erwin, and L. Y. Dyrenforth. 1938. Arthus phenomenon from mosquito bites. Southern Med. J., 31:590–595.

Brown, E. A. 1944. Insects and allergy. Ann. Allerg. 2:235–246.

Buckley, E. E., and N. Porges. 1956. Venoms. Washington, D. C., Amer. Ass. Advance. Sci. Publ. No. 44.

Campbell, A. C. P., A. M. Drennan, and T. Rettie. 1935. The relationship of the eosinophile leucocyte to allergy and anaphylaxis. J. Path. Bact., 40:537–548.

Caro, M. R., V. J. Derbes, and R. C. Jung. 1957. Skin responses to the sting of the
imported fire ant (Solenopsis saevissima). Arch. Derm., 75:475–488.

Cavanaugh, D. C., and R. Randall. 1959. The role of multiplication of Pasteurella pestis
in mononuclear phagocytes in the pathogenesis of flea-borne plague. J. Immun.,
83:348–363.

Cavili, G. W. K., P. L. Robertson, and F. B. Whitfield. 1964. Venom and venom apparatus of the bull ant, Myrmecia gulosa (Fabr.). Science, 146:79–80.

Cebra, J. J. 1961. Studies on the combining sites of the protein antigen silk fibroin. I.
Characterization of the fibroin-rabbit antifibroin system. J. Immun., 86:190–196.

Cervera, E. 1936. Suero anti-Alacranico. Bol. Ofic. Sanit. Panamer., 15:142–149.

Cherney, L. S., C. M. Wheeler, and A. C. Reed. 1939. Flea-antigen in prevention of flea
bites. Amer. J. Trop. Med., 19:327–332.

Chobot, R. 1947. Food allergy. In Allergy in Theory and Practice. Cooke, R. A., ed.
Philadelphia, W. B. Saunders Co., pp. 469–474.

Cloudsley-Thompson, J. L. 1958. Spiders, Scorpions, Centipedes, and Mites. New York,
Pergamon Press.

Coleman, W. P., and V. J. Derbes. 1964. Anaphylactic reactions from shellfish. Derma-
tologia Tropica, 3:91–94.

Cornwall, J., and W. Patton. 1914. Some observations on the salivary secretions of the
common blood sucking insects and ticks. Indian J. Med. Res., 2:569–593.

Crewe, W., and R. M. Gordon. 1949. The histology of the lesions caused by the sting of
the hive-bee (Apis mellifica). Ann. Trop. Med. Parasit., 43:341–344.

D'Amour, F. E., F. E. Becker, and W. Van Riper. 1936. Black widow spider. Quart.
Rev. Biol., 11:123–160.

Day, M. F., and D. F. Waterhouse. 1953. Functions of salivary glands. In Insect Physiology. Roeder, K. D., ed. New York, John Wiley and Sons, Inc., pp. 308–310.

De Buck, A. 1937. Some observations on the salivary and stomach secretion of Anopheles and other mosquitoes. Proc. Roy. Acad. Amsterdam, 40:217–223.

Del Pozo, E. C. 1956. Mechanism of pharmacological actions of scorpion venoms. In
Venoms. Buckley, E. E., and Porges, N., eds. Washington, D. C., Amer. Ass. Advanc.
Sci. Publ. No. 44, pp. 123–192.

De Meillon, B. 1949. The relationship between ectoparasite and host. IV. Host reactions
to the bites of arthropods. The Leech, August 1949: 43–46.

Denny, W. F., C. J. Dillaha, and P. N. Morgan. 1964. Hemotoxic effects of Loxosceles
reclusus venom: In vivo and in vitro studies. J. Lab. Clin. Med., 64:291–298.

Dickerson, G., and M. M. J. Lavoipierre. 1959. Studies on the methods of feeding of
blood-sucking arthropods. II. The method of feeding adopted by the bedbug Cimex
lectularius, when obtaining a blood-meal from the mammalian host. Ann. Trop. Med.
Parasit., 53:347–357.

Dienes, L., and T. B. Mallory. 1932. Histologic studies of hypersensitive reactions.
Amer. J. Path., 8:689–710.

Dillaha, C. J., G. T. Jansen, W. M. Honeycut, and C. R. Hayden. 1963. The gangrenous
bite of the brown recluse spider in Arkansas. J. Arkansas Med. Soc., 60:91–94.

——— G. T. Jansen, W. M. Honeycutt, and C. R. Hayden. 1964. North American loxoscelism. Necrotic bite of the brown recluse spider. J. A. M. A., 188:33–36.

Diniz, C. R., and J. M. Goncalves. 1956. Some chemical and pharmacological properties
of Brazilian scorpion venoms. In Venoms. Buckley, E. E., and Porges, N., eds. Washington, D.C., Amer. Ass. Advance. Sci. Publ. No. 44, pp. 131–139.

Dubin, N., J. D. Reese, and L. A. Seamans. 1948. Attempt to produce protection against
mosquitoes by active immunization. J. Immun., 58:293–297.

Efrati, P. 1949. Poisoning by scorpion stings in Israel. Amer. J. Trop. Med., 29:249–257.

Eisen, H. N. 1959. Hypersensitivity to simple chemicals. In Cellular and Humoral
Aspects of the Hypersensitive State. Lawrence, H. S., ed. New York, Harper and
Row, pp. 89–122.

Fairbairn, H., and J. Williamson. 1956. The composition of tsetse fly saliva. I. A histochemical analysis. Ann. Trop. Med. Parasit., 50:322–333.

Favilli, G. 1956. Occurrence of spreading factors and some properties of hyaluronidases
in animal parasites and venoms. In Venoms. Buckley, E. E., and Porges, N., eds.
Washington, D.C., Amer. Ass. Advance. Sci. Publ. No. 44, pp. 281–289.

Feinberg, A. R., S. M. Feinberg, and C. Benaim-Pinto. 1956. Asthma and rhinitis from insect allergens. I. Clinical importance. J. Allerg., 27:437–444.

Feingold, Ben F. 1964. Clinical and immunological aspects of hypersensitivity to flea bites. *In* Proceedings of the First International Congress of Parasitology, Vol. 2. Corradetti, A., ed., Oxford, Pergamon Press, pp. 1089–1090.

———— and B. W. Hudson, 1960. Unpublished data.

———— and E. Benjamini. 1961. Allergy to flea bites: Clinical and experimental observations. Ann. Allerg. 19:1275–1289.

———— E. Benjamini, and M. Shimizu. 1964. Induction of delayed and immediate types of skin reactivity in guinea pigs by variation in dosages of antigens. Ann. Allerg., 22:279–291.

Finlayson, M. H, 1936. Knoppie-spider bite. S. Afr. Med. J., 10:43.

———— and K. Hollow. 1945. The treatment of spider-bite in South Africa by specific sera. S. Afr. Med. J., 19:431–433.

Foot, N. C. 1922. Pathology of the dermatitis caused by *Megalopyge opercularis*, a Texan caterpillar. J. Exp. Med., 35:737–753.

Foubert, E. L., and R. A. Stier. 1958. Antigenic relationships between honeybees, wasps, yellow hornets, black hornets, and yellowjackets. J. Allerg., 29:13–23.

Fox, I., and N. S. Berman. 1960. A preliminary report on biting mosquitoes in Puerto Rico together with some experimental work on natural and acquired sensitivity of man to insect bites. Biol. Ass. Med. Puerto Rico, 52:89–94.

———— W. B. Knight, and L. G. Bayona. 1963. Antigenic relationship among mosquitoes and sand flies demonstrated by agar-gel tests. J. Allerg., 34:196–202.

Frankland, A. W. 1953. Locust sensitivity. Ann. Allerg., 11:445–453.

Frontali, N., and A. Grasso. 1964. Separation of three toxicologically different protein components from the venom of the spider *Latrodectus tredecimguttatus*. Arch. Biochem. Biophys., 106:213–218.

Geigy, R., and M. Huber. 1959. Demonstration of trehalose in the vector of African trypanosomiasis: the tsetse fly. Acta Trop. (Basel), 16:225–262.

Gell, P. G. H. 1959. Cytologic events in hypersensitivity reactions. *In* Cellular and Humoral Aspects of the Hypersensitive State. Lawrence, H. S., ed. New York, Harper and Row, pp. 43–62.

Gilmer, P. M. 1924. A comparative study of the poison-apparatus of certain lepidopterous larvae. Ann. Entom. Soc. Amer., 18:203–239.

Glenn, W. G., and F. W. Whittemore. 1962. Intergeneric relationship among various scorpion venoms. Science, 135:434–435.

Goldman, L. 1956. Parasitic infections of the skin. Pediat. Clin. N. Amer., 3:625–637.

———— 1963. Tick bite granuloma: Failure of prevention of lesion by excision of tick bite area. Amer. J. Trop. Med. Hyg., 12:246–248.

———— E. Rockwell, and D. F. Richfield. 1925. Histopathological studies on cutaneous reactions to the bites of various arthropods. Amer. J. Trop. Med. Hyg., 1:514–525.

———— P. Johnson, and J. Ramsey. 1952. The insect bite reaction. I. The mechanism. J. Invest. Derm., 18:403–417.

———— F. Sawyer, A. Levine, J. Goldman, S. Goldman, and J. Spinanger. 1960. Investigative studies of skin irritations from caterpillars. J. Invest. Derm., 34:67–78.

Gordon, R. M., and W. Crewe. 1948. The mechanism by which mosquitoes and tsetseflies obtain their blood meal, the histology of the lesions produced, and the subsequent reactions of the mammalian host; together with some observations on the feeding of *Chrysops* and *Cimex*. Ann. Trop. Med. Parasit., 42:334–356.

———— and W. H. R. Lumsden. 1939. Study of the behaviour of the mouthparts of mosquitoes when taking up blood from living tissue; together with some observations on the ingestion of microfilariae. Ann. Trop. Med. Parasit., 33:259–278.

Goren, S. 1950. The scorpions of Turkey and antiscorpion serum. Turk. Z. Hyg. Exp. Biol., 10:81–95.

Gregson, J. D. 1960. Morphology and functioning of the mouthparts of *Dermacentor andersoni* Stiles. Acta Trop. (Basel), 17:47–79.

Griffiths, R. B., and R. M. Gordon. 1952. An apparatus which enables the process of feeding by mosquitoes to be observed in the tissue of a live rodent; together with an account of the ejection of saliva and its significance in malaria. Ann. Trop. Med. Parasit., 46:311–319.

Haberman, E. 1965. Recent studies on hymenoptera venom. *In* Recent Advances of Pharmacology of Toxins. Proceedings of the Second International Pharmacology

Meeting, Prague, August 1963. Rašková, H., and Vaněček, J., eds. Oxford, Pergamon Press, Vol. 9, pp. 53–62.

———— and M. M. A. El-Karemi. 1956. Antibody formation by protein components of bee venom. Nature (London), 178:1349.

———— and J. Jentsch. 1966. Über die Struktur des toxischen Bienengiftpeptids Melittin und deren Beziehung zur pharmakologischen Wirkung. Naunyn-Schmiedebergs Arch. Exp. Path. Pharm., 253:40–41.

Hartman, M. M. 1946. Flea bite reactions. Clinical and experimental observations and effect of histamine-azoprotein therapy. Ann. Allerg., 4:131–136.

Hase, A. 1916. Weitere Beobachtungen über die Lauseplage. Zbl. Bakt. [Orig.], 77:153–163.

Hatoff, A. 1946. Desensitization to insect bites. J. A. M. A., 130:850–854.

Hecht, O. 1928. Über die Sprosspilze der Oesophagusausstulpungen und über die Giftigverkung der Speicheldrüsen von Stechmücken. Arch. Schiffs. Tropenhyg., 32:561–575.

———— 1929. Die Hautreaktionen auf Insektenstiche als allergische Erscheinungen. Arch. Schiffs.Tropenhyg., 33:364–366.

———— 1933. Hautreaktionen auf die Stiche blutsaugender Insekten und Milben als allergische Erscheinungen. Z. Haut. Geschlechtskr., 44:241–255.

———— 1943a. Estudios comparativos de algunas reacciones alergicas contra las picaduras de insectos. Experiencias obteinidas con pulgas, zacudos y simulidos en Venezuela. Rev. Sanid. Asist. Soc., 8:392–407.

———— 1943b. Las reacciones da la piel contra las picaduras de insectos como fenomenos alergicos. Rev. Sanid. Asist. Soc., 8:945–959.

Heilesen, B. 1949. Studies on mosquito bites. Acta Allerg. (Kobenhavn), 2:245–267.

Herms, W. B., and M. T. James. 1961. Medical Entomology, 5th Ed., New York, The Macmillan Co.

Hindle, E. 1914. Flies in Relation to Disease. Blood Sucking Flies. Cambridge, Cambridge University Press.

Hodgson, N. B. 1955. Bee venom. Its components and their properties. Bee World, 36:217–222.

Holdstock, D. J., A. P. Mathias, and M. Schachter. 1957. A comparative study of kinin, kallidin, and bradykinin. Brit. J. Pharmacol., 12:149–158.

Horen, P. W. 1963. Arachnidism in the United States. J. A. M. A., 185:839–843.

Hudson, A., J. A. McKiel, A. S. West, and T. K. R. Bourns. 1958. Reaction to mosquito bites. Mosquito News, 18:249–252.

———— L. Bowman, and C. W. M. Orr. 1960. Effect of absence of saliva on blood feeding by mosquitoes. Science, 131:1730–1731.

Hudson, B. W., Ben F. Feingold, and L. Kartman. 1960a. Allergy to flea bites. I. Experimental induction of flea-bite sensitivity in guinea pigs. Exp. Parasit., 9:18–24.

———— B. F. Feingold, and L. Kartman. 1960b. Allergy to flea bites. II. Investigations of flea bite sensitivity in humans. Exp. Parasit., 9:151–157.

Insect Allergy Committee of the American Academy of Allergy. 1965. Insect-sting allergy. J. A. M. A., 193:115–120.

Insect Allergy Committee Report. 1966. American Academy of Allergy Report, February, 1966.

Janssen, W. A., W. D. Lawton, G. M. Fukui, and M. J. Surgalla. 1963. The pathogenesis of plague. I. A study of correlation between virulence and relative phagocytosis resistance of some strains of Pasteurella pestis. J. Infect. Dis., 113:139–149.

Jamieson, H. C. 1938. The housefly as a cause of nasal allergy. J. Allerg., 9:273–274.

Jaques, R. 1956. The hyaluronidase content of animal venoms. In Venoms. Buckley, E. E., and Porges, N., eds. Washington, D.C., Amer. Ass. Advance. Sci. Publ. No. 44, pp. 291–293.

———— and M. Schachter. 1954. The presence of histamine, 5-hydroxytryptamine and a potent, slow contracting substance in wasp venom. Brit. J. Pharmacol., 9:53–58.

Jensen, O. M. 1962. Sudden death due to stings from bees and wasps. Acta Path. Microbiol. Scand., 54:9–29.

Johnson, R. M., and H. L. Stahnke. 1960. Chromatographic comparison of scorpion venoms. Nature (London), 132:895–896.

Jones, D. L., and J. H. Miller. 1959. Pathology of the dermatitis produced by the urticating caterpillar, Automeris io. Arch. Derm., 79:81–85.

Jones, J. P. 1961. Public health significance of Triatoma protracta Uhler in Sierra

Nevada foothill areas. State of California Department of Public Health Bureau of Vector Control Bulletin, pp. 1–70.

Jones, T. D., and J. R. Mote. 1934. The phases of foreign protein sensitization in human beings. New Eng. J. Med., 210:120–123.

Kailin, L. W. 1965. Interim report of the committee on insect allergy. J. Allerg., 36:190–192.

Kaiser, E., and H. Michl. 1958. Die Biochemie der tierischen Gifte. Vienna, Franz Deuticke.

Kaplan, M. H., and L. Dienes. 1958. The cellular response in form of delayed- and immediate-type skin reactions in the guinea pig. *In* Mechanisms of Hypersensitivity, Henry Ford Hospital Intern. Symposium. Shaffer, J. H., Lo Grippo, G. A., and Chase, M. W., eds. Boston, Little, Brown and Co., pp. 435–449.

Kartman, L. 1964. Insect allergy and arthropod-borne infection: A hypothesis. *In* Proceedings of the First International Congress of Parasitology, Vol. 2. Corradetti, A., ed. Oxford, Pergamon Press, pp. 1092–1093.

——— 1965. Insect allergy and arthropod-borne infection: A hypothesis. Zoonoses Res. (in press).

Keegan, H. L. 1955. Effectiveness of *Latrodectus tredecimguttatus* antivenin in protecting laboratory mice against effects of intraperitoneal injections of *Latrodectus mactans* venom. Amer. J. Trop. Med. Hyg., 4:762–764.

——— 1956. Antivenins available for treatment of envenomation by poisonous snakes, scorpions and spiders. *In* Venoms. Buckley, E. E., and Porges, N., eds. Washington, D.C., Amer. Ass. Advance. Sci. Publ. No. 44, pp. 413–438.

——— 1963. Caterpillars and moths as public health problems. *In* Venomous and Poisonous Animals and Noxious Plants of the Pacific Region. Keegan, H. L., and MacFarlane, W. V., eds. New York, The MacMillan Co., pp. 165–170.

——— R. A. Hedeen, and F. W. Whittemore. 1960. Seasonal variation in venom of black widow spiders. Amer. J. Trop. Med. Hyg., 9:477–479.

Kemper, H. 1929. Beobachtungen über den Stech- und Saugakt der Bettwanze und seine Wirkung auf die menschliche Haut. Z. Desinfekt., 21:61–67.

——— 1958. Experimentalle Untersuchungen über die Wirkung von Raupenhaaren auf die menschliche Haut. *In* Proceedings of the 10th International Congress of Entomology, Montreal, 1956. Vol. 3. Becker, E. C., ed. Ottawa, Mortimer, Ltd., pp. 719–723.

Kern, R. A. 1938. Asthma due to sensitization to a mushroom fly (*Aphichaeta agarici*). J. Allerg., 9:604–606.

Kikuth, W., and L. Mudrow. 1939a. Die Entwicklung der Sporozoiten von *P. cathemerium* im Kanarienvogel. Zbl. Bakt. [Orig.], 145:81–88.

——— and L. Mudrow. 1939b. Frühstadien der Vogelmalariaparasiten nach Sporozoiteninfektion. Klin. Wschr., 18:1443–1444.

Kissileff, A. 1938. The dog flea as a causative agent in summer eczema. J. Amer. Vet. Med. Ass., 46:21–27.

——— 1962. Relationship of dog fleas to dermatitis. Small Animal Clinician, 2:132–135.

Koegel, A. 1924. Präzipitations und Anaphylaxie Versuche mit Parasitenextracten (Larven von *Hypoderma bovis*, *Gastrophilus equi* und *Gastrophilus haemorrhoidalis*). Berlin. München. Tierärztl. Wschr., 75:945–954.

Langlois, C., S. Schulman, and C. E. Arbesman. 1963a. Immunologic studies of caddis fly. IV. Hemagglutination and gel precipitation studies of extracts. J. Allerg., 34:235–241.

——— S. Shulman, and C. E. Arbesman. 1963b. Immunologic studies of caddis fly. V. Cross reaction with other insects. J. Allerg., 34:385–394.

——— S. Shulman, and C. E. Arbesman. 1965a. The allergic response to stinging insects. II. Immunologic studies of human sera from allergic individuals. J. Allerg., 36:12–22.

——— S. Shulman, and C. F. Arbesman. 1965b. The allergic response to stinging insects. III. The specificity of venom sac antigens. J. Allerg., 36:109–120.

Larrivee, D. H., E. Benjamini, Ben F. Feingold, and M. Shimizu. 1964. Histologic studies of guinea pig skin: Different stages of allergic reactivity to flea bites. Exp. Parasit., 15:491–502.

Lavoipierre, M. M. J., and R. F. Riek. 1955. Observations on the feeding habits of Argasid ticks and on the effect of their bites on laboratory animals, together with a note on the production of coxal fluid by several of the species studied. Ann. Trop. Med. Parasit., 49:96–113.

—— G. Dickerson, and R. M. Gordon. 1959. Studies on the methods of feeding of blood-sucking arthropods. I. The manner in which triatomine bugs obtain their blood-meal as observed in tissues of the living rodent, with some remarks on the effects of the bite on human volunteers. Ann. Trop. Med. Parasit., 53:235–250.

Lawlor, W. K. 1949. Immunological studies of antigens extracted from mosquitoes and their application in taxonomy. Ph.D. Thesis, School of Hygiene and Public Health, Johns Hopkins University, Baltimore, Maryland.

Lebez, D., Z. Maretić, and J. Kristan. 1965. Studies on labeled animal poisons. I. Distribution of P^{32}-labeled *Latrodectus tredecimguttatus* venom in the guinea pig. Toxicon, 2:251–253.

Leclercq, M. 1950. À propos des accidents graves par piqûres d'Hyménoptères. Rev. Med. Liège, 5:750–753.

—— 1961. Les accidents allergiques provoqués par les insectes. Rev. Med. Liège, 26:109–115.

—— 1963. Les piqûres d'insectes venimeux. Les différents types d'accidents et leur thérapeutique. Ann. Soc. Belg. Med. Trop., 1:53–60.

—— 1965. Nouvel exemple de réaction allergique grave après piqûe de gûepe. Rev. Med. Liège, 20:141.

Lessenden, C. M., and L. K. Zimmer. 1960. Brown spider bites. J. Kansas Med. Soc., 61:379–385.

Lester, H. M. O., and L. Lloyd. 1928. Notes on the process of digestion in tsetse flies. Bull. Entom. Res., 19:39–60.

Litt, M. 1964. Eosinophils and antigen-antibody reactions. Ann. N. Y. Acad. Sci., 116:964–985.

Loveless, M. H. 1960. Sudden death from insect venom allergy reported often mistaken for coronary. Medical Tribune, September 5, 1960.

—— 1962. Immunization in wasp-stings allergy through venom-repositories and periodic insect stings. J. Immun., 89:204–215.

—— 1966. Antibody of atopy and serum disease in man. *In* Annual Review of Pharmacology. Vol. 6. Elliott, H. W., Cutting, W. S., and Dreisbach, R. H. eds. Palo Alto, California, Annual Reviews Inc., pp. 309–326.

—— and W. R. Fackler. 1956. Wasp venom allergy and immunity. Ann. Allerg., 14:347–366.

—— and T. M. Nall. 1965. Use of polistes venom in petrolatum: Arlacel repositories to immunize against yellow jacket wasp-sting allergy. J. Immun., 94:785–793.

Macchiavello, A. 1947a. Cutaneous arachnoidism or gangrenous spot of Chile. Puerto Rico J. Public Health Trop. Med., 22:425–466.

—— 1947b. Cutaneous arachnoidism experimentally produced with the glandular poison of *Loxosceles laeta*. Puerto Rico J. Public Health Trop. Med., 23:266–279.

Mackinnon, J. E., and J. Witkind. 1953. Arachnidismo necrotico. Ann Fac. Med. Montevideo Univ., 38:75–100.

MacLaren, W. R., Ben C. Eisenberg, D. E. Frank, and J. Kessler. 1960. Reactions to insect allergens. The incidence of response to testing among allergic and nonallergic persons. Calif. Med., 93:224–226.

Magalhães, O. 1947. Soro anti-escorpionico. Mem. Inst. Oswaldo Cruz, 45:847-851.

Maksianovich, M. I. 1939. The venom of *Latrodectus tredecimguttatus* as an antigen. The efficacy of the antitoxin in animal experiments. (In Russian with French summary). Med. Parazit. (Moskva), 8:51–63.

Manalang, C. 1931. Origin of the irritating substance in mosquito bite. Philippine J. Sci., 46:39–45.

Maretić, Z., and M. Stanic. 1954. The health problem of arachnidism. Bull. W. H. O., 11:1007–1022.

—— H. W. Levi, and L. R. Levi. 1964. The theridiid spider *Steatoda paykulliana*, poisonous to mammals. Toxicon, 2:149–154.

Markow, H. 1960. Food allergy. *In* Fundamentals of Modern Allergy. Prigal, S. J., ed. New York, McGraw-Hill Book Co., Inc., pp. 412–417.

Marshall, T. K. 1957. Wasp and bee stings. Practitioner, 179:712–722.

Marzan, B. 1955. Pathologic reactions associated with bite of *Latrodectus tredecimguttatus*. Observations in experimental animals. Arch. Path. (Chicago), 59:727–728.

Master, R. W. P., S. Srinivasa Rao, and P. D. Soman. 1963. Electrophoretic separation of biologically active constituents of scorpion venoms. Biochim. Biophys. Acta, 71:422–428.

Mathias, A. P., and M. Schachter. 1958. The chromatographic behavior of wasp venom, kinin, kallidin, and bradykinin. Brit. J. Pharmacol., 13:326–329.

Mazzotti, L., and M. A. Bravo-Becherelle. 1963. Scorpionism in the Mexican Republic. *In* Venomous and Poisonous Animals and Noxious Plants of the Pacific Region. Keegan, H. L., and MacFarlane, W. V., eds. New York, The Macmillan Co., pp. 119–131.

McCormick, W. F. 1963. Fatal anaphylactic reactions to wasp stings. Amer. J. Clin. Path., 39:485–491.

McCrone, J. D., and M. L. Netzloff. 1965. An immunological and electrophoretical comparison of the venoms of the North American *Latrodectus* spiders. Toxicon, 3:107–110.

McGovern, J. P., G. B. Barkin, T. R. McElhenney, and R. Wende. 1961. *Megalopyge opercularis*. Observations of its life history, of its sting in man, and report of an epidemic. J. A. M. A., 175:1155–1158.

McIvor, B. C., and L. S. Cherney. 1941. Studies in insect bite desensitization. Amer. J. Trop. Med., 21:493–497.

————— and L. S. Cherney. 1943. Clinical use of flea-antigen in patients hypersensitive to flea bites. Amer. J. Trop. Med., 23:377–379.

McKiel, J. A. 1955. Reactions to mosquito bites. Studies of causation and remedial measures. Ph.D. Thesis, Queen's University, Kingston, Ontario.

————— 1959. Sensitization to mosquito bites. Canad. J. Zool., 37:341–351.

————— and J. C. Clunie. 1960. Chromatographic fractionation of the non-dialyzable portion of mosquito extract and intracutaneous reactions of mosquito-bite-sensitive subjects to the separated components. Canad. J. Zool., 38:479–487.

————— and A. S. West. 1961a. Nature and causation of insect bite reactions. Pediat. Clin. N. Amer., 8:795–816.

————— and A. S. West. 1961b. Effects of repeated exposures of hypersensitive humans and laboratory rabbits to mosquito antigens. Canad. J. Zool., 39:597–603.

Mellanby, K. 1944. The development of symptoms, parasitic infection, and immunity in human scabies. Parasitology, 35:197–206.

————— 1946. Man's reaction to mosquito bites. Nature (London) 158:554.

Metcalf, R. L. 1945. The physiology of the salivary glands of *Anopheles quadrimaculatus*. J. Nat. Malar. Soc., 4:271–278.

Michaeli, D. 1967. Unpublished data.

————— E. Benjamini, J. D. Young, and Ben F. Feingold. 1965a. Biochemical studies on hypersensitivity to flea bites. *In* Proceedings of the 12th International Congress of Entomology, London. Freeman, P., ed., Vol. 12, p. 832.

————— E. Benjamini, F. P. de Buren, D. H. Larrivee, and Ben F. Feingold. 1965b. The role of collagen in the induction of hypersensitivity to flea bites. J. Immun., 95:162–170.

————— E. Benjamini, R. C. Miner, and Ben F. Feingold. 1966. *In vitro* studies on the role of collagen in the induction of hypersensitivity to flea bites. J. Immun., 97:402–406.

Micks, D. W. 1952. Clinical effects of the sting of the "pus caterpillar" (*Megalopyge opercularis* S. and A.) on man. Texas Rep. Biol. Med., 10:399–405.

Miller, D. G. 1956. Massive anaphylaxis from insect stings. *In* Venoms. Buckley, E. E., and Porges, N., eds. Washington, D.C., Amer. Ass. Advance., Sci. Publ. No. 44. pp. 117–121.

Miranda, F., and S. Lissitzky. 1961. Scorpamins: The toxic proteins of scorpion venoms. Nature (London), 190:443–444.

————— H. Rochat, and S. Lissitzky. 1960. Sur la neurotoxine du venin des scorpions. I. Purification à partir du venin de deux espèces de scorpions nord-africains. Bull. Soc. Chim. Biol. (Paris), 42:379–391.

————— H. Rochat, and S. Lissitsky. 1961. Sur la neurotoxine du venin des scorpions. II. Utilisation de l'électrophorèse sur papier pour l'orientation et le contrôle de la purification. Bull. Soc. Chim. Biol. (Paris), 43:945–952.

————— H. Rochat, C. Rochat, and S. Lissitzky. 1966a. Complexes moleculaires présentés par les neurotoxines animals. I. Neurotoxine des venin de scorpions (*Androctonus australis* Hector, et *Buthus occitanus tunetanus*). Toxicon, 4:123–144.

————— H. Rochat, C. Rochat, and S. Lissitzky. 1966b. Essais de purification des neurotoxines du venin d'un scorpion d'Amerique du Sud (*Tityus serrulatus* L. et M.) par des methodes chromatographiques. Toxicon, 4:145–152.

Mohammed, A. H. 1950. Blood sugar response to Egyptian scorpions. Nature (London), 166:734–735.

—— and M. M. A. El-Karemi. 1961. Immunity of bee keepers to some constituents of bee venom: phospholipase-A antibodies. Nature (London), 189:837–838.

—— and K. Zaki. 1961. Effect of bee venom on concentration of blood glucose and liver glycogen in rabbits. Nature (London), 191:605–606.

—— H. Rohayem, and O. Zaky. 1954. The action of scorpion toxin on blood sodium and potassium. J. Trop. Med. Hyg., 57:85–87.

Moore, W., and A. D. Hirschfelder. 1919. An investigation on the louse problem. Res. Pub. Univ. Minnesota, Vol. 7, Minneapolis, University of Minnesota.

Morse, E. S. 1897. Acquired immunity from insect stings. Nature (London), 55:533.

Mote, J. R., and T. D. Jones. 1936. The development of foreign sensitization in human beings. J. Immun., 30:149–167.

Mueller, H. L. 1965. Insect allergy, *In* Immunological Diseases. Samter, M., ed. Boston, Little, Brown and Co., pp. 682–689.

—— and L. W. Hill. 1953. Allergic reactions to bee and wasp stings. New Eng. J. Med., 249:726–731.

Muller, G. H. 1961. Flea allergy dermatitis. Small Animal Clinician, June 1961.

Nelson, W. A., and A. R. Bainborough. 1963. Development in sheep of resistance to the ked *Melophagus ovinus* (L). III. Histopathology of sheep skin as a clue to the nature of resistance. Exp. Parasit., 13:118–127.

Nitzan, M., and A. Shulov. 1966. Electrophoretic patterns of the venoms of six species of Israeli scorpions. Toxicon, 4:17–23.

O'Connor, R., and W. Rosenbrook. 1963. The venom of the mud-dauber wasps. I. *Sceliphron caementarium*: Preliminary separation and free amino acid content. Canad. J. Biochem. Physiol., 41:1943–1948.

—— W. Rosenbrook, Jr., and R. Erickson. 1964. Disc electrophoresis of Hymenoptera venoms and body proteins. Science, 145:1320–1321.

Oda, M., and T. T. Puck. 1961. Interaction of mammalian cells with antibodies. J. Exp. Med., 113:599–610.

Ordman, D. 1958. Desensitization to bee stings by intracutaneous injections of whole-bee extract. Brit. Med. J., 2:352–355.

Orr, C. W. M., A. Hudson, and A. S. West. 1961. The salivary glands of *Aedes aegypti*. Histological-histochemical studies. Canad. J. Zool., 39:265–272.

Ovary, Z. 1958. Immediate reactions in the skin of experimental animals provoked by antibody-antigen interaction. *In* Progress in Allergy, Vol. 5. Kallos, P. ed. Basel, S. Karger, pp. 459–508.

Parlato, J. S. 1929. A case of coryza and asthma due to sand flies (caddis flies). J. Allerg., 1:35–42.

—— 1930. The sand fly (caddis fly) as an exciting cause of allergic coryza and asthma. II. Its relative frequency. J. Allerg., 1:307–312.

—— 1932. Emanations of flies as exciting causes of allergic coryza and asthma. J. Allerg., 3:125–138.

Parrish, H. M. 1963. Analysis of 460 fatalities from venomous animals in the United States. Amer. J. Med. Sci., 425:129–141.

Patterson, R. A. 1960. Physiological action of scorpion venom. Amer. J. Trop. Med. Hyg., 9:410–414.

—— 1962. Pharmacologic action of scorpion venom on intestinal smooth muscle. Toxic. Appl. Pharmacol., 4:710–719.

Pavan, M. 1958. Biochemical aspects of insect poisons. *In* Proceedings of the Fourth International Congress of Biochemistry, Vienna, 1958, Vol. 12. Hoffmann, O., ed. London, Pergamon Press, pp. 15–36.

Pawlowsky, E. N., and A. K. Shtein. 1928. Experimentelle Untersuchungen über die Wirkung der wirksammen Bestandteil der Mücke *Culex pipiens* auf die Menschenhaut. Z. Parasitenk., 1:484–488.

Perlman, F. 1958. Insects as inhalant allergens. J. Allerg., 29:302–328.

—— 1961. Insect allergens: Their interrelationship and differences. J. Allerg., 32:93–101.

—— 1962. Insect allergens as injectants. Severe reactions to bites and stings of arthropods. Calif. Med., 96:1–10.

———— 1964. Arthropods as causes of allergy. *In* Sensitivity Chest Diseases. Harris, M. C., and Shure, N., eds. Philadelphia, F. A. Davis Co., pp. 157–168.

Pirosky, I., and J. W. Abalos. 1963. Spiders of the genus *Latrodectus* in Argentina. Latrodectism and *Latrodectus* antivenin. *In* Venomous and Poisonous Animals and Noxious Plants of the Pacific Region. Keegan, H. L., and McFarlane, W. V., eds. New York, The Macmillan Co., pp. 137–140.

———— R. Sampayo, and C. Franceschi. 1942. Suero anti-Latrodectus. I. Obtencion y purificacion. Rev. Inst. Bact. Buenos Aires, 11:83–93.

Plescia, O. J., W. Braun, and E. Cora-Figueroa. 1966. Specificity of antibodies against a trinucleotide. Fed. Proc., 25:725.

Potter, J. M., and W. T. Northey. 1962. An immunological evaluation of scorpion venoms. Amer. J. Trop. Med. Hyg., 11:712–716.

Prince, H. E., and P. G. Secrest, Jr. 1939. Use of whole bee extract in sensitization to bees, wasps and ants. J. Allerg., 10:379–381.

Pruzansky, J., A. R. Feinberg, G. Schick, and S. M. Feinberg. 1958. Antigenic relationships in insect extracts. Proc. Soc. Exp. Biol. Med., 97:312–314.

Raffel, S. 1951. Pathogenesis of the allergic reaction. *In* Premier Congrès International D'allergie. Grumbach, A. S., ed. Basel, S. Karger, pp. 333–341.

———— 1961. Immunity, 2nd Ed. New York, Appleton-Century-Crofts.

Randel, H. W., and G. B. Doan. 1956. Caterpillar urticaria in the Panama Canal Zone: Report of five cases. *In* Venoms. Buckley, E. E., and Porges, N., eds. Washington, D.C., Amer. Ass. Advance. Sci. Publ. No. 44, pp. 111–116.

Randolph, H. 1934. Allergic response to dust of insect origin. J. A. M. A., 103:560–562.

Rapp, D., S. Shulman, and C. E. Arbesman. 1962. Immunologic studies of the caddis fly. I. Preparation and characterization of extracts. J. Allerg., 33:97–111.

Riek, R. F. 1958. Studies on the reactions of animals to infestation with ticks. III. The reactions of laboratory animals to repeated sublethal doses of egg extracts of *Haemaphysalis bispinosa* Neumann. Aust. J. Agric. Res., 9:830–841.

———— 1959. Studies on the reactions of animals to infestation with ticks. IV. The protein components of tick extracts. Aust. J. Agric. Res., 10:604–613.

———— 1962. Studies on the reactions of animals to infestation with ticks. VI. Resistance of cattle to infestation with the tick *Boophilus microplus*. Aust. J. Agric. Res., 13:532–550.

Rockwell, E. M., and P. Johnson. 1952. The insect bite reaction. II. Evolution of the allergic reaction. J. Invest. Derm., 19:137–155.

Rosenbrook, W., Jr., and R. O'Connor. 1964. The venom of the mud-dauber wasp. III. *Sceliphron caementarium*: General character. Canad. J. Biochem., 42:1567–1575.

Roxburgh, A. C. 1927. The treatment of insect bites and stings. Lancet, 212:1146.

Sabrosky, C. W. 1952. Introducing the insects. *In* Insects. Yearbook of Agriculture, 1952. Washington, D.C., U.S. Dept. Agric., pp. 1–7.

Salvin, S. B. 1958. Occurrence of delayed hypersensitivity during development of Arthus type hypersensitivity. J. Exp. Med., 107:109–124.

Sampayo, R. R. L. 1943. Toxic action of *Latrodectus mactans* bite and its treatment. Amer. J. Trop. Med., 23:537–543.

Samter, M. 1949. The response of eosinophils in guinea pigs to sensitization, anaphylaxis, and various drugs. Blood, 4:217–246.

———— 1965. Eosinophils. *In* Immunological Diseases. Samter, M., ed. Boston, Little, Brown and Co., pp. 241–245.

Savory, T. 1964. Arachnida. New York, Academic Press, Inc.

Schachter, M. 1963. Kinins of different origins. *In* Structure and function of biologically active peptides: Bradykinin, kallidin, and congeners. Ann. N. Y., Acad. Sci., 104:108–116.

———— and E. M. Thain. 1954. Chemical and pharmacological properties of the potent, slow contracting substance (kinin) in wasp venom. Brit. J. Pharmacol., 9:352–359.

Schaudinn, F. 1904. Generations und Wirtswechsel bei Trypanosoma und Spirochaete. Arbeiten aus den kaiserlichen Gesundheitsamte (Berlin), 20:387–439.

Schenone, H., and F. Prats. 1961. Arachnidism by *Loxosceles laeta*. Arch. Derm., 83:139–142.

Schottler, W. H. A. 1954. On the toxicity of scorpion venom. Amer. J. Trop. Med. Hyg., 3:172–178.

Schwartz, H. J. 1965. Skin sensitivity in insect allergy. J. A. M. A., 194:113–115.

Sehon, A. H., and L. Gyenes. 1966. Antibodies in nontreated patients and antibodies developed during treatment. *In* Immunological Diseases. Samter, M., ed. Boston, Little, Brown and Co., pp. 519–538.

Sergent, E. 1936. Préparation d'un serum contre le venin de scorpion. Ann. Inst. Pasteur (Paris), 57:240–243.

——— 1949. Douze années de serotherapie antiscorpionique. Ann. Inst. Pasteur (Paris), 76:50–52.

Shulman, S. 1967. Allergic responses to insects. *In* Annual Review of Entomology. Smith, R. F., and Mittler, T. E., eds. Palo Alto, California, Annual Reviews Inc., Vol. 12, pp. 323–346.

——— D. Rapp, P. Bronson, and C. E. Arbesman. 1962. Immunologic studies of caddis fly. II. Isolation of the allergenic fractions of caddis fly extract. J. Allerg., 33:438–447.

——— P. Bronson, and C. E. Arbesman. 1963. Immunologic studies of caddis fly. III. Physical and chemical characterization of the major antigen. J. Allerg., 34:1–7.

——— F. Bigelsen, R. Lang, and C. Arbesman. 1966a. The allergic response to stinging insects: Biochemical and immunologic studies on bee venom and other bee body preparations. J. Immun., 96:29–38.

——— F. Bigelsen, and C. Arbesman. 1966b. Immunologic properties of bee venom. J. Allerg., 36:217.

Shulov, A. 1939. The venom of the scorpion *Buthus quinquestriatus* and the preparation of anti-serum. Trans. Roy. Soc. Trop. Med. Hyg., 33:253–256.

——— D. Flesh, C. Geriscter, Z. Eshkol, and G. Schillinger. 1960. The anti-scorpion serum prepared by use of fresh venom and the assessment of its efficacy against scorpion stings. Int. Ass. Microbiol. Soc., Sect. Biol. Standardization, 5:419–424.

Simon, F. A., and F. M. Rackman. 1934. The development of hypersensitiveness in man following intradermal injection of antigen. J. Allerg., 5:439–450.

Snodgrass, R. E. 1944. The feeding apparatus for biting and sucking insects affecting man and animals. In Smithsonian Misc. Coll., 104(7), Publ. No 3773. Washington, D.C., Smithsonian Institute.

——— 1948. The feeding organs of Arachnida, including mites and ticks. *In* Smithsonian Misc. Coll. 110(10), Publ. No. 3944. Washington, D.C., Smithsonian Institute.

Stahnke, H. L. 1950. The Arizona scorpion problem. Arizona Med., 7:23–29,

——— 1966. The Treatment of Venomous Bites and Stings, Rev. Ed. Tempe, Arizona, Arizona State University Press.

Sternberg, L. 1929. A case of asthma caused by *Cimex Lectularius*. Med. J. Rec., 129:622.

Swellengrebel, N. H., and M. M. Sterman. 1961. Animal Parasitism. Princeton, New Jersey, D. Van Nostrand Co., Inc.

Terr, A. I., and J. A. McLean 1964. Studies on insect sting hypersensitivity. J. Allerg., 35:127–133.

Tezner, O. 1934. Sofortreaktion und Spätreaktion als allergische hautproben, ihre theoretische und praktische Bedeutung. Jahrb. Kinderheilk., 142:69–101.

Theodor, O. 1935. A study of the reaction of *Phlebotomus* bites with some remarks on "harara." Trans. Roy. Soc. Trop. Med. Hyg., 29:273–284.

Thompson, F. 1933. About bee venom. Lancet, 2:446–448.

Trager, W. 1939a. Acquired immunity to ticks. J. Parasit., 25:57–81.

——— 1939b. Further observations on acquired immunity to the tick *Dermacentor variabilis* Say. J. Parasit., 25:137–139.

——— 1940. A note on the problem of acquired immunity to argasid ticks. J. Parasit., 26:71–74.

Tulga, T. 1960. Cross-reactions between anti-scorpion (*Buthus quinquestriatus*) and anti-scorpion (*Prionurus crassicauda*) sera. Turk. Hij. Tecr. Biyol. Derg. (Turk. Bull. Hyg. Exp. Biol.), 20:191–203.

United States Public Health Service. 1966. Personal communication. San Francisco Field Station, Communicable Diseases Center, U. S. Public Health Service.

Usinger, R. L. 1966. Monograph of Cimicidae. Entomological Society of America, Thomas Say Foundation, Vol. 7, pp. 1–585.

Valle, J. R., Z. P. Picarelli, and J. H. Prado. 1954. Histamine content and pharmacological properties of crude extracts from setae of urticating caterpillars. Arch. Int., Pharmacodyn., 98:324–334.

Vazquez-Colon, A., and W. B. Elliott. 1966. The response of rat liver mitochondria to treatment with bee venom. Toxicon, 4:61–63.

Vellard, J. 1936. Le venin des araignées. Monogr. Inst. Pasteur. Paris, Masson et Cie.

Vermeil, C. 1959. Sur l'utilisation des scorpions morts pour la préparation du serum antiscorpionique. Arch. Inst. Pasteur (Algerie), 37:385–386.

Waterhouse, A. T. 1914. Bee sting anaphylaxis. Lancet, 2:946.

Waterman, J. A. 1938. Some notes on scorpion poisoning in Trinidad. Trans. Roy. Soc. Trop. Med. Hyg., 31:607–624.

Weidner, H. 1937. Beitrage zu einer Monographie der Raupen mit Gifthaaren. Z. Angew. Entomol., 23:432–484.

Weinberg, M., and P. Sequin. 1914. Recherches biologiques sur l'eosinophile. Ann. Inst. Pasteur (Paris), 28:470–508.

Weiser, R. S. 1957. Mechanism of immunological tissue injury. J. Allerg., 28:475–488.

Welsh, J. H. 1964. Composition and mode of action of some invertebrate venoms. In Annual Review of Pharmacology, Vol. 4. Cutting, W. C., Dreisbach, R. H., Elliott, H. W., eds. Palo Alto, California, Annual Reviews Inc., pp. 293–304.

Whittemore, F. W., and H. L. Keegan. 1963. Medically important scorpions in the Pacific area. In Venomous and Poisonous Animals and Noxious Plants of the Pacific Region. Keegan, H. L., and MacFarlane, W. V., eds. New York, The Macmillan Co., pp. 107–110.

———— H. L. Keegan, and J. L. Borowitz. 1961. Studies of scorpion antivenins. Bull. W. H. O., 25:185–188.

Wiener, S. 1956. The Australian red back spider (Latrodectus hasseltii): I. Preparation of antiserum by the use of venom adsorbed on aluminium phosphate. Med. J. Aust., 1:739–742.

———— 1961a. The Sydney funnel-web spider (Atrax robustus): III. The neutralization of venom by haemolymph. Med. J. Aust., 1:449–451.

———— 1961b. Red back spider antivenene. Med. J. Aust., 2:41–44.

———— 1961c. Red back spider bite in Australia. An analysis of 167 cases. Med. J. Aust., 2:44–49.

———— 1961d. Observations on the venom of the Sydney funnel-web spider (Atrax robustus). Med. J. Aust., 2:693–699.

———— 1963. Antigenic and electrophoretic properties of funnel-web spider (Atrax robustus) venom. In Venomous and Poisonous Animals and Noxious Plants of the Pacific Region. Keegan, H. L., and McFarlane, W. V., eds. New York, The Macmillan Co. pp. 141–151.

———— and A. Fraser. 1956. Red back spider bite treated with antivenene. Med. J. Aust., 1:858.

Williamson, J. 1956. The composition of tsetse fly saliva. II. Analysis of amino acids and sugars by paper partition chromatography. Ann. Trop. Med. Parasit., 50:334–344.

Wilson, A. B., and A. N. Clements. 1965. The nature of the skin reaction to mosquito bites in laboratory animals. Int. Arch. Allerg., 26:294–314.

Wilson, H. W. 1913. Preliminary report of a case of sensitization to the May-fly (Ephemera). J. A. M. A., 61:1618.

Wiseman, R. D., W. G Woodin, H. C. Miller, and M. A. Myers. 1959. Insect allergy as a possible cause of inhalant sensitivity. J. Allerg., 30:191–197.

Wittich, F. W. 1940a. The nature of various mill dust allergens. J. Lancet, 60:418–442.

———— 1940b. Allergic rhinitis and asthma due to sensitization to the mexican bean weevil (Zabrotes subfasciatus Boh). J. Allerg., 12:42–45.

Wood, S. F. 1942. Reactions of man to the feeding of reduviid bugs. J. Parasit., 28:43–49.

Yorke, W., and J. W. S. MacFie. 1924. The action of the salivary secretion of mosquitoes and Glossina tachinoides on human blood. Ann. Trop. Med. Parasit., 18:103–108.

Young, J. D., E. Benjamini, Ben F. Feingold, and H. Noller. 1963. Allergy to flea bites. V. Preliminary results of fractionation, characterization, and assay for allergenic activity of material derived from the oral secretion of the cat flea, Ctenocephalides felis felis. Exp. Parasit., 13:155–166.

Ziprkowsky, L., E. Hofshi, and A. S. Tahori. 1959. Caterpillar dermatitis. Israel Med. J., 18:26–31.

7

Immunity: Diagnosis and Prophylaxis

Evaluation of the Immune State by Immunologic Techniques

IRVING G. KAGAN

National Communicable Disease Center, Health Services and Mental Health
Administration, Public Health Service, U.S. Department of Health, Education, and
Welfare, Atlanta, Georgia

INTRODUCTION 1138
SEROLOGIC REACTIONS AND THE IMMUNE STATE 1139
Serologic tests with living parasites 1139
Gel-diffusion reactions and the immune response 1141
Mucosal extracts and resistance 1141
Immunoglobulins and parasitic infections 1142
HYPERSENSITIVITY AND THE IMMUNE STATE 1143
Immediate hypersensitivity 1144
Reaginic-like antibody in parasitic infections 1146
Prausnitz-Küstner antibody 1147
Passive cutaneous anaphylactic antibodies
    in parasitic diseases 1148
General allergic immediate-type reactions
    in parasitic infections 1148
DELAYED HYPERSENSITIVITY 1149
Delayed skin reactions in parasitic diseases 1150
Lymphocyte migration 1151
Lymphocyte transformation 1152
Target-cell destruction 1152
Cytophilic antibodies 1153
Delayed hypersensitivity and parasitic diseases 1153
Cellular immunity 1154
CONCLUSION 1155
REFERENCES 1156

1137

INTRODUCTION

Evaluation of immunity by *in vitro* methods would be very useful in both clinical and experimental parasitology. The study of immunity against parasitic species has centered around *in vivo* methods. A common protocol in experimental helminth infections is to challenge the host animal with a second infection and to determine on necropsy whether the parasites of the second infection developed. If the number of worms recovered in challenged animals is significantly less than the number of worms recovered from control animals (singly infected hosts), the challenged animals can be characterized as immune or resistant.

Indirect methods have been used with varying degrees of success to initiate the immune state in a host. Some of these are: (1) vaccination with extractions of worms or metabolic product antigens, (2) infection with irradiated larvae, (3) infection abbreviated by chemotherapy, (4) infection initiated with related organisms or attenuated strains, (5) stimulation of the host by the transfer of sensitized cells, and (6) passive transfer of specific antisera.

Characteristics indicative of host immunity are the lack of parasitemia or tissue invasion in protozoan infections, and in helminth infections the inhibition of egg production, expulsion of worms, stunting of worm growth, inhibition of larval development, the self-cure phenomenon (Stoll, 1958), and an ability to withstand the "toxic" manifestations of infection.

Evaluation of the resistant status of the host by serologic methods has not been as intensively studied. In response to infection, a host will develop antibodies which can be detected and quantitated by a variety of serologic tests. Demonstration of antibodies in the serum of the infected animal is an indication of antigenic experience with the parasite; however, in a number of carefully made studies, demonstration of antibodies in response to nematode and trematode infections has not been correlated with immunity (Soulsby, 1962).

For example, an animal infected with the roundworm *Haemonchus contortus* will develop an excellent serologic response which can be measured by complement-fixation (CF), indirect hemagglutination (IHA), and agar-gel diffusion methods. The titer, however, develops after immunity or self-cure has taken place and will persist when the immunity in the host is suppressed with antihistaminic drugs (Soulsby, 1960). Soulsby (1962), in an excellent review of antigen-antibody reactions in helminth infections, concluded that "despite the extensive work which has been done on various serological manifestations of nematode infections, no convincing evidence exists to date to show that antibodies detected by numerous serological tests play any functional part in immunity."

Attempts to relate circulating antibodies to acquired resistance in schistosome infections have also been unsuccessful (Vogel and Minning, 1953;

Kagan, 1958, 1966; Smithers, 1962; Jachowski et al., 1963). In no instance has there been conclusive evidence that immunity can be conferred by passive transfer of hyperimmune serum. In the few reports of passive transfer of schistosome resistance, experiments using proper controls with absorbed immune sera have not been made.

Humoral involvement in cestode immunity has been convincingly demonstrated. Both "early" and "late" immunities have been characterized for *Cysticercus fasciolaris* infections in the rat (Campbell, 1938a,b,c). Resistance against infection when manifested at the intestinal level or when the larvae are established in the liver or other tissues has also been demonstrated for *Echinococcus granulosus* (Gemmell, 1962) and *Hymenolepis nana* infections (Bailey, 1951; Weinmann, 1966). Antibodies are involved in these reactions since resistance can be mediated by passive transfer (Miller and Gardiner, 1934), but identification and specific characterization of the antibodies have not been carried out.

"The immunity mechanisms to protozoan infections are complex and varied so that rules and general laws can be applied only to more general phenomena" (Maekelt, 1966). Many antibodies have been demonstrated for protozoan infections, but humoral antibodies detected by serologic tests have, in general, been shown to be unrelated to immunity. The interaction of antibodies and immunity to protozoan species is complex. In cutaneous leishmaniasis, circulating antibody appears to play no role in the development of immunity and resistance. In visceral leishmaniasis, antibody can be readily demonstrated during infection. Whether the antibodies are involved in resistance to the parasite has not been demonstrated. In malaria, humoral involvement in resistance has been demonstrated by the passive transfer of hyperimmune globulin to susceptible individuals (Cohen and McGregor, 1963), but in experimental infections in monkeys, antibody titers in the complement-fixation test or the fluorescent-antibody test have not been correlated with resistance (Targett and Voller, 1965).

SEROLOGIC REACTIONS AND THE IMMUNE STATE

Serologic tests with living parasites

Although the antigenic components of individual helminth and protozoan parasites have not yet been sufficiently purified to detect the functional serologic antibodies by direct serologic tests, *in vitro* techniques have been used to detect precipitin antibodies in the sera of infected animals. Since the biologic activity of these antibodies affects viability and infectivity, and since the antibodies develop late in the course of infection, an association between antibodies and immunity in the host has been established.

In vitro manifestations of immune sera on parasitic species are reviewed by Weinstein (1967). Immobilizing antibodies have been described for the protozoa *E. histolytica* (Cole and Kent, 1953; Biagi and Buentello, 1961), *Balantidium coli* (Zamon, 1962), and *T. cruzi* (Adler, 1958). The *in vitro* microprecipitin phenomenon (Sarles and Taliaferro, 1936) has been demonstrated with larvae of *Nippostrongylus brasiliensis* (Sarles, 1938), *Ancylostoma caninum* (Otto, 1940), *Trichinella spiralis* (Mauss, 1940; Oliver-González, 1940), *Ascaridia galli* (Sadun, 1949), *Heterakis spumosa* (Smith, 1953), the hexacanth embryos of *Taenia saginata* (Silverman, 1955), *Spirometra mansonoides* (Mueller, 1961), *Echinococcus granulosus* (Schulz and Ismagilova, 1962), *Oesophagostomum radiatum* (Douvres, 1962), and other nematode and cestode larvae.

Labzoffsky et al. (1964) studied sera from three human cases of trichinosis and from serial bleedings of experimentally infected rabbits. Sera from infected rabbits were positive in 4 days with the fluorescent antibody (FA) test, in 8 to 10 days with the CF test, and in 3 to 4 weeks with the microprecipitin test. *In vitro* reactions with larvae of the nematode *H. contortus* incubated in sera of resistant sheep showed that the fourth- and early fifth-stage larvae were adversely affected by these sera (Silverman, 1965). There is similar evidence with other parasitic nematodes: Thorson (1954) incubated larvae of *N. brasiliensis* in immune serum and reported reduction in infectivity, as did Otto (1940) with larvae of *Ancylostoma caninum*, and Mauss (1940) with larvae of *T. spiralis*. Weinmann (1966) reported that larvae of the cestode *Hymenolepis nana* were killed by immune serum *in vitro*. Second-stage larvae of the nematode *Ascaris suum* implanted in diffusion chambers in the peritoneal cavity of immune and nonimmune mice showed growth retardation only in the immune animals (Crandall and Arean, 1964). Blacklock and Gordon (1927) observed that the maggot *Cordylobia anthropophaga*, which did not develop in the skin of immune guinea pigs, was killed by precipitates which developed inside the gut of the larval insect. However, larvae of some species are neither killed nor developmentally inhibited in immune serum; for example, the larvae of the insect-parasitizing nematode *Neoaplectana glaseri* developed normally in spite of precipitates present on and around them in culture medium which contained sera from rabbits injected with these worms (Jackson, 1961).

A number of *in vitro* tests with schistosome life cycle stages have been described, such as the miracidial immobilization test (Senterfit, 1953; Kagan, 1955), the "Cercarienhüllenreaktion" (CHR) (Vogel and Minning, 1949a,b), and the circumoval precipitin reaction (COP) (Oliver-González, 1954). The correlation of these *in vitro* reactions with acquired immunity against these blood flukes (trematodes) has not been demonstrated. Miracidial immobilization antibodies occur late in infection and do not appear to be related to protection (Senterfit, 1958); CHR antibodies also occur late in infection and have not been related to protection (Kagan and Pellegrino, 1961). The COP titer does not rise in the challenged animal, and the COP test is negative with sera from unisexual infections (Bruijning, 1964). Since infections with male worms of *Schistosoma japonicum* confer protection in experimentally infected monkeys (Vogel and Minning, 1953), the absence of activity in the COP test may be significant. Jachowski et al. (1963) concluded that in experimentally infected monkeys the COP antibodies were not related to immunity.

Gel-diffusion reactions and the immune response

Precipitin antibodies can also be demonstrated in gel-diffusion tests. The various gel-diffusion techniques employed today (Kagan, 1961; Biguet et al, 1965a) have been of value in delineating the complexity of the sera and antigens employed in experimental studies. Only a few limited studies have attempted to correlate a specific band with some type of biologic activity. Sera from sheep which undergo the self-cure phenomenon when infected with the nematode *Haemonchus contortus* show at least five antigen-antibody lines with an extract prepared from exsheathing fluid of third-stage larvae (Soulsby and Stewart, 1960). Circumstantial evidence indicates that one of these components is associated with the antigen that stimulates the self-cure reaction. If this component could be sufficiently purified for use in the test, the self-cure reaction could be monitored. To date this purification has not been accomplished.

Specific precipitates from the reaction between mucosal extracts of sheep infected with *Oesophagostomum columbianum* and an extract of third-stage larvae of this parasite were observed by Dobson (1966a) in agar-gel plates. These lines develop only with sera from sheep which have been infected twice with this nematode (Dobson, 1966b).

Detailed analyses of the development of immunoelectrophoretic bands during the course of infection have been made with *T. spiralis* infections (Biguet et al., 1965b) and with schistosome infections (Capron et al., 1966). Although none of these studies has correlated the development of these bands with that of resistance, the assay system for future studies of this type is available.

Mucosal extracts and resistance

The review by Pierce (1959) on mucosal antibodies is more meaningful today because of the development of a large body of literature on the biologic activity of immunoglobulin. In his review the only evidence for stimulation of local production of antibody by a parasitic protozoan was for the species *Trichomonas foetus*. Douvres (1962) reported that mucosal extracts from calves immune to *Oesophagostomum radiatum* produced precipitates around larvae cultured in these extracts, but larvae cultured in the sera from immune hosts did not develop precipitates. Dobson (1966c) isolated antibody from intestinal mucus of sheep infected with *O. columbianum*, and was able to demonstrate this antibody in agar-gel plates and in passive cutaneous anaphylaxis (PCA) reactions. Weinmann (1966) incubated day-old worms of *Hymenolepis nana* in sera and mucosal extracts of normal and immune mice. Neither immune nor normal serum had any effect on the viability or infectivity of the incubated immature worms. Worms incubated in mucosal extracts were adversely affected. Incubation in normal mucosal extract for three hours killed 5 percent of the worms and infectivity was slightly reduced (5 of 9 mice became infected); immune mucosal extract killed 30 percent of the worms in three hours and reduced the infectivity to zero percent (none of the mice became infected).

Deleterious effects on growth of *Ascaridia galli* cultured in intestinal mucus extracts were investigated by Ackert (1942). He found a direct relationship between the age of the chicken host, the development of resistance against this nematode parasite, and the number of goblet cells in the intestinal epithelium. Dobson (1966b) also reported a correlation between duration of infection in sheep with *O. columbianum* and the occurrence and number of globule leukocytes in the intestinal tract.

Immunoglobulins and parasitic infections

In recent years a body of information has developed on the structure and function of the immunoglobulins (Franklin, 1964; Janeway et al., 1967). At least five classes of immunoglobulin in man are recognized: IgG, IgA, IgM, IgD, and IgE. The immunoglobulin subclasses are differentiated on the basis of the biologic, immunologic, and physiochemical specificities of their heavy chains. Normal serum contains approximately 1.26 gram percent of IgG, 0.12 gram percent of IgM, 0.39 gram percent of IgA, and trace amounts of IgD and IgE. In electrophoretic separation, the different immunoglobulins migrate with distinctive mobilities and can thus be identified. The role of the subclasses of immunoglobulins in parasitic infections has been studied in only a few laboratories.

Smithers (1967) and Remington (1967) reviewed some of the work on the alterations in immunoglobulin classes during parasitic infections. Striking increases in IgM antibody are noted in trypanosome infections (Mattern et al., 1961). Increases in both IgM and IgG occur in malaria (Abele et al., 1965; Tobie et al., 1966). Remington and Miller (1966) have studied the role of IgG and IgM in differentiating congenital from acquired toxoplasmosis. Crandall et al., (1967), using the fluorescent-antibody technique with specific anti-IgG, -IgM, and -IgA conjugates, studied the cells in the intestines of rabbits infected with *T. spiralis*. An apparent increase in cells containing IgM was detected early in the infection, and as the infection matured, the proportion of cells containing IgG increased. The antibody which developed against the *T. spiralis* organism was of the IgM and IgG type; there was no anti-IgA type observed. Maddison et al. (1968a) fractionated sera from patients with amoebiasis and showed that IgG was reactive in all the serodiagnostic tests for *E. histolytica*. Reaginic activity assayed by PCA tests in the monkey was associated with IgA and IgG. Kagan et al. (1968) fractionated sera from patients with infections of *T. spiralis* and *E. granulosus* and characterized the immunoglobulins active in diagnostic tests. In sera from patients with *T. spiralis*, the fluorescent-antibody test measured IgM antibody, whereas the latex and bentonite flocculation tests measure both IgM and IgG antibodies. In sera from patients with echinococcosis, the IgG antibody was the most active in all serodiagnostic tests.

The biologic role of IgG and IgM has been extensively studied since immunologic methods for their isolation and purification have become available. IgA antibody is more difficult to isolate, but it merits special consideration due to the fact that high concentrations of this immunoglobulin are associated with mucosal surfaces (Tomasi et al., 1965), with tears (Chodirker and Tomasi, 1963), and with gastrointestinal and nasal secretions (Remington et al., 1964). Circulating IgA differs from tissue IgA by the absence of a "transfer piece" (South et al., 1966). Tissue IgA may be produced locally by immunologically competent cells. In cestode infections in particular, the intestinal mucosa is a barrier to penetration of the hexacanth embryo in the resistant host. Assays for noncirculating IgA antibody in saliva (Ishizaka et al., 1964) or nasal mucosa (Brandzaeg et al., 1967) may be a way of evaluating the degree of resistance of a particular host.

If IgA antibody at the mucosal surface is in part responsible for maintaining an immune state in a resistant host, this supposition may explain why mucosal extracts are so active in *in vitro* tests. It may also explain why relatively large doses of hyperimmune serum are required to transfer immunity passively to *N. brasiliensis* in the rat (3 ml per 100 g of body weight, as reported by Urquhart et al., 1965). South et al. (1966) showed that detecting labeled IgA at tissue sites requires exceedingly large doses of serum when the serum is administered intravenously, since very little reaches the intestinal surface from the vascular system. Barth et al. (1966) induced nonspecific anaphylaxis in rats and found that the action of immune serum in initiating the self-cure mechanism against *N. brasiliensis* was enhanced. The anaphylactic reaction initiated a "leak lesion" in the sensitized gut, which allowed the passage of immunoglobulins from the capillaries to the mucosal surfaces. The role of IgA immunoglobulin, especially in cestode immunity, is not well understood and merits further study.

Wilson (1966) showed that a specific immunoglobulin class was active in providing protection but not in producing skin-sensitizing or precipitin antibodies. In guinea pigs infected with the nematode *Dictyocaulus viviparus*, the γ_1 electrophoretic fraction of the sera conferred passive immunity to noninfected recipients. Sera from immunized animals contained skin-sensitizing and precipitin antibodies, but the animals did not develop any γ_1 antibody; sera from such animals were not protective.

HYPERSENSITIVITY AND THE IMMUNE STATE

Humphrey and White (1963) defined hypersensitivity or allergy "as a specifically induced altered reactivity in which there is evidence for an underlying immunological mechanism." Two types of mechanisms are recognized: humoral or immediate hypersensitivity, exemplified by atopic disease, and cellular or delayed hypersensitivity. The tuberculin reaction is the classical example of the latter.

Hypersensitivity and infection with parasitic worms are closely linked in man (Andrews, 1962). Eosinophilia in a differential blood count immediately raises the possibility of a parasitic infection. Immediate-type skin reactions are demonstrable in a number of helminthic infections. Ascariasis is associated with asthma and urticaria, filariasis with lymphadenopathy, and anaphylaxis has been recorded in patients with ruptured hydatid cysts. Delayed hypersensitivity in some of the helminthic infections, as well as in protozoan conditions such as toxoplasmosis and leishmaniasis, is demonstrable by delayed skin tests. The association of infection with development of a hypersensitive state is well-established, but the relationship of hypersensitivity and immunity is not. The volume of literature on hypersensitivity is growing rapidly, but further information on the role of the lymphoid cells must be obtained before the processes of immunity can be fully understood.

Immediate hypersensitivity

Immediate hypersensitivity (Crowle, 1964) is associated with serum antibodies or antigen-antibody complexes. Clinical symptoms may vary from mild urticaria to the severe manifestations of the Arthus reaction, serum sickness, or anaphylaxis. There is no sharp delineation between the last three types of reactions, since the basic mechanism is the interaction of antibody with antigen which results in complexes which in one way or another cause cellular changes.

In the anaphylactic reaction, antibodies with selected affinities attach to various cells in the body. The antibody which attaches to the mast cell and sensitizes it has been actively studied. The presence of specific antigen at the surface of the sensitized mast cell in the presence of specific antibody leads to its disruption (degranulation) and the release of pharmacologically active substances such as histamine, 5-hydroxytryptamine (serotonin), slow-reacting substance (SRS-A), and bradykinin. These substances produce changes in the body, such as extravasation of fluid and smooth muscle contraction, which are characteristic of local or systemic anaphylaxis. The Schultz-Dale reaction, which utilizes the contraction of smooth uterine muscle, is a technique for studying anaphylaxis.

In the Arthus reaction the antigen is deposited in the skin, and the tissue changes are caused by the interaction of antibody with antigen and complement. The reaction is characterized by inflammatory, necrotizing, and degenerative types of focal tissue injury which is mediated by antigen-antibody complexes. The antigen-antibody complex is toxic by itself, has greatest activity in slight antigen excess, has tissue affinity, and can interact with complement. The biologic activity of the complex is dependent on the property of the antibody and not of the antigen. Polymorphonuclear cells are attracted to the site and then attempt to destroy the complexes by phagocytosis. Necrosis of the tissue due to the release of acid proteases by the polymorphonuclear cells takes place after a few days.

Injection with a foreign protein, such as horse serum, into a host sensitized to this protein will, after a latent period of several days, stimulate the formation of antibodies to the injected material. The antibodies combine with the free antigen circulating in the host, and the antigen-antibody complexes are deposited on glomeruli in the kidneys, in arteries, or in the heart. The clinical syndrome which results is called serum sickness.

Immediate hypersensitivity can be studied by the Prausnitz-Küstner (PK) skin test, by passive systemic anaphylaxis reactions (Patterson et al., 1965; Ogilvie et al., 1966), and by passive cutaneous anaphylaxis (PCA) reactions (Ovary, 1964). In the passive systemic reaction, serum containing cell-sensitizing (reaginic) antibody is injected intravenously into a homologous recipient, and after a suitable latent period (24 to 72 hours), antigen is administered by the same route. The ensuing antigen-antibody reaction results in release of histamine, increased vascular permeability, and smooth muscle contraction. In the PCA reaction, reaginic serum is injected intradermally, and after a latent period varying from 3 to 72 hours, antigen is introduced either systemically or locally accompanied by a suitable dye. The antigen-antibody reaction with its release of pharmacologically reactive substances enhances permeability of the capillaries of the skin, permitting extravasation of plasma proteins and visualization of the process by leakage of the dye into adjacent areas of the skin surrounding the sensitized area. The reaction can be quantitated, and its intensity is directly proportional to the quantity of antigen and antibody.

Reaginic properties have been attributed to IgG, IgA, IgM, and IgE immunoglobulins in man. They may well be heterogeneous in nature (Fireman et al., 1967). In the guinea pig and mouse, such activity is associated with the electrophoretically fast-moving γ_1 component of IgG (Ovary et al., 1963); in the rabbit and rat (Barth and Fahey, 1965), the component has an electrophoretic mobility between IgG and IgM (Zvaifler and Becker, 1966; Binaghi et al., 1964). Though the ability of reaginic serum to be fixed passively by skin is generally considered to be species-specific, some abnormalities have been reported: Dog reagin is able to be fixed to the skin of man and primates, while human reagin is incapable of being fixed to the skin of the dog (Patterson et al., 1965).

"Blocking antibody" is an immunoglobulin that inhibits the anaphylactic reaction by competing for absorption sites on the tissue cells. Blocking antibody may also be an immunoglobulin which does not attach to cells but which combines preferentially with antigen to prevent the anaphylaxis reaction.

Reaginic-like antibody in parasitic infections

With the development of the passive cutaneous anaphylaxis technique (Ovary, 1964), assays for reagin-like or homocytotrophic antibody became possible. The role of this antibody in *Nippostrongylus brasiliensis* infections has been extensively studied. Ogilvie (1964, 1967) characterized the component as appearing 19 to 25 days after infection in the rat. The antibody appears in the infected host when the egg counts fall and the immune response is initiated. Reinfection of the immune host is associated with a rise in reagin-like antibody. The antibody is stimulated by the living worm and cannot be produced by vaccination. In later studies, Jones and Ogilvie (1967) found that the injection of a small amount of a saline extract of adult worms neutralized the immunizing effect of passive transfer of reaginic serum. Fractionation of the immune serum on a Sephadex* G-200 column indicated that the antibody was intermediate in molecular size between 7S and 19S globulin and could not be related to IgG or IgA of rat serum by immunoelectrophoresis. Fractionation of the adult worm antigen on a Sephadex G-200 column resulted in the isolation of a protein with a molecular weight of approximately 12,000 to 17,000 as the allergen. The small size of the molecule and the fact that reagin antibody can only be stimulated by living worms suggest that the allergen may be an enzyme or metabolic product of the worm (Smithers, 1967).

An antigen related to the rat homocytotrophic antibody was detected in culture fluids of adult *N. brasiliensis* worms by Wilson (1967). The antigen, with a molecular weight between 12,000 and 15,000, showed a mobility on preparative agar-gel electrophoresis resembling that of a rat IgA globulin. Reaginic antibody was assayed in immune lactating mothers and newborn rats. Reagins were never detected in the circulation of the young rats, although immunity was transferred in the colostrum. Although the evidence is not convincing, reagins may not be related to worm elimination in the rat (Jones and Ogilvie, 1967). In further studies by Ogilvie and Jones (1967), neonatal thymectomy suppressed both reagin production and resistance to the parasite, suggesting that mechanisms other than immediate hypersensitivity were operative in the immune response. Wilson et al. (1967) found that rats thymectomized at birth showed normal development of infection and parasite egg production, as did sham-operated controls. PCA titers in rats (anaphylactic antibody) were depressed in the thymectomized animals but, in spite of this, the thymectomized rats resisted a second infection almost as well as did sham-operated rats with high rat PCA titers.

Homocytotrophic (reaginic) antibody has been studied in rabbits infected with schistosome cercariae. This antibody appears 7 to 12 weeks following infection, persists at high titers for 3 to 6 weeks, and then disappears. The antibody titer rises upon reinfection (Zvaifler et al., 1966). Antischistosomal reaginic antibodies were detected in humans and chimpanzees and

* Use of trade names is for identification only and does not constitute endorsement by the Public Health Service or by the U.S. Department of Health, Education, and Welfare.

were successfully transferred to rhesus monkeys by Sadun et al. (1966). Ogilvie et al. (1966) demonstrated reaginic-like antibodies in the sera of rats and monkeys infected with *Schistosoma mansoni*. Reaginic serum protected rats from reinfection if the cercariae were placed directly over the impregnated area 3 days later.

In our own studies on homocytotrophic antibody in the rat infected with *Schistosoma mansoni*, we were able to confirm the studies of Ogilvie et al. (1966). The antibody was found to be present 3 to 4 weeks after infection and to disappear 12 weeks after infection. This period coincides with the initiation of a self-cure mechanism in the rat which results in a drastic diminution in the worm burden (Smithers and Terry, 1965).

Although reagins of *S. mansoni* are protective in rats infected with this parasite, they are not protective in the skin of the monkey (Ogilvie et al., 1966). This observation was confirmed in monkeys injected intradermally with reaginic sera and exposed to cercariae of *S. japonicum* (Hsü and Hsü, 1966).

The presence of reagin-like or homocytotrophic antibody when an immune state is initiated in a host is not proof of association, but this interesting phenomenon also warrants further study. Smithers (1967) believes that the evidence obtained to date militates against involvement of reagins in any protective function in schistosome infections.

Prausnitz-Küstner antibody

The detection of reaginic antibody in man is accomplished by performing the Prausnitz-Küstner (PK) skin test. Serum from a hypersensitive patient is injected intradermally into the skin of a nonreactive individual. Seventy-two hours later the site is challenged with specific antigen. Reaginic antibody, if present, attaches to the skin of the subject and, upon challenge, combines with antigen to induce a wheal and a flare reaction. Nonreagin or precipitin antibody will diffuse away from the skin during the latent 72-hour period between injection and challenge.

Attempts to substitute the skin of the rhesus monkey for the skin of man in the test (Layton et al., 1962; Layton, 1965) indicate that antibody from human atopic patients with various inherited allergic tendencies can be detected in PK tests in a wide range of primates. In addition, Patterson et al. (1965) were able to demonstrate passive systemic sensitization in the monkey, and the *in vitro* experiments of Goodfriend et al. (1966) utilized monkey tissue. Rose et al. (1964) concluded that monkey skin is less sensitive than human skin. This finding was confirmed by Ishizaka et al. (1967), who tested purified reaginic IgE in *Macaca irus*. Our findings (Maddison et al., 1968b) in amoebiasis also suggest this lack of sensitivity, as monkey skin fixed only two sera from 29 patients with active clinical amoebiasis who had given positive immediate-type intradermal reactions. PK tests in man with the sera from this group have not been studied.

The role of PK antibody in resistance to parasitic infections has not been evaluated. PK antibodies have been detected in the serum of man infected with ascariasis (Rackemann and Stevens, 1927), hydatid disease (Graña, 1945), diphyllobothriasis (Brunner, 1928), paragonimiasis (Yokogawa et al., 1957), filariasis (Kagan, 1963), and schistosomiasis (Taliaferro and Taliaferro, 1931; Guerra et al., 1945; Coker and Oliver-González, 1956; Mendes and Amato Neto, 1963). PK tests in the monkey will allow further study of this antibody, provided the limitations of sensitivity of monkey skin is taken into account.

Passive cutaneous anaphylactic antibodies in parasitic diseases

The passive cutaneous anaphylactic (PCA) antibody differs from the PK antibody in that it fixes to heterologous skin. The guinea pig is the animal usually used in studies of this antibody. Antibody in the mucosal extracts of sheep infected with *Oesophagostomum columbianum* was reactive in PCA tests carried out in guinea pigs. The antigen employed was an extract of third-stage larvae of *O. columbianum*. Mucosal extracts of animals infected twice gave the strongest response (Dobson, 1966c).

PCA antibodies in rats infected with larvae of *Toxocara canis* appeared after 12 days and were active in the skin of guinea pigs. After 24 days, reagin-like antibodies active in the skin of the rat were detected (Dobson et al., 1967). Ivey and Slanga (1965) and Ivey (1965) utilized the PCA reaction to assay antibody to *Toxocara canis* and *Trichinella spiralis* in experimental infections. Bray and Lainson (1965) were able to demonstrate PCA antibodies in sera of man and monkeys infected with leishmania. PCA antibodies were demonstrated in the sera of monkeys, dogs, and humans infected with filariasis. Although the tests in the guinea pig skin were quite sensitive, they were not specific, since sera from *Brugia pahangi* and *B. malayi* infections reacted with *Wuchereria bancrofti* antigen (Guest et al., 1966).

In studies on amoebiasis by Maddison et al. (1968a), PCA antibodies were found to correlate well with hemagglutination and fluorescent-antibody titers in patients with clinical disease. Reaginic antibodies assayed in monkey skin did not show this correlation. Kagan et al. (1968) demonstrated that in trichinosis sera, PCA antibodies did not correlate with bentonite flocculation test titers.

General allergic immediate-type reactions in parasitic infections

Anaphylactic reactions have been demonstrated in guinea pigs and in mice infected with *T. spiralis* (Sharp and Olson, 1962; Briggs, 1963a; Briggs and DeGuisti, 1966), in guinea pigs infected with *Ascaris* (Sprent, 1950), and in rats infected with *N. brasiliensis* (Urquhart et al., 1965; Jones and Ogilvie, 1967). Injection of antigen into the skin of sensitized animals leads to mast cell degranulation in hosts infected with *T. spiralis* (Briggs, 1963b; Bloebaum and Olson, 1965) and *Strongyloides ratti* (Goldgraber and Lewert, 1965). Whur (1966) reported that challenge of the rat infected with *N. brasiliensis* resulted in degranulation of the mast cells in the intestine but not of the intestinal globule leukocytes.

Both the Shwartzman and Arthus reactions were reported in experimental animals (guinea pigs and rabbits) with extracts of *Paragonimus ohirai* (Araki, 1959). Japanese workers have extensively studied immediate-type hypersensitivity in experimental animals and in man infected with *Ascaris lumbricoides*. Ikeda (1951, 1952a, b) demonstrated Shwartzman activity and Arthus and Schultz-Dale reactivity with extracts of *A. lumbricoides* in experimentally infected guinea pigs. *Ascaris* allergen was isolated from serum, mothers' milk, ascitic fluid, spinal fluid, tears, nasal mucosa, saliva, and urine of infected individuals. The allergic reactions were induced by carbohydrate extracts of the parasite, and they were specific, since sensitized animals did not react to *Ancylostoma* extracts. PK antibodies were also demonstrated in the sera of children. Nakajima (1954) purified "*Ascaris* toxin" and showed it to be a protein. The most comprehensive studies were made by Matsumura (1963) and his colleagues. PCA antibodies were demonstrated in the serum of infected animals. No correlation was reported between PK and hemagglutinating antibody in infected adults. In studies on immediate hypersensitivity, the Matsumura group showed that blood platelet agglutination was related to immediate hypersensitivity, that epigastric pain in man could be induced with *Ascaris* body fluid, and that antihistamines alleviated such pain within 15 to 20 minutes.

Although varying degrees of immediate hypersensitivity can be demonstrated in animals infected with parasitic infections, a strong correlation with protective immunity has not been demonstrated.

DELAYED HYPERSENSITIVITY

A brief description of the principles of delayed hypersensitivity and the methods for their study are included in this chapter, since the author is of the opinion that when such investigations are undertaken on a larger scale, the immune mechanisms of parasitic infections will be greatly elucidated.

In contrast with immediate hypersensitivity in which humoral antibody reacts with antigen, delayed hypersensitivity is characterized by the presence of immunologically competent (immunocompetent) cells possessing a specific capacity for the antigen. The phenomenon has been associated with infections, neoplastic and autoimmune diseases, and transplantation hypersensitivities. Delayed hypersensitivity can be passively transferred to a normal isogenic recipient by means of sensitized lymphocytes, but not by serum (Coe et al., 1966). Cellular antibody is the sensitizing factor of the immunocompetent cells. There is evidence of an RNA "transfer factor" (Thor, 1967) which is capable of conveying the immunospecific information

to normal lymphoid cells, thus stimulating them to produce antibody
(Crowle, 1964); in addition, circulating cytophilic antibody may in some
instances play a cell-sensitizing role (Boyden, 1964; Jonas et al., 1965).

The studies of immunocompetent cells by *in vitro* methods and of their
association with delayed hypersensitivity are new fields. Although some concepts are vague and apparent anomalies are still unresolved, a greater understanding of the mechanisms of cellular immunity is being gained. The majority of the studies with parasitic materials in the area of delayed hypersensitivity has been concerned with cell transfer and histologic studies. There
have been only a few reports of *in vitro* studies with immunocompetent cells
(Soulsby, 1967).

Delayed skin reactions in parasitic diseases

Animals which have developed cellular or delayed hypersensitivity demonstrate skin reactivity that requires 48 hours to develop (i.e., delayed skin
reaction). Inflammation at the site of antigen inoculation is predominantly
made up of mononuclear cells. The host shows no detectable circulating antibody, and sensitivity can be transferred only with cells.

The behavior of the antigenic stimulus in cellular hypersensitivity differs
from antibody hypersensitivity in that local injection of antigen into the skin
is not associated with increased capillary permeability or polymorphonuclear
leukocytic invasion of the site. The principal cell types observed to accumu-
late are lymphocytes and macrophages. The macrophages of the sensitized
animal have an increased capacity for phagocytosis. Both lymphocytes and
macrophages from sensitized animals show increased susceptibility to the
physiologic effects of homologous antigen. Steroids can suppress the manifestations of delayed hypersensitivity, whereas they have a negligible effect
on the development of immediate hypersensitivity. Cortisone, however, inhibits the immediate hypersensitivity responses of trichinella-infected mice
to exogenous antigens. (Briggs and DeGuisti, 1966). Rynes et al. (1967)
have been able to transfer immediate hypersensitivity by lymphocytes from
the blood of ragweed-sensitive patients to normal individuals.

Helminth skin-test antigens usually confer an immediate histaminic-type
of wheal and flare in individuals infected with various parasitic diseases. In
addition to the immediate type of skin test, individuals infected with hydatid
cysts almost without exception show a delayed type of skin reactivity
(Kagan et al., 1966). Early workers (Graña, 1945; Grinblat, 1945) believed
that the delayed-type skin test was more specific than the immediate reaction. In schistosomiasis (Taliaferro and Taliaferro, 1931) and in trichinosis
(Bachman, 1928a, b), delayed skin responses occur, but the significance or
prevalence of this response has not been extensively studied. Skin test reactions for toxoplasmosis, leishmaniasis, Chagas' disease, and mycotic infections are invariably of the tuberculin delayed-type.

In a recent evaluation of a skin-test antigen in patients infected with

Entamoeba histolytica (Maddison et al., 1968b), both immediate and delayed skin tests were observed. Patients with amoebic liver abscess showed both reactions; patients with intestinal amoebiasis showed predominantly immediate responses. Nine asymptomatic individuals living in the endemic area reacted; one reacted with an immediate response, two with immediate and delayed responses, and six with delayed responses. These results suggested that the immediate response was associated with acute disease and the late response with past tissue invasion and chronic disease.

The relationship of skin reactivity and immunity in man has been studied in leishmaniasis. In cutaneous leishmaniasis (infection with *Leishmania tropica*), the skin test becomes positive early in the infection and is not associated with the development of immunity (Adler, 1963). In systemic kala-azar (systemic infection with *L. donovani*) a positive skin test develops only after cure and denotes immunity to reinfection (Manson-Bahr, 1963). In a study carried out in Kenya by Southgate and Manson-Bahr (1967), 14 individuals were challenged with a dermotropic ground-squirrel strain of *L. donovani*. All were immune to reinfection. All the skin-test positive subjects developed Arthus reactions. Unfortunately, histologic studies were not made to determine the cell type in the exudate observed.

Lymphocyte migration

The specific inhibition of cell migration by antigen was first described by Rich and Lewis (1932), who demonstrated that tuberculin inhibited the migration of cells taken from animals with delayed hypersensitivity to tuberculin. David et al. (1964a), using the same antigenic system, showed that circulating antibody played no part in the reaction. A comparatively small number of sensitized cells, when mixed with normal cells, confers sensitivity on the latter (David et al., 1964b). They also demonstrated that in contrast to the reactivity of circulating antibodies in immunized animals, both carrier protein and hapten are essential for inhibiting the migration of cells from guinea pigs hypersensitive to DNP-conjugated protein (David et al., 1964c). *In vitro* tests for delayed hypersensitivity also require the presence of the carrier protein (Benacerraf and Levine, 1962).

Some disparity exists among the types of cells reported in migration studies. Dumonde (1967) suggests that in guinea pig peritoneal exudates "the visible effect of the antigen is on the macrophages, whereas lymphocytes are free to emigrate and do not interfere with the inhibition of macrophage migration." Bloom and Bennett (1966) found in similar cell populations that lymphocytes alone do not migrate, but they concluded that lymphocytes are the immunologically competent cells whereas the macrophages are the indicators. The cell-migration technique has been applied to sensitized cells from various sites in several species of animals, including peripheral lymphocytes (Søborg and Bendixen, 1967) and lymph node cells from man (Thor, 1967).

A cell-migration inhibiting substance was found by Bloom and Bennett

(1966) to be produced by sensitized exudate lymphocytes only when specifically stimulated by antigen. Thor (1967) was able to confer sensitivity to normal cells with extracts of RNA from lymph node cells of sensitive donors.

Although these findings appear difficult to interpret, they may well be related to differences in the functional roles of lymphocytes which cannot be differentiated morphologically but which may actually be different classes of cells, i.e., which look alike but have different immunologic activities.

Lymphocyte transformation

Peripheral lymphocytes from sensitive individuals, when cultured in the presence of specific antigen, undergo transformation into blast cells showing mitotic division. This method has been used to assess immediate-type hypersensitivity in atopy (Wiener and Brasch, 1965; Lichtenstein et al., 1967) and drug allergies (Gill, 1967; Kunz et al., 1967; Halpern et al., 1967). A similar lymphocyte transformation was observed in cells from humans following their immunization against tetanus and smallpox (Caron, 1967). Mills (1965) suggested that the transformation of lymph node lymphocytes from sensitized guinea pigs was specifically related to their state of delayed hypersensitivity to either tuberculin or ovalbumin.

Nonsensitized peripheral leukocytes can undergo transformation when stimulated by phytohemagglutinin (PHA) (Nowell, 1960) or staphylococcal filtrate. Therefore, the prerequisites of a reliable test are meticulous technique and the use of control cultures without antigen for each test lot of sensitized cells (Halpern et al., 1967). In addition, the concentration of antigen used to stimulate the sensitized lymphocytes is critical—the reaction is inhibited if the sensitized cells are obtained from a patient on steroid therapy.

Histocompatibility antigens also induce lymphocyte proliferation in mixed peripheral leukocyte cultures of unrelated individuals (Bain et al., 1964). Lymphocyte transformation is a significant indicator of the homograft reaction in that a high rate of blast transformation in cultures of donor-recipient mixed leukocytes is a sign of the onset of graft rejection (Rubin et al., 1964; Oppenheim et al., 1965).

Target-cell destruction

Rosenau and Moon (1966) have shown that sensitized lymphocytes can cause destruction of monolayer cultures of homologous target cells. Their experimental model was the mouse. Lymphocytes were obtained from the spleens of BALB/c mice sensitized to homologous tissue culture cells of C3H mouse origin. They related this destruction reaction to functional modification of the sensitized lymphocytes. The reaction is inhibited by pretreatment of the sensitized cells with puromycin (Calabresi et al., 1967), further indicating that protein synthesis in the sensitized cells plays a part in the cellular immunity.

The technique has been applied to studies of diseases such as autoimmunity and tumor immunity, as well as homograft reaction (Rosenau and Moon, 1966). Application of this phenomenon to the study of parasitic infection is limited at present by the absence of suitable techniques for culturing parasite tissues.

Cytophilic antibodies

Boyden and Sorkin (1960) demonstrated circulating cytophilic antibody in rabbits immunized with human serum albumin (HSA). This antibody had an affinity for normal rabbit spleen cells, conferring upon them an ability to adsorb I^{131}-HSA. Results of further experiments suggest an association between the presence of cytophilic antibody and delayed hypersensitivity (Boyden, 1964). Jonas et al. (1965) found that the macrophage-cytophilic antibody in guinea pigs immunized with Freund's complete adjuvant, β-lactoglobulin, and sheep red blood cells did not sensitize any type of cell other than macrophages. The antibody was associated with the slow-moving γ_2 component of IgG and thus was distinct from the γ_1-type anaphylactic antibody.

Gordon (1967a) has hypothesized that histiocyte (macrophage) cytophilic antibody may be implicated in the target-cell destruction reaction, and suggests that this antigen-specific type of cellular immunity, as well as the nonspecific reaction of macrophages, may play a role in defense mechanisms against parasitic infections.

Delayed hypersensitivity and parasitic diseases

Kim's recent studies (Kim, 1966; Kim et al., 1967a,b) with *Trichinella spiralis* in the guinea pig showed that typical delayed hypersensitivity reactions could be manifested in sensitized animals. Delayed skin reactions were observed from 4 to 28 hours after inoculation of antigen. A perivascular infiltration of predominantly mononuclear cells was observed at the skin test site. Transfer of the hypersensitive state to normal recipients was accomplished by means of splenic and lymph node cells. The transfer of sensitized cells to recipient animals accelerated the development of PCA antibodies in skin-tested animals. Larsh et al. (1964a,b; 1966) suggested that delayed hypersensitivity may be involved in the mechanisms that bring about expulsion of adult worms in the intestines of infected mice. Expulsion of worms was mediated by the transfer of peritoneal exudate cells. Gordon (1967b) was critical of Larsh's study for not having a proper assay for delayed hypersensitivity (skin test) and for not having a proper control group of animals that received exudate cells. C. A. Crandall (1965) was not able to confer immunity to *Ascaris suum* by transfer of splenic or exudate cells. However, she was able to demonstrate the transfer of immunity by parabiotic union of mice.

Dineen and Wagland (1966) injected lymph node cells from isogenic strains of guinea pigs resistant to *Trichostrongylus colubriformis* into normal recipients and were able to demonstrate that node cells transferred protection to the recipients by inhibiting development of the fourth-stage larvae of the parasite. In previous studies (Wagland and Dineen, 1965), transfer of serum from resistant guinea pigs into virgin recipients was not effective. Miller (1967) reported the transfer of immunity to *Ancylostoma caninum* in puppies by serum and lymphoid cells. Recent studies by Lang (1967) and Lang et al. (1967) on acquired immunity to *Fasciola hepatica* in white mice suggest that delayed hypersensitivity was part of the mechanism of immunity. The transfer of immunity against *Hymenolepis nana* with spleen cells was reported by Friedberg et al. (1967).

Organisms that parasitize macrophages generally initiate a state of delayed hypersensitivity in the host (Mackaness, 1967). Frenkel (1967) was able to transfer immunity to *Besnoitia jellisoni* and *Toxoplasma gondii* to isogenic irradiated tolerant hamsters with cells of spleen and lymph node origin. Cells of the bone marrow, thymus, liver, and kidney were ineffective. Lymphoid cells of an immune irradiated donor were likewise nonreactive.

Although one would expect adoptive transfer in leishmaniasis, Adler and Nelken (1965) were unsuccessful in transferring sensitivity with blood leukocytes from a highly allergic human donor to four recipients. It is regrettable that differential counts were not made, and in light of more recent *in vitro* lymphocyte tests, it would have been of interest to determine whether the donors' lymphocytes were indeed sensitive to extracts of *L. tropica* before being transferred. Bray and Lainson (1965) were also unsuccessful in transferring hypersensitivity from man to man or monkey to monkey with washed blood leukocytes.

Cellular immunity

Comprehensive studies on the cellular aspects of immunity were recently reviewed by Soulsby (1967). Studies that were carried out in Soulsby's laboratory with *in vitro* manifestations of lymphoid cells that adhere to the surfaces of antibody-sensitized larvae of *A. suum* were reviewed. Antibody-sensitized, third-stage larvae did not attract lymphocytes from lymph nodes or splenic sources. Transformed lymphocytes, blast cells, or cells which had been cultured for 3 to 6 days in the presence of *Ascaris suum* antigens adhered avidly to sensitized larvae. The lymphocyte cells exposed to antigen were reactive in fluorescent-antibody tests with anti-*A. suum* conjugated globulin. The immunoglobulin responsible for the sensitization of the surface of the larvae appeared on immunoelectrophoretic analysis to be in the macroglobulin fraction and was sensitive to 2-mercaptoethanol treatment.

Similar studies of adsorption of immune globulin to larvae and adults of *T. spiralis* were reported by Gadea et al. (1967).

Adherence of cells to the surface of sensitized larvae is not specific to lymphocytes, since the granulocytic series of cells also attach. Crandall and Arean (1967) report that peritoneal macrophages adhere to the cuticle of larvae placed in the peritoneal cavity of mice immune to *Ascaris*. The adherence of granulocytes to *Ascaris* larvae appears to be completely nonspecific, whereas the adhesion of lymphocytic cells is mediated by specific antibody.

Soulsby (1967) was able to demonstrate that lymphoid cells transformed by phytohemagglutinin also attach to larvae, but to a lesser extent than antigen-transformed cells do. Evidence is also presented that lymphocytes obtained from the peripheral blood of man can also be transformed by PHA and *Ascaris* antigen. Miggiano et al. (1966) isolated lymphoid cells from the peripheral circulation of individuals infected with *Echinococcus granulosus*. These cells, when cultured in 20 percent calf or human serum, underwent blast transformation in the presence of hydatid antigen.

Cells of the nonlymphocytic series also play a role in infection. Chemotactic response of polymorphonuclear leukocytes to *T. spiralis* and *A. suum* extracts in an *in vitro* system was reported by R. B. Crandall (1965).

Much additional work must be done to delineate the role of delayed hypersensitivity in parasitic infections. Larsh (1967) reviewed some of the recent work on delayed (cellular) hypersensitivity in parasitic infections. Delayed hypersensitivity can operate in the presence of immediate hypersensitivity. The two types of responses can be separated, and the assay tools are now available for their evaluation.

CONCLUSION

Although parasitologists have alluded to the role of cellular factors in parasitic immunity, preoccupation with antibodies has blocked effective work in this area. As the multitude of antibodies elicited by infection with parasites is described and characterized, it is becoming more and more evident that immunity or resistance in most parasitic diseases is not mediated by these antibodies. The task ahead lies in sorting out the cellular factors involved. The methods for working with the lymphoid-macrophage system are now available. Workers in parasitic immunity have all the tools of the immunochemist at their disposal. The *in vitro* techniques for working with lymphocytes are exquisitely sensitive and lend themselves to analysis of the minute amounts of antigenic fractions that can be obtained from chromatography and gel filtration columns and preparative electrophoresis. Isogenic strains of mice, rats, and guinea pigs are available for adoptive transfer studies. I believe we will come to grips in the near future with the mechanisms of protection in parasite infections through the study of immediate and, especially, delayed hypersensitivity reactions.

REFERENCES

Abele, D. C., J. E. Tobie, G. J. Hill, P. G. Contacos, and C. B. Evans. 1965 Alternations in serum proteins and 19S antibody production during the course of induced malarial infections in man. Amer. J. Trop. Med., 14: 191-197.

Ackert, J. E. 1942. Natural resistance to helminthic infections. J. Parasit., 28: 1-24.

Adler, S. 1958. The action of specific serum on a strain of *Trypanosoma cruzi*. Ann. Trop. Med. Parasit., 52: 282-301.

——— 1963. Immune Phenomenon in Leishmaniasis. *In* Immunity to Protozoa. Garnham, P. C. C., Pierce, A. E., and Roitt, I., eds. Oxford, Blackwell Scientific Publications, pp. 235-245.

——— and D. Nelken. 1965. Attempts to transfer delayed hypersensitivity to *Leishmania tropica* by leukocytes and whole blood. Trans. Roy. Soc. Trop. Med. Hyg., 59: 59-63.

Andrews, J. M. 1962. Parasitism and allergy. J. Parasit., 48: 3-12.

Araki, M. 1959. Immunological studies of *Paragonimus ohirai* Miyazaki, 1939. Fukuoka Acta Medica, 50: 2180-2181.

Bachman, G. W. 1928a. An intradermal reaction in experimental trichiniasis. Preliminary Report. J. Prevent. Med., 2: 169-173.

——— 1928b. An intradermal reaction in experimental trichiniasis. Final Report. J. Prevent. Med., 2: 513-523.

Bailey, W. S. 1951. Host-tissue reactions to initial and superimposed infections with *Hymenolepis nana* var. *fraterna*. J. Parasit., 37: 440-444.

Bain, B., M. R. Vas, and L. Lowenstein. 1964. The development of large immature mononuclear cells in mixed leukocyte cultures. Blood, 23: 108-128.

Barth, E. E. E., W. F. H. Jarrett, and G. M. Urquhart. 1966. Studies on the mechanism of self-cure reaction in rats infected with *Nippostrongylus brasiliensis*. Immunology, 10:459-464.

Barth, W. F., and J. L. Fahey. 1965. Heterologous and homologous skin-sensitizing activity of mouse 7S γ_1- and 7S γ_2-globulins. Nature (London), 206: 730-731.

Benacerraf, B., and B. B. Levine. 1962. Immunological specificity of delayed and immediate hypersensitivity reactions. J. Exp. Med., 115: 1026-1036.

Biagi, F. F., and L. Buentello. 1961. Immobilization reaction for the diagnosis of amebiasis. Exp. Parasit., 11: 188-190.

Biguet, J., F. Rosé, A. Capron, and P. Tran Van Ky. 1965a. Contribution de l'analyse immunoélectrophoretique à la connaissance des antigènes vermineux. Incidences pratiques sur leur standardisation, leur purification et le diagnostic des helminthiases par immuno-électrophorèse. Rev. Immun. (Paris), 29: 5-30.

——— P. Tran Van Ky, Y. Moschetto, and D. Gnamey-Koffy. 1965b. Contribution à l'étude de la structure antigènique des larves de *Trichinella* spiralis et des precipitines expérimentales du lapin. Wiad. Parazyt., 11: 299-315.

Binaghi, R. A., B. Benacerraf, K. J. Bloch, and F. M. Kourilsky. 1964. Properties of rat anaphylactic antibody. J. Immun., 92: 927-933.

Blacklock, D. B., and R. M. Gordon. 1927. The experimental production of immunity against metazoan parasites and an investigation of its nature. Ann. Trop. Med. Parasit., 21: 181-224.

Bloebaum, A. P., and L. J. Olson. 1965. Effect of *Trichinella spiralis* extracts on guinea pig mast cells. J. Parasit., 51 (Sec. 2): 38.

Bloom, B. R., and B. Bennett. 1966. Mechanism of a reaction *in vitro* associated with delayed-type hypersensitivity. Science, 153: 80-82.

Boyden, S. V. 1964. Cytophilic antibody in guinea pigs with delayed-type hypersensitivity. Immunology, 7: 474-483.

——— and E. Sorkin. 1960. The adsorption of antigen by spleen cells previously treated with antiserum in vitro. Immunology, 3: 272-283.

Brandzaeg, P., I. Fjellanger, and S. T. Gjeruldsen. 1967. Localization of immunoglobulins in human nasal mucosa. Immunochemistry, 4: 57-60.

Bray, R. S., and R. Lainson. 1965. Failure to transfer hypersensitivity to *Leishmania* by injection of leucocytes. Trans. Roy. Soc. Trop. Med. Hyg., 59: 221-222.

Briggs, N. T. 1963a. Hypersensitivity in murine trichinosis: Some responses of *Trichinella*-infected mice to antigen and 5-hydroxytryptophan. Ann. N.Y. Acad. Sci., 113: 456-466.

———— 1963b. Immunological injury of mast cells in mice actively and passively sensitized to antigens from *Trichinella spiralis*. J. Infect. Dis., 113: 22-32.

———— and D. L. DeGuisti. 1966. Generalized allergic reactions in *Trichinella*-infected mice: The temporal association of host immunity and sensitivity to exogenous antigens. Amer. J. Trop. Med., 15: 919-929.

Bruijning, C. F. A. 1964. The circumoval precipitate reaction in experimental schistosomiasis II. Trop. Geogr. Med., 16: 256-262.

Brunner, M. 1928. Immunological studies in human parasitic infestation. 1. Intradermal testing with parasitic extracts as an aid in the diagnosis of parasitic infestation. J. Immun., 15: 83-101.

Calabresi, P., K. T. Brunner, and J. Mavel. 1967. Inhibition by puromycin *in vitro* of cell-bound immunity induced by tumor homografts. Fed. Proc., 26(Abstr. 1233):478.

Campbell, D. H. 1938a. The specific protective property of serum from rats infected with *Cysticercus crassicollis*. J. Immun., 35: 195-204.

———— 1938b. The specific absorbability of protective antibodies against *Cysticercus crassicollis* in rats and *Cysticercus pisiformis* in rabbits from infected and artificially immunized animals. J. Immun., 35: 205-216.

———— 1938c. Further studies on the "non-absorbable" protective property in serum from rats infected with *Cysticercus crassicollis*. J. Immun., 35: 465-476.

Capron, A., A. Vernes, J. Biguet, F. Rosé, A. Clay, and L. Adenis. 1966. Les précipitines sériques dans les bilharzioses humaines et expérimentales à *Schistosoma mansoni*, *S. haematobium* and *S. japonicum*. Ann. Parasit. Hum. Comp. (Paris), 41: 123-187.

Caron, G. A. 1967. The effect of antigens in combination on lymphocyte transformation *in vitro*. Int. Arch. Allerg., 31: 521-528.

Chodirker, W. B., and T. B. Tomasi, Jr. 1963. Gamma globulins: Quantitative relationships in human serum and nonvascular fluids. Science, 142: 1080-1081.

Coe, J. E., J. D. Feldman, and S. Lee. 1966. Immunological competence of thoracic duct cells 1. Delayed hypersensitivity. J. Exp. Med., 123: 267-281.

Cohen, S., and I. A. McGregor. 1963. Gamma globulin and acquired immunity to malaria. *In* Immunity to Protozoa. Garnham, P. C. C., Pierce, A. E., and Roitt, I., eds. Oxford, Blackwell Scientific Publications, pp. 123-159.

Coker, C. M., and J. Oliver-González. 1956. Studies on immunity to schistosomiasis—Passive transfer of anti-egg antibody in humans. Amer. J. Trop. Med., 5: 385.

Cole, B. A, and J. F. Kent. 1953. Immobilization of *Entamoeba histolytica in vitro* by antiserum produced in the rabbit. Proc. Soc. Exp. Biol. Med., 83: 811-814.

Crandall, C. A 1965. Studies on the transfer of immunity to *Ascaris suum* in mice by serum, parabiotic union, and cells. J. Parasit., 51: 405-408.

———— and V. M. Arean. 1964. In vivo studies of *Ascaris suum* larvae planted in diffusion chambers in immune and non-immune mice. J. Parasit., 50: 685-688.

———— and V. M. Arean. 1967. Electron microscope observations on the cuticle and submicroscopic binding of antibody in *Ascaris suum* larvae. J. Parasit., 53: 105-109.

Crandall, R. B. 1965. Chemotactic response of polymorphonuclear leukocytes to *Trichinella spiralis* and *Ascaris suum* extracts. J. Parasit., 51: 397-404.

———— J. J. Cebra, and C. A. Crandall. 1967. The relative proportions of IgG-, IgA- and IgM-containing cells in rabbit tissues during experimental trichinosis. Immunology, 12: 147-158.

Crowle, A. J. 1964. Delayed hypersensitivity and its allergic implications. Ann. Allerg., 22: 215-228.

David, J. R., S. Al-Askari, H. S. Lawrence, and L. Thomas. 1964a. Delayed hypersensitivity *in vitro* I. The specificity of inhibition of cell migration by antigens. J. Immun. 93: 264-273.

———— H. S. Lawrence, and L. Thomas. 1964b. Delayed hypersensitivity *in vitro*. II. Effect of sensitized cells on normal cells in the presence of antigen. J. Immun., 93: 274-278.

———— H. S. Lawrence, and L. Thomas. 1964c. Delayed hypersensitivity *in vitro*. III. The specificity of hapten-protein conjugates in the inhibition of cell migration. J. Immun., 93: 279-282.

Dineen, J. K., and B. M. Wagland. 1966. The cellular transfer of immunity to *Tricho-*

strongylus colubriformis in an isogenic strain of guinea pig. II. The relative suscepti-bility of the larval and adult stages of the parasite to immunological attack. Immunol-ogy, 11: 47-57.

Dobson, C. 1966a. Precipitating antibodies in extracts from mucosa and tunica muscu-laris of the alimentary tract of sheep infected with *Oesophagostomum columbianun*. J. Parasit., 52: 1037-1038.

——— 1966b. Studies on the immunity of sheep to *Oesophagostomum columbianum*: The nature and fate of the globule leucocyte. Aust. J. Agric. Res., 17: 955-966.

——— 1966c. The demonstration of antibodies in the intestinal mucus of sheep infected with *Oesophagostomum columbianum* by means of the percutaneous anaphylaxis test. Aust. J. Biol. Sci., 19: 339-340.

——— R. W. Campbell, and A. I. Webb. 1967. Anaphylactic and reagin-like antibody in rats infected with *Toxocara canis* larvae. J. Parasit., 53: 209.

Douvres, F. W. 1962. The "in vitro" cultivation of *Oesophagostomum radiatum,* the nodular worm of cattle. II. The use of this technique to study immune responses of host tissue extracts against the developing nematode. J. Parasit., 48: 852-864.

Dumonde, D. C. 1967. The role of the macrophage in delayed hypersensitivity. Brit. Med. Bull., 23: 9-14.

Fireman, P., M. Boesman, and D. Gitlin. 1967. Heterogeneity of skin-sensitizing anti-bodies. J. Allerg., 40: 259-268.

Franklin, E. C. 1964. The immune globulins—Their structure and function and some techniques for their isolation. Progr. Allerg., 8: 58-148.

Frenkel, J. K. 1967. Adoptive immunity to intracellular infection. J. Immun., 98: 1309-1319.

Friedberg, W., B. R. Neas, D. N. Faulkner, and M. H. Friedberg. 1967. Immunity to *Hymenolepis nana*: Transfer by spleen cells. J. Parasit., 53: 895-896.

Gadea, D., L. L. A. Moore, and J. Oliver-González. 1967. Adsorption of globulin to the cuticle of larvae and adults of *Trichinella spiralis*. Amer. J. Trop. Med., 16: 750-751.

Gemmell, M. A. 1962. Natural and acquired immunity factors inhibiting penetration of some hexacanth embryos through the intestinal barrier. Nature (London), 194: 701-702.

Gill, F. A. 1967. The association of increased spontaneous lymphocyte transformation *in vitro* with clinical manifestations of drug hypersensitivity. J. Immun., 98: 778-785.

Goldgraber, M. B., and R. M. Lewert. 1965. Immunological injury of mast cells and connective tissue in mice infected with *Strongyloides ratti*. J. Parasit., 51: 169-174.

Goodfriend, L., B. A. Kovacs, and B. Rose. 1966. *In vitro* sensitization of monkey lung fragments with human ragweed atopic serum. Int. Arch. Allerg., 30: 511-518.

Gordon, B. L. 1967a. The case for cytophilic antibodies in cellular immunity. Ann. Allerg., 25: 1-5.

——— 1967b. Functional immunity to nematode disease: A review. Ann. Allerg., 25: 137-144.

Graña, A. 1945. Alergia y diagnostico biologico de la hidatidosis. Arch. Uruguay Med. Cirug. Espec., 26: 538-559.

Grinblat, S. 1945. Estudio sobre el valor de la reacción de Casoni complemtada con la prueba de Michailow para el diagnostico de la equinococcosis. Rev. Asoc. Med. Argent., 59: 17-26.

Guerra, P., M. Mayer, and J. Di Prisco. 1945. La especificidad de las intradermo-reacciones con antigenos de *Schistosoma mansoni* y *Fasciola hepatica* por el métado de Prausnitz-Küstner. Rev. Sanid. Asist. Soc., 10: 51-63.

Guest, M. F., M. M. Wong, and L. K. Chin. 1966. Passive cutaneous anaphylaxis using a microfilarial antigen-antibody system. Presented at Laboratory Meeting of the Malaysian Society of Parasitology, Kuala Lumpur, Malaysia.

Halpern, B., N. T. Ky, and N. Amache. 1967. Diagnosis of drug allergy *in vitro* with the lymphocyte transformation test. J. Allerg., 40: 168-181.

Hsü, H. F., and S. Y. Li Hsü. 1966. Reagin-like antibody in rhesus monkeys immune to *Schistosoma japonicum*. Z. Tropenmed. Parasit., 17: 166-176.

Humphrey, J. H., and R. G. White. 1963. Immunology for Students of Medicine. Oxford, Blackwell Scientific Publications.

Ikeda, T. 1951. Experimental studies on allergenicity and antigenicity of ascaris extract. Report I. Igaku Kenkyuu (Jap. J. Med. Sci.), 21: 1481-1495.

——— 1952a. Experimental studies on allergenicity and antigenicity of ascaris extract. Report II. Igaku Kenkyuu (Jap. J. Med. Sci.), 22: 66-81.

—— 1952b. Experimental studies on allergenicity and antigenicity of ascaris extract. Report III. Igaku Kenkyuu (Jap. J. Med. Sci.), 22: 82-97.

Ishizaka, K., E. G. Dennis, and M. Hornbrook. 1964. Presence of reagin in saliva. J. Allerg, 35:143-148.

—— T. Ishizaka, and C. E. Arbesman. 1967. Induction of passive cutaneous anaphylaxis in monkeys by human γ E antibody. J. Allerg., 39: 254-264.

Ivey, M. H. 1965. Immediate hypersensitivity and serological responses in guinea pigs infected with *Toxocara canis* or *Trichinella spiralis*. Amer. J. Trop. Med., 14: 1044-1051.

—— and R. Slanga. 1965. An evaluation of passive cutaneous anaphylactic reactions with *Trichinella* and *Toxocara* antibody-antigen systems. Amer. J. Trop. Med. 14: 1052-1056.

Jachowski, L. A., R. I. Anderson, and E. H. Sadun. 1963. Serologic reactions to *Schistosoma mansoni* 1. Quantitative studies of experimentally infected monkeys (*Macaca mulatta*). Amer. J. Hyg., 77: 137-145.

Jackson, G. J. 1961. The parasite nematode, *Neoaplectana glaseri,* in axenic culture. 1. Effects of antibodies and anthelminthics. Exp. Parasit., 11: 241-247.

Janeway, C., F. S. Rosen, E. Merler, and C. A. Alper. 1967. The Gamma Globulins. Boston, Little, Brown and Co.

Jonas, W. E., B. W. Gurner, D. S. Nelson, and R. R. A. Coombs. 1965. Passive sensitization of tissue cells. 1. Passive sensitization of macrophages by guinea-pig cytophilic antibody. Int. Arch. Allerg., 28: 86-104.

Jones, V. E., and B. M. Ogilvie. 1967. Reaginic antibodies and immunity to *Nippostrongylus brasiliensis* in the rat. II. Some properties of the antibodies and antigens. Immunology, 12: 583-597.

Kagan, I. G. 1955. Studies on the serology of schistosomiasis 1. The *in vitro* activity of cercariae and miracidia in serum of experimental natural and immunized hosts. Exp. Parasit., 4: 361-376.

—— 1958. Contributions to the immunology and serology of schistosomiasis. Rice Institute Pamphlet No. 45, pp. 151-183.

—— 1961. Gel diffusion techniques for the analysis of parasitic material. Proc. Helminth. Soc. (Washington), 28: 97-102.

—— 1963. A review of immunologic methods for the diagnosis of filariasis. J. Parasit., 49: 773-798.

—— 1966. Mechanisms of immunity in trematode infection. *In* Biology of Parasites. Soulsby, E. J. L., ed. New York, Academic Press, Inc., pp. 277-299.

—— and J. Pellegrino. 1961. A critical review of immunological methods for the diagnosis of bilharziasis. Bull. W.H.O., 25: 611-674.

—— J. J. Osimani, J. C. Varela, and D. S. Allain. 1966. Evaluation of intradermal and serologic tests for the diagnosis of hydatid disease. Amer. J. Trop. Med., 15: 172-179.

—— S. E. Maddison, and L. Norman. 1968. Reactivity of human immunoglobulins in echinococcosis and trichinosis. Amer. J. Trop. Med., 17: 79-85.

Kim, C. W. 1966. Delayed hypersensitivity to larval antigens of *Trichinella spiralis*. J. Infect. Dis., 116: 208-214.

—— H. Savel, and L. D. Hamilton. 1967a. Delayed hypersensitivity to *Trichinella spiralis* I. Transfer of delayed hypersensitivity by lymph node cells. J. Immun., 99: 1150-1155.

—— M. P. Jamuar, and L. D. Hamilton. 1967b. Delayed hypersensitivity to *Trichinella spiralis*. II. Antibody response in recipients after transfer of delayed hypersensitivity. J. Immun., 99: 1156-1161.

Kunz, M. L., R. E. Reisman, and C. E. Arbesman. 1967. Evaluation of penicillin hypersensitivity by two newer immunologic procedures. J. Allerg., 40: 135-144.

Labzoffsky, N. A., R. K. Baratawidjaja, E. Kuitunen, F. N. Lewis, D. A. Kavelman, and L. P. Morrissey. 1964. Immunofluorescence as an aid in the early diagnosis of trichinosis. Canad. Med. Ass. J., 90: 920-921.

Lang, B. Z. 1967. Host-parasite relationships of *Fasciola hepatica* in the white mouse. II. Studies on acquired immunity. J. Parasit., 53: 21-30.

—— J. E. Larsh, Jr., N. F. Weatherly, and H. T. Goulson. 1967. Demonstration of immunity to *Fasciola hepatica* in recipient mice given peritoneal exudate cells. J. Parasit., 53: 208-209.

Larsh, J. E., Jr. 1967. Delayed cellular hypersensitivity in parasitic infections. Amer. J. Trop. Med., 16: 735-745.

———— H. T. Goulson, and N. F. Weatherly. 1964a. Studies on delayed (cellular) hypersensitivity in mice infected with *Trichinella spiralis*. I. Transfer of lymph node cells. J. Elisha Mitchell Sci. Soc., 80: 133-135.

———— H. T. Goulson, and N. F. Weatherly. 1964b. Studies on delayed (cellular) hypersensitivity in mice infected with *Trichinella spiralis*. II. Transfer of peritoneal exudate cells. J. Parasit., 50: 496-498.

———— G. J. Race, H. T. Goulson, and N. F. Weatherly. 1966. Studies on delayed (cellular) hypersensitivity in mice infected with *Trichinella spiralis* III. Serologic and histopathologic findings in recipients given peritoneal exudate cells. J. Parasit., 52: 146-156.

Layton, L. 1965. Passive transfer of human atopic allergies into lemurs, lorises, pottos, and galagos: Possible primate-ordinal specificity of acceptance of passive sensitization by human atopic reagin. J. Allerg., 36: 523-531.

———— S. Lee, and E. Yamanaka. 1962. Allergen testing on monkeys passively sensitized by hay fever and asthma reagins of human sera. Nature (London), 193: 988-999.

Lichtenstein, L. M., P. S. Norman, and J. T. Connell. 1967. Comparison between skin-sensitizing antibody titers and leucocyte sensitivity measurements as an index of the severity of ragweed hay fever. J. Aller., 40: 160-167.

Mackaness, G. B. 1967. The relationship of delayed hypersensitivity to acquired cellular resistance. Brit. Med. Bull., 23: 52-54.

Maddison, S. E., I. G. Kagan, and L. Norman. 1968a. Reactivity of human immunoglobulins in amebiasis. J. Immun., 100: 217-226.

———— I. G. Kagan and R. Elsdon-Dew. 1968b. Comparison of intradermal and serological tests for the diagnosis of amebiasis. Amer. J. Trop. Med., 17: 540-547.

Maekelt, G. A. 1966. Immunity mechanisms to protozoa. *In* Biology of Parasites. Soulsby, E. J. L., ed. New York, Academic Press, Inc., pp. 321-334.

Manson-Bahr, P. E. C. 1963. Active immunization in leishmaniasis. *In* Immunity to Protozoa. Garnham, P. C. C., Pierce, A. E., and Roitt, I., eds. Oxford, Blackwell Scientific Publications, pp. 759-774.

Matsumura, T. 1963. Ascaris allergy. Gunma J. Med. Sci., 12: 186-226.

Mattern, P. R., R. Masseyeff, R. Michel, and P. Peretti. 1961. Étude immunochemique de la ß₂ macroglobuline des serums de malades atteints de trypanosomiase Africaine à *T. gambiense*. Ann. Inst. Pasteur (Paris), 101: 382-388.

Mauss, E. A. 1940. The *in vitro* effect of immune serum upon *Trichinella spiralis* larvae. Amer. J. Hyg., 32: 80-83.

Mendes, E., and V. Amato Neto. 1963. Alguns aspectos imunológicos relativos à esquistossomiase mansonica: Prova da transferência passiva de anticorpos e prova das precipitinas. Hospital (Rio de Janeiro), 64: 1289-1293.

Miggiano, V. C., S. Ferrari, and F. Ingrao. 1966. *In vitro* stimulation of human peripheral leucocytes with *Echinococcus granulosus* antigens. (Preliminary communication.) Boll. Ist. Sieroter. (Milan), 45: 585-588.

Miller, H. M., and M. L. Gardiner. 1934. Further studies on passive immunity to a metazoan parasite, *Cysticercus fasciolaris*. Amer. J. Hyg., 20: 424-431.

Miller, T. A. 1967. Transfer of immunity to *Ancylostoma caninum* infection in pups by serum and lymphoid cells. Immunology, 12: 231-241.

Mills, J. A. 1965. Lymphocyte response to antigen *in vitro*. Clin. Res., 13: 289.

Mueller, J. F. 1961. The laboratory propagation of *Spirometra mansonoides* as an experimental tool. V. Behavior of the sparganum in and out of the mouse host, and formation of immune precipitates. J. Parasit., 47: 879-881.

Nakajima, M. 1954. Biochemical studies on the nature of ascaris toxin. Yokohama Med. Bull., 5: 10-20.

Nowell, P. C. 1960. Phytohemagglutinin: An initiator of mitosis in cultures of normal human leukocytes. Cancer Res., 20: 462-468.

Ogilvie, B. M. 1964. Reagin-like antibodies in animals immune to helminth parasites. Nature (London), 204: 91-92.

———— 1967. Reagin-like antibodies in rats infected with the nematode parasite *Nippostrongylus brasiliensis*. Immunology, 12: 113-131.

———— and V. E. Jones. 1967. Reaginic antibodies and immunity to *Nippostrongylus brasiliensis* in the rat. 1. The effect of thymectomy, neonatal infections, and splenectomy. Parasitology, 57: 335-349.

———— S. R. Smithers, and R. J. Terry. 1966. Reagin-like antibodies in experimental infection of *Schistosoma mansoni* and the passive transfer of resistance. Nature (London), 209: 1221-1223.

Oliver-González, J. 1940. The *in vitro* action of immune serum on the larvae and adults of *Trichinella spiralis*. J. Infect. Dis., 67: 292-300.

—— 1954. Anti-egg precipitin in the serum of humans infected with *Schistosoma mansoni*. J. Infect. Dis., 95: 86-91.

Oppenheim, J. J., J. Whang, and E. Frei. 1965. The effect of skin homograft rejection on recipient and donor mild leucocyte cultures. J. Exp. Med., 122: 651-664, 1965.

Otto, G. F. 1940. A serum antibody in dogs actively immunized against the hookworm, *Ancylostoma caninum*. Amer. J. Hyg., 31: 23-37.

Ovary, Z. 1964. Passive cutaneous anaphylaxis. *In* Immunologic Methods. Ackroyd, J. F., ed. Oxford, Blackwell Scientific Publications, pp. 259-283.

—— B. Benecerraf, and K. J. Bloch. 1963. Properties of guinea pig 7S antibodies. II. Identification of antibodies involved in passive cutaneous and systemic anaphylaxis. J. Exp. Med., 117: 951-964.

Patterson, R., J. N. Fink, E. T. Nishimura, and J. J. Pruzansky. 1965. The passive transfer of immediate type hypersensitivity from man to other primates. J. Clin. Invest., 44: 140-148.

Pierce, A. E. 1959. Specific antibodies at mucous surfaces. 1959. Vet. Rev. Ann., 5: 17-36.

Rackemann, F. M., and A. H Stevens. 1927. Skin tests to extracts of *Echinococcus* and *Ascaris*. J. Immun., 13: 389-394.

Remington, J. S. 1967. Characterization of antibodies to parasites. *In* Immunologic Aspects of Parasitic Infections. Pan American Health Organization Scientific Publication No. 150.

—— and M. J. Miller. 1966. 19S and 7S anti-toxoplasma antibodies in the diagnosis of acute congenital and acquired toxoplasmosis. Proc. Soc. Exp. Biol. Med., 121: 357-363.

—— K. L. Vosti, A. Lietze, and A. L. Zimmerman. 1964. Serum proteins and antibody activity in human nasal secretions. J. Clin. Invest., 43:1613-1624.

Rich, A. R., and M. R. Lewis. 1932. Nature of allergy in tuberculosis as revealed by tissue culture studies. Bull. Hopkins Hosp., 50: 115-131.

Rose, N. R., J. H. Kent, R. E. Reisman, and C. E. Arbesman. 1964. Demonstration of human reagin in the monkey. 1. Passive sensitization of monkey skin with sera of untreated atopic patients. J. Allerg., 35: 520-534.

Rosenau, W., and H. D. Moon. 1966. Studies on the mechanism of the cytolytic effect of sensitized lymphocytes. J. Immun., 96: 80-84.

Rubin, A. L., K. H. Stenzel, K. Hirschhorn, and F. Bach. 1964. Histocompatibility and immunologic competence in renal homotransplantation. Science, 143: 815-816.

Rynes, S. E., C. F. Milon, and H. C. Leopold. 1967. Transfer of immediate hypersensitivity by lymphocytes from blood of ragweed-sensitive patients. J. Allerg., 39: 139-147.

Sadun, E. H. 1949. The antibody basis of immunity in chickens to *Ascaridia galli*. Amer. J. Hyg., 49: 101-116.

—— F. von Lichtenberg, R. L. Hickman, J. I. Bruce, J. H. Smith, and M. J. Schoenbechler. 1966. Schistosomiasis mansoni in the chimpanzee: Parasitologic, clinical, serologic, pathologic, and radiologic observations. Amer. J. Trop. Med., 15: 496-506.

Sarles, M. P. 1938. The *in vitro* action of immune rat serum in the nematode, *Nippostrongylus muris*. J. Infect. Dis., 62: 337-348.

—— and W. H. Taliaferro. 1936. The local points of defense and the passive transfer of acquired immunity to *Nippostrongylus muris* in rats. J. Infect. Dis., 59: 207-220.

Schulz, R. S., and R. G. Ismagilova. 1962. A new immunological reaction in hydatidosis. Vestnik Selskokhozyaistvennoi Nauki (Alma-Ata), 6: 45-49.

Senterfit, L. B. 1953. Immobilization of *Schistosoma mansoni* miracidia by immune serum. Proc. Soc. Exp. Biol. Med., 84: 5-7.

—— 1958. Immobilization of the miracidia of *Schistosoma mansoni* by immune sera. 1. The nature of the reaction as studied in hamster sera. Amer. J. Hyg., 68: 140-147.

Sharp, A. D., and L. J. Olson. 1962. Hypersensitivity responses in *Toxocara-*, *Ascaris-*, and *Trichinella*-infected guinea pigs to homologous and heterologous challenge. J. Parasit., 48: 362-367.

Silverman, P. H. 1955. A technique for studying the *in vitro* effect of serum on activated taeniid hexacanth embryos. Nature (London), 176: 598-599.

—— 1965. Some immunologic aspects of parasitic helminth infections. Amer. Zool., 5: 153-163.

Smith, P. E. 1953. Life history and host-parasite relations of *Heterakis spumosa,* a nematode parasite in the colon of the rat. Amer. J. Hyg., 57: 194-221.

Smithers, S. R. 1962. Stimulation of acquired resistance to *Schistosoma mansoni* in monkeys: Role of eggs and worms. Exp. Parasit., 12: 263-273.

———— 1967. The induction and nature of antibody response to parasites. *In* Immunologic Aspects of Parasitic Infections. Pan American Health Organization Scientific Publication No. 150, pp. 43-49.

———— and R. J. Terry. 1965. Acquired resistance to experimental infection of *Schistosoma mansoni* in the albino rat. Parasitology, 55: 711-717.

Søborg, M., and G. Bendixen. 1967. Human lymphocyte migration as a parameter of hypersensitivity. Acta Med. Scand., 181: 247-256.

Soulsby, E. J. L. 1960. Immunity to helminths—Recent advances. Vet. Rec., 72: 322-327.

———— 1962. Antigen-antibody reactions in helminth infections. *In* Advances in Immunology, Vol. 2. Taliaferro, W. H., and Humphrey, J. H., eds. New York, Academic Press, Inc., pp. 265-308.

———— 1967. Lymphocyte, macrophage, and other cell reactions to parasites. *In* Immunologic Aspects of Parasitic Infections. Pan American Health Organization Scientific Publication No. 150, pp. 66-84.

———— and D. F. Stewart. 1960. Serological studies of the self-cure reaction in sheep infected with *Haemonchus contortus*. Aust. J. Agric. Res., 11: 595-603.

South, M. A., M. D. Cooper, F. A. Wollheim, R. Hong, and R. A. Good. 1966. The IgA system. 1. Studies of the transport and immunochemistry of IgA in the saliva. J. Exp. Med., 123: 615-627.

Southgate, B. A., and P. E. C. Manson-Bahr. 1967. Studies in the epidemiology of East African leishmaniasis. 4. The significance of the positive leishmanin test. J. Trop. Med. Hyg., 70: 29-33.

Sprent, J. F. A. 1950. On the toxic and allergic manifestations caused by the tissues and fluids of *Ascaris*. II. Effect of different chemical fractions on worm-free, infected and sensitized guinea pigs. J. Infect. Dis., 86: 146-158.

Stoll, N. R. 1958. The induction of self-cure and protection with special reference to experimental vaccination against *Haemonchus*. Rice Institute Pamphlet No. 45, pp. 184-208.

Taliaferro, W. H., and L. G. Taliaferro. 1931. Skin reactions in persons infected with *Schistosoma mansoni*. Puerto Rico J. Public Health Trop. Med., 7: 23-35.

Targett, G. A. T., and A. Voller. 1965. Studies on antibody levels during vaccination of rhesus monkeys against *Plasmodium knowlesi*. Brit. Med. J., 2: 1104-1106.

Thor, D. E. 1967. Delayed hypersensitivity in man: A correlate *in vitro* and transfer by an RNA extract. Science, 157: 1567-1569.

Thorson, R. E. 1954. Effect of immune serum from rats on infective larvae of *Nippostrongylus muris*. Exp. Parasit., 3: 9-15.

Tobie, J. E., D. C. Abele, S. M. Wolff, P. G. Contacos, and C. B. Evans. 1966. Serum immunoglobulin levels in human malaria and their relationship to antibody production. J. Immun., 97: 498-505.

Tomasi, T. B., Jr., E. M. Tan, A. Soloman, and R. A. Prendergast. 1965. Characteristics of an immune system common to certain external secretions. J. Exp. Med., 121: 101-124.

Urquhart, G. M., W. Mulligan, R. M. Eadie, and F. W. Jennings. 1965. Immunological studies on *Nippostrongylus brasiliensis* infection in the rat: The role of local anaphylaxis. Exp. Parasit., 17: 210-217.

Vogel, H., and W. Minning. 1949a. Hüllenbildung bei Bilharzia-Cercarien im Serum Bilharzia-infizierter Tiere und Menschen. Zbl. Bakt. [Orig.], 153: 91-105.

———— and W. Minning. 1949b. Weitere Beobachtungen über die Cercarienhüllenreaktion, eine Seropräzipitation mit lebenden Bilharzia-Cercarien. Z. Tropenmed. Parasit., 1: 378-386.

———— and W. Minning. 1953. Über die erworbene Resistenz von *Macacus rhesus* gegenüber *Schistosoma japonicum*. Z. Tropenmed. Parasit., 4: 418-505.

Wagland, B. M., and J. K. Dineen. 1965. The cellular transfer of immunity to *Trichostrongylus colubriformis* in an isogenic strain of guinea pig. Aust. J. Exp. Biol. Med. Sci., 43: 429-438.

Weinmann, C. J. 1966. Immunity mechanisms in cestode infections. *In* Biology of Parasites. Soulsby, E. J. L., ed. New York, Academic Press, Inc., pp. 301-320.

Weinstein, P. P. 1967. Immunologic aspects of parasitic infections. *In* Immunologic Aspects of Parasitic Infections. Pan American Health Organization Scientific Publication No. 150, pp. 91-99.

Whur, P. 1966. Mast cell and globule leucocyte response to *Nippostrongylus brasiliensis* infection and to induced anaphylaxis. Int. Arch. Allerg., 30: 351-359.

Wiener, S., and J. Brasch. 1965. The mitogenic effect of grass-pollen extract. Med. J. Aust., 1: 148-149.

Wilson, R. J. M. 1966. γ₁-antibodies in guinea pigs infected with the cattle lungworm Immunology, 11: 199-209.

——— 1967. Homocytotrophic antibody response to the nematode *Nippostrongylus brasiliensis* in the rat—Studies on the worm antigen. J. Parasit., 53: 752-762.

——— V. E. Jones, and S. Leskowitz. 1967. Thymectomy and anaphylactic antibody in rats infected with *Nippostrongylus brasiliensis*. Nature (London), 213: 398-399.

Yokogawa, M., H. Yoshimura, T. Oshima, and M. Kihata. 1957. Immunological study on paragonimiasis. III. Passive transfer (P-K) experiments in human skins. Kiseichugaku Zasshi (Jap. J. Parasit.), 6: 449-457.

Zamon, V. 1962. An immobilization reaction against *Balantidium coli*. Nature (London), 194: 404-405.

Zvaifler, N. J., and E. L. Becker. 1966. Rabbit anaphylactic antibody. J. Exp. Med, 123: 935-950.

——— E. Sadun, and E. L. Becker. 1966. Anaphylactic (reaginic) antibodies in helminthic infections. Clin. Res., 14: 336.

Vaccination: Progress and Problems

PAUL H. SILVERMAN

Department of Zoology, University of Illinois, Urbana, Illinois

INTRODUCTION

Prophylactic immunization as a means of controlling parasitic infections in man and his domestic animals has not, until recently, played a major role in veterinary or medical practice, nor in the planning of research programs which were aimed at the development of control measures. For example, the relationship of the macroscopic helminths to disease has been known since recorded history, yet the recognition of resistance to infection and the application of this finding in attempts to induce protection against these parasites is only recent.

This situation contrasts strongly with the early history of bacteriology and virology. Thucydides (460–404 B.C.), the historian of the Peloponnesian War, commented on the well-known fact that survivors of the plague were never known to suffer from the disease again and were important as nurses to the ill. Smallpox vaccination traces its history to early observations in Asia that survivors of childhood infection remained unaffected during subsequent recurrent epidemics. The introduction of heterologous cowpox vaccine as a safe and effective human immunizing agent by Jenner (circa 1796) is well-known. Finally, the development of vaccines against anthrax and rabies by Pasteur and against diphtheria by Roux and Yersin in the latter part of the nineteenth century followed very shortly the isolation or demonstration of an infectious organism as the causative disease agent.

The only similar situation in the field of parasitic diseases is that of dermal leishmaniasis (Oriental sore) caused by the protozoan, *Leishmania tropica*. It has long been known that people who recovered from a case of Oriental sore never developed another. For this reason, the practice became established of inoculating, by scarification, material from an active sore into a site in children (particularly females) where the cosmetic effects would be less noticeable.

In the central Asian republics of the U.S.S.R., prophylactic vaccination is widely practiced, using material obtained from cultures of a zoonotic strain of *L. tropica* isolated from wild gerbils (*see* Manson-Bahr, 1963; Stauber, 1963). Unfortunately, very little detailed information on the preparation and effectiveness of this living vaccine is available.

One of the earliest reports of parasitic immunity observed under laboratory conditions is that of Theobald Smith (1910), who recognized the development of immunity to the sporozoan protozoa, *Eimeria stiedae*, in rabbits. Since Smith's report, the research on the mechanisms of resistance to coccidiosis, which has included numerous attempts to stimulate resistance by means of dead antigenic material prepared from various stages in the life cycle of the parasite, has not been successful. Active immunity in avian or rabbit coccidiosis, as in the case of the leishmanias, has been produced only through the use of living material (Horton-Smith et al., 1963).

Although the use of dead material was equally unsuccessful in early attempts to confer resistance to trypanosomiasis, it was eventually found that such antigenic preparations could be used to stimulate an apparent sterile immunity (Soltys, 1964). Soltys found that:

> Success in immunizing rabbits, rats, and sheep with dead trypanosomes depends on the method of killing trypanosomes, the frequency of inoculations and the strain used for immunization. Positive results were obtained when trypanosomes were killed by formalin or by freezing and thawing five times. Negative results were obtained when trypanosomes were killed by 56°C for half an hour.

This statement on the quality of antigen and frequency of vaccination may well be applied to all the parasitic vaccination studies which have been undertaken with dead antigens. It underlines the importance of testing a wide variety of experimental immunization procedures and antigen preparation methods before negative results are conclusively accepted.

In the case of malaria, the most important protozoan parasite of man, acquired immunity and the possibility of prophylactic immunization are now being seriously considered (Sadun et al., 1966; Goodman, 1966). In areas of hyperendemic malaria, the necessity of several years of exposure to constant reinfection in order to acquire a level of resistance sufficient to suppress acute manifestations of the disease suggests formidable practical problems in the development of a vaccine (Cohen and McGregor, 1963). Nevertheless, encouraging results by Targett and Fulton (1965) with trophozoite antigens of simian malaria, Richards (1966) with sporozoite antigens of avian malaria, and the serotherapeutic success of Cohen and McGregor (1963) using concentrated gamma-globulin to treat children with high parasitemias of *Plasmodium falciparum* led workers to give greater significance to the immunologic response to this infection and its possible use in control. With the development of drug resistance by the plasmodia and insecticide resistance by the mosquito vectors, the need for an immunologic approach is further emphasized.

Among the first workers to recognize the phenomenon of acquired resistance to helminths was Stoll (1928, 1929, 1958). His discovery of acquired immunity in sheep to the stomach worm, *Haemonchus contortus*, along with his suggestion that it was similar to the resistance following bacterial infections, did not gain immediate acceptance by parasitologists. Today the picture is quite different. Stoll (1961) openly and rhetorically asked, "The worms: can we vaccinate against them?" His qualified affirmative answer is based largely on the work carried out with parasitic nematodes.

Jarrett et al. (1959) introduced the first commercially produced vaccine against *Dictyocaulus viviparus*, the lung worm of cattle. The vaccine, which consists of living infective larvae attenuated by ionizing irradiation, has been in use since 1959 and has proved to be safe and effective (Poynter and Terry, 1966). However, this technique has not been found to be so successful when applied to other helminth species. The reasons for this are not clearly understood, but the inconsistency in results has emphasized the needs for a better understanding of the mechanism of resistance and for the isolation of the functional antigens involved. Progress toward this aim has been slow but encouraging (Silverman, 1965a).

Resistance to the larval stages of tapeworms was first described by Miller (1931) and Campbell (1936). The role of functional antigens associated with different stages and different activities is strongly confirmed by the recent work of Gemmel (1965a,b, 1966), who investigated the use of heterologous activated hexacanth embryos as a living vaccine in sheep against *Echinococcus granulosus*. The importance of transitory antigens associated with early penetration and establishment of the parasite is also apparent from studies with schistosomes, the blood fluke of man and domestic animals (*see* Sadun, 1963; Silverman, 1966).

ACTIVE IMMUNIZATION

The details of specific host-parasite relationships and the present status of studies on immunity to protozoa and helminths are summarized in the preceding chapters. It is the purpose of this contribution to deal with some of the factors which are *common* to the process of prophylactic immunization. My thesis is that vaccination procedures, either alone or in association with biologic or chemotherapeutic measures, can make a useful and significant contribution to the control and treatment of parasitic infections. Furthermore, as already indicated, it is becoming increasingly clear that protozoan and metazoan parasites stimulate the same kinds of immune reactions that are known to occur in response to bacteria and viruses. The hypothesis that unless natural infection readily induces resistance, it is not possible to stimulate it artificially, no longer appears tenable when one considers parasitic infections.

Many of the puzzling phenomena concerning the apparent lack of immunity to natural infection with parasites can be shown to be due to the changing antigenic character of metamorphosing parasites, to subthreshold stimulation by transitory functional antigens, or to other factors associated with the complex nature of parasitic infections. The research challenge is the unraveling of the qualitative and quantitative mechanisms by which recognition of and resistance to parasites can be enhanced through artificial or natural means. The pessimistic promulgations which have been broadcast on this subject are inevitably based on negative data. As Schad (1966) has pointed out, negative data do not rule out immunologic explanations in the case of inhibiting interactions between heterologous parasites. Neither do they rule out interactions between host and parasite.

ANTIGENS

Stage-specific antigens

Protozoa. The results of passive transfer of gamma-globulin to parasitized children from adults with many years of exposure to malaria in an hyperendemic area suggest that immunoglobulin "may act upon mature intracellular parasites or inactivate merozoites liberated from red blood cells" (Cohen and McGregor, 1963). Subsequent to passive transfer of protective sera, the rapid fall in trophozoites after schizogony is followed by an increase in gametocytes which appear to be unaffected by immune sera.

Richards (1966), interested in active immunization against malaria, used sporozoite antigens of avian species. He observed that immunized animals which were completely resistant to challenge with sporozoites could still be infected by the erythrocytic stages when these were injected directly into the blood stream.

The observations of Cohen and McGregor (1963) and Richards (1966) are illustrative of a phenomenon characteristic of parasitic infections, i.e., the diversity of antigenicity associated with various stages of a parasite occurring in the same host. The fact that immunity develops naturally only after many years of exposure suggests that the replicating blood stages are poor antigens in stimulating resistance to reinfection. The highly effective immunity obtained experimentally by Richards (1966) with sporozoites raises the question of whether the minimal exposure in nature (apparently less than 30 minutes) of this immunogenic stage is below the immunologic threshold required for the stimulation of active immunity in the host.

Evidence of stage-specific antigens in the case of fowl coccidiosis has been reported by Horton-Smith and his co-workers (1963). They found that second-generation merozoites and the subsequent gametocytes were poor in their ability to stimulate resistance to reinfection with challenge doses of second-generation merozoites. After three or four repeated infections with second-generation merozoites, the birds become resistant, but were shown to be completely susceptible to oral challenge with oocysts. No evidence of protection was found against schizogony or gametogony. It was concluded that exposure to both the sporozoites and schizogony were necessary in the natural stimulation of resistance. In both fowls and rabbits, the primary and probably most important immunologic barrier to parasite development appears to be at the sporozoite stage. Schizogony is seemingly suppressed entirely by the host's resistant response after development of immunity.

Helminths. The immunogenic stages which have been identified as important sources of functional antigen (i.e., resistance stimulating) in natural helminth infections elaborate substances during early infection and development of the metazoan parasite (*see* Silverman, 1965a, 1966).

Infection with parasitic nematodes is initiated by second- or third-stage infective larvae. In animals which have developed resistance as a result of repeated exposure to reinfection with third-stage larvae, the stage at which resistance is directed is the molting fourth-stage larva and, to a lesser extent, the molting fifth-stage. The adult worm does not appear to be as important as a source of resistance-stimulating antigen nor to be as adversely affected by the resistance response as the larvae. For this reason, animals which are resistant to *reinfection* may still maintain a worm burden of adult stages.

The existence of stage-specific antigens raises a number of important problems from the viewpoint of helminth vaccination and helps to explain the failure of some vaccination attempts which utilized the most readily available, but inappropriate, adult worm antigens. It appears that functional antigens may be associated with the somatic tissues of certain larval stages or may be secreted or excreted as toxins or metabolic products. To date, such antigens have been obtained only from actively metabolizing parasites. After the parasite stage(s) responsible for elaborating the resistance-stimulating antigens have been determined, techniques for collecting and standardizing the appropriate antigens must be developed.

Strain-specific antigens

Although much emphasis has been placed on evidence of strain- and species-specific immunity, a growing body of data suggests that there are many biologically important cross-reactions and basic species antigens that transcend strain variations. Gray (1965), in an extensive study of *Trypanosoma brucei* transmitted by two species of tsetse flies to goats and rabbits, followed the development of serologic substrains. He found that a common basic strain antigen persisted throughout the variants, and the trypanosomes eventually reverted to the basic strain in the absence of antibody, i.e., in the invertebrate host. Brown and Brown (1965) observed a similar phenomenon with monkey malaria.

Of even greater interest are the experimental findings of Nussenzweig et al. (1966), who induced a high degree of protection in mice to *Plasmodium vinckei* by prior infection with *P. chabaudi*. Voller et al. (1966) have also reported on cross-immunity between several species of monkey malaria. In contrast, the coccidia remain distinguished by their apparently high degree of species specificity (Horton-Smith et al., 1963).

Among the helminths, numerous examples of immune cross-reactions between species have been reported, and no evidence of intraspecific strain specificity has been reported. Although research workers have postulated strain differences to explain failures to reproduce experimental results in different laboratories by different workers using the same helminth species, other explanations seem more overriding. The age and sex of host animals, size of inoculum, site and route of immunizing injections, and type of adjuvant have varied greatly and could account for all the differences which have been described. Strain differences of immunogenic importance might exist amongst helminths, but the evidence to date is inconclusive.

The ability of some phylogenetically widely separated species to induce protective reactions (*see* Schad, 1966) is illustrated in the work of Silverman et al. (1962), who found that antigens prepared from *Haemonchus contortus* stimulated a highly significant degree of resistance in guinea pigs to infection with *Dictyocaulus viviparus*. On the other hand, *H. contortus* antigen had no apparent effect in protecting guinea pigs when challenged with *Trichostrongylus colubriformis*. The inability to predict where and how the useful antigens for potential vaccines might be obtained should encourage research workers to cast their nets widely. In our laboratory, Jakstys (1969) has found serologic cross-reactions between antigens of the free-living nematode, *Caenorhabditis briggsae*, and the parasitic nematode, *Haemonchus contortus*. Lehnert (1967) also has demonstrated similar reactions between *Ascaris suum* and *C. briggsae*.

In many invertebrates, numerous activities such as molting have been found to have common physiologic and biochemical mechanisms. Molting hormones in the class Insecta can be prepared from one order of insects and shown to be active in all respects in other insect orders. In those cases where chemical characterization of insect hormones has been completed, little difference has been found when distinct insect species are used as sources of hormone. If molting fluids of helminths are important functional antigens, there is no reason to believe that they will be species-specific, since specificity seems to offer little selective value if the analogy with insect hormones is valid.

It is obviously too much to expect that a single nonspecific antigen will be found that is active in stimulating protection against a whole spectrum of parasite species; on the other hand, there is enough presumptive evidence so that the concept of common antigens within limited groups might have useful applications.

Living organisms

Immunizing procedures for parasitic infections have been investigated using living (homologous and heterologous) organisms, attenuated organisms, and dead antigen vaccines.

Although living organisms have been used to vaccinate against certain parasitic diseases, e.g., fowl coccidiosis, human dermal leishmaniasis, monkey schistosomiasis, and bovine lung worm (Jarrett et al., 1959; Manson-Bahr, 1963; Sadun, 1963), many problems are inherent in this approach. The use of living organisms, such as sporulated oocysts, schistosome cercariae, or infective nematode larvae, as a source of antigen requires the maintenance of infected snails or other invertebrate intermediate hosts, or of infected dogs, sheep, cattle, or flocks of birds, according to the host requirements of particular parasite species.

As Lumsden (1965) has pointed out in the case of trypanosomes, the continuous syringe passage from host to host in the laboratory of the blood stages of strains of parasites that in nature normally pass through invertebrate vectors tends to result in strains that are fundamentally altered in morphology, susceptibility to drugs, infectivity to arthropod vectors, and antigenic characteristics. The situation is further complicated by the evidence that the artificial maintenance of the Tsetse fly vector of trypanosomes can have a considerable effect on the infection of this intermediate host (Weitz, 1964). However, an important advantage in using the arthropod vector hosts is that although the antigenic character of trypanosomes alters during their vertebrate host stage, when they are passed through the invertebrate host they revert to the antigenic variant of the original parent strain (Gray, 1965). The experiences with trypanosomes emphasize the need to work with cyclically transmitted parasites when this is the natural mode of infection.

Presumably, similar considerations apply to other arthropod-vectored parasites such as malaria, and from the viewpoint of providing a source of relevant and effective antigen(s) for potential vaccines, these considerations greatly complicate antigen production. This is particularly so when the need becomes apparent for large quantities of arthropods for the production of particular parasite stages (such as sporozoite antigens) for an effective malarial vaccine.

In the case of the live vaccine against fowl coccidiosis, the maintenance of numerous monospecific strains in infected birds has been successfully established for commercial production. A mixture of eight species of sporulated oocysts (*Eimeria tenella, E. necatrix, E. hagani, E. acervulina, E. maxima, E. brunetti, E. praecox, E. mivati*) is available* to be used in drinking water, and it is claimed that under controlled conditions of feed and litter management, sufficient immunity against both cecal and intestinal coccidiosis results from the initial infection and subsequent controlled reinfection to protect birds without producing undue pathologic effects. If symptoms warrant, treatment with coccidiostats such as sulfaquinoxaline or sulfamethazine are recommended.

Although insufficient evidence is available for drawing firm conclusions, there are enough indications to suggest that the physiology of the infected host has an influence on the virulence, physiology, and antigenicity of the parasite. How this effect is translated into variations of protection-stimulating antigens in infected laboratory animals is still unclear but requires early investigation.

The regular production of third-stage larvae of the lung worm of cattle, *Dictyocaulus viviparus*, using calves as donor animals, has been successfully operating since 1959 (*see* Poynter et al., 1960). The complexity of such an operation makes standardization almost impossible. However, the use of the normal host with its selective pressures in both the production of lung worm larvae and, as described above, fowl coccidial oocysts seems to ensure that an adequately antigenic organism is produced. Compensation for variations in parasites harvested from infection of any single host is provided by pooling material from a number of donor animals. Even with all of its complexities and its dependence upon the maintenance of groups of infected donor animals, this approach has proved to be amenable to veterinary commercial production methods; however, it has obvious limitations, especially when human parasites are considered.

In vitro cultivation

The *in vitro* cultivation of bacteria and viruses in cell-free media or tissue cultures has long provided the basis for antigen production for bacterial and viral vaccines. The standardization of both *in vitro* production techniques and the resultant harvested antigens has been the foundation of successful microbial vaccines.

* Coccivac®, Dorn and Mitchell Laboratories, Inc., Opelika, Alabama.

Similarly, it has become acutely apparent that cultivation techniques must be developed to maintain parasitic protozoa and metazoa *in vitro* before significant steps in the evolution of parasite vaccines can take place. The problem areas include diverse and formidable challenges such as mammalian erythrocyte and tissue culture maintenance, insect tissue culture, and cultivation of intact metazoan helminths. As great as the problems are, encouraging results have been reported for the *in vitro* maintenance of erythrocytic stages of rodent, simian, and human plasmodia (Geiman et al., 1966; Polet, 1966; Trager, 1966), for the exoerythrocytic stages of avian malaria (Huff, 1966), for the *in vitro* culture of the mosquito phase of avian malaria (Ball, 1966), for the intracellular stages of leishmania, for both the intra- and extracellular stages of trypanosomes and toxoplasma (*see* Zuckerman, 1966), and for the early intracellular stages of coccidia (Strout et al., 1965). Berntzen (1966) has made important technologic contributions toward the goal of maintaining cestode and nematode helminths *in vitro* through successive generations (*see also* Silverman, 1965b).

The need for intensive research in these areas cannot be overemphasized. The number of technologic problems to be resolved are enormous; however, the potential effect of readily available *in vitro* culture methods for parasites is immense. This would be useful not only from the immunologic aspect, but also as a tool for examining many facets of the host-parasite relationship. So far, the development of cultivation methods for parasitologic research has attracted a relatively small number of workers. It is to be hoped that extensive exploration of all types of culture techniques as they may be applied to protozoan and metazoan parasites will be increased. The problem of finding suitable tissue media for parasites may not be as difficult as anticipated. Strout et al. (1965) found, for example, that the sporozoites of the fowl coccidian, *Eimeria acervulina*, showed little requirement for specific cell species and underwent development in chicken, mouse, and human cells. Shumard and co-workers (1967, personal communication) have found that sporozoites of the fowl coccidian, *Eimeria tenella*, will develop in cultures of bovine cells. The possibility of continuous culture of the trophozoite stages of tissue and hemotropic parasites now seems an exciting feasibility. The lack of host specificity as observed in the *in vitro* cultures raises many interesting questions and suggests the use of cultured immunologically competent cells to test the role of the host response in determining host specificity.

The use of *in vitro* tissue culture methods for producing attenuated strains of parasites is another possibility and has been suggested by the work of Weiss and DeGiusti (1964, 1966). Working with a mouse strain of *P. berghei*, they found that after passage through rats and tissue culture in a medium containing lamb serum, the plasmodium became modified so that when reinoculated into susceptible mice, it stimulated sterile immunity without apparently establishing a primary patent infection. The further application of this technique to other hemotropic parasites appears warranted.

Sanders and Wallace (1966) found that trypanosomes which have been attentuated by a level of x-irradiation that prevented infection of rats with the still motile protozoa were capable of stimulating an apparent sterile immunity. These results suggest support for the work of Thillet and Chandler (1957), who found that the metabolic products collected from *in vitro* culture fluids were effective immunizing antigens. It seems, therefore, that somatic constituents alone are not effective by themselves.

Silverman, Poynter, and Podger (1962) and, more recently, Silverman, Alger, and Hansen (1966) have used antigens produced in *in vitro* cultures by the histotropic stages of nematodes for immunization procedures. For those nematodes so far examined, chemically defined media have been utilized. The opportunity of using these model systems is worthy of more attention, since little is known of the *in vitro* culture factors which affect the quality and quantity of antigen production. The best conditions for harvesting such material and the exploration of suitable methods for concentrating and storing functional antigens need to be determined. The development of serologic and biochemical standards for assessing antigenicity is one of the most immediate challenges.

The further development of *in vitro* culture methods, preferably continuous culture procedures, will require research into many fundamental problems. These include an analysis of the factors which, in nature, trigger the intrinsic biologic clock mechanisms and signal the initiation of physiologic and morphologic changes associated with growth, development, and metamorphosis of the various parasitic stages (*see* Rogers, 1962). These factors include specific enzymes or biologic substances elaborated by the host, physicochemical conditions, gas-phase interrelationships, and temperature effects. Optimal concentration of parasites in culture media and the need to alter conditions at critical times must be determined. An attempt to simulate the conditions of vertebrate or invertebrate host environment does not always prove to be the most profitable approach. Other, sometimes surprising, culture materials have been found to be useful. Jackson (1962), for example, found that a medium similar to that designed by Trager (1957) for the leptomonad or insect-inhabiting stage of *Leishmania tarentolae* was a suitable culture environment for the nematode, *Neoaplectana glaseri*; Hansen et al. (1966) found that a medium designed for the free-living nematode, *Caenorhabditis briggsae* was suitable for the parasitic helminth, *Haemonchus contortus*.

Quality of parasite antigens

In a report (1965) of a World Health Organization Expert Committee on Immunology and Parasitic Diseases, the following recommendations were made:

> The logical and probably necessary first step toward achieving immunological measures of host resistance and immunological means of inducing or increasing that resistance is the definition of antigens related to critical stages of parasite development. Field testing with crude preparations of multiple antigens is not likely to add significantly to our knowledge of the pathogenesis of parasitic diseases. If essential components of the parasite, preferably those in contact with

the host environment, can be isolated and found antigenic, they would serve as the best possible test and immunizing agents. The urgent necessity for such studies has emerged from the discussion in many places in the report and especially in the following areas:

(1) the differentiation in various parasitic diseases between
  (a) non-protective antigens (which may be useful in diagnosis) and
  (b) protective antigens (necessary in immunoprophylaxis and possibly also in diagnosis);
(2) the search for antigens common to parasites and the tissues of their particular host species;
(3) the chemical nature of the antigens secreted at natural orifices in helminths, as these may possibly be involved in protective immunity;
(4) antigenic analysis of moulting fluids of helminths;
(5) morphological and physiological studies in helminths that would lead to identification of antigenic structures, e.g., in the cuticle;
(6) the characterization of anti-enzymes, inasmuch as parasite enzymes are important in penetration and migration.

The recommendations of the W.H.O. Expert Committee allude to important qualitative aspects of parasite antigens which bear on potential vaccines. First of all, the functional antigens which appear to be important in stimulating resistance seem to be characterized by low antigenicity. The reasons for this are unknown, but speculation has centered on the enzymatic nature of these antigens. It is known that proteins which fulfill similar functions in different species may be chemically similar and this may account, at least in part, for reduced antigenicity. For this and other reasons, the need to isolate and concentrate functional antigens is a primary objective. The mosaic of antigens which are elaborated by or extracted from parasites contains a wide variety of potentially immunogenic material, and the serologic characterization of such mosaics is of little significance unless the data are closely correlated with *in vivo* protection tests. Unfortunately, very few critical studies of this type have been undertaken, but the work of Mills and Kent (1965) with *Trichinella spiralis* serves as an outstanding example of the critical studies. Another promising approach is the one used by Rhodes et al. (1965), who partially purified the enzyme, malic dehydrogenase, from *Ascaris suum* and found that it conferred some protection when injected into guinea pigs.

Secondly, the reference by the W.H.O. committee to antigens common to parasites and hosts touches on the analysis of the evolution of host-parasite relationships which affect the ability of hosts to recognize parasite antigens. Damian (1964), in an excellent review, proposed the concept of "eclipsed antigens" for an antigenic determinant of parasite origin which resembles an antigenic determinant of its host. There is considerable evidence from studies on microbes and parasites that eclipsed antigens are widespread. Obviously, if important components of potentially functional antigens become eclipsed, then the ability of a host to recognize them and to produce appropriate antibodies is lessened. Damian underlined the evolutionary forces selecting both hosts and parasite. Cogently, he proposed that one of the most effective defense mechanisms operating against the complete selection of eclipsed parasite antigens is host-antigenic polymorphism. The parasite, under this scheme, would overwhelm nonreactive hosts and select from host populations survivors with alternative antigenic states. That such polymorphic antigenic potential exists in vertebrate hosts is evident from many examples. As Schad (1966) pointed out, where such eclipsed antigens are evident, it might be possible to enhance recognition by using antigens from closely related parasites. In Schad's review, a number of reports are summarized indicating that heterologous species may interfere with a competing parasite within the same host by an immunologic mechanism even when homologous antigenicity is low or absent.

IMMUNIZING PROCEDURES

Adjuvants and routes of inoculation

It is repeatedly emphasized in reports of successful immunization procedures that adjuvants enhance the protection-stimulating effect of the crude antigen (e.g., Silverman et al., 1962; Targett and Fulton, 1965; Richards, 1966). Freund et al. (1945), using adjuvanted dead trophozoite preparations of *P. knowlesi*, successfully immunized monkeys. However, when Heidelberger et al. (1946a, b), in a series of heroic human experiments, tried to use nonadjuvanted trophozoites of *P. vivax*, they were unable to demonstrate any immunity either to the injected erythrocyte stage of the parasite or to challenge infections by mosquito bite. The omission of adjuvant appears to have been an important factor. This has been recently illustrated by the work of Targett and Fulton (1965), who found that when they omitted adjuvant and vaccinated with antigen alone, no protection was conferred in monkeys to *P. knowlesi*.

The use of adjuvants as an accepted means of enhancing antigenicity, whether it be for the induction of resistance or the production of antisera, is testimony that the poor quality of parasitic antigens is recognized by research workers. In spite of the obvious importance of adjuvants, no critical studies on the relative merits and effects of various adjuvants have been reported.

Freund's complete adjuvant consists of a stabilized emulsion of mineral oil and mycobacteria. It has obvious limitations for human use, although its efficacy is unrivaled in enhancing antigenicity. The mineral oil component is a potential carcinogenic agent, and the injection of mycobacteria would interfere with tuberculosis tests, in addition to producing unwelcome lesions. In an attempt to find useful alternatives, Silverman (1963) compared the adjuvant effects of sodium alginate, water in oil and oil in water emulsions, aluminum hydroxide, and Freund's preparation. Using nematode antigens, it was found that aluminum hydroxide, although not quite as effective as Freund's preparation, enhanced the production of more specific antisera and stimulated minimal host tissue reactions. The adjuvant was found to be effective in enhancing the production of resistance (Silverman et al., 1962).

Other adjuvants such as cholesterol and saponin (Richards, 1966) have been used to good advantage with parasitic antigens. The advantages of various adjuvants for specific antigens cannot be predicted, and experimental work to determine optimal combinations will have to be undertaken for each test material. The implications and importance of adjuvants for vaccines must not be underestimated.

Recently, Schelling (1966), using ovalbumin, the lipopolysaccharide of *Escherichia coli* bacteria, and somatic and metabolic antigens of the parasitic nematode, *Haemonchus contortus*, compared the effect of various routes of injection on the antibody response in rabbits. All three antigens were adjuvanted with sodium alginate, and comparable quantities were used for each injection. The intravenous, intramuscular, intradermal, and intraperitoneal routes of injection were tested for each antigen, and two injections were given within an 18-day interval. Antibody titers were measured by the tanned-cell passive hemagglutination technique, and all sera were subjected to treatment with 2-mercaptoethanol to distinguish between 19S and 7S globulins. The serum titers measured in response to the injection of ovalbumin and the *H. contortus* antigens were found to be entirely due to 7S gamma-globulin, and the intravenous and intramuscular routes consistently elicited the highest antibody titers and sustained the longest duration of antibody production. The primary antibody response to *E. coli* lipopolysaccharide was found to be 19S globulin, and the most effective route of injection proved to be the intradermal route. This work suggests that the efficacy of an injection route depends to some degree on the type of antibody elicited.

The importance of injection routes and adjuvants can be better appreciated when more information on protective antibodies is available. Cohen and McGregor (1963) showed that the protective properties of human immune serum were associated with the 7S gamma-globulin fraction. As Tobie et al. (1966) pointed out in their study on immunoglobulins in human malaria, for the induction of 7S antibody the antigen dose requirement was at least 50 times as great as that for 19S antibody. Similar studies on other parasitic infections are needed to determine both the qualitative and quantitative thresholds required for the protective immune response.

Antigen-antibody complexes

In recent years, immunologists have been investigating the role of soluble antigen-antibody complexes in stimulating an immune response. It has been found, for example, that in several types of hypersensitivity reactions the *in vitro*-formed complex is much more active than the antigen alone. Further studies have shown that such complexes form *in vivo* and are capable of initiating biologic reactions which could not be produced either by antigen or antibody alone. These phenomena were reviewed by Weigle (1961), who also summarized some of the work which suggests that the complexes may be operating either as a stable unit or that they may be effecting their activity by a process of dissociation and reassociation. The mechanism of action is not clearly understood; however, it is obvious that such complexes are formed in nature and that preformed *in vitro* complexes (in the proper proportion of antigen to antibody) result in a greatly enhanced antigenicity. The use of preformed *in vitro* antigen-antibody complexes as a natural adjuvanting procedure for parasite antigens is strongly suggested.

Stumberg (1933), after the demonstration by Stoll (1929) that sheep acquire resistance to *Haemonchus contortus*, examined the sera of resistant and infected animals. By means of an anaphylactic test in guinea pigs, he found evidence which strongly suggested that *H. contortus* antigen occurred in the serum of sheep. The possible role of soluble antigen-antibody complexes was the subject of recent studies by Ristic (1966) and his co-workers on *Babesia* and *Plasmodium*. They have found serum-soluble antigens which can be used for the diagnosis of the disease and which, when used as immunizing agents, confer protection on dogs challenged with babesiosis (Sibinovic, 1966) or chickens challenged with malaria (Todorovic et al., 1966). A possible explanation for the presence of antigens in the serum is that they represent antigen-antibody complexes consisting of parasite metabolites and host antibody. These are exciting results which ought to be further pursued with vigor, and they suggest similar lines of inquiry for other parasitic infections.

Quantitative factors

The existence of immunologic thresholds in animals has long been established in the field of bacteriology (*see* Wilson and Miles, 1964). Below a certain minimum quantity of whole bacilli or bacterial polysaccharide or protein antigen, no immunologic response is induced. During the induction period of the primary response, it appears necessary to maintain a minimum level of circulating antigen in the serum. The threshold necessary must be maintained either by a sufficiently large single inoculation or by a series of multiple injections. On the other hand, too much antigen can induce unresponsiveness in the form of immunologic paralysis. Immunologic paralysis inhibits an animal from responding to an antigen for varying lengths of times (i.e., from weeks to months). However, following recovery from immunologic paralysis, the animal can respond normally to the original immunologically paralyzing antigen if stimulated at an appropriate threshold level.

In a critical study of quantitative factors affecting the primary response Mitchison (1964), using bovine serum albumin as an antigen in mice, found two dosage zones, one low and one high, at which immunologic paralysis rather than antibody production was induced. He also found dramatic differences when adjuvant was used, when multiple injections were given, or when the interval between injections was reduced. With respect to the secondary complex, additional observations by Mitchison (1964) and Makela and Mitchison (1965) may explain the puzzling reports that prior immunization with parasite antigens exacerbated the challenge infection over that seen in the controls. Studying the quantitative effects of bovine and human serum albumin on the ability of primed cells to respond to a second antigenic stimulus and using adoptively transferred cells in syngenic hosts, they found that as little as 10^{-3} μg of BSA was needed to stimulate a secondary response. At higher dose ranges (10^5 μg), the proliferation of immunocytes and synthesis of antibody were inhibited. The significance of these results in terms of attempts to immunize artificially against parasites is obvious. Tests with potential functional antigens must be planned over a range of dosage levels and using varying schedules.

In addition, a determination of the most appropriate size of challenge dose and how it is to be administered must be considered. Little definitive information is available on the rate and number of infective stages which host animals are apt to be exposed to in nature. Thus, a single massive dose of the infective stage of a parasite presented to an experimentally immunized animal might completely overwhelm the immune response and suggest that no immunity has been established. On the other hand, in nature, the animal may never encounter more than a small number of infective stages presented at intervals in the form of a "trickle" challenge. Indeed, much more information is needed, e.g., on the number of sporozoites, infective nematode larvae, or trematode cercariae, to which hosts are exposed under normal epidemiologic conditions.

The effects of small quantities of "good" antigens on the type of immune response have been studied by Salvin and Smith (1959, 1960). Using a variety of protein antigens and purified diphtheria toxoid, they found that in guinea pigs after injection with very low doses of antigen, a delayed hypersensitivity reaction was observed but no circulating antibody was detected. Further stimulation of the sensitized guinea pig with the specific homologous antigen resulted in an anamnestic response during which both circulating antibody and Arthus-type hypersensitivity developed. These data support the suggestion that delayed hypersensitivity is an intermediate stage in the formation of circulating antibody. The delayed hypersensitivity reaction has often been reported as a result of infection with parasites or inoculation with parasite antigens. This would tend to suggest that in terms of the model proposed by Salvin and Smith, the host animal was only partially immunized, and that further stimulation would be necessary for a complete circulating antibody response. During natural infection, the inadequacy of antigenic stimulation for the production of circulating antibody because of qualitative and quantitative reasons may explain why resistance is slow in developing and why serologic tests yield low titers. The transitory nature of functional antigens contributes to the difficulty in obtaining a minimum immunologic threshold. Conceivably, the number of parasites required to produce sufficient antigen during the induction phase may be of such an order that the concurrent pathologic stress adversely affects antibody synthesis by the host.

STANDARDIZATION

Criteria

The aim of vaccination against microbial infectious diseases is to prevent disease and mortality. The fact that populations immunized against polio continue to excrete virulent viruses or that clostridial spores can be isolated from symptomless hosts is accepted by microbiologists as a sign of successful vaccination. Reduction in morbidity and mortality are the main criteria used in assessing the potency of vaccines against poliomyelitis, diphtheria, tetanus, pertussis, erysipelas, cholera, pneumonia, smallpox, and rabies. It is not necessary to demonstrate that the protected host is completely free of the infectious agent, i.e., that sterile immunity exists.

Unfortunately, the same criteria have not always been applicable to studies on parasite vaccines. In many protozoan and metazoan parasitic infections, the disease tends to be chronic in nature rather than acute, so the lethal end-points are difficult to establish. A wide variety of criteria are described in the preceding chapters, and most of them deal with reduction in degree of parasitization instead of mortality. The use of reduced parasitization as an index of partial or complete immunity is fraught with many problems, and more subtle criteria for assessing different levels of host morbidity and parasite inhibition must be established. Furthermore, on the basis of data related to dosage loads in nature (referred to earlier), a more reasonable assessment of the levels of immunity to be attained can be determined.

The expectation that vaccination will lead to parasite-free individuals is unrealistic on the basis of present evidence. In fact, in certain epidemiologic situations, this might be unwise. It appears that the maintenance of a very low level of nonpathogenic parasitization may be desirable, since this may help to maintain an adequate level of resistance by providing a constant source of antigenic stimulation. The aim at this stage appears to be best illustrated by the case of adults in hyperendemic malarious areas who have developed resistance and show very few parasites in their circulating erythrocytes. When such persons are removed from their native environments for long periods of time and then return, they suffer a fresh but mild malaria attack. Similarly, domestic animals which develop resistance to helminth infections during the summer and autumn apparently lose some of this immunity during the winter when transmission of infective larvae is at a low ebb. As a result, the animals become reinfected with low levels of parasites in the spring, but quickly regain their previous state of resistance.

Potency and safety

The establishment of potency standards for widely used vaccines has occupied microbiologists for many years. A wide range of techniques and standards has been used and is accepted on an international basis (*see* World Health Organization Tech. Rep. Ser. No. 222, 1961). In general, potency is measured by comparison of an unknown vaccine preparation with a known antigen or standard antiserum in a laboratory-animal protection test. Potency testing may use natural routes or highly artificial routes of challenge, i.e., intraperitoneal or intracerebral inoculation. The important factor is that the test measures the same kind of immunity that it is desired to induce. The actual units are arbitrary, but some reference standard must always be available. The range for effective vaccine doses can be fairly wide but must provide some margin of error so that effective doses do not become ineffective because of too little stimulation or result in immunologic paralysis because of too much antigen.

Several widely used microbial vaccines have not yet been standardized because they depend on living organisms. With biologic products such as yellow fever, smallpox, and B.C.G. vaccines, direct tests on animals in order to indicate potency have to be carried out. It is perhaps needless to point out that in all cases the ability to store vaccine material until potency and safety factors have been established is a prerequisite. So-called shelf-life studies become important in providing for an adequate period of potency and safety testing and in allowing for distribution to the user.

The question of safety standards becomes particularly important when living organisms are used for vaccination. In the case of attenuation by passage through abnormal hosts, by irradiation, or by *in vitro* cultivation, each batch must be tested to ensure that attenuation has been effected so that potential pathogens can be eliminated. In the case of certain organisms such as infective nematode larvae that are reared in highly contaminated fecal media, it is necessary to ensure that the cleansing process has removed the potentially infective microbes that might be present in association with the larvae. In this regard, the problem is further complicated by the fact that bacteria and viruses can survive in the intestine of the nematode even after extensive cleansing of the cuticular surfaces.

For reasons of potency and safety standardization and to provide for maximal shelf life, dead vaccines offer many advantages over live ones. Undoubtedly, the process of research to produce dead vaccines by isolating and enhancing the activity of the functional antigens is a long and tedious one. Nevertheless, though there is much justification for the use of living vaccines, the attempt to understand the immune mechanisms and to produce standardized immunologic products must continue.

CONCLUSION

One of the striking impressions gained from a review of the literature in the fields of microbial and parasitic immunity and vaccination is the similarity of problems. These common problems are found at every level of study of host-parasite relations, infection and transmission, *in vitro* cultivation, serologic evaluation, antigen preparations, immunization, and parasite selection and evolution, to name only a few areas of obvious common interest. In this regard, bacteriologists, virologists, and parasitologists concerned with immune mechanisms and prophylactic immunization have much to learn from one another. Also, the theoretically inclined immunologist working with model systems and artificial antigens provides a source of new insight and ideas for experimentation with the crude parasite antigens so far available.

Immunoparasitologists have too often in the past focused narrowly on single organisms or on a limited group of parasites. Papers published on the immune response of one species of parasite often refer to literature related only to that species and ignore relevant work done on other even closely related organisms. As a result, a mystique of parasite "exceptionalisms" has developed with the implication that each host-parasite relationship is unique.

Quantitative phenomena related to antigenic stimulation and the development of resistance cannot always be conveniently studied with all parasites, and guidelines must be sought from whatever source available. Similarly, information on the effects of adjuvants, routes of inoculation, immunization schedules, and the qualitative alterations to antigens which lead to an enhanced host immune response or immune paralysis are of interest, no matter what the source of antigen used for such studies may be.

Basic to the approach outlined in this chapter are the convictions that a host immune response is a normal reaction to parasitism and that wherever such immune responses have protective value, it should be possible to stimulate immunity artificially. The opportunity to review the literature afforded by the occasion of writing this chapter has further deepened this conviction.

REFERENCES

Ball, G. H. 1966. Adaptation of the malarial parasite, particularly to its insect host. *In* Host-Parasite Relationships. McCauley, J. E., ed. Corvallis, Oregon State University Press, pp. 73-96.

Berntzen, A. K. 1966. A controlled culture environment for axenic growth of parasites. Ann. N.Y. Acad. Sci., 139: 176-189.

Brown, K. N., and I. N. Brown. 1965. Immunity of malaria: Antigenic variation in chronic infections of *Plasmodium knowlesi*. Nature (London), 208: 1286-1288.

Campbell, D. H. 1936. Active immunization of albino rats with protein fractions from *Taenia taeniaeformis* and its larval form *Cysticercus fasciolarus*. Amer. J. Hyg., 23: 104-113.

Cohen, S., and I. A. McGregor. 1963. Gamma globulin and acquired immunity to malaria. *In* Immunity to Protozoa. Garnham, P. C. C., Pierce, A. E., and Roitt, I., eds. Oxford, Blackwell Scientific Publications, pp. 123-159.

Damian, R. T. 1964. Molecular mimicry: Antigen sharing by parasite and host and its consequences. Amer. Naturalist, 98: 129-149.

Freund, J., K. J. Thompson, H. E. Sommer, A. W. Walter, and E. L. Schenkein. 1945. Immunization of rhesus monkeys against malarial infection (*P. knowlesi*) with killed parasites and adjuvants. Science, 102: 202-204.

Geiman, Q. M., W. A. Siddiqui, and J. V. Schnell. 1966. *In vitro* studies on erythrocytic stages of plasmodia; medium improvement and results with seven species of malarial parasites. *In* Research in Malaria. Military Med. 131 (Suppl.): 1015-1025.

Gemmell, M. A. 1965a. Immunological responses of the mammalian host against tapeworm infections. II. Species specificity of hexacanth embryos in protecting rabbits against *Taenia pisiformis*. Immunology, 8: 270-280.

────── 1965b. Immunological responses of the mammalian host against tapeworm infections. II. Species specificity of hexacanth embryos in protecting sheep against *Taenia ovis*. Immunology, 8: 281-290.

────── 1966. Immunological responses of the mammalian host against tapeworm infections. IV. Species specificity of hexacanth embryos in protecting sheep against *Echinococcus granulosus*. Immunology, 11: 325-335.

Goodman, H. C. 1966. Comments on immunization. *In* Research in Malaria. Military Med., 131 (Suppl.): 1265-1268.

Gray, A. R. 1965. Antigenic variation in a strain of *Trypanosoma brucei* transmitted by *Glossina morsitans* and *G. palpalis*. J. Gen. Microbiol., 41: 195-214.

Hansen, E. L., P. H. Silverman, and E. J. Buecher, Jr. 1966. Development of *Haemonchus contortus* in media designed for studies on *Caenorhabditis briggsae*. J. Parasit., 52: 137-140.

Heidelberger, M., W. A. Coates, and M. M. Mayer. 1946a. Studies in human malaria. II. Attempts to influence relapsing vivax malaria by treatment of patients with vaccine (*Pl. vivax*). J. Immun., 53: 101-107.

────── C. Prout, J. A. Hindle, and A. S. Rose. 1946b. Studies in human malaria. III. An attempt at vaccination of paretics against blood-borne infection with *Pl. vivax*. J. Immun., 53: 109-112.

Horton-Smith, C., P. L. Long, A. E. Pierce, and M. E. Rose. 1963. Immunity to coccidia in domestic animals. *In* Immunity to Protozoa. Garnham, P. C. C., Pierce, A. E., and Roitt, I., eds. Oxford, Blackwell Scientific Publications, pp. 273-295.

Huff, C. G. 1966. Comments on cultivation. *In* Research in Malaria. Military Med., 131 (Suppl.): 1032-1033.

Jackson, G. J. 1962. The parasitic nematode, *Neoaplectana glaseri,* in axenic culture. II. Initial results with defined media. Exp. Parasit., 12: 25-32.

Jakstys, B. P., and P. H. Silverman. 1969. The effect of heterologous antibody on *Haemonchus contortus* development *in vitro*. J. Parasit., 55: 486-492.

Jarrett, W. F. H., F. W. Jennings, W. I. M. McIntyre, W. Mulligan, N. C. C. Sharp, and G. M Urquhart. 1959. Immunological studies on *Dictyocaulus viviparus* infection in calves: double vaccination with irradiated larvae. Amer. J. Vet. Res., 20: 522-526.

Lehnert, J. P. 1967. Studies on the biology and immunology of *Ascaris suum* in mice. Ph. D. Thesis. University of Illinois, Urbana, Illinois.

Lumsden, W. H. R. 1965. Biological aspects of trypanosomiasis research. *In* Advances in Parasitology, Vol. 3. Dawes, B., ed. New York, Academic Press, Inc., pp. 1-57.

Makela, O., and N. A. Mitchison. 1965. The effect of antigen dosage on the response of adoptively transferred cells. Immunology, 8: 549-556.

Manson-Bahr, P. E. C. 1963. Active immunization in leishmaniasis. *In* Immunity to Protozoa. Garnham, P. C. C., Pierce, A. E., and Roitt, I., eds. Oxford, Blackwell Scientific Publications, pp. 246-252.

Miller, H. M. 1931. The production of artificial immunity in the albino rat to a metazoan parasite. J. Prevent. Med., 5: 429-452.

Mills, C. K., and N. H. Kent. 1965. Excretions and secretions of *Trichinella spiralis* and their role in immunity. Exp. Parasit., 16: 300-310.

Mitchison, N. A. 1964. Induction of immunological paralysis in two zones of dosage. Proc. Roy. Soc. [Biol.], 161: 275-292.

Nussenzweig, R. A., M. Yoeli, and H. Most. 1966. Studies on the protective effect of *Plasmodium chabaudi* infection in mice upon subsequent infection with another rodent malaria species, *Plasmodium vinckei*. *In* Research in Malaria. Military Med., 131 (Suppl.): 1237-1242.

Polet, H. 1966. *In vitro* cultivation of erythrocytic forms of *Plasmodium knowlesi* and *Plasmodium berghei*. *In* Research in Malaria. Military Med., 131 (Suppl.): 1026-1031.

Poynter, D., and R. J. Terry. 1966. Practical vaccination against bovine parasitic bronchitis. *In* Proceedings of the First International Congress of Parasitology, Vol. 1. Corradetti, A., ed. New York, Pergamon Press, pp. 110-111.

────── B. V. Jones, A. R. M. Nelson, R. Peacock, J. Robinson, P. H. Silverman, and R. J. Terry. 1960. Recent experiences with vaccination. Vet. Rec., 72: 1078-1086.

Rhodes, M. B., D. P. Nayak, G. W. Kelley, Jr., and C. L. Marsh. 1965. Studies in helminth enzymology. IV. Immune responses to malic dehydrogenase from *Ascaris suum*. J. Parasit., 16: 373-381.

Richards, W. H. G. 1966. Active immunization of chicks against *Plasmodium galli-naceum* by inactivated homologous sporozoites and erythrocytic parasites. Nature (London), 212: 1492-1494.

Ristic, M. 1966. The vertebrate developmental cycle of *Babesia* and *Theileria*. *In* Biology of Parasites. Soulsby, E. J. L., ed. New York, Academic Press, Inc., pp. 127-141.

Rogers, W. P. 1962. The Nature of Parasitism, Vol. 2. New York, Academic Press, Inc.

Sadun, E. H. 1963. Immunization in schistosomiasis by previous exposure to homologous and heterologous cercariae by inoculation of preparations from schistosomes and by exposure to irradiated cercariae. Ann. N.Y. Acad. Sci., 113: 418-439.

—— R. L. Hickman, B. T. Wellde, A. P. Moon, and I. O. K. Udeozo. 1966. Active and passive immunization of chimpanzees infected with West African and Southeast Asian strains of *Plasmodium falciparum*. *In* Research in Malaria. Military Med., 131 (Suppl.): 1250-1262.

Salven, S. B., and R. F. Smith. 1959. Delayed hypersensitivity and the anamnestic response. J. Immunol., 84: 449-457.

—— and R. F. Smith. 1960. The specificity of allergic reactions. I. Delayed versus Arthus hypersensitivity. J. Exp. Med., 111: 465-483.

Sanders, A., and F. G. Wallace. 1966. Immunization of rats with irradiated *Trypanosoma lewisi*. Exp. Parasit., 18: 301-304.

Schad, G. A. 1966. Immunity, competition, and natural regulation of helminth populations. Amer. Naturalist, 100: 359-364.

Schelling, M. A. E. 1966. The effect of route of injection upon the development of circulating antibody in response to a variety of antigens. M.S. Thesis, University of Illinois, Urbana, Illinois.

Shumard, R. 1967. Personal communication.

Sibinovic, S. K. H. 1966. Immunogenic properties of purified antigens isolated from the serum of horses, dogs and rats with acute babesiosis. Ph.D. Thesis, University of Illinois, Urbana, Illinois.

Silverman, P. H. 1963. *In vitro* cultivation and serological techniques in parasitology. *In* Techniques in Parasitology. Taylor, A. E., ed. Oxford, Blackwell Scientific Publications, pp. 45-67.

—— 1965a. Some immunologic aspects of parasitic helminth infections. Amer. Zoologist, 5: 153-163.

—— 1965b. *In vitro* cultivation procedures for parasitic helminths. *In* Advances in Parasitology, Vol. 3. Dawes, B., ed. New York, Academic Press, Inc., pp. 159-222.

—— 1966. A concept of host-parasite immunologic relationships. *In* Host-Parasite Relationships. McCauley, J. E., ed. Corvallis, Oregon State University Press, pp. 117-126.

—— D. Poynter, and K. R. Podger. 1962. Studies on larval antigens derived by cultivation of some parasitic nematodes in simple media; protection tests in laboratory animals. J. Parasit., 48: 562-571.

—— N. E. Alger, and E. L. Hansen. 1966. Axenic helminth cultures and their use for the production of antiparasitic vaccines. Ann. N.Y. Acad. Sci., 139: 124-142.

Smith, T. 1910. A protective reaction of the host in intestinal coccidiosis of the rabbit. J. Med. Res., 23: 407-415.

Soltys, M. A. 1964. Immunity in trypanosomiasis. V. Immunization of animals with dead trypanosomes. Parasitology, 54: 585-591.

Stauber, L. 1963. Immunity to leishmania. Ann. N.Y. Acad. Sci., 113: 409-417.

Stoll, N. R. 1928. The occurrence of self-cure and protection in typical nematode parasitism. J. Parasit., 15: 147-148.

—— 1929. Studies with the strongyloid nematode, *Haemonchus contortus*. I. Acquired resistance of hosts under natural reinfection conditions out-of-doors. Amer. J. Hyg., 10: 384-418.

—— 1958. The induction of self-cure and protection with special reference to experimental vaccination against *Haemonchus*. Rich Institute Pamphlet No. 45, pp. 184-208.

—— 1961. The worms: Can we vaccinate against them? Amer. J. Trop. Med. Hyg., 10: 298-303.

Strout, R. G., J. Colis, S. C. Smith, and W. R. Dunlop. 1965. *In vitro* cultivation of *Eimeria acervulina* (coccidia). Exp. Parasit., 17: 241-246.

Stumberg, J. E. 1933. The detection of proteins of the nematode *Haemonchus contortus* in the sera of infected sheep and goats. Amer. J. Hyg., 18: 247-265.

Targett, G. A. T., and J. D. Fulton. 1965. Immunization of rhesus monkeys against *Plasmodium knowlesi* malaria. Exp. Parasit., 17: 180-193.

Thillet, G. J., and A. C. Chandler. 1957. Immunization against *Trypanosoma lewisi* in rats by injection of metabolic products. Science, 125: 246-347.

Tobie, J. E., D. C. Abele, S. M Wolff, P. G. Contacos, and C. B. Evans. 1966. Serum immunoglobulin levels in human malaria and their relationship to antibody production. J. Immun., 97: 498-505.

Todorovic, R., D. Ferris, and M. Ristic. 1966. Serologic and immunogenic properties of serum soluble antigens of *Plasmodium gallinaceum*. Report, 41st Annual Meeting, Amer. Soc. Parasit., San Juan, Puerto Rico.

Trager, W. 1957. Nutrition of a hemoflagellate (*Leishmania tarentolae*) having an interchangeable requirement for choline or pyridoxal. J. Protozool., 4: 269-276.

———— 1966. Comments on cultivation. *In* Research in Malaria. Military Med., 131 (Suppl.): 1034-1035.

Voller, A., P. C. C. Garnham, and G. A. T. Targett. 1966. Cross immunity in monkey malaria. J. Trop. Med. Hyg., 69: 121-123.

Weigle, W. O. 1961. Fate and biological action of antigen-antibody complexes. *In* Advances in Immunology, Vol. 1. Taliaferro, W. H., and Humphrey, J. H., eds. New York, Academic Press, Inc., pp. 283-317.

Weiss, M. L. and D. L. DeGiusti. 1964. The effect of different sera in the culture medium on the behavior of *Plasmodium berghei* following serial passage through tissue culture. J. Protozool., 11: 224-228.

———— and D. L. DeGiusti. 1966. Active immunization against *Plasmodium berghei* in mice. Amer. J. Trop. Med. Hyg., 15: 472-482.

Weitz, B. 1964. The reaction of trypanosomes to their environment. *In* Microbial Behavior *In Vivo* and *In Vitro*. Smith, H., and Taylor, J., eds., New York, Cambridge University Press, pp. 112-121.

Wilson, G. S., and A. L. Miles. 1964. Principles of Bacteriology and Immunity, 5th ed., Vol. 2. Baltimore, The Williams and Wilkins Co.

World Health Organization Expert Committee. 1961. Biological Standardization. W.H.O. Tech. Rep. Ser. No. 222, pp. 1-54.

World Health Organization Expert Committee. 1965. Immunology and Parasitic Diseases. W.H.O. Tech. Rep. Ser. No. 315, pp. 1-64.

Zuckerman, A. 1966. Recent studies on factors involved in malarial anemia. *In* Research in Malaria. Military Med., 131 (Suppl.): 1201-1216.

INDEX

Pig *(cont.)*
  balantidiasis, 463
  malaria, 344
  nematodes, 932
  trichomoniasis, 486
Pigeon
  antibody transfer from mother, 304
  helminths, 410
  malaria, 341, 363
  precipitin production, 312
  trichomoniasis, 471, 510, 511
Pinworms, 918, 922
Pituitary hormones, toxoplasmosis and, 879
Plague, flea-rodent relationship and, 1087
Plasma cell numbers, bursectomy and, 310
Plasmodium, 331 ff., 767 ff., 1178. *See also* Malaria.
  berghei, 332, 333, 702, 745, 776, 794 ff. 1173
    acquired immunity to, 356
    anemia and, 358
    Babesia and, 854
    erythrocytes and, 351, 353
    hemagglutination and, 359
    innate immunity to, 340, 343
    interactions, 363
    in lower mammals, 794 ff.
    sporozoites, 340
    yoelii, 787
  brasilianum, 770, 781
  cathemerium, 333, 774
    in blackbird, 337
    innate immunity to, 339, 342, 349, 350
    interactions, 362
  chabaudi, 333, 794, 802, 820, 1170
  circumflexum, 332, 333
    acquired immunity to, 355
    ecology and, 336-37
    innate immunity to, 339, 349, 350
    segmentation, 361
  coatneyi, 770, 771, 778, 786
  cynomolgi, 332, 356, 769, 770, 773 ff.
    bastianellii, 770, 775, 778, 786, 787
    ceylonensis, 770, 778, 786
    cyclopis, 770
    cynomolgi, 770
  elongatum, 331, 339, 340
  eylesi, 771
  falciparum, 771 ff., 779, 781, 782, 787, 1167
  fallax, 333, 338-39
  fieldi, 770, 771
  fragile, 770, 777, 778, 786
  gallinaceum, 331, 332, 775, 787, 837
    acquired immunity to 355, 356
    innate immunity to, 338 ff., 343, 349
    segmentation, 361
  girardi, 768
  gonderi, 769, 770
  hylobati, 771
  inopinatum, 794

  inui, 769, 770, 778, 786
  jefferyi, 771
  juxtanucleare, 363
  knowlesi, 355, 770, 776 ff., 786, 803, 820, 1176
  kochi, 768
  lemuris, 768
  lophurae, 332
    acquired immunity to, 355, 356
    agglutinins to, 355
    duck complement and, 320
    immunopathology, 357 ff.
    innate immunity to, 342-44, 349-51
    interactions, 362, 363
    sporozoites of, 339
  malariae, 771, 782, 783, 786
  metastaticum, 794
  nucelophilum, 361
  ovale, 771, 772, 775, 778, 782
  pitheci, 771
  reichenowi, 771, 778
  relictum, 333
    in aves, 339, 341
    host specificity to, 350
    immunopathology, 357
    interactions, 362, 363
  rouxi, 361
  schwetzi, 771, 778
  shortti, 770, 778, 786
  simiovale, 770, 778
  simium, 769, 770, 771
  vaughani, 361
  vinckei, 333, 794, 802 ff., 816, 1170
  vivax, 770 ff., 778, 780, 783, 785, 787, 1176
  youngi, 771
Platyhelminthes. *See* Cestodes; Trematodes.
Plerocercoids, 1028
Pleurodema dibronii, 605
Plistophora culicis, 774
Plodia interpunctella, 1122
Pneumonia, nematodes and, 948
Polistes, 1103, 1105
  exclamans, 1103
  fuscatus, 1103, 1105
Polyadenylic acid, 409
Polycytidylic acid, 409
Polymers, 317
  schistomiasis and, 988
Polymorphonuclear leukocytes, nematodes and, 936
Polynesia, *Wuchereria bancrofti* in, 972
Polysaccharide
  Chagas' disease and, 649, 657
  nematodes and, 932
  trichomonads and, 482, 520, 521
Porcupine, leishmaniasis of, 741
Potency of vaccine, 1180-81
Potus flavus, 741
Poultry. *See also* Aves; Chickens.
  coccidiosis, 371 ff.